T0140578

Lecture Notes in Computer Science   11071

Commenced Publication in 1973
Founding and Former Series Editors:
Gerhard Goos, Juris Hartmanis, and Jan van Leeuwen

Editorial Board

David Hutchison
  Lancaster University, Lancaster, UK
Takeo Kanade
  Carnegie Mellon University, Pittsburgh, PA, USA
Josef Kittler
  University of Surrey, Guildford, UK
Jon M. Kleinberg
  Cornell University, Ithaca, NY, USA
Friedemann Mattern
  ETH Zurich, Zurich, Switzerland
John C. Mitchell
  Stanford University, Stanford, CA, USA
Moni Naor
  Weizmann Institute of Science, Rehovot, Israel
C. Pandu Rangan
  Indian Institute of Technology Madras, Chennai, India
Bernhard Steffen
  TU Dortmund University, Dortmund, Germany
Demetri Terzopoulos
  University of California, Los Angeles, CA, USA
Doug Tygar
  University of California, Berkeley, CA, USA
Gerhard Weikum
  Max Planck Institute for Informatics, Saarbrücken, Germany

More information about this series at http://www.springer.com/series/7412

Alejandro F. Frangi · Julia A. Schnabel
Christos Davatzikos · Carlos Alberola-López
Gabor Fichtinger (Eds.)

Medical Image Computing and Computer Assisted Intervention – MICCAI 2018

21st International Conference
Granada, Spain, September 16–20, 2018
Proceedings, Part II

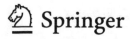 Springer

Editors
Alejandro F. Frangi ⓘ
University of Leeds
Leeds
UK

Carlos Alberola-López ⓘ
Universidad de Valladolid
Valladolid
Spain

Julia A. Schnabel
King's College London
London
UK

Gabor Fichtinger
Queen's University
Kingston, ON
Canada

Christos Davatzikos ⓘ
University of Pennsylvania
Philadelphia, PA
USA

ISSN 0302-9743   ISSN 1611-3349   (electronic)
Lecture Notes in Computer Science
ISBN 978-3-030-00933-5   ISBN 978-3-030-00934-2   (eBook)
https://doi.org/10.1007/978-3-030-00934-2

Library of Congress Control Number: 2018909526

LNCS Sublibrary: SL6 – Image Processing, Computer Vision, Pattern Recognition, and Graphics

© Springer Nature Switzerland AG 2018
This work is subject to copyright. All rights are reserved by the Publisher, whether the whole or part of the material is concerned, specifically the rights of translation, reprinting, reuse of illustrations, recitation, broadcasting, reproduction on microfilms or in any other physical way, and transmission or information storage and retrieval, electronic adaptation, computer software, or by similar or dissimilar methodology now known or hereafter developed.
The use of general descriptive names, registered names, trademarks, service marks, etc. in this publication does not imply, even in the absence of a specific statement, that such names are exempt from the relevant protective laws and regulations and therefore free for general use.
The publisher, the authors and the editors are safe to assume that the advice and information in this book are believed to be true and accurate at the date of publication. Neither the publisher nor the authors or the editors give a warranty, express or implied, with respect to the material contained herein or for any errors or omissions that may have been made. The publisher remains neutral with regard to jurisdictional claims in published maps and institutional affiliations.

This Springer imprint is published by the registered company Springer Nature Switzerland AG
The registered company address is: Gewerbestrasse 11, 6330 Cham, Switzerland

Preface

We are very pleased to present the conference proceedings for the 21st International Conference on Medical Image Computing and Computer Assisted Intervention (MICCAI), which was successfully held at the Granada Conference Center, September 16–20, 2018 in Granada, Spain.

The conference also featured 40 workshops, 14 tutorials, and ten challenges held on September 16 or 20. For the first time, we had events co-located or endorsed by other societies. The two-day Visual Computing in Biology and Medicine (VCBM) Workshop partnered with EUROGRAPHICS[1], the one-day Biomedical Workshop Biomedical Information Processing and Analysis: A Latin American perspective partnered with SIPAIM[2], and the one-day MICCAI Workshop on Computational Diffusion on MRI was endorsed by ISMRM[3]. This year, at the time of writing this preface, the MICCAI 2018 conference had over 1,400 firm registrations for the main conference featuring the most recent work in the fields of:

- Reconstruction and Image Quality
- Machine Learning and Statistical Analysis
- Registration and Image Guidance
- Optical and Histology Applications
- Cardiac, Chest and Abdominal Applications
- fMRI and Diffusion Imaging
- Neuroimaging
- Computer-Assisted Intervention
- Segmentation

This was the largest MICCAI conference to date, with, for the first time, four volumes of *Lecture Notes in Computer Science* (LNCS) proceedings for the main conference, selected after a thorough double-blind peer-review process organized in several phases as further described below. Following the example set by the previous program chairs of MICCAI 2017, we employed the Conference Managing Toolkit (CMT)[4] for paper submissions and double-blind peer-reviews, the Toronto Paper Matching System (TPMS)[5] for automatic paper assignment to area chairs and reviewers, and Researcher.CC[6] to handle conflicts between authors, area chairs, and reviewers.

---

[1] https://www.eg.org.

[2] http://www.sipaim.org/.

[3] https://www.ismrm.org/.

[4] https://cmt.research.microsoft.com.

[5] http://torontopapermatching.org.

[6] http://researcher.cc.

In total, a record 1,068 full submissions (ca. 33% more than the previous year) were received and sent out to peer-review, from 1,335 original intentions to submit. Of those submissions, 80% were considered as pure Medical Image Computing (MIC), 14% as pure Computer-Assisted Intervention (CAI), and 6% as MICCAI papers that fitted into both MIC and CAI areas. The MICCAI 2018 Program Committee (PC) had a total of 58 area chairs, with 45% from Europe, 43% from the Americas, 9% from Australasia, and 3% from the Middle East. We maintained an excellent gender balance with 43% women scientists on the PC.

Using TPMS scoring and CMT, each area chair was assigned between 18 and 20 manuscripts using TPMS, for each of which they suggested 9–15 potential reviewers. Subsequently, 600 invited reviewers were asked to bid for the manuscripts they had been suggested for. Final reviewer allocations via CMT took PC suggestions, reviewer bidding, and TPMS scores into account, allocating 5–6 papers per reviewer. Based on the double-blind reviews, 173 papers (16%) were directly accepted and 314 papers (30%) were directly rejected – these decisions were confirmed by the handling area chair. The remaining 579 papers (54%) were invited for rebuttal. Two further area chairs were added using CMT and TPMS scores to each of these remaining manuscripts, who then independently scored these to accept or reject, based on the reviews, rebuttal, and manuscript, resulting in clear paper decisions using majority voting: 199 further manuscripts were accepted, and 380 rejected.

The overall manuscript acceptance rate was 34.9%. Two PC teleconferences were held on May 14, 2018, in two different time zones to confirm the final results and collect PC feedback on the peer-review process (with over 74% PC attendance rate). For the MICCAI 2018 proceedings, the 372 accepted papers[7] have been organized in four volumes as follows:

- Volume LNCS 11070 includes: Image Quality and Artefacts (15 manuscripts), Image Reconstruction Methods (31), Machine Learning in Medical Imaging (22), Statistical Analysis for Medical Imaging (10), and Image Registration Methods (21)
- Volume LNCS 11071 includes: Optical and Histology Applications (46); and Cardiac, Chest, and Abdominal Applications (59)
- Volume LNCS 11072 includes: fMRI and Diffusion Imaging (45); Neuroimaging and Brain Segmentation (37)
- Volume LNCS 11073 includes: Computer-Assisted Intervention (39) grouped into image-guided interventions and surgery; surgical planning, simulation and work flow analysis; and visualization and augmented reality; and Image Segmentation Methods (47) grouped into general segmentation methods; multi-organ segmentation; abdominal, cardiac, chest, and other segmentation applications.

We would like to thank everyone who contributed greatly to the success of MICCAI 2018 and the quality of its proceedings. These include the MICCAI Society, for support and insightful comments; and our sponsors for financial support and their presence on site. We are especially grateful to all members of the Program Committee for their diligent work in the reviewer assignments and final paper selection, as well as the 600

---

[7] One paper was withdrawn.

reviewers for their support during the entire process. Finally, and most importantly, we thank all authors, co-authors, students, and supervisors, for submitting and presenting their high-quality work which made MICCAI 2018 a greatly enjoyable, informative, and successful event. We are especially indebted to those reviewers and PC members who helped us resolve last-minute missing reviews at a very short notice.

We are looking forward to seeing you in Shenzhen, China, at MICCAI 2019!

August 2018

Julia A. Schnabel
Christos Davatzikos
Gabor Fichtinger
Alejandro F. Frangi
Carlos Alberola-López
Alberto Gomez Herrero
Spyridon Bakas
Antonio R. Porras

Organization

Organizing Committee

General Chair and Program Co-chair

Alejandro F. Frangi   University of Leeds, UK

General Co-chair

Carlos Alberola-López   Universidad de Valladolid, Spain

Associate to General Chairs

Antonio R. Porras   Children's National Medical Center, Washington D.C., USA

Program Chair

Julia A. Schnabel   King's College London, UK

Program Co-chairs

Christos Davatzikos   University of Pennsylvania, USA
Gabor Fichtinger   Queen's University, Canada

Associates to Program Chairs

Spyridon Bakas   University of Pennsylvania, USA
Alberto Gomez Herrero   King's College London, UK

Tutorial and Educational Chair

Anne Martel   University of Toronto, Canada

Tutorial and Educational Co-chairs

Miguel González-Ballester   Universitat Pompeu Fabra, Spain
Marius Linguraru   Children's National Medical Center, Washington D.C., USA
Kensaku Mori   Nagoya University, Japan
Carl-Fredrik Westin   Harvard Medical School, USA

Workshop and Challenge Chair

Danail Stoyanov   University College London, UK

Workshop and Challenge Co-chairs

Hervé Delingette   Inria, France
Lena Maier-Hein   German Cancer Research Center, Germany
Zeike A. Taylor   University of Leeds, UK

Keynote Lecture Chair

Josien Pluim   TU Eindhoven, The Netherlands

Keynote Lecture Co-chairs

Matthias Harders   ETH Zurich, Switzerland
Septimiu Salcudean   The University of British Columbia, Canada

Corporate Affairs Chair

Terry Peters   Western University, Canada

Corporate Affairs Co-chairs

Hayit Greenspan   Tel Aviv University, Israel
Despina Kontos   University of Pennsylvania, USA
Guy Shechter   Philips, USA

Student Activities Facilitator

Demian Wasserman   Inria, France

Student Activities Co-facilitator

Karim Lekadir   Universitat Pompeu-Fabra, Spain

Communications Officer

Pedro Lopes   University of Leeds, UK

Conference Management

DEKON Group

Program Committee

Ali Gooya   University of Sheffield, UK
Amber Simpson   Memorial Sloan Kettering Cancer Center, USA
Andrew King   King's College London, UK
Bennett Landman   Vanderbilt University, USA
Bernhard Kainz   Imperial College London, UK
Burak Acar   Bogazici University, Turkey

Carola Schoenlieb	Cambridge University, UK
Caroline Essert	University of Strasbourg/ICUBE, France
Christian Wachinger	Ludwig Maximilian University of Munich, Germany
Christos Bergeles	King's College London, UK
Daphne Yu	Siemens Healthineers, USA
Duygu Tosun	University of California at San Francisco, USA
Emanuele Trucco	University of Dundee, UK
Ender Konukoglu	ETH Zurich, Switzerland
Enzo Ferrante	CONICET/Universidad Nacional del Litoral, Argentina
Erik Meijering	Erasmus University Medical Center, The Netherlands
Gozde Unal	Istanbul Technical University, Turkey
Guido Gerig	New York University, USA
Gustavo Carneiro	University of Adelaide, Australia
Hassan Rivaz	Concordia University, Canada
Herve Lombaert	ETS Montreal, Canada
Hongliang Ren	National University of Singapore, Singapore
Ingerid Reinertsen	SINTEF, Norway
Ipek Oguz	University of Pennsylvania/Vanderbilt University, USA
Ivana Isgum	University Medical Center Utrecht, The Netherlands
Juan Eugenio Iglesias	University College London, UK
Kayhan Batmanghelich	University of Pittsburgh/Carnegie Mellon University, USA
Laura Igual	Universitat de Barcelona, Spain
Lauren O'Donnell	Harvard University, USA
Le Lu	Ping An Technology US Research Labs, USA
Li Cheng	A*STAR Singapore, Singapore
Lilla Zöllei	Massachusetts General Hospital, USA
Linwei Wang	Rochester Institute of Technology, USA
Marc Niethammer	University of North Carolina at Chapel Hill, USA
Marius Staring	Leiden University Medical Center, The Netherlands
Marleen de Bruijne	Erasmus MC Rotterdam/University of Copenhagen, The Netherlands/Denmark
Marta Kersten	Concordia University, Canada
Mattias Heinrich	University of Luebeck, Germany
Meritxell Bach Cuadra	University of Lausanne, Switzerland
Miaomiao Zhang	Washington University in St. Louis, USA
Moti Freiman	Philips Healthcare, Israel
Nasir Rajpoot	University of Warwick, UK
Nassir Navab	Technical University of Munich, Germany
Pallavi Tiwari	Case Western Reserve University, USA
Pingkun Yan	Rensselaer Polytechnic Institute, USA
Purang Abolmaesumi	University of British Columbia, Canada
Ragini Verma	University of Pennsylvania, USA
Raphael Sznitman	University of Bern, Switzerland
Sandrine Voros	University of Grenoble, France

Sotirios Tsaftaris	University of Edinburgh, UK
Stamatia Giannarou	Imperial College London, UK
Stefanie Speidel	National Center for Tumor Diseases (NCT) Dresden, Germany
Stefanie Demirci	Technical University of Munich, Germany
Tammy Riklin Raviv	Ben-Gurion University, Israel
Tanveer Syeda-Mahmood	IBM Research, USA
Ulas Bagci	University of Central Florida, USA
Vamsi Ithapu	University of Wisconsin-Madison, USA
Yanwu Xu	Baidu Inc., China

Scientific Review Committee

Amir Abdi	Martin Benning
Ehsan Adeli	Aïcha BenTaieb
Iman Aganj	Ruth Bergman
Ola Ahmad	Alessandro Bevilacqua
Amr Ahmed	Ryoma Bise
Shazia Akbar	Isabelle Bloch
Alireza Akhondi-asl	Sebastian Bodenstedt
Saad Ullah Akram	Hrvoje Bogunovic
Amir Alansary	Gerda Bortsova
Shadi Albarqouni	Sylvain Bouix
Luis Alvarez	Felix Bragman
Deepak Anand	Christopher Bridge
Elsa Angelini	Tom Brosch
Rahman Attar	Aurelien Bustin
Chloé Audigier	Irène Buvat
Angelica Aviles-Rivero	Cesar Caballero-Gaudes
Ruqayya Awan	Ryan Cabeen
Suyash Awate	Nathan Cahill
Dogu Baran Aydogan	Jinzheng Cai
Shekoofeh Azizi	Weidong Cai
Katja Bühler	Tian Cao
Junjie Bai	Valentina Carapella
Wenjia Bai	M. Jorge Cardoso
Daniel Balfour	Daniel Castro
Walid Barhoumi	Daniel Coelho de Castro
Sarah Barman	Philippe C. Cattin
Michael Barrow	Juan Cerrolaza
Deepti Bathula	Suheyla Cetin Karayumak
Christian F. Baumgartner	Matthieu Chabanas
Pierre-Louis Bazin	Jayasree Chakraborty
Delaram Behnami	Rudrasis Chakraborty
Erik Bekkers	Rajib Chakravorty
Rami Ben-Ari	Vimal Chandran

Catie Chang
Pierre Chatelain
Akshay Chaudhari
Antong Chen
Chao Chen
Geng Chen
Hao Chen
Jianxu Chen
Jingyun Chen
Min Chen
Xin Chen
Yang Chen
Yuncong Chen
Jiezhi Cheng
Jun Cheng
Veronika Cheplygina
Farida Cheriet
Minqi Chong
Daan Christiaens
Serkan Cimen
Francesco Ciompi
Cedric Clouchoux
James Clough
Dana Cobzas
Noel Codella
Toby Collins
Olivier Commowick
Sailesh Conjeti
Pierre-Henri Conze
Tessa Cook
Timothy Cootes
Pierrick Coupé
Alessandro Crimi
Adrian Dalca
Sune Darkner
Dhritiman Das
Johan Debayle
Farah Deeba
Silvana Dellepiane
Adrien Depeursinge
Maria Deprez
Christian Desrosiers
Blake Dewey
Jwala Dhamala
Qi Dou
Karen Drukker

Lei Du
Lixin Duan
Florian Dubost
Nicolas Duchateau
James Duncan
Luc Duong
Nicha Dvornek
Oleh Dzyubachyk
Zach Eaton-Rosen
Mehran Ebrahimi
Matthias J. Ehrhardt
Ahmet Ekin
Ayman El-Baz
Randy Ellis
Mohammed Elmogy
Marius Erdt
Guray Erus
Marco Esposito
Joset Etzel
Jingfan Fan
Yong Fan
Aly Farag
Mohsen Farzi
Anahita Fathi Kazerooni
Hamid Fehri
Xinyang Feng
Olena Filatova
James Fishbaugh
Tom Fletcher
Germain Forestier
Denis Fortun
Alfred Franz
Muhammad Moazam Fraz
Wolfgang Freysinger
Jurgen Fripp
Huazhu Fu
Yang Fu
Bernhard Fuerst
Gareth Funka-Lea
Isabel Funke
Jan Funke
Francesca Galassi
Linlin Gao
Mingchen Gao
Yue Gao
Zhifan Gao

Utpal Garain
Mona Garvin
Aimilia Gastounioti
Romane Gauriau
Bao Ge
Sandesh Ghimire
Ali Gholipour
Rémi Giraud
Ben Glocker
Ehsan Golkar
Polina Golland
Yuanhao Gong
German Gonzalez
Pietro Gori
Alejandro Granados
Sasa Grbic
Enrico Grisan
Andrey Gritsenko
Abhijit Guha Roy
Yanrong Guo
Yong Guo
Vikash Gupta
Benjamin Gutierrez Becker
Séverine Habert
Ilker Hacihaliloglu
Stathis Hadjidemetriou
Ghassan Hamarneh
Adam Harrison
Grant Haskins
Charles Hatt
Tiancheng He
Mehdi Hedjazi Moghari
Tobias Heimann
Christoph Hennersperger
Alfredo Hernandez
Monica Hernandez
Moises Hernandez Fernandez
Carlos Hernandez-Matas
Matthew Holden
Yi Hong
Nicolas Honnorat
Benjamin Hou
Yipeng Hu
Heng Huang
Junzhou Huang
Weilin Huang

Xiaolei Huang
Yawen Huang
Henkjan Huisman
Yuankai Huo
Sarfaraz Hussein
Jana Hutter
Seong Jae Hwang
Atsushi Imiya
Amir Jamaludin
Faraz Janan
Uditha Jarayathne
Xi Jiang
Jieqing Jiao
Dakai Jin
Yueming Jin
Bano Jordan
Anand Joshi
Shantanu Joshi
Leo Joskowicz
Christoph Jud
Siva Teja Kakileti
Jayashree Kalpathy-Cramer
Ali Kamen
Neerav Karani
Anees Kazi
Eric Kerfoot
Erwan Kerrien
Farzad Khalvati
Hassan Khan
Bishesh Khanal
Ron Kikinis
Hyo-Eun Kim
Hyunwoo Kim
Jinman Kim
Minjeong Kim
Benjamin Kimia
Kivanc Kose
Julia Krüger
Pavitra Krishnaswamy
Frithjof Kruggel
Elizabeth Krupinski
Sofia Ira Ktena
Arjan Kuijper
Ashnil Kumar
Neeraj Kumar
Punithakumar Kumaradevan

Manuela Kunz
Jin Tae Kwak
Alexander Ladikos
Rodney Lalonde
Pablo Lamata
Catherine Laporte
Carole Lartizien
Toni Lassila
Andras Lasso
Matthieu Le
Maria J. Ledesma-Carbayo
Hansang Lee
Jong-Hwan Lee
Soochahn Lee
Etienne Léger
Beatrice Lentes
Wee Kheng Leow
Nikolas Lessmann
Annan Li
Gang Li
Ruoyu Li
Wenqi Li
Xiang Li
Yuanwei Li
Chunfeng Lian
Jianming Liang
Hongen Liao
Ruizhi Liao
Roxane Licandro
Lanfen Lin
Claudia Lindner
Cristian Linte
Feng Liu
Hui Liu
Jianfei Liu
Jundong Liu
Kefei Liu
Mingxia Liu
Sidong Liu
Marco Lorenzi
Xiongbiao Luo
Jinglei Lv
Ilwoo Lyu
Omar M. Rijal
Pablo Márquez Neila
Henning Müller

Kai Ma
Khushhall Chandra Mahajan
Dwarikanath Mahapatra
Andreas Maier
Klaus H. Maier-Hein
Sokratis Makrogiannis
Grégoire Malandain
Anand Malpani
Jose Manjon
Tommaso Mansi
Awais Mansoor
Anne Martel
Diana Mateus
Arnaldo Mayer
Jamie McClelland
Stephen McKenna
Ronak Mehta
Raphael Meier
Qier Meng
Yu Meng
Bjoern Menze
Liang Mi
Shun Miao
Abhishek Midya
Zhe Min
Rashika Mishra
Marc Modat
Norliza Mohd Noor
Mehdi Moradi
Rodrigo Moreno
Kensaku Mori
Aliasghar Mortazi
Peter Mountney
Arrate Muñoz-Barrutia
Anirban Mukhopadhyay
Arya Nabavi
Layan Nahlawi
Ana Ineyda Namburete
Valery Naranjo
Peter Neher
Hannes Nickisch
Dong Nie
Lipeng Ning
Jack Noble
Vincent Noblet
Alexey Novikov

Ilkay Oksuz
Ozan Oktay
John Onofrey
Eliza Orasanu
Felipe Orihuela-Espina
Jose Orlando
Yusuf Osmanlioglu
David Owen
Cristina Oyarzun Laura
Jose-Antonio Pérez-Carrasco
Danielle Pace
J. Blas Pagador
Akshay Pai
Xenophon Papademetris
Bartlomiej Papiez
Toufiq Parag
Magdalini Paschali
Angshuman Paul
Christian Payer
Jialin Peng
Tingying Peng
Xavier Pennec
Sérgio Pereira
Mehran Pesteie
Loic Peter
Igor Peterlik
Simon Pezold
Micha Pfeifer
Dzung Pham
Renzo Phellan
Pramod Pisharady
Josien Pluim
Kilian Pohl
Jean-Baptiste Poline
Alison Pouch
Prateek Prasanna
Philip Pratt
Raphael Prevost
Esther Puyol Anton
Yuchuan Qiao
Gwénolé Quellec
Pradeep Reddy Raamana
Julia Rackerseder
Hedyeh Rafii-Tari
Mehdi Rahim
Kashif Rajpoot

Parnesh Raniga
Yogesh Rathi
Saima Rathore
Nishant Ravikumar
Shan E. Ahmed Raza
Islem Rekik
Beatriz Remeseiro
Markus Rempfler
Mauricio Reyes
Constantino Reyes-Aldasoro
Nicola Rieke
Laurent Risser
Leticia Rittner
Yong Man Ro
Emma Robinson
Rafael Rodrigues
Marc-Michel Rohé
Robert Rohling
Karl Rohr
Plantefeve Rosalie
Holger Roth
Su Ruan
Danny Ruijters
Juan Ruiz-Alzola
Mert Sabuncu
Frank Sachse
Farhang Sahba
Septimiu Salcudean
Gerard Sanroma
Emine Saritas
Imari Sato
Alexander Schlaefer
Jerome Schmid
Caitlin Schneider
Jessica Schrouff
Thomas Schultz
Suman Sedai
Biswa Sengupta
Ortal Senouf
Maxime Sermesant
Carmen Serrano
Amit Sethi
Muhammad Shaban
Reuben Shamir
Yeqin Shao
Li Shen

Bibo Shi
Kuangyu Shi
Hoo-Chang Shin
Russell Shinohara
Viviana Siless
Carlos A. Silva
Matthew Sinclair
Vivek Singh
Korsuk Sirinukunwattana
Ihor Smal
Michal Sofka
Jure Sokolic
Hessam Sokooti
Ahmed Soliman
Stefan Sommer
Diego Sona
Yang Song
Aristeidis Sotiras
Jamshid Sourati
Rachel Sparks
Ziga Spiclin
Lawrence Staib
Ralf Stauder
Darko Stern
Colin Studholme
Martin Styner
Heung-Il Suk
Jian Sun
Xu Sun
Kyunghyun Sung
Nima Tajbakhsh
Sylvain Takerkart
Chaowei Tan
Jeremy Tan
Mingkui Tan
Hui Tang
Min Tang
Youbao Tang
Yuxing Tang
Christine Tanner
Qian Tao
Giacomo Tarroni
Zeike Taylor
Kim Han Thung
Yanmei Tie
Daniel Toth

Nicolas Toussaint
Jocelyne Troccaz
Tomasz Trzcinski
Ahmet Tuysuzoglu
Andru Twinanda
Carole Twining
Eranga Ukwatta
Mathias Unberath
Tamas Ungi
Martin Urschler
Maria Vakalopoulou
Vanya Valindria
Koen Van Leemput
Hien Van Nguyen
Gijs van Tulder
S. Swaroop Vedula
Harini Veeraraghavan
Miguel Vega
Anant Vemuri
Gopalkrishna Veni
Archana Venkataraman
François-Xavier Vialard
Pierre-Frederic Villard
Satish Viswanath
Wolf-Dieter Vogl
Ingmar Voigt
Tomaz Vrtovec
Bo Wang
Guotai Wang
Jiazhuo Wang
Liansheng Wang
Manning Wang
Sheng Wang
Yalin Wang
Zhe Wang
Simon Warfield
Chong-Yaw Wee
Juergen Weese
Benzheng Wei
Wolfgang Wein
William Wells
Rene Werner
Daniel Wesierski
Matthias Wilms
Adam Wittek
Jelmer Wolterink

Ken C. L. Wong
Jonghye Woo
Pengxiang Wu
Tobias Wuerfl
Yong Xia
Yiming Xiao
Weidi Xie
Yuanpu Xie
Fangxu Xing
Fuyong Xing
Tao Xiong
Daguang Xu
Yan Xu
Zheng Xu
Zhoubing Xu
Ziyue Xu
Wufeng Xue
Jingwen Yan
Ke Yan
Yuguang Yan
Zhennan Yan
Dong Yang
Guang Yang
Xiao Yang
Xin Yang
Jianhua Yao
Jiawen Yao
Xiaohui Yao
Chuyang Ye
Menglong Ye
Jingru Yi
Jinhua Yu
Lequan Yu
Weimin Yu
Yixuan Yuan
Evangelia Zacharaki
Ernesto Zacur

Guillaume Zahnd
Marco Zenati
Ke Zeng
Oliver Zettinig
Daoqiang Zhang
Fan Zhang
Han Zhang
Heye Zhang
Jiong Zhang
Jun Zhang
Lichi Zhang
Lin Zhang
Ling Zhang
Mingli Zhang
Pin Zhang
Shu Zhang
Tong Zhang
Yong Zhang
Yunyan Zhang
Zizhao Zhang
Qingyu Zhao
Shijie Zhao
Yitian Zhao
Guoyan Zheng
Yalin Zheng
Yinqiang Zheng
Zichun Zhong
Luping Zhou
Zhiguo Zhou
Dajiang Zhu
Wentao Zhu
Xiaofeng Zhu
Xiahai Zhuang
Aneeq Zia
Veronika Zimmer
Majd Zreik
Reyer Zwiggelaar

Mentorship Program (Mentors)

Stephen Aylward   Kitware Inc., USA
Christian Barillot   IRISA/CNRS/University of Rennes, France
Kayhan Batmanghelich   University of Pittsburgh/Carnegie Mellon University,
                         USA
Christos Bergeles   King's College London, UK

Marleen de Bruijne — Erasmus Medical Center Rotterdam/University of Copenhagen, The Netherlands/Denmark

Cheng Li — University of Alberta, Canada

Stefanie Demirci — Technical University of Munich, Germany

Simon Duchesne — University of Laval, Canada

Enzo Ferrante — CONICET/Universidad Nacional del Litoral, Argentina

Alejandro F. Frangi — University of Leeds, UK

Miguel A. González-Ballester — Universitat Pompeu Fabra, Spain

Stamatia (Matina) Giannarou — Imperial College London, UK

Juan Eugenio Iglesias-Gonzalez — University College London, UK

Laura Igual — Universitat de Barcelona, Spain

Leo Joskowicz — The Hebrew University of Jerusalem, Israel

Bernhard Kainz — Imperial College London, UK

Shuo Li — University of Western Ontario, Canada

Marius G. Linguraru — Children's National Health System/George Washington University, USA

Le Lu — Ping An Technology US Research Labs, USA

Tommaso Mansi — Siemens Healthineers, USA

Anne Martel — Sunnybrook Research Institute, USA

Kensaku Mori — Nagoya University, Japan

Parvin Mousavi — Queen's University, Canada

Nassir Navab — Technical University of Munich/Johns Hopkins University, USA

Marc Niethammer — University of North Carolina at Chapel Hill, USA

Ipek Oguz — University of Pennsylvania/Vanderbilt University, USA

Josien Pluim — Eindhoven University of Technology, The Netherlands

Jerry L. Prince — Johns Hopkins University, USA

Nicola Rieke — NVIDIA Corp./Technical University of Munich, Germany

Daniel Rueckert — Imperial College London, UK

Julia A. Schnabel — King's College London, UK

Raphael Sznitman — University of Bern, Switzerland

Jocelyne Troccaz — CNRS/University of Grenoble, France

Gozde Unal — Istanbul Technical University, Turkey

Max A. Viergever — Utrecht University/University Medical Center Utrecht, The Netherlands

Linwei Wang — Rochester Institute of Technology, USA

Yanwu Xu — Baidu Inc., China

Miaomiao Zhang — Lehigh University, USA

Guoyan Zheng — University of Bern, Switzerland

Lilla Zöllei — Massachusetts General Hospital, USA

Sponsors and Funders

Platinum Sponsors

- NVIDIA Inc.
- Siemens Healthineers GmbH

Gold Sponsors

- Guangzhou Shiyuan Electronics Co. Ltd.
- Subtle Medical Inc.

Silver Sponsors

- Arterys Inc.
- Claron Technology Inc.
- ImSight Inc.
- ImFusion GmbH
- Medtronic Plc

Bronze Sponsors

- Depwise Inc.
- Carl Zeiss AG

Travel Bursary Support

- MICCAI Society
- National Institutes of Health, USA
- EPSRC-NIHR Medical Image Analysis Network (EP/N026993/1), UK

Contents – Part II

Optical and Histology Applications: Histology Applications

Optical and Histology Applications: Microscopy Applications

Optical and Histology Applications: Optical Coherence Tomography and Other Optical Imaging Applications

**Cardiac, Chest and Abdominal Applications:
Cardiac Imaging Applications**

Cardiac, Chest and Abdominal Applications: Colorectal, Kidney and Liver Imaging Applications

**Cardiac, Chest and Abdominal Applications: Lung
Imaging Applications**

**Cardiac, Chest and Abdominal Applications: Breast
Imaging Applications**

Cardiac, Chest and Abdominal Applications:
Other Abdominal Applications

Optical and Histology Applications:
Optical Imaging Applications

Instance Segmentation and Tracking with Cosine Embeddings and Recurrent Hourglass Networks

Christian Payer[1]([✉]) [iD], Darko Štern[2] [iD], Thomas Neff[1] [iD], Horst Bischof[1] [iD], and Martin Urschler[2,3] [iD]

[1] Institute of Computer Graphics and Vision, Graz University of Technology, Graz, Austria
christian.payer@icg.tugraz.at
[2] Ludwig Boltzmann Institute for Clinical Forensic Imaging, Graz, Austria
[3] BioTechMed-Graz, Graz, Austria

Abstract. Different to semantic segmentation, instance segmentation assigns unique labels to each individual instance of the same class. In this work, we propose a novel recurrent fully convolutional network architecture for tracking such instance segmentations over time. The network architecture incorporates convolutional gated recurrent units (ConvGRU) into a stacked hourglass network to utilize temporal video information. Furthermore, we train the network with a novel embedding loss based on cosine similarities, such that the network predicts unique embeddings for every instance throughout videos. Afterwards, these embeddings are clustered among subsequent video frames to create the final tracked instance segmentations. We evaluate the recurrent hourglass network by segmenting left ventricles in MR videos of the heart, where it outperforms a network that does not incorporate video information. Furthermore, we show applicability of the cosine embedding loss for segmenting leaf instances on still images of plants. Finally, we evaluate the framework for instance segmentation and tracking on six datasets of the ISBI celltracking challenge, where it shows state-of-the-art performance.

Keywords: Cell · Tracking · Segmentation · Instances · Recurrent Video · Embeddings

1 Introduction

Instance segmentation plays an important role in biomedical imaging tasks like cell migration, but also in computer vision based tasks like scene understanding. It is considerably more difficult than semantic segmentation (e.g., [10]), since instance segmentation does not only assign class labels to pixels, but also distinguishes between instances within each class, e.g., each individual person on an image from a surveillance camera is assigned a unique ID.

This work was supported by the Austrian Science Fund (FWF): P28078-N33.

© Springer Nature Switzerland AG 2018
A. F. Frangi et al. (Eds.): MICCAI 2018, LNCS 11071, pp. 3–11, 2018.
https://doi.org/10.1007/978-3-030-00934-2_1

Mainly due to the high performance of the U-Net [12], semantic segmentation has been successfully used as a first step in medical instance segmentation tasks, e.g., cell tracking. However, for instances to be separated as connected components during postprocessing, borders of instances have to be treated with special care. In the computer vision community, many methods for instance segmentation have in common that they solely segment one instance at a time. In [4], all instances are first detected and independently segmented, while in [11], recurrent networks are used to memorize which instances were already segmented. Segmenting solely one instance at a time can be problematic when hundreds of instances are visible in the image, as often is the case with e.g., cell instance segmentation. Recent methods are segmenting each instance simultaneously, by predicting embeddings for all pixels at once [5,8]. These embeddings have similar values within an instance, but differ among instances. In the task of cell segmentation and tracking, temporal information is an important cue to establish coherence between frames, thus preserving instances throughout videos. Despite improvements of instance segmentation using embeddings, to the best of our knowledge, combining them with temporal information for tracking instance segmentations has not been presented.

In this paper, we propose to use recurrent fully convolutional networks for embedding-based instance segmentation and tracking. To memorize temporal information, we integrate convolutional gated recurrent units (ConvGRU [2]) into a stacked hourglass network [9]. Furthermore, we use a novel embedding loss based on cosine similarities, where we exploit the four color map theorem [1], by requiring only neighboring instances to have different embeddings.

2   Instance Segmentation and Tracking

Figure 1 shows our proposed framework on a cell instance segmentation and tracking example. To distinguish cell instances, they are represented as embeddings at different time points. By representing temporal sequences of embeddings in a recurrent hourglass network, a predictor can be learnt from the data, which allows tracking of embeddings also in the case of mitosis events. To finally generate instance segmentations, clustering of the predicted embeddings is performed.

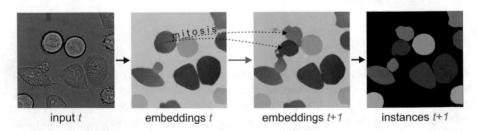

input t embeddings t embeddings $t+1$ instances $t+1$

Fig. 1. Overview of our proposed framework showing input image, propagation of cosine embeddings from frame t to frame $t + 1$ (three randomly chosen embedding dimensions as RGB channels), and resulting clustered instances.

2.1   Recurrent Stacked Hourglass Network

We modify the stacked hourglass architecture [9] by integrating ConvGRU [2] to propagate temporal information, as shown in Fig. 2. Differently from the original stacked hourglass network, we use single convolution layers with 3×3 filters and 64 outputs for all blocks in the contracting and expanding paths, while we use ConvGRU with 3×3 filters and 64 outputs in between paths. As proposed by [9], we also stack two hourglasses in a row to improve network predictions. Therefore, we concatenate the output of the first hourglass with the input image to use it as input for the second hourglass. We apply the loss function on the outputs of both hourglasses, while we only use the outputs of the second hourglass for the clustering of embeddings.

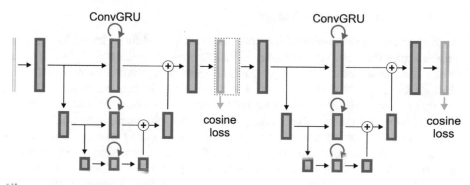

Fig. 2. Overview of the recurrent stacked hourglass network with two hourglasses and three levels. Yellow bars: input; blue boxes: convolutions; red boxes: ConvGRU; dashed black box: concatenation; green boxes: embeddings.

2.2   Cosine Embedding Loss

We let the network predict a d-dimensional embedding vector $e_p \in \mathbb{R}^d$ for each pixel p of the image. To separate instances $i \in \mathbb{I}$, firstly, embeddings of pixels $p \in \mathbb{S}^{(i)}$ belonging to the same instance i need to be similar, and secondly, embeddings of $\mathbb{S}^{(i)}$ need to be dissimilar to embeddings of pixels $p \in \mathbb{S}^{(j)}$ of other instances $j \neq i$. Here, we treat background as an independent instance. Following from the four color map theorem [1], only neighboring instances need to have different embeddings. Thus, we relax the need of dissimilarity between different instances only to the neighboring ones, i.e., $\mathbb{N}^{(i)} = \bigcup_j \mathbb{S}^{(j)}$ for all instances $j \neq i$ within pixel-wise distance $r_\mathbb{N}$ to instance i. This relaxation simplifies the problem by assigning only a limited number of different embeddings to a possibly large number of different instances.

We compare two embeddings with the cosine similarity

$$\cos(e_1, e_2) = \frac{e_1 \cdot e_2}{\|e_1\| \|e_2\|}, \tag{1}$$

which ranges from -1 to 1, while -1 indicates the vectors have the opposite, 0 orthogonal, and 1 the same direction. We define the cosine embedding loss as

$$L = \frac{1}{|\mathbb{I}|} \sum_{i \in \mathbb{I}} \left(1 - \frac{1}{|\mathbb{S}^{(i)}|} \sum_{p \in \mathbb{S}^{(i)}} \cos(\bar{e}^{(i)}, e_p) \right) + \left(\frac{1}{|\mathbb{N}^{(i)}|} \sum_{p \in \mathbb{N}^{(i)}} \cos(\bar{e}^{(i)}, e_p)^2 \right), \quad (2)$$

where the mean embedding of instance i is defined as $\bar{e}^{(i)} = \frac{1}{|\mathbb{S}^{(i)}|} \sum_{p \in \mathbb{S}^{(i)}} e_p$. By minimizing L, the first term urges embeddings e_p of pixels $p \in \mathbb{S}^{(i)}$ to have the same direction as the mean $\bar{e}^{(i)}$, which is the case when $\cos(\bar{e}^{(i)}, e_p) \approx 1$, while the second term pushes embeddings e_p of pixels $p \in \mathbb{N}^{(i)}$ to be orthogonal to the mean $\bar{e}^{(i)}$, i.e., $\cos(\bar{e}^{(i)}, e_p) \approx 0$.

2.3 Clustering of Embeddings

To get the final segmentations from the predicted embeddings, individual groups of embeddings that describe different instances need to be identified. As the number of instances is not known, we perform this grouping with the clustering algorithm HDBSCAN [3] that estimates the number of clusters automatically. For each dataset, two HDBSCAN parameters have to be adjusted: minimal points m_{pts} and minimal cluster size m_{clSize}. To simplify clustering and still be able to detect splitting of instances, we cluster only overlapping pairs of consecutive frames at a time. Since our embedding loss allows same embeddings for different instances that are far apart, we use both image coordinates and value of the embeddings as data points for the clustering algorithm. After identifying the embedding clusters with HDBSCAN and filtering clusters that are smaller than t_{size}, the final segmented instances for each frame pair are obtained.

For merging the segmented instances in overlapping frame pairs, we identify same instances by the highest intersection over union (IoU) between each segmented instance in the overlapping frame. The resulting segmentations are then upsampled back to the original image size, generating the final segmented and tracked instances.

3 Experimental Setup and Results

We train the networks with TensorFlow[1] and perform on-the-fly data augmentation with SimpleITK[2]. We use hourglass networks with seven levels and an input size of 256×256, while we scale the input images to fit. All recurrent networks are trained on sequences of ten frames. We refer to the supplementary material for individual training and augmentation parameters, as well as individual values of parameter described in Sect. 2.

Left Ventricle Segmentation: To show that our proposed recurrent stacked hourglass network is able to incorporate temporal information, we perform

---

[1] https://www.tensorflow.org/.
[2] http://www.simpleitk.org/.

semantic segmentation on videos of short-axis MR slices of the heart from the left ventricle segmentation challenge [14]. We compare the recurrent network with a non-recurrent version, where we replace each ConvGRU with a convolution layer to keep the network complexity the same. Since outer slices do not contain parts of the left ventricle, the networks are evaluated on the three central slices that contain both left ventricle myocardium and blood cavity (see Fig. 3a). We train the networks with a softmax cross entropy loss to segment three labels, i.e., background, myocardium, and blood cavity. We use a three-fold cross-validation setup, where we randomly split datasets of 96 patients into three equally sized folds. Table 1a shows the IoU for our internal cross-validation of both recurrent and non-recurrent stacked hourglass networks.

Leaf Instance Segmentation: We show that the cosine embedding loss and the subsequent clustering are suitable for instance segmentation without temporal information, by evaluating on the A1 dataset of the CVPPP challenge for segmenting individual plant leaves [7] (see Fig. 3b). We use the non-recurrent version of the proposed network from the previous experiment to predict embeddings with 32 dimensions. Consequently, the clustering is also performed on single images. As we were not able to provide results on the challenge test set in time before finalizing this paper, we report results of an internal three-fold cross-validation of the 128 training images. In consensus with [13], we report the symmetric best Dice (SBD) and the absolute difference in count ($|DiC|$) and compare to other methods in Table 1b.

Cell Instance Tracking: As our main experiment, we show applicability of our full framework for instance segmentation and tracking by evaluating six different datasets of cell microscopy videos from the ISBI celltracking challenge [15]. Each celltracking dataset consists of two annotated training videos and two testing videos with image sizes ranging from 512×512 to 1200×1024 and with 48 to 138 frames. We refer to [6] for additional imaging and video parameters. As the instance IDs in groundtruth images are consistent throughout the whole video only for tracking, but not for segmentation, we merge both tracking and segmentation groundtruth for each frame to have consistent instance IDs. Furthermore to learn the background embeddings, we only use the frames on which every cell is segmented. With hyperparameters determined on the two annotated training videos from each dataset, we train the networks for predicting embeddings of size 16 on both videos for our challenge submission.

To compete in the tracking metric of the challenge, the framework is required to identify the parent ID of each cell. As the framework is able to identify splitting cells and to assign new instance IDs (i.e., mitosis as seen on Fig. 1), the parent ID of each newly created instance is determined as the instance with the highest IoU in previous frames. We further postprocess the cells' family tree to be consistent with the evaluation criteria, e.g., an instance ID may not be used after splitting into children. The results in comparison to the top performing methods are presented in Table 2.

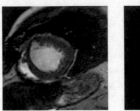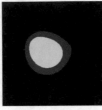

(a) Heart MRI input and segmentation.

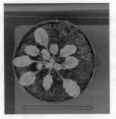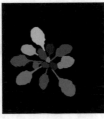

(b) Plant leaves input and instances.

Fig. 3. Qualitative results of the left ventricle segmentation and the CVPPP leaf instance segmentation. The images on the left side show example inputs, the images on the right side show the predicted segmentations.

Table 1. Quantitative results of the left ventricle segmentation and the CVPPP leaf instance segmentation. Values show mean ± standard deviation. Note that we report our results for both datasets based on a three-fold cross-validation setup. Thus, they are not directly comparable to other published results. IoU: intersection over union; myo: myocardium; cav: blood cavity; SBD: symmetric best Dice; |DiC|: absolute difference in count.

(a) Quantitative results of the heart MRI left ventricle segmentation.

	IoU_{myo}	IoU_{cav}
non-recurrent	78.3 ± 9.2	89.1 ± 7.7
recurrent	$\mathbf{79.4 \pm 8.5}$	$\mathbf{89.4 \pm 7.2}$

(b) Quantitative results of the CVPPP leaf instance segmentation. Values taken from [13].

	SBD	|DiC|
RIS+CRF	66.6 ± 8.7	1.1 ± 0.9
MSU	66.7 ± 7.6	2.3 ± 1.6
Nottingham	68.3 ± 6.3	3.8 ± 2.0
Wageningen	71.1 ± 6.2	2.2 ± 1.6
IPK	74.4 ± 4.3	2.6 ± 1.8
IS+RA [11]	$\mathbf{84.9 \pm 4.8}$	$\mathbf{0.8 \pm 1.0}$
Ours	84.5 ± 5.5	1.5 ± 1.2

4 Discussion and Conclusion

Up to our knowledge, we are the first to present a method that incorporates temporal information into a network to allow tracking of embeddings for instance segmentation. We perform three experiments to show different aspects of our novel method, i.e., temporal segmentation, instance segmentation, and combined instance segmentation and tracking. Thus, we demonstrate the wide applicability of our approach.

We use the left ventricle segmentation experiment to show that our novel recurrent stacked hourglass network can be used for incorporating temporal information. It can be seen from the results of the experiment that incorporating ConvGRU between contracting and expanding path deeply inside the architecture improves over the baseline stacked hourglass network. Nevertheless, since we simplified the evaluation protocol of the challenge, the results of the experiment should not be directly compared to other reported results. Moreover,

Table 2. Quantitative results of the celltracking datasets for overall performance (OP), segmentation (SEG), and tracking (TRA), as described in [15].

		DIC-HeLa	Fluo-MSC	Fluo-GOWT1	Fluo-HeLa	PhC-U373	Fluo-SIM+	
OP	1st	0.864	0.759	0.951	0.942	0.951	0.882	Ours
	2nd	0.828	0.676	0.914	0.940	0.896	0.878	BGU-IL (1–2)
	3rd	0.629	0.658	0.902	0.928	0.895	0.874	CUNI-CZ
			5th 0.631		11th 0.829	4th 0.888	9th 0.810	CVUT-CZ
SEG	1st	0.814	0.645	0.927	0.903	0.920	0.802	FR-Be-GE
	2nd	0.776	0.590	0.893	0.893	0.832	0.791	FR-Ro-GE
	3rd	0.464	0.582	0.887	0.869	0.826	0.781	HD-Har-GE
			5th 0.496	4th 0.880	10th 0.749	5th 0.793	8th 0.718	KIT-GE
TRA	1st	0.915	0.873	0.976	0.991	0.983	0.975	KTH-SE (1–4)
	2nd	0.881	0.765	0.947	0.987	0.981	0.961	LEID-NL
	3rd	0.797	0.763	0.925	0.986	0.977	0.957	
					12th 0.909		10th 0.902	

benefits of such deep incorporation compared to having recurrent layers on other positions in the network [11] remain to be shown.

This paper also contributes with a novel embedding loss based on cosine similarities. Most of the methods that use embeddings for differentiating between instance segmentations are based on maximizing distances of embeddings in the Euclidean space, e.g., [8]. When using such embedding losses, we observed problems when combining them with recurrent networks, presumably due to unrestricted embedding values. To overcome these problems, we use cosine similarities that normalize embeddings. The only other work that suggests cosine similarities for instance segmentation with embeddings is the unpublished work of [5]. However, compared to their embedding loss that takes all instances into account, our novel loss focuses only on neighboring ones, which can be beneficial for optimization in the case of a large number of instances. We evaluate our novel loss on the CVPPP challenge dedicated to instance segmentation from still images. While waiting for the results of the competition, our method evaluated with three-fold cross-validation shows to be in line with the currently leading method, and has a significant margin to the second best. Moreover, compared to the leading method [11], the architecture of our method is considerably simpler.

In our main experiment for segmentation and tracking of instances, we evaluate our method on the ISBI celltracking challenge, showing large variability in visual appearance, size and number of cells. Our method achieves two first and two second places among the six submitted datasets in the tracking metric. For the dataset DIC-HeLa, having a dense layout of cells as seen in Fig. 1, we outperform all other methods in both tracking and segmentation metrics. On the dataset Fluo-GOWT1 we rank overall second. On the datasets Fluo-HeLa and Flou-SIM+, which consist of images with small cells, our method does not perform well due to the need to downsample images for the network to process them. When the downsampling results in drastic reduction of cell sizes, our method fails to create instance segmentations, thus explaining the not satisfying performance also in tracking. To increase the resolution and consequently improve segmentation and tracking, we could split the input image into multiple smaller parts, similarly as done in [12].

In conclusion, our work has shown that embeddings for instance segmentation can be successfully combined with recurrent networks incorporating temporal information to perform instance tracking. In future work, we will investigate the possibility of incorporating the required clustering step inside of a single end-to-end trained network, which could simplify the framework and further improve the segmentation and tracking results.

References

1. Appel, K., Haken, W.: Every planar map is four colorable. Bull. Am. Math. Soc. **82**(5), 711–712 (1976)
2. Ballas, N., Yao, L., Pal, C., Courville, A.: Delving deeper into convolutional networks for learning video representations. In: International Conference on Learning Representations. CoRR, abs:1511.06432 (2016)
3. Campello, R.J.G.B., Moulavi, D., Zimek, A., Sander, J.: Hierarchical density estimates for data clustering, visualization, and outlier detection. ACM Trans. Knowl. Discov. Data **10**(1), 5:1–5:51 (2015)
4. He, K., Gkioxari, G., Dollár, P., Girshick, R.: Mask R-CNN. In: Proceedings of the International Conference on Computer Vision, pp. 2980–2988 (2017)
5. Kong, S., Fowlkes, C.: Recurrent pixel embedding for instance grouping. CoRR, abs:1712.08273 (2017)
6. Maška, M., Ulman, V., Svoboda, D., Matula, P., Matula, P., Ederra, C., et al.: A benchmark for comparison of cell tracking algorithms. Bioinformatics **30**(11), 1609–1617 (2014)
7. Minervini, M., Fischbach, A., Scharr, H., Tsaftaris, S.A.: Finely-grained annotated datasets for image-based plant phenotyping. Pattern Recogn. Lett. **81**, 80–89 (2016)
8. Newell, A., Huang, Z., Deng, J.: Associative embedding: end-to-end learning for joint detection and grouping. In: Advances in Neural Information Processing Systems, pp. 2277–2287. Curran Associates, Inc. (2017)
9. Newell, A., Yang, K., Deng, J.: Stacked hourglass networks for human pose estimation. In: Leibe, B., Matas, J., Sebe, N., Welling, M. (eds.) ECCV 2016. LNCS, vol. 9912, pp. 483–499. Springer, Cham (2016). https://doi.org/10.1007/978-3-319-46484-8_29
10. Payer, C., Štern, D., Bischof, H., Urschler, M.: Multi-label whole heart segmentation using CNNs and anatomical label configurations. In: Pop, M., et al. (eds.) STACOM 2017. LNCS, vol. 10663, pp. 190–198. Springer, Cham (2018). https://doi.org/10.1007/978-3-319-75541-0_20
11. Ren, M., Zemel, R.S.: End-to-end instance segmentation with recurrent attention. In: Proceedings of the Computer Vision and Pattern Recognition, pp. 6656–6664 (2017)
12. Ronneberger, O., Fischer, P., Brox, T.: U-Net: convolutional networks for biomedical image segmentation. In: Navab, N., Hornegger, J., Wells, W.M., Frangi, A.F. (eds.) MICCAI 2015. LNCS, vol. 9351, pp. 234–241. Springer, Cham (2015). https://doi.org/10.1007/978-3-319-24574-4_28

13. Scharr, H., et al.: Leaf segmentation in plant phenotyping: a collation study. Mach. Vis. Appl. **27**(4), 585–606 (2016)
14. Suinesiaputra, A., Cowan, B.R., Al-Agamy, A.O., Elattar, M.A., Ayache, N., et al.: A collaborative resource to build consensus for automated left ventricular segmentation of cardiac MR images. Med. Image Anal. **18**(1), 50–62 (2014)
15. Ulman, V., Maška, M., Magnusson, K.E., Ronneberger, O., Haubold, C., Harder, N.: An objective comparison of cell-tracking algorithms. Nat. Methods **14**(12), 1141–1152 (2017)

Skin Lesion Classification in Dermoscopy Images Using Synergic Deep Learning

Jianpeng Zhang[1], Yutong Xie[1], Qi Wu[2], and Yong Xia[1(✉)]

[1] School of Computer Science and Engineering, Northwestern Polytechnical
University, Xi'an 710072, People's Republic of China
yxia@nwpu.edu.cn
[2] School of Computer Science, University of Adelaide, Adelaide, SA 5005, Australia

Abstract. Automated skin lesion classification in the dermoscopy images is an essential way to improve diagnostic performance and reduce melanoma deaths. Although deep learning has shown proven advantages over traditional methods, which rely on handcrafted features, in image classification, it remains challenging to classify skin lesions due to the significant intra-class variation and inter-class similarity. In this paper, we propose a synergic deep learning (SDL) model to address this issue, which not only uses dual deep convolutional neural networks (DCNNs) but also enables them to mutually learn from each other. Specifically, we concatenate the image representation learned by both DCNNs as the input of a synergic network, which has a fully connected structure and predicts whether the pair of input images belong to the same class. We train the SDL model in the end-to-end manner under the supervision of the classification error in each DCNN and the synergic error. We evaluated our SDL model on the ISIC 2016 Skin Lesion Classification dataset and achieved the state-of-the-art performance.

1 Introduction

Skin cancer is one of the most common form of cancers in the United States and many other countries, with 5 million cases occurring annually [1]. Dermoscopy, a recent technique of visual inspection that both magnifies the skin and eliminates surface reflection, is one of the essential means to improve diagnostic performance and reduce melanoma deaths [2]. Classifying the melanoma in dermoscopy images is a significant and challenging task in the computer-aided diagnosis.

Recently, deep learning has led to tremendous success in skin lesion classification [3–5]. Ge et al. [3] demonstrated the effectiveness of cross-modality learning of deep convolutional neural networks (DCNNs) by jointly using the dermoscopy and clinical skin images. Yu et al. [4] proposed to leverage very deep DCNNs for automated melanoma recognition in dermoscopy images in two steps – segmentation and classification. Esteva et al. [5] trained a DCNN using 129,450 clinical images for the diagnose of the malignant carcinomas and malignant melanomas and achieved the performance that matches the performance of

© Springer Nature Switzerland AG 2018
A. F. Frangi et al. (Eds.): MICCAI 2018, LNCS 11071, pp. 12–20, 2018.
https://doi.org/10.1007/978-3-030-00934-2_2

21 board-certified dermatologists. Despite the achievements, this task remains challenging due to two reasons. First, deep neural network models may overfit the training data, as there is usually a relative small dermoscopy image dataset and this relates to the work required in acquiring the image data and then in image annotation [6]. Second, the intra-class variation and inter-class similarity pose even greater challenges to the differentiation of malignant skin lesions from benign ones [4]. As shown in Fig. 1, there is a big visual difference between the benign skin lesions (a) and (b) and between malignant lesions (c) and (d). Nevertheless, the benign skin lesions (a) and (b) are similar to the malignant lesions (c) and (d), respectively, in both shape and color.

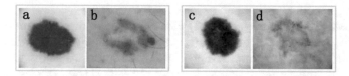

Fig. 1. Examples show the intra-class variation and inter-class similarity in skin lesion classification: (a, b) benign skin lesions, and (c, d) malignant skin lesions

To address the first issue, pre-trained deep models have been adopted, since it has been widely recognized that the image representation ability learned from large-scale datasets, such as ImageNet, can be efficiently transferred to generic visual recognition tasks, where the training data is limited [7–9]. However, it is still difficult to well address the second issue, despite some attempts reported in [4,10]. Since hard cases (see Fig. 1) may provide more discriminatory information than easy ones [11], we, inspired by the biometrical authentication, suggest using dual DCNNs to learn from pairs of images such that the misclassification of a hard case leads to a synergic error, which can then be used to further supervise the training of both DCNN components.

Specifically, we propose a synergic deep learning (SDL) model for skin lesion classification in dermoscopy images, which consists of dual pre-trained DCNNs and a synergic network. The main uniqueness of this model includes: (1) the dual DCNNs learn the image representation simultaneously from pairs of images, including two similar images in different categories and two dissimilar images in the same category; (2) the synergic network, which has a fully connected structure, takes the concatenation the image representation learned by both DCNNs as an input and predicts whether the pair of images belong to the same class; (3) the end-to-end training of the model is supervised by both the classification error in each DCNN and the synergic error; and (4) the synergic error, which occurs when at least one DCNN misclassify an image, enables dual DCNNs to mutually facilitate each other during the learning. We evaluated our SDL model on the ISIC 2016 Skin Lesion Classification dataset [2] and achieved an accuracy of 85.75% and an average precision of 0.664, which is the current state-of-the-art.

2   Datasets

The ISIC 2016 Skin Lesion Classification dataset [2], released by the International Skin Imaging Collaboration (ISIC), is made up of 900 training and 379 test images which are screened for both privacy and quality assurance. Lesions in dermoscopic images are all paired with a gold standard (definitive) malignancy diagnosis, i.e. benign or malignant. The training set is comprised of 727 benign lesion images and 173 malignant lesion images, and the test set consists of 304 benign and 75 malignant ones.

3   Method

The proposed SDL model (see Fig. 2) consists of three modules: an input layer, dual DCNN components (DCNN-A/B) and a synergic network. The input layer takes a pair of images as input. Each DCNN component serves to learn independently the images representation under the supervision of class labels. The synergic network verifies whether the input image pair belongs to the same category or not and gives the corrective feedback if a synergic error occurs. We now delve into each of the three modules.

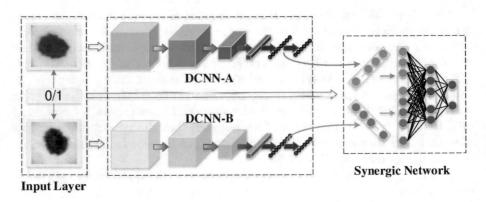

Fig. 2. Architecture of the proposed SDL model which has an input layer, dual DCNN components (DCNN-A/B) and a synergic network.

3.1   Input Layer

Different from traditional DCNNs, the proposed SDL model accepts a pair of images as an input, which are randomly selected from the training set. Each image, together with its class label, is put into a DCNN component, and each pair of images has a corresponding synergic label that is fed into the synergic network. To unify the image size, we resized each image to $224 \times 224 \times 3$ using the bicubic interpolation.

3.2   Dual DCNN Components

Although a DCNN with any structures can be embedded in the SDL model as a DCNN component, we chose a pre-trained residual network with 50 learnable layer (ResNet-50) [12] for both DCNN components, due to the trade-off between the image classification performance and the number of parameters. To adapt ResNet-50 to our problem, we replaced the original classification layer with a fully connected layer of 1024 neurons, a fully connected layer of K (the number of classes) neurons and a softmax layer, and initialized the parameters of these layers by sampling a uniform distribution $U(-0.05, 0.05)$. Then, we used an image sequence $\boldsymbol{X} = \{\boldsymbol{x}_1, \boldsymbol{x}_2, ..., \boldsymbol{x}_M\}$ and a corresponding class label sequence $\boldsymbol{Y} = \{y_1, y_2, ..., y_M\}$ to fine-tune each DCNN component, aiming to find a set of parameters $\boldsymbol{\theta}$ that minimizes the following cross-entropy loss

$$l(\boldsymbol{\theta}) = -\frac{1}{M}[\sum_{i=1}^{M}\sum_{j=1}^{K} 1\{y_i = j\}logp(y_i = j|\boldsymbol{x_i}; \boldsymbol{\theta})] \tag{1}$$

We adopted the mini-batch stochastic gradient descent (mini-batch SGD) algorithm with a batch size of 32 as the optimizer. The obtained parameter sets for DCNN-A and DCNN-B are denoted by $\boldsymbol{\theta}^{(A)}$ and $\boldsymbol{\theta}^{(B)}$, respectively, which are not shared between two DCNNs during the optimization.

3.3   Synergic Network

The synergic network consists of an embedding layer, a fully connected learning layer and an output layer (see Fig. 2). Let a pair of images $(\boldsymbol{x}_i, \boldsymbol{x}_j)$ be an input of the dual DCNNs. We defined the output of the penultimate fully connected layer in DCNN-A and DCNN-B during the forward computing as the deep feature learned on image $\boldsymbol{x}_i, \boldsymbol{x}_j$, formally shown as follows

$$\begin{aligned} \boldsymbol{f}_i &= \mathcal{F}(\boldsymbol{\theta}^{(A)}, \boldsymbol{x}_i) \\ \boldsymbol{f}_j &= \mathcal{F}(\boldsymbol{\theta}^{(B)}, \boldsymbol{x}_j) \end{aligned} \tag{2}$$

Then, we concatenated the deep features learned on both images as an input of the synergic network, denoted by $\boldsymbol{f}_{ioj}$, and defined the expected output, i.e. the synergic label of the image pair, as

$$y_S(\boldsymbol{x}_i, \boldsymbol{x}_j) = \begin{cases} 1 & if \quad y_i = y_j \\ 0 & if \quad y_i \neq y_j \end{cases}. \tag{3}$$

To avoid the unbalance data problem, we set the percentage of intra-class image pairs is about 45%-55% in each batch. It is convenient to monitor the synergic signal by adding another sigmoid layer and using the following binary cross entropy loss

$$l^{(S)}(\boldsymbol{\theta}^{(S)}) = y_S logp(y_S = 0|\boldsymbol{f}_{ioj}; \boldsymbol{\theta}^{(S)}) + (1 - y_S)logp(y_S = 1|\boldsymbol{f}_{ioj}; \boldsymbol{\theta}^{(S)}) \tag{4}$$

where $\boldsymbol{\theta}^{(S)}$ is the parameters of the synergic network. If one DCNN makes a correct decision, the mistake made by the other DCNN leads to a synergic error that serves as an extra force to learn the discriminative representation. The synergic network enables dual DCNNs to mutually facilitate each other during the training process.

3.4 Training and Testing

We applied data augmentation (DA), including the random rotation and horizontal and vertical flips, to the training data, aiming to enlarge the dataset and hence alleviate the overfitting of our model. We denoted two image batches as $\boldsymbol{X}_A = \{\boldsymbol{x}_{A1}, \boldsymbol{x}_{A2}, ..., \boldsymbol{x}_{AM}\}$, $\boldsymbol{X}_B = \{\boldsymbol{x}_{B1}, \boldsymbol{x}_{B2}, ..., \boldsymbol{x}_{BM}\}$, corresponding classification labels as $\boldsymbol{Y}_A$, $\boldsymbol{Y}_B$, and the synergic label as $\boldsymbol{Y}_S$. After the forward computation of both DCNNs, we have two sets of deep features $\boldsymbol{F}_A$ and $\boldsymbol{F}_B$. Then, we concatenated the corresponding pair of deep feature maps, and obtained $\boldsymbol{F}_{A \circ B} = \{\boldsymbol{f}_{A1 \circ B1}, \boldsymbol{f}_{A2 \circ B2}, ..., \boldsymbol{f}_{AM \circ BM}\}$, which was used as the input of the synergic network. Next, we computed the two classification losses $l^{(A)}(\boldsymbol{\theta}^{(A)})$, $l^{(B)}(\boldsymbol{\theta}^{(B)})$ and synergic loss $l^{(S)}(\boldsymbol{\theta}^{(S)})$ which are all cross-entropy loss. The parameters of each DCNN component and the synergic network are updated as

$$\boldsymbol{\theta}^{(A)}(t+1) = \boldsymbol{\theta}^{(A)}(t) - \eta(t) \cdot \Delta^{(A)}$$
$$\boldsymbol{\theta}^{(B)}(t+1) = \boldsymbol{\theta}^{(B)}(t) - \eta(t) \cdot \Delta^{(B)} \tag{5}$$
$$\boldsymbol{\theta}^{(S)}(t+1) = \boldsymbol{\theta}^{(S)}(t) - \eta(t) \cdot \Delta^{(S)}$$

where $\Delta^{(A)} = \frac{\partial l^{(A)}(\boldsymbol{\theta}^{(A)})}{\partial \boldsymbol{\theta}^{(A)}} + \lambda \Delta^{(S)}$, $\Delta^{(B)} = \frac{\partial l^{(B)}(\boldsymbol{\theta}^{(B)})}{\partial \boldsymbol{\theta}^{(B)}} + \lambda \Delta^{(S)}$, $\Delta^{(S)} = \frac{\partial l^{(S)}(\boldsymbol{\theta}^{(S)})}{\partial \boldsymbol{\theta}^{(S)}}$, λ represents the trade-off between subversion of classification error and synergic error, t is the index of iteration and $\eta(t) = \frac{\eta(0)}{1+10^{-4} \times t}$ is a variable learning rate scheme with an initialization $\eta(0) = 0.0001$. We empirically set the maximum iteration number to 100,000, the hyper parameter λ to 3.

At the testing stage, let the probabilistic prediction given by both DCNN components be denoted by $\boldsymbol{P}^{(i)} = (p_1^{(i)}, p_2^{(i)}, ..., p_K^{(i)})$, i=1, 2. The corresponding class label given by the SDL model is

$$\underset{j}{argmax}\{\sum_{i=1}^{2} p_1^{(i)}, ..., \sum_{i=1}^{2} p_j^{(i)}, ..., \sum_{i=1}^{2} p_K^{(i)}\} \tag{6}$$

4   Results

Comparison to the Ensemble Learning: Figure 3 shows the receiver operating characteristic (ROC) curves and area under the ROC curve (AUC value) obtained by applying the ensemble of two ResNet-50 (ResNet-50^2) and proposed SDL model without DA to the test set, respectively. It reveals that our SDL model (red curves) outperforms ResNet-50^2 (blue curves). More comprehensively, we give the average precision (AP), classification accuracy (Acc) and

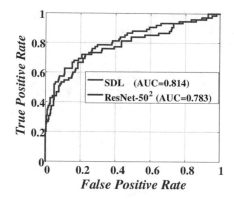

Fig. 3. ROC curves and AUC values of the proposed SDL model and ResNet-50[2].

Table 1. Performance of ResNet-50, ResNet-50[2] and SDL with or without DA.

Methods	DA	AP	Acc	AUC
ResNet-50	N	0.6102	0.8496	0.7742
	Y	0.6224	0.8522	0.7829
ResNet-50[2]	N	0.6115	0.8443	0.7826
	Y	0.6308	0.8549	0.7968
SDL	N	0.6536	0.8522	0.8139
	Y	**0.6644**	**0.8575**	**0.8179**

AUC value of ResNet-50, ResNet-50[2] and the proposed SDL model on the test set with or without DA in Table 1. It shows that SDL performs steadily better than ResNet-50 and ResNet-50[2] regarding three evaluation metrics no matter using or not using DA. It clearly demonstrates that the synergic learning strategy makes a big contribution to higher performance of the SDL model, compared with ResNet-50[2] without synergic learning.

Comparison to the State-of-the-Art Methods: Table 2 shows the performance of the proposed SDL model and the top five challenge records [1], which were ranked based on AP, a more suitable evaluation metric for unbalanced binary classification [13]. Among these six solutions, our SDL model achieved the highest AP, highest Acc and second highest AUC. The 1st place method [4] leveraged a segmentation network to extract lesion objects based on the segmented results, for helping the classification network focus on more representative and specific regions. Without using segmentation, the SDL model still achieved a higher performance in skin lesion classification by using synergic learning strategy.

---

[1] https://challenge.kitware.com/#phase/5667455bcad3a56fac786791.

Table 2. Performance of the proposed SDL model and the top five challenge records in the leaderboard. Note that AP is the only evaluation metric, according to which all participants were ranked.

Methods	$AP(*)$	Acc	AUC
SDL	**0.664**	**0.858**	0.818
CUMED [4]	0.637	0.855	0.804
GTDL	0.619	0.813	0.802
BF-TB	0.598	0.834	**0.826**
ThrunLab	0.563	0.786	0.796
Jordan Yap	0.559	0.844	0.775

5   Discussion

Stability Interval of Hyper Parameter λ: The hyper parameter λ is important in the propose SDL model. Figure 4 shows the variation of the AP of SDL over λ. It reveals that, as λ increases, the AP of SDL monotonically increases when λ is less than 3 and monotonically decreases otherwise in the validation set. Therefore, we suggest setting the value of λ to 3 for better performance.

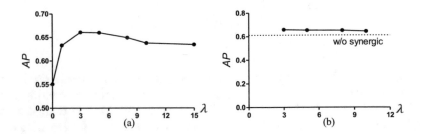

Fig. 4. Variation of the AP of our SDL model (without DA) on the validation set (a) and test set (b) over λ.

Synergic Learning and Ensemble Learning: The proposed SDL model can be easily extended to the SDL^n model, in which there are n DCNN components and C_n^2 synergic networks. Different from the ensemble learning, the synergic learning enables n DCNNs to mutually learn from each other. Hence, the SDL^n model benefits from not only the ensemble of multiple DCNNs, but also the synergic learning strategy. We plotted the AP and relative time-cost (TC) of the SDL^n model versus the number of DCNN components in Fig. 5. The relative TC is defined as the ratio between the training time of SDL^n and the training time of the single ResNet-50. It shows that, with the increase of DCNN components, the TC grows significantly and monotonically, whereas the improvement of AP

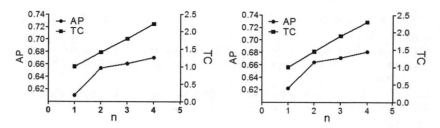

Fig. 5. Performance-time curve of the SDL^n model in the test set (left: without DA, right: with DA) when n changes from 1 to 4 (n = 1 represents single ResNet-50).

is first sharply and then becomes slowly when using more than two DCNNs. Therefore, taking the computational complexity into consideration, we suggest using the SDL^2 and SDL^3 models.

6 Conclusion

In this paper, we propose a synergic deep learning (SDL) model to address the challenge caused by the intra-class variation and inter-class similarity for skin lesion classification. The SDL model simultaneously uses dual DCNNs with a synergic network to enable dual DCNNs to mutually learn from each other. Our results on the ISIC 2016 Skin Lesion Classification dataset show that the proposed SDL model achieves the state-of-the-art performance in the skin lesion classification task.

Acknowledgments. This work was supported in part by the National Natural Science Foundation of China under Grants 61771397 and 61471297.

References

1. Siegel, R.L., Miller, K.D., Jemal, A.: Cancer statistics, 2016. CA Cancer J. Clin. **66**(1), 7–30 (2016)
2. Gutman, D., et al.: Skin Lesion Analysis toward Melanoma Detection: A Challenge at the International Symposium on Biomedical Imaging (ISBI) (2016). arXiv:1605.01397
3. Ge, Z., Demyanov, S., Chakravorty, R., Bowling, A., Garnavi, R.: Skin disease recognition using deep saliency features and multimodal learning of dermoscopy and clinical images. In: Descoteaux, M., Maier-Hein, L., Franz, A., Jannin, P., Collins, D.L., Duchesne, S. (eds.) MICCAI 2017. LNCS, vol. 10435, pp. 250–258. Springer, Cham (2017). https://doi.org/10.1007/978-3-319-66179-7_29
4. Yu, L., Chen, H., Dou, Q., Qin, J., Heng, P.A.: Automated melanoma recognition in dermoscopy images via very deep residual networks. IEEE Trans. Med. Imaging **36**(4), 994–1004 (2017)
5. Esteva, A.: Dermatologist-level classification of skin cancer with deep neural networks. Nat. Res. **542**(7639), 115–118 (2017)

6. Weese, J., Lorenz, C.: Four challenges in medical image analysis from an industrial perspective. Med. Image Anal. **33**, 44–49 (2016)
7. Oquab, M., Bottou, L., Laptev, I., Sivic, J.: Learning and transfering mid-level image representations using convolutional neural networks. In: CVPR, pp. 1717–1724 (2014)
8. Zhou, Z., Shin, J., Zhang, L., Liang J.: Fine-tuning convolutional neural networks for biomedical image analysis: actively and incrementally. In: CVPR, pp. 4761–4772 (2017)
9. Xie, Y., Xia, Y., Zhang, J., Feng, D.D., Fulham, M., Cai, W.: Transferable multi-model ensemble for benign-malignant lung nodule classification on chest CT. In: Descoteaux, M., Maier-Hein, L., Franz, A., Jannin, P., Collins, D.L., Duchesne, S. (eds.) MICCAI 2017. LNCS, vol. 10435, pp. 656–664. Springer, Cham (2017). https://doi.org/10.1007/978-3-319-66179-7_75
10. Song, Y., et al.: Large margin local estimate with applications to medical image classification. IEEE Trans. Med. Imaging **34**(6), 1362–1377 (2015)
11. Bengio, Y., Collobert, R., Weston, J.: Curriculum learning. In: ICML, pp. 41–48 (2016)
12. He, K., Zhang, X., Ren, S., Sun, J.: Deep residual learning for image recognition. In: CVPR, pp. 770–778 (2016)
13. Yuan, Y., Su, W., Zhu, M.: Threshold-free measures for assessing the performance of medical screening tests. Front. Public Health **3**, 57 (2015)

SLSDeep: Skin Lesion Segmentation Based on Dilated Residual and Pyramid Pooling Networks

Md. Mostafa Kamal Sarker[1]($\boxtimes$), Hatem A. Rashwan[1], Farhan Akram[2],
Syeda Furruka Banu[3], Adel Saleh[1], Vivek Kumar Singh[1],
Forhad U. H. Chowdhury[4], Saddam Abdulwahab[1], Santiago Romani[1],
Petia Radeva[5], and Domenec Puig[1]

[1] DEIM, Universitat Rovira i Virgili, Tarragona, Spain
mdmostafakamal.sarker@urv.cat
[2] Imaging Informatics Division, Bioinformatics Institute, Singapore, Singapore
[3] ETSEQ, Universitat Rovira i Virgili, Tarragona, Spain
[4] Liverpool School of Tropical Medicine, Liverpool, UK
[5] Department of Mathematics, University of Barcelona, Barcelona, Spain

Abstract. Skin lesion segmentation (SLS) in dermoscopic images is a crucial task for automated diagnosis of melanoma. In this paper, we present a robust deep learning SLS model represented as an encoder-decoder network. The encoder network is constructed by dilated residual layers, in turn, a pyramid pooling network followed by three convolution layers is used for the decoder. Unlike the traditional methods employing a cross-entropy loss, we formulated a new loss function by combining both Negative Log Likelihood (NLL) and End Point Error (EPE) to accurately segment the boundaries of melanoma regions. The robustness of the proposed model was evaluated on two public databases: ISBI 2016 and 2017 for skin lesion analysis towards melanoma detection challenge. The proposed model outperforms the state-of-the-art methods in terms of the segmentation accuracy. Moreover, it is capable of segmenting about 100 images of a 384 × 384 size per second on a recent GPU.

Keywords: Skin lesion segmentation melanoma
Deep learning · Dilated residual networks · Pyramid pooling

1 Introduction

According to the Skin Cancer Foundation statistics, the percentage of both melanoma and non-melanoma skin cancers is rapidly being increased over the last few years [18]. Dermoscopy, non-invasive dermatology imaging methods, can help the dermatologists to inspect the pigmented skin lesions and diagnose malignant melanoma at an initial-stage [11]. Even the professional dermatologists can not properly classify the melanoma only by relying on their perception and vision. Sometimes human tiredness and other distractions during visual diagnosis can

© Springer Nature Switzerland AG 2018
A. F. Frangi et al. (Eds.): MICCAI 2018, LNCS 11071, pp. 21–29, 2018.
https://doi.org/10.1007/978-3-030-00934-2_3

also yield a high number of false positives. Therefore, a Computer-Aided Diagnosis (CAD) system is needed to assist the dermatologists to properly analyze the dermoscopic images and accurately segment the melanomas. Many melanoma segmentation approaches have been proposed in the literature. An overview on numerous melanoma segmentation techniques is presented in [25]. However, this task is still a challenge, since the dermoscopic images have various complexities including different sizes and shapes, fuzzy boundaries, different colors and the presence of hair [7].

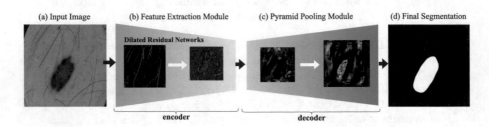

Fig. 1. Architecture of the proposed skin lesion segmentation network.

In last few decades, many approaches have been proposed to cope with the aforementioned challenges. Most of them are based on thresholding, edge-based, region-based active contour models, clustering and supervised learning [4]. However, these methods are unreliable when dermoscopic images are inhomogeneous or lesions have fuzzy or blurred boundaries [4]. Furthermore, their performance relies on efficient pre-processing algorithms, such as illumination correction and hair removal, which badly affect the generalizability of these models.

Recently, deep learning methods applied to image analysis, specially Convolutional Neural Networks (CNNs) have been used to solve the image segmentation problem [14]. These CNN-based methods can automatically learn features from raw pixels to distinguish between background and foreground objects to attain the final segmentation. Most of these approaches generally are based on encoder-decoder networks [14]. The encoder networks are used for extracting the features from the input images, in turn the decoder ones used to construct the segmented image. The U-net network proposed in [17] has been particularly designed for biomedical image segmentation based on the concept of Fully Convolutional Networks (FCN) [14]. The U-net model reuses the feature maps of the encoder layers to the corresponding decoders and concatenates them to upsampled decoder feature maps, which are also called "skip-connections". The U-Net model for SLS outperformed many classical clustering techniques [13].

In addition, the deep residual network (ResNet) model [23] is a 50-layers network designed for segmentation tasks. ResNet blocks are used to boost the overall depth of the networks and allow more accurate segmentation depending on more significant image features. Moreover, Dilated Residual Networks (DRNs) proposed in [22] increase the resolution of the ResNet blocks's output by replacing a subset of interior subsampling layers by dilation [21]. DRNs outperform the normal ResNet without adding algorithmic complexity to the model. DRNs are able to represent both tiny and large image features. Furthermore, a Pyramid Pooling Network (PPN) that is able to extract additional contextual information based on a multi-scale scheme is proposed for image segmentation [26].

Inspired by the success of the aforementioned deep models for semantic segmentation, we propose a model combining skip-connections, dilated residual and pyramid pooling networks for SLS with different improvements. In our model, the encoder network depends on DRNs layers, in turn the decoder depends on a PPN layer along with their corresponding connecting layers. More features can be extracted from the input dermoscopic images by combining DRNs with PPN, in turn it also enhances the performance of the final network. Finally, our SLS segmentation model uses a new loss function, which combines Negative Log Likelihood (NLL) and End Point Error (EPE) [1]. Mainly, cross-entropy is used for multi-class segmentation models, however it is not as useful as NLL in binary class segmentation. Thus, in such melanoma segmentation, we propose to use NLL as a loss function. In addition, for preserving the melanoma boundaries, EPE is used as a content loss function. Consequently, this paper aims at developing an automated deep SLS model with two main contributions:

- An encoder-decoder network for efficient SLS without any pre- and post-processing algorithms based on dilated residual and pyramid pooling networks to enclose coarse-to-fine features of dermoscopic images.
- A new loss function that is a combination of Negative Log Likelihood and End Point Error for properly detecting the melanoma with weak edges.

2 Proposed Model

2.1 Network Architecture

Figure 1 shows the architecture of the proposed SLSDeep model with DRNs [27] and PPN [9]. The network contains two-fold architecture: encoder and decoder. Regarding the encoder phase, the first layer is a 3×3 convolutional layer followed by 3×3 max pooling with stride 2.0 that generates 64 feature maps. This layer uses ReLU as an activation and batch normalization to speed-up the training steps with a random initialization. Following, four pre-trained DRNs blocks are then used to extract 256, 512, 1024 and 2048 feature maps, respectively as shown in Fig. 2. The first, third, and fourth DRNs layers are with stride 1.0, in turn the second one is with stride 2.0. Thus, the size of final output of encoder is $1/8$ of the input image (e.g. in our model, the input image is in 384×384 and the output feature maps of the encoder is 48×48). For global contextual prior, average pooling is used before feeding to fully connected layers in image classification [20]. However, it is not sufficient to extract necessary information from our skin lesion images. Therefore, we do not use average pooling at the end of the encoder and directly fed the output feature maps to the decoder network.

On the other hand, for the decoder network, we use the concept of PPN for producing multi-scale (coarse-to-fine) feature maps and then all scales are

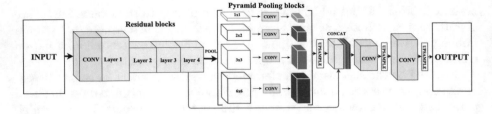

Fig. 2. Architecture of the encoder-decoder network.

concatenated together to get more robust feature maps. PPN use a hierarchical global prior of variant size feature maps in multi-scales with different spatial filters as shown in Fig. 2. In this paper, the used PPN layer extracts feature maps using four pyramid scales with rescaling sizes of $1 \times 1, 2 \times 2, 3 \times 3$ and 6×6. A convolutional layer with a 1×1 kernel in every pyramid level is used for generating 1024 feature maps. The low-dimension feature maps are then upsampled based on bilinear interpolation to get the same size of the input feature maps. The input and four feature maps are finally concatenated to produce 6144 feature maps (i.e., 4×1024 feature maps concatenated with the input 2048 feature maps). Sequentially, two 3×3 convolutional layers are followed by two upsampling layers. Finally, a softmax function (i.e. normalized exponential function) is utilized as logistic function for producing the final segmentation map. A ReLU activation with batch normalization is used in the two convolutional layers [10]. Moreover, in order to avoid the overfitting problem, the dropout function with a ratio of 0.5 [19] is used before the second upsampling layer.

The skip connections between all layers of the encoder and decoder were tested during the experiments. However, the best results were provided when only one connection was skipped between the last layer of the encoder and the output of PPN layer of the decoder. The details of the encoder and decoder architectures are given in the supplementary materials.

2.2 Loss Function

Most of the traditional deep learning methods commonly employ cross-entropy as a loss function for segmentation [17]. Since the melanoma is mostly a small part of a dermoscopic image, the minimization of cross-entropy tends to be biased towards the background. To cope with this challenge, we propose a new loss function by combining objective and content losses: NLL and EPE, respectively. In order to fit a log linear probability model to a set of binary labeled classes, the NLL that is our objective loss function is minimized.

Let $v \in \{0, 1\}$ be a true label for binary classification and $p = Pr(v = 1)$ a probability estimate, the NLL of the binary classifier can be defined as:

$$L_{nll}(v, p) = -\log Pr(v|p) = -(v \log(p) + (1 - v) \log(1 - p)). \tag{1}$$

In order to maximize Peak Signal-to-Noise Ratio, a content loss function based on an end-point error proposed in [1] is used for preserving the melanoma boundaries. In EPE, We compared the magnitude and orientation of the edges of the predicted mask with the correct one. Let M a generated mask and G the corresponding ground-truth, then the EPE can be defined as:

$$L_{epe} = \sqrt{(M_x - G_x)^2 + (M_y - G_y)^2}, \tag{2}$$

where (M_x, M_y) and (G_x, G_y) are the first derivatives of M and G, respectively in x and y directions.

Thus, our final loss function combining the NLL and EPE can be defined as:

$$L_{total} = L_{nll} + \alpha L_{epe}, \tag{3}$$

where $\alpha < 1$ is a weighted coefficient. In this work, we use $\alpha = 0.5$.

3   Experimental Setup and Evaluation

Database: To test the robustness of the proposed model, it was evaluated on two public benchmark datasets of dermoscopy images for skin lesion analysis: **ISBI 2016** [6] and **ISBI 2017** [8]. The datasets images are captured by different devices at various top clinical centers around the world. In ISBI 2016 dataset, training and testing part contain 900 and 379 annotated images, respectively. The size of the images ranges from 542×718 to 2848×4288 pixels. In turn, ISBI 2017 dataset is divided into training, validation and testing parts with 2000, 150 and 600 images, respectively.

Evaluation Metrics: We used the evaluation metrics of ISBI 2016 and 2017 challenges for evaluating the segmentation performances including Specificity(SPE), Sensitivity(SEN), Jaccard index(JAC), Dice coefficient(DIC) and Accuracy(ACC) detailed in [6,8].

Implementation: The proposed model is implemented on an open source deep learning library named PyTorch [15]. For optimization algorithm, we used Adam [12] for adjusting learning rate, which depends on first and second order moments of the gradient. We used a "poly" learning rate policy [5] and selected a base learning rate of 0.001 and 0.01 for encoder and decoder, respectively with a power of 0.9. For data augmentation, we selected random scale between 0.5 and 1.5, random rotation between -10 and 10 degrees. The "batchsize" is set to 16 for training and the epochs to 100. All the experiments are executed on NVIDIA TITAN X with 12GB memory taking around 20 hours to train the network.

Evaluation and Results: Since the size of the given images is very large, we resized the input images to 384×384 pixels for training our model. In this work, we tested different sizes and the 384×384 size yields the best results. In order to separately assess the different contributions of this model, the resulting segmentation for the proposed model with different variations have been computed: (a) The SLSDeep model without the content loss EPE (SLSDeep-EPE), (b) the proposed method with skip connections of all encoder and decoder layers (SLSDeep+ASC) and (c) the final proposed model (SLSDeep) with NLL and EPE loss functions and only one skip connection between the last layer of the encoder and the PPN layer. Quantitative results on ISBI'2016 and ISBI'2017 datasets are shown in Table 1. Regarding ISBI'2016, we compared the SLSDeep and its variations to the four top methods: ExB, [16, 23, 24] providing the best results according to [8]. The segmentation results of our model SLSDeep with its variations (SLSDeep-EPE and SLSDeep+ASC) provided better results than the other four evaluated methods on the ISBI'2016 in terms of the five aforementioned evaluation metrics. SLSDeep yields the best results among the three variations. In addition, for the DIC score, our model, SLSDeep, improved the results with around 3.5%, while the JAC score was significantly improved with 8%. The SLSDeep yielded results with an overall accuracy of more than 98%. Furthermore, SLSDeep on the ISBI'2017 provided segmentation results with improvements of 3% and 2% in terms of DIC and JAC scores, respectively. Again SLSDeep outperformed the three top methods of the ISBI'2017 benchmark, [2, 3, 24], in terms of ACC, DIC and JAC scores. However, [24] yielded the best SEN score with just a 0.9% improvement than our model. The SLSDeep-EPE and SLSDeep+ASC provided reasonable results, however their results were worse than the other tested methods in terms of ACC, DIC, JAC and SEN. However, SLSDeep-EPE yields the highest SPE with a 0.1% and 0.3% more than MResNet-Seg [3] and SLSDeep, respectively. Using the EPE function with the final SLSDeep model significantly improved the DIC and JAC scores of 3% and 5%, respectively, on ISBI'2016 and of 5% and 8%, respectively, with ISBI'2017. In addition, SLSDeep with only one skip connections yields better results than SLSDeep+ASC on both ISBI datasets.

Table 1. Performance evaluation on the ISBI challenges dataset

Challenges	Methods	ACC	DIC	JAC	SEN	SPE
ISBI 2016	ExB	0.953	0.910	0.843	0.910	0.965
	CUMED [23]	0.949	0.897	0.829	0.911	0.957
	Rahman et al. [16]	0.952	0.895	0.822	0.880	0.969
	Yuan et al. [24]	0.955	0.912	0.847	0.918	0.966
	SLSDeep	**0.984**	**0.955**	**0.913**	**0.945**	**0.992**
	SLSDeep-EPE	0.973	0.919	0.850	0.890	0.990
	SLSDeep+ASC	0.975	0.930	0.869	0.952	0.979
ISBI 2017	Yuan et al. [24]	0.934	0.849	0.765	**0.825**	0.975
	Berseth et al. [2]	0.932	0.847	0.762	0.820	0.978
	MResNet-Seg [3]	0.934	0.844	0.760	0.802	0.985
	SLSDeep	**0.936**	**0.878**	**0.782**	0.816	0.983
	SLSDeep-EPE	0.913	0.826	0.704	0.729	**0.986**
	SLSDeep+ASC	0.906	0.850	0.739	0.808	0.905

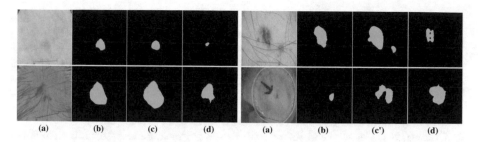

Fig. 3. Segmentation results: (a) input image, (b) ground truth and (c) correct segmentation by our model, (c') incorrect segmentation by our model, (d) segmentation by Yuan et al. [24] model.

Qualitative results of four examples from the ISBI'2017 dataset are shown in Fig. 3. For the first and second examples (on the top- and down-left side), the lesions were properly detected, although the color of the lesion area is very similar to the rest of the skin. In addition, the lesion area was accurately segmented regardless the unclear melanoma edges. Regarding the third example (on the top-right side), SLSDeep properly segmented the lesion area; however a small false region having similar melanoma features was also detected. The last example is very tricky, since the lesion shown is very small. However, the SLSDeep model was able to detect it, but with a large false negative region.

4   Conclusions

This paper proposed a novel deep learning skin lesion segmentation model based on training an encoder-decoder network. The encoder network used the dilated ResNet layers with downsampling to extract the features of the input image, in turn convolutional layers with pyramid pooling and upsampling are used to reconstruct the segmented image. This approach outperforms, in terms of skin lesion segmentation, the literature evaluated on two ISBI'2016 and ISBI'2017 datasets. The quantitative results show that SLSDeep is a robust segmentation technique based on different evaluation metrics: accuracy, Dice coefficient, Jaccard index and specificity. In addition, qualitative results show promising skin lesion segmentation. Future work aims at applying the proposed model to various medical applications to prove its versatility.

Acknowledgement. This research is funded by the program Marti Franques under the agreement between Universitat Rovira i Virgili and Fundació Catalunya La Pedrera.

References

1. Baker, S., Scharstein, D., Lewis, J., Roth, S., Black, M.J., Szeliski, R.: A database and evaluation methodology for optical flow. IJCV **92**(1), 1–31 (2011)
2. Berseth, M.: ISIC 2017-skin lesion analysis towards melanoma detection. arXiv preprint arXiv:1703.00523 (2017)

3. Bi, L., Kim, J., Ahn, E., Feng, D.: Automatic skin lesion analysis using large-scale dermoscopy images and deep residual networks. preprint arXiv:1703.04197 (2017)
4. Celebi, M.E., Wen, Q., Iyatomi, H., Shimizu, K., Zhou, H., Schaefer, G.: A state-of-the-art survey on lesion border detection in dermoscopy images. In: Dermoscopy Image Analysis, pp. 97–129 (2015)
5. Chen, L.C., Papandreou, G., Kokkinos, I., Murphy, K., Yuille, A.L.: DeepLab: semantic image segmentation with deep convolutional nets, atrous convolution, and fully connected CRFs. arXiv preprint arXiv:1606.00915 (2016)
6. Codella, N.C., et al.: Skin lesion analysis toward melanoma detection: a challenge at the 2017 international symposium on biomedical imaging (ISBI), hosted by the international skin imaging collaboration (ISIC). arXiv preprint arXiv:1710.05006 (2017)
7. Day, G.R., Barbour, R.H.: Automated melanoma diagnosis: where are we at? Skin Res. Technol. **6**(1), 1–5 (2000)
8. Gutman, D., et al.: Skin lesion analysis toward melanoma detection: a challenge at the international symposium on biomedical imaging (ISBI) 2016, hosted by the international skin imaging collaboration (ISIC). arXiv preprint arXiv:1605.01397 (2016)
9. He, K., Zhang, X., Ren, S., Sun, J.: Spatial pyramid pooling in deep convolutional networks for visual recognition. IEEE Trans. PAMI **37**(9), 1904–1916 (2015)
10. Ioffe, S., Szegedy, C.: Batch normalization: accelerating deep network training by reducing internal covariate shift. In: ICML, pp. 448–456 (2015)
11. Kardynal, A., Olszewska, M.: Modern non-invasive diagnostic techniques in the detection of early cutaneous melanoma. J. Dermatol. Case Rep. **8**(1), 1 (2014)
12. Kingma, D.P., Ba, J.: Adam: a method for stochastic optimization. arXiv preprint arXiv:1412.6980 (2014)
13. Lin, B.S., Michael, K., Kalra, S., Tizhoosh, H.: Skin lesion segmentation: U-nets versus clustering. arXiv preprint arXiv:1710.01248 (2017)
14. Long, J., Shelhamer, E., Darrell, T.: Fully convolutional networks for semantic segmentation. In: Proceedings of CVPR, pp. 3431–3440 (2015)
15. Paszke, A., Gross, S., Chintala, S., Chanan, G.: Pytorch (2017)
16. Rahman, M., Alpaslan, N., Bhattacharya, P.: Developing a retrieval based diagnostic aid for automated melanoma recognition of dermoscopic images. In: Applied Imagery Pattern Recognition Workshop (AIPR), pp. 1–7. IEEE (2016)
17. Ronneberger, O., Fischer, P., Brox, T.: U-Net: convolutional networks for biomedical image segmentation. In: Navab, N., Hornegger, J., Wells, W.M., Frangi, A.F. (eds.) MICCAI 2015. LNCS, vol. 9351, pp. 234–241. Springer, Cham (2015). https://doi.org/10.1007/978-3-319-24574-4_28
18. Siegel, R.L., Miller, K.D., Jemal, A.: Cancer statistics, 2017. CA Cancer J. Clin. **67**(1), 7–30 (2017). https://doi.org/10.3322/caac.21387
19. Srivastava, N., Hinton, G., Krizhevsky, A., Sutskever, I., Salakhutdinov, R.: Dropout: a simple way to prevent neural networks from overfitting. J. Mach. Learn. Res. **15**(1), 1929–1958 (2014)
20. Szegedy, C., et al.: Going deeper with convolutions. In: CVPR (2015)
21. Yu, F., Koltun, V.: Multi-scale context aggregation by dilated convolutions. arXiv preprint arXiv:1511.07122 (2015)
22. Yu, F., Koltun, V., Funkhouser, T.: Dilated residual networks. In: Computer Vision and Pattern Recognition, vol. 1 (2017)
23. Yu, L., Chen, H., Dou, Q., Qin, J., Heng, P.A.: Automated melanoma recognition in dermoscopy images via very deep residual networks. TMI **36**(4), 994–1004 (2017)

24. Yuan, Y., Chao, M., Lo, Y.C.: Automatic skin lesion segmentation with fully convolutional-deconvolutional networks. arXiv preprint arXiv:1703.05165 (2017)
25. Zhang, X.: Melanoma segmentation based on deep learning. Comput. Assist. Surg. **22**(sup1), 267–277 (2017)
26. Zhao, H., Shi, J., Qi, X., Wang, X., Jia, J.: Pyramid scene parsing network. In: IEEE Conference on CVPR, pp. 2881–2890 (2017)
27. Zhou, B., Zhao, H., Puig, X., Fidler, S., Barriuso, A., Torralba, A.: Scene parsing through ADE20K dataset. In: Proceedings of the IEEE Conference CVPR (2017)

β-Hemolysis Detection on Cultured Blood Agar Plates by Convolutional Neural Networks

Mattia Savardi, Sergio Benini, and Alberto Signoroni(✉)

Department of Information Engineering, University of Brescia, Brescia, Italy
alberto.signoroni@unibs.it

Abstract. The recent introduction of Full Laboratory Automation (FLA) systems in Clinical Microbiology opens to the availability of huge streams of high definition diagnostic images representing bacteria colonies on culturing plates. In this context, the presence of β-hemolysis is a key diagnostic sign to assess the presence and virulence of pathogens like streptococci and to characterize major respiratory tract infections. Since it can manifest in a high variety of shapes, dimensions and intensities, obtaining a reliable automated detection of β-hemolysis is a challenging task, never been tackled so far in its real complexity. To this aim, here we follow a deep learning approach operating on a database of 1500 fully annotated dual-light (top-lit and back-lit) blood agar plate images collected from FLA systems operating in ordinary clinical conditions. Patch-based training and test sets are obtained with the help of an ad-hoc, total recall, region proposal technique. A DenseNet Convolutional Neural Network architecture, dimensioned and trained to classify patch candidates, achieves a 98.9% precision with a recall of 98.9%, leading to an overall 90% precision and 99% recall on a plate basis, where false negative occurrence needs to be minimized. Being the first approach able to detect β-hemolysis on a whole plate basis, the obtained results open new opportunities for supporting diagnostic decisions, with an expected high impact on the efficiency and accuracy of the laboratory workflow.

Keywords: Digital Microbiology Imaging
Full Laboratory Automation · Beta-hemolysis detection
Convolutional Neural Networks · Image classification

1 Introduction

Clinical microbiology is tasked with providing diagnosis and treatment of infectious diseases. The ability to achieve accurate diagnoses in standardized and reproducible conditions is of utmost importance in order to provide appropriate and fast treatment. The gold standard for bacteria identification in the workflow of Clinical Microbiology Laboratories (CML) is bacteria culturing on agar plates. Since traditionally performed almost totally manually, this requires

© Springer Nature Switzerland AG 2018
A. F. Frangi et al. (Eds.): MICCAI 2018, LNCS 11071, pp. 30–38, 2018.
https://doi.org/10.1007/978-3-030-00934-2_4

labor-intensive pre-analytical phases with critical aspects arising with respect to both intra- and inter-laboratory repeatability. Nevertheless, new groundbreaking trends related to the recent diffusion of Full Laboratory Automation (FLA) systems started deeply changing working habits in many clinical microbiology facilities worldwide [1,2]. A single FLA plant is able to process even thousands of plates per day, generating huge flows of high-resolution digital images (taken during and after plate incubation) to be read on diagnostic workstations. As a consequence, the new field of Digital Microbiology Imaging (DMI) involves high expectations related to the solution of a variety of visual interpretation challenges aimed at supporting and improving the accuracy and speed of the clinical procedures and decisions in CMLs. In this work we focus on the automated detection of one of the main diagnostically relevant features for the assessment of human infections, that is the identification of phatogens' β-hemolytic activity.

1.1 Problem Definition

β-hemolysis is an effect caused by certain bacteria species growing on blood agar plates that leads to the dissolution of the blood substrate surrounding the colony. The produced visual effect is a yellowish halo visible by holding the plate against the light [3] or on back-lit images acquired by FLA systems under proper plate illumination settings. In many clinical microbiology protocols, β-hemolysis has high impact and it is the (almost) first step of a chain that needs a high sensitivity. This is true especially in throat swabs culture, and when it is important to address streptococci. Moreover, there is a diagnostically relevant information about virulence (see for instance *E. Coli* [4]) that is promptly available from hemolytic activity assessment which is not possible or difficult to achieve by other diagnostic procedures. However, to accurately distinguish β-hemolysis with the naked eye in all possible manifestations is difficult even for a skilled microbiologist. This requires caution and experience and, especially under high labs load, it is an error prone procedure. In Fig. 1 some examples of negative (a–f) and positive (g–p) cases are shown. In the first line of positive examples (g–l) β-hemolysis is easily recognizable, even if appearing in a variety of different morphological forms and textures: in the middle of a confluence growth (g), over a written portion of the plate (h), or forming multiple rings (i) or in heavy mixed situations inside big confluences (l). These situations and their variability configure a first main challenge (we refer to it as *Multiform Challenge, MC*) for a machine which is asked to reliably classify images, usually well interpretable by a microbiologist, by containing false positives (FP) while maintaining a high recall. A second challenge (we refer to it as *Detectability Challenge, DC*) occurs in cases with soft hemolysis like in (m, n) and particularly in diagnostically relevant cases when early detection by humans start being difficult due to the presence of very thin halos (check for example (b) with respect to (o)), or when β-hemolysis is barely visible because hidden under the colony (see (p)). In this case both humans and machine-based techniques are particularly committed to prevent false negatives (FN) by maintaining a suitable degree of precision.

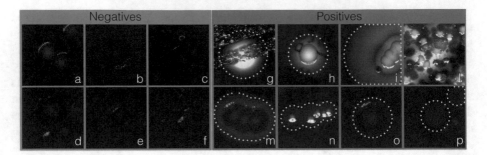

Fig. 1. Negative and positive β-hemolysis examples on blood agar plates. The dotted yellow line highlights the β-hemolytic regions.

1.2 Related Work and Contribution

So far, there has been only one and very recent work dealing with the problem of automated detection of hemolysis on agar plates [5], where a machine-learning method based on hand-crafted features is able to accurately classify hemolysis on image patches representing single colonies. On the one hand, this previous work does not handle detection on a whole plate basis and is not even able to handle most of the frequently occurring range of cases exemplified in Fig. 1 (under-the-colony, within confluences, very thin halo, over the written part cases) which characterize the clinical problem in its real complexity. On the other hand, classification in [5] comprises α-hemolysis (which generates a brownish halo), which is however virtually absent and of no diagnostic interest for the throat-swab clinical context considered in our work.

Deep learning (DL) approaches, especially those based on Convolutional Neural Networks (CNN), have recently been shown to outperform feature-based machine learning solutions whenever difficult visual tasks and large datasets are involved. Applications of deep learning to medical image analysis started to appear consistently only very recently and nowadays are rapidly spreading [6]. Concerning DL methods in the field of DMI, Ferrari et al. [7] already proposed a system for bacterial colony counting, while Turra et al. [8] started investigating bacterial species identification by using hyper-spectral images. More in general, DL detection methods in Computer Assisted Diagnosis (CAD) contexts have been recently proposed for classification of skin cancer [9], cells and mitosis detection [10,11], and mammographic lesions [12], to name a few.

In this work, by exploiting a dataset created for the purpose (as described in Sect. 2), we present a β-hemolysis detection technique, based on a region proposal stage (Sect. 3.1) followed by a CNN (Sect. 3.2) which classifies image patches as β-hemolytic or not. Our system is able to effectively cope with the highly diversified behaviour that β-hemolysis displays in the considered CML procedures involving throat swab cultures finalized to respiratory tract infections identification. Our approach overcomes all the limitations of [5] thus resulting the first one capable to work in real complexity conditions (i.e., facing both the above defined challenges MC and DC). We eventually validate the effectiveness of the method according to both patch-based and whole-plate tests to evaluate the quality of the classification stage and of the overall system, respectively (Sect. 4).

2   Throat Swab Culture Dataset

We collected a dataset from 1,500 culture plates coming from routine lab screening tests and produced by the inoculation of throat swab samples on REMEL 5% sheep blood agar media. Images came from a WASPLab FLA system (by Copan Diagnostics Inc.) which acquires, by linear scanning, 16-mega-pixel RGB color images. For each plate we retrieved both back-light and top-light acquisitions. The ground truth data for the training process consists in throat swab (1,200 plates), randomly selected from a one week of work in a medium size lab, and comprises the segmentation maps produced for the purpose by expert microbiologists that delineated β-hemolytic regions. This dataset is composed of 160 positive plates and 1,040 negative ones. In order to create a blind test-set for the overall evaluation of the system, we labelled another batch composed of 300 new plates acquired two weeks after with respect to the training one. In this case we only required specialists to give information accounting for the presence or not of β-hemolysis. In this case we had a proportion of 51 positive plates and 249 negative ones.

From the image database an image patch dataset can be created by considering 150×150 pixel patches extracted from the 1200 fully annotated plate images, labeling them as positives if at least one pixel from the delineated β-hemolytic regions falls inside a 100×100 pixel region centered with respect to the patch. Every patch is taken with a 33% of overlap so that every portion of the image falls inside the 100-pixel region. We choose 150 pixels as patch dimension as a good trade-off between the colony dimensions and the required computational effort. To the above patches extracted on a regular grid basis, we added all the patches generated by the differential region proposal approach that we explain in Sect. 3.1, resized to 150×150 pixels if needed, where again each patch is labeled negative or positive according to the same rule above. This is done to add more examples similar to those that will be encountered during test-time, when only patches coming from the region proposal are considered. At the same time, the use of a sliding window guarantees to collect a suitable amount of training material, being the region proposal tailored to the reduction of the analyzed patches. Moreover, since following natural CML proportions, negative patches would be about 50 times more than the positive ones, we randomly sample just a portion of them, from each plate, until the patch dataset results balanced. Finally, the full set of patches (about 160k in total) is further divided on a plate basis in two additional sets for the CNN training (70%) and validation (30%) processes.

3   β-Hemolysis Detection Method

In this section, we describe our approach to β-hemolysis detection, consisting of a patch extraction (region proposal) phase followed by a classification stage

based on a specific CNN architecture. An overall scheme of the proposed solution
is depicted in Fig. 2.

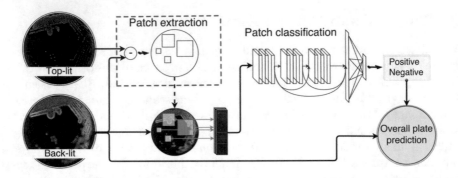

Fig. 2. The overall system for β-hemolysis detection.

3.1 Patch Extraction

In a common scenario the plate is covered by colony growth only in a minor-
ity portion with respect to the whole substrate. Moreover hemolysis usually
involve (with few exceptions) only a small portion of the growth. This is why a
sliding window patch extraction mechanisms for hemolysis detection and classification would be highly inefficient. To significantly increase the computational
efficiency of our method we exploit the physical effect that hemolysis produces
i.e., an erosion of the blood film, which results in a region in which more light
is transmitted from below when acquired back-lit. Thus we adopt a region
proposal solution which works on a differential image obtained by subtracting the back-lit image from the top-lit one. We process this image by bilateral
filter denoising and morphological filtering in order to produce a map composed of high probability β-hemolytic blobs. Specifically, this map is obtained
as $max(|Img_{top} - Img_{back}|, t) \bullet K$, where $\bullet$ is a morphological closure operating
on the denoised differential image with a circular 5×5 structuring kernel K,
and where t is a parameter impacting on the recall of the patch-proposal that
mainly depends on the FLA illumination settings and plate manufacturer. All
the parameters, including t, are tuned by using the patch database so as to produce a 100% recall region proposal (no FNs). As a last step we use this map to
create a list of possible hemolytic regions to be extracted from the back-light
plate for the subsequent classification phase. In particular 150×150 patches are
created with smaller regions in their centre or by subdivision of larger regions.

3.2 Patch Classification

For the patch-classification phase we need a state-of-the-art CNN architecture
particularly suited to be used on datasets with similar dimension and complexity

to ours. This is why we selected DenseNet [13] which is composed of a fully-interconnected series of layers that ensure maximum information flow and force an efficient use of the learned representation (Fig. 2 top-right). DenseNet exposes two parameters: the number of layers L which controls the vertical scale, while the growth rate k accounts for the horizontal scale (i.e., the number of filters). Moreover, to increase the computational efficiency we add a bottleneck layer before each convolutional layer (solution referred to as DenseNet-BC). We train the network from scratch following Xavier weight initialization. In this case in fact, due to the new type of images, fine-tuning approaches would lead to no performance improvement. We adopt Adam as optimizer, Keras framework with TensorFlow, and a Nvidia GPU. We perform 120 training epochs with an initial learning rate set to 0.01 and factor-two reduction on plateaus.

4   Results and Discussion

After a quantitative assessment of the complexity reduction factor produced by the region proposal method, we evaluate the obtained detection performance according to two different criteria: (1) *Patch-based*: we consider the ability to correctly identify and classify patches that present β-hemolysis from negative ones. This metric is useful to evaluate and guide CNN hyper-parameter tuning and training, and accounts for the high performance of the implemented solution in response to both MC and DC challenges. (2) *Plate-based*: we investigate the ability to correctly classify the whole plate, which is the ultimate clinically relevant target.

Patch Extraction. The adopted region proposal allows to extract image patches containing all regions with a high probability of β-hemolysis occurrence. Following the parameter selection described in Sect. 3.1 we indeed obtained no FN, with a concurrent 20× reduction in the number of patches to classify with respect to the sliding window generation used for dataset creation (Sect. 2).

Patch Classification. In Table 1 we report some results obtained with different configurations of DenseNet. We achieve best result with a medium capacity model, either using or not the bottleneck layer BC. This can be explained observing that medium-sized models have a number of trainable parameters which is more compatible to the dimension of our dataset. Bigger models tend to overfit and prevent to reach a good generalization. The adoption of conventional radiometric and geometric data augmentation techniques accounts for an improvement of about 0.2% already included in the final score. In Fig. 3(a) we show the confusion matrix of the best classifier (BC-Medium). FN errors are mainly due to borderline cases, which are also very difficult to discriminate to the naked eye, while FP patches are typically caused by light reflections creating misleading color effects on the plate. In the additional material we included both correctly classified patches as well as FP and FN cases. Results are very promising with both recall and precision approaching 99%. This demonstrates a highly satisfactory response to both the *MC* and *DC* challenges defined in Sect. 1.1. In Fig. 3(b), we show the CNN internal representation of the last hidden layer by using a reduced dimensionality visualization based on t-SNE, where a random portion of the validation patches is taken in input. This allows to appreciate the good level of separability of the two classes (with isolated rare exceptions).

Table 1. DenseNet models comparison on patch classification task (L is the depth and k the growth-rate as in [13]).

Model	Parameters (10^6)	Accuracy
Small (L$=$13, k$=$12)	0.085	0.964
Medium (L$=$22, k$=$24)	0.961	0.989
Big (L$=$40, k$=$24)	4.182	0.968
BC-Small (L$=$13, k$=$12)	0.071	0.988
BC-Medium (L$=$22, k$=$24)	0.688	**0.990**
BC-Big (L$=$40, k$=$24)	1.906	0.954

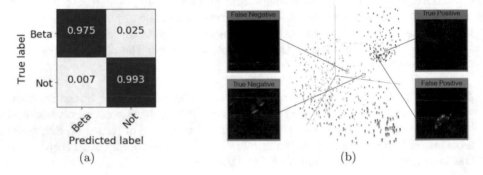

(a)   (b)

Fig. 3. (a) Normalized confusion matrix of the patch-based classifier. (b) T-SNE visualization of the last CNN hidden layer for β-hemolysis discrimination.

Plate Classification. We now apply the proposed pipeline to the 300 unseen plates (blind test-set). Without any post-processing we reach 83% precision and 99% recall with only 3 FN plates with a single and very light β-hemolytic colony in challenging conditions (in our cases near the plate border or below a colony). All the images of FN plates are given in the additional material, with TP, TN and FP meaningful examples as well. By using instead one third of the blind test-set to tune the classification threshold, and test again on the remaining, we reach a 90% precision with the same recall.

Finally, we compare our solution against the one in [5], using their publicly available plate based test-set. In a fair comparison, which requires the exclusion of all the colonies grown over the written portion, we reach almost the same recall of 96% with a significantly increased precision by 12% up to 87%. Beyond this improvement, our method handles β-hemolysis detection inside confluences (not considered in [5]) and over the usually large written plate portions as well, thus standing as a system able to better cope with the real problem complexity.

5   Conclusion

We presented a fully automatic method for β-hemolysis detection on blood agar plate images. We operated with a complexity reduction region proposal and with a representation learning approach based on DenseNet CNN for the classification of both single patches and full plates. Our solution evidenced highly satisfactory performance on a blind test-set and overcomes performance and functional limitations of a previous work. As a next step, we would like to integrate our method in a diagnostic workflow with the microbiologist-in-the-loop. Our feeling is that thanks to the achievements reached on both the multiform and detectability challenges, further impact can be expected in terms of consistency and efficiency as suggested in [14], where the combination of deep leaning predictions with the human diagnostic activity led to significantly improve the total error rate.

References

1. Bourbeau, P.P., Ledeboer, N.A.: Automation in clinical microbiology. J. Clin. Microbiol. **51**(6), 1658–1665 (2013)
2. Doern, C., Holfelder, M.: Automation and design of the clinical microbiology laboratory. Manual of Clinical Microbiology (2015)
3. Hogg, S.: Essential Microbiology. Wiley, Chichester (2005)
4. Jorgensen, J., Pfaller, M., Carroll, K.: Manual of Clinical Microbiology, 11th edn. ASM Press, Washington (2015)
5. Savardi, M., Ferrari, A., Signoroni, A.: Automatic hemolysis identification on aligned dual-lighting images of cultured blood agar plates. Comput. Methods Programs Biomed. **156**, 13–24 (2017)
6. Litjens, G., et al.: A survey on deep learning in medical image analysis. Med. Image Anal. **42**, 60–88 (2017)
7. Ferrari, A., Lombardi, S., Signoroni, A.: Bacterial colony counting by convolutional neural networks. In: Proceedings of the IEEE Engineering in Medicine and Biology Society Conference, pp. 7458–7461 (2015)
8. Turra, G., Arrigoni, S., Signoroni, A.: CNN-based identification of hyperspectral bacterial signatures for digital microbiology. In: Battiato, S., Gallo, G., Schettini, R., Stanco, F. (eds.) ICIAP 2017. LNCS, vol. 10485, pp. 500–510. Springer, Cham (2017). https://doi.org/10.1007/978-3-319-68548-9_46
9. Esteva, A., et al.: Dermatologist-level classification of skin cancer with deep neural networks. Nature **542**(7639), 115 (2017)
10. Xie, Y., Xing, F., Shi, X., Kong, X., Su, H., Yang, L.: Efficient and robust cell detection: A structured regression approach. Med. Image Anal. **44**, 245–254 (2018)
11. Li, C., Wang, X., Liu, W., Latecki, L.J.: Deepmitosis: mitosis detection via deep detection, verification and segmentation networks. Med. Image Anal. **45**, 121–133 (2018)

12. Kooi, T., et al.: Large scale deep learning for computer aided detection of mammographic lesions. Med. Image Anal. **35**, 303–312 (2017)
13. Huang, G., Liu, Z., Weinberger, K.Q., van der Maaten, L.: Densely connected convolutional networks. In: Proceedings of the IEEE Conference on Computer Vision and Pattern Recognition, vol. 1, p. 3 (2017)
14. Wang, D., Khosla, A., Gargeya, R., Irshad, H., Beck, A.H.: Deep learning for identifying metastatic breast cancer. arXiv preprint arXiv:1606.05718 (2016)

A Pixel-Wise Distance Regression Approach for Joint Retinal Optical Disc and Fovea Detection

Maria Ines Meyer[1]([✉]), Adrian Galdran[1]([✉]), Ana Maria Mendonça[1,2], and Aurélio Campilho[1,2]

[1] INESC-TEC - Institute for Systems and Computer Engineering, Technology and Science, Porto, Portugal
{maria.i.meyer,adrian.galdran}@inesctec.pt
[2] Faculdade de Engenharia da Universidade do Porto, Porto, Portugal
{amendon,campilho}@fe.up.pt

Abstract. This paper introduces a novel strategy for the task of simultaneously locating two key anatomical landmarks in retinal images of the eye fundus, namely the optic disc and the fovea. For that, instead of attempting to classify each pixel as belonging to the background, the optic disc, or the fovea center, which would lead to a highly class-imbalanced setting, the problem is reformulated as a pixelwise regression task. The regressed quantity consists of the distance from the closest landmark of interest. A Fully-Convolutional Deep Neural Network is optimized to predict this distance for each image location, implicitly casting the problem into a per-pixel Multi-Task Learning approach by which a globally consistent distribution of distances across the entire image can be learned. Once trained, the two minimal distances predicted by the model are selected as the locations of the optic disc and the fovea. The joint learning of every pixel position relative to the optic disc and the fovea favors an automatic understanding of the overall anatomical distribution. This results in an effective technique that can detect both locations simultaneously, as opposed to previous methods that handle both tasks separately. Comprehensive experimental results on a large public dataset validate the proposed approach.

Keywords: Optic Disk Detection · Fovea detection · Retinal Image Analysis

1 Introduction

Among the landmarks of interest in the human retina, the fovea (a small depression in the macula center) and the optic disc (the location where the optic nerve and blood vessels leave the retina) are key for diagnostic purposes. Consequently, plenty of research has addressed their automatic location in the past [3,6,10].

Most previous work approaches either the problem of detecting the optic disc (OD) or the fovea. In the OD case, several techniques leverage the knowledge that

© Springer Nature Switzerland AG 2018
A. F. Frangi et al. (Eds.): MICCAI 2018, LNCS 11071, pp. 39–47, 2018.
https://doi.org/10.1007/978-3-030-00934-2_5

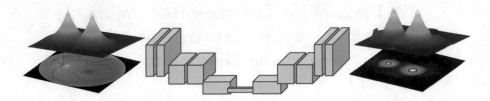

Fig. 1. Proposed approach for joint OD and fovea detection via regressing a distance map from both landmarks to every other pixel in the image.

retinal vessels originate on it in order to find its center. This is typically achieved by extracting geometrical and orientation information from the vascular tree [5]. Fuzzy convergence algorithms [7], Hough transforms [9], and matched-filtering approaches [8] have also been reported for the task of OD location.

Regarding fovea detection, in [6] authors proposed to pre-detect a region likely to contain the fovea based on constraints on its anatomical position relative to OD and blood vessels, with a subsequent thresholding stage to refine its location.

Several other works have reported results on both tasks, although solved in separate stages. The method introduced in [14] analyzed the intensity differences around the OD center to identify it, followed by a template matching technique to locate the fovea. Template matching was also proposed in [16], coupled with directional matched filters. The method in [11] devised a cost function based on a set of global and local anatomical features that was then minimized to yield the most likely locations of OD, fovea and vascular arch. The same authors redefined in [10] both tasks as regression problems, applying a k-NN strategy to estimate OD and fovea location.

Fewer work has addressed the location of both anatomical landmarks simultaneously. In [3] a super-elliptical convergence index filter was applied for this purpose, while in [2] two Convolutional Neural Networks (CNN) were built, the first one aiming at locating a region of interest around both the OD and the fovea, and the second one refining these predictions.

The main contribution of this work is a new strategy for jointly detecting the OD and the fovea. In contrast with previous techniques, the proposed method does not attempt to directly detect only OD and fovea centers. Instead, the distance to both locations is regressed for every pixel in a retinal image, as illustrated in Fig. 1. This regression problem can be effectively solved by means of a Fully-Convolutional Neural Network. This strategy poses a multi-task-like problem, on which information of every pixel contributes to generate a globally consistent prediction map where likelihood of OD and fovea locations are maximized.

2   Joint Optic Disc and Fovea Detection Methodology

Next, the motivation for considering joint OD and fovea detection as a pixel-based distance regression problem and the methodology to solve it are detailed.

2.1   Casting the Problem into a Pixel-Wise Regression Task

In order to solve the joint detection of the OD and the fovea on retinal images, we implicitly adopt a Multi-Task Learning (MTL) approach. MTL is known to be an effective regularizing technique for machine learning models with a large quantity of parameters to be learned, which are typically prone to overfitting.

MTL can be described as a strategy to improve generalization of machine learning models based on solving simultaneously two or more related tasks. It has been observed that this approach can improve learning of abstract representations, which can be mutually useful for the range of tasks to be solved [13].

Jointly detecting the OD and the fovea can be considered as a pixelwise classification problem, where there are three classes: background, OD location, and fovea location. However, under this configuration, the resulting problem becomes highly skewed in terms of examples for each class. A straightforward MTL-like solution would consist on designing two sub-tasks, which would be defined by binary classification problems, and solve them jointly. Nevertheless, this approach would still suffer from a class imbalance issue that would complicate substantially the optimization of a model in this setting.

In this paper, a pixel-wise MTL-like strategy is adopted. Instead of attempting to classify each pixel into two or three classes, we reformulate the problem as regressing the distance from each image location to the closest of both retinal landmarks of interest. For this, we first define the *Bi-Distance Map* $\mathcal{B}(x,y)$ for each pixel location $(x,y) \in \Omega$, being $\Omega \subset \mathbb{R}^2$ the image domain on which a retinal image $I(x,y)$ is defined. Given the location of the OD (x_{od}, y_{od}) and the fovea (x_{fov}, y_{fov}), $\mathcal{B}(x,y)$ is defined as follows:

$$\mathcal{B}(x,y) = \min \left(\sqrt{(x - x_{od})^2 + (y - y_{od})^2}, \sqrt{(x - x_{fov})^2 + (y - y_{fov})^2} \right). \quad (1)$$

From the Bi-Distance Map definition, a normalized form, bounded in $[0, 1]$, can be easily built:

$$\mathcal{B}^N(x,y) = \left(1 - \frac{\mathcal{B}(x,y)}{\max\limits_{\Omega} \mathcal{B}(x,y)} \right)^{\gamma}, \quad (2)$$

where γ is a decay parameter governing the spread of $\mathcal{B}^N$ across the image domain. The effect of modifying the decay parameter γ on the normalized Bi-Distance Map is shown in Fig. 2.

The goal of the model designed in the next sub-section will be to produce an accurate estimate of $\mathcal{B}^N(x,y)$ simultaneously for every pixel. By casting the initial classification problem into a pixel-wise regression task, the model is required

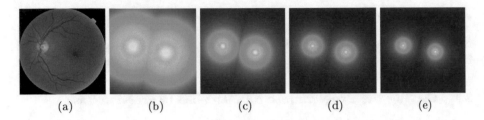

(a)   (b)   (c)   (d)   (e)

Fig. 2. (a) Retinal Image with **O** or **F** marked green and blue respectively. (b)–(f) Normalized Bi-Distance Maps for different decays parameters: $\gamma \in \{1, 3, 5, 7\}$.

to solve a different task on each location, implicitly turning the regression of Eq. (1) into a hierarchical multi-task technique: (1) at a high-level, for each pixel location the model needs to predict which landmark, the OD or the fovea, is closest to it, and (2) at a low-level, for each pixel location the model is required to produce an estimate of the distance to the closest landmark.

Hence, each pixel poses two independent but deeply related goals, effectively regularizing the initial problem, and favoring a globally consistent solution.

2.2   A Fully-Convolutional Deep Neural Network for Distance Regression

In recent years, Convolutional Neural Networks (CNNs) have attained a remarkable success in medical image analysis problems. Although CNNs were initially employed for image classification tasks, subsequent advances allowed the application of convolutional architectures for detection and segmentation tasks. For the latter, a CNN is reformulated to produce pixel-wise classification based on the ideas of *Fully-Convolutional Neural Networks* (F-CNN) and *skip connections*, which enable the coupling of coarse and fine layers of a CNN. In our case, the goal is also to assign a single prediction to each pixel, similarly to a segmentation problem. However, this prediction should not match a discrete set of categories, but rather be a continuous value in $[0, 1]$.

According to the above considerations, our approach is to build on successful F-CNN architectures tailored for segmentation problems, but modifying the loss function to perform distance regression. A popular F-CNN architecture is U-net, introduced in [12]. In U-Net, a contracting sub-network is coupled with a symmetric upsampling sub-network in such a way that the representation produced by the final layer of the upsampling path matches the dimensions of the second last layer. This representation is then fused with the one coming from the corresponding layer in the contracting section. This process is iterated until the output of the upsampling path shares dimensionality with the initial input. This results in a U-shaped architecture, whereby the output feature maps of the contracting sub-network are effectively combined with the output from the upsampling sub-network, providing multi-scale context to the model. The U-Net based architecture employed in this paper is illustrated in Fig. 3.

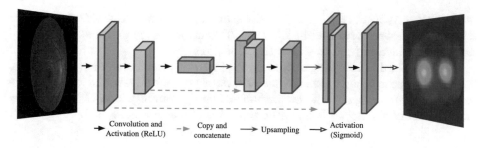

Fig. 3. The proposed F-CNN architecture for Normalized Bi-Distance Map Regression.

Regarding the objective function employed to optimize the model $\mathcal{U}_\theta$, the goal is to predict, for each pixel (x, y), $\mathcal{B}^N(x, y)$ as defined in Eq. (2). Given the smooth nature of $\mathcal{B}^N(x, y)$, we select a standard $\mathcal{L}^2$ loss for this task:

$$\mathcal{L}_{reg}(\theta) = \frac{1}{M} \sum_{x,y \in \Omega} \|\mathcal{U}_\theta(x, y) - \mathcal{B}^N(x, y)\|^2, \tag{3}$$

where M is the number of pixels within a retinal image.

The above loss is backpropagated to update iteratively the weights θ, with mini-batch stochastic gradient descent using the Adam optimizer. The initial learning rate was $\alpha = 0.01$, and it was halved whenever the loss monitored on the validation set was not observed to be improving [1].

2.3   Optic Disc and the Fovea Assignment

The output of the above model is a smooth prediction on distances to both landmarks of interest. Out of this, a Laplacian-of-Gaussian operator was applied in order to extract the two most prominent maxima.

Even if the outlined technique can find the locations of both landmarks, it is unable to specify which of them corresponds to the OD and which one to the fovea. Fortunately, this can be easily solved by a simple local intensity analysis around the two detected maxima produced by U_θ. Specifically, the region around the OD is typically brighter, whereas the fovea is generally darker than the rest of the image. As such, the predicted locations were examined in a local neighborhood of the original images, and the mean red intensity extracted. The region with higher average intensity was selected as belonging to the OD.

3   Experimental Evaluation

3.1   Data

The model was trained and evaluated on the Messidor dataset [4]. Messidor comprises 1200 retinal images of varying resolutions (2240×1488, 1440×960,

---

[1] An implementation can be found at github.com/minesmeyer/od-fovea-regression.

and 2304 × 1536 pixels). The locations of the fovea and the OD for 1136 of these images were provided in [6]. The OD centroids were extracted from these segmentations and used to define their location.

The available 1136 images were divided into two sets containing 568 images, and the proposed model was trained alternately on one subset and tested on the other one, reporting average performance. During training, 20% of the data was separated and employed to monitor the value of the loss in Eq. (3).

3.2   Evaluation Approach

In order to provide a standardized and fair comparison to prior work, we adopt the evaluation approach from [6]. Accordingly, we calculated the Euclidean distance between the ground-truth OD and fovea coordinates and their predicted positions. Predictions falling within a certain distance of the ground-truth are considered successful. This distance is set as a multiple of the OD radius R, and different distances are considered: $(1/8)R$, $(1/4)R$, $(1/2)R$ and $1R$.

Since R varies between images with different resolutions, a separate R was set for each of the three resolutions in the dataset. Namely, $R = 68$ for resolution 1440 × 960, $R = 103$ for resolution 2240 × 1488 and $R = 109$ for resolution 2304 × 1536. Following [6,9], we also compute the mean euclidean distance $(\bar{D})$ between predicted and ground-truth positions normalized by the FOV diameter $(\bar{D}_{FOV} = (D(p_{exp}, p_{real})/d_{FOV} \cdot 100))$ and by the OD radius $(\bar{D}_R = (D(p_{exp}, p_{real})/R \cdot 100))$.

3.3   Quantitative Evaluation

Initially, the decay parameter γ defined in Eq. (2) was varied in the range of $\{1, 2, \ldots, 9\}$ with the goal of estimating the most appropriate value. In order to avoid contaminating the training data, we performed this experiment on an independent dataset provided in [1], which contains 413 retinal fundus images and corresponding annotations for OD and fovea centers. The resulting mean distances for both landmarks are presented in Fig. 4. From this experiment, we selected $\gamma = 7$ as a good decay parameter, since it achieved a low error in combination with the lowest standard deviations in both tasks.

After fixing $\gamma = 7$, we proceed to train on the Messidor dataset as specified in the previous section. Table 1 presents the obtained results in comparison to the state-of-the-art in terms of R criteria and average normalized Euclidean distances. When considering the median values of $\bar{D}_{FOV}$ and $\bar{D}_R$, OD and fovea detection reached a mean/median of $\bar{D}_R = 15.01/9.87$ and $\bar{D}_{FOV} = 0.94/0.70$ respectively, which comes close to human observer performance. The proposed technique achieves a high detection performance in the two tasks, and surpasses other state of the art methods in fovea detection for $1/2R$ and $1R$ criteria.

The generalization ability of the model was evaluated by means of a cross-dataset experiment on the DRIVE dataset [15]. Results for OD detection in this case were well-aligned with current techniques, meeting the $1R$ criterion in 97.5% of the cases. It is worth noting that the method failed only in one image,

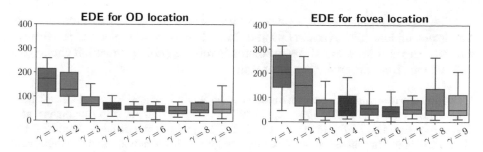

Fig. 4. Euclidean Distance Error (EDE) distributions in pixels for varying decay parameters.

Table 1. Performance comparison of the proposed model on OD and fovea detection.

Optic disc detection	No. images	1/8R	1/4R	1/2R	1R	$\bar{D}_{FOV}$	$\bar{D}_R$
Al-Bander et al. [2]	1200	–	83.6	95.00	97.00	–	–
Yu et al. [16]	1200	–	–	99.08	98.24	–	–
Marin et al. [9]	1200	87.33	97.75	99.50	99.75	–	7.03
Proposed Approach	**1136**	**65.58**	**93.57**	**97.10**	**98.94**	**1.12**	**15.01**
Fovea detection							
Gegundez-Arias et al. [6]	800	82.00	94.25	95.88	96.50	1.41	–
Yu et al. [16]	800	23.63	64.88	94.00	98.00	2.34	–
Niemeijer et al. [10]	800	76.88	93.25	96.00	97.38	1.87	–
Dashtbozorg et al. [3]	1200	–	66.50	93.75	98.87	–	–
Al-Bander et al. [2]	1200	–	66.80	91.40	96.60	–	–
Proposed Approach	**1136**	**70.33**	**94.01**	**97.71**	**99.74**	**0.94**	**12.55**
Human observer [6]	800	94.38	98.50	99.88	99.88	0.52	–

which contains a highly degenerated OD. Excluding this fail case, the method achieved a mean normalized distance $\bar{D}_{FOV}$ from the OD centroid of 2.99.

4 Conclusions and Future Work

A novel approach for jointly detecting the OD and fovea centers has been presented. The proposed technique is based on regressing the distance from each pixel to the closest of both landmarks. A F-CNN is optimized to solve this task, achieving competitive results in OD detection and surpassing the current state-of-the-art in fovea location.

The idea of replacing single-point landmark location by distance map regression is not limited to the task of OD and fovea detection. Therefore, in the future, different medical image analysis problems involving similar detection challenges may benefit from an analogous approach.

Acknowledgments. This work is funded by the North Portugal Regional Operational Programme (NORTE 2020), under the PORTUGAL 2020 Partnership Agreement, and the European Regional Development Fund (ERDF), within the project "NanoSTIMA: Macro-to-Nano Human Sensing: Towards Integrated Multimodal Health Monitoring and Analytics/NORTE-01-0145-FEDER-000016". The Titan Xp used for this research was donated by the NVIDIA Corporation.

References

1. IDRiD - Indian Diabetic Retinopahty Image Dataset (2018). https://idrid.grand-challenge.org/
2. Al-Bander, B., Al-Nuaimy, W., Williams, B.M., Zheng, Y.: Multiscale sequential convolutional neural networks for simultaneous detection of fovea and optic disc. Biomed. Signal Process. Control. **40**, 91–101 (2018)
3. Dashtbozorg, B., Zhang, J., Huang, F., ter Haar Romeny, B.M.: Automatic optic disc and fovea detection in retinal images using super-elliptical convergence index filters. In: Campilho, A., Karray, F. (eds.) ICIAR 2016. LNCS, vol. 9730, pp. 697–706. Springer, Cham (2016). https://doi.org/10.1007/978-3-319-41501-7_78
4. Decencière, E., et al.: Feedback on a publicly distributed database: the Messidor database. Image Anal. Ster. **33**(3), 231–234 (2014)
5. Foracchia, M., Grisan, E., Ruggeri, A.: Detection of optic disc in retinal images by means of a geometrical model of vessel structure. IEEE Trans. Med. Imaging **23**(10), 1189–1195 (2004)
6. Gegundez-Arias, M.E., Marin, D., Bravo, J.M., Suero, A.: Locating the fovea center position in digital fundus images using thresholding and feature extraction techniques. Comput. Med. Imaging Graph. **37**, 386–393 (2013)
7. Hoover, A., Goldbaum, M.: Locating the optic nerve in a retinal image using the fuzzy convergence of the blood vessels. IEEE Trans. Med. Imaging **22**(8), 951–958 (2003)
8. Lalonde, M., Beaulieu, M., Gagnon, L.: Fast and robust optic disc detection using pyramidal decomposition and hausdorff-based template matching. IEEE Trans. Med. Imaging **20**(11), 1193–1200 (2001)
9. Marin, D., Gegundez-Arias, M.E., Suero, A., Bravo, J.M.: Obtaining optic disc center and pixel region by automatic thresholding methods on morphologically processed fundus images. Comput. Methods Programs Biomed. **118**(2), 173–185 (2015)
10. Niemeijer, M., Abràmoff, M.D., van Ginneken, B.: Fast detection of the optic disc and fovea in color fundus photographs. Med. Image Anal. **13**(6), 859–870 (2009)
11. Niemeijer, M., Abràmoff, M.D., Van Ginneken, B.: Segmentation of the optic disc, macula and vascular arch in fundus photographs. IEEE Trans. Med. Imaging **26**(1), 116–127 (2007)
12. Ronneberger, O., Fischer, P., Brox, T.: U-Net: convolutional networks for biomedical image segmentation. In: Navab, N., Hornegger, J., Wells, W.M., Frangi, A.F. (eds.) MICCAI 2015. LNCS, vol. 9351, pp. 234–241. Springer, Cham (2015). https://doi.org/10.1007/978-3-319-24574-4_28. arXiv:1505.04597

13. Ruder, S.: An overview of multi-task learning in deep neural networks, June 2017. http://arxiv.org/abs/1706.05098
14. Sinthanayothin, C., Boyce, J.F., Cook, H.L., Williamson, T.H.: Automated localisation of the optic disc, fovea and retinal blood vessels from digital color fundus images. Br. J. Ophthalmol. **4**(83), 902–910 (1999)
15. Staal, J., Abramoff, M., Niemeijer, M., Viergever, M., van Ginneken, B.: Ridge based vessel segmentation in color images of the retina. IEEE Trans. Med. Imaging **23**(4), 501–509 (2004)
16. Yu, H., et al.: Fast localization of optic disc and fovea in retinal images for eye disease screening. In: SPIE Medical Imaging, p. 796317 (2011)

Deep Random Walk for Drusen Segmentation from Fundus Images

Fang Yan[1], Jia Cui[1], Yu Wang[1], Hong Liu[1,2], Hui Liu[3], Benzheng Wei[4],
Yilong Yin[5], and Yuanjie Zheng[1,2,6,7(✉)]

[1] School of Information Science and Engineering, Shandong Normal University,
Jinan, China
yjzheng@sdnu.edu.cn
[2] Shandong Provincial Key Lab for Distributed Computer Software Novel
Technology, Jinan, China
[3] Department of Biomedical Engineer, Dalian University of Technology,
Dalian, China
[4] College of Science and Technology, Shandong University of Traditional Chinese
Medicine, Jinan, China
[5] School of Computer Science and Technology, Shandong University, Jinan, China
[6] Institute of Biomedical Sciences, Shandong Normal University, Jinan, China
[7] Key Lab of Intelligent Computing and Information Security in Universities
of Shandong, Jinan, China

Abstract. This paper presents a deep random walk technique for drusen
segmentation from fundus images. It is formulated as a deep learning
architecture which learns deep representations from fundus images and
specify an optimal pixel-pixel affinity. Specifically, the proposed architecture is mainly composed of three parts: a deep feature extraction module
to learn both semantic-level and low-level representation of image, an
affinity learning module to get pixel-pixel affinities for formulating the
transition matrix of random walk and a random walk module which propagates manual labels. The power of our technique comes from the fact
that the learning procedures for deep image representations and pixel-
pixel affinities are driven by the random walk process. The accuracy of
our proposed algorithm surpasses state-of-the-art drusen segmentation
techniques as validated on the public STARE and DRIVE databases.

Keywords: Drusen segmentation · Retinal fundus images
Deep feature extraction · Affinity learning · Random walk

1 Introduction

Drusen are a kind of degenerative disease that occurs in choroidal retina. They
are caused by abnormal deposition of metabolites from retinal pigment epithe-
lium(RPE) cells. Moreover, drusen are the main manifestations of age-related
macular degeneration(AMD), at the same time they are also the major causes of
blindness in the elderly [1]. Longitudinal studies show that eyes with larger size

© Springer Nature Switzerland AG 2018
A. F. Frangi et al. (Eds.): MICCAI 2018, LNCS 11071, pp. 48–55, 2018.
https://doi.org/10.1007/978-3-030-00934-2_6

or number of drusen are more likely to cause degeneration of pigment epithe-lial cells, leading to a decline of central vision [2,3]. Therefore, the evaluation of the areas, locations and quantity of drusen from retinal fundus images is of great significance in the clinic especially in the remote screening and diagnosis of AMD.

The main challenges for drusen segmentation lie in three factors that are color or brightness, shape and boundary fuzziness of drusen. For color or brightness, drusen in yellowish-white which is close to the color of fundus image and optic disc. Moreover, drusen also present the characteristic of uneven brightness and the interference of factors such as blood vessels, which have a great impact on the accuracy of the segmentation. In the aspect of shape, drusen often present irregular shapes or circles, and have obvious changes in size, scattering in the vascular arch. For the boundary fuzziness, there is no obvious boundary for soft drusen, which increase difficulty for segmentation accuracy [4–6]. The deep feature extraction module used in this paper can effectively improve the accuracy in view of the semantic features and the low-level features.

There are a variety of drusen segmentation technologies in the field of oph-thalmology image research. In this paper, we mainly extract semantic features from fundus images based on the characteristics of drusen, and then acquire classified labels via random walk to detect the locations and areas of drusen. There are various techniques for drusen segmentation approaches, for instance, in frequency domain [7], thresholding methods [8], and feature extraction [3]. Specially, in the aspect of feature extraction, many features have been used in the previous work, such as the image gray value [6,9], Hessian features and intensity histogram, total variation features [5], etc. For deep learning semantic segmentation methods, lots of networks have tried in improving accuracy, like traditional method [10], fully convolutional networks (FCNs) [11], deep convolu-tional nets (SegNet) [12], multi-path refinement networks (RefineNet) [13], etc. Though most of the existing methods can be used as good references in drusen segmentation, there are still some restrictive problems. First, most drusen seg-mentation methods still use manual feature and cannot get deeper and lower-level information. Second, semantic segmentation is easy to make results smooth. Third, this kind of methods are rarely applied in drusen segmentation now.

In this article, we propose a novel deep random walk network for the imple-mentation of drusen segmentation from retinal fundus images. It extracts the semantic-level and low-level features of patches which are generated from fun-dus images as training data to the net, and then constructs a translation matrix storing pixel-pixel affinities. Inspired by random walk methods, the framework structs an end-to-end training network combining the stochastic initial status of the input image with pixel-pixel affinities. Specifically, we obtain the feature maps across an encoder-decoder structure and a refined fully convolutional net-work, and the whole structures can be jointly optimized. Therefore, the progress not only reduces the parameters, but also preserves the edges information under the condition that the spatial information is not lost, which finally improves the accuracy.

The proposed method can effectively solve challenges above in dealing with drusen segmentation problems, and specific advantages are as follows. Firstly, compared with traditional approaches extracting manual features, we combine semantic information representations with low-level feature extraction method which makes up for the lack of edge smoothing in the process of semantic feature extraction. This is crucial to drusen photos because of characteristics of images themselves. Secondly, the application of random walk approach which is matrix multiplication in mathematics can guarantee the implementation of back propagation algorithm in training process. Finally, the integration of feature descriptions, pixel-level affinities learning and random walk to do classification can be jointly optimized to form an end-to-end network. This results in the dimensionality of parameters space reduced. Based on above advantages, the experiments also prove that our method can improve the accuracy of drusen segmentation.

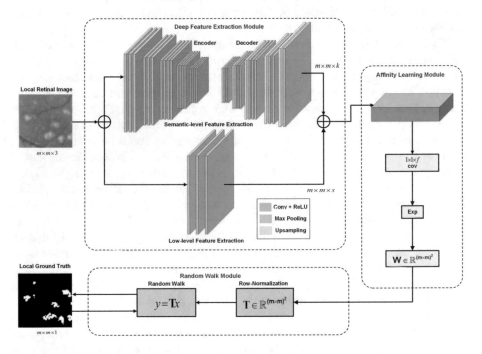

Fig. 1. The architecture of our proposed drusen segmentation method. Deep random walk networks contain 3 modules for deep feature extraction, affinity learning and random walk for drusen segmentation, respectively.

2   Deep Random Walk Networks

The proposed deep random walk networks aim to detect and segment locations and areas of drusen from retinal fundus images. Given color fundus images and corresponding ground truth as training materials, we divide them into patches whose size is $m \times m$ in order to solve the problem of fewer medical samples. When selecting training data, n patches were sampled stochastically from drusen and non-drusen regions. We represent the training data as $\{S_1, S_2, \ldots, S_n\}$, and n denotes the number of training images.

Three main modules of deep random walk architecture were integrated to extract both semantic-level and low-level features and construct transition matrix which represents relationship between pixels. Figure 1 shows a schematic illustration of our framework. Deep feature extraction module aims at semantic and low level information's extraction. Affinity learning Module formulates the transition matrix of random walk. And the random walk module aims to acquire manual labels. Random walk is a form of matrix multiplication in mathematics. This form helps to optimize the three modules in the network and achieves end-to-end training process using the stochastic gradient descent. The detailed description is as follows.

2.1 Deep Feature Extraction Module

The feature extraction module consists of two branches, a semantic-level feature extraction branch which learns deep information based semantic features and a low-level feature extraction branch which acquires detailed features such as sharper edges to improve accuracy. Then the obtained descriptions of image features can be used to represent pixel-pixel affinities in affinity learning module.

For semantic-level feature extraction branch, we get dense feature maps through a encoder and decoder network corresponding to SegNet [12] which considers fundus image patches as training input. Different from SegNet, we obtain feature maps via encoder and decoder network and put the dense representations to affinity learning module to acquire relationships between pixels and then detect drusen in random walk module instead of soft-max classifier. The encoder network transforming the input fundus patches to downsampled feature representations is idential to the VGG16 network [14]. Moreover, it is composed by 13 convolutional layers related to the first 13 convolutional layers in VGG16 network and 5 max pooling layers which carry out with 2×2 windows and the stride is 2. Specially, an element-wise rectified-linear non-linearity(ReLU) $max(0,x)$ is applied before the max pooling layer. The decoder network upsamples the feature maps learnt from the encoder network using upsampling layers and convolutional layers. In order to reduce the loss of spatial resolution, it is needful to transform max pooling indices from encoder network to upsampling layers in decoder network.

For low-level feature extraction branch, it consists of 3 convolutional layers, each of which followed by non-linear "ReLU" layers. The goal of this branch is to acquire low-level information such as sharper edges missed in front branch for the encoder and decoder networks sometimes result in overly smooth. The detailed illustration is shown in [15].

Compared to the structure of [15], the semantic-level network is in parallel action with low-level network instead of the concatenation. The output of semantic-level network is $m \times m \times k$, where m denotes the length of the input square patch and k represents the number of features. Similarly, the output of low-level network is $m \times m \times s$, where s is the number of feature maps.

2.2   Affinity Learning Module

The target of the affinity learning module is to construct a transformation matrix which learns the information of pairwise pixel-pixel and is required in the random walk module. According to the semantic-level and low-level features obtained from the feature extraction module, we integrate the two feature maps into a matrix denoted as $m \times m \times (k + s)$. Then a new weight matrix $(N_n \times f)$ is generated via computing relationships between neihoboring-pixel pairs, where N_n represents the total number of neighboring affinities and f is equal to $2(k+s)$. The neighborhood can be defined as 4-connection in this paper.

The affinity learning module consists of a $1 \times 1 \times f$ convolutional layer and an exponential layer which normalize the obtained matrix W. Moreover, matrix W will be a sparse weight matrix after transformation to $m^2 \times m^2$ and via a limited threshold computing in order to reduce the complexity.

2.3   Random Walk Module

Random walk can be expressed as a form of $y = T \times x$, where T storing the weight of pixel-pixel affinities is called the transformation matrix denoted as $m^2 \times m^2$ via row-normalization of W, and x is the initial state recorded as $m^2 \times 1$. Here we can understand each pixel in the segmented image as a node in the space, and the relationships between each pair of nodes can be represented by weight values. This work, we take the initial value of x via the given initial segmentation using [6], and get the final stable potential via matrix multiplication. Finally, the segmented image are obtained via the softmax layer [16].

During testing, random walk algorithm converts the initial potential energy of image segmentation to the final potential energy via iterations. Furthermore, the terminational condition is that the energy of the image tends to be stable, which is to say the vector x is no longer changing. A detailed proof and deduction are presented in [16].

3   Implementation

We implemented the deep random walk network using Caffe, and carried training and testing process on a NVIDIA GTX 1080Ti graphics card. When in the training time, the fixed learning rate was 0.001 and the momentum was 0.9. The overall training phase was 30 epochs.

4   Experiment

4.1   Dataset

We evaluated the proposed deep architecture in two public datasets: STARE and DRIVE. The STARE dataset contains of 400 retinal fundus images, each of which has a size of 700×605. We selected 46 images containing drusen from 63 diseased images to verify our ideas, where we used 20 images for training and 26 images for testing. The DRIVE dataset includes 40 retinal fundus images, and each of them is 768×584. 9 photos were chosen to test our network. As shown in [3], the ground truth is marked manually via the computer drawing tool.

We make the number increase to $28,800$ after augmentation by applying 18 rotations, 16 stretching effects and 5 bias fields on training images. In addition, we train our network with patches extracted from the training images, for which the number is nearly $2,880,000$ taking patches with each size of which is 64×64. It is worth noting that it is allowed to be covered when selecting training patches in the same one eye image. In the prediction stage, we use a sliding window of 64×64 to take tiles, and the stride is 64. Therefore, this is a non-covered selection.

Table 1. Accuracy evaluation in dataset STARE and DRIVE.

Method	%Se	%Spe	%Acc
Our method	92.02	97.30	97.13
HALT [17]	90.13	94.37	94.89
Liu *et al.* [18]	84.00	87.94	88.38
Ren *et al.* [3]	90.12	96.84	96.56
Zheng *et al.* [6]	87.49	89.82	90.27

4.2   Evaluation and Result

The common evaluation methods of drusen segmentation are sensitivity(Se), specificity(Spe), and accuracy(Acc) [19], where Se refers to the rate of true positive detection, Spe represents the rate of false positive detection, and Acc measures the ration of the total correctly identified piexls [3,5]. According to the three evaluation indexes, we run our algorithm on public dataset STARE and DRIVE, and compare the results with four classical drusen segmentation approaches which are HALT [17], Liu *et al.* [18], Ren *et al.* [3] and Zheng *et al.* [6]. As the results shown in Table 1, our network can resolve the challenges of drusen segmentation better than other state-of-the-art techniques because the learned deep features can help to deal with color similarity of drusen to other tissues and drusen variations in shape and size. Moreover, the random walk process achieves precise segmentation at fuzzy drusen boundaries.

Figure 2 shows the segmentation results on three classifical photos from the STARE dataset with large drusen, vague small and large drusen, and small sparse drusen. The results of drusen segmentation are satisfying because of the areas and locations are successfully detected. Our algorithm acquired satisfied segmented results due to the deep random walk network which extracts the semantic-level and low-level features.

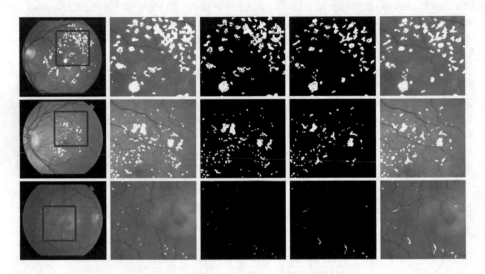

Fig. 2. Segmentation results of different drusen types from the STARE dataset. From left to right: the entire original fundus image, drusen region in the retinal color image, ground truth, segmented image, result of our algorithm.

5   Conclusion

In this work, we introduced a deep random walk network for drusen segmentation from fundus images. Our technique formulated as a deep learning architecture extracts the semantic-level and low-level feature maps to construct pixel-pixel affinities. Inspired by the random walk method, our structure constructs an end-to-end training network and the accuracy of our proposed algorithm surpasses state-of-the-art drusen segmentation techniques. Our future work would include experimenting with other frameworks in order to alternate to the deep random walk network. In addition, we would like to extend our net to other domains such as matting and so on.

Acknowledgements. This work was made possible through support from Natural Science Foundation of China (NSFC) (61572300) and Taishan Scholar Program of Shandong Province in China (TSHW201502038).

References

1. Brandon, L., Hoover, A.: Drusen detection in a retinal image using multi-level analysis. In: Ellis, R.E., Peters, T.M. (eds.) MICCAI 2003. LNCS, vol. 2878, pp. 618–625. Springer, Heidelberg (2003). https://doi.org/10.1007/978-3-540-39899-8_76

2. Sarks, S.H., Arnold, J.J., Killingsworth, M.C., Sarks, J.P.: Early drusen formation in the normal and aging eye and their relation to age related maculopathy: a clinicopathological study. Br. J. Ophthalmol. **83**(3), 358–368 (1999)

3. Ren, X., et al.: Drusen segmentation from retinal images via supervised feature learning. IEEE Access **PP**(99), 1 (2017)

4. Schlanitz, F.G., et al.: Performance of drusen detection by spectral-domain optical coherence tomography. Investig. Ophthalmol. Vis. Sci. **51**(12), 6715 (2010)

5. Zheng, Y., Wang, H., Wu, J., Gao, J.: Multiscale analysis revisited: detection of drusen and vessel in digital retinal images. In: IEEE International Symposium on Biomedical Imaging: From Nano To Macro, pp. 689–692 (2011)

6. Zheng, Y., Vanderbeek, B., Daniel, E., Stambolian, D.: An automated drusen detection system for classifying age-related macular degeneration with color fundus photographs. In: IEEE International Symposium on Biomedical Imaging, pp. 1448–1451 (2013)

7. Barriga, E.S., et al.: Multi-scale am-fm for lesion phenotyping on age-related macular degeneration. In: IEEE International Symposium on Computer-Based Medical Systems, pp. 1–5 (2009)

8. Shin, D.S., Javornik, N.B., Berger, J.W.: Computer-assisted, interactive fundus image processing for macular drusen quantitation. Ophthalmology **106**(6), 1119–25 (1999)

9. Smith, R.T.: Automated detection of macular drusen using geometric background leveling and threshold selection. Arch. Ophthalmol. **123**(2), 200–206 (2005)

10. Shotton, J., et al.: Real-time human pose recognition in parts from single depth images. Commun. ACM **56**(1), 1297–1304 (2011)

11. Long, J., Shelhamer, E., Darrell, T.: Fully convolutional networks for semantic segmentation. In: Computer Vision and Pattern Recognition, pp. 3431–3440 (2015)

12. Badrinarayanan, V., Kendall, A., Cipolla, R.: Segnet: A deep convolutional encoder-decoder architecture for scene segmentation. IEEE Trans. Pattern Anal. Mach. Intell. **PP**(99), 1 (2017)

13. Lin, G., Milan, A., Shen, C., Reid, I.D.: Refinenet: multi-path refinement networks for high-resolution semantic segmentation. In: CVPR, vol. 1, no. 2, 5 p. (2017)

14. Simonyan, K., Zisserman, A.: Very deep convolutional networks for large-scale image recognition. Comput. Sci. arXiv preprint arXiv:1409.1556 (2014)

15. Xu, N., Price, B., Cohen, S., Huang, T.: Deep image matting. In: IEEE Conference on Computer Vision and Pattern Recognition, pp. 311–320 (2017)

16. Bertasius, G., Torresani, L., Yu, S.X., Shi, J.: Convolutional random walk networks for semantic image segmentation, pp. 6137–6145 (2016)

17. Rapantzikos, K., Zervakis, M., Balas, K.: Detection and segmentation of drusen deposits on human retina: potential in the diagnosis of age-related macular degeneration. Med. Image Anal. **7**(1), 95–108 (2003)

18. Liu, H., Xu, Y., Wong, D.W.K., Liu, J.: Effective drusen segmentation from fundus images for age-related macular degeneration screening. In: Asian Conference on Computer Vision, pp. 483–498 (2014)

19. Briggs, D.A.H.: Handling uncertainty in cost-effectiveness models. Pharmacoeconomics **17**(5), 479 (2000)

Retinal Artery and Vein Classification via Dominant Sets Clustering-Based Vascular Topology Estimation

Yitian Zhao[1]([⊠]), Jianyang Xie[1,2], Pan Su[3], Yalin Zheng[4], Yonghuai Liu[5],
Jun Cheng[1], and Jiang Liu[1]

[1] Cixi Institute of Biomedical Engineering, Ningbo Institute of Industrial
Technology, Chinese Academy of Sciences, Cixi, China
yitian.zhao@nimte.ac.cn
[2] School of Optics and Electronics, Beijing Institute of Technology, Beijing, China
[3] School of Control and Computer Engineering,
North China Electric Power University, Baoding, China
[4] Department of Eye and Vision Science, Liverpool University, Liverpool, UK
[5] Department of Computer Science, Aberystwyth University, Aberystwyth, UK

Abstract. The classification of the retinal vascular tree into arteries
and veins is important in understanding the relation between vascular
changes and a wide spectrum of diseases. In this paper, we have proposed
a novel framework that is capable of making the artery/vein (A/V) distinction in retinal color fundus images. We have successfully adapted
the concept of *dominant sets clustering* and formalize the retinal vessel
topology estimation and the A/V classification problem as a pairwise
clustering problem. Dominant sets clustering is a graph-theoretic approach that has been proven to work well in data clustering. The proposed
approach has been applied to three public databases (INSPIRE, DRIVE
and VICAVR) and achieved high accuracies of 91.0%, 91.2%, and 91.0%,
respectively. Furthermore, we have made manual annotations of vessel
topologies from these databases, and this annotation will be released
for public access to facilitate other researchers in the community to do
research in the same and related topics.

Keywords: Artery/vein classification · Dominant sets · Vessel
Topology

1 Introduction

Automated analysis of retinal vascular structure is very important to support
examination, diagnosis and treatment of eye disease [1,2]. Vascular changes in the
eye fundus images, such as the arteriolar constriction or arteriovenous nicking,
are also associated with diabetes, cardiovascular diseases and hypertension [3].
Arteriolar-to-Venular Ratio (AVR) is considered to be an important characteristic sign of a wide spectrum of diseases [4]. Low AVR, i.e., narrowing in arteries

© Springer Nature Switzerland AG 2018
A. F. Frangi et al. (Eds.): MICCAI 2018, LNCS 11071, pp. 56–64, 2018.
https://doi.org/10.1007/978-3-030-00934-2_7

and widening of veins, is a direct biomarker for diabetic retinopathy. By contrast, a high AVR has been associated with higher cholesterol levels and inflammatory markers [5]. However, manual annotation of the artery and vein vessels is time consuming and prone to human errors. An automated method for classification of vessels as arteries or veins is indispensable.

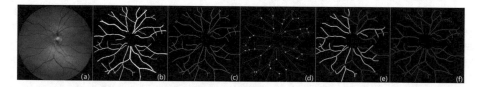

Fig. 1. Overview of the proposed method. (a) Original image. (b) Extracted vessels. (c) Skeletonized vessels. (d) Graph generated with significant nodes overlaid. (e) Estimated vascular network topology. (f) Classified arteries and veins, where arteries are shown in red and veins in blue.

The task of separating vascular network into arteries and veins appear to be understudied. Martinez-Perez et al. [6] proposed a semi-automatic retinal vessel analysis method that is capable of measuring and quantifying the geometrical and topological properties of retinal vessels. Vazquez et al. [3] combined color-based clustering and vessel tracking to differentiate arteries and veins. A tracking strategy based on the minimal path approach is employed to support the resulting classification by voting. Dashtbozorg et al. [7] proposed a graph-based method for A/V classification. Graph nodes and intensity feature analysis were undertaken to establish the artery/vein distinction. Estrada et al. [5] utilized a global likelihood model to capture the structural plausibility of each vessel, and employed a graph-theoretic method of estimating the overall vessel topology with domain-specific knowledge to accurately classify the A/V types. Huang et al. [8] introduced four new features to avoid distortions resulted from lightness inhomogeneity, and the accuracy of the A/V classification is improved by using a linear discriminate analysis classifier.

Numerous factors can cause the aforementioned A/V classification methods to return inaccurate results. Several methods [3,6,8,9] rely on precise segmentation results: any ambiguity in distinguishing between small and midsized vessels makes the subsequent A/V classification a very difficult computational task. On the other hand, pathological conditions and intensity inhomogenities also affect the performance of A/V classification techniques [7,8]. To address these problems, we propose a novel Dominant Sets-based A/V classification method (DoS) based on vessel topological features. The underlying vessel topology reveals how the different vessels are anatomically connected to each other, and is able to identify and differentiate the structure of individual vessels from the entire vessel network. The concept of dominant sets clustering [10,11] was introduced to tackle the problem of vessel topology estimation and A/V classification.

2   Method

Figure 1 shows a graphical overview of the proposed method.

2.1   Graph Generation

Our proposed topology estimation approach can be applied either on manual annotations or automated segmentation results. The method proposed in [1] was employed to automatically segment the retinal vessel. An iterative morphology thinning operation [12] is performed on the extracted vessels to obtain a single-pixel-wide skeleton map. The vascular bifurcations/crossovers, and vessel ends (terminal points) can be extracted from the skeleton map by locating intersection points (pixels with more than two neighbors) and terminal points (pixels with one neighbor). All the intersection points and their neighbors may then be removed from the skeleton map, in order to obtain an image with clearly separated vessel segments. A vessel graph can be generated by linking first and last nodes in the same vessel segment. The generated graph usually includes misrepresentations of the vessels: typical errors are *node splitting, missing link* and *false link*. Correction of these errors can be achieved by using the strategy proposed in [7]. Red dots in Fig. 1(d) indicate terminal points, green triangle bifurcations, and blue squares intersection or crossover points.

2.2   Dominant Sets Clustering-Based Topology Estimation

The topology reconstruction can be achieved by breaking down the graph nodes into four categories (node degrees 2–5): connecting points (2), bifurcation points (3, 4), and crossing/meeting points (3, 4, 5). The number in the bracket indicates the possible number of links connected to each node (node degree). The method proposed by Dashtbozorg et al. [7] is used to handle cases of nodes of degrees 2–3. For nodes of degrees 4 and 5, a classification method based on dominant sets clustering is proposed. The nodes to be classified are represented as an undirected edge-weighted graph with $G = (V, E, \omega)$.

Since we are only taking into account of the pixels around the connecting point, we have $|V| \leq 5$. The edge set $E \subseteq V \times V$ indicates all the possible connections. $\omega : E \to R_+^*$ is the positive weight function. The symmetric matrix $A = (a_{ij})$ is used to represent the graph G with a weighted adjacency matrix. This non-negative adjacency matrix is defined as:

$$a_{ij} = \begin{cases} \omega(i,j) \text{ , if } (i,j) \in E \land i \neq j \\ 0 \qquad \text{ , otherwise.} \end{cases} \tag{1}$$

The concept of dominant set is similar to that of maximum clique. In an undirected edge-weighted graph, the weights of edges within a dominant set should be large, representing high internal homogeneity or similarity, while the weights of those linking to the dominant set from outside it will be small [13]. Let $S \subseteq V$ be a nonempty subset of nodes, $i \in S$, and $j \notin S$. Intuitively, the similarity between nodes j and i can be defined as:

$$\phi_S(i,j) = a_{ij} - \frac{1}{|S|} \sum_{k \in S} a_{ik} \tag{2}$$

It is worth noticing that $\phi_S(i,j)$ can be either positive or negative. $\frac{1}{|S|}\sum_{j\in S}a_{ij}$ is the average weighted degree of i with regard to S. It can be observed that $\frac{1}{|S|}\sum_{j\in S}a_{ij}=0$ for any $S : |S|=1 \wedge S \subseteq V$, hence $\phi_{\{i\}}(i,j)=a_{ij}$. For each node $i \in S$, the weight of i with regard to S is assigned as:

$$\omega_s(i) = \begin{cases} 1 & \text{if } |S|=1 \\ \sum_{j\in S\setminus\{i\}} \phi_{S\setminus\{i\}}(j,i)\omega_{S\setminus\{i\}}(j) & \text{otherwise.} \end{cases} \quad (3)$$

where $S\setminus\{i\}$ indicates the node set S excluding the node i. $\omega_S(i)$ demonstrates the overall similarity between node i and the nodes of $S\setminus\{i\}$.

A subset of nodes $S, S \in V$ is called a *dominant set* if the set S satisfies the following two conditions: (a) $\omega_S(i) > 0,$ for all $i \in S$; and (b) $\omega_{S\cup\{i\}}(i) < 0,$ for all $i \notin S$ [11]. It is evident from the above properties that (a) a dominant set is defined by high internal homogeneity, whereas (b) defines the degree of external incoherence. One can find a dominant set by first localizing a solution of the program:

$$\begin{aligned} \text{maximize } f(\mathbf{x}) &= \mathbf{x}'A\mathbf{x} \\ \text{subject to } \mathbf{x} &\in \Delta \end{aligned} \quad (4)$$

where $\mathbf{x}'$ denotes the transposition of $\mathbf{x}$, $\Delta \subset \mathbb{R}^{|V|}$, and

$$\Delta = \left\{ \sum_{k=1}^{|V|} x_k = 1, \text{ and } x_k \geq 0 \text{ for all } k = 1\cdots|V| \right\}$$

A strict local solution to the standard quadratic program $\mathbf{x}$ indicates a dominant set S of G, where $x_k > 0$ means that the according node $i_k \in S$. As suggested in [10,11], an effective optimization approach for solving Eqn. (4) is given by the so-called *replicator dynamics*:

$$x_k^{(t+1)} = x_k^{(t)} \frac{(A\mathbf{x}^{(t)})_i}{\mathbf{x}^{(t)'}A\mathbf{x}^{(t)}}, \quad (5)$$

where $k = 1, 2, \cdots, |V|$. It has been proven that for any initialization of $\mathbf{x} \in \Delta$, its trajectory will remain in Δ with the increase of iteration t. Since A is symmetric, the objective function $f(x)$ in Eqn. (4) is either strictly increasing, or constant. In practice, the stop criteria of Eqn. (5) can be set either as a maximal number of iteration $t$of iterations or a minimal increment of $f(x)$ over two consecutive iterations.

In the reconstruction of a vascular network topology, the dominant set is a good method of identifying branches of the vascular tree with nodes whose degree is above 3. In general, the weights of edges within a vessel segment should be large, representing high internal homogeneity, or similarity. By contrast, the weights of edges will be small for two or more different vessel segments, because those on the edges connecting the vessel ends represent high inhomogeneities [10]. Intuitively, the identification of vessel branches is more likely to be carried out by finding the most "dominant" vessel branch first and then finding the second most "dominant" vessel branch (and so on). Therefore, dominant set clustering is adopted in this step to determine the most "dominant" vessel branch pixels around each connecting point and assign them to one vessel segment. The remaining pixels are then assigned to the other vessel segment. Practically, for each vessel segment, a feature vector of 23 features is derived for each vessel segment to generate the symmetric matrix A, and these features are listed in Table 1.

2.3   Artery/Vein Classification

After estimating the vessel topology, the complete vessel network is separated into several *subgraphs* with individual labels. The final goal is to assign these labels to one of two classes: artery and vein. Again, the features listed in Table 1 and the DoS classifier are utilized to classify these individual labels into two clusters, A and B. For each subgraph v, the probability of its being A is computed by the number of vessel pixels classified by DoS as A: $P_A^v = n_A^v/(n_A^v + n_B^v)$, where n_A^v is the number of pixels classified as A, and n_B^v is the number of pixels classified as B. For each subgraph, the higher probability is used to define whether the subgraph is assignable to category A or B. Cluster A and B are then assigned as artery and vein, respectively, based on their average intensity in the green channel: a higher average intensity is classified as artery and lower as vein.

Table 1. List of feature vectors for classification.

No.	Features
1–6	Mean and stand deviation of the intensities within the segment in RGB channels
7–8	Mean and stand deviation of the orientations of each centerline pixels
9–10	Mean and stand deviation of the curvatures of each centerline pixels
11–12	Mean and stand deviation of the vessel diameters of each vessel segment
13–18	Mean and stand deviation of the intensities of centerline pixel under a Gaussian blurring ($\sigma = 4$) in RGB channels
19–23	Entropy of intensity in RGB channels, orientation and curvature of each centerline pixels

3   Experimental Results

The proposed topology estimation and A/V classification method was evaluated on three publicly available datasets: INSPIRE [14], AV-DRIVE [15], and VICAVR [16]. All of these datasets have manual annotations on A/V classification, but no manual annotations of vessel topology were made on these datasets. Therefore, an expert was asked to manually label the topological information of the vascular structure on all the images from these datasets. Each vessel tree is marked with a distinct color, as shown in the second column of Fig. 2.

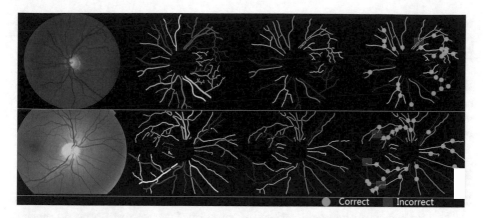

Fig. 2. Examples of vascular topology estimation performances. From left to right column: original image; manual annotations; results from the proposed topology estimation, and the highlighted correct and incorrect connections.

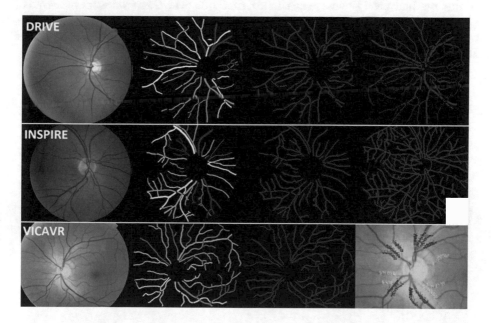

Fig. 3. A/V classification results on three different datasets. From left to right column: original image; vessel topology; A/V classification results of the proposed method; and corresponding manual annotations.

3.1 Topology Estimation

The two right-hand columns of Fig. 2 illustrate the results of our vascular topology estimation method. Compared with the manual annotations shown in the second column of Fig. 2, it is clear from visual inspection that our method is able to trace most vascular structures correctly: only a few crossing points were incorrectly traced, as shown in the last column of Fig. 2 - the pink squares indicate the incorrectly traced significant points.

To facilitate better observation of the performance of the proposed method, the percentage of the relevant significant points (connecting, bifurcation, and crossing points) that were correctly identified (average accuracy): was calculated as 91.5%, 92.8%, and 88.9% in INSPIRE, AV-DRIVE, and VICAVR, respectively.

3.2   A/V Classification

Figure 3 shows the A/V classification performances of the DoS classifier on sample images based on their topological information. Overall, our proposed method correctly distinguished most of the A/V labels on all three datasets, when compared with the corresponding manual annotations. In order to better demonstrate the superiority of the proposed method, Table 2 reports the comparison of our method with the state-of-the-art methods over three datasets in terms of pixel-wise sensitivity (Se), specificity (Sp), and accuracy (Acc). It is clear that our method outperforms all the compared methods on all datasets, except that the sp score on DRIVE dataset is 0.2% lower than [5].

Table 2. Performances of different A/V classification methods on three datasets.

	INSPIRE			DRIVE[a]		VICAVR[b]
	Se	Sp	Acc	Se	Sp	Acc
Niemeijer et al. [4]	78.0%	78.0%		80.0%	80.0%	-
Vazquez et al. [3]	-	-	-	-	-	88.8%
Dashbozorg et al. [7]	91.0%	86.0%	84.9%	90.0%	84.0%	89.8%
Estrada et al. [5]	91.5%	90.2%	90.9%	91.7%	**91.7%**	-
Huang et al. [8]	-	-	85.1%	-	-	90.6%
DoS	**91.8%**	**90.2%**	**91.0%**	**91.9%**	91.5%	**91.0%**

[a]The compared methods only reported their performances on **Se** and **Sp** on DRIVE.
[b]The compared methods only reported their performances on **Acc** on VICAVR.

Table 3. Classification results by different classifiers on INSPIRE dataset.

	LDA	QDA	kNN	SVM	DoS
Se	89.6%	90.6%	87.3%	89.9%	**91.8%**
Sp	84.6%	88.4%	82.6%	88.2%	**90.2%**
Acc	85.1%	89.2%	83.5%	88.6%	**91.0%**

To highlight the relative performance of our DoS classifier, we also employed commonly-used classifiers, namely linear discriminant analysis (LDA), quadratic discriminant analysis (QDA), support vector machine (SVM) and k-nearest neighbor (kNN) for A/V classification based on the topology-assigned structures derived from images from the INSPIRE dataset, with the same feature vectors as listed in Table 1. It can be seen from Table 3 that our method clearly outperforms the compared classification methods.

4 Conclusions

Development of the proposed framework was motivated by medical demands for a tool to measure vascular changes from the retinal vessel network. In this paper, we have proposed a novel artery/vein classification method based on vascular topological characteristics. We utilized the underlying vessel topology to better distinguish arteries from veins. The concept of dominant set clustering was adapted and formalized for topology estimation and A/V classification, as a pairwise clustering problem. The proposed method accurately classified the vessel types on three publicly accessible retinal datasets, outperforming several existing methods. The significance of our method is that it is capable of classifying the whole vascular network, and does not restrict itself to specific regions of interest. Future work will focus on the AVR calculation based on the proposed methodology.

Acknowledgment. This work was supported National Natural Science Foundation of China (61601029, 61602322), Grant of Ningbo 3315 Innovation Team, and China Association for Science and Technology (2016QNRC001).

References

1. Zhao, Y., Rada, L., Chen, K., Zheng, Y.: Automated vessel segmentation using infinite perimeter active contour model with hybrid region information with application to retinal images. IEEE Trans. Med. Imaging **34**(9), 1797–1807 (2015)
2. Zhao, Y., et al.: Automatic 2-d/3-d vessel enhancement in multiple modality images using a weighted symmetry filter. IEEE Trans. Med. Imaging **37**(2), 438–450 (2018)
3. Vázquez, S.G., Cancela, B., Barreira, N., Coll de Tuero, G., Antònia Barceló, M., Saez, M.: Improving retinal artery and vein classification by means of a minimal path approach. Mach. Vis. Appl. **24**(5), 919–930 (2013)
4. Niemeijer, M., Xu, X., Dumitrescu, A., van Ginneken, B., Folk, J., Abràmoff, M.: Automated measurement of the arteriolar-to-venular width ratio in digital color fundus photographs. IEEE Trans. Med. Imaging **30**(11), 1941–1950 (2011)
5. Estrada, R., Tomasi, C., Schmidler, S., Farsiu, S.: Tree topology estimation. IEEE Trans. Pattern Anal. Mach. Intell. **37**(8), 1688–1701 (2015)
6. Martínez-Pérez, M., et al.: Retinal vascular tree morphology: a semi-automatic quantification. IEEE Trans. Biomed. Eng. **49**(8), 912–917 (2002)
7. Dashtbozorg, B., Mendonça, A.M., Campilho, A.: An automatic graph-based approach for artery/vein classification in retinal images. IEEE Trans. Image Process. **23**(3), 1073–1083 (2014)

8. Huang, F., Dashtbozorg, B., Haar Romeny, B.: Artery/vein classification using reflection features in retina fundus images. Mach. Vis. Appl. **29**(1), 23–34 (2018)
9. Rothaus, K., Jiang, X., Rhiem, P.: Separation of the retinal vascular graph in arteries and veins based upon structural knowledge. Image Vis. Comput. **27**(7), 864–875 (2009)
10. Pavan, M., Pelillo, M.: Dominant sets and hierarchical clustering. In: Proceedings of 9th IEEE International Conference on Computer Vision, pp. 362–369 (2003)
11. Pavan, M., Pelillo, M.: Dominant sets and pairwise clustering. IEEE Trans. Pattern Anal. Mach. Intell. **29**(1), 167–172 (2007)
12. Bankhead, P., McGeown, J., Curtis, T.: Fast retinal vessel detection and measurement using wavelets and edge location refinement. PLoS ONE **7**, e32435 (2009)
13. Zemene, E., Pelillo, M.: Interactive image segmentation using constrained dominant sets. In: European Conference on Computer Vision, pp. 278–294 (2016)
14. INSPIRE. http://webeye.ophth.uiowa.edu/component/k2/item/270
15. Qureshi, T., Habib, M., Hunter, A., Al-Diri, B.: A manually-labeled, artery/vein classified benchmark for the drive dataset. In: Proceedings of IEEE 26th International Symposium on Computer-Based Medical Systems, pp. 485–488 (2013)
16. VICAVR. http://www.varpa.es/vicavr.html

Towards a Glaucoma Risk Index Based on Simulated Hemodynamics from Fundus Images

José Ignacio Orlando[1(✉)], João Barbosa Breda[2], Karel van Keer[2],
Matthew B. Blaschko[3], Pablo J. Blanco[4], and Carlos A. Bulant[1]

[1] CONICET - Pladema Institute, UNICEN, Tandil, Argentina
jiorlando@conicet.gov.ar
[2] Research Group Ophthalmology, KU Leuven, Leuven, Belgium
[3] ESAT-PSI, KU Leuven, Leuven, Belgium
[4] National Laboratory for Scientific Computing, LNCC/MCTIC, Petrópolis, Brazil

Abstract. Glaucoma is the leading cause of irreversible but preventable blindness in the world. Its major treatable risk factor is the intra-ocular pressure, although other biomarkers are being explored to improve the understanding of the pathophysiology of the disease. It has been recently observed that glaucoma induces changes in the ocular hemodynamics. However, its effects on the functional behavior of the retinal arterioles have not been studied yet. In this paper we propose a first approach for characterizing those changes using computational hemodynamics. The retinal blood flow is simulated using a 0D model for a steady, incompressible non Newtonian fluid in rigid domains. The simulation is performed on patient-specific arterial trees extracted from fundus images. We also propose a novel feature representation technique to comprise the outcomes of the simulation stage into a fixed length feature vector that can be used for classification studies. Our experiments on a new database of fundus images show that our approach is able to capture representative changes in the hemodynamics of glaucomatous patients. Code and data are publicly available in https://ignaciorlando.github.io.

1 Introduction

Glaucoma is a neurodegenerative condition that is the leading cause of irreversible but preventable blindness [1]. The disease is characterized by the interruption in the communication between the retinal photoreceptors and the brain, preventing visual signals to be carried to the brain via the optic nerve [1]. These progressive changes are asymptomatic until advanced stages of the disease, when undiagnosed patients notice the disease when a considerable amount of visual field has been lost. The major treatable glaucoma risk factor is the intra-ocular

Electronic supplementary material The online version of this chapter (https://doi.org/10.1007/978-3-030-00934-2_8) contains supplementary material, which is available to authorized users.

© Springer Nature Switzerland AG 2018
A. F. Frangi et al. (Eds.): MICCAI 2018, LNCS 11071, pp. 65–73, 2018.
https://doi.org/10.1007/978-3-030-00934-2_8

pressure (IOP), although individuals with high IOP might not develop glaucoma, and subjects with normal IOP values can develop it [2]. Hence, alternative genetic, vascular, anatomical or systemic factors are being extensively studied to better understand the pathophysiology of glaucoma [2,3].

The ocular hemodynamics has long been observed to be affected by glaucoma [2,4] through imaging modalities such as color Doppler imaging or laser Doppler flowmetry, among others [4]. These tools provide non-invasive measurements of hemodynamic parameters from ocular vascular structures such as the central retinal artery (CRA), the ophthalmic artery (OA) or the retinal capillary network. In turn, the analysis of the hemodynamic characteristics of the retinal arterioles and venules, easily accessible through fundus photography, has been limited despite the availability of this imaging modality for several decades.

In this paper, we propose a first approach to characterize the hemodynamics of the retinal microvasculature of glaucomatous and control subjects based on computer simulations performed on vascular networks extracted from fundus images (Fig. 1). Our method is based on patient-specific graph representations of the arterial network that are used as the topological vascular substrate to build 0D models, which account for the steady, incompressible flow of a non Newtonian fluid (the blood) in rigid domains. Although simpler than fully 3D [5] or 2D [6] blood flow models, 0D models (also known as lumped parameter models) are computationally cheaper and, thus, enable the simulation of blood flow in large networks of vessels [7]. Similar modeling approaches have been used before in the context of retinal hemodynamics simulation. In [7], the blood hematocrit is incorporated as transport species in the model, considering constant cross-sectional radius per vessel segment in a network of arteries and veins of a mouse model. More recently, 0D modeling has been applied in [8] for characterizing abnormal changes due to diabetic retinopathy. Although the simulation approach is similar to ours, a Newtonian fluid model was used in [8]. Furthermore, instead of using the whole retinal network, the numerical experiments have been performed in a single vascular bifurcation, which was manually isolated for each image. As a further novel aspect of the present study, the simulation outcomes are summarized in a fixed-length feature vector using a novel technique inspired in the bag of words [9] technique for feature representation. This allows the characterization approach to be applied in combination with linear classifiers to study its relationship with the presence/absence of the disease. We empirically validate this approach on a new database, namely LES-AV, comprising 22 fundus photographs with available manual segmentations of the retinal vessels and their expert classification into arteries and veins.

In summary, the key contributions of this study are: (i) a computational workflow for quantifying patient-specific hemodynamics non-invasively; (ii) a feature representation technique to comprise the simulated outcomes into a fixed length feature vector; (iii) a first pilot study showing that glaucomatous patients exhibit changes in the hemodynamic variables with respect to control subjects; and (iv) a new database of fundus images that is released, jointly with code and implementation details, in https://ignaciorlando.github.io.

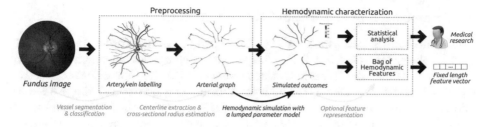

Fig. 1. Proposed method for characterizing patient-specific retinal hemodynamics.

2   Materials and Methods

The experiments were conducted on a new database of color fundus images, called LES-AV, comprising 22 images/patients with resolutions of 30° FOV and 1444×1620 pixels (21 images), and 45° FOV and 1958×2196 pixels (one image), with each pixel $= 6\,\mu$m. Demographic data about the groups are provided in Sect. 3 and the supplementary materials.

2.1   Preprocessing

Patient-specific segmentations of the retinal vasculature must be first retrieved from a fundus image, and subsequently classified into arteries and veins. Although several methods have been introduced for this purpose [10], we follow a semiautomatic approach to ensure a proper input for the simulation step. Hence, a first coarse segmentation of the vessels is obtained using a fully convolutional neural network [11] (see supplementary materials for details). The segmentation is then manually refined to improve the vessel profiles and their connectivity, and each structure is manually labelled as artery or vein. Subsequently, the arteries are taken and their corresponding centerlines are automatically identified using a skeletonization method [12]. The result is a binary mask T with N_I connected components. Since the vasculature is observed as a 2D projection of the original 3D structure in a fundus image, the vessels in the optic disc (OD) are generally overlapped with each other, making unfeasible the identification of the roots of the trees in any realistic scenario. To mitigate this issue, the arterial segments inside the OD are removed from T, and a root pixel I_t is automatically chosen for each connected component $T_t \in T$, such that I_t corresponds to the closest pixel to the OD center. Subsequently, each tree T_t is modeled as a graph structure $G_t = \langle I_t, \mathcal{V}_t, \mathcal{E}_t \rangle$, where each node $v_j \in \mathcal{V}_t$ is a set of branching pixels in T_t, and each edge $e_{(i,j)} \in \mathcal{E}_t$ is a segment of centerline pixels connecting two branching points v_i and v_j. The pixels in the skeletonized arterial trees are automatically classified as part of a node or an edge in G_t by analyzing their neighborhood. Finally, the cross-sectional lumen radius at each centerline pixel is estimated from the segmentation using the Euclidean transform [13].

2.2   Simulation of the Retinal Hemodynamics

The simulation is performed on a patient-specific computational mesh associated to the graphs G_t (Sect. 2.1). This structure comprises the key information required by the model to perform the simulation: (a) the topological connectivity of the arterial segments, through their branching points; (b) the pixel-wise information of the arterial radius, r_i, $i = \{1, ..., N\}$, with N the number of centerline pixels (a computational node per pixel is considered); (c) the root points, which are the network inlets I_t, $t = 1, ..., N_I$; and the network outlets O_m, $m = 1, ..., N_O$.

A steady state 0D model is used to describe the incompressible flow of a non-Newtonian fluid in non-compliant vessels. Such a model is ideal for this scenario, as it allows to efficiently analyze different simulations, and provides physiologically reasonable coarse descriptions of the hemodynamics in vascular networks. The non Newtonian properties of the blood are incorporated by expressing the viscosity as a function of the vessel cross-sectional radius, to describe the Fahraeus-Lindqvist effect [14]. As a result of the simulation process, the blood pressure (P_i) and the blood flow rate Q_i are computed at each computational node (i). The governing 0D equations are detailed below.

The standard mass conservation and pressure continuity junction model is used at each bifurcation point, where node i branches to nodes j and k (Eq. (1)).

Given an arterial segment of M pixels length, $M - 1$ lumped parameter elements are used, where the mass conservation and the hydraulic analogue of the Ohm's law are considered. Then, for an element formed by nodes i and $i + 1$ (Eq. (2)), the resistance to the flow at each segment is modeled with the Poiseuille's law: $R_{i,i+1} = 8\mu L / \pi r_{i,i+1}^4$ where L is the segment length, $r_{i,i+1} = (r_i + r_{i+1})/2$ is the average radius and $\mu = \mu(r_{i,i+1})$ is the blood viscosity, which is assumed to be a function of the arterial radius (since $r < 150\,\mu m$), see the supplementary materials.

$$\begin{cases} Q_i & = Q_j + Q_k, \\ P_i & = P_j = P_k. \end{cases} \tag{1}$$

$$\begin{cases} Q_{i+1} & = Q_i, \\ Q_{i+1} & = \dfrac{P_i - P_{i+1}}{R_{i,i+1}}. \end{cases} \tag{2}$$

Regarding boundary conditions, the pressure and flow rates, are prescribed at the inlet and outlets, respectively:

$$\begin{cases} P_{I_l} = P_0, & \forall l = 1, \ldots, N_I, \\ Q_{O_m} = \beta r_{O_m}^\gamma, & \forall m = 1, \ldots, N_O. \end{cases} \tag{3}$$

The pressure at all the inlets is set to the mean CRA pressure, P_0, while the flow at the outlets is set to the value given by Murray's law, which relates the flow rate to the outlet radius to the power of γ. Specifically, we set $\gamma = 2.66$ [15], and putting $\beta = Q_T / \sum_m r_{O_m}^\gamma$ ensures the total retinal flow Q_T.

The inlet pressure is set to the mean value of normotensive patients (i.e. $P_0 = 62.22$ mmHg). Due to the lack of consensus on normal values for Q_T [16], we proposed three scenarios, namely $Q_T^{SC1} = 30, Q_T^{SC2} = 45.6, Q_T^{SC3} = 80 \, \mu l/m$, which represent the mean (SC2) and extreme values (SC1 and SC3) for healthy subjects. These values are preset for any given subject, without using patient-specific parameters. Further details about the physiological considerations of the parameters choice are provided in the supplementary materials.

The resulting real linear system of equations is solved using LAPACK dgles function through a QR factorization within a custom C++ source code. After solving the system, for each centerline pixel i in the network G, a feature vector $\mathbf{F}_i$ is computed, comprising: the flow rate Q_i, the blood pressure P_i, the mean cross sectional velocity $v_i = Q_i/(\pi r_i^2)$, the Poiseuille's resistance R_i, the Reynolds number $\mathrm{Re}_i = \rho 2 r_i v_i / \mu_i$ and the wall shear stress $\mathrm{WSS}_i = 4\mu_i Q_i/(\pi r_i^3)$. Here, $\rho = 1.040$ g/cm^3 is the blood density. At bifurcation points, the variables assume the value of the last computational node of the parent artery.

2.3 Bag of Hemodynamic Features (BoHF)

One key aspect of the functional characterization is how to construct a feature vector $\mathbf{F}$ for discriminating control subjects from diseased. As $\mathbf{F}_i$ is given for every centerline pixel i, it is necessary to find an alternative feature representation with a fixed length, suitable e.g. for linear discriminant analysis. To this end, we propose a new technique inspired by the Bag of Words (BoW) method [9], named as Bag of Hemodynamic Features (BoHF).

Our analysis is focused on three relevant structures for the graph $G^{(u)}$ of the u-th subject: the terminal and the bifurcation points, and the arterial segments. For every pixel i being a terminal or a bifurcation point, the vector $\tilde{\mathbf{F}}_i$ is used. However, for a given arterial segment $s \in \mathcal{E}$, the average vector $\tilde{\mathbf{F}}_s$ over the pixels enclosed by the segment is used as a summary statistic. This allows our representation to lower its variance and to normalize for the length of an arterial segment. The resulting vectors associated to each arterial segment, bifurcation and terminal points are collected into a set, denoted X.

Let $S = \{(X^{(u)}, y^{(u)})\}, u \in \{1, ..., n\}$ be a training set of n samples, where $X^{(u)}$ is the set of summary statistics at arterial segments, bifurcation and terminal points described above, and $y^{(u)} \in \mathcal{L} = \{-1, +1\}$ is its associated binary label (e.g. healthy or glaucomatous). Since the size of $X^{(u)}$ varies from one subject to another, our purpose is to map it into a feature vector $\mathbf{x}^{(u)} \in \mathbb{R}^d$, with d fixed. In the traditional BoW approach, the $\mathbf{x}$ vectors are histograms of *codewords* (analogous to words in text documents), and are obtained based on a *codebook* $\mathcal{C}$ (analogous to a word dictionary). $\mathcal{C}$ must be designed such that it summarizes the most representative characteristics of each class in $\mathcal{L}$. Let us denote by S_{-1} and S_{+1} the set of negative and positive samples in S, respectively. A codebook $\mathcal{C} = \{\mathcal{C}_{-1}, \mathcal{C}_{+1}\}$ can be automatically learned by applying k-means clustering in the p-dimensional feature space of each subset $S_{(\cdot)}$. The centroids of each of the learned k clusters can be then taken as the codewords, resulting in a set of k codewords for each class ($|\mathcal{C}| = d = 2k$). Hence, the feature vector $\mathbf{x}$ can be obtained such that the j-th position in $\mathbf{x}$ corresponds to the number of nearest neighbors in $X^{(u)}$ to the j-th code in $\mathcal{C}$. If the codewords are representative of each label group, it is expected that the samples belonging to the positive/negative class will have higher/lower values in the last k positions of $\mathbf{x}$.

Finally, the discrimination of glaucomatous patients from control subjects can be posed as a binary classification problem that can be tackled using any binary classification algorithm, e.g. ℓ_2 regularized logistic regression. The linear discriminant function of the logistic regression model $f(\mathbf{x}) = \langle \beta, \mathbf{x} \rangle$ with parameters β is obtained by solving: $\hat{\beta} = \arg\min_{\beta} \left[\lambda \|\beta\|_2^2 + \sum_{u=0}^{n} \log(1 + e^{-y^{(u)} \langle \beta, \mathbf{x}^{(u)} \rangle}) \right]$.

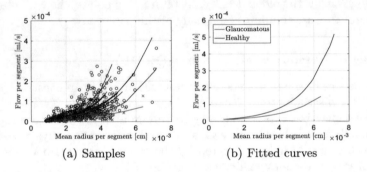

(a) Samples   (b) Fitted curves

Fig. 2. Mean radius vs. flow rate per segment for healthy (black) and glaucomatous (red) subjects in the LES-AV database. (a) Samples per image and fitted curves for each individual. (b) Fitted curves for each group. The SC1 and SC3 were used for the glaucomatous and healthy groups, respectively.

3   Results

The computational simulations of all scenarios resulted in mean values of pressure drop (ΔP to inlet, P_0) and blood velocity (v) consistent with previous studies in the human retinal circulation [6].

The ability of the BoHF to capture the hemodynamic changes in the glaucomatous (G) from normal (H) subjects was empirically assessed using ℓ_2 regularized logistic regression on LES-AV, in a leave-one-out cross-validation setting. The SC2 simulations were used for all the cases to avoid any bias in the classification performance. The values of $k \in \{2, ..., 15\}$ (BoHF length) and $\lambda \in 10^i, i \in \{-3, ..., 0, ..., 5\}$ (regularization parameter) were fixed to the values that maximized the accuracy in a held-out validation set randomly sampled from the training set. The features were centered to zero mean and unit variance using the training sets mean and standard deviation. The resulting area under the ROC curve was 0.70248, with an accuracy of 68.18%.

The hemodynamic quantities obtained using the outcomes of SC1 and SC3 for the G and H groups, respectively, are in line with clinical observations. Figure 2(a) shows the flow vs. mean radius per segment for all subjects. The exponential curves fitted for each group are depicted in Fig. 2(b). The variables are correlated (Spearman's $\rho = 0.71$, $p \ll 0.01$), which is consistent with the literature [6].

Finally, statistical analysis at a confidence level of 99% were performed on a per-patient and a per-measurement basis. On the former (Table 1), we focused on the age, sex and number of segments (NoS). The differences in the mean values of the NoS and the age were not significant (Wilcoxon test, $p > 0.1$). Moreover, the patient diagnosis was independent from the sex (χ^2 test, $p = 1$).

Table 1. Summary of statistics at a per-patient level. None of the variables present statistically significant differences between groups ($p \gg 0.01$).

Variable/ Group	All ($n = 22$)	Healthy ($n = 11$)	Glaucomatous ($n = 11$)
NoS	33.27 ± 13.72	37.91 ± 16.78	28.64 ± 8.15
Age [years]	71.36 ± 9.98	68.64 ± 9.24	74.09 ± 10.36
Sex (Males)	12	6	6

Table 2. Summary of statistics at a per-measurement level (terminals, bifurcations and arterial segments). (*) points statistically significant differences between groups ($p \ll 0.01$). (†) reached $p = 0.02$.

Variable/ Group	All ($n = 1466$)	Healthy ($n = 836$)	Glaucomatous ($n = 630$)
ΔP [mmHg]*	6.94 ± 7.40	8.08 ± 8.12	5.43 ± 5.99
v [cm/s]*	2.26 ± 1.84	2.61 ± 2.03	1.79 ± 1.41
r [cm]	0.003 ± 0.001	0.003 ± 0.001	0.003 ± 0.001
Age [years]*	72.08 ± 9.68	70.83 ± 9.74	73.74 ± 9.35
Sex (Males)†	763	413	350

On a per-measurement basis (Table 2), all the arterial segments, terminal and bifurcations points were considered as separate measurements. The analysis was focused on the ΔP, v, r, age and sex. The differences in the mean value of ΔP and v were larger in the H group, while the age was larger in the G group ($p \ll 0.01$) (two tailed Wilcoxon test). The r was lower in the G group, although not significant ($p = 0.31$). As in the per-patient analysis, the diagnostic was independent from the sex (χ^2 test, $p = 0.02$). The Pearson correlation coefficient between age vs. ΔP and age vs. v was close to zero and not significant, suggesting that the age is not an influential factor for the comparison of the means.

4   Discussion

We have presented a first approach to characterize the retinal hemodynamics of glaucoma patients using computational fluid-dynamics. To the best of our knowledge, this is the first study in which the relationship between glaucoma and simulated hemodynamic outcomes of the retinal arterioles are studied.

The arterial radius was previously observed to be smaller in glaucoma patients than in normal subjects [17], a setting that is consistent with our data.

On the other hand, in-vivo velocity measurements in the CRA of affected patients was shown to be lower than in control subjects [18]. Under these considerations, we have used SC1 for the G group and SC3 for the H group in our first pilot study, resulting in a simulated behavior that is in line with existing observations made on other measurable vessels (i.e. $G(v) < H(v)$) [18]. Moreover, this rendered physiologically correct values of Δp in the retinal network.

The classification experiment based on BoHF and the unbiased SC2 outcomes showed an AUC different than random for identifying the glaucomatous patients, indicating that the tool is able to preserve the variations in the hemodynamics of the arteries affected by the disease. Future efforts will be focused on incorporating the venous network and also modeling of the IOP, which is relevant for clinical studies [19]. Also, the incorporation of a deep learning based method for simultaneous segmentation and classification of the vasculature will be explored in order to allow a more efficient characterization of larger populations.

Finally, our MATLAB/C++/python code and the LES-AV database are publicly released. To the best of our knowledge, our data set is the first in providing not only the segmentations of the arterio-venous structures but also diagnostics and clinical parameters at an image level.

Acknowledgements. This work is funded by ANPCyT PICTs 2016-0116 and start-up 2015-0006, the FWO through project G0A2716N, and a NVIDIA Hardware Grant. JIO is now with OPTIMA, Medical University of Vienna, Austria.

References

1. Tham, Y.C., et al.: Global prevalence of glaucoma and projections of glaucoma burden through 2040: a systematic review and meta-analysis. Ophthalmology **121**(11), 2081–2090 (2014)
2. Harris, A., et al.: Ocular hemodynamics and glaucoma: the role of mathematical modeling. Eur. J. Ophthalmol. **23**, 139–146 (2013)
3. Barbosa-Breda, J., et al.: Clinical metabolomics and glaucoma. Ophthalmic Res. **59**(1), 1–6 (2018)
4. Abegão Pinto, L., et al.: Ocular blood flow in glaucoma-the Leuven Eye Study. Acta Ophthalmol. **94**(6), 592–598 (2016)
5. Lu, Y., et al.: Computational fluid dynamics assisted characterization of parafoveal hemodynamics in normal and diabetic eyes using adaptive optics scanning laser ophthalmoscopy. Biomed. Opt. Express **7**(12), 4958 (2016)
6. Liu, D., et al.: Image-based blood flow simulation in the retinal circulation. In: Vander Sloten, J., Verdonck, P., Nyssen, M., Haueisen, J. (eds.) ECIFMBE 2008. IFMBE Proceedings, vol. 22, pp. 1963–1966. Springer, Heidelberg (2009). https://doi.org/10.1007/978-3-540-89208-3_468
7. Ganesan, P., He, S., Xu, H.: Analysis of retinal circulation using an image-based network model of retinal vasculature. Microvasc. Res. **80**(1), 99–109 (2010)
8. Caliva, F., et al.: Hemodynamics in the retinal vasculature during the progression of diabetic retinopathy. JMO **1**(4), 6–15 (2017)
9. Li, F.-F., Perona, P.: A Bayesian hierarchical model for learning natural scene categories. In: CVPR, vol. 2, pp. 524–531. IEEE (2005)

10. Moccia, S., et al.: Blood vessel segmentation algorithms-review of methods, datasets and evaluation metrics. CMPB **158**, 71–91 (2018)
11. Giancardo, L., Roberts, K., Zhao, Z.: Representation learning for retinal vasculature embeddings. In: Cardoso, M.J., et al. (eds.) FIFI/OMIA -2017. LNCS, vol. 10554, pp. 243–250. Springer, Cham (2017). https://doi.org/10.1007/978-3-319-67561-9_28
12. Rumpf, M., Telea, A.: A continuous skeletonization method based on level sets. In: Eurographics/IEEE VGTC Symposium on Visualization, pp. 151–159 (2002)
13. Maurer, C.R., Qi, R., Raghavan, V.: A linear time algorithm for computing exact Euclidean distance transforms of binary images in arbitrary dimensions. IEEE PAMI **25**(2), 265–270 (2003)
14. Pries, A.R., Secomb, T.W., Gaehtgens, P.: Biophysical aspects of blood flow in the microvasculature. Cardiovasc. Res. **32**(4), 654–667 (1996)
15. Blanco, P., Queiroz, R., Feijóo, R.: A computational approach to generate concurrent arterial networks in vascular territories. Int. J. Numer. Method Biomed. Eng. **29**, 601–614 (2013)
16. Pournaras, C.J., Riva, C.E.: Retinal blood flow evaluation. Ophthalmologica **229**(2), 61–74 (2013)
17. Mitchell, P., et al.: Retinal vessel diameter and open-angle glaucoma: the Blue Mountains Eye Study. Ophthalmology **112**(2), 245–250 (2005)
18. Abegão Pinto, L., Vandewalle, E., Stalmans, I.: Disturbed correlation between arterial resistance and pulsatility in glaucoma patients. Acta Ophthalmol. **90**(3), e214–e220 (2012)
19. Abegão Pinto, L., et al.: Lack of spontaneous venous pulsation: possible risk indicator in normal tension glaucoma? Acta Ophthalmol. **91**(6), 514–520 (2013)

A Framework for Identifying Diabetic Retinopathy Based on Anti-noise Detection and Attention-Based Fusion

Zhiwen Lin[1], Ruoqian Guo[1], Yanjie Wang[1], Bian Wu[2], Tingting Chen[1], Wenzhe Wang[1], Danny Z. Chen[3], and Jian Wu[1(✉)]

[1] College of Computer Science and Technology,
Zhejiang University, Hangzhou, China
wujian2000@zju.edu.cn
[2] Data Science and AI Lab, WeDoctor Group Limited, Hangzhou, China
[3] Department of Computer Science and Engineering, University of Notre Dame,
Notre Dame, IN 46556, USA

Abstract. Automatic diagnosis of diabetic retinopathy (DR) using retinal fundus images is a challenging problem because images of low grade DR may contain only a few tiny lesions which are difficult to perceive even to human experts. Using annotations in the form of lesion bounding boxes may help solve the problem by deep learning models, but fully annotated samples of this type are usually expensive to obtain. Missing annotated samples (i.e., true lesions but not included in annotations) are noise and can affect learning models negatively. Besides, how to utilize lesion information for identifying DR should be considered carefully because different types of lesions may be used to distinguish different DR grades. In this paper, we propose a new framework for unifying lesion detection and DR identification. Our lesion detection model first determines the missing annotated samples to reduce their impact on the model, and extracts lesion information. Our attention-based network then fuses original images and lesion information to identify DR. Experimental results show that our detection model can considerably reduce the impact of missing annotation and our attention-based network can learn weights between the original images and lesion information for distinguishing different DR grades. Our approach outperforms state-of-the-art methods on two grand challenge retina datasets, EyePACS and Messidor.

1 Introduction

Diabetic retinopathy (DR) is one of the most severe complications of diabetes, which can cause vision loss or even blindness. DR can be identified by ophthalmologists based on the type and count of lesions. Usually, the severity of DR is rated on a scale of 0 to 4: normal, mild, moderate, severe, and proliferative. As shown in Fig. 1(b), grades 1 to 3 are classified as non-proliferative

---

Z. Lin, R. Guo, Y. Wang—These authors contributed equally to this work.

© Springer Nature Switzerland AG 2018
A. F. Frangi et al. (Eds.): MICCAI 2018, LNCS 11071, pp. 74–82, 2018.
https://doi.org/10.1007/978-3-030-00934-2_9

DR (NPDR), which can be identified by the amount of lesions including microaneurysm (MA), hemorrhages (HE), and Exudate (EXU). Grade 4 is proliferative DR (PDR) whose lesions (such as retinal neovascularization (RNV)) are different from those of other grades. Ophthalmologists can identify the presence of DR by examining digital retinal fundus images, but this is a time-consuming and manual-intensive process. Thus, it is important to develop an automatic method to assist DR diagnosis for better efficiency and reducing expert labor.

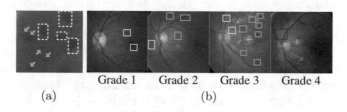

(a)   Grade 1   Grade 2   Grade 3   Grade 4

(b)

Fig. 1. (a) Missing annotated lesions in images. Yellow dotted boxes are ophthalmologists' notes and blue arrows indicate missing annotation. (b) DR grades can be identified by the types and count of lesions (yellow: MA, blue: HE, green: EXU, and red: RNV). The lesions for Grade 4 are different from those of other grades.

There are mainly two kinds of machine learning methods for identifying DR. The first kind uses image-level labels to train a classification model that distinguishes DR grades directly. Kumar et al. [7] tackled this task as abnormality detection using a mixture model. Recently, deep learning techniques, such as convolution neural networks (CNN), have been employed to identify DR [5][3]. Wang et al. [11] used CNN feature maps to find the more important locations, thus improving the performance. But, tiny lesions (e.g., MA and HE) may be neglected by these methods with only image-level labels, affecting prediction accuracy, especially for DR grades 1 and 2. The second kind of methods first detects lesions for further processing. Dai et al. [2] tried to detect lesions using clinical reports. van Grinsven et al. [4] sped up model training by selective data sampling for HE detection. Seoud et al. [9] used hand-crafted features to detect retinal lesions and identify DR grade. Yang et al. [13] gave a two-stage framework for both lesion detection and DR grading using annotation of locations including MA, HE, and EXU.

Fusing lesion information to identify DR can effectively help the models perform better. However, there are still other difficulties to handle: (i) A common problem is that usually not all lesions are annotated. In retinal fundus images, the amount of MA and HE is often relatively large, and experts may miss quite some lesions (e.g., see Fig. 1(a)). Note that the missing annotated lesions are treated as negative samples (i.e., background) and thus are "noise" to the model. (ii) Not all kinds of lesions are beneficial to distinguishing all DR grades. For example, DR grade 4 (PDR) can be identified using RNV lesions, but has no direct relationship with MA and HE lesions (see Fig. 1(b)). If we fuse the information of these two types of lesions directly, it may be noisy information to detecting PDR and affect the model's performance.

To handle these difficulties, we develop a new framework for identifying DR using retinal fundus images based on annotation that includes DR grades and bounding boxes of MA and HE lesions (possibly with a few missing annotated lesions). We first extract lesion information into a *lesion map* by a detection model, and then fuse it with the original image for DR identification. To deal with noisy negative samples induced by missing annotated lesions, our detection model uses center loss [12], which can cluster the features of similar samples around a feature center called *Lesion Center*. We also propose a sampling method, called *Center-Sample*, to find noisy negative samples by measuring their features' similarity to the Lesion Center and reduce their sampling probabilities. Besides, we adapt center loss from classification tasks to detection tasks efficiently, which makes the model more discriminative and robust. In the classification stage, we integrate feature maps of the original images and lesion maps using an *Attention Fusion Network (AFN)*. AFN can learn the weights between the original images and lesion maps when identifying different DR grades to reduce the interference of unnecessary lesion information on classification. We evaluate our framework using datasets collected from a local hospital and two public datasets, EyePACS and Messidor. Experimental results show that our Center-Sample mechanism can effectively determine noisy samples and achieve promising performance. Our AFN can utilize lesion information well and outperform the state-of-the-art methods on the two public datasets.

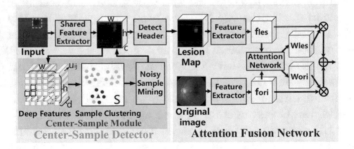

Fig. 2. The Center-Sample Detector (left) predicts the probabilities of the lesions using the anti-noise Center-Sample Module. Then *AFN* (right) uses the original image and detection model output as input to identify DR (f_{les} and f_{ori} are feature maps, W_{les} and W_{ori} are attention weights).

2   Method

This section presents the key components of our approach, the *Center-Sample* detector and *Attention Fusion Network*. As shown in Fig. 2, the detection model predicts the probabilities of the lesions in the entire image. Then *AFN* uses both the original image and detection model output as input to identify DR grades.

2.1   Center-Sample Detector

The Center-Sample detector aims to detect n types of lesions (here, $n = 2$, for MA and HE) in a fundus image. Figure 2 gives an overview of the Center-Sample detector, which composes of three main parts: shared feature extractor, classification/bounding box detecting header, and *Noisy Sample Mining* module.

The first two parts form the main network for lesion detection to predict the lesion probability map. Their main structures are adapted from SSD [8]. The backbone until conv4_3 is used as feature extractor, and the detect headers are the same as SSD. The third part includes two components: *Sample Clustering* for clustering similar samples and *Noisy Sample Mining* for determining the noisy samples and reducing their sampling weight.

Sample Clustering. Here we show how to adapt *center loss* in classification tasks to detection tasks and how to cluster similar samples using center loss. This component begins by taking the feature map from the shared feature extractor, which is a tensor of size $h \times w \times c$. We transform it to a feature map u of size $h \times w \times d$ ($d \ll c$) by adding 1×1 convolution layers after the shared feature extractor. Each position u_{ij} in u is a d-D vector, called *deep feature*, as shown in Fig. 2. That is, u_{ij} is a feature vector mapped from a corresponding position patch f_{ij} in the original image to a high-dimensional feature space S, where f_{ij} denotes the receptive field of u_{ij}. We assign each u_{ij} with a label indicating whether a lesion is in the corresponding position and (if yes) which type of lesion it is (in Fig. 2, different colors are for different labels). Thus, there are totally $n + 1$ label classes including background (no lesion in corresponding location) and n classes of lesions. We treat background as negative samples and the n classes of lesions as positive samples. Then, we average the deep features u_{ij} of each class to obtain $n + 1$ feature centers (the centers of positive labels are called *lesion centers*), and make the u_{ij} cluster around their corresponding center in the space S using center loss [12] (in Fig. 2, the triangles denote the centers): $\mathcal{L}_C = \frac{1}{2} \sum_{i=1}^{w} \sum_{j=1}^{h} ||u_{ij} - c_{y_{ij}}||_2^2$, where $y_{ij} \in [0, n]$ is the corresponding label of u_{ij} in location (i, j), and $c_{y_{ij}} \in \mathbb{R}^d$ is the center of the y_{ij}-th class. During the detection training phase, we minimize $\mathcal{L}_C$ and simultaneously update the feature centers using the SGD algorithm in each iteration, to make the u_{ij} cluster to the center $c_{y_{ij}}$. Note that the deep features u_{ij} of noisy negative samples become closer to the corresponding lesion center $c_{y_{ij}}$ than true negative samples after several iterations.

Noisy Sample Mining. In the Noisy Sample Mining module, we reduce the impact of noisy negative samples by down-weighting them. First, for each u_{ij}

labeled as a negative sample, we select the minimum $\mathcal{L}2$ distance between u_{ij} and all *lesion centers*, denoted by $min\text{-}dist_{ij}$ and sort all elements in $min\text{-}dist$ in increasing order. Then, the sampling probability $P(u_{ij})$ is assigned as:

$$P(u_{ij}) = \begin{cases} 0 & 0 < r_{ij} < t_l \\ (\frac{r_{ij}-t_l}{t_u-t_l})^{\gamma} & t_l \leq r_{ij} < t_u \\ 1 & r_{ij} \geq t_u \end{cases} \tag{1}$$

where r_{ij} is the rank of u_{ij} in $min\text{-}dist$. Note that u_{ij} is close to lesion centers if r_{ij} is small. The lower bound t_l and upper bound t_u of sampling ranking and γ are three hyper-parameters. If $r_{ij} < t_u$, then u_{ij} shall be a noisy sample with high probability and we ignore it by setting the sampling probability to 0. $P(u_{ij})$ is set to 1.0 when $r_{ij} > t_u$ for treating u_{ij} as a true negative sample. γ smoothly adjusts the sampling probability between ranks t_l and t_u. We treat the summation of $\mathcal{L}_C$ and detection loss in [8] as multi-task loss for robustness. In [12], center loss is required for a comparable large batch size for stable center gradient computing, but in our method, a large number of deep features ensures the stability in small batch size.

During the training phase, we train the model with cropped patches of the original images that include lesions. During the inference phase, a whole image is fed to the trained model, and the output is a tensor M of size $h \times w \times n$, where every n-D vector M_{ij} in M denotes the maximum probability among all Anchor Boxes in this position for each lesion. We take this tensor, called *Lesion Map*, as the input of the *Attention Fusion Network*.

2.2 Attention Fusion Network

As stated in Sect. 1, some lesion information can be noise to identifying certain DR grades. To resolve this issue, we propose an information fusion method based on attention mechanism [1], called *Attention Fusion Network (AFN)*. AFN can produce the weights based on the original images and lesion maps to reduce the impact of unneeded lesion information for identifying different DR grades. AFN contains two feature extractors and an attention network (see Fig. 2). The scaled original images and lesion maps are the inputs of two separate feature extractors, respectively. We extract feature maps f_{ori} and f_{les} using these two CNNs. Then, f_{ori} and f_{les} are concatenated on channel dimension as the input of the attention network.

The attention network consists of a 3×3 Conv, a ReLU, a dropout, a 1×1 Conv, and a Sigmoid layer. It produces two weight maps W_{ori} and W_{les}, which have the same shape as the feature maps f_{ori} and f_{les}, respectively. Then, we compute the weighted sum $f(i,j,c)$ of the two feature maps as follows:

$$f(i,j,c) = W_{ori}(i,j,c) \circ f_{ori}(i,j,c) + W_{les}(i,j,c) \circ f_{les}(i,j,c) \tag{2}$$

where $\circ$ denotes element-wise product. The weights W_{ori} and W_{les} are computed as $W(i,j,c) = \frac{1}{1+e^{-h(i,j,c)}}$, where $h(i,j,c)$ is the last layer output before Sigmoid produced by the attention network. $W(i, j, c)$ reflects the importance of the feature at position (i, j) and channel c. The final output is produced by performing a softmax operation on $f(i, j, c)$ to get the probabilities of all grades.

3 Experiments

In this section, we evaluate Center-Sample detector and AFN on various datasets.

3.1 Evaluating Center-Sample Detector

Dataset and Evaluation Metric. A private dataset was provided by a local hospital, which contains 13k abnormal (more severe than grade of 0) fundus images of size about 2000×2000. Lesion bounding boxes were annotated by ophthalmologists, including 25 k MA and 34 k HE lesions, with about 26% missing annotated lesions. The common metric for object detection mAP is used as the evaluation metric since it reflects the precision and recall of each lesion.

Implementation Details. In our experiments, we select MA and HE lesions as the detection targets since other types of lesions are clear even in compressed images (512×512). During training, we train the model with cropped patches (300×300) which include annotated lesions from the original images. Random flips are applied as data augmentation. We use SGD (momentum $= 0.9$, weight decay $= 10^{-5}$) as the optimizer and batch size is 16. The learning rate is initialized to 10^{-3} and divided by 10 after 50k iterations. When training the Center-Sample detector, we first use center loss and detection loss as multi-task loss for pre-training. Then the Center-Sample mechanism is included after 10k training steps. t_l and t_u are set to 1st and 5th percentile among all deep features in one batch.

Results and Analysis. We evaluate the effects of the Center-Sample components by adding them to the detection model one by one. Table 1 shows that the base detection network (*BaseNet*), which is similar to SSD, gives mAP $= 41.7\%$. After using Center Loss as one part of multi-task loss, it raises to 42.2%. The Center-Sample strategy further adds 1.4% to it, with the final mAP $= 43.6\%$. Note that common detectors like SSD lack mechanisms to address the missing annotation issue. The results show the robustness of our proposed method. Figure 3 visualizes some regions where deep features are close to lesion centers.

3.2 Evaluating the Attention Fusion Network

Datasets and Evaluation Metric. The private dataset used (which is different from the one for evaluating Center-Sample above) contains 40k fundus images, with 31k/3k/4k/1.1k/1k images for DR grades 0 to 4 respectively, rated by ophthalmologists. The EyePACS dataset gives 35k/11k/43k images for train/val/test sets, respectively. The Messidor dataset has 1.2 k retinal images with different criteria for DR grades 0 to 3. For the EyePACS dataset and the private dataset, we adopt the quadratic weighted kappa score which can effectively reflect the performance of the model on an unbalanced dataset. For the Messidor dataset, we refer to the experimental methods [11] and conduct tasks of referable v.s. non-referable and normal v.s. abnormal, with AUC as the metric.

Implementation Details. We use two ResNet-18 [6] as the feature extractors for both inputs. The preprocessing includes cropping the images and resizing them to 224×224. Random rotations/crops/flips are used as data augmentation. AFN is trained with the SGD algorithm. All models are trained for 300k iterations with the initial learning rate$=10^{-5}$ and divided by 10 at iterations 120k and 200k. Weight decay and momentum are set to 0.1 and 0.9.

Fig. 3. Missing annotated samples determined by the Center-Sample module.

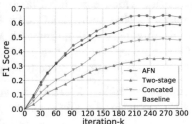

Fig. 4. F1 scores of DR grade 4 with different algorithms on the validation set.

Table 1. Results of the Center-Sample components.

BaseNet	√	√	√
Center Loss		√	√
Center-Sample			√
mAP(%)	41.7	42.2	**43.6**

Table 2. Results on private dataset.

Algorithms	kappa	acc.
Baseline	0.786	0.843
Two-stage	0.804	0.849
Concated	0.823	0.854
AFN	**0.875**	**0.873**

Results on the Private Dataset. We evaluate AFN and several models on the private dataset as shown in Table 2. Baseline only employs scaled original images as input to ResNet-18 for training. We re-implement the feature fusion method in [13], called Two-stage. Another fusion method that concatenates lesion maps and scaled images on channel dimension (called Concated) is compared, since both these inputs equally contribute to identifying DR with this method. Our approach outperforms the other methods considerably. Note that the Two-stage method performs not as well as in the original paper [13] on our dataset, possibly for the following reasons. (a) The Two-stage method cannot identify grade 4 well,

Table 3. Kappa on the EyePACS.

Algorithms	val	test
Min-pooling*	0.860	0.849
o_O	0.854	0.844
Zoom-in-Net [11]	0.865	0.854
AFN	**0.871**	**0.859**

*https://www.kaggle.com/c/
diabetic-retinopathy-detection/
leaderboard

Table 4. AUC for referral/normal tasks

Method	referral	normal
Comp. CAD [10]	0.910	0.876
DSF-RF_{cara} [9]	0.916	0.899
Zoom-in-Net [11]	0.957	0.921
AFN	**0.968**	**0.935**

because MA and HE lesions might be noisy information for grade 4. (b) There are some unannotated lesions in our dataset. We visualize F1 scores of identifying PDR (grade 4) in Fig. 4, which shows AFN has similar ability as Baseline to determine PDR, and other models perform better than Baseline as a whole but worse in PDR identification. This shows the lesion maps of MA and HE are useless noisy information for PDR and our AFN can reduce the impact.

Results on EyePACS and Messidor. We use the Center-Sample detector trained on the private datasets to produce EyePACS and Messidor's lesion maps. Table 3 shows that AFN obtains kappa scores of 0.857 and 0.849 on the val/test sets, respectively. Since the size of Messidor is quite small for training CNNs from scratch, we fine-tune AFN using weights pre-trained on EyePACS. Table 4 shows the results of proposed approach compared with previous studies. To our best knowledge, we achieve state-of-the-art results on both public datasets.

4 Conclusions

In this paper, we proposed a new framework unifying lesion detection and DR grade identification. With the Center-Sample detector, we can use low quality annotated data to train an effective model, and employ center loss to make the model more discriminative and robust. Further, using a new information fusion method based on attention mechanism, we achieve better DR identification. Experiments showed that our approach outperforms state-of-the-art methods.

Acknowledgement. D.Z. Chen's research was supported in part by NSF Grant CCF-1617735. The authors would like to thank the RealDoctor AI Research Center.

References

1. Chen, L.C., Yang, Y., Wang, J., Xu, W., Yuille, A.L.: Attention to scale: Scale-aware semantic image segmentation. In: CVPR, pp. 3640–3649 (2016)
2. Dai, L., et al.: Retinal microaneurysm detection using clinical report guided multi-sieving CNN. In: Descoteaux, M., Maier-Hein, L., Franz, A., Jannin, P., Collins, D.L., Duchesne, S. (eds.) MICCAI 2017. LNCS, vol. 10435, pp. 525–532. Springer, Cham (2017). https://doi.org/10.1007/978-3-319-66179-7_60
3. Gargeya, R., Leng, T.: Automated identification of diabetic retinopathy using deep learning. Ophthalmology **124**(7), 962–969 (2017)
4. van Grinsven, M.J.J.P., van Ginneken, B., Hoyng, C.B., Theelen, T., Sanchez, C.I.: Fast convolutional neural network training using selective data sampling: application to hemorrhage detection in color fundus images. IEEE Trans. Med. Imaging **35**(5), 1273–1284 (2016)
5. Gulshan, V., et al.: Development and validation of a deep learning algorithm for detection of diabetic retinopathy in retinal fundus photographs. JAMA **316**(22), 2402 (2016)
6. He, K., Zhang, X., Ren, S., Sun, J.: Deep residual learning for image recognition. In: CVPR, pp. 770–778 (2015)
7. Kumar, N., Rajwade, A.V., Chandran, S., Awate, S.P.: Kernel generalized-gaussian mixture model for robust abnormality detection. In: Descoteaux, M., Maier-Hein, L., Franz, A., Jannin, P., Collins, D.L., Duchesne, S. (eds.) MICCAI 2017. LNCS, vol. 10435, pp. 21–29. Springer, Cham (2017). https://doi.org/10.1007/978-3-319-66179-7_3
8. Liu, W., et al.: SSD: single shot multibox detector. In: Leibe, B., Matas, J., Sebe, N., Welling, M. (eds.) ECCV 2016. LNCS, vol. 9905, pp. 21–37. Springer, Cham (2016). https://doi.org/10.1007/978-3-319-46448-0_2
9. Seoud, L., Hurtut, T., Chelbi, J., Cheriet, F., Langlois, J.M.P.: Red lesion detection using dynamic shape features for diabetic retinopathy screening. IEEE Trans. Med. Imaging **35**(4), 1116–1126 (2015)
10. Sánchez, C.I., Niemeijer, M., Dumitrescu, A.V., Suttorpschulten, M.S., Abràmoff, M.D., Van, G.B.: Evaluation of a computer-aided diagnosis system for diabetic retinopathy screening on public data. IOVS **52**(7), 4866 (2011)
11. Wang, Z., Yin, Y., Shi, J., Fang, W., Li, H., Wang, X.: Zoom-in-net: deep mining lesions for diabetic retinopathy detection. In: Descoteaux, M., Maier-Hein, L., Franz, A., Jannin, P., Collins, D.L., Duchesne, S. (eds.) MICCAI 2017. LNCS, vol. 10435, pp. 267–275. Springer, Cham (2017). https://doi.org/10.1007/978-3-319-66179-7_31
12. Wen, Y., Zhang, K., Li, Z., Qiao, Y.: A discriminative feature learning approach for deep face recognition. In: Leibe, B., Matas, J., Sebe, N., Welling, M. (eds.) ECCV 2016. LNCS, vol. 9911, pp. 499–515. Springer, Cham (2016). https://doi.org/10.1007/978-3-319-46478-7_31
13. Yang, Y., Li, T., Li, W., Wu, H., Fan, W., Zhang, W.: Lesion detection and grading of diabetic retinopathy via two-stages deep convolutional neural networks. In: Descoteaux, M., Maier-Hein, L., Franz, A., Jannin, P., Collins, D.L., Duchesne, S. (eds.) MICCAI 2017. LNCS, vol. 10435, pp. 533–540. Springer, Cham (2017). https://doi.org/10.1007/978-3-319-66179-7_61

Deep Supervision with Additional Labels for Retinal Vessel Segmentation Task

Yishuo Zhang and Albert C. S. Chung[✉]

Lo Kwee-Seong Medical Image Analysis Laboratory, Department of Computer Science and Engineering, The Hong Kong University of Science and Technology, Hong Kong, China
ys.zhang@connect.ust.hk, achung@cse.ust.hk

Abstract. Automatic analysis of retinal fundus images is of vital importance in diagnosis tasks of retinopathy. Segmenting vessels accurately is a fundamental step in analysing retinal images. However, it is usually difficult due to various imaging conditions, low image contrast and the appearance of pathologies such as micro-aneurysms. In this paper, we propose a novel method with deep neural networks to solve this problem. We utilize U-net with residual connection to detect vessels. To achieve better accuracy, we introduce an edge-aware mechanism, in which we convert the original task into a multi-class task by adding additional labels on boundary areas. In this way, the network will pay more attention to the boundary areas of vessels and achieve a better performance, especially in tiny vessels detecting. Besides, side output layers are applied in order to give deep supervision and therefore help convergence. We train and evaluate our model on three databases: DRIVE, STARE, and CHASEDB1. Experimental results show that our method has a comparable performance with AUC of 97.99% on DRIVE and an efficient running time compared to the state-of-the-art methods.

1 Introduction

Retinal vessels are commonly analysed in the diagnosis and treatment of various ophthalmological diseases. For example, retinal vascular structures are correlated to the severity of diabetic retinopathy [5], which is a cause of blindness globally. Thus, the precise segmentation of retinal vessels is of vital importance. However, this task is often extremely challenging due to the following factors [1]: 1. The shape and width of vessel vary, which cannot be represented by a simple pattern; 2. The resolution, contrast and local intensity change among different fundus images, increasing the difficulty of segmenting; 3. Other structures, like optical disks and lesions, can be interference factors; 4. Extremely thin vessels are hard to detect due to the low contrast and noise.

In recent years, a variety of methods have been proposed to solve retinal vessel segmentation tasks, including unsupervised methods [9] and supervised methods [11]. Although promising performances have been shown, there is still some room for improvement. As we mentioned before, tiny capillaries are hard

© Springer Nature Switzerland AG 2018
A. F. Frangi et al. (Eds.): MICCAI 2018, LNCS 11071, pp. 83–91, 2018.
https://doi.org/10.1007/978-3-030-00934-2_10

to find and missing these can lead to low sensitivity. Besides, methods that need less running time are preferred in clinical practice. In this paper, we aim to design a more effective and efficient method to tackle these problems.

The emergence of deep learning methods provides a powerful tool for computer vision tasks and these kinds of methods have outperformed other methods in many areas. By stacking convolutional layers and pooling layers, networks can gain the capacity to learn the very complicated representation of features. U-net, proposed in [12], can deal with image patches in an end-to-end manner and therefore is widely used in medical image segmentation.

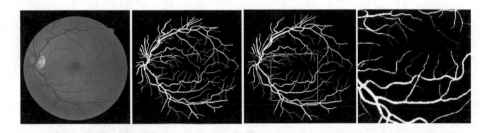

Fig. 1. Images sampled from datasets. From left to right: original fundus image, ground truth, output of a single trained U-net and zoomed segment inside the green rectangle in the third image. In the last image, blue regions denote false negative, while red regions denote false positive.

We analyse the output of a single trained U-net model as shown in Fig. 1. Most mislabelled pixels come from boundaries between foreground and background. Regarding thick vessels, the background areas around vessels are easy to be labelled as positive. However regarding very thin vessels, many of these are ignored by networks and labelled as background. To tackle this problem, we process the ground truth, by labelling the boundary, thick vessels and thin vessels as different classes, which forces the networks to pay different extra attention to error-prone regions. This operation makes the original task become a harder task. If the new task can be solved by our method perfectly, then so could the original task. Besides, we also utilize deep supervision to help networks converge.

Our main contributions are as follows:

1. Introducing a deep supervision mechanism into U-net, which helps networks learn a better semantically representation;
2. Separating thin vessels from thick vessels during the progress of training;
3. Applying an edge-aware mechanism by labelling the boundary region to extra classes, making the network focus on the boundaries of vessels and therefore get finer edges in the segmentation result.

2   Proposed Method

2.1   U-Net

The architecture of U-net is illustrated in Fig. 2. The left-hand part consists of four blocks, each of which contains stacked convolutional layers (Conv) to learn hierarchical features. The size of the input feature maps is halved after each stage, implemented by a Conv layer with a stride of 2. In contrast, the number of feature channels increases when the depth increases, in order to learn more complicated representations. The right-hand part has a similar structure to the left part. The size of input feature maps is doubled after each stage by a deconvolution layer to reconstruct spatial information.

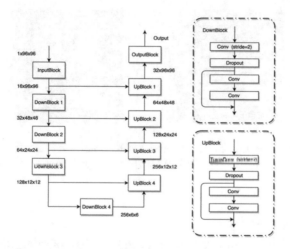

Fig. 2. Architecture of a simple U-net. We annotate shapes about feature maps of each block in the format of 'Channels, Width, Height'. Inner structures of DownBlock and UpBlock are shown on the right, where each Conv layer is followed by two unseen layers: a BatchNorm layer and a ReLU layer.

To utilize feature learned by earlier layers at subsequent layers, feature maps from the left-hand blocks will be fed into the corresponding right-hand blocks. In this way, networks can gain detailed information which may be lost in former downsampling operations but useful for fine boundary prediction. To improve the robustness and help convergence, we apply a residual connection [3] inside each block, which adds feature maps before Conv layers to the output maps pixelwisely. We also leverage Dropout and BatchNorm inside each block to reduce overfitting and gradient vanishing respectively.

2.2   Additional Label

Additional labels are added to the original ground truth before training, which converts this task into a multi-class segmentation task. Firstly, we distinguish thick vessels from thin vessels (with a width of 1 or 2 pixels), implemented by an opening operation. Then, we locate the pixels near to the vessel by a dilation operation and label them to the additional class. Therefore, we have 5 classes, which are 0 (other background pixels), 1 (background near thick vessels), 2 (background near thin vessels), 3 (thick vessel) and 4 (thin vessel) (Fig. 3).

The objective of this is to force the networks to treat background pixels differently. As we reported above, the boundary region is easy to be mislabelled. We separate these classes so that we can give more supervision in crucial areas by modifying the class weight in the loss function but not influencing others. Boundary classes have heavier weights in the loss function, which means that these classes will attract a higher penalty if labelled wrongly.

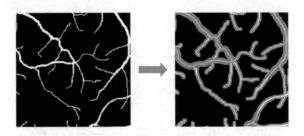

Fig. 3. Generated new multi-class ground truth, where different classes are shown in different colours: 0 (black), 1 (green), 2 (orange), 3 (grey) and 4 (white).

2.3 Deep Supervision

Deep supervision [6] is employed to solve the problem of information loss during forward propagation and improve detailed accuracy. This mechanism is beneficial because it gives semantic representations to the intermediate layers. We implement it by adding four side output layers as shown in Fig. 4. The output of each side layer is compared with the ground truth to calculate auxiliary losses. Final prediction maps are generated by fusing the outputs of all four side layers.

We employ cross-entropy as loss function and calculate it for the final output as well as each side output. Owing to the amounts of different classes being imbalanced, we add a class-balanced weight for each class to correct imbalances. As we discussed before, pixels of boundaries around thick vessels and pixels of thin vessels should be given relatively heavier weights.

$$CE(pred, target) = -\sum_i weight_i \times target_i \times log(pred_i). \tag{1}$$

The total loss is defined as below, comprising of loss of fused output, losses of side outputs and L-2 regular term.

$$Loss = CE(fuse, GT) + \sum_3^n CE(side_i, GT) + \frac{\lambda}{2}\|w\|^2. \tag{2}$$

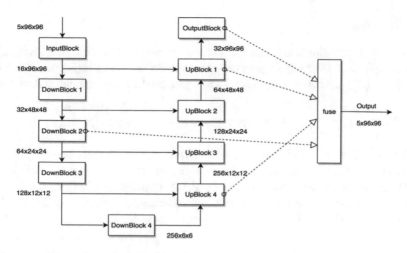

Fig. 4. Diagram of our proposed method.

3 Experiments

We implement our model with PyTorch library. Stochastic gradient descent algorithm (SGD) with momentum is utilized to optimize our model. The learning rate is set to 0.01 initially and halved every 100 epochs. We train the whole model for 200 epochs on a single NVIDIA GPU (GeForce Titan X). The training progress takes nearly 10 h.

3.1 Datasets

We evaluate our method on three public datasets: DRIVE [13], STARE [4] and CHASEDB1 [2], each of which contains images with two labelled masks annotated by different experts. We take the first labelled mask as ground truth for training and testing. The second labelled masks are used for comparison between our model and a human observer. The DRIVE dataset contains 20 training images and 20 testing images; thus, we take them as the training set and testing set respectively. STARE and CHASEDB1 datasets contain 20 and 28 images, respectively. As these two datasets are not divided for training and testing, we perform a four-fold cross-validation, following [10].

Before feeding the original image into networks, some preprocessing operations are performed. We employ contrast-limited adaptive histogram equalization (CLAHE) to enhance the image and increase contrast. Then the whole images are cropped into patches with the size of 96 * 96 pixels. To augment the training data, we perform the flip, affine transformation, and noising operations randomly. In addition, the lightness and contrast of the original images are changed randomly to improve the robustness of the model.

3.2 Results

A vessel segmentation task can be viewed as an unbalanced pixel-wise classification task. For evaluation purpose, measurements including Specificity (Sp), Sensitivity (Se) and Accuracy (Acc) are computed. They are defined as below:

$$Sp = \frac{TN}{TN + FP}, Se = \frac{TP}{TP + FN}, Acc = \frac{TP + TN}{TP + FP + TN + FN}, \quad (3)$$

Here TP, FN, TN, FP denote true positive, false negative, true negative and false positive, respectively. Additionally, a better metric, area under the receiver operating characteristic (ROC) curve (AUC), is used. We believe that AUC is more suitable for measuring an unbalanced situation. A perfect classifier should have an AUC value of 1.

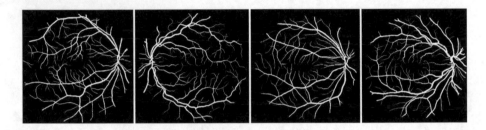

Fig. 5. Examples of our experiment output.

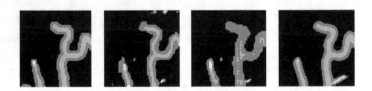

Fig. 6. Comparison between side output and ground truth. From left to right: Ground Truth, 2 side outputs, and final prediction.

We have three observations: 1. Even if the side output cannot locate the vessel, they can locate the boundary region, which can help to find the vessel in final output precisely as a guide. 2. As the resolution of the side output is lower, the tiny vessel may be missed but the boundary region is more distinct and easier to find. This shows mutual promotion between the additional label and deep supervision. 3. The boundary of the boundary region is not refined, but it does not affect the prediction because we will take all of the boundary regions as background (Figs. 5 and 6).

Table 1. Performance comparison with simple U-net on dataset DRIVE

Methods	AUC of all vessels	AUC of thick vessels	AUC of thin vessels
Simple U-net	0.9736	0.9830	0.8678
Our method	0.9799	0.9897	0.9589

To validate the effect of our idea, we perform comparison experiments with a simple U-net. With additional label and well-designed deep supervision, our method has better capabilities of detecting vessels, especially for capillaries. AUC of thin vessels has been increased by 9.11%, as shown in Table 1.

3.3   Comparison

We report performances of our method in respect to the aforementioned metrics, compared with other state-of-the-art methods, as shown in Tables 2 and 3.

Table 2. Performance comparison on the DRIVE dataset

Methods	Acc	Sp	Se	AUC
2nd Observer	0.9472	0.9730	0.7760	N.A
Fraz et al. [2]	0.9480	**0.9807**	0.7406	0.9747
Liskowski et al. [8]	**0.9535**	**0.9807**	0.7811	0.9790
Mo et al. [10]	0.9521	0.9780	0.7779	0.9782
Leopold et al. [7]	0.9106	0.9573	0.6963	0.8268
Our method	0.9504	0.9618	**0.8723**	**0.9799**

Table 3. Performance comparison on STARE and CHASEDB1 datasets

Methods	STARE				CHASEDB1			
	Acc	Sp	Se	AUC	Acc	Sp	Se	AUC
2nd Observer	0.9353	0.9387	**0.8951**	N.A	0.9560	0.9793	0.7425	N.A.
Fraz et al. [2]	0.9534	0.9763	0.7548	0.9768	0.9468	0.9711	0.7224	0.9712
Liskowski et al. [8]	**0.9729**	0.9862	0.8554	**0.9928**	0.9628	0.9836	0.7816	0.9823
Mo et al. [10]	0.9674	0.9844	0.8147	0.9885	0.9599	0.9816	0.7661	0.9812
Leopold et al. [7]	0.9045	0.9472	0.6433	0.7952	0.8936	0.8961	**0.8618**	0.8790
Our method	0.9712	**0.9901**	0.7673	0.9882	**0.9770**	**0.9909**	0.7670	**0.9900**

We have highlighted the highest scores for each column. Our method achieves the highest Sensitivity on the DRIVE dataset and the highest Specificity on the other two datasets. Due to the differences of inherent errors among datasets and the class imbalance, we prefer using AUC as an equatable metric for comparison. Our method has the best performance on the DRIVE and CHASEDB1 datasets in terms of AUC.

Table 4. Time comparison with other methods

Method	Training time (h)	Running time (s)
Liskowski et al. [8]	8	92
Mo et al. [10]	10	0.4
Our method	10	0.9

In terms of running time, our method is also computationally efficient when compared to other methods (Table 4). Our proposed method can deal with an image size of 584*565 in 1.2 s, much faster than the method proposed in [8]. This benefit is obtained from our method by using the U-net architecture which works from patch to patch, instead of using a patch to predict the central pixel alone. The method proposed in [10] is a little faster than ours, as their network has less up-sampling layers. However, removing up-sampling leads to a decrease in fine prediction and especially sensitivity. By overall consideration, we choose proper numbers of layers as used in our presented method, which can achieve the best performance with highly acceptable running time.

4   Conclusion

In this paper, we propose a novel deep neural network to segment retinal vessel. To give more importance to boundary pixels, we label thick vessels, thin vessels and boundaries into different classes, which makes a multi-class segmentation task. We use a U-net with residual connections to perform the segmentation task. Deep supervision is introduced to help the network learn better features and semantic information. Our method offers a good performance and efficient running time compared to other state-of-the-art methods, which can give high efficacy in clinical applications.

References

1. Fraz, M.M., et al.: An approach to localize the retinal blood vessels using bit planes and centerline detection. Comput. Methods Programs Biomed. **108**(2), 600–616 (2012)
2. Fraz, M.M., et al.: An ensemble classification-based approach applied to retinal blood vessel segmentation. IEEE Trans. Biomed. Eng. **59**(9), 2538–2548 (2012)
3. He, K., Zhang, X., Ren, S., Sun, J.: Deep residual learning for image recognition. In: Proceedings of the IEEE Conference on Computer Vision and Pattern Recognition, pp. 770–778 (2016)

4. Hoover, A., Kouznetsova, V., Goldbaum, M.: Locating blood vessels in retinal images by piecewise threshold probing of a matched filter response. IEEE Trans. Med. Imaging **19**(3), 203–210 (2000)
5. Jelinek, H., Cree, M.J.: Automated Image Detection of Retinal Pathology. CRC Press, Boca Raton (2009)
6. Lee, C.Y., Xie, S., Gallagher, P., Zhang, Z., Tu, Z.: Deeply-supervised nets. In: Artificial Intelligence and Statistics, pp. 562–570 (2015)
7. Leopold, H.A., Orchard, J., Zelek, J.S., Lakshminarayanan, V.: Pixelbnn: augmenting the pixelcnn with batch normalization and the presentation of a fast architecture for retinal vessel segmentation. arXiv preprint arXiv:1712.06742 (2017)
8. Liskowski, P., Krawiec, K.: Segmenting retinal blood vessels with deep neural networks. IEEE Trans. Med. Imaging **35**(11), 2369–2380 (2016)
9. Marín, D., Aquino, A., Gegúndez-Arias, M.E., Bravo, J.M.: A new supervised method for blood vessel segmentation in retinal images by using gray-level and moment invariants-based features. IEEE Trans. Med. Imaging **30**(1), 146–158 (2011)
10. Mo, J., Zhang, L.: Multi-level deep supervised networks for retinal vessel segmentation. Int. J. Comput. Assist. Radiol. Surg. **12**(12), 2181–2193 (2017)
11. Orlando, J.I., Blaschko, M.: Learning fully-connected CRFs for blood vessel segmentation in retinal images. In: Golland, P., Hata, N., Barillot, C., Hornegger, J., Howe, R. (eds.) MICCAI 2014. LNCS, vol. 8673, pp. 634–641. Springer, Cham (2014). https://doi.org/10.1007/978-3-319-10404-1_79
12. Ronneberger, O., Fischer, P., Brox, T.: U-Net: convolutional networks for biomedical image segmentation. In: Navab, N., Hornegger, J., Wells, W.M., Frangi, A.F. (eds.) MICCAI 2015. LNCS, vol. 9351, pp. 234–241. Springer, Cham (2015). https://doi.org/10.1007/978-3-319-24574-4_28
13. Staal, J., Abràmoff, M.D., Niemeijer, M., Viergever, M.A., Van Ginneken, B.: Ridge-based vessel segmentation in color images of the retina. IEEE Trans. Med.Imaging **23**(4), 501–509 (2004)

A Multi-task Network to Detect Junctions in Retinal Vasculature

Fatmatülzehra Uslu$^{(\boxtimes)}$ (ID) and Anil Anthony Bharath

BICV Group, Bioengineering Department, Imperial College London, London, UK
fzehrauslu@gmail.com, a.bharath@imperial.ac.uk

Abstract. Junctions in the retinal vasculature are key points to be able to extract its topology, but they vary in appearance, depending on vessel density, width and branching/crossing angles. The complexity of junction patterns is usually accompanied by a scarcity of labels, which discourages the usage of very deep networks for their detection. We propose a multi-task network, generating labels for vessel interior, centerline, edges and junction patterns, to provide additional information to facilitate junction detection. After the initial detection of potential junctions in junction-selective probability maps, candidate locations are re-examined in centerline probability maps to verify if they connect at least 3 branches. The experiments on the DRIVE and IOSTAR showed that our method outperformed a recent study in which a popular deep network was trained as a classifier to find junctions. Moreover, the proposed approach is applicable to unseen datasets with the same degree of success, after training it only once.

Keywords: Restricted Boltzmann machines · Deep networks
Bifurcation · Crossing · Fundus images

1 Introduction

The variations on geometry and topology of retinal vasculature can give information about the health of the eye. Junctions in the retinal vasculature represent important landmarks to extract retinal vessel topology, and can also facilitate image registration. The appearance of junctions in fundus images can vary markedly depending on branching angles, vessel widths and junction sizes, somewhat complicating their detection.

Several previous studies have made use of algorithms designed to work on binary vessel maps, usually on vessel skeletons [3,4,6,10]. Generally, these methods relied on examining the intersection numbers in the skeletons [4] accompanied with vessel widths, lengths and branching angles [6]. However, the skeletons can misrepresent vessel topology due to either/both gaps in vessels in segmented vessel maps or, missing or false vessels in these maps.

Recently, deep learning methods have been frequently used for medical image analysis. However, they have been rarely applied to junction detection in retinal

© Springer Nature Switzerland AG 2018
A. F. Frangi et al. (Eds.): MICCAI 2018, LNCS 11071, pp. 92–100, 2018.
https://doi.org/10.1007/978-3-030-00934-2_11

vasculature. As far as we are aware, the only study is Pratt *et al.*'s [10], where a popular network was trained as a classifier to identify image patches with junctions. The image patches contained vessel skeletons, generated from binary vessel maps. The major factor restricting the application of deep architectures on this task seems the shortage of training data. The number of publicly accessible image datasets is only two [1], as far as we are aware. Also, the task is extremely skewed, where the fraction of junction pixels in a fundus image is lower than 10^{-4} [1]. These factors – and primarily the imbalanced nature of the junction presence – complicate the training of deep networks containing a large number of parameters.

In this study, we introduce a multi-task network for junction detection on fundus images, which can deal with the shortage of labeled data and highly skewed nature of the task. We also present a junction probability map, which significantly facilitates finding junctions by removing possible variations in vessel thickness. Experiments on the DRIVE and IOSTAR show our method outperformed Pratt *et al.*'s method [10], despite operating directly on fundus images.

2   Method

Our method has three stages: (i) training our multi-task network, (ii) initial junction search and (iii) refined junction search.

2.1   Learning Junction Patterns with Multi-task Network

The amount of labeled data for junction locations in retinal vasculature is not sufficient to successfully train a deep network with many parameters. In contrast, vessel segmentation has been realized by deep networks in increasing numbers of studies [12]. In order to deal with the shortage of labeled data for the junction detection, we propose a multi-task network, which simultaneously generates label patches for vessel interior, centerline, edge locations and junction patterns.

The proposed network for this task is a fully connected network, which is initialized with weights learned by training a stack of Restricted Boltzmann Machines (RBMs) [8] on five types of image patches: fundus image patches, label patches for vessel interior, centerline, edges and junction patterns. Label patches can be combined, as suggested by Li *et al.* [9], to generate a likelihood map for the whole fundus image (see Fig. 1). After initialization, the network is trained patch-wise with the l_2 loss function in Eq. (1):

$$\mathcal{L} = ||\mathcal{V}_i^p - \tilde{\mathcal{V}}_i^p||_2 + ||\mathcal{V}_c^p - \tilde{\mathcal{V}}_c^p||_2 + ||\mathcal{V}_e^p - \tilde{\mathcal{V}}_e^p||_2 + ||\mathcal{V}_j^p - \tilde{\mathcal{V}}_j^p||_2 \tag{1}$$

where $\tilde{\mathcal{V}}_i^p$, $\tilde{\mathcal{V}}_c^p$, $\tilde{\mathcal{V}}_e^p$ and $\tilde{\mathcal{V}}_j^p$ respectively represent estimates of ground truth label patches for vessel interior ($\mathcal{V}_i^p$), centerline ($\mathcal{V}_c^p$), edges ($\mathcal{V}_e^p$) and junction patterns ($\mathcal{V}_j^p$) by the network.

One key advantage of this network is that – despite the ability to perform more than one task – it has relatively fewer parameters, slightly over one million, than those of many state-of-the-art networks. For example, *Res*16 [7] has

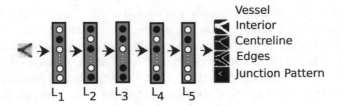

Fig. 1. The generation of junction pattern label patches with a fully connected network with 5 hidden layers.

over eleven million parameters, which was used by Pratt *et al.* to classify image patches with junctions [10]. Also, pretraining can provide a good initialization for the network parameters and facilitate training of the network in the face of the scarcity of labeled data.

2.2   Initial Junction Search

The junction probability maps produced by our method, shown in Figs. 2(b) and (e), demonstrate significantly larger probabilities in the presence of junctions, but can also yield occasional weak responses to the centrelines of larger vessels. The center regions of the junction patterns on the maps appear to be

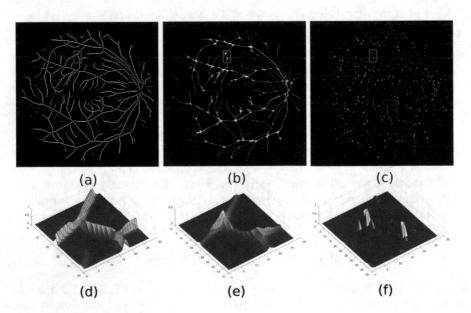

Fig. 2. (a) A centerline probability map generated by the proposed method for the 19th image in the DRIVE test set. (b) Its junction probability map (c) The map is generated after multiplying eigenvalues calculated on the junction probability map in (b). (d)–(f) 3D visualization of regions framed in red in (a)–(c).

blob-like and can be detected by eigen-analysis on Hessian decomposition [5] of junction probability maps. Bright blob-like structures have negative eigenvalues with similar magnitudes; $|\overrightarrow{E_1}| \simeq |\overrightarrow{E_2}|$ [5].

Because the magnitude of junction probabilities can vary depending on the network's recognition ability for these structures, we normalize eigenvalues locally in the range of $[0, 1]$ to make the detection of junction centers more immune to variations on junction probabilities. Simply multiplying normalized eigenvalues for each pixel is observed to generate greater values for junctions than those for vessel centerlines, as demonstrated in Figs. 2(c) and (f). This map is thresholded to locate junctions, but yields some false positives. The following section will describe a method to eliminate these false positives.

2.3 Refined Junction Search

We count branch numbers on our vessel centerline probability maps, demonstrated in Figs. 2(a) and (d), to remove false positives obtained in the initial search. In contrast to previous studies counting intersection numbers in vessel skeletons to identify junction locations [4], we use centerline probability maps to avoid mistakes, which can occur due to further processing of segmented vessel maps. For example, skeletonization may lead to false branches [4].

We locate four circles centered at potential junctions obtained in the previous step, and decide on branch numbers by calculating the most repetitive and largest intersection number over the circles (see Fig. 3). The reason for using multiple circles is to reduce the possibility of detecting false branches in the centerline probability maps.

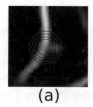
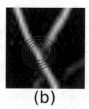

(a)   (b)

Fig. 3. Two examples from refined junction search: a falsely detected location with two branches in (a) is eliminated and the location with three branches in (b) is kept despite having lower centerline probabilities near the junction center.

3 Experimental Setup and Material

Parameter Settings: The proposed network consists of the input layer with 256 units, 5 hidden layers with 400 units in each layer and the output layer with 1024 units. The size of an input image patch and that of a label patch are 16 by 16 pixels.

The initialization of network weights in pretraining was made by sampling from a normal distribution $\mathcal{N}(0, 0.001)$. After training the network for 50 epochs with a learning rate of 0.005, a momentum of 0.5 for the first 5 epochs and that of 0.9 for the rest of pretraining, as recommended in [8], we finetuned the weights for 120 epochs with a learning rate of 0.08.

The parameters for junction detection (initial and refined search) were as follows. Radii of circles were 3 to 6 pixels. Threshold for junction probability map was 0.3 and that for centerline probability maps to calculate branch number was 0.1.

Performance Evaluation: We used precision, recall and F_1 score for performance evaluation, similar to [1,3,14], and accepted junctions estimated in the distance of 5 pixels to actual junctions true. These metrics are calculated with the following definitions over the entire set of junctions in a dataset: $Recall = \frac{TP}{TP+FN}$, $Precision = \frac{TP}{TP+FP}$ and $F_1 score = \frac{2 \cdot Recall \cdot Precision}{Recall+Precision}$, where TP, FN and FP respectively denote the number of correctly labeled junctions, that of missed junctions and that of mistakenly labeled junctions.

Material: We evaluated the performance of our method on two fundus image datasets, which are captured by different image modalities. The DRIVE [13] is the most popular dataset for the evaluation of retinal vessel segmentation methods, which contains 40 images with a resolution of 768×584 pixels, acquired with a nonmydriatic CCD camera. The IOSTAR [1] consists of 24 scanning laser ophthalmoscope (SLO) images. Both datasets have ground truth vessel maps and junction locations [1][1], and are publicly available. The number of junctions per image, including both bifurcations and crossings, is roughly 130 for the DRIVE and 78 for IOSTAR.

Training Data Preparation: We obtained ground truth labels for, respectively, vessel centerline and edges by applying a simple thinning and edge detection method to ground truth vessel maps. Later, we generated junction pattern labels by using ground truth centerline maps: we firstly located masks of 5×5 pixels centered at ground truth junction locations then removed centerline labels outside these masks. The training dataset contains the last 20 images in the DRIVE and test set includes the first 20 images, which are separated by authors in [13]. We prepared 18,000 mini-batches, each contains 100 training samples. Because the network was only trained with the DRIVE dataset, there was no need for preparing a training set for IOSTAR.

---

[1] The ground truth data is available at http://retinacheck.org/datasets.

4   Results

We evaluated the performance of the proposed method on the DRIVE test set and the complete set of IOSTAR. Similar to Pratt *et al.*'s training [10], we trained our network with only the DRIVE training set. The reason for this is that the number of ground truth junctions per image in IOSTAR is almost half that given for the DRIVE dataset. We also assessed the performance of our method on ground truth vessel maps, to make a fair performance comparison with previous methods that utilize these maps. Table 1 presents our findings and compares them with those of previously reported methods.

Table 1. The performance comparison for junction detection.

		Input image type	DRIVE			IOSTAR		
			Precision	Recall	F_1 score	Precision	Recall	F_1 score
Our method	Initial search*	Ground truth vessel maps	0.25	0.84	0.38	0.26	0.88	0.40
	Refined search*	Ground truth vessel maps	0.63	**0.77**	**0.69**	**0.74**	**0.82**	**0.78**
	Initial search	Fundus images	0.29	0.85	0.43	0.17	0.87	0.29
	Refined search	Fundus images	0.65	0.69	0.67	0.52	0.67	0.59
	Pratt *et al.* [10]**	Ground truth vessel maps	0.74	0.57	0.64	0.52	0.54	0.53
	BICROS [1]	Fundus images & Vessel maps segmented with [11]	**0.75**	0.61	0.67	0.47	0.60	0.52
		Fundus images & Vessel maps segmented with [2]	**0.75**	0.61	0.66	0.67	0.57	0.61

*Junctions labeled by [1] but not corresponding to any junctions in the ground truth vessel maps of the DRIVE were ignored during the performance evaluation. No refinement were performed for the junction labels in IOSTAR.
**The result for the DRIVE belongs to the experiment where the network was trained on GRADE 1 and tested on $G1A2$ [1].

According to the table, recall rates at the initial search for both datasets are over 0.84 regardless of image type (e.g. ground truth or fundus image), which indicates that junction probability maps have a high potential for the detection of almost 90% of junctions in the ground truth data. However, precision at this stage is low because of the large number of false positives generated with the eigen-analysis. The refined search eliminates many of these false positives, with precision values increasing from 0.26 up to 0.74 (in the IOSTAR dataset) when ground truth images are input, and from 0.29 up to 0.65 (in the DRIVE dataset) when fundus images are input. Due to the elimination of some true positives at this stage, recall rates can drop for both image types; however, this is observed to be less recognizable when ground truth images are input.

Considering input image types, the performance of the network is found to be better at ground truth images, particularly for IOSTAR with a 0.19 increase on F_1 score for fundus images. However, we did not observe significant performance difference between the DRIVE and IOSTAR cases, which indicates the generalization ability of our method for unseen datasets even if they are captured by different imaging modalities.

Regarding the usage of a deep network, the most relevant study to ours is Pratt *et al.*'s [10], where a deep network was trained with vessel skeletons produced from ground truth vessel maps as a classifier to identify image patches carrying any types of junctions; then, local maxima in selected patches were labelled as junction locations. Although their tolerance distance to actual junctions, 10 pixels, is two times larger than ours, our recall and F_1 score on the DRIVE and all the three metrics on IOSTAR are significantly larger than their findings. Moreover, the performance we obtained on fundus images for the same metrics, particularly for recall, was found to be still better than their performance on both datasets.

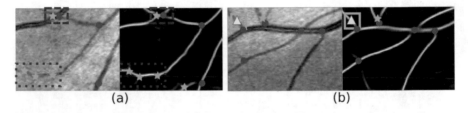

Fig. 4. Example results from our junction detection on a fundus image in the DRIVE, where each image pair contains a fundus image patch and its centerline probability map from left to right. Pink discs, green stars and yellow rectangles respectively show correctly detected, mistakenly detected and missing junctions. See the text for an explanation of the red dashed line, blue dotted line and green solid line rectangles.

BICROS [1] combined two approaches: one relying on orientation scores obtained from fundus images and the other finding branches on skeletons generated from segmented vessel maps. Because of using different segmentation methods, their performance varies depending on suitability of segmentation methods to imaging modality [1]. However, the approach we propose yielded better recall rates than theirs, regardless of imaging modalities and input image types.

Precision rates reported by Pratt *et al.* [10] and obtained with BICROS [1] appear to be larger, particularly for the DRIVE, than ours. However, it should be noted that our method is not designed to differentiate crossings from bifurcations, and errors can occur if crossing vessels have large width [4]. This situation can be observed inside the red dashed line rectangle in Fig. 4(a), where a crossing is represented with two joints. Also, some unlabeled junctions in ground truth data can reduce precision. False positives inside the blue dotted line rectangle in Fig. 4(a) seem to be good candidates for junctions. On the other hand, our method can fail to detect a few junctions if they are not represented with sufficient probabilities in centerline probability maps. The green solid line square in Fig. 4(b) shows a junction missed by our method; but it is not easily seen by the naked eye.

5   Conclusion

Although deep networks have recently become the method of choice for medical image segmentation, their application is limited to those with large amounts of labeled data for the desired task. In order to deal with the scarcity of labeled data for junction detection in fundus images as a prior step to bifurcation and crossing classification, we propose a multi-task deep network. This network can produce probability maps of vessel interior, centerline, edges and junctions. Because of learning various descriptions of retinal vasculature, the network was found to confidently indicate junction locations. Potential junction locations suggested by the junction probability maps were reassessed by simply counting branch numbers on centerline probability maps.

We evaluated the performance of our network on the DRIVE test set and IOSTAR after training the network with the DRIVE training set once. We found that the proposed approach outperformed previous approaches for the junction detection task. Moreover, the performance of the proposed approach appeared to be better than that of a similar method due to Pratt *et al.* [10], which used a popular deep network to identify junctions. Our findings suggest that the proposed method can be used for unseen retinal datasets, even if they have slightly different characteristics, without retraining the network.

References

1. Abbasi-Sureshjani, S., Smit-Ockeloen, I., Bekkers, E., Dashtbozorg, B., ter Haar Romeny, B.: Automatic detection of vascular bifurcations and crossings in retinal images using orientation scores. In: The IEEE International Symposium on Biomedical Imaging (ISBI), pp. 189–192. IEEE (2016)
2. Abbasi-Sureshjani, S., Smit-Ockeloen, I., Zhang, J., Ter Haar Romeny, B.: Biologically-inspired supervised vasculature segmentation in SLO retinal fundus images. In: Kamel, M., Campilho, A. (eds.) ICIAR 2015. LNCS, vol. 9164, pp. 325–334. Springer, Cham (2015). https://doi.org/10.1007/978-3-319-20801-5_35
3. Azzopardi, G., Petkov, N.: Automatic detection of vascular bifurcations in segmented retinal images using trainable COSFIRE filters. Pattern Recogn. Lett. **34**(8), 922–933 (2013)
4. Calvo, D., Ortega, M., Penedo, M.G., Rouco, J.: Automatic detection and characterisation of retinal vessel tree bifurcations and crossovers in eye fundus images. Comput. Methods Programs Biomed. **103**(1), 28–38 (2011)

5. Frangi, A.F., Niessen, W.J., Vincken, K.L., Viergever, M.A.: Multiscale vessel enhancement filtering. In: Wells, W.M., Colchester, A., Delp, S. (eds.) MICCAI 1998. LNCS, vol. 1496, pp. 130–137. Springer, Heidelberg (1998). https://doi.org/10.1007/BFb0056195

6. Hamad, H., Tegolo, D., Valenti, C.: Automatic detection and classification of retinal vascular landmarks. Image Anal. Stereol. **33**(3), 189–200 (2014)

7. He, K., Zhang, X., Ren, S., Sun, J.: Deep residual learning for image recognition. In: The IEEE Conference on Computer Vision and Pattern Recognition, pp. 770–778 (2016)

8. Hinton, G.E.: A practical guide to training restricted Boltzmann machines. In: Montavon, G., Orr, G.B., Müller, K.-R. (eds.) Neural Networks: Tricks of the Trade. LNCS, vol. 7700, pp. 599–619. Springer, Heidelberg (2012). https://doi.org/10.1007/978-3-642-35289-8_32

9. Li, Q., Feng, B., Xie, L., Liang, P., Zhang, H., Wang, T.: A cross-modality learning approach for vessel segmentation in retinal images. IEEE Trans. Med. Imaging **35**(1), 109–118 (2016)

10. Pratt, H., et al.: Automatic detection and distinction of retinal vessel bifurcations and crossings in colour fundus photography. J. Imaging **4**(1), 4 (2017)

11. Soares, J.V., Leandro, J.J., Cesar, R.M., Jelinek, H.F., Cree, M.J.: Retinal vessel segmentation using the 2-D Gabor wavelet and supervised classification. IEEE Trans. Med. Imaging **25**(9), 1214–1222 (2006)

12. Srinidhi, C.L., Aparna, P., Rajan, J.: Recent advancements in retinal vessel segmentation. J. Med. Syst. **41**(4), 70 (2017)

13. Staal, J., Abràmoff, M.D., Niemeijer, M., Viergever, M.A., Van Ginneken, B.: Ridge-based vessel segmentation in color images of the retina. IEEE Trans. Med. Imaging **23**(4), 501–509 (2004)

14. Zhang, H., Yang, Y., Shen, H.: Line junction detection without prior-delineation of curvilinear structure in biomedical images. IEEE Access **6**, 2016–2027 (2018)

A Multitask Learning Architecture for Simultaneous Segmentation of Bright and Red Lesions in Fundus Images

Clément Playout[1(✉)], Renaud Duval[2], and Farida Cheriet[1]

[1] LIV4D, École Polytechnique de Montréal, Montreal, Canada
`clement.playout@polymtl.ca`
[2] CUO-Hôpital Maisonneuve Rosemont, Montreal, Canada

Abstract. Recent CNN architectures have established state-of-the-art results in a large range of medical imaging applications. We propose an extension to the U-Net architecture relying on multi-task learning: while keeping a single encoding module, multiple decoding modules are used for concurrent segmentation tasks. We propose improvements of the encoding module based on the latest CNN developments: residual connections at every scale, mixed pooling for spatial compression and large kernels for convolutions at the lowest scale. We also use dense connections within the different scales based on multi-size pooling regions. We use this new architecture to jointly detect and segment red and bright retinal lesions which are essential biomarkers of diabetic retinopathy. Each of the two categories is handled by a specialized decoding module. Segmentation outputs are refined with conditional random fields (CRF) as RNN and the network is trained end-to-end with an effective Kappa-based function loss. Preliminary results on a public dataset in the segmentation task on red (resp. bright) lesions shows a sensitivity of 66,9% (resp. 75,3%) and a specificity of 99,8% (resp. 99,9%).

1 Introduction

Diabetic retinopathy (DR) is a potential consequence of diabetes, affecting nearly 34% of the diabetic population. The disease progresses through stages characterized mainly by the lesions observed in the retina. In 2D fundus, those lesions can be regrouped in two categories according to their appearance: bright (such as exudates and cotton wool spots) and red (such as hemorrhages and microaneurysms). Most of the literature on DR lesion segmentation proposes three main stages: candidates detection, candidates classification and refinement of the segmentation. This approach is used for example for red lesion detection in [1] using handcrafted features. Deep learning has been used in [2] for hemorrhage detection. For bright lesions, detection and segmentation usually rely on unsupervised methods, as in [3]. Nonetheless, clinical assessment requires detection of all types of lesions. This hypothesis stems from the empirical observation of the labeling process done by medical experts on fundus images. Each salient region

© Springer Nature Switzerland AG 2018
A. F. Frangi et al. (Eds.): MICCAI 2018, LNCS 11071, pp. 101–108, 2018.
https://doi.org/10.1007/978-3-030-00934-2_12

is classified according to its specific content but also to the context of the entire image (like the presence of other lesions). An automatic decision system can learn implicitly the DR grading by using a model as a black box. However, to reproduce the protocol used by the grader the decision should rely on an explicit full detection of lesions. Meanwhile, the capacity of CNNs to segment medical images obtained from multiple modalities through multitasking has been demonstrated in [4]. Even for a single modality, multitasking is well suited for jointly segmenting different types of lesions. This approach provides several advantages, especially shorter inference times and the ability to train a single architecture to independently perform multiple highly specialized tasks that share a common basis.

To our knowledge, there are no methods based on fully convolutional approaches used for joint lesions segmentations. To address this gap, this paper focuses on segmenting bright and red lesions with a single deep multitask architecture, without the need of blood vessels nor optic disc removal. We propose a novel network based on recent developments of CNNs, like Residual Connections, Global Convolution and Mixed-pooling. We also introduce Dense Pooling Connections, a new type of connection that is designed to reinforce the robustness to noise by aggregating maximum activations within multiple regions. We prove a performance improvement in comparison with existing architecture.

2 Methods

Overview. We train a novel CNN architecture with patches randomly extracted from normalized images. The architecture extends the U-Net [5] with multi-task learning. Improvement of the descending part (the encoder) of U-Net is proposed as well as a new training strategy. The features from the encoder are shared by two decoders respectively specialized respectively in bright and red lesions segmentation.

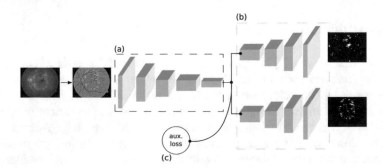

Fig. 1. The network is fed patches from the normalized images. (a) The *encoding module* uses a generic set of parameters shared by the two tasks. (b) The *decoding modules* are task-specific. An auxiliary cost (c) is added at the end of the encoding module; it is trained only to predict the presence of lesions.

2.1 Multitask Architecture

Multitask learning was introduced in [6] as a way to improve generalization. Part of the model is shared across independent tasks, while each task has its specifics parameters. Figure 1 shows our global architecture and Fig. 2 describes the encoding module in detail. The intuition behind multi-task learning in our case is that information needed for bright and red lesions segmentation is common to both tasks (for example, anatomical features of the retina).

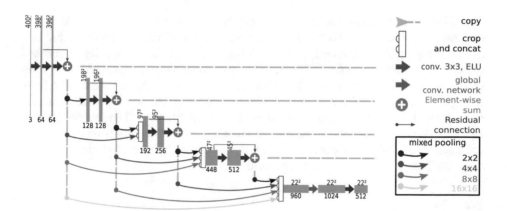

Fig. 2. Decoding module used with residual connections at every level, dense pooling connections and global convolutional network.

Mixed Pooling: Each max-pooling is replaced by mixed-pooling layer [7]. For an input tensor x composed of N channels and a vector a (trainable parameter), the mixed-pooling layer computes:

$$f_{mix}(x_n) = a_n \cdot f_{max}(x_n) + (1 - a_n) \cdot f_{avg}(x_n) \text{ with } n \in \{1, ..., N\} \quad (1)$$

We use one scalar ($a_n \in [0, 1]$) per layer/channel, for an efficient combination without drastically increasing the number of parameters of the model (N additional parameters per pooling layer).

Residual Connection: At each resolution level, the two 3×3 convolutions of the original U-Net are extended to become residual blocks as introduced in [8]. The motivation is to prevent the degradation problem observed in large models by allowing the blocks to possibly become identity mappings.

Dense Pooling Connections: We introduce dense pooling connections through multiple resolution levels. Each level is connected to those beneath it. Pooling operations with various pooling sizes guarantee spatial resolution consistency. We make the hypothesis that pooling operations over successively larger regions reinforce scale and translation invariance while reducing sensitivity to noise as more and more context is added. At the lowest level, for a given field of view, every previous levels transmit a combination of its maximal and average activation. The aggregation of those data should facilitate discrimination between relevant features and local noise.

Global Convolutional Network: At the lowest scale of the network, we use convolutions with large kernels following the implementation recently proposed in [9]. This further aggregates the contextual information.

Task Specific Decoders. The decoding modules used are the same as in the original U-Net design. We use two decoding modules, each specialized for one lesion category. Near the end of the training, we also added two fully connected Conditional Random Fields (CRFs). CRFs were originally introduced by [10]. We use the softmax output of each decoding module as the unary potential. The pairwise potential consists in a weighted sum of two Gaussian kernels that "control" the appearance and the smoothness of the segmentation. The parameters of the kernels are trained with the rest of the network, according to the proposed method in [11] which implements the CRF as an additional RNN layer on top of a traditional convolutional architecture.

2.2   Training

Each task is associated with its specific cost function. We also use an auxiliary cost trained to detect whether a lesion is present or not in the patch. This helps the encoding module to focus on distinguishing between an actual lesion and other biomarkers. During training, the objective function C_{global} is the weighted sum of each cost:

$$C_{global} = \lambda_{bright} \cdot C_{bright} + \lambda_{red} \cdot C_{red} + \lambda_{aux} \cdot C_{aux} \qquad (2)$$

Training is performed in three stages. In the first stage, the network is trained with a log-likelihood based cost $(\mathcal{L}(\theta \mid x) = -\frac{1}{D} \sum_i^D \log P(Y = y^{(i)} | x^{(i)}, \theta))$.

In the second stage, we change the objective function to a Kappa-based one. Cohen's Kappa (κ) coefficient measures the agreement between two raters. As it takes into account the possibility of agreement occurring by chance, this coefficient is well suited for distinguishing highly unbalanced classes as in our case. The core idea of the κ coefficient is to quantify the difference between the accuracy ρ_{acc} and the probability of pure chance agreement ρ_{chance}:

$$\kappa = \frac{\rho_{acc} - \rho_{chance}}{1 - \rho_{chance}} \qquad (3)$$

As the accuracy is not a differentiable measure, we use soft approximation to model it. The output of the softmax, y_{proba}, approximates the predicted label, y_{pred}, which is valid for high-confidence predictions as y_{proba} tends to y_{pred} encoded in a one-hot vector. This is why we initially train the network with the likelihood $\mathcal{L}$, in order to obtain this high level of confidence.

Table 1. Training stages

Stage	C_{aux}	C_{red}	C_{bright}	λ_{bright}	λ_{red}	λ_{aux}	CRF	Epochs	Encoder trained
I	$\mathcal{L}$	$\mathcal{L}$	$\mathcal{L}$	0.5	0.5	0.1	No	10	Yes
II	$\mathcal{L}$	κ	κ	0.5	0.5	0.1	No	90	Yes
III	–	κ	κ	1.0	1.0	–	Yes	20	No

The third training stage adds the CRFs after the two decoders. The auxiliary cost is discarded and only the weights of the two decoding modules are updated. Table 1 summarizes the parameters for the training stages.

As an optimizer, we use the Adadelta algorithm introduced in [12]. The weights update policy is:

$$\Delta x_t = -\nu \frac{\sqrt{E[\Delta x^2]_{t-1} + \epsilon}}{\sqrt{E[g^2]_t + \epsilon}} g_t \qquad (4)$$

Where $E[\Delta x^2]$ and $E[g^2]$ are the running averages characterized by a parameter γ. We use $\gamma = 0.95$ (a high value counter-balances the noise introduced by small batch sizes). As Adadelta is designed to remove the need of an explicit learning rate, in the original paper [12] ν is fixed and equal to 1. Nonetheless, as it was also originally suggested, we found that dividing ν by 10 every 20 epochs drastically helps the convergence, as shown in Fig. 3.

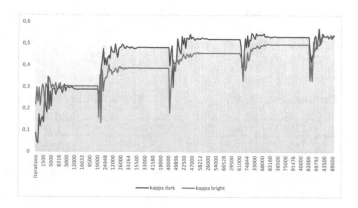

Fig. 3. Evolution of the κ metric on the validation set. The jump observed every 20000 iterations corresponds to the decrease of ν (One epoch $\sim$ 1000 iterations)

3 Experiments

We mainly used the publicly available DIARETDB1 database [13], which provides 89 fundus images from DR patients. As this database was designed for lesion detection rather than segmentation, we refined the lesions boundaries manually, and an ophthalmologist validated them. 61 images were used for test and validation (8 images from the recommended test set were randomly selected for the validation set). The training set was composed of 28 images from DIARETDB1, supplemented by 17 images with lesions from a private database and 18 healthy images extracted from the e-ophtha database [14], giving a total of 63 training images. A simple preprocessing step was applied to normalize the illumination and we increased the dataset using data augmentation. We applied geometrical (translation, rotation, shearing and elastic distortion) and color (brightness, contrast, gamma, HSV saturation/value) transformations to the input images. For each image, a random combination of those operations was applied. The parameters of each transformation were also randomly sampled at each epoch. We thereby ensured that the network never saw the exact same patch twice. The network was fed patches of size 400 × 400. Between 8 and 10 patches were randomly extracted per image, with a prior distribution to favor patches centered on a lesion. We used a weights decay rate of 0.0005 and a batch size of 2.

4   Results and Discussion

We tested our model by comparing it with the original U-Net architecture (one decoder, three classes), and with another model similar to the U-Net but with two decoding modules. We refer to these latter networks as U-Net and U-Net2; we trained them with the same strategy as our proposed network. Sensitivity and specificity were measured pixel-wise and averaged over the test set. Tables 2 and 3 provide the segmentation performance results. The quality of the segmentation was also evaluated in a patch-wise manner, as this corresponds to what the network actually "sees". Patches were of size 400 × 400. We averaged the κ and

Table 2. Pixel-wise sensitivity

Model	Red (%)	Bright (%)
Our model	66,91	**75,35**
Our model (no CRF)	**68.58**	71.98
U-Net2	67.97	71.12
U-Net	–	58.47

Table 3. Pixel-wise specificity

Model	Red (%)	Bright (%)
Our model	99.82	99.86
Our model (no CRF)	99.83	**99.92**
U-Net2	**99.91**	98.99
U-Net	–	99.87

Table 4. κ coefficient measured on a patch-based level.

Model	Red (%)	Bright (%)
Our model	45.71	68,86
Our model (no CRF)	**51.97**	**77.56**
U-Net2	24.26	73.26
U-Net	–	54,77

Table 5. Dice coefficient measured on a patch-based level.

Model	Red (%)	Bright (%)
Our model	59.80	78.97
Our model (no CRF)	**65.63**	**82.99**
U-Net2	37.46	79.77
U-Net	–	82.63

the Dice coefficient s, measured per patch, to get averages per image κ_{image} and s_{image}. To get global values, we then averaged each κ_{image} and s_{image} over the entire test set (see Tables 4 and 5).

The results are encouraging with regard to the proposed network's segmentation performance in comparison with both U-Net and U-Net2. The U-Net gave satisfactory results in bright lesions segmentation but was completely unable to predict red lesions. This gives strong support in favor of multitasking, as specialized branches appear to be able to capture features that a single branch cannot (at least for the same number of training epochs). Nonetheless, we also observe that our results tend to globally worsen with the CRFs. Visual inspection shows that the CRFs tend to add tiny false positive red lesions, near the vessels. In addition, the CRFs are well suited for hard exudates but tend to miss the boundaries of soft ones. The inference time was approximately 1 s per image, running on NVIDIA GTX 1070 Ti hardware. Obtaining a fast and complete segmentation of the image constitutes an important first step toward our ultimate goal of constituting an extensive, fully labelled fundus image database. This process will be greatly accelerated using our model. We also plan to assess the capacity of grading DR using features obtained directly from the encoding module and output segmentation results. Indeed, the inferior results of the basic U-Net as compared to the multi-task networks suggests that in those, encoded features are highly representative of the abnormalities observed in the images.

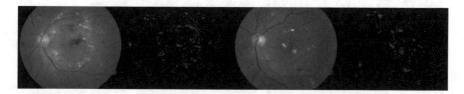

Fig. 4. Some results showing good performance overall but with over-segmentation of red lesions (false positives). One source of errors (observable in the first image) comes from laser coagulation marks, similar to small hemorrhages.

5   Conclusion

We have proposed a novel CNN architecture to jointly segment bright and red lesions in fundus images. We have highlighted the value of a multitask learning approach, as opposed to single task classification. The present work opens the door to many possibilities, from clinical assistance (computer-assisted lesion identification) to DR grading methods that do not rely on a "black-box" approach.

References

1. Seoud, L., Hurtut, T., Chelbi, J., Cheriet, F., Langlois, J.M.P.: Red lesion detection using dynamic shape features for diabetic retinopathy screening. IEEE Trans. Med. Imaging **35**(4), 1116–1126 (2016)
2. van Grinsven, M.J.J.P., van Ginneken, B., Hoyng, C.B., Theelen, T., Sánchez, C.I.: Fast convolutional neural network training using selective data sampling: application to hemorrhage detection in color fundus images. IEEE Trans. Med. Imaging **35**(5), 1273–1284 (2016)
3. Vanithamani, R., Renee Christina, R.: Exudates in detection and classification of diabetic retinopathy. In: Abraham, A., Cherukuri, A.K., Madureira, A.M., Muda, A.K. (eds.) SoCPaR 2016. AISC, vol. 614, pp. 252–261. Springer, Cham (2018). https://doi.org/10.1007/978-3-319-60618-7_25
4. Moeskops, P., et al.: Deep learning for multi-task medical image segmentation in multiple modalities. In: Ourselin, S., Joskowicz, L., Sabuncu, M.R., Unal, G., Wells, W. (eds.) MICCAI 2016. LNCS, vol. 9901, pp. 478–486. Springer, Cham (2016). https://doi.org/10.1007/978-3-319-46723-8_55
5. Ronneberger, O., Fischer, P., Brox, T.: U-Net: convolutional networks for biomedical image segmentation. In: Navab, N., Hornegger, J., Wells, W.M., Frangi, A.F. (eds.) MICCAI 2015. LNCS, vol. 9351, pp. 234–241. Springer, Cham (2015). https://doi.org/10.1007/978-3-319-24574-4_28
6. Caruana, R.: Multitask learning. Mach. Learn. **28**(1), 41–75 (1997)
7. Yu, D., Wang, H., Chen, P., Wei, Z.: Mixed pooling for convolutional neural networks. In: Miao, D., Pedrycz, W., Ślęzak, D., Peters, G., Hu, Q., Wang, R. (eds.) RSKT 2014. LNCS (LNAI), vol. 8818, pp. 364–375. Springer, Cham (2014). https://doi.org/10.1007/978-3-319-11740-9_34
8. He, K., Zhang, X., Ren, S., Sun, J.: Deep residual learning for image recognition. In: 2016 IEEE Conference on Computer Vision and Pattern Recognition (CVPR), pp. 770–778, June 2016
9. Peng, C., Zhang, X., Yu, G., Luo, G., Sun, J.: Large kernel matters - improve semantic segmentation by global convolutional network. CoRR abs/1703.02719 (2017)
10. Krähenbühl, P., Koltun, V.: Efficient inference in fully connected CRFs with Gaussian edge potentials. CoRR abs/1210.5644 (2012)
11. Zheng, S., et al.: Conditional random fields as recurrent neural networks. In: 2015 IEEE International Conference on Computer Vision (ICCV), pp. 1529–1537, December 2015
12. Zeiler, M.D.: ADADELTA: an adaptive learning rate method. CoRR abs/1212.5701 (2012)
13. Kauppi, T., et al.: DIARETDB1 diabetic retinopathy database and evaluation protocol (01 2007)
14. Decencière, E., et al.: TeleOphta: machine learning and image processing methods for teleophthalmology. IRBM **34**(2), 196–203 (2013). Special issue: ANR TECSAN: Technologies for Health and Autonomy

Uniqueness-Driven Saliency Analysis for Automated Lesion Detection with Applications to Retinal Diseases

Yitian Zhao[1]([✉]), Yalin Zheng[2], Yifan Zhao[3], Yonghuai Liu[4], Zhili Chen[5], Peng Liu[1], and Jiang Liu[1]

[1] Cixi Institute of Biomedical Engineering, Ningbo Institute of Industrial Technology, Chinese Academy of Sciences, Cixi, China
yitian.zhao@nimte.ac.cn
[2] Department of Eye and Vision Science, Liverpool University, Liverpool, England
[3] School of Aerospace, Transport and Manufacturing, Cranfield University, Cranfield, England
[4] Department of Computer Science, Aberystwyth University, Aberystwyth, Wales
[5] School of Information and Control Engineering, Shenyang Jianzhu University, Shenyang, China

Abstract. Saliency is important in medical image analysis in terms of detection and segmentation tasks. We propose a new method to extract uniqueness-driven saliency based on the uniqueness of intensity and spatial distributions within the images. The main novelty of this new saliency feature is that it is powerful in the detection of different types of lesions in different types of images without the need of tuning parameters for different problems. To evaluate its effectiveness, we have applied our method to the detection lesions of retinal images. Four different types of lesions: exudate, hemorrhage, microaneurysms and leakage from 7 independent public retinal image datasets of diabetic retinopathy and malarial retinopathy, were studied and the experimental results show that the proposed method is superior to the state-of-the-art methods.

Keywords: Saliency · Uniqueness · Computer aided-diagnosis Retinopathy

1 Introduction

The accurate identification of suspicious regions such as lesions in medical images is significant in the development of computer aided-diagnosis systems. Many different strategies have been developed towards automated detection of lesions in addressing different problems. However, these strategies often work on single type of lesions with careful parameter optimization and are unlikely to work for other types of lesions without problem specific optimization. It is therefore essential to develop generic algorithms that can have accurate and reliable performance in the detection of multiple lesions without handcrafted parameters.

© Springer Nature Switzerland AG 2018
A. F. Frangi et al. (Eds.): MICCAI 2018, LNCS 11071, pp. 109–118, 2018.
https://doi.org/10.1007/978-3-030-00934-2_13

In this work, we propose a new uniqueness-driven saliency approach for the detection of different types of lesions. The concept of saliency is that an object stands out relative to its neighbors by virtue of its uniqueness or rarity features [1,2]. Saliency plays an important role in describing the tendency of those regions that may contain consequential matters for diagnostic purposes to draw the attention of human experts [3]. To evaluate its effectiveness, we aim to segment four different types of retinal lesions related to diabetic and malarial retinopathy: exudates (EX), microaneurysms (MA), and hemorrhages (HA) in retinal color fundus (CF) images [4], and leakage (LK) in fluorescein angiogram (FA) [3]. MA and HM are referred to as dark lesion while EX and LK as bright lesion.

Diabetic retinopathy (DR) is a leading cause of vision impairment and loss in the working age population, and early diagnosis of DR is important for the prevention of vision loss [4]. The severity of DR is usually determined based on feature-based grading by identifying features such as MA, HA and EX in color fundus images, and thus automated detection of these features is essential in the automated diagnosis of DR [5,6]. On the other hand, malarial retinopathy is believed as the surrogate for the differential diagnosis of cerebral malaria, which is still a major cause of death and disability in children in sub-Saharan Africa [3], and LK in angiography is an important sign to determine the activities and development of lesions. Manual grading of these lesions is impractical given the scale of the problem and the shortage of trained professionals. Automated detection of these lesions is ideal to the early diagnosis and prevention of these challenges in a cost-effective way. However, the challenges are still open to be addressed [7].

A particular strength of the proposed method compared to previous work is that it has undergone rigorous quantitative evaluation on seven independent publicly available datasets including CF and FA images. The experimental results demonstrate its effectiveness and potential for wider medical applications.

2   Method

This work was inspired by the findings of Perazzi et al. [8] that the *uniqueness* of a component may be used to reveal the rarity of an image component. The relative intensity or spatial distribution of intensity are commonly used properties to investigate saliency [1,8]. In particular, Cheng et al. [1] suggest that the spatial variance of color can measure whether an element is salient: a lower variance usually implies more salient.

Saliency at Coarse Scale: In order to reduce the computational cost, saliency is first derived from superpixels of an image under consideration by using the SLIC superpixel algorithm with default parameter settings [9]. Without loss of generality, we assume that N superpixels are generated, the color of any superpixel i and j, $1 \leq i, j \leq N$, are c_i, c_j while their positions are p_i and p_j. The uniqueness saliency U_i of superpixel i is then defined by combining the uniqueness in both the intensity and the spatial distribution domains:

$$\mathbf{U}_i = \mathcal{I}_i \cdot \exp(-k \cdot \mathcal{D}_i), \tag{1}$$

where $\mathcal{I}_i$ and $\mathcal{D}_i$ indicates the uniqueness of superpixel i in the intensity and spatial distribution domain respectively. Here an exponential function is employed to emphasize $\mathcal{D}_i$ that is of higher significance and greater diagnostic capability than the intensity measurement $\mathcal{I}_i$ [8]. The parameter k represents the strength of the spatial weighting, and is set as 6 and -6 for dark and bright lesion detection, respectively. The uniqueness in the intensity domain I_i of superpixel i can be obtained by computing the rarity compared to all the other superpixels j:

$$\mathcal{I}_i = \sum_{j=1}^{N} \|\mathbf{c}_i - \mathbf{c}_j\|^2 \cdot w^I(\mathbf{p}_i, \mathbf{p}_j). \tag{2}$$

The local weighting function $w^I(\mathbf{p}_i, \mathbf{p}_j)$ is introduced here so that global and local contrast can be effectively combined with control over the influence radius. A standard Gaussian function is utilized to generate the local contrast in terms of geometric distances between superpixel i and j: $w^I(\mathbf{p}_i, \mathbf{p}_j) = \frac{1}{\mathbf{Z}_i^I} \exp\{-\frac{\|\mathbf{p}_i - \mathbf{p}_j\|^2}{2\sigma_p^2}\}$, where standard deviation $\sigma_{\mathbf{p}}$ controls the range of the uniqueness operator from 0 to 1 (where 1 = global uniqueness). The normalization term $\mathbf{Z}_i^I$ ensure that $\sum_{j=1}^{N} w^I(\mathbf{p}_i, \mathbf{p}_j) = 1$. Equation (1) is decomposed by factoring out:

$$\mathcal{I}_i = \mathbf{c}_i^2 \underbrace{\sum_{i=1}^{N} w^I(\mathbf{p}_i, \mathbf{p}_j)}_{1} - 2\mathbf{c}_i \underbrace{\sum_{j-1}^{N} \mathbf{c}_j w^I(\mathbf{p}_i, \mathbf{p}_j)}_{\text{Gaussian blur } \mathbf{c}_j} + \underbrace{\sum_{j=1}^{N} \mathbf{c}_j^2 w^I(\mathbf{p}_i, \mathbf{p}_j)}_{\text{Gaussian blur } \mathbf{c}_j^2}. \tag{3}$$

It can be seen that $\sum_{j=1}^{N} \mathbf{c}_j w^I(\mathbf{p}_i, \mathbf{p}_j)$ of second and third term can be regarded as the Gaussian blurring kernel on intensity $\mathbf{c}_j$ and its square $\mathbf{c}_j^2$, respectively. Similarly, the uniqueness of spatial distribution $\mathcal{D}_i$ can be computed as:

$$\mathcal{D}_i = \sum_{j=1}^{N} \|\mathbf{p}_j - \mu_i\|^2 \cdot w^D(\mathbf{c}_i, \mathbf{c}_j), \tag{4}$$

where $\mu_i = \sum_{j=1}^{N} \mathbf{p}_j w^D(\mathbf{c}_i, \mathbf{c}_j)$ defines the weighted mean position of color $\mathbf{c}_i$, $w^D(\mathbf{c}_i, \mathbf{c}_j)$ indicates the similarity between color $\mathbf{c}_i$ and $\mathbf{c}_j$. Similar to Eq. (2), the color similarity weight is also a Gaussian $w^D(\mathbf{c}_i, \mathbf{c}_j) = \frac{1}{\mathbf{Z}_i^D} \exp\{-\frac{\|\mathbf{c}_i - \mathbf{c}_j\|^2}{2\sigma_c^2}\}$, where

$\mathbf{Z}_i^D$ can be defined similar to $\mathbf{Z}_i^I$ while σ_c controls the sensitivity of the spatial distribution: larger values of σ_c indicate increased values of spatial distribution, and vice versa. Equation (4) can be expanded as:

$$\mathcal{D}_i = \sum_{j=1}^{N} \mathbf{p}_j^2 w^D(\mathbf{c}_i, \mathbf{c}_j) - 2\mu_i \underbrace{\sum_{j=1}^{N} \mathbf{p}_j w^D(\mathbf{c}_i, \mathbf{c}_j)}_{\mu_i} + \mu_i{}^2 \underbrace{\sum_{j=1}^{N} w^D(\mathbf{c}_i, \mathbf{c}_j)}_{1}$$

$$= \underbrace{\sum_{j=1}^{N} \mathbf{p}_j^2 w^D(\mathbf{c}_i, \mathbf{c}_j)}_{\text{Gaussian blur } \mathbf{p}_j^2} - \underbrace{\mu_i^2}_{\text{blur } \mathbf{p}_j} . \tag{5}$$

Again, both terms $\sum_{j=1}^{N} \mathbf{p}_j w^D(\mathbf{c}_i, \mathbf{c}_j)$ and μ_i^2 can be effectively evaluated by Gaussian blurring. After determining $\mathcal{I}_i$ and $\mathcal{D}_i$, the uniqueness-based saliency $\mathcal{U}_i$ can be calculated by using Eq. (1).

Saliency at Fine Scale: After coarse level estimation, the saliency at each pixel is temporarily assigned the saliency value of the superpixel it belongs to. Further refinement is made by introducing the concept of bilateral filter. That is, $S_u = \sum_{v=1}^{M} w_{uv} \mathbf{U}_v$, where M is the total number of pixels in the image, $\mathbf{U}$ is the saliency map at coarse scale, and the Gaussian weight w_{uv} is defined as $w_{uv} = \frac{1}{Z_u} \exp(-\frac{1}{2}\alpha \|\mathbf{c}_u - \mathbf{c}_v\|^2 + \beta \|\mathbf{p}_u - \mathbf{p}_v\|^2)$, where Z_u can be defined similar to Z_i^D. In other words, a weighted Gaussian filter which concerns both color and position is applied on the saliency map $\mathbf{U}$ at coarse scale, in order to achieve the translation of per-superpixel saliency to per-pixel saliency. The trade-off between intensity and position is controlled by α and β, which in the present work were both set to 0.01. The result is that, the final saliency map highlights salient object regions of interest by suppressing the background of the image.

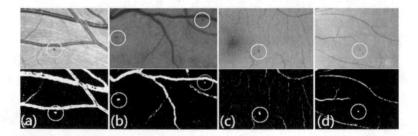

Fig. 1. Illustrative **microaneurysm** detection result on example images from four datasets: (a) RC-RGB-MA; (b) DiaretDB1; (c) ROC; (d) e-ophtha. The yellow circles indicate the location of MAs.

Table 1. Microaneurysms detection result: sensitivities of different methods at the predefined rates of false positives per image in four different datasets.

Dataset	Method	1/8	1/4	1/2	1	2	4	8	FS
e-ophtha	Dashtbozorg et al. [10]	0.358	0.417	0.471	0.522	0.558	0.605	0.638	0.510
	Zhang et al. [11]	0.170	0.240	0.320	0.440	0.540	0.630	0.740	0.440
	Proposed	0.325	0.387	0.443	0.501	0.551	0.637	0.738	**0.512**
ROC	Wang et al. [12]	0.273	0.379	0.398	0.481	0.545	0.576	0.598	0.464
	Dai et al. [13]	0.219	0.257	0.338	0.429	0.528	0.598	0.662	0.433
	Proposed	0.254	0.335	0.388	0.420	0.540	0.630	0.725	**0.472**
DiaretDB1	Seoud et al. [5]	0.140	0.175	0.250	0.323	0.440	0.546	0.642	0.359
	Dai et al. [13]	0.035	0.058	0.112	0.254	0.427	0.607	0.755	0.321
	Proposed	0.163	0.201	0.279	0.365	0.501	0.612	0.723	**0.406**
RC-RGB-MA	Dashtbozorg et al. [10]	0.541	0.591	0.618	0.662	0.697	0.704	0.714	0.647
	Proposed	0.512	0.588	0.621	0.673	0.704	0.735	0.741	**0.653**

3   Experimental Evaluation

In practice, the large vessels and the optic disc may also be detected as ROIs, as these regions in retinal images are conspicuous objects, as shown in Figs. 1, 2, 3 and 4. To detect the exact lesions there is a need to remove them from the produced saliency map. In this work, the vessel segmentation outlined in [14] and the optic disc detection method discussed in [15] were employed.

We have thoroughly evaluated the proposed method on seven publicly available retinal image datasets. These are: the Retina Check project managed by Eindhoven University of Technology (RC-RGB-MA) [10]; the DiaretDB1 [16]; the Retinopathy Online Challenge training set (ROC) [4]; the e-ophtha [17]; the Messidor [18]; the Diabetic Macular Edema (DME-DUKE) [19] dataset collected by Duke University; and the Malarial Retinopathy dataset collected by the University of Liverpool (LIMA) [3].

3.1   Dark Lesion Detection

A large number of studies, i.e., ([5,6,11]) have detected lesions on prevalence of performance defined at image level, and it is difficult to categorize the pixels as true positives and false negatives. In this study, the sensitivity values against the average number of false positives per image (FPI) was used to measure the MA detection performance [4], and sensitivity values for FPI rates of 1/8, 1/4, 1/2, 1, 2, 4, and 8 were used. A final score (FS) was computed by averaging the sensitivity values obtained at each of these seven predefined FPIs [20].

Figure 1 shows that the proposed method has successfully detected the MA regions as salient. Table 1 compares the performances of MA detection of the proposed method and existing methods in terms of sensitivity against FPI on the e-ophtha, ROC, DiaretDB1, and RC-RGB-MA datasets. Due to the page limit, we provide readers with the performance from only two most recent MA detection methods: this is not intended to be taken as exhaustive. As can be observed, the proposed method outperforms both the state-of-the-art methods on all four datasets in terms of final score.

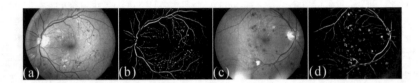

Fig. 2. Illustrative **hemorrhage** detection results on two randomly-selected DiaretDB1 images. (a) (c) Green channel images; (b) (d) Proposed saliency map.

Table 2. Hemorrhages detection performance: sensitivity scores at image level and pixel level on the **DiaretDB1** dataset.

	Quellec et al. [21]	Gondal et al. [22]	Zhou et al. [23]	Proposed
Image level	0.947	0.972	0.944	0.981
Pixel level	0.710	0.720	-	0.788

The ability of the proposed method to detect hemorrhages is demonstrated in Fig. 2. Evaluation was undertaken at image and pixel level respectively. At the image level, the intention is to reveal whether hemorrhage in an image can be detected or not. At the pixel level, the goal is to judge the detection accuracy in terms of overlapping. Table 2 demonstrates the sensitivity values achieved by the proposed method and the selected competitors over the DiaretDB1 dataset. It can be seen that the proposed method achieves the best performance at both image level and lesion level.

3.2 Bright Lesion Detection

We have evaluated the exudate detection method using three datasets: DiaretDB1, e-ophtha, and Messidor. Both the DiaretDB1 and the e-ophtha datasets provide a lesion map generated by experts, while the Messidor dataset provides a DR diagnostic for each image, but without manual annotation on exudate contours. However, Messidor contains information on the risk of macular edema, and the presence of exudates has been used to grade the risk of macular edema. Therefore, it is an important resource given the number of images available for the validation of the presence of exudate. Figure 3 indicates the proposed saliency detection method with application to exudate detection. Table 3 shows the evaluation results obtained by the proposed method and four state-of-the-art exudate detection methods: the area under the receiver operating characteristics curve (AUC) is employed to measure the performances. As can be observed, the proposed method achieves the best AUC scores, with scores of 0.952, 0.950, and 0.941, respectively in DiaretDB1, e-ophtha, and Messidor. It is worth noting that the AUC scores were computed at image level (presence of exudate).

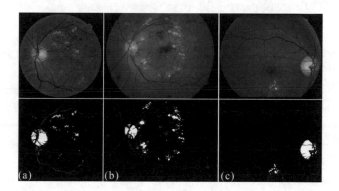

Fig. 3. Exudate detection results of the proposed method on example images from three datasets: (a) Messidor; (b) DiaretDB1; (c) e-ophtha.

Table 3. Exudates detection performance: AUC scores on three datasets. Note that, the validation on the Messidor was performed in at the image level.

	Zhang et al. [11]	Giancardo et al. [6]	Roychowdhury et al. [24]	Quellec et al. [21]	Proposed
DiaretDB1	0.950	0.930	0.870	0.809	0.952
e-ophtha	0.950	0.870	-	-	0.950
Messidor	0.930	0.900	0.904	-	0.941

In this work, the performance of the proposed method on leakage detection was obtained on two FA image datasets: DME-DUKE with DR pathology, and LIMA with MR pathology. Table 4 shows the performances of different methods in detecting leakage sites in terms of sensitivity, specificity, and AUC at the pixel level. It can be observed that the performances of our proposed method are better than those of the compared methods.

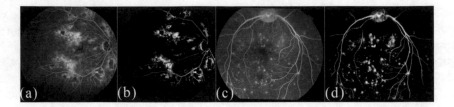

Fig. 4. Leakage detection results on example images from the DUKE-DME and LIMA datasets. (a), (c) Original images; (b), (d) Proposed saliency map.

Table 4. Leakage detection performance at pixel level: sensitivity, specificity, and AUC scores over DME-DUKE, and LIMA datasets.

	DME-DUKE			LIMA		
	Sensitivity	Specificity	AUC	Sensitivity	Specificity	AUC
Rabbani et al. [19]	0.69	0.91	0.80	0.81	0.87	0.84
Zhao et al. [3]	0.78	0.94	0.86	0.93	0.96	0.94
Proposed	0.81	0.93	0.87	0.95	0.95	0.95

4   Conclusions

Development of the proposed framework was motivated by medical demands for a tool to measure various types of lesions in retinal images. The accurate detection of retinal lesions is a challenging problem due to image intensity inhomogeneity and the irregular shapes of lesions, with substantial variability in appearance. To address this problem, a novel saliency detection method is proposed, based on the uniqueness feature derived from the intensity and spatial distribution of components of the image. To the best of our knowledge, this is the first work on the automated detection of hemorrhages, microaneurysms, exudate, and leakage from both retinal color fundus images and fluorescein angiograms. The experimental results, based on seven publicly accessible DR and MR datasets, show that our method outperforms the most recently proposed methods. The proposed method is not only capable of identifying the presence of lesions in an image, but also has the ability to measure the size of such lesions.

Acknowledgment. This work was supported National Natural Science Foundation of China (61601029, 61572076), Grant of Ningbo 3315 Innovation Team, and China Association for Science and Technology (2016QNRC001).

References

1. Cheng, M., Zhang, G., Mitra, N., Huang, X., Hu, S.: Global contrast based salient region detection. In: Proceedings IEEE International CVPR, pp. 409–416 (2011)
2. Fu, H., Cao, X., Tu, Z.: Cluster-based co-saliency detection. IEEE Trans. Image Process. **22**(10), 3766–3778 (2013)
3. Zhao, Y., et al.: Intensity and compactness enabled saliency estimation for leakage detection in diabetic and malarial retinopathy. IEEE Trans. Med. Imag. **36**(1), 51–63 (2017)
4. Niemeijer, M., van Ginneken, B., Abramoff, M.D., et al.: Retinopathy online challenge: automatic detection of microaneurysms in digital color fundus photographs. IEEE Trans. Med. Imag **29**(1), 185–195 (2010)
5. Seoud, L., Hurtut, T., Chelbi, J., Cheriet, F., Pierre Langlois, J.M.: Red lesion detection using dynamic shape features for diabetic retinopathy screening. IEEE Trans. Med. Imag **35**(4), 1116–1126 (2016)
6. Giancardo, L., et al.: Exudate-based diabetic macular edema detection in fundus images using publicly available datasets. Med. Image Anal. **16**(1), 216–226 (2012)
7. Pereira, C., Gonçalves, L., Ferreira, M.: Exudate segmentation in fundus images using an ant colony optimization approach. Inf. Sci. **296**, 14–24 (2015)
8. Perazzi, F., Pritch, Y., Hornung, A.: Saliency filters: contrast based filtering for salient region detection. In: CVPR (2012)
9. Achanta, R., Shaji, A., Smith, K., Lucchi, A., Fua, P.: Slic superpixels compared to state-of-the-art superpixel methods. IEEE Trans. Pattern Anal. Mach. Intell. **34**, 2274–2282 (2012)
10. Dashtbozorg, B., Zhang, J., ter Haar Romeny, B.M.: Retinal microaneurysms detection using local convergence index features. CoRR, abs/1707.06865 (2017)
11. Zhang, X., et al.: Exudate detection in color retinal images for mass screening of diabetic retinopathy. Med. Image Anal. **18**(7), 1026–1043 (2014)
12. Wang, S., Tang, H., et al.: Localizing microaneurysms in fundus images through singular spectrum analysis. IEEE Trans. Biomed. Eng. **64**, 990–1002 (2017)
13. Dai, B., Wu, X., Bu, W.: Retinal microaneurysms detection using gradient vector analysis and class imbalance classification. PLOS ONE **11**, 1–23 (2016)
14. Zhao, Y., Rada, L., Chen, K., Harding, S., Zheng, Y.: Automated vessel segmentation using infinite perimeter active contour model with hybrid region information with application. IEEE Trans. Med. Imag. **34**(9), 1797–1807 (2015)
15. Cheng, J., et al.: Superpixel classification based optic disc and optic cup segmentation for glaucoma screening. IEEE Trans. Med. Imag **32**, 1019–1032 (2013)
16. Kalesnykiene, V., et al.: Diaretdb1 diabetic retinopathy database and evaluation protocol. In: Proceedings Conference on MIUA (2007)
17. Decencire, E., et al.: TeleOphta: machine learning and image processing methods for teleophthalmology. IRBM **34**(2), 196–203 (2013)
18. Kandemir, M., Hamprecht, F.A.: Computer-aided diagnosis from weak supervision: a benchmarking study. Comput. Med. Imag. Graph. **42**, 44–50 (2015)
19. Rabbani, H., Allingham, M., Mettu, P., Cousins, S., Farsiu, S.: Fully automatic segmentation of fluorescein leakage in subjects with diabetic macular edema. Invest. Ophthalmol. Vis. Sci. **56**(3), 1482–1492 (2015)
20. Antal, B., et al.: An ensemble-based system for microaneurysm detection and diabetic retinopathy grading. IEEE Trans. Biomed. Eng. **59**(6), 1720–1726 (2012)
21. Quellec, G., Charrière, K., Boudi, Y., Cochener, B., Lamard, M.: Deep image mining for diabetic retinopathy screening. Med. Image Anal. **39**, 178–193 (2017)

22. Gondal, W., et al.: Weakly-supervised localization of diabetic retinopathy lesions in retinal fundus images. CoRR, abs/1706.09634 (2017)
23. Zhou, L., et al.: Automatic hemorrhage detection in color fundus images based on gradual removal of vascular branches. In: Proceedings on ICIP, pp. 399–403 (2016)
24. Roychowdhury, S., Parhi, K.K.: DREAM: diabetic retinopathy analysis using machine learning. IEEE J. Biomed. Health Inform **18**(5), 1717–1728 (2014)

Multiscale Network Followed Network Model for Retinal Vessel Segmentation

Yicheng Wu[1], Yong Xia[1(✉)], Yang Song[2], Yanning Zhang[1], and Weidong Cai[2]

[1] School of Computer Science and Engineering, Northwestern Polytechnical University, Xi'an 710072, People's Republic of China
yxia@nwpu.edu.cn
[2] School of Information Technologies, University of Sydney, Sydney, NSW 2006, Australia

Abstract. The shape of retinal blood vessels plays a critical role in the early diagnosis of diabetic retinopathy. However, it remains challenging to segment accurately the blood vessels, particularly the capillaries, in color retinal images. In this paper, we propose the multiscale network followed network (MS-NFN) model to address this issue. This model consists of an 'up-pool' NFN submodel and a 'pool-up' NFN submodel, in which max-pooling layers and up-sampling layers can generate multiscale feature maps. In each NFN, the first multiscale network converts an image patch into a probabilistic retinal vessel map, and the following multiscale network further refines the map. The refined probabilistic retinal vessel maps produced by both NFNs are averaged to construct the segmentation result. We evaluated this model on the digital retinal images for vessel extraction (DRIVE) dataset and the child heart and health study (CHASE_DB1) dataset. Our results indicate that the NFN structure we designed is able to produce performance gain and the proposed MS-NFN model achieved the state-of-the-art retinal vessel segmentation accuracy on both datasets.

Keywords: Retinal vessel segmentation · Network followed network Fully convolutional network

1 Introduction

Diabetic retinopathy (DR) is one of the major ocular health problems worldwide, the leading cause of visual impairment in the working-age population in developed countries [1]. The early diagnosis of DR, in which retina vessel segmentation plays an important role, is critical for best patient care.

A number of automated retinal vessel segmentation algorithms have been published in the literature. Many of them formulate the segmentation into a retinal pixel classification problem, in which various visual features are extracted to characterize each pixel. As an typical example, Lupascu et al. [2] jointly employed filters with different scales and directions to extract 41-dimensional

© Springer Nature Switzerland AG 2018
A. F. Frangi et al. (Eds.): MICCAI 2018, LNCS 11071, pp. 119–126, 2018.
https://doi.org/10.1007/978-3-030-00934-2_14

visual features and applied the AdaBoosted decision trees to those features for vessel segmentation. Meanwhile, the prior knowledge about retinal vessels is indispensable to address the difficulties caused by intensity inhomogeneity and low contrast. For instance, Staal et al. [3] introduced the vessel centerlines and other heuristics to the segmentation process, and Lam et al. [4] incorporated the shape prior into vessels detection.

Recent years have witnessed the success of deep learning in medical image processing, including the retinal vessel segmentation. Liskowski et al. [5] trained a deep neural network using the augmented blood vessel data at variable scales for vessel segmentation. Li et al. [6] adopted an auto-encoder to initialize the neural network for vessel segmentation without preprocessing retinal images. Ronneberger et al. [7] proposed a fully convolutional network (FCN) called U-Net to segment retinal vessels.

Despite their success, these algorithms still generate less accurate segmentation of retinal vessels, particularly the capillaries, which have smaller diameter and lower contrast than major arteries and veins in retinal images. Since the regions that contain vessels with different diameters have diverse visual appearance (see Fig. 1), we suggest applying multiscale models to segment multiwidth retinal vessels. Furthermore, although deep convolutional neural networks (DCNNs) have a strong ability to learn image representations, they can hardly incorporate the spatial information of pixels into the pixel classification process, resulting in poor connectedness of the segmented retinal vessels. Traditionally, we can apply a conditional random field (CRF) to the pixel features learned by a DCNN to address this drawback, but this makes it impossible to learn pixel features and the classifier in a unified network.

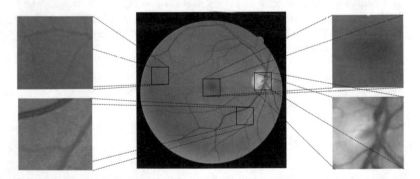

Fig. 1. A fundus retinal image: (upper right) the macular area, (bottom right) optic disc region, (upper left) low contrast patch and (bottom left) high contrast patch.

Therefore, we propose a multiscale network followed network (MS-NFN) model for blood vessel segmentation in color retinal images. The main uniqueness of this model includes: (1) there are an 'up-pool' NFN submodel, in which up-sampling layers are in front of max-pooling layers, and a 'pool-up' NFN submodel, in which max-pooling layers are in front of up-sampling layers; (2) each NFN submodel consists of two identical multiscale networks: one, with an auxiliary loss, converts an image patch into a probabilistic retinal vessel map, and the other further refines the map. Each multiscale network has a U-Net structure, in which up-sampling layers and max-pooling layers generate multiscale feature maps. The refined probabilistic retinal vessel maps produced by both NFNs are averaged to construct the segmentation result. We evaluated our MS-NFN model on the digital retinal images for vessel extraction (DRIVE) dataset [3] against eight algorithms and on the child heart and health study (CHASE_DB1) dataset [8,9] against five algorithms, and achieved the current state-of-the-art performance.

2   Datasets

The DRIVE dataset comes from a diabetic retinopathy screening program initiated in Netherlands. It consists of 20 training and 20 testing fundus retinal color images of size 584×565. These images were taken by optical camera from 400 diabetic subjects, whose ages are 25–90 years. Among them, 33 images do not have any pathological manifestations and the rest have very small signs of diabetes. Each image is equipped with the mask and ground truth from the manual segmentation of two experts.

The CHASE_DB1 dataset consists of 28 retinal images taken from both eyes of 14 school children. Usually, the first 20 images are used for training and the rest 8 images are for testing [6]. The size of each image is 999×960. The binary field of view (FOV) mask and segmentation ground truth were obtained by manual methods [10].

3   Method

The proposed MS-NFN model (see Fig. 2) can be applied to retinal vessel segmentation in five steps: (1) retinal image preprocessing, (2) patch extraction, (3) feeding each patch simultaneously into the 'up-pool' NFN and 'pool-up' NFN for segmentation, (4) averaging the output of both NFNs, and (5) segmentation result reconstruction. We now delve into the major steps.

3.1   Images Pre-processing and Patch Extraction

Each color retinal image is converted into an intensity image to avoid the impact of hue and saturation. Then, the contrast limited adaptive histogram equalization (CLAHE) algorithm [11] and gamma adjusting algorithm are used to improve image contrast and suppress noise. Next, partly overlapped patches of size 48×48 are randomly extracted in each image, resulting in 190,000 patches from the DRIVE dataset and 400,000 patches from the CHASE_DB1 dataset for training our model.

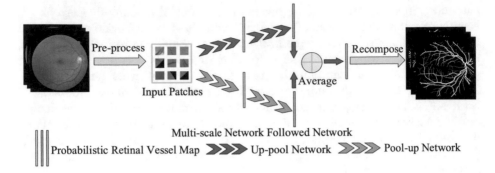

Fig. 2. Illustration of the MS-NFN model-based retinal vessel segmentation

3.2   Training Two NFN Models

Extracted patches are fed into two NFN submodels for independent training. Each NFN (see Fig. 3) consists of two identical multiscale networks: the first network inputs an extracted patch and outputs the probabilistic map of retinal vessels, and the second network inputs the probabilistic vessel map generated by the first one and then outputs a refined probabilistic vessel map. The NFN is trained in an 'end-to-end' manner to minimize the cross entropy loss L_1. The first network also has an auxiliary cross entropy loss L_2, which is added to the back propagated error with a weight of $\lambda = 0.8$. The mini-batch stochastic gradient descent (mini-batch SGD) algorithm with a batch size of 32 is adopted as the optimizer. The maximum iteration number is empirically set to 100 and the learning rate is set to 0.01.

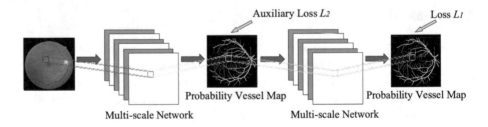

Fig. 3. Illustration of the NFN submodel-based patch segmentation.

The 'up-pool' NFN consists of two multiscale 'up-pool' networks (see Fig. 4 (top)), each having a symmetrical architecture and containing consequently an up-sampling and max-pooling module, a U-Net module [7], and another up-sampling and max-pooling module. Similarly, the 'pool-up' NFN consists of two multiscale 'pool-up' networks (see Fig. 4 (bottom)), each containing consequently a max-pooling and up-sampling module, a U-Net module, and another max-pooling and up-sampling module.

3.3   Testing the MS-NFN Model

Each test image is first pre-processed using the method described in the Subsect. 3.1. Then, partly overlapped patches of size 48×48 are extracted with a stride of 5 along both horizontal and vertical directions. Next, each patch is fed into two NFN submodels for segmentation, and the obtained probabilistic vessel maps are averaged. Since the patches are heavily overlapped, each pixel may appear in multiple patches, and its probabilistic values in these patches are further averaged. Finally, the averaged probabilistic vessel map is binarized with a threshold 0.5 to form the retinal vessel segmentation result.

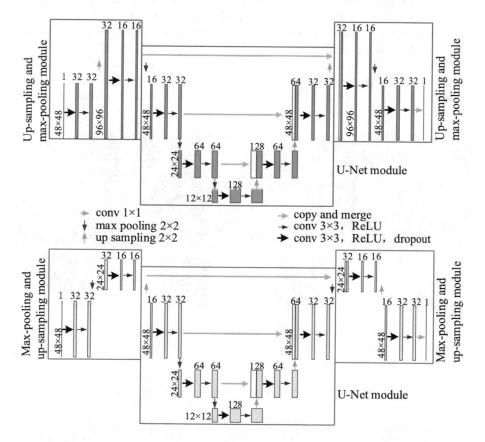

Fig. 4. Architecture of the 'up-pool' network (top) and 'pool-up' network (bottom)

4   Results

Performance Gain Caused by NFN: To demonstrate the performance gain caused by the NFN structure, we implemented a MS model, which has a similar architecture to MS-NFN except that each NFN is replaced with a single multiscale network. Figures 5 and 6 show an example test image from DRIVE and CHASE_DB1, respectively, together with the segmentation results obtained by using the MS model and proposed MS-NFN model, and the ground truth. It reveals that our MS-NFN model, with the NFN structure, can detect more retinal vessels than the MS model.

Comparison to Existing Methods: Tables 1 and 2 give the average accuracy, specificity, sensitivity and area under the ROC curve (AUC) obtained by applying several existing retinal vessel segmentation methods, the MS model, and the proposed MS-NFN model to the DRIVE dataset and CHASE_DB1 dataset, respectively. It shows that the overall performance of our MS-NFN model is superior to those competing methods on both datasets. Particularly, our method achieved a substantially improved AUC value (i.e., 0.60% higher than the second best AUC on DRIVE and 1.09% higher than the second best AUC on CHASE_DB1). Considering the size of each retinal image, such improvement leads to a large number of retinal vessel pixels being correctly classified.

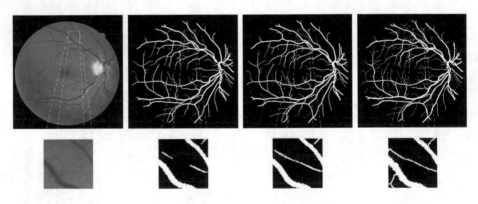

Fig. 5. A test image from the DRIVE dataset (1st column), the segmentation results obtained by using the MS model (2nd column) and our MS-NFN model (3rd column), and ground truth (4th column).

Table 1. Performance of nine segmentation methods on the dataset.

Method	AUC (%)	Accuracy (%)	Specificity (%)	Sensitivity (%)
Fraz et al. [8] (2012)	97.47	94.80	98.07	74.06
Mapayi et al. [12] (2015)	97.11	95.00	96.68	74.28
Azzopardi et al. [13] (2015)	96.14	94.42	97.04	76.55
Roychowdhury et al. [14] (2015)	96.72	94.94	97.82	73.95
Li et al. [6] (2016)	97.38	95.27	98.16	75.69
Orlando et al. [15] (2017)	95.07	N.A	96.84	78.97
Dasgupta et al. [16] (2017)	97.44	95.33	98.01	76.91
MS Model	*97.98*	*95.62*	*97.99*	*79.34*
Proposed (MS-NFN)	*98.07*	*95.67*	*98.19*	*78.44*

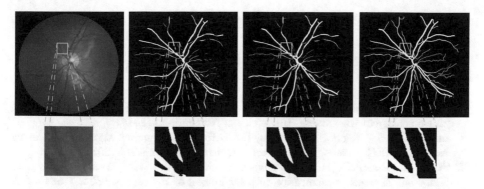

Fig. 6. A test image from the CHASE_DB1 dataset (1st column), the segmentation results obtained by using the MS model (2nd column) and our MS-NFN model (3rd column), and ground truth (4th column).

Table 2. Performance of six segmentation methods on the CHASE_DB1 dataset.

Method	AUC (%)	Accuracy (%)	Specificity (%)	Sensitivity (%)
Fraz et al. [8] (2012)	97.12	94.69	97.11	72.24
Azzopardi et al. [14] (2015)	94.87	93.87	95.87	75.85
Li et al. [6] (2016)	97.16	95.81	97.93	75.07
Orlando et al. [15] (2017)	95.24	N.A	97.12	72.77
MS Model	98.07	96.26	98.85	70.36
Proposed (MS NFN)	98.25	96.37	98.47	75.38

Computational Complexity: It took more than 16 h to train the proposed MS-NFN model on the DRIVE dataset and more than 30 h to train it on the CHASE_DB1 dataset (Intel Xeon E5-2640 V4 CPU, NVIDIA Titan Xp GPU, 512 GB Memory, and Keras 1.1.0). However, applying our MS-NFN model to retinal vessel segmentation is relatively fast, as it took less than 10 s to segment a 584×565 retinal image on average.

5   Conclusions

We propose the MS-NFN model for retinal vessel segmentation and evaluated it on the DRIVE and CHASE_DB1 datasets. Our results indicate that the NFN structure we designed is able to produce performance gain and the proposed MS-NFN model achieved, to our knowledge, the most accurate retinal vessel segmentation on both datasets.

Acknowledgements. This work was supported in part by the National Natural Science Foundation of China under Grants 61771397 and 61471297, in part by the China Postdoctoral Science Foundation under Grant 2017M623245, in part by the Fundamental Research Funds for the Central Universities under Grant 3102018zy031, and in part by the Australian Research Council (ARC) Grants. We also appreciate the efforts devoted to collect and share the DRIVE and CHASE_DB1 datasets for retinal vessel segmentation.

References

1. Saker, S.: Diabetic retinopathy: in vitro and clinical studies of mechanisms and pharmacological treatments. University of Nottingham (2016)
2. Lupascu, C.A., Tegolo, D., Trucco, E.: FABC: retinal vessel segmentation using AdaBoost. IEEE Trans. Inf. Technol. Biomed. **14**, 1267–1274 (2010)
3. Staal, J., Abràmoff, M.D., Niemeijer, M., Viergever, M.A., Van Ginneken, B.: Ridge-based vessel segmentation in color images of the retina. IEEE Trans. Med. Imaging **23**, 501–509 (2004)
4. Lam, B.S.Y., Yan, H.: A novel vessel segmentation algorithm for pathological retina images based on the divergence of vector fields. IEEE Trans. Med. Imaging **27**, 237–246 (2008)
5. Liskowski, P., Krawiec, K.: Segmenting retinal blood vessels with deep neural networks. IEEE Trans. Med. Imaging **35**, 2369–2380 (2016)
6. Li, Q., Feng, B., Xie, L.P., Liang, P., Zhang, H., Wang, T.: A cross-modality learning approach for vessel segmentation in retinal images. IEEE Trans. Med. Imaging **35**, 109–118 (2016)
7. Ronneberger, O., Fischer, P., Brox, T.: U-Net: convolutional networks for biomedical image segmentation. In: Navab, N., Hornegger, J., Wells, W.M., Frangi, A.F. (eds.) MICCAI 2015. LNCS, vol. 9351, pp. 234–241. Springer, Cham (2015). https://doi.org/10.1007/978-3-319-24574-4_28
8. Fraz, M.M.: An ensemble classification-based approach applied to retinal blood vessel segmentation. IEEE Trans. Biomed. Eng. **59**, 2538–2548 (2012)
9. Owen, C.G.: Measuring retinal vessel tortuosity in 10-year-old children: validation of the Computer-assisted image analysis of the retina (CAIAR) program. Invest. Ophthalmol. Vis. Sci. **50**, 2004–2010 (2009)
10. Soares, J.V.B., Leandro, J.J.G., Cesar, R.M., Jelinek, H.F., Cree, M.J.: Retinal vessel segmentation using the 2-D Gabor wavelet and supervised classification. IEEE Trans. Med. Imaging **25**, 1214–1222 (2006)
11. Setiawan, A.W., Mengko, T.R., Santoso, O.S., Suksmono, A.B.: Color retinal image enhancement using CLAHE. In: ICISS, pp. 1–3. IEEE, Jakarta (2013)
12. Mapayi, T., Viriri, S., Tapamo, J.R.: Adaptive thresholding technique for retinal vessel segmentation based on GLCM-energy information. Comput. Math. Methods Med. **2015**, 597475 (2015)
13. Azzopardi, G., Strisciuglio, N., Vento, M., Petkov, N.: Trainable COSFIRE filters for vessel delineation with application to retinal images. Med. Image Anal. **19**, 46 (2015)
14. Roychowdhury, S., Koozekanani, D., Parhi, K.: Blood vessel segmentation of fundus images by major vessel extraction and sub-image classification. IEEE J. Biomed. Health Inform. **19**, 1118–1128 (2015)
15. Orlando, J., Prokofyeva, E., Blaschko, M.: A discriminatively trained fully connected conditional random field model for blood vessel segmentation in fundus images. IEEE Trans. Biomed. Eng. **64**, 16–27 (2017)
16. Dasgupta, A., Singh, S.: A fully convolutional neural network based structured prediction approach towards the retinal vessel segmentation. In: IEEE 14th ISBI, pp. 248–251. IEEE, Melbourne (2017)

Optical and Histology Applications:
Histology Applications

Predicting Cancer with a Recurrent Visual Attention Model for Histopathology Images

Aïcha BenTaieb[(⊠)] and Ghassan Hamarneh

School of Computing Science, Simon Fraser University, Burnaby, Canada
{abentaie,hamarneh}@sfu.ca

Abstract. Automatically recognizing cancers from multi-gigapixel whole slide histopathology images is one of the challenges facing machine and deep learning based solutions for digital pathology. Currently, most automatic systems for histopathology are not scalable to large images and hence require a patch-based representation; a sub-optimal solution as it results in important additional computational costs but more importantly in the loss of contextual information. We present a novel attention-based model for predicting cancer from histopathology whole slide images. The proposed model is capable of attending to the most discriminative regions of an image by adaptively selecting a limited sequence of locations and only processing the selected areas of tissues. We demonstrate the utility of the proposed model on the slide-based prediction of macro and micro metastases in sentinel lymph nodes of breast cancer patients. We achieve competitive results with state-of-the-art convolutional networks while automatically identifying discriminative areas of tissues.

1 Introduction

Cancers are primarily diagnosed from the visual analysis of digitized or physical histology slides of tumor biopsies [4]. Growing access to large datasets of digitized histopathology images has led to the emergence of computational models where the aim is to reduce experts workload and improve cancer treatment procedures [6]. Recently, convolutional neural networks (CNN) have become the state-of-the-art for many histopathology image classification tasks. However, CNNs are not the best suited for large scale (i.e. millions of pixels) multi-resolution histopathology whole slide images (WSI). Finding adequate and computationally efficient solutions to automatically analyze WSI remains an open challenge.

A standard approach for analyzing WSI consists of sampling patches from areas of interest and training a supervised model to predict a desired output (e.g., a class label) for each patch independently [6]. The trained model can then be applied to patches densely extracted from an unseen WSI where the final slide prediction is the result of an aggregation of all patch predictions. Such patch based representation comes with different shortcomings: (i) processing

© Springer Nature Switzerland AG 2018
A. F. Frangi et al. (Eds.): MICCAI 2018, LNCS 11071, pp. 129–137, 2018.
https://doi.org/10.1007/978-3-030-00934-2_15

all patches of a WSI is computationally inefficient (as most tissue areas are diagnostically irrelevant) and almost always unfeasible; (ii) randomly sampled patches can result in the loss of relevant information and often involve using finer-level annotations (i.e. segmentation masks) to guide the patch extraction; and (iii) using independently analyzed patches implies a loss of context.

Different works were proposed to improve patch-based representations. Mainly, these works present different aggregation strategies and encode global context. For instance, weakly-supervised models based on multiple instance learning [7] or structured latent representations [3] have been proposed to show the importance of identifying discriminative regions when training a prediction model. To capture context (without increasing patch size), pyramid representations where patches are extracted at different magnifications can be leveraged. For instance, Bejnardi et al. [2] proposed a patch-based model consisting of a cascaded CNN architecture where features from patches extracted at increasing scales are aggregated to classify breast cancer tissue slides. Another strategy for capturing spatial context from patch-based representations is to use recurrent networks. Agarwalla et al. [1] used 2D LSTMs to aggregate features from neighbouring patches in a WSI. While these works indirectly impose more context in the training of a patch-based prediction model, they rely on an initial random selection of patches that does not prevent from an eventual loss of information and most importantly requires processing all patches independently. In this work, we attempt to leverage spatial context while selecting discriminative areas. Studies on experts visual diagnostic procedure [4] showed that over time, experts make fewer fixations and perform less examinations of non-diagnostic areas. We hypothesize that patch-based analysis of tissue slides should be a sequential process in which a prediction model identifies where to focus given the context of the entire tissue and the history of previously seen regions without other forms of annotation than the slide level class.

To design such system, we take inspiration from visual attention models [8]. A number of recent studies have demonstrated that visual content can be captured through a sequence of spatial 'glimpses' [9] describing parts of an image. Focusing computational resources on parts of a scene has the interesting property of substantially reducing the task complexity as objects of interest can be placed in the center of the glimpse. Existing visual attention systems were introduced for analyzing natural scene images [9] but their utility for large scale images has not been demonstrated yet.

We propose a system to analyze whole slide histopathology images and predict the presence of cancer while automatically learning to focus on discriminative areas (Fig. 1). We assume the system should be able to predict normal vs abnormal slides from a limited set of observations or glimpses. Locations and scales at which glimpses are extracted should be automatically inferred. Decisions about the central locations of glimpses should be based on the global context of a given tissue slide as well as the memory of all previously observed glimpses. The slide level class prediction should be based on information integrated from all observed glimpses as well as the global context. Finally, through time, the system should learn to make decisions about the class of a tissue slide using a limited set of glimpses.

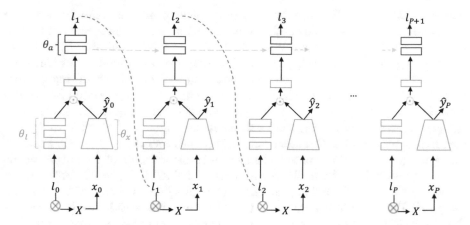

Fig. 1. Proposed recurrent visual attention model for classifying histopathology images. Grey dashed lines represent temporal connections while solid black lines describe the information flow between components within one time-step. The model includes three primary components composed of dense (rectangular boxes) or convolutional (trapezoid) layers. X is an input whole slide image, $\{x_0, \ldots, x_P\}$ is the sequence of glimpses with their corresponding location parameters $\{l_0, \ldots, l_P\}$. The system contains three main components parameterized by θ_x, θ_l and θ_a. $\odot$ represents the Hadamard product and $\otimes$ is a matrix multiplication. The model sequentially predicts a class label $\hat{y}$ for the tissue slide given the sequence of glimpses.

2   Method

Given a whole slide histopathology image X, our goal is to identify a set of locations $\{l_0, l_1, \ldots, l_P\}$ from which to extract glimpses $\{x_0, x_1, \ldots, x_P\}$ that are discriminative of a given class Y (e.g. presence or absence of metastatic cancer). To this end, we propose a sequential system structured around a recurrent neural network equipped with an attention memory and an appearance description of the tissue at different locations.

At each time step, the system receives a location l_p that defines the extraction of a corresponding glimpse x_p. A location network θ_l forms a feature representation of a given location and an appearance network θ_x generates a feature representation for a given glimpse. These feature representations are aggregated to form part of the input to the attention network θ_a. Given a sequence $\{x_0, x_1, \ldots, x_P\}$ of P extracted glimpses, the system parameterized by $\theta = \{\theta_l, \theta_x, \theta_a\}$ predicts a probability score $Q(Y|\{x_0, x_1, \ldots, x_P\}; \theta)$ for the slide-level label Y. The attention network is the recurrent component of the model and uses information from the glimpses and their corresponding location parameters to update its internal representation of the input and outputs the next location parameters. Figure 1 is a graphical representation of this sequential procedure.

Spatial Attention: The spatial attention mechanism consists of extracting a glimpse x_p from a tissue slide and is a modification of the read mechanism introduced in [8]. Given an input tissue slide $X \in \mathcal{R}^{H \times W \times 3}$ of size $H \times W$, we apply two grids (one for each axis of the image) of two-dimensional Gaussian filters, where each filter response corresponds to a pixel in the resulting glimpse $x_p \in \mathcal{R}^{h \times w \times 3}$ of size $h \times w$. The attention mechanism is represented by parameters $l = \{\mu_w, \mu_h, \sigma_w^2, \sigma_h^2, \delta_w, \delta_h\}$ that describe the centers of the Gaussians (i.e. the grid center coordinates), their variances (i.e. amount of blurring to apply), and strides between the Gaussian centers (i.e. the scale of the glimpse). Parameters l are dynamically computed as an affine transformation of the output of the recurrent network θ_a. Formally, the glimpse is defined by $x_p = A_p^x X A_p^{yT}$, where A_p^x and A_p^y are the Gaussian grid matrices applied on each axis of the original image X. To integrate the entire context of a given tissue slide, we initialize the first location parameters l_0 such that the resulting glimpse x_0 corresponds to a coarse representation of the tissue slide (i.e. lowest magnification) re-sized to the desired glimpse size $h \times w$.

Combining Appearance and Spatial Information: Given a glimpse x_p and its corresponding location parameters l_p, we construct a fixed-dimensional feature vector comprising appearance and spatial information about the current glimpse. We denote the appearance-based features obtained for a given glimpse by $f_x(x_p; \theta_x)$ and the features computed for the corresponding location parameters by $f_l(l_p; \theta_l)$. We used a CNN to represent f_x and a fully connected layer for f_l. The outputs of both networks are fused to obtain a joint representation that captures spatial and appearance features using $g_p = \sigma(f_l(l_p; \theta_l) \odot f_x(x_p; \theta_x))$, where g_p is the output joint feature vector, σ corresponds to the logistic sigmoid function, and $\odot$ is the Hadamard product. By combining appearance and spatial features, the system integrates features related to "where" and "what" patterns to seek for when predicting the next glimpse location parameters.

Recurrent Attention: The recurrent component of the system aggregates information extracted from all individual glimpses and their corresponding locations. It receives as input the joint spatial and appearance representation (i.e. g_p) and maintains an internal state summarizing information extracted from the sequence of past glimpses. At each step p, the recurrent attention network updates its internal state (formed by the hidden units of the network) based on the incoming feature representation g_p and outputs a prediction for the next location l_{p+1} to focus on at time step $p + 1$. The spatial attention parameters l_p are formed as a linear function of the internal state of the network.

Objective Function: The system is trained by minimizing a loss function comprised of a classification loss term and auxiliary regularization terms that guide the attention mechanism. The total loss $\mathcal{L}(.)$ is given by:

$$\mathcal{L}(\mathcal{D}; \theta) = \mathcal{L}_c(\mathcal{D}; \theta) + \mathcal{L}_p(\mathcal{D}; \theta) + \mathcal{L}_a(\mathcal{D}; \theta) + \mathcal{L}_l(\mathcal{D}; \theta) \qquad (1)$$

where $\mathcal{D} = \{(X^{(i)}, Y^{(i)})\}_{i=1}^N$ is a training set of N tissue slides $X^{(i)}$ and their corresponding labels $Y^{(i)}$ and $\theta = \{\theta_a, \theta_x, \theta_l\}$ represent the system's parameters.

Tissue Slide Classification: The slide-level classification loss $\mathcal{L}_c$ is defined as the cross entropy between the final slide-level predicted label $\hat{Y}$ and the true label $Y^{(i)}$. To obtain a slide-level prediction, we combine the feature representations of all glimpses $f_x(x_{[1:P]}; \theta_x)$ using a non-linear function represented by a fully connected layer. This layer is then fed to another linear layer that generates final predictions $Q(Y^{(i)}|x_{[1:P]}^{(i)}; \theta)$. The slide-level loss is computed using $\mathcal{L}_c(\mathcal{D}; \theta) = \sum_{i=1}^N \log Q(\hat{Y} = Y^{(i)}|x_{[1:P]}^{(i)}; \theta)$.

Discriminative Attention and Selective Exploration: We observed that adding a patch-level classification loss facilitates training by enforcing the model to attend to discriminative tissue areas. $\mathcal{L}_p$ corresponds to a classification cross entropy loss between each predicted patch-level label $\hat{y}_p$ and the ground truth slide label $Y^{(i)}$. The goal here is not to leverage other forms of annotations but to encourage finding discriminative regions in a weakly supervised setting. Feature representations of each attended patch $f_x(x_p; \theta_x)$ are used to compute the patch-level loss by $\mathcal{L}_p(\mathcal{D}; \theta) = \sum_{i=1}^N \sum_{p=1}^P \log Q(\hat{y}_p = Y^{(i)}|x_p^{(i)}; \theta)$, where $Q(\hat{y}_p^{(i)}|x_p^{(i)}; \theta)$ represents the probabilities obtained from a fully-connected layer applied to the patch-level features $f_x(x_p; \theta_x)$ with the sigmoid activation.

We also observed that after seeing the coarse image representation x_0, it becomes harder to attend to other areas as the rich contextual representation is often enough to discriminate between simple cases (e.g. benign vs macro-metastases). To encourage the system to explore different locations and scales, we introduce a regularization term that serves two ends. First, we encourage the system to gradually approach the most discriminative regions and scales by favouring glimpses with high prediction probabilities for the ground truth class using $\mathcal{L}_a$. Second, we encourage exploration by enforcing large differences between successive predicted centers μ_w and μ_h using $\mathcal{L}_l$. Formally, we define:

$$\mathcal{L}_a(\mathcal{D}; \theta) = -\sum_{i=1}^N \sum_{p=2}^P Q(y_p^{(i)}|x_p^{(i)}; \theta) - \left(\frac{1}{p-1}\sum_{k=1}^{p-1} Q(y_k^{(i)}|x_k^{(i)}; \theta)\right) \quad (2)$$

$$\mathcal{L}_l(\mathcal{D}; \theta) = \gamma \sum_{i=1}^N \sum_{p=1}^P \exp(-|l_p - l_{p+1}|), \quad (3)$$

where the hyper-parameter γ enables us to control how much exploration the system performs by being linearly annealed from one to zero during training. At inference, given an unseen tissue slide, the model extracts a sequence of glimpses to attend to the most discriminative regions. The final prediction score for the slide is computed using the aggregated features $f_x(x_{[1:P]}^{(i)}; \theta_x)$.

3   Experiments

We tested the system on the publicly available Camelyon16 dataset [5] where the task is to predict benign from metastatic cases of lymph nodes tissue slides.

Table 1. Evaluation of different patch-based models for WSI classification. Columns represent: patch level (ACC-P) and WSI level (ACC-WSI) accuracy, area under ROC curve (AUC), precision (PREC) and recall (REC).

Method	ACC-P	ACC-WSI	AUC	PREC	REC
Wang et al. [10]	0.98	–	**0.96**	–	–
LSVM [3]	0.89 ± 0.2	0.84 ± 0.2	0.75	0.87	0.69
Dense Patches	0.84 ± 0.2	0.76 ± 0.3	0.72	0.94	0.66
Proposed 1 Glimpse - $\mathcal{L}_c$	0.81 ± 0.2	0.79 ± 0.2	0.68	0.60	0.48
Proposed 3 Glimpses - $\mathcal{L}_c$	0.84 ± 0.1	0.80 ± 0.2	0.85	0.69	0.64
Proposed 5 Glimpses - $\mathcal{L}_c$	0.81 ± 0.1	0.78 ± 0.2	0.83	0.65	0.62
Proposed 3 Glimpses - $\mathcal{L}_c + \mathcal{L}_p$	0.87 ± 0.2	0.86 ± 0.2	0.84	0.81	0.78
Proposed 3 Glimpses - $\mathcal{L}_c + \mathcal{L}_p + \mathcal{L}_a$	$\mathbf{0.97 \pm 0.1}$	$\mathbf{0.95 \pm 0.2}$	0.95	**0.98**	**0.82**

The dataset contains a total of 400 WSI and we used the same dataset splits as the ones released by the challenge organizers for training (270) and test (130).

Typically histopathology images contain billions of pixels but only a few portion of the slide contains biological tissues. To reduce the amount of computation, we remove all unnecessary background pixels using a simple threshold on the pixel intensity values and crop all slides around the tissue. Although the total size is reduced, in practice, performing the matrix multiplication for the spatial attention at the highest magnification level of a slide, is computationally unfeasible with standard resources. Instead, we opt for processing images at the intermediate 20x magnification using tiles covering as much context as possible. A tile size of 5000×5000 pixels (Fig. 2) was the largest we could process. To predict a class label for a slide, we apply the system on all 20x tiles and let it decide at which scale and location to attend. We use the average of the probabilities obtained after attention to get a final slide prediction. The total run-time was on average less than 4s per slide.

Table 1 reports the performance of the model against different baselines. Wang et al. [10], the winners of the challenge, used the Inception CNN architecture to train a patch-based classifier on randomly sampled patches at 40x magnification. To obtain slide level predictions, the output probabilities of the patch-based CNN are used to predict a heatmap. Statistical features are extracted from the resulting heatmap (e.g. morphology and geometry features) and used to train a random forest classifier that outputs the final predicted slide label. We also compared against the latent structured SVM model presented in [3]. To train this model, we extracted patches at two magnification levels (20x and 40x) and used a pre-trained Inception CNN model to extract features for each patch. The latent structured model uses a hierarchical representation of patches at both magnifications to identify the most discriminative patches while training the classifier. We also trained the Inception CNN model using densely sampled patches from each whole slide image at magnification 20x. Given the high ratio of positives to negatives, we leveraged the segmentation masks of tumors to train this baseline and dynamically sampled tumor patches. Finally, we tested the following configurations of our system: (i) different number of glimpses and (ii) different combinations of the proposed loss terms in Eq. (1).

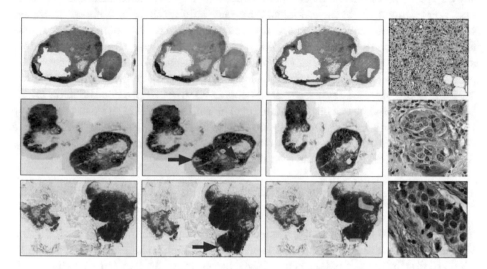

Fig. 2. Qualitative evaluation of the attention model. Rows represent different cases of macro to micro metastases. Columns from left to right are the downsampled WSI, the cyan overlay of the ground truth tumor mask with red arrows pointing at micro-metastasis, the yellow overlay of the attended glimpses and the glimpse with highest prediction score showing how glimpses are automatically extracted at different scales.

We tested the performance of the system using different numbers of glimpses (i.e., 1, 3 or 5 glimpses per tile). On average, after background removal, we obtain ∼14 tiles per tissue slide. Thus, the final performance results reported in Table 1 correspond to an aggregation of 14 (case of 1 glimpse per tile) to 70 glimpses. In contrast, all other automatic systems were trained with thousands of patches. We obtained best results using 3 glimpses (i.e., 85% AUC vs 68% and 83% for 1 and 5 glimpses when training with $\mathcal{L}_c$ only). We also observed that using 1 glimpse (i.e., 14 attention patches per slide) resulted in a 4% drop in AUC only. Note that this is most likely specific to this particular dataset in which macro-metastatic tissues contain large amounts of abnormality and are thus easily discriminated from benign tissues. However, this also shows the utility of identifying discriminative locations when training prediction systems.

We also tested the impact of the different loss terms in Eq. (1). In general, the patch-level loss $\mathcal{L}_p$ resulted in improving the attention on positive cases which is reflected by the improved recall scores (i.e., from 64% to 78% with 3 glimpses). Finally, adding the attention regularization terms $\mathcal{L}_a$ and $\mathcal{L}_l$ primarily helped facilitate convergence (i.e. reduced the convergence time by ∼15%) and improved the final AUC, precision and recall. Note that our final AUC is 1%

lower than [10], however, our aim in this work is to demonstrate how attention can be leveraged in histopathology by selectively choosing where to focus.

In Fig. 2 we show examples of glimpses. Comparing the attended areas to the ground truth masks of metastatic tissues (columns 3 and 2 respectively) shows that the attention mechanism is able to identify discriminative patterns and solely focus on those regions. The last column in Fig. 2 shows glimpses with the highest prediction score for each WSI class and demonstrates that the system learns patterns from different scales. The last row in Fig. 2 shows a failure example on a challenging case of micro-metastases. In this case, the model was correctly able to identify discriminative patterns (the yellow overlay on images of column 3 shows the attention areas used to predict the slide label) but unable to predict the correct slide level class. Given the high ratio of negative to positive tissue in micro-metastatic patches, this may indicate that a more complex aggregation strategy (instead of the simple linear aggregation) for the different attended glimpses may be necessary.

4   Conclusion

We hypothesized that enforcing a selective attention mechanism when predicting the presence of cancer within a tissue slide would enable the prediction system to identify discriminative patterns and integrate context. To test our hypothesis, we proposed a prediction model that integrates a recurrent attention mechanism. Experiments on a dataset of breast tissue images showed that the proposed model is capable of selectively attending to discriminative regions of tissues and accurately identifying abnormal areas with a limited sequence of visual glimpses.

Acknowledgements. We thank NVIDIA Corporation for GPU donation and The Natural Sciences and Engineering Research Council of Canada (NSERC) for funding.

References

1. Agarwalla, A., Shaban, M., Rajpoot, N.M.: Representation-aggregation networks for segmentation of multi-gigapixel histology images. arXiv preprint arXiv:1707.08814 (2017)
2. Bejnordi, B.E., et al.: Context-aware stacked convolutional neural networks for classification of breast carcinomas in whole-slide histopathology images. MedIA 4(4), 044504 (2017)
3. BenTaieb, A., et al.: A structured latent model for ovarian carcinoma subtyping from histopathology slides. MedIA 39, 194–205 (2017)
4. Brunye, T.T., et al.: Eye movements as an index of pathologist visual expertise: a pilot study. PloS one 9(8), e103447 (2014)
5. Golden, J.A.: Deep learning algorithms for detection of lymph node metastases from breast cancer: helping artificial intelligence be seen. JAMA 318(22), 2184–2186 (2017)
6. Komura, D., Ishikawa, S.: Machine learning methods for histopathological image analysis. arXiv preprint arXiv:1709.00786 (2017)

7. Mercan, C., et al.: Multi-instance multi-label learning for multi-class classification of whole slide breast histopathology images. IEEE TMI **37**(1), 316–325 (2018)
8. Mnih, V., et al.: Recurrent models of visual attention. In: NIPS, pp. 2204–2212 (2014)
9. Sermanet, P., Frome, A., Real, E.: Attention for fine-grained categorization. arXiv preprint arXiv:1412.7054 (2014)
10. Wang, D., et al.: Deep learning for identifying metastatic breast cancer. arXiv preprint arXiv:1606.05718 (2016)

A Deep Model with Shape-Preserving Loss for Gland Instance Segmentation

Zengqiang Yan[1]([✉]), Xin Yang[2], and Kwang-Ting Tim Cheng[1]

[1] Department of Computer Science and Engineering,
The Hong Kong University of Science and Technology, Kowloon, Hong Kong
z.yan@connect.ust.hk
[2] School of Electronic Information and Communications,
Huazhong University of Science and Technology, Wuhan, China

Abstract. Segmenting gland instance in histology images requires not only separating glands from a complex background but also identifying each gland individually via accurate boundary detection. This is a very challenging task due to lots of noises from the background, tiny gaps between adjacent glands, and the "coalescence" problem arising from adhesive gland instances. State-of-the-art methods adopted multi-channel/multi-task deep models to separately accomplish pixelwise gland segmentation and boundary detection, yielding a high model complexity and difficulties in training. In this paper, we present a unified deep model with a new shape-preserving loss which facilities the training for both pixel-wise gland segmentation and boundary detection simultaneously. The proposed shape-preserving loss helps significantly reduce the model complexity and make the training process more controllable. Compared with the current state-of-the-art methods, the proposed deep model with the shape-preserving loss achieves the best overall performance on the 2015 MICCAI Gland Challenge dataset. In addition, the flexibility of integrating the proposed shape-preserving loss into any learning based medical image segmentation networks offers great potential for further performance improvement of other applications.

Keywords: Deep convolutional neural network
Gland instance segmentation · Shape-preserving loss
Histology image analysis

1 Introduction

Accurate gland instance segmentation from histology images is a crucial step for pathologists to quantitatively analyze the malignancy degree of adenocarcinomas for further diagnosis [1]. However, manual annotation of gland instances is time consuming given the large size of a histology image and a large number of glands in an image. Therefore, accurate and automatic methods for gland instance segmentation are in great demand. Gland instance segmentation consists of two

© Springer Nature Switzerland AG 2018
A. F. Frangi et al. (Eds.): MICCAI 2018, LNCS 11071, pp. 138–146, 2018.
https://doi.org/10.1007/978-3-030-00934-2_16

sub-tasks: (1) gland segmentation which separates glands from the background and (2) boundary detection so as to identify each gland individually, as shown in Fig. 1. In practice, gland instance segmentation is a challenging task due to the following two unique characteristics. First, the appearances of glands vary significantly in different histology image patches (or even within a single patch), as shown in Fig. 1. Large appearance variations make the pixel-wise gland segmentation problem very challenging. Second, some gland instances are very close to each other or even share one entity borders, making it hard to identify gland instances individually and preserve the shape of each gland.

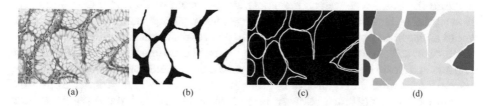

    (a)   (b)   (c)   (d)

Fig. 1. Gland instance segmentation problem: (a) histology image patch, (b) gland segmentation, (c) boundary detection and (d) ground-truth gland instance segmentation (different colors represent different gland instances). Gland instance segmentation can be regarded as the combination of boundary detection and gland segmentation.

Several methods have been proposed for accurate gland instance segmentation. Xu *et al.* [2,3] proposed multi-channel deep neural networks to extract gland region, boundaries and location cues separately. The results from different channels were fused to produce the final gland instance segmentation result. In their methods, different channels and the fusion module were implemented using different deep learning architectures and were pre-trained separately. While achieving the best performance so far on the 2015 MICCAI Gland Challenge dataset, the method incurs a high model complexity and complicated training process. Chen *et al.* [4] formulated the gland instance segmentation problem as a multi-task learning problem. The model contains two branches trained using the manual annotations for gland segmentation and the manually generated boundary maps for boundary detection separately.

Different from the complicated multi-channel/-task deep models, we propose a shape-preserving loss which enables a single deep model to jointly learn pixel-wise gland segmentation and boundary detection simultaneously. The proposed shape-preserving loss mainly consists of two parts: (1) a pixel-wise cross-entropy loss for gland segmentation and (2) a shape similarity loss for gland boundary detection. Experimental results demonstrate that the deep model trained by the shape-preserving loss outperforms the state-of-the-art methods on the public gland segmentation dataset. In addition, the great flexibility of the shape-preserving loss for integration into any deep learning models is a significant benefit.

2   Method

A straightforward solution to learn a unified deep model for both gland segmentation and boundary detection is to minimize pixel-wise cross-entropy losses between: (1) detected gland pixels and annotated gland pixels (gland segmentation), (2) detected gland boundaries and annotated boundaries (gland boundary detection). However, learning a boundary detector via pixel-wise cross-entropy loss utilizes only information of individual pixels with little consideration of global shape information of an entire boundary segment. In addition, it is often very challenging to precisely localize gland boundary pixels due to the ambiguity at gland boundaries as well as low contrast, as shown in Fig. 2(a). Consequently, directly using the pixel-wise cross-entropy loss for gland instance segmentation would suffer from poor performance on shape preservation. Increasing the importance of boundary pixels could partially solve the problem while it would also degrade the gland segmentation performance due to numerous holes in gland segmentation results. Therefore, it is difficult for the pixel-wise cross-entropy loss to balance the importance between boundary detection and gland segmentation in the training process. In this section, we first present a novel shape-preserving loss to enable a unified deep model for both accurate and efficient boundary detection and gland segmentation followed by the corresponding deep model.

2.1   Shape-Preserving Loss

The proposed shape-preserving loss consists of two losses: (1) a shape similarity loss [5] which is able to detect boundary segments with similar geometric shapes as manual annotations while allows certain boundary location variations arising from low intensity contrast and ambiguities of boundaries; and (2) a weighted pixel-wise cross-entropy loss for close and/or adhesive gland segmentation. In the following, we describe each loss in more details.

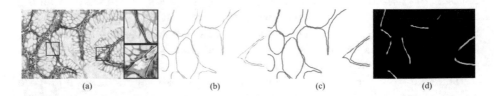

Fig. 2. Shape-preserving loss construction: (a) histology patch by remapping the annotated boundaries, (b) boundary segmentation map, (c) searching range map and (d) weight map background pixels between close glands. In the boundary segmentation map, different boundary segments are assigned with different colors. In the weight map, the intensity of each pixel represents its weight (0∼1.0).

Shape Similarity Loss. Given a manual annotation, we first generate the corresponding boundary map and segment the whole boundary map into boundary segments (by default the length is in the range of $[16, 24]$ pixels) as shown in Fig. 2(b). For each boundary segment l_i, as shown in Fig. 2(c) a 3-pixel searching range is assigned to find the corresponding boundary segment s_i in the output segmentation map. As the 3-pixel searching range allows limited location variation between l_i and s_i, the measurement is less restrictive and more efficient compared to the pixel-wise cross-entropy measurement. Then, the shape similarity is measured based on the curve fitting method. Given l_i and s_i, we adopt a curve (cubic function) fitting method to obtain their approximated curve functions $f(l_i) = a_1x^3 + b_1x^2 + c_1x + d_1$ and $f(s_i) = a_2x^3 + b_2x^2 + c_2x + d_2$. The shape similarity between l_i and s_i is defined as

$$ss_i = \left| \frac{< F_1, F_2 >}{|F_1||F_2|} \right| \in [0, 1], \tag{1}$$

where $F_1 = [a_1, b_1, c_1]$, $F_2 = [a_2, b_2, c_2]$, $<>$ is the dot product operation and $||$ measures the length of the vector. Furthermore, if $|s_i| < 0.9 \cdot |l_i|$ or $|s_i| > 1.2 \cdot |l_i|$, the shape similarity ss_i is manually set as 0. Based on the shape similarity measurement, the shape similarity loss L_s for pixels in the generated segmentation map located within the 3-pixel searching range is constructed as $L_s = w_s \cdot (1 - ss)$, where w_s is set to 4 to increase the importance of the shape similarity loss in the overall loss calculation.

Weighted Pixel-Wise Cross-Entropy Loss. To better identify close and/or adhesive gland instances individually and inspired by the weight matrix in the *U-Net* model [6], we construct a weight matrix W which effectively increases the importance of those background pixels between close gland instances. For each background pixel i, the weight $w(i)$ is defined as

$$w(i) = 1 + w_0 \cdot \frac{1}{1 + e^{d_1(i) + d_2(i) - \mu}}, \tag{2}$$

where d_1 denotes the distance to the nearest gland and d_2 is the distance to the second nearest gland. In our experiments we set $w_0 = 6$ and $\mu = 15$ pixels.

Accordingly, the shape-preserving loss L can be formulated as

$$L = W \cdot L_p \cdot (1 + L_s), \tag{3}$$

where L_p is the overall pixel-wise cross-entropy loss for gland segmentation.

2.2 Deep Convolutional Neural Network

In terms of the deep learning architecture, we design the deep model with reference to the *HED* model [7,8] which was proposed for edge/contour detection. Since the deep model has multiple side outputs, the model is able to learn accurate boundary detection by the first several side outputs and accurate pixel-wise gland segmentation by the last few side outputs. As the shape-preserving loss re-balances the importance between boundary detection and pixel-wise gland segmentation, the training process is controllable and is able to converge quickly.

3   Evaluation and Discussion

We evaluated the proposed deep model on the 2015 MICCAI Gland Challenge dataset [9]. Three officially provided metrics are used for the performance evaluation: (1) the F1 score, (2) the object-level dice score and (3) the object-level Hausdorff distance. We compared our method with three state-of-the-art methods, *i.e.* Chen *et al.* [4] which achieved the best results in the 2015 MICCAI Gland Segmentation Challenge and the multi-channel deep models proposed by Xu *et al.* [2,3] which reported the best performance so far on this dataset. Table 1 shows the comparison results among these methods. Based on the construction of the proposed shape-preserving loss, the deep model is able to identify different glands individually which helps achieve the best performance in the F1 score. As the shape similarity measurement in the shape-preserving loss allows limited boundary location variation, the performance of the deep model in terms of the object-level dice score would be slightly influenced. Since the radius of the searching range adopted is set to only 3 pixels, the influence would be relatively limited and the deep model can still achieve top results. Similarly, as the shape similarity measurement is different from the definition of the Hausdorff distance, the performance may also be influenced. In short, the deep model with the proposed shape-preserving loss achieves the best overall performance (Fig. 3).

Exemplar segmentation results are shown in Fig. 4. Compared to the manual annotations, the deep model can effectively segment different glands individually and preserve shapes of glands accurately. Although boundaries of the segmented glands are slightly different from those annotated boundaries at the pixel-wise

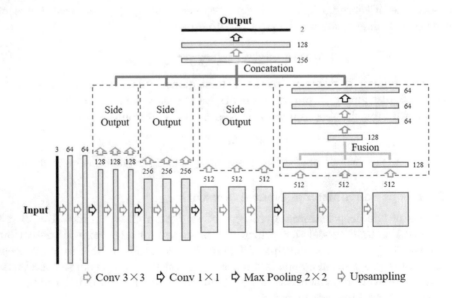

⇨ Conv 3×3   ⇨ Conv 1×1   ⇨ Max Pooling 2×2   ⇨ Upsampling

Fig. 3. The overview of the proposed deep model trained by the shape-preserving loss.

Table 1. Comparison results among different methods on the public dataset.

Method	F1 Score		ObjectDice		ObjectHausdorff	
	Part A	Part B	Part A	Part B	Part A	Part B
Ours	**0.924**	**0.844**	0.902	**0.840**	49.881	**106.075**
Xu [2]	0.893	0.843	**0.908**	0.833	**44.129**	116.821
Xu [3]	0.858	0.771	0.888	0.815	54.202	129.930
Chen [4]	0.912	0.716	0.897	0.781	45.418	160.347

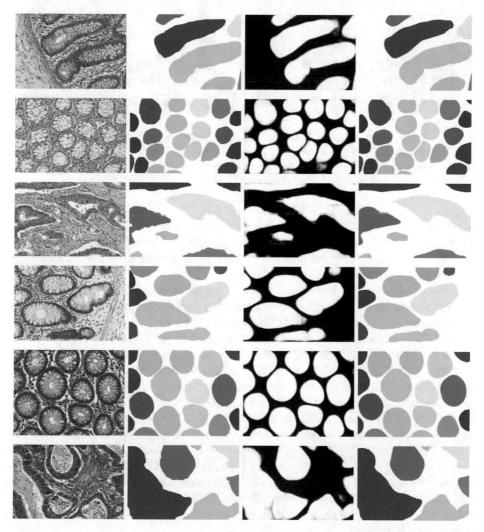

Fig. 4. Exemplar segmentation results obtained by the proposed deep model. For each row, from left to right: raw histology patch, manual annotation, generated probability map and the output segmentation map. In both manual annotation and output segmentation map, different glands are assigned with different colors.

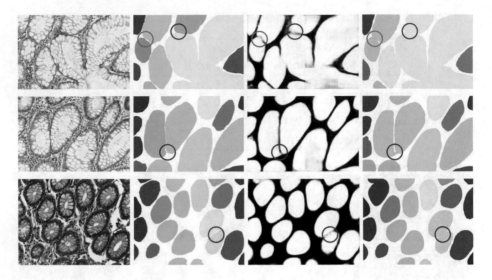

Fig. 5. Challenging cases in dealing with close boundaries. For each row, from left to right: raw histology patch, manual annotation, generated probability map and the output segmentation map. In both manual annotation and output segmentation map, different glands are assigned with different colors.

level, the shapes of different glands are well preserved, which is quite important for further diagnosis. In dealing with close glands, due to the constructed weight matrix, the deep model can effectively separate close glands although the gaps between close glands are slightly enlarged.

Several challenging cases are shown in Fig. 5. As we adopt a new shape similarity measurement instead of the pixel-wise cross-entropy measurement, the deep model should be able to detect boundaries more effectively. However, as we directly adopt the Otsu thresholding method to generate final segmentation maps for evaluation, some background pixels may not be successfully identified although the probability values are relatively lower than those neighboring gland pixels. One possible way to solve the problem is to search for an optimal threshold to generate the final segmentation map or to utilize an adaptive local thresholding scheme. These solutions will be explored in our future work as post-processing for performance improvement. Another issue is caused by the curve fitting method in the shape similarity measurement as shown in the second row of Fig. 5. Since the lengths of l_i and s_i in (1) are not required to be exactly the same, it is possible that although most boundary pixels are correctly identified, two glands may be wrongly connected by some discrete pixels. One solution to address the problem is to reduce the default length in the boundary segmentation process as discussed in Sect. 2.1.

Exemplar failure cases are shown in Fig. 6. The main reason for these failures is the shortage of corresponding training samples. One interesting observation is that although the deep model fails to identify some glands, the boundaries of

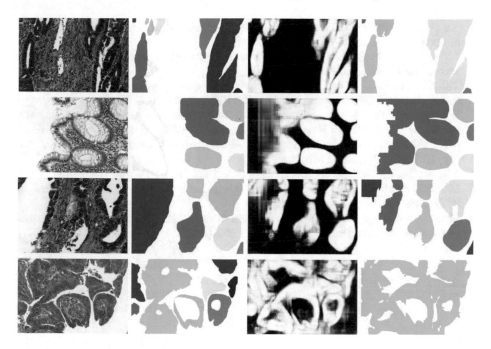

Fig. 6. Exemplar bad results generated by the proposed deep model. For each row, from left to right: raw histology patch, manual annotation, generated probability map and the output segmentation map. In both manual annotation and output segmentation map, different glands are assigned with different colors.

most segmented glands are quite similar to those annotated boundaries, which demonstrates the effectiveness of the proposed loss in shape preservation.

4   Conclusion

In this paper, we propose a deep model with a new shape-preserving loss that achieves the best overall performance on gland instance segmentation. Compared to the current best-known multi-channel/-task deep models, the shape-preserving loss enables one single deep model to generate accurate gland instance segmentation, which could largely reduce the model complexity and could be utilized in any other deep learning models for medical image segmentation.

References

1. Fleming, M., et al.: Colorectal carcinoma: pathologic aspects. J. Gastrointest. Oncol. **3**(3), 153–173 (2012)
2. Xu, Y., et al.: Gland instance segmentation using deep multichannel neural networks. IEEE Trans. Med. Imaging **64**(12), 2901–2912 (2017)

3. Xu, Y., et al.: Gland instance segmentation by deep multichannel neural networks. arXiv preprint arXiv:1607.04889 (2016)
4. Chen, H., et al.: DCAN: deep contour-aware networks for accurate gland segmentation. In: CVPR, pp. 2487–2496 (2016)
5. Yan, Z., et al.: A skeletal similarity metric for quality evaluation of retinal vessel segmentation. IEEE Trans. Med. Imaging **37**(4), 1045–1057 (2017)
6. Ronneberger, O., Fischer, P., Brox, T.: U-Net: convolutional networks for biomedical image segmentation. In: Navab, N., Hornegger, J., Wells, W.M., Frangi, A.F. (eds.) MICCAI 2015. LNCS, vol. 9351, pp. 234–241. Springer, Cham (2015). https://doi.org/10.1007/978-3-319-24574-4_28
7. Xie, S., Tu, Z.: Holistically-nested edge detection. In: ICCV, pp. 1395–1403 (2015)
8. Liu, Y., et al.: Richer convolutional features for edge detection. In: CVPR, pp. 5872–5881 (2017)
9. Sirinukunwattana, K.: Gland segmentation in colon histology images: the GlaS challenge contest. Med. Image Anal. **35**, 489–502 (2017)

Model-Based Refinement of Nonlinear Registrations in 3D Histology Reconstruction

Juan Eugenio Iglesias[1]([⊠]), Marco Lorenzi[2], Sebastiano Ferraris[1], Loïc Peter[5],
Marc Modat[1], Allison Stevens[3], Bruce Fischl[3,4], and Tom Vercauteren[5]

[1] Medical Physics and Biomedical Engineering,
University College London, London, UK
[2] Epione Team, INRIA Sophia Antipolis, Sophia Antipolis Cedex, France
[3] Martinos Center for Biomedical Imaging, Harvard Medical School
and Massachusetts General Hospital, Boston, USA
[4] MIT Computer Science and Artificial Intelligence Laboratory, Cambridge, USA
[5] Wellcome EPSRC Centre for Interventional and Surgical Sciences (WEISS),
University College London, London, UK

Abstract. Recovering the 3D structure of a stack of histological sections
(3D histology reconstruction) requires a linearly aligned reference volume
in order to minimize z-shift and "banana effect". Reconstruction can then
be achieved by computing 2D registrations between each section and its
corresponding resampled slice in the volume. However, these registrations are often inaccurate due to their inter-modality nature and to the
strongly nonlinear deformations introduced by histological processing.
Here we introduce a probabilistic model of spatial deformations to efficiently refine these registrations, without the need to revisit the imaging
data. Our method takes as input a set of nonlinear registrations between
pairs of 2D images (within or across modalities), and uses Bayesian inference to estimate the most likely spanning tree of latent transformations
that generated the measured deformations. Results on synthetic and real
data show that our algorithm can effectively 3D reconstruct the histology
while being robust to z-shift and banana effect. An implementation of the
approach, which is compatible with a wide array of existing registration
methods, is available at JEI's website: www.jeiglesias.com.

1 Introduction

Combining histology with mm-scale volumetric images finds multiple applications in areas such as atlas building (e.g., [1]) or modeling the relationship
between the information at micro- and macro-scale (e.g., [2]). Combining the two
modalities requires histology reconstruction, i.e., registration of 2D histological
sections to volumes to recover the lost 3D structure. The role of the reference
volume is critical in reconstruction; in its absence, one can only resort to pairwise

M. Modat and T. Vercauteren—Currently with the School of Biomedical Engineering
and Imaging Science, King's College London.

© Springer Nature Switzerland AG 2018
A. F. Frangi et al. (Eds.): MICCAI 2018, LNCS 11071, pp. 147–155, 2018.
https://doi.org/10.1007/978-3-030-00934-2_17

registration of the histological sections [3], which leads to z-shift (accumulation of registration errors) and banana effect (straightening of curved structures). In the remainder we assume that a reference volume is always available.

Most reconstruction methods assume that the nonlinear deformations in the histological sections occur within plane. Then, reconstruction can be decoupled into estimating a 3D transformation (often linear) between the histological stack and the volume, and estimating a set of nonlinear 2D transformations between each section and the corresponding resampled plane in the registered volume. An intermediate modality is sometimes used to estimate the 3D transformation; e.g., blockface photographs can be stacked and linearly registered to the reference volume [4]. Otherwise, the two problems can be solved iteratively, i.e., optimizing a 3D transformation with the 2D deformations fixed, and vice versa [5].

If the 3D registration is fixed, any 2D, nonlinear, intermodality registration algorithm can be used to align the histological sections to the corresponding resampled slices in the reference volume. However, this baseline approach often yields jagged reconstructions, as this registration problem is difficult to solve due to two reasons: the large and slice-varying differences in intensity and contrast profiles between the modalities; and the extensive geometric distortion introduced by sectioning and mounting of the tissue – including folding and tears.

Smoother, more accurate reconstructions, can be obtained by considering neighboring sections when computing the 2D registrations, e.g., a section is deformed to match not only the corresponding resampled slice, but also the sections right above and below [1]. This approach unfortunately inherits the efficiency limitations of coordinate descent, and is thus computationally expensive: it requires many passes over each slice, and the use of a cost function with three channels. For instance, 20–25 reconstruction iterations were required on average in [1], hence running 60–70 times slower than the baseline approach.

A faster alternative is to first compute 2D nonlinear registrations between neighboring histological sections, and then use them regularize the 2D transformations between the histology and the reference volume. Since images are not revisited to update registrations, such approaches are computationally efficient. For example, poor linear registrations between neighboring sections are corrected by registration to other neighbors in [6]. Other approaches seek smoothness in the z direction with low-pass filtering in linear [5,6] or nonlinear transformation spaces [7]. However, the optimality of such *ad hoc* approaches is unclear; e.g., early stopping is required in [7] as it converges to a solution with banana effect.

Here we present a probabilistic model in the space of 2D nonlinear spatial deformations, which accommodates measurements (2D registrations) between arbitrary pairs of sections and slices, neighboring or not, within or across modalities. The measurements are assumed to be noisy observations of compositions of latent transformations, which interconnect all the images in the two datasets through a spanning tree. We then use Bayesian inference to estimate the most likely latent transformations that generated the observations. Compared to previous works: 1. We explicitly optimize a principled objective function, which achieves smooth registrations while minimizing z-shift and banana effect;

2. Model parameters are estimated in inference (no parameter tuning required); and 3. Thanks to approximate composition of stationary velocity fields (SVF) [8], the latent transformations can be globally and efficiently optimized for fixed model parameters.

2   Methods

2.1   Probabilistic Framework

Let $\{H_n(\boldsymbol{x})\}_{n=1,...,N}$ be a stack of N histological sections, where $\boldsymbol{x} \in \Omega$ represents the pixel locations over a discrete, 2D image domain Ω. Let $\{M_n(\boldsymbol{x})\}_{n=1,...,N}$ be the corresponding slices of the reference volume, which we will henceforth assume to be an MRI scan. We further assume that the MRI and histological stack have been linearly aligned (e.g., with [5]). Let $\{\mathcal{T}_n\}_{n=1,...,2N-1}$ be a set of $2N - 1$ latent, noise-free, nonlinear, diffeormorphic spatial transformations, which yield a spanning tree interconnecting all the images in the two datasets. Although our algorithm is independent of the choice of tree, we use for convenience the convention in Fig. 1a: $\mathcal{T}_n$, for $n \leq N$, registers histological section n to MRI slice n (i.e., maps coordinates from MRI space to histology); and $\mathcal{T}_{N+n}$ maps MRI slice n to MRI slice $n + 1$, thereby modeling the banana effect and z-shift.

Now, let $\{\mathcal{R}_k\}_{k=1,...,K}$ be a set of K diffeomorphic transformations between pairs of images in the dataset (*any* pair, within or across modalities), estimated with an image registration method. $\mathcal{R}_k$ can be seen as a noisy version of a transformation equal to the composition of a subset of (possibly inverted) latent transformations of the spanning tree $\{\mathcal{T}_n\}$. In general, K will be several times larger than N, and we can use Bayesian inference to estimate the latent transformations $\{\mathcal{T}_n\}$ that most likely generated the observed registrations $\{\mathcal{R}_k\}$.

Our choice of modeling nonlinear spatial transformation with diffeomorphisms is motivated by the Log-Euclidean framework, in which transformations are parameterized in the Lie group of SVFs [8]. Let $\{\boldsymbol{T}_n\}$ and $\{\boldsymbol{R}_k\}$ be the SVFs of the transformations, whose Lie exponentials are the corresponding diffeomorphisms $\{\mathcal{T}_n\}$ and $\{\mathcal{R}_k\}$, i.e., $\mathcal{T}_n = \exp[\boldsymbol{T}_n]$ and $\mathcal{R}_k = \exp[\boldsymbol{R}_k]$. Then, it follows (one-parameter subgroup property) that the inverse of a transformation is equivalent to its negation in the Log-space, i.e., $\mathcal{T}_n^{-1} = \exp[-\boldsymbol{T}_n]$. Moreover, the composition of diffeomorphisms parameterized by SVFs is given by $\boldsymbol{T}_n \oplus \boldsymbol{T}_{n'} = \log[\exp(\boldsymbol{T}_n) \circ \exp(\boldsymbol{T}_{n'})]$, whose analytical solution is provided by the Baker-Campbell-Hausdorff (BCH) series. By truncating the Lie bracket and considering only its first order terms, the BCH series can be approximated by: $\mathcal{T}_n \circ \mathcal{T}_{n'} \approx \exp[\boldsymbol{T}_n + \boldsymbol{T}_{n'}]$. While this approximation theoretically only holds for relatively small deformations, it is commonplace in state-of-the-art registration methods (e.g., [9]), and also enables us to globally optimize the objective function with respect to the transformations in inference – see Sect. 2.2 below.

To model the noise in the registrations, we choose an isotropic Gaussian model in the Log-space, which, despite its simplicity, works well in practice (e.g., [8]). Henceforth, we will assume that $\boldsymbol{T}_n$ and $\boldsymbol{R}_k$ are shaped as $|\Omega| \times 1$ vectors. Then, the SVFs of the registrations are independent and distributed as:

$$\boldsymbol{R}_k \sim \mathcal{N}\left(\sum_{n=1}^{2N-1} w_{k,n}\boldsymbol{T}_n, \sigma_k^2 \boldsymbol{I}\right),$$

where $\mathcal{N}$ is the Gaussian distribution; σ_k^2 is the variance of the kth measurement; $\boldsymbol{I}$ is the identity matrix; and $W := (w_{k,n})$, with $w_{k,n} \in \{-1, 0, 1\}$, is a matrix encoding the latent transformations that the registrations $\{\mathcal{R}_k\}$ traverse. Therefore, $\boldsymbol{R}_k$ is a Gaussian distribution centered on the concatenation of latent transformations corresponding to the measurement. More specifically, $w_{k,n} = 1$ if $\mathcal{T}_n$ is part of the path traversed by $\mathcal{R}_k$ with positive orientation, $w_{k,n} = -1$ if it is part of it with negative orientation, and $w_{k,n} = 0$ otherwise. Therefore, if a measurement estimates a transform from MRI slice n' to MRI slice $n'' \geq n'$, then $w_{k,n} = 1$, for $n' + N \leq n < n'' + N$, and 0 otherwise. If the measurement is from MRI slice n' to histological section n'', then $w_{k,n''} = 1$ needs to be added to W. And if the measurement is between histological sections n' and n'', then we need to set $w_{k,n'} = -1$ in W, as well (see example in Fig. 1b).

The probabilistic framework is completed by a model for σ_k^2. A simple choice that we found to work well in practice is:

$$\sigma_k^2 = c_k \sigma_c^2 + d_k \sigma_d^2,$$

where $c_k = 1$ when transformation k is across modalities (0 otherwise); d_k is the number of sections or slices that $\mathcal{R}_k$ traverses; and σ_c^2 and σ_d^2 are the associated variance parameters, which will be estimated in inference – details below.

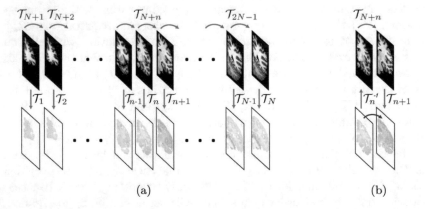

(a)   (b)

Fig. 1. (a) Latent transformations $\{\mathcal{T}_n\}$ connecting the MRI and histological sections in the proposed model. A transformation between any pair of images can be written as the composition of a subset of (possibly inverted) transformations in $\{\mathcal{T}_n\}$. For example, the transformation represented by the red arrow in (b) can be written as: $\mathcal{T}_n^{-1} \circ \mathcal{T}_{N+n} \circ \mathcal{T}_{n+1}$ – or, in log-Euclidean framework, approximated as $\exp[-\boldsymbol{T}_n + \boldsymbol{T}_{N+n} + \boldsymbol{T}_{n+1}]$.

2.2   Inference: Proposed Method

In a fully Bayesian approach, one would optimize the posterior probability of the first N transformations $\{\mathcal{T}_n\}_{n=1,\ldots,N}$ given the observations $\{\boldsymbol{R}_k\}$. However, computing such a posterior requires marginalizing over the remaining $N-1$ transformations and the variances σ_c^2, σ_d^2. A much simpler and faster inference algorithm can be derived by maximizing the joint posterior of all latent transforms $\{\mathcal{T}_n\}_{n=1,\ldots,2N-1}$ and variances $[\sigma_c^2, \sigma_d^2]^{\mathrm{T}}$, which is a good approximation because: 1. the uncertainty in the intramodality transformations ($n \leq N$) is much lower than that in the intermodality transformations ($n > N$); and 2. the two noise parameters can be accurately estimated, given residuals at $K|\Omega|$ locations. Using Bayes' rule and taking logarithm, we obtain the cost function:

$$
\operatorname*{argmax}_{\{\boldsymbol{T}_n\}, \sigma_c^2, \sigma_d^2} p(\{\boldsymbol{T}_n\}, \sigma_c^2, \sigma_d^2 | \{\boldsymbol{R}_k\}) = \operatorname*{argmax}_{\{\boldsymbol{T}_n\}, \sigma_c^2, \sigma_d^2} p(\{\boldsymbol{R}_k\} | \{\boldsymbol{T}_n\}, \sigma_c^2, \sigma_d^2)
$$

$$
= \operatorname*{argmin}_{\{\boldsymbol{T}_n\}, \sigma_c^2, \sigma_d^2} \sum_{k=1}^{K} \left[|\Omega| \log \left[2\pi \left(c_k \sigma_c^2 + d_k \sigma_d^2 \right) \right] + \frac{\| \boldsymbol{R}_k - \sum_{n=1}^{2N-1} w_{k,n} \boldsymbol{T}_n \|^2}{2 \left(c_k \sigma_c^2 + d_k \sigma_d^2 \right)} \right], \quad (1)
$$

which we alternately minimize with respect to $\{\boldsymbol{T}_n\}$ and $[\sigma_c^2, \sigma_d^2]^{\mathrm{T}}$.

Update for the Transformations: Since we approximate composition by addition in the space of SVFs, optimizing Eq. 1 with respect to $\{\boldsymbol{T}_n\}$ is just a weighted least squares problem, with a closed form expression for its global optimum. Moreover, and since W does not depend on pixel locations, the solution is given by a location-independent set of regression coefficients:

$$
\boldsymbol{T}_n \leftarrow \sum_{k=1}^{K} z_{n,k} \boldsymbol{R}_k, \quad \text{with} \quad Z = \left(W^{\mathrm{T}} \operatorname{diag}(1/\sigma_k^2) W \right)^{-1} W^{\mathrm{T}} \operatorname{diag}(1/\sigma_k^2), \quad (2)
$$

where $Z := (z_{n,k})$ is the matrix of regression coefficients. We note that *all* measurements can impact the estimation of every deformation.

Update for the Variances: We update the variances σ_c^2 and σ_d^2 simultaneously using a quasi-Newton method (L-BFGS). The gradient of the cost in Eq. 1 is:

$$
\nabla_\sigma \mathcal{C} = \sum_{k=1}^{K} \left(\frac{|\Omega|}{c_k \sigma_c^2 + d_k \sigma_d^2} - \frac{E_k}{2(c_k \sigma_c^2 + d_k \sigma_d^2)^2} \right) [c_k, d_k]^{\mathrm{T}}, \quad (3)
$$

where $E_k = \| \boldsymbol{R}_k - \sum_{n=1}^{2N-1} w_{k,n} \boldsymbol{T}_n \|^2$ is the energy of the kth residual.

Practical Implementation: We initialize the $\{\mathcal{T}_n\}$ with direct measurements, i.e., registrations $\{\mathcal{R}_k\}$ that map the same pairs of images as $\{\mathcal{T}_n\}$. Next, we compute the average squared error $S = (K|\Omega|)^{-1} \sum_k E_k$, and initialize $\sigma_c^2 = 3S$, $\sigma_d^2 = S/3$, such that $\sigma_c^2 \approx 10\sigma_d^2$. Finally, we iterate between updating $\{\mathcal{T}_n\}$ (with Eq. 2) and $[\sigma_c^2, \sigma_d^2]^{\mathrm{T}}$ (numerically with the gradient in Eq. 3). The algorithm often converges in 3–4 iterations (approximately an hour, including registrations).

3   Experiments and Results

3.1   Data

We validated our method quantitatively on a synthetic dataset, and qualitatively on a real dataset. The synthetic dataset consists of 100 randomly selected cases from the publicly available, multimodal IXI dataset (`brain-development.org/ixi-dataset`). After skull stripping with ROBEX [10], we generated synthetic 2D deformation fields independently for each slice, and applied them to the T2 images to simulate the geometric distortion of the histological processing. Then, we used the T1 volume as reference to recover the deformation in the T2 slices. The synthetic fields were created by composing a random similarity transformation with a nonlinear deformation; the latter was computed as the integration of a random SVF generated as smoothed Gaussian noise.

The real dataset consists of the Allen atlas [11], publicly available at http:// atlas.brain-map.org. This dataset includes a multiecho flash MRI scan acquired on a 7 T scanner at 200 µm resolution, and 679 Nissl-stained, 50 µm thick, coronal, histological sections of a left hemisphere. Manual segmentations of 862 brain structures are available for a subset of 106 sections. We downsampled the images from 1 µm to 200 µm to match the resolution of the MRI. We used the algorithm in [5] to linearly align the MRI and the stack of histological sections.

3.2   Experiments on Synthetic Dataset

We computed all registrations with NiftyReg, using the SVF parametrization ("-vel") [9]. We affinely prealigned each distorted T2 slice to its T1 counterpart, in order to keep $\{R_k\}$ as small as possible – and hence minimize the error in the approximation in the BCH series. We computed the following registrations: 1. intermodality, between corresponding T1 and T2 slices; 2. intramodality, between each T1 slice and up to four slices right above; and 3. intramodality, between each T2 slice and up to four slices right above. The intermodality registrations used mutual information and 8 pixel control point spacing. Within modalities, we used local normalized cross correlation and 4 pixel spacing (since it is more reliable than intermodality). We then used the proposed method to recover the deformations, using between 0 and 4 intramodality neighbors – where 0 corresponds to the baseline approach, i.e., slice-wise, intermodality registration.

Figure 2a shows the root mean square (RMS) error of the registration, whereas Fig. 2b shows sample outputs of the method. The baseline approach produces very jagged contours around the cortex and ventricles. The proposed approach, on the other hand, produces smoother registrations that yield a reduction of approximately 25% in the RMS error when two neighbors are used. When a higher number of neighbors are considered, the results are still smooth, but z-shift starts to accumulate, leading to higher RMS error; see for instance the hypointense area on the hippocampus in the example in Fig. 2b (blue arrow).

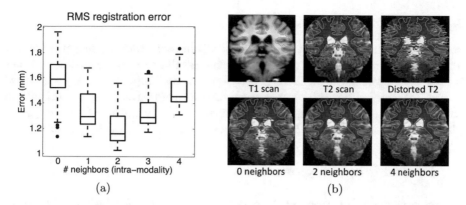

Fig. 2. (a) Box plot for RMS registration errors in synthetic dataset. The central mark is the median; the box edges are the first and third quartile; whiskers extend to the most extreme data points not considered outliers (marked as dots). (b) A sample coronal slice from the synthetic dataset, distorted and subsequently corrected with the baseline (i.e., 0 intramodality neighbors) and proposed method (with 2 and 4 neighbors). We have superimposed the contour of the lateral ventricles (red) and white matter surface (green), manually delineated on the T1 slice. The blue arrow marks an area with z-shift.

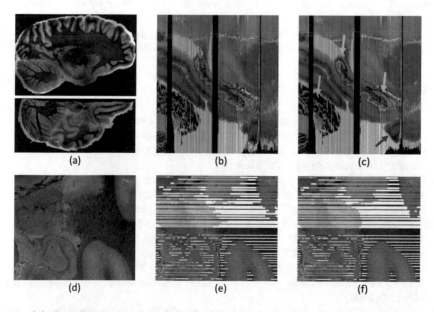

Fig. 3. (a) Sample slices of the *ex vivo* MRI of the Allen atlas. (b) Close-up of hippocampus, with histological reconstruction computed with the baseline approach. (c) Same region, reconstructed with the proposed method. (d) Close-up of axial MRI slice. (e) Reconstruction of manual segmentations with baseline approach. (f) Reconstruction with our method. The color map can be found on the Allen Institute website.

3.3   Experiments on Allen Dataset

For the Allen data, we used two neighbors within each stack, as suggested by the results on the synthetic dataset. Qualitative results are shown in Fig. 3. Much crisper reconstruction is achieved in areas such as the hippocampus (green arrows in Fig. 3c), cerebellum (blue) or cortical area 36 (red). Likewise, segmentations are more accurately propagated in areas such as the nuclei of the amygdala (different shades of green if Fig. 3e–f) and cortical regions (shades of pink).

4   Discussion and Conclusion

We have presented a probabilistic model for refining deformation fields in 3D histology reconstruction based on SVFs, and thus directly compatible with many widespread registration methods. Our model also serves as a starting point for future work in four main directions: 1. Inspecting better approximations to the composition of transformations; 2. Considering more realistic models for the registration errors, which account for their spatial correlation; 3. Investigating other noise models, which are more robust to outliers; and 4. Integrating an intensity homogenization model in the framework to correct for uneven section staining. The presented method is available at JEI's site: www.jeiglesias.com.

Acknowledgement. Supported by the ERC (Starting Grant 677697, awarded to JEI), Wellcome Trust (WT101957) and EPSRC (NS/A000027/1).

References

1. Adler, D.H., et al.: Histology-derived volumetric annotation of the human hippocampal subfields in postmortem MRI. Neuroimage **84**, 505–523 (2014)
2. Stikov, N., et al.: In vivo histology of the myelin g-ratio with magnetic resonance imaging. Neuroimage **118**, 397–405 (2015)
3. Ourselin, S., Roche, A., Prima, S., Ayache, N.: Block matching: a general framework to improve robustness of rigid registration of medical images. In: Delp, S.L., DiGoia, A.M., Jaramaz, B. (eds.) MICCAI 2000. LNCS, vol. 1935, pp. 557–566. Springer, Heidelberg (2000). https://doi.org/10.1007/978-3-540-40899-4_57
4. Amunts, K., et al.: BigBrain: an ultrahigh-resolution 3D human brain model. Science **340**(6139), 1472–1475 (2013)
5. Malandain, G., Bardinet, E., Nelissen, K., Vanduffel, W.: Fusion of autoradiographs with an MR volume using 2-D and 3-D linear transformations. NeuroImage **23**(1), 111–127 (2004)
6. Yushkevich, P., et al.: 3D mouse brain reconstruction from histology using a coarse-to-fine approach. In: Pluim, J.P.W., Likar, B., Gerritsen, F.A. (eds.) WBIR 2006. LNCS, vol. 4057, pp. 230–237. Springer, Heidelberg (2006). https://doi.org/10.1007/11784012_28
7. Casero, R., et al.: Transformation diffusion reconstruction of 3D histology volumes from 2D image stacks. Med. Image Anal. **38**, 184–204 (2017)

8. Arsigny, V., Commowick, O., Pennec, X., Ayache, N.: A log-euclidean framework for statistics on diffeomorphisms. In: Larsen, R., Nielsen, M., Sporring, J. (eds.) MICCAI 2006. LNCS, vol. 4190, pp. 924–931. Springer, Heidelberg (2006). https:// doi.org/10.1007/11866565_113
9. Modat, M., Daga, P., Cardoso, M.J., Ourselin, S., Ridgway, G.R., Ashburner, J.: Parametric non-rigid registration using a stationary velocity field. In: Mathematical Methods in Biomedical Image Analysis, pp. 145–150 (2012)
10. Iglesias, J.E., Liu, C.Y., Thompson, P.M., Tu, Z.: Robust brain extraction across datasets and comparison with publicly available methods. IEEE Trans. Med. Imaging **30**(9), 1617–1634 (2011)
11. Ding, S.L., et al.: Comprehensive cellular-resolution atlas of the adult human brain. J. Comp. Neurol. **524**(16), 3127–3481 (2016)

Invasive Cancer Detection Utilizing Compressed Convolutional Neural Network and Transfer Learning

Bin Kong[1], Shanhui Sun[2(✉)], Xin Wang[2], Qi Song[2], and Shaoting Zhang[1(✉)]

[1] Department of Computer Science, UNC Charlotte, Charlotte, NC, USA
szhang16@uncc.edu
[2] CuraCloud Corporation, Seattle, WA, USA
shanhuis@curacloudcorp.com

Abstract. Identification of invasive cancer in Whole Slide Images (WSIs) is crucial for tumor staging as well as treatment planning. However, the precise manual delineation of tumor regions is challenging, tedious and time-consuming. Thus, automatic invasive cancer detection in WSIs is of significant importance. Recently, Convolutional Neural Network (CNN) based approaches advanced invasive cancer detection. However, computation burdens of these approaches become barriers in clinical applications. In this work, we propose to detect invasive cancer employing a lightweight network in a fully convolution fashion without model ensembles. In order to improve the small network's detection accuracy, we utilized the "soft labels" of a large capacity network to supervise its training process. Additionally, we adopt a teacher guided loss to help the small network better learn from the intermediate layers of the high capacity network. With this suite of approaches, our network is extremely efficient as well as accurate. The proposed method is validated on two large scale WSI datasets. Our approach is performed in an average time of 0.6 and 3.6 min per WSI with a single GPU on our gastric cancer dataset and CAMELYON16, respectively, about 5 times faster than Google Inception V3. We achieved an average FROC of 81.1% and 85.6% respectively, which are on par with Google Inception V3. The proposed method requires less high performance computing resources than state-of-the-art methods, which makes the invasive cancer diagnosis more applicable in the clinical usage.

1 Introduction

Invasive cancer is one of the leading worldwide health problems and the second killer in the United States [13]. Early diagnosis of invasive cancers with timely treatment can significantly reduce the mortality rate. Traditionally, the cancer regions of Whole Slide Images (WSIs) are delineated by experienced pathologists for histological analysis. However, precise delineation of the tumor regions and identification of the nuclei for pathologists are time-consuming and error-prone. Thus, Computer-aided diagnosis (CAD) methods are required to assist

© Springer Nature Switzerland AG 2018
A. F. Frangi et al. (Eds.): MICCAI 2018, LNCS 11071, pp. 156–164, 2018.
https://doi.org/10.1007/978-3-030-00934-2_18

pathologists' diagnostic tasks. However, WSI has a large image resolution up to $200,000 \times 100,000$ pixels and traditional methods are usually limited to only small regions of the WSIs considering the computational burden.

Recently, with deep learning becoming the methodology of choice [1,5], many work focus on applying these powerful techniques on directly analyzing WSIs. In the context of WSI cancer detection, the common practice is to extract patches of fixed size (e.g., 256×256) in a sliding window fashion and feed them to a neural network for prediction. In [16], GoogleNet [14] is utilized as the detector. Kong et al. [6] extended this approach considering neighborhood context information decoded using a recurrent neural network. Using model ensembles (i.e., several Inception V3 models [15]), Liu et al. [8] brings the detection result to 88.5% in terms of average FROC on CAMELYON16 [1] dataset. The above deep learning based methods face the common problem: the computation is expensive which becomes barriers to clinical deployment.

One of the most challenging problems for WSI image analytics is handling large scale images (e.g., 2 GB). High performance computing resources such as cloud computing and HPC machines mitigate the computational challenges. However, they either have a data traffic problem or are not always available due to high cost. Thus, high accuracy and efficiency become essential for deploying WSI invasive cancer diagnosis software into the clinical applications. In the previous work, there is few focusing on both accuracy and computation efficiency in computer-aided WSI cancer diagnosis. Resource efficiency in neural network study such as network compression is an active research topic. Product quantization [17], hashing, Huffman coding, and low bit networks [10] have been studied but they sacrifice accuracy.

How to make the invasive cancer detection system as efficient as possible while maintaining the accuracy? We answer this question with a suite of training and inference techniques: (1) For efficiency we design a small capacity network based on depthwise separable convolution [1]; (2) To improve accuracy, we refine the small capacity network learning from a large capacity network on the same training dataset. We enforced the logits layer of the small capacity network has a close response as logits layer of the large capacity network. A similar approach was investigated in work [2]. In addition to that, we use an additional teacher guided loss to help the small network better learn from the intermediate layers of the high capacity network; (3) To further speed up the computation in the inference stage, we avoid the procedure of frequently extracting small patches in a sliding window fashion but instead, we convert the model into a fully convolution network (a network does not have multilayer perceptron layers). As a result, our method is 5 times faster compared to one of the popular and state-of-the-art benchmark solutions without sacrificing accuracy.

In summary, the major contributions of this work are as follows: (1) We designed a multi-stage deep learning based approach to locate invasive cancer regions with discriminative local cues; (2) Instead of relying on histological level annotation such as nuclei centers and cell masks, the proposed method auto-

---

[1] https://camelyon16.grand-challenge.org/.

matically learn to identify these regions based on the regional annotation, which are much easier to obtain. Thus, our approach is extremely scalable. (3) We designed a novel method to shrink the large capacity network while maintaining its accuracy. (4) Our method is extensively validated on two large scale WSI dataset: gastric cancer dataset and CAMELYON16. The results demonstrate its superior performance in both its efficiency and accuracy.

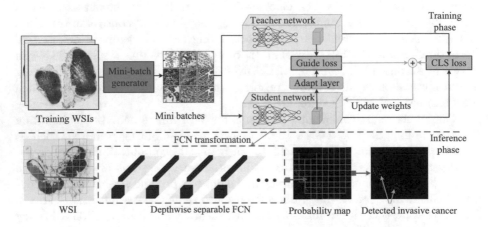

Fig. 1. Overview of the proposed framework. The above part indicates the training phase and below part indicates inference phase. Note that we only illustrate proposed transfer learning method in the training phase.

2   Methodology

2.1   Overview

Figure 1 shows an overview of our proposed method. The method is derived from detection by performing patch classification (normal patches vs cancer patches) via a sliding window. However, it is different from the traditional method of detection by performing classification. The base network is a small capacity network proposed for solving patch classification problem with a faster inference speed than a large capacity network.

This small network is trained on the training patches. The small capacity network has weak learning capability due to small number of learnable weights and may cause under-fitting and lower inference accuracy than the large capacity network in the inference stage. To solve this problem, we enforce the small capacity network learning the "useful knowledge" from the high capacity network in order to improve inference accuracy. Thus, we first train a high capacity network on the same training set. Then, we distill small capacity network's weights in a fine-tuning stage discussed in Sect. 2.3. In the inference stage, we convert multilayer perceptron layers (fully connected layers) of the network into fully convolution layers (fcn layers). This change allows the network using arbitrary sized tiles so that we can use large tiles resulting in faster speed. The output probability map is post-processed and detection results are produced from it using a method similar to [8].

The training objective function can be denoted as follows:

$$L = \frac{1}{|\mathbb{S}|} \sum_{x \in \mathbb{S}} (L_{cls}(x) + \lambda L_{guide}(x)) + \gamma L_{reg} \tag{1}$$

where $\mathbb{S}$ is the training patches. L_{cls} denotes the classification loss, comprising of the softmax loss using the hard ground truth label of the training patch and the regression loss using the soft probability label from the large capacity network. We will discuss it in detail in Sect. 2.3. L_{guide} is the teacher guided loss, which will be elaborated in Sect. 2.3. L_{reg} denotes the regularization penalty term which punishes large weights. Finally, λ and γ are balancing hyper-parameters to control the weights of difference losses, which are cross-validated in our experiments.

2.2   Small Capacity Network

To reduce the model's capacity, we utilized depthwise separable convolution in our small capacity network architecture. Depthwise separable convolution (depthwise convolution + pointwise convolution) is proposed in [1] and replaces convolution layers. Each kernel in a depthwise convolution layer performs convolution operation on only a single channel of input feature maps. To incorporate cross-channel information and change the number of output feature maps, pointwise convolution (i.e., 1×1 convolution) is applied after depthwise convolution. The depthwise separable convolution in [3] obtains a large factor of reduction in terms of computation comparing to corresponding convolution operations.

2.3   Transfer Learning from Large Capacity Network

We utilized a large capacity network (deep and wide network with more weights) to "teach" the small capacity network and adapt the model moving towards large network's manifold resulting logits of two networks being closer. We use the knowledge of both the output (probability) and intermediate layers (feature) in the large capacity network to teach the small capacity network.

Transfer Learning from the Probability: The network distilling technique proposed in [2] serves this transfer learning task. The softmax layer transforms the logit z_i for each class into the corresponding probability p_i:

$$p_i = \frac{\exp(z_i/T)}{\sum_{j \in \{0,1\}} \exp(z_j/T)} \tag{2}$$

where $i = 0$ and $i = 1$ represent negative and positive labels, respectively. T is the temperature which controls the softness of the probability distribution over the label. A higher temperature $T > 1$ produces soft probabilities distribution over classes, which helps the transfer learning. We used soft regression loss ($L_{soft} = ||p_i - \hat{p}_i||^2$, where p_i and $\hat{p}_i$ are the probabilities produced by the small and large capacity networks, respectively) to enforce small capacity network's outputs to match the large capacity network's outputs. We pre-trained the large capacity network using $T = 2$. In transfer learning, large capacity network's weights are fixed, and $T = 2$ is used in both small and large networks. In prediction, $T = 1$ is used.

We additionally use the hard ground truth label of the training patch to supervise the training. Then, the total classification loss is as follows:

$$L_{cls} = L_{hard} + \beta L_{soft} \tag{3}$$

where L_{hard} denotes the softmax (hard) loss. Hyper-paramter β controls the weights of hard and soft losses, which is cross-validated in our experiments.

Feature Adaptation from the Intermediate Layers: Romero et al. [11] demonstrated that the features learned in the intermediate layers of large capacity networks can be efficiently used to guide the student network to learn effective representations and improve the accuracy of the student network. Inspired by this idea, we apply the L2 distance between feature of the teacher network F_{tea} and the student network F_{stu}, which we name as teacher guided loss:

$$L_{guide} = ||F_{tea} - F_{stu}||^2 \tag{4}$$

While applying teacher guided loss, it is required that shape of the feature map dimension from teacher network should be the same as the student network. However, these two features are from different networks and the shape can be different. Thus, we use an adaptation layer (we use a fully connected layer) to map the feature from the student network to the same shape of the teacher network.

2.4   Efficient Inference

In most of popular WSI detection solutions such as [8,16], fixed-size patch based classification is performed in a sliding window fashion. The number of forward computation is linear to the number of evaluated patches. The memory cannot hold all patches so that frequent I/O operations have to be performed. This is the major source of the computational bottleneck. Inspired by [9], we replace all the fully connected layers in the small capacity network using equivalent convolutional layers. After the transformation, the FCN can take a significantly larger image if the memory allows. Let $size_p$ be the input image size used in a classification network before FCN transformation. After FCN transformation, the output of the network is a 2D probability map. The resolution of the probability map is scaled due to strided convolution and pooling operations. Let d be the scale factor. We assume that n layers (either convolution or pooling) have stride values >1 (i.e. stride $= 2$ in our implementation). Thus the scale factor $d = 2^n$. A pixel location $\mathbf{x}_o$ in the probability map corresponds to the center $\mathbf{x}_i$ of a patch with size $size_p$ in the input image. Centers displace d pixels from each other. $\mathbf{x}_i$ is computed as $\boldsymbol{x}_i = d \cdot \boldsymbol{x}_o + \lfloor (size_p - 1)/2 \rfloor$.

3   Experiment and Discussion

Datasets: Our experiments are conducted on gastric cancer dataset, acquired from our collaborative hospital. The invasive cancer regions were carefully delineated by the experts. It includes 204 training WSI (117 normal and 87 tumor) and 68 testing WSIs (29 tumor and 39 normal) with average testing image size 107595×161490. We additionally validated our approach on the CAMELYON16 dataset. It includes 270 training WSIs (160 normal and 110 tumor images), and 129 testing WSIs (80 normal and 49 tumor images) with average testing image size 64548×43633.

Experimental Setting and Implementations: We used Inception V3 as the teacher network (large capacity network) in transfer learning. To train the teacher network, we re-implemented the method in [8]. The patch size for the teacher network is 299×299. The patch size for the student network is 224×224. In the transfer learning, we randomly generated mini batches of patch size 299×299 for the teacher network and crop a 224×224 patch from it for the student network. We augment the training samples using random rotation, flipping and color jittering. We developed our approach using deep learning toolbox Caffe [4]. The inference part is implemented in C++ and validated on a standard workstation with a Nvidia Tesla M40 (12 GB GPU memory). To hide the I/O latency, we prefetch image patches into the memory in one thread and the network inference is implemented in another two threads. Note that this data prefetch scheme is applied to all investigated approaches. Besides this, we don't have other implementation optimization. In addition, all the experiments were conducted on the highest magnification (40×). For the student network, we use a normal convolutional layer followed by 13 depthwise separable convolutional (3×3 depthwise separable convolutional layer followed by 1×1 convolutional layer), 1 average pooling (7×7) and 1 fully connected layers. The number of convolution filters for the first to the last convolutional layers (including depthwise separable convolutional layers) are 32, 64, 128, 128, 256, 256, 512, 512, 512, 512, 512, 512, 960 and 960, respectively. We use average FROC (Ave. FROC, $[0, 1]$) [12] to evaluate detection performance. It is an average sensitivity at 6 false positive rates: $1/4$, $1/2$, 1, 2, 4, and 8 per WSI.

Table 1. Comparison for different detection approaches in terms of computation time and Ave. FROC. They are Inception V3, Inception V3 with FCN (IF), student network (S), student network with FCN (SF), distilled student network with FCN (DSF), and distilled student network with both FCN and teacher guided loss (DSFG, the final proposed network).

Methods		I	IF	S	SF	DSF	DSFG
Gastric cancer	Time (mins.)	3.8	2.3	1.5	0.6	0.6	0.6
	Ave. FROC	0.806	0.813	0.768	0.773	0.801	0.811
CAMELYON16	Time (mins.)	17.0	9.1	7.8	3.6	3.6	3.6
	Ave. FROC	0.857	0.859	0.809	0.815	0.847	0.856

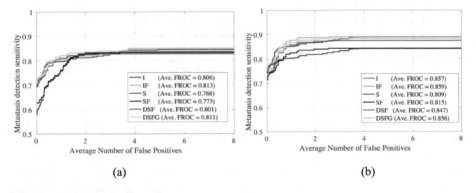

(a)   (b)

Fig. 2. Experimental results of the methods on the (a) gastric cancer and (b) CAMELYON16 datasets

Results and Analysis: We compared Inception V3 network (method I) using explicitly sliding window fashion proposed in [8], Inception V3 with our fully convolution (method IF) implementation, student network using explicitly sliding window (method S), student network with fully convolution (method SF), distilled student network with fully convolution (method DSF), and our final proposed approach: distilled student network with both FCN and teacher guided loss (DSFG). The stride of the sliding window is 128. The explicitly sliding window based method is the most widely used method and it achieved the state-of-the-art results [8,16]. Note that the original Inception V3 in [8] utilized 8 ensembled models. However, for a fair comparison here, we only used one single model. Due to GPU memory limitation, for the FCN based methods (IF, SF, DSF, and DSFG), we partition the WSI into several blocks with overlaps and stitch the probability maps to a single one accordingly after the inferences. In the method IF, we used a block 1451×1451 with an overlap of 267 pixels. In methods SF, DSF, DSFG, we used a block 1792×1792 with an overlap of 192 pixels.

Table 1 and Fig. 2 illustrate comparisons of these methods in terms of computation time and Ave. FROC. Fully convolution based detection significantly speeds up the inference compared to the corresponding sliding window approach. The method IF is 1.7 and 1.9 times faster than the method I for gastric cancer and CAMELYON16 datasets, respectively. The method SF is 2.5 and 2.2 times faster than the method S for gastric cancer and CAMELYON16 datasets, respectively. Note that small capacity model (SF) is about 2.5 and 2.2 times faster than the large capacity model (IF) for gastric cancer and CAMELYON16 datasets, respectively. In addition, we observed that the small capacity model reduced Ave. FROC of about 4% and 5% for gastric cancer and CAMELYON16 datasets, respectively. However, once the small network gained knowledge from transfer learning, the detection accuracy of it became close to the large model. For CAMELYON16 dataset, we observed that single Inception V3 model cause Ave. FROC decreasing to 85.7% from 88.5% reported in [8]. This drop is expected because ensembled models reduced model variance and overfitting. However, this result has been state-of-the-art accuracy among single model based methods. Lin et al. developed an efficient inference algorithm and in their study [7], they reported 15 min per WSI on CAMELYON16. While we achieved a much faster computation time, the validation is performed in different hardware and software environments.

These experiments demonstrate that we could keep the same detection accuracy compared to the method I and improve the efficiency significantly (5 times faster than the method I) via model "compression" and transfer learning. Our proposed model is more memory efficient and costs only 12 MB memory in contrast to the 84 MB required in the method I.

4   Conclusion

State-of-the-art deep CNN based invasive cancer detection methods have pushed the accuracy boundary closer to clinical application, however, the computation and memory burdens are barriers in real clinical setups. We proposed a new framework to keep high detection accuracy with efficient computation and memory usage. Particularly, we improved detection accuracy of a utilized small capacity network using a large capacity network pre-trained on the same data set, who taught the small network having similar prediction power. In addition, the proposed method requires less high performance computing resources and runs much faster than state-of-the-art methods. Thus, we expect that our work will become more applicable in the clinical usage.

Acknowledgements. This work is partially supported by the National Science Foundation under grant IIP-1439695, ABI-1661280 and CNS-1629913.

References

1. Chollet, F., et al.: Xception: deep learning with depthwise separable convolutions. In: CVPR, pp. 1251–1258 (2017)
2. Hinton, G., et al.: Distilling the knowledge in a neural network. arXiv preprint arXiv:1503.02531 (2015)
3. Howard, A., et al.: Mobilenets: efficient convolutional neural networks for mobile vision applications. arXiv preprint arXiv:1704.04861 (2017)
4. Jia, Y., et al.: Caffe: convolutional architecture for fast feature embedding. In: ACMMM, pp. 675–678. ACM (2014)
5. Kong, B., Zhan, Y., Shin, M., Denny, T., Zhang, S.: Recognizing end-diastole and end-systole frames via deep temporal regression network. In: Ourselin, S., Joskowicz, L., Sabuncu, M.R., Unal, G., Wells, W. (eds.) MICCAI 2016. LNCS, vol. 9902, pp. 264–272. Springer, Cham (2016). https://doi.org/10.1007/978-3-319-46726-9_31
6. Kong, B., Wang, X., Li, Z., Song, Q., Zhang, S.: Cancer metastasis detection via spatially structured deep network. In: Niethammer, M., et al. (eds.) IPMI 2017. LNCS, vol. 10265, pp. 236–248. Springer, Cham (2017). https://doi.org/10.1007/978-3-319-59050-9_19
7. Lin, H., et al.: Scannet: a fast and dense scanning framework for metastatic breast cancer detection from whole-slide images. arXiv preprint arXiv:1707.09597 (2017)
8. Liu, Y., et al.: Detecting cancer metastases on gigapixel pathology images. arXiv preprint arXiv:1703.02442 (2017)
9. Long, J., et al.: Fully convolutional networks for semantic segmentation. In: CVPR, pp. 3431–3440 (2015)
10. Rastegari, M., Ordonez, V., Redmon, J., Farhadi, A.: XNOR-net: imagenet classification using binary convolutional neural networks. In: Leibe, B., Matas, J., Sebe, N., Welling, M. (eds.) ECCV 2016. LNCS, vol. 9908, pp. 525–542. Springer, Cham (2016). https://doi.org/10.1007/978-3-319-46493-0_32
11. Romero, A., et al.: Fitnets: hints for thin deep nets. arXiv preprint arXiv:1412.6550 (2014)
12. Shiraishi, J.: Computer-aided diagnostic scheme for the detection of lung nodules on chest radiographs: localized search method based on anatomical classification. Med. Phys. **33**(7), 2642–2653 (2006)
13. Siegel, R.L., et al.: Cancer statistics, 2017. CA Cancer J. Clin. **67**(1), 7–30 (2017). https://doi.org/10.3322/caac.21387
14. Szegedy, C., et al.: Going deeper with convolutions. In: CVPR, pp. 1–9 (2015)
15. Szegedy, C., et al.: Rethinking the inception architecture for computer vision. In: CVPR, pp. 2818–2826 (2016)
16. Wang, D., et al.: Deep learning for identifying metastatic breast cancer. arXiv preprint arXiv:1606.05718 (2016)
17. Wu, J., et al.: Quantized convolutional neural networks for mobile devices. In: CVPR, pp. 4820–4828 (2016)

Which Way Round? A Study on the Performance of Stain-Translation for Segmenting Arbitrarily Dyed Histological Images

Michael Gadermayr[1]([✉]), Vitus Appel[1], Barbara M. Klinkhammer[2],
Peter Boor[2], and Dorit Merhof[1]

[1] Institute of Imaging and Computer Vision, RWTH Aachen University,
Aachen, Germany
`Michael.Gadermayr@lfb.rwth-aachen.de`
[2] Institute Pathology, University Hospital Aachen, RWTH Aachen University,
Aachen, Germany

Abstract. Image-to-image translation based on convolutional neural networks recently gained popularity. Especially approaches relying on generative adversarial networks facilitating unpaired training open new opportunities for image analysis. Making use of an unpaired image-to-image translation approach, we propose a methodology to perform stain-independent segmentation of histological whole slide images requiring annotated training data for one single stain only. In this experimental study, we propose and investigate two different pipelines for performing stain-independent segmentation, which are evaluated with three different stain combinations showing different degrees of difficulty. Whereas one pipeline directly translates the images to be evaluated and uses a segmentation model trained on original data, the other "way round" translates the training data in order to finally segment the original images. The results exhibit good performance especially for the first approach and provide evidence that the direction of translation plays a crucial role considering the final segmentation accuracy.

Keywords: Histology · Adversarial network · Segmentation · Kidney

1 Motivation

Image-to-image translation gained popularity during the last few years generating highly attractive and realistic output [8,9,14]. The majority of approaches require image pairs for training the image-to-image transformation models and make use of single fully-convolutional networks (FCNs) [9] or adversarial networks (ANs) [8]. Recently, the so-called cycleGAN [14] was introduced which eliminates the restriction of corresponding image pairs for training the network.

© Springer Nature Switzerland AG 2018
A. F. Frangi et al. (Eds.): MICCAI 2018, LNCS 11071, pp. 165–173, 2018.
https://doi.org/10.1007/978-3-030-00934-2_19

The authors proposed a generative adversarial network (GAN) relying on a cycle-consistency loss which is combined with the discriminator loss (GAN loss) to perform circular trainings. That means, translations from domain A to domain B and back to domain A and the same vice versa are conducted. This GAN architecture exhibits excellent performance in image-to-image translation applications, based on unpaired training. As image pairs often cannot be obtained (or are at least difficult and/or expensive to achieve), this architecture opens up entirely new opportunities especially in the field of biomedical image analysis.

In this work, we investigate the applicability of image-to-image translation for image-level domain adaptation showing the following advantages: (1) image-to-image translation allows completely unsupervised domain adaptation. (2) The domain adaptation model can be trained independently of the underlying segmentation or classification problem which increases flexibility and saves computation time in case of more than one segmentation and domain adaptation tasks (compared to other methods incorporating both steps into one architecture [10]). (3) Domain adaptation is completely transparent as the intermediate representation is an image and (4) domain adaptation is typically utilized to adapt quite similar domains [3]. Domain pairs considered in image-to-image translation on the other hand are often highly divergent considering color as well as texture. Despite all of these advantages, one problem of the cycleGAN formulation is that there is no guarantee that the objects' outline is kept stable during the adaptation process. Problems can especially occur if the underlying distribution of the objects' shapes are dissimilar between the domains. In this case, it is very likely that GAN training leads to changed shapes as otherwise the discriminator could easily distinguish between real and fake images. If the objects' shapes are changed during GAN training, a segmentation of the fake data and subsequently a transfer of the segmentation mask to the real image cannot be conducted without losing segmentation accuracy.

Due to the dissemination of digital whole slide scanners generating large amounts of digital histological image data, image analysis in this field has recently gained significant importance. Considered applications mostly consist of segmentation [2,4], classification [1,7,12] and regression tasks [13]. For segmentation, especially FCNs [2,11] yielded excellent performances. However, problems arise if the underlying distribution between training and testing data is dissimilar, which could be introduced by various aspects, such as inter-subject variability, dye variations, different staining protocols or pathological modifications [5]. Although FCNs are capable to learn variability if sufficient (and the right) training data is available, annotating whole slide images (WSIs) for all potential combination of characteristics is definitely not feasible due to the large number of degrees-of-freedom. The authors of previous work [6] proposed a pipeline to perform stain-independent segmentation by registering an arbitrarily dyed WSI with a differently stained WSI for which a trained model exists in order to directly transfer the obtained segmentation mask. Although this strategy allows a segmentation of arbitrarily stained WSIs, it requires for consecutive slices (which show similar image content but are in general not available).

The authors also showed that the registration step and the fact that consecutive slices do not show exactly the same content constitute limiting factors considering segmentation accuracy.

Contributions: To tackle the problem of a large range of different stains, (1) we propose two stain-independent segmentation approaches (P1, P2) for the analysis of histological image data (Fig. 1). We consider a scenario where annotated training data is available for one staining protocol only (S_T). Both pipelines consist of completely separate segmentation and GAN-based stain-translation stages which learn to convert between an arbitrary stain (S_U) and the stain for which annotated data is available (S_T). In case of P1, the input images to be segmented are adapted to match the stain of the training data, whereas in case of P2, the training data is adapted in order to train a segmentation model which fits the images to be segmented. (2) We investigate if stain-translation based on image-to-image translation can be performed effectively for stain-independently segmenting WSIs. (3) As the characteristics and the segmentation-difficulty of the individual stains differ, we expect dissimilar performances on the two pipelines and therefore pose the question for the "best way round". There exists only one related publication which focusses on stain-independent segmentation of WSIs [6]. Compared to this work, the proposed method does not require consecutively cut slices which are in general not available. Evaluation is performed based on a segmentation task in renal histopathology. Particularly, we segment the so called glomeruli exhibiting probably the most relevant renal structure (Fig. 2).

2   Methods

We propose two stain-independent segmentation pipelines (P1, P2) consisting of a separate stain-translation and a segmentation stage. Supposed we have annotated training WSIs available for a domain S_T where the domain corresponds to a specific staining protocol. For another domain S_U, there are only non-annotated WSIs available. In the following, focus is on obtaining segmentation masks for new images of the domain without available annotations (S_U, Fig. 1) by making use of two different pipelines. For both pipelines, first a stain-translation GAN (cycleGAN [14]) is trained (Fig. 1, right) consisting, inter alia, of the two generators G_U and G_T converting from S_T to S_U and vice versa.

Pipeline 1 (P1): For P1, the segmentation model M_T is trained with original (S_T) training data. The input images to be segmented are first stain-adapted using model G_T, then segmented based on model M_T and finally the output masks obtained for the stain-adapted fake images are directly transferred to the original images (as shown in Fig. 1, P1). An advantage of P1 is, that the segmentation model can be trained independently of the stain-translation model which improved efficiency in case of more than one adaptation and segmentation tasks.

Pipeline 2 (P2): The training data is stain-adapted utilizing model G_U to translate it from S_T to S_U before training the segmentation model M_U based on fake S_U image data. This model is directly utilized to segment the original (S_U) images without the need for adapting them (Fig. 1, P2). An advantage of P2 is, that during testing only one network is needed (and no stain-translation is performed) improving segmentation efficiency.

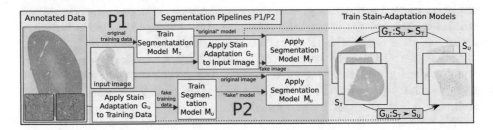

Fig. 1. Outline of the proposed stain-independent segmentation approaches (P1 & P2): In case of P1, the input image is adapted and finally segmented with the model M_T trained on original data (S_T). In case of P2, the training data is adapted before training the segmentation model M_U which is finally used to segment the original data (S_U).

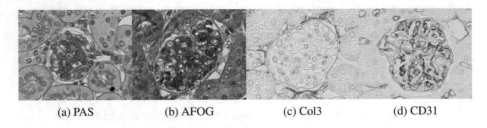

(a) PAS   (b) AFOG   (c) Col3   (d) CD31

Fig. 2. Example patches from renal tissue showing a glomerulus dyed with four different staining protocols.

Considerations: Due to the final segmentation task, we do not only need to generate realistic images, but also corresponding image pairs (i.e. the objects' masks need to be similar). For example, if the generator creates images with displaced objects, they could look realistic and could potentially also be inversely translated to satisfy the cycle consistency. Such data, however, would be useless for our segmentation task. For this purpose, in case of both pipelines, the following two assumptions need to hold. (a) Firstly, the objects' shapes need to be stain-invariant, i.e. the outline of the objects-of-interest must not depend on the staining protocol. This is because in case of changing shapes between the stains, the GAN would need to change the objects' shape as well. As a result, the unchanged corresponding annotations which are reused either for obtaining the final mask (P1) or for training the segmentation model (P2) would no longer be adequate. (b) Secondly, obviously information on the outline of the objects-of-interest need to be available in both stainings to facilitate image-to-image translation.

For the considered image data sets, both conditions hold true [6], as can also be assessed based on Fig. 2. Therefore, we expect that cycleGAN is capable to maintain the underlying objects' shape and to perform appropriate stain-translation. Evaluation is performed by assessing the finally obtained segmentation scores.

2.1 Stain-Translation Model and Sampling Strategies

For training the stain-translation cycleGAN model, first patches are extracted from source domain S_U as well as from target domain S_T WSIs. The target domain corresponds to the stain which should be finally segmented whereas the source domain corresponds to the stain for which training data for segmentation is available. A patch extraction is required, because due to the large size of the WSIs in the range of gigapixels, a holistic processing of complete images is not feasible. Training patches with a size of 512×512 pixels are extracted from the original WSIs. For each data set, we extract 1500 of these patches. To account for the sparsity of the glomeruli, we consider uniform sampling of training patches as well as an equally weighted mixture of uniformly sampled patches (750) and patches containing glomeruli (750). Uniform sampling in both domains is referred to as T_{rand}, 50%/50% sampling in the PAS domain combined with uniform sampling in the other as $T_{50/rand}$ and 50%/50% sampling in both domains is referred to as T_{50}. The first two scenarios are completely unsupervised (as non-PAS domain data is uniformly sampled) whereas the last is not completely unsupervised. With these patches, a cycleGAN based on the GAN-loss $\mathcal{L}_{GAN}$, the cycle-loss $\mathcal{L}_{cyc}$ as well as the identity loss $\mathcal{L}_{id}$ is trained [14] (with corresponding weights $w_{id} = 1, w_{cyc} = 1, w_{GAN} = 1$). Apart from a U-Net based generator network [11] and an initial identity loss only (w_{id} is only used to stabilize training at the beginning of training and is set to zero after five epochs), the standard configuration based on the patch-wise CNN discriminator is utilized [14])[1].

2.2 Segmentation Model and Evaluation Details

For segmentation, we rely on an established fully-convolutional network architecture, specifically the so-called U-Net [11] which was successfully applied for segmenting kidney pathology [4]. For taking the distribution of objects into account (the glomeruli are small, sparse objects covering only approximately 2% of the renal tissue area) training patches are not randomly extracted. Instead, as suggested in [4], 50% of the patches are extracted in object-containing-area (to obtain class balance) whereas the other 50% are randomly extracted (to include regions far away from the objects-of-interest).

---

[1] We use the provided PyTorch reference implementation [14].

The experimental study investigates WSIs showing renal tissue of mouse kidney. Images are captured by the whole slide scanner model C9600-12, by Hamamatsu with a 40× objective lens. As suggested in previous work [4], the second highest resolution (20× magnification) is used for both segmentation and stain-translation. We consider a scenario where manually annotated WSIs dyed with periodic acid Schiff (PAS) are available for training the segmentation model. For adaptation and finally for stain-independent segmentation, we consider WSIs dyed with Acid Fuchsin Orange G (AFOG), a cluster-of-differentiation stain (CD31) and a stain focused on highlighting Collagen III (Col3). The overall data set consists of 23 PAS, 12 AFOG, 12 Col3 and 12 CD31 WSIs, respectively. 10 of the 12 AFOG, Col3 and CD31 images are used for training the stain-translation model and two are employed for evaluation. All 23 PAS WSIs are utilized for training the segmentation network. For segmentation, we rely on the original U-Net architecture [11]. Batch-size is set to one and L2-normalization is applied. Besides standard data augmentation (rotation, flipping), moderate non-linear deformations are applied similar to [4]. Training is conducted with 4,566 patches (492 × 492 pixels) extracted from all 23 PAS-stained WSIs. For evaluating the final segmentation performance, the evaluation WSIs (which are not used for training) for each of the stainings AFOG, CD31 and Col3 are manually annotated.

3 Results

The mean Dice similarity coefficients (DSCs) including standard deviations, precision as well as recall are provided in Fig. 3. We notice that P1 generally exhibits higher DSCs compared to P2. P1 also shows stable DSCs with lower standard deviations and rather balanced recall and precision. Considering the different

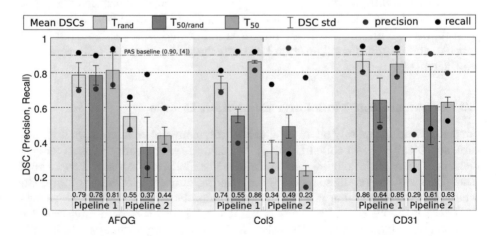

Fig. 3. Segmentation results (DSC, Precision, Recall) individually shown for the two pipelines, the three training configurations and the three stain modalities. PAS baseline indicates the DSC obtained for segmenting original PAS stained images [4].

training strategies, either T_{50} or T_{rand} shows the best rates. The strategy based on different sampling strategies in the two domains $T_{50/rand}$ performs worst. Regarding the three stain combinations, we notice similar rates (between 0.81 and 0.86) in case of T_{50} compared to more divergent DSCs between 0.74 and 0.86 in case of T_{rand}. The overall best DSC is obtained for CD31 in combination with T_{rand}. Figure 4 shows example images after the stain-translation process. We notice that the translation process generally results in highly realistic fake images. We also do not notice any significant changes of the shape of the glomeruli which would automatically lead to degraded final segmentations (in Fig. 3).

4   Discussion

Making use of unpaired image-to-image translation, we propose a methodology to facilitate stain independent segmentation of WSIs relying on unsupervised image-level domain adaptation. A crucial outcome is given by the divergent segmentation performances considering the two proposed and investigated pipelines. It proved to be highly advantageous to translate the WSIs to the PAS staining before segmenting the images and not translating the training images to the target stain (i.e. the stain to be segmented). A reason for this behavior could be given by weakly translated images in case of converted PAS patches. Visual assessment (Fig. 4) indicates that PAS-to-any translation leads to even visually indistinguishable fake images. Thus we are confident that this is not the limiting factor here. Therefore, we assume that this is because the PAS stained images are easier to segment (there is mostly a distinct change in color distribution in

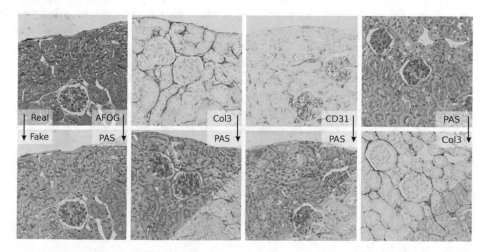

Fig. 4. Example translations as well as overlays of the real and the corresponding fake images (see bottom-right corners). The fake images look highly realistic and do not show any significant changes in objects' morphology.

case of the glomeruli) and a translation from PAS to a more difficult-to-segment staining leads to a loss of discriminative information. In opposite, if the difficult-to-segment image is converted to an easier-to-segment image, the GAN visually makes a segmentation task even easier. This hypothesis is also supported by the fact that Col3, which is visually most difficult to segment and which exhibits the lowest average DCSs, shows the most significant decrease with P2. Consequently, P1 could be considered as a multi-stage segmentation approach first facilitating the segmentation task using GAN-based stain-conversion followed by segmenting the easy-to-segment image data. In case of P1, we observe that the DSCs (at least in case of T_{rand} and T_{50}) are similar for all stainings whereas strong differences are observed in case of P2. The GAN is obviously able to perform stain-translation similarly well for all stain combinations (see P1 results), although the segmentation networks show divergent outcomes for the different stains (see P2 results). This again demonstrates the high effectiveness of the image translation stage indicating that the limiting factor is rather given by the segmentation network. Considering the different training set strategies, we notice that the approaches considering similar distributions in both domains perform best (T_{rand} and T_{50}). A dissimilar distribution ($T_{50/rand}$) partly leads to a transformation of glomerulus-like samples to fake-glomeruli which are finally also segmented as glomerulus tissue in case of P1. In previous work on registration-based segmentation [6], WSIs stained with CD31 were investigated. While this reference approach reaches 0.83 and also exhibits higher variance, here we obtain DSCs of 0.85 and 0.86, respectively. With our novel method, the inconvenient requirement of consecutive slides can also be circumvented.

To conclude, we introduced two pipelines to enable a stain-independent segmentation of histopathological image data requiring for annotated data for one single stain only. The pipeline based on translating the image to be segmented showed excellent performance and distinctly outperformed the other way round for all configurations. Fortunately, "the best way round" not only delivers the most accurate results, but also constitutes the more flexible method as it allows to arbitrarily combine pre-trained segmentation and translation models. Extended analysis indicates that actually segmentation and not translation is the limiting factor here. Therefore we expect that a pre-selection of special high-quality (and thereby easy-to-segment) slides for training the stain-translation model can boost the overall performance even further by facilitating the segmentation task.

Acknowledgement. This work was supported by the German Research Foundation (DFG) under grant no. ME3737/3-1.

References

1. Barker, J., Hoogi, A., Depeursinge, A., Rubin, D.L.: Automated classification of brain tumor type in whole-slide digital pathology images using local representative tiles. Med. Image Anal. **30**, 60–71 (2016)
2. BenTaieb, A., Hamarneh, G.: Topology aware fully convolutional networks for histology gland segmentation. In: Proceedings of the International Conference on Medical Image Computing and Computer-Assisted Intervention (MICCAI), pp. 460–468 (2016)
3. Chopra, S., Balakrishnan, S., Gopalan, R.: DLID: deep learning for domain adaptation by interpolating between domains. In: Proceedings of the International Conference on Machine Learning (ICML) (2013)
4. Gadermayr, M., Dombrowski, A., Klinkhammer, B.M., Boor, P., Merhof, D.: CNN cascades for segmenting whole slide images of the kidney. CoRR, https://arxiv.org/abs/1708.00251 (2017)
5. Gadermayr, M., Strauch, M., Klinkhammer, B.M., Djudjaj, S., Boor, P., Merhof, D.: Domain adaptive classification for compensating variability in histopathological whole slide images. In: Campilho, A., Karray, F. (eds.) ICIAR 2016. LNCS, vol. 9730, pp. 616–622. Springer, Cham (2016). https://doi.org/10.1007/978-3-319-41501-7_69
6. Gupta, L., Klinkhammer, B.M., Boor, P., Merhof, D., Gadermayr, M.: Stain independent segmentation of whole slide images: a case study in renal histology. In: Proceedings of the IEEE International Symposium on Biomedical Imaging (ISBI) (2018)
7. Hou, L., Samaras, D., Kuru, T.M., Gao, Y., Davis, J.E., Saltz, J.H.: Patch-based convolutional neural network for whole slide tissue image classification. In: Proceedings of the International Conference on Computer Vision (CVPR) (2016)
8. Isola, P., Zhu, J.Y., Zhou, T., Efros, A.A.: Image-to-image translation with conditional adversarial networks. In: Proceedings of the International Conference on Computer Vision and Pattern Recognition (CVPR) (2017)
9. Johnson, J., Alahi, A., Fei-Fei, L.: Perceptual losses for real-time style transfer and super-resolution. In: Proceedings of the European Conference on Computer Vision (ECCV) (2016)
10. Kamnitsas, K., et al: Unsupervised domain adaptation in brain lesion segmentation with adversarial networks. In: Proceedings of the International Conference on Information Processing in Medical Imaging (IPMI), pp. 597–609 (2017)
11. Ronneberger, O., Fischer, P., Brox, T.: U-Net: convolutional networks for biomedical image segmentation. In: Navab, N., Hornegger, J., Wells, W.M., Frangi, A.F. (eds.) MICCAI 2015. LNCS, vol. 9351, pp. 234–241. Springer, Cham (2015). https://doi.org/10.1007/978-3-319-24574-4_28
12. Sertel, O., Kong, J., Shimada, H., Catalyurek, U., Saltz, J., Gurcan, M.: Computer-aided prognosis of neuroblastoma on whole-slide images: classification of stromal development. Pattern Recognit. **42**(6), 1093–1103 (2009)
13. Veta, M., van Diest, P.J., Pluim, J.P.W.: Cutting out the middleman: measuring nuclear area in histopathology slides without segmentation. In: Ourselin, S., Joskowicz, L., Sabuncu, M.R., Unal, G., Wells, W. (eds.) MICCAI 2016. LNCS, vol. 9901, pp. 632–639. Springer, Cham (2016). https://doi.org/10.1007/978-3-319-46723-8_73
14. Zhu, J.Y., Park, T., Isola, P., Efros, A.A.: Unpaired image-to-image translation using cycle-consistent adversarial networks. In: Proceedings of the International Conference on Computer Vision (ICCV) (2017)

Graph CNN for Survival Analysis on Whole Slide Pathological Images

Ruoyu Li[1,2], Jiawen Yao[1,2], Xinliang Zhu[1,2], Yeqing Li[1,2],
and Junzhou Huang[1,2(✉)]

[1] Department of Computer Science and Engineering,
The University of Texas at Arlington, Arlington, TX 76019, USA
jzhuang@uta.edu
[2] Tencent AI Lab, Shenzhen 518057, China

Abstract. Deep neural networks have been used in survival prediction by providing high-quality features. However, few works have noticed the significant role of topological features of whole slide pathological images (WSI). Learning topological features on WSIs requires dense computations. Besides, the optimal topological representation of WSIs is still ambiguous. Moreover, how to fully utilize the topological features of WSI in survival prediction is an open question. Therefore, we propose to model WSI as graph and then develop a graph convolutional neural network (graph CNN) with attention learning that better serves the survival prediction by rendering the optimal graph representations of WSIs. Extensive experiments on real lung and brain carcinoma WSIs have demonstrated its effectiveness.

1 Introduction

Survival analysis is generally a set of statistical models where the output is the elapsed time until a certain event occurs. The event can range from vehicle part failure to adverse drug reaction. Clinical trials are aimed to assess different treatment regimes with the biological death as primary event of interest to observe. An accurate estimate of survival probability provides invaluable information for clinical interventions.

The Cox proportional hazards model [3] is most popular in survival analysis. However, the classical Cox model and its early followers overly simplified the patient's survival probability as linear mapping from covariates. Recently, Katzman *et al.* designed a fully connected network (DeepSurv [9]) to learn the nonlinear survival functions. Although it was showed that neural networks outperformed the linear Cox model [4], it cannot directly learn from pathological images. Along with the success of convolutional neural networks (CNNs) on generic images, pathological image, as well as CT and MRI [14], have become ideal data sources for training DL-based survival models. Among them, whole

This work was partially supported by NSF IIS-1423056, CMMI-1434401, CNS-1405985, IIS-1718853 and the NSF CAREER grant IIS-1553687.

© Springer Nature Switzerland AG 2018
A. F. Frangi et al. (Eds.): MICCAI 2018, LNCS 11071, pp. 174–182, 2018.
https://doi.org/10.1007/978-3-030-00934-2_20

slide image (WSI) [12] is one of the most valuable data formats due to the massive multi-level pathological information on nidus and its surrounding tissues.

WSISA [21] was the first trial of moving survival prediction onto whole slide pathological images. To have a efficient approach on WSIs, a patch sampling on WSIs is inevitable. However, their DeepConvSurv model was trained on clustered patch samples separately. Consequently, the features extracted were over-localized for WSIs because the receptive field is constrained within physical area corresponding to a single patch $(0.063\,mm^2)$. The pathological sections of nidus from patients contain more than the regions of interest (e.g tumor cells), therefore, the representations from random patch may not strongly correspond to the disease. Furthermore, it has been widely recognized that the topological properties of instances on pathological images are crucial in medical tasks, e.g. cell subtype classification and cancer classification. While, WSISA is neither able to learn global topological representations of WSIs nor to construct feature maps upon given topological structures.

Graph is widely employed to represent topological structures. However, modeling a WSI as graph is not straightforward. Cell-graph [6] is infeasible for WSIs due to its huge number of cells and the many possible noisy nodes (isolated cells). The intermediate patch-wise features are a good option to construct graph with, balancing efficiency and granularity. However, applying CNNs on graph-structured data is still difficult.

In the paper, we propose a graph convolutional neural network (GCN) based survival analysis model (DeepGraphSurv) where global topological features of WSI and local patch features are naturally integrated via spectral graph convolution operators. The contributions are summarized as: (1) learn both local and global representations of WSIs simultaneously: local patch features are integrated with global topological structures through convolution; (2) task-driven adaptive graphs induce better representations of WSI; (3) introducing graph attention mechanism reduces randomness of patch sampling and therefore increases model robustness. As far as we know, DeepGraphSurv is the first GCN based survival prediction model with WSIs as input. Extensive experiments on cancer patient WSI datasets demonstrate that our model outperforms the state-of-the-art models by providing more accurate survival risk predictions.

2 Methodology

Graph Construction on WSI: Given a set of sampled patch images $\mathbf{P} = \{\mathbf{P_i}\}$ from WSI, we have to dump those patches from the margin areas which contains few cells, therefore, the cardinality $\|\mathbf{P}\|$ differs by WSI. Consequently, the graphs we construct for WSIs are of different sizes. Given patches as vertices, vertex features are generated by the VGG-16 network pre-trained on ImageNet. Due to the lack of patch labels, we cannot fine-tune the network on WSI patches. We will introduce how graph CNN model mitigates this deficiency in next section. Graph edges were constructed by thresholding the Euclidean distances between patch pairs, which were calculated using the 128 features compressed from the

VGG-16 outputs with patches as input. Compressions are committed separately on train and test sets by principal component analysis (PCA).

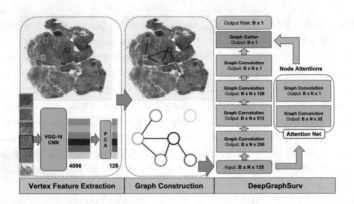

Fig. 1. The architecture of DeepGraphSurv. An example of graph with 6 nodes on WSI constructed based on the 128 compressed VGG-16 features from 6 random patches. In real experiments, we sample 1000+ patches (as graph nodes) on WSI.

Spectral Graph Convolution. Given a graph $\mathcal{G} = (V, E)$, its normalized graph Laplacian $L = I - D^{-1/2}AD^{-1/2}$, where A is the adjacency matrix and D is the degree matrix of $\mathcal{G}$. The graph on WSI is irregular with $\Delta(\mathcal{G}) \gg \delta(\mathcal{G})$. A spectral convolutional filter built based on spectral graph theory [1,2,20] is more applicable to irregular WSI graph. It was proved that a spectrum formed by smooth frequency components leads to a localized spatial kernel. Furthermore, [5] formulated kernel as a Kth order polynomial of diagonal Λ, and $diag(\Lambda)$ is the spectrum of graph Laplacian L:

$$g_\theta(\Lambda^K) = \sum_{k=0}^{K-1} \theta_k \Lambda^k. \tag{1}$$

Based on theorem from [2], spectral convolution on graph $\mathcal{G}$ with vertex features $X \in \mathrm{R}^{N \times F}$ as layer input is formulated as:

$$Y = ReLU\big(g_\theta(L^K)X\big). \tag{2}$$

ReLU is activation function. Output $Y \in \mathrm{R}^{N \times F}$ is a graph of identical number of vertices with convolved features. The learning complexity of K-localized kernel is $\mathcal{O}(K)$. To have a fast filtering, [5] used Chebyshev expansion as approximation of $g_\theta(L)$, Recursive calculation of $g_\theta(L^K)$ reduces the time cost from $\mathcal{O}(KN^2)$ to $\mathcal{O}(KS)$, S ($\ll N^2$) is the count of nonzeros in L. Sparseness of L was enforced by edge thresholding when graph construction. Initial WSI graph $\mathcal{G}$ was built upon compressed patch features. The VGG-16 feature network was not fine-tuned on WSI patches due to the lack of patch labels. Patient-wise censored survival label is absolutely infeasible for a patch-wise training. Therefore, the initial graph may not correctly represent the topological structures between patches on WSI.

Survival-Specific Graph. The deficiency of initial graph results from the insufficiently trained feature network. It has two problems: (1) network used irrelevant supervision (i.e ImageNet label); (2) network was not fine-tuned on pathological images. It would be better, if the patch features could be fine-tuned with survival censor labels. To achieve it, we design a separate graph $\tilde{\mathcal{G}}$ and $\tilde{L}$ to describe the specific survival-related topological relationship between WSI patches [13, 15]. $\tilde{L}$ is learned individually on each WSI. Direct learning of $\tilde{L}$ is impractical because of the graph size and the uniqueness of topology on WSIs. Instead of learning and storing graph edges, we learn the Mahalanobis distance metrics M for evaluating edge connectivity. If d is the dimensionality of feature, the learning complexity is reduced from $\mathcal{O}(N^2)$ to $\mathcal{O}(d^2)$. Because there is no priors on metrics, M has to be randomly initialized. To accelerate the convergence, we keep initial graph as regularization term for survival-specific graph. The final graph Laplacian in convolution will be $\mathcal{L}(M, X) = \tilde{L}(M, X) + \beta L$. β is trade-off coefficient. With survival-specific graph, the proposed graph convolution is formulated as:

$$Y = ReLU\big(g_\theta(\mathcal{L}(M, X)^K)X\big). \qquad (3)$$

Afterwards, there is a feature transform operator parameterized as $W \in \mathrm{R}^{F_{in} \times F_{out}}$ and bias $b \in \mathrm{R}^{F_{out}}$ applied to output Y: $Y' = YW + b$. This reparameterization on activations will lead to a better imitation of CNNs, whose output features are mappings of all input feature dimensions. Model parameters $\{M, \theta\}$ get updated by back-propagation w.r.t. survival loss, which promises fine-tuned features and graphs optimized for survival analysis purpose.

Graph Attention Mechanism. Generally, there are merely a few local regions of interest (RoIs) on WSIs matter in survival analysis. Random sampling cannot guarantee patches are all from RoIs. Attention mechanism provides an adaptive patch selection by learning "importance" on them. In DeepGraphSurv, there is a parallel network to learn attention on nodes conditioned on node features. The network consists of two proposed GCN layers (Eq. 3). The outputs of attention network are node attention values: $\alpha = f'_{attn}(X)$. Given learned attentions, the output risk R for X on graph $\mathcal{G}(V, E)$ is the weighted sum of Y_n of each node n:

$$R = \sum_n f'_{attn}(X)_n Y_n, \quad n \in \{0, \cdots, \|V\|\}. \qquad (4)$$

As shown above, in graph gather layer (Fig. 1), the learned attentions are multiplied onto the node-wise predictions when aggregating attentive graph outputs. The attention network will be trained jointly with the prediction network. Different from previous DL-based survival models that basically act as feature extractor [21], DeepGraphSurv directly generates predicted risks. We integrated regression of survival risk with graph feature learning on WSIs. The loss function is negative Cox log partial likelihood for censored survival data:

$$L(\mathbf{R}) = \sum_{i \in \{i : S_i = 1\}} \big(-R_i + \log \sum_{j \in \{j : T_j >= T_i\}} \exp(R_j)\big). \qquad (5)$$

S_i, T_i are respectively the censor status and the survival time of i-th patient. The fine-tuned patch features and the survival-specific graphs of WSIs are accessible at each proposed GCN layer, while the later layers offer more high-level topology-aware features of WSI.

3   Experiment

3.1   Dataset

As to the raw data source, we utilized the whole slide pathological images from a generic cancer patient dataset TCGA, publicly released by The Cancer Genome Atlas project [8]. The research studied what and how errors in DNA trigger the occurrence of 33 cancer subtypes. We tested our model on two cancer subtypes from TCGA data: glioblastoma multiforme (GBM) and lung squamous cell carcinoma (LUSC). Besides, NLST (National Lung Screening Trials [10]) employed 53,454 heavy smokers of age 55 to 74 with at least 30-year smoking history as high risk group for lung cancer survival analysis. We also committed an experiment on a subset of NLST database that consists of both squamous-cell carcinoma (SCC) and adenocarcinoma (ADC) patients' WSIs to evaluate the performance of our model on mixed cancer subtype dataset. Some quantitative facts of WSI used in the experiments are listed in Table 1.

Table 1. Dataset Statistics. Some patients may have multiple WSIs on record. Avg. size is the mean image size of WSI on disk.

Database	Cancer Subtype	No. Patient	No. WSI	Quality	Avg. Size
TCGA	LUSC	463	535	Medium	0.72 GB
TCGA	GBM	365	491	Low	0.50 GB
NLST	ADC & SCC	263	425	High	0.74 GB

3.2   State-of-the-Art Methods

The baseline survival methods include: LASSO-Cox model [18], BoostCI [17] and Multi-Task Learning model for Survival Analysis (MTLSA) [16]. However, their effectiveness largely depends on the quality of hand-crafted features. Moreover, they were entirely not designed for WSI based survival analysis. For a fair comparison, we first feed those models with the features extracted by CellProfiler [11], e.g cell shape and textures, sampled and averaged over patch images. Then, we feed them with the WSI features generated by DeepGraphSurv from the same group of patient in order to demonstrate the gain of performance brought by the fine-tuned topology-aware WSI features only.

Besides classical models, we compared DeepGraphSurv with the state-of-the-art deep learning based survival models on WSI. WSISA [21] worked on clustered patches from WSIs, however, they simply neglected the topological relationship of the instances on WSI, which is also of great importance on survival analysis. Graph CNNs have recognized power of mining structured features on graph data. We concatenate the latest spectral GCN model [5], working on pre-trained fixed graphs, with a Cox regression as one of comparison methods in order to confirm the advantages brought by adding proposed survival-specific graphs onto GCN.

3.3   Result and Discussion

As far as we know, DeepGraphSurv is the first survival model that used attention scheme. Figure 2 shows that, after 40 epoch, the regions of high attention on a WSI have correctly highlighted the most of RoIs annotated by medical experts. This interpreted part of global structural knowledge we have discovered on WSI.

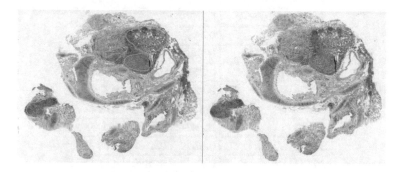

Fig. 2. Left: annotation of RoIs; Right: learned attention map. The yellow color marks the regions of high attention values on WSI. (Best viewed in color)

The concordance probability (C-index) is the fraction of all pairs of patients whose predicted survival times are correctly ordered as all censored patients that can be reasonably ordered. Forming survival order as graph $\mathcal{G}_t(\mathcal{D}, \mathcal{E})$ whose edge $\mathcal{E}_{i,j}$ implies $T_i < T_j$, the C-index is: $C(\mathcal{D}, \mathcal{G}_t, f(x)) = \frac{1}{\|\mathcal{E}\|} \sum_{\mathcal{E}_{i,j}} \mathbf{1}_{f(x_i)<f(x_j)}$, where $\mathbf{1}_{f(x_i)<f(x_j)}$ is the indicator function: $\mathbf{1}_{a<b} = 1$ if $a < b$, otherwise 0. $f(x_i)$ is the predicted risk of x_i. When a patient has multiple WSIs, the predicted risks were first averaged for the patient before calculating C-index.

The C-index results are reported in Table 2. Training and testing sets were randomly splitted and separately prepared. The classical survival models, e.g LASSO-Cox, cannot perform well was because they only utilize hand-crafted features. Possible issues include: (1) patches are partial representations of WSI; (2) the data quality of patch may vary. Consequently, the features collected from random patches brought noisy and biased representations of WSI. Moreover, the features from CellProfiler are general descriptors of pathological images. After feeding them with the WSI features generated by DeepGraphSurv, the C-index were largely lifted by 0.04 on average on NLST and LUSC. This outcome showed that the features fine-tuned with survival labels are indeed better representations of WSI for survival analysis purpose.

However, we also observe that, due to the lower image quality, only using fine-tuned patch features cannot improve prediction on GBM data. DeepGraphSurv generates predictions by encoding patch features with their topological structure via convolution. When patch features are unreliable, topological structure of WSI instances makes more sense in recognition of survival patterns. This may explain the lift by DeepGraphSurv compared to [5,21] who learn little from topology.

Table 2. C-index Table. ⋆ indicates that the model was trained and tested with the features generated by DeepGraphSurv.

Model	LUSC	GBM	NLST
LASSO-Cox [18]	0.5280	0.5574	0.4738
LASSO-Cox⋆	**0.5663**	0.5165	**0.5663**
BoostCI [17]	0.5633	0.5543	0.5705
BoostCI⋆	**0.5800**	0.5130	**0.5716**
EnCox [19]	0.5216	0.5597	0.4883
EnCox⋆	**0.5740**	0.5231	**0.5742**
RSF [7]	0.5066	0.5570	0.5964
RSF⋆	**0.5492**	0.5193	0.5491
MTLSA [16]	0.5386	0.5787	0.6042
MTLSA⋆	0.5247	0.5630	0.5573
WSISA [21]	0.6380	0.5760	0.6539
GCN-Cox [5]	0.6280	0.5901	0.6845
DeepGraphSurv	**0.6606**	**0.6215**	**0.7066**

The previous GCN [5] outperformed WSISA [21] on most of datasets because it can aggregate node features as graph representation of WSI according to graph structure, while [21] cannot. However, [5] still worked on unsupervised graphs obtained with noisy VGG-16 features. DeepGraphSurv conducted convolution on the fine-tuned survival-specific graphs that were trained to represent the survival-related topological structures on each individual WSI. This improved C-index by another 0.03 on average, which again verified that the topological features trained in supervised way work better than that learned from unsupervised approaches.

4   Conclusion

Survival prediction is a useful clinical intervention tool, although it cannot act as expected in many scenarios. Efficient mining of survival-related structured features on whole slide images is a promising solution of boosting survival analysis.

In this paper, we suggested to model WSI as graph and proposed DeepGraph-Surv to learn global topological representations of WSI. Instead of unsupervised graph, DeepGraphSurv creatively utilized a survival-specific graph trained under supervision of survival labels. The effectiveness of our model has been confirmed by improved accuracy of risk ranking on multiple cancer patient datasets across carcinoma subtypes.

References

1. Chen, P.Y., Zhang, B., Al Hasan, M.: Incremental eigenpair computation for graph laplacian matrices: theory and applications. Soc. Netw. Anal. Min. **8**(1), 4 (2018)
2. Chung, F.R.: Spectral Graph Theory, no. 92. American Mathematical Society, Providence (1997)
3. Cox, D.R.: Regression models and life-tables. J. R. Stat. Society. Ser. B (Methodological) **34**, 187–220 (1972)
4. Dave, V.S., Al Hasan, M., Zhang, B., Reddy, C.K.: Predicting interval time for reciprocal link creation using survival analysis. Soc. Netw. Anal. Min. **8**(1), 16 (2018)
5. Defferrard, M., Bresson, X., Vandergheynst, P.: Convolutional neural networks on graphs with fast localized spectral filtering. In: Advances in Neural Information Processing Systems, pp. 3837–3845 (2016)
6. Gunduz, C., Yener, B., Gultekin, S.H.: The cell graphs of cancer. Bioinformatics **20**(suppl_1), i145–i151 (2004)
7. Kalbfleisch, J.D., Prentice, R.L.: The Statistical Analysis of Failure Time Data, vol. 360. Wiley, Hoboken (2011)
8. Kandoth, C., et al.: Mutational landscape and significance across 12 major cancer types. Nature **502**(7471), 333–339 (2013)
9. Katzman, J., Shaham, U., Cloninger, A., Bates, J., Jiang, T., Kluger, Y.: Deep survival: a deep cox proportional hazards network. arXiv preprint arXiv:1606.00931 (2016)
10. Kramer, B.S., Berg, C.D., Aberle, D.R., Prorok, P.C.: Lung cancer screening with low-dose helical CT: results from the national lung screening trial (NLST). J. Med. Screen **18**(3), 109–111 (2011)
11. Lamprecht, M.R., Sabatini, D.M., Carpenter, A.E., et al.: Cellprofiler^{TM}: free, versatile software for automated biological image analysis. Biotechniques **42**(1), 71 (2007)
12. Li, R., Huang, J.: Fast regions-of-interest detection in whole slide histopathology images. In: Wu, G., Coupé, P., Zhan, Y., Munsell, B., Rueckert, D. (eds.) Patch-MI 2015. LNCS, vol. 9467, pp. 120–127. Springer, Cham (2015). https://doi.org/10.1007/978-3-319-28194-0_15
13. Li, R., Huang, J.: Learning graph while training: an evolving graph convolutional neural network. arXiv preprint arXiv:1708.04675 (2017)
14. Li, R., Li, Y., Fang, R., Zhang, S., Pan, H., Huang, J.: Fast preconditioning for accelerated multi-contrast MRI reconstruction. In: Navab, N., Hornegger, J., Wells, W.M., Frangi, A.F. (eds.) MICCAI 2015. LNCS, vol. 9350, pp. 700–707. Springer, Cham (2015). https://doi.org/10.1007/978-3-319-24571-3_84
15. Li, R., Wang, S., Zhu, F., Huang, J.: Adaptive graph convolutional neural networks. arXiv preprint arXiv:1801.03226 (2018)

16. Li, Y., Wang, J., Ye, J., Reddy, C.K.: A multi-task learning formulation for survival analysis. In: Proceedings of the 22nd ACM SIGKDD International Conference on Knowledge Discovery and Data Mining, pp. 1715–1724 (2016)
17. Mayr, A., Schmid, M.: Boosting the concordance index for survival data-a unified framework to derive and evaluate biomarker combinations. PloS one **9**(1), e84483 (2014)
18. Tibshirani, R., et al.: The lasso method for variable selection in the cox model. Stat. Med. **16**(4), 385–395 (1997)
19. Yang, Y., Zou, H.: A cocktail algorithm for solving the elastic net penalized cox's regression in high dimensions. Stat. Interface **6**(2), 167–173 (2013)
20. Zhang, B., Hasan, M.A.: Name disambiguation in anonymized graphs using network embedding. In: Proceedings of the 26th ACM International on Conference on Information and Knowledge Management (2017)
21. Zhu, X., Yao, J., Zhu, F., Huang, J.: Wsisa: making survival prediction from whole slide histopathological images. In: IEEE Conference on Computer Vision and Pattern Recognition, pp. 7234–7242 (2017)

Fully Automated Blind Color Deconvolution of Histopathological Images

Natalia Hidalgo-Gavira[1], Javier Mateos[1(✉)], Miguel Vega[2], Rafael Molina[1], and Aggelos K. Katsaggelos[3]

[1] Dpto. de Ciencias de la Computación e I. A., Universidad de Granada, Granada, Spain
jmd@decsai.ugr.es

[2] Dpto. de Lenguajes y Sistemas Informáticos, Universidad de Granada, Granada, Spain

[3] Department of Electrical Engineering and Computer Science, Northwestern University, Evanston, IL, USA

Abstract. Most whole-slide histological images are stained with hematoxylin and eosin dyes. Slide stain separation or color deconvolution is a crucial step within the digital pathology workflow. In this paper, the blind color deconvolution problem is formulated within the Bayesian framework. Our model takes into account both spatial relations among image pixels and similarity to a given reference color-vector matrix. Using Variational Bayes inference, an efficient new blind color deconvolution method is proposed which provides a fully automated procedure to estimate all the unknowns in the problem. A comparison with classical and current state-of-the-art color deconvolution algorithms, using real images with known ground truth hematoxylin and eosin values, has been carried out demonstrating the superiority of the proposed approach.

Keywords: Blind color deconvolution · Histopathological images
Bayesian modelling and inference · Variational Bayes

1 Introduction

In digital brightfield microscopy, tissues are usually stained before digitization and evaluation, with hematoxylin and eosin (H&E) being the most widely used stains. Color deconvolution (CD) aims at separating a color image into the concentration of each stain present in it. This is not an easy task since the exact spectral profile of the stains varies from one image to another [10]. Hence, the stain color-vector matrix, which relates the color image and the stain concentrations, often needs to be estimated for each slide. Once the stain color-vectors

This work was supported in part by the Spanish Ministerio de Economía y Competitividad under contract DPI2016-77869-C2-2-R.

© Springer Nature Switzerland AG 2018

A. F. Frangi et al. (Eds.): MICCAI 2018, LNCS 11071, pp. 183–191, 2018.
https://doi.org/10.1007/978-3-030-00934-2_21

are calculated, the color of different images can be normalized to a target image for an easier evaluation. This is usually done by replacing the stain vectors with the target stain vectors obtained from the reference slide, and converting the calculated concentrations back to an RGB image.

One of the first CD methods was proposed by Ruifrok et al. [9]. The values for the stain vector of each dye were obtained by measuring the relative absorption of each color from single-stained images. While these standard values are frequently used, they have a strong dependence on the experimental setting utilized in [9]. In [6] H&E color-vector are obtained from the two largest singular values of the SVD decomposition of the optical density matrix. McCann et al. [7] extend the method in [6] by adjusting the contrast of the eosin channel and including a weak interaction between eosin and hematoxylin in the pixels of the hematoxylin channel where eosin values were changed. The algorithm is tested on a set of three H&E images that were stained and destained to create H-only and E-only images that are used as ground-truth separated images for the H&E image. In [4] the stain color-vectors are estimated by projecting the input color image in the Maxwellian chromaticity plane to form clusters, each one corresponding to one stained tissue type. In [5] color normalization is performed by first deconvolving both source and target images, applying a non-linear mapping of the source to the target image channels and recombining the mapped channels into the normalized source image. In [8] the CD problem is formulated as a blind source separation problem tackled by Non-negative Matrix Factorization (NMF) and Independent Component Analysis (ICA). Vahadane et al. [11] and Xu et al. [13] independently extend the NMF in [8] with regularization and sparsity terms since they assume that most pixels contain one type of biological material. The use of Non-negative Least Squares (NNLS) instead of NMF is proposed in [3]. Alsubaie et al. [1] propose using ICA in the wavelets domain where the independence condition among sources is relaxed. All these methods depend on parameters that need to be manually adjusted for an optimal deconvolution.

In this paper we propose a novel fully automated CD method that simultaneously estimates the color-vector matrix, the concentration of the stains, and all required model parameters. In our Bayesian blind CD problem formulation we introduce a smoothness prior model on the stain concentrations which helps reduce the acquisition noise and takes into account the spatial correlation between adjacent pixels. Despite the variability among images, the color-vector matrices are often assumed to be close to a commonly accepted standard matrix. Our Bayesian modelling allows us to include this additional prior knowledge on the sought after solution.

The rest of the paper is organized as follows: in Sect. 2 we mathematically formulate the blind CD of histopathological images problem. This problem is approached using the Bayesian framework in Sect. 3. In this section we also carry out Bayesian inference to estimate the color-vector matrix, concentrations, and model parameters in a fully automated manner. In Sect. 4 the proposed method is evaluated in a set of H&E stained images and its performance is compared with other classical and state-of-the-art CD methods. Finally, Sect. 5 concludes the paper.

2   Problem Formulation

The RGB intensity image detected by a brightfield microscope observing a stained histological specimen's slide is the $(M \times N) \times 3$ matrix, $\mathbf{I}$, with columns $\mathbf{i}_c = (i_{1c}, \ldots, i_{MNc})^{\mathrm{T}}, c \in \{R, G, B\}$ and MN the number of pixels. According to the monochromatic Beer-Lambert law [9], the *Optical Density* (OD) for channel c of the slide, $\mathbf{y}_c \in \mathbb{R}^{MN \times 1}$, is $\mathbf{y}_c = -\log_{10}(\mathbf{i}_c / \mathbf{i}_c^0)$, where $\mathbf{i}_c^0$ denotes the incident light, and the division operation and $\log_{10}(\cdot)$ function are computed element-wise. For a slide stained using n_s stains the observed OD image $\mathbf{Y} = [\mathbf{y}_R, \mathbf{y}_G, \mathbf{y}_B] \in \mathbb{R}^{MN \times 3}$ can be obtained from

$$\mathbf{Y}^{\mathrm{T}} = \mathbf{M}\mathbf{C}^{\mathrm{T}} + \mathbf{N}^{\mathrm{T}}, \tag{1}$$

where $\mathbf{N}$ is the capture noise matrix of size $MN \times 3$ with i.i.d. $\mathcal{N}(0, \beta^{-1})$ components, $\mathbf{C} \in \mathbb{R}^{MN \times n_s}$ is the stain concentration matrix

$$\mathbf{C} = \begin{bmatrix} c_{11} & \cdots & c_{1n_s} \\ \vdots & \vdots & \vdots \\ c_{MN1} & \cdots & c_{MNn_s} \end{bmatrix} = \begin{bmatrix} \mathbf{c}_{1,:}^{\mathrm{T}} \\ \vdots \\ \mathbf{c}_{MN,:}^{\mathrm{T}} \end{bmatrix} = \begin{bmatrix} \mathbf{c}_1 \cdots \mathbf{c}_{n_s} \end{bmatrix}, \tag{2}$$

with i-th row $\mathbf{c}_{i,:}^{\mathrm{T}} = (c_{i1}, \ldots, c_{in_s})$, $i = 1, \ldots, MN$ and columns $\mathbf{c}_s = (c_{1s}, \ldots, c_{MNs})^{\mathrm{T}}, s \in \{1, \ldots, n_s\}$ and $\mathbf{M} \in \mathbb{R}^{3 \times n_s}$ is the normalized stains' specific color-vector matrix. Each column in matrix $\mathbf{M}$ is a unit $\ell 2$ norm stain color-vector containing the relative RGB color composition of the corresponding stain. *Color Deconvolution* (CD) is a technique that allows to obtain the stain concentration matrix, $\mathbf{C}$, and the color-vector matrix, $\mathbf{M}$, from the observed optical densities, $\mathbf{Y}$. In the following section we will use Bayesian modeling and inference to estimate $\mathbf{M}$ and $\mathbf{C}$ as well as the model parameters.

3   Bayesian Modelling and Inference

Following the degradation model in (1), we have

$$\mathrm{p}(\mathbf{Y}|\mathbf{M}, \mathbf{C}, \beta) = \prod_{i=1}^{MN} \mathrm{p}(\mathbf{y}_{i,:}|\mathbf{M}, \mathbf{c}_{i,:}, \beta) = \prod_{i=1}^{MN} \mathcal{N}(\mathbf{y}_{i,:}|\mathbf{M}\mathbf{c}_{i,:}, \beta^{-1}\mathbf{I}_{3 \times 3}). \tag{3}$$

The stain concentrations at each pixel on the image are expected to have values similar to the ones of the surrounding pixels. So, we impose smoothing prior models on the concentrations $\mathbf{c}_s$, $s = 1, \ldots, n_s$, that is, on the columns of $\mathbf{C}$, as the Gaussian distributions of the form

$$\mathrm{p}(\mathbf{C}|\boldsymbol{\alpha}) = \prod_{s=1}^{n_s} \mathrm{p}(\mathbf{c}_s|\alpha_s) \propto \prod_{s=1}^{n_s} \alpha_s^{\frac{MN}{2}} \exp\left(-\frac{1}{2}\alpha_s \mathbf{c}_s^{\mathrm{T}} \mathbf{F}^{\mathrm{T}} \mathbf{F} \mathbf{c}_s\right), \tag{4}$$

where $\mathbf{F} \in \mathbb{R}^{MN \times MN}$ is a smoothing filter and α_s, $s = 1, \ldots, n_s$, controls the amount of smoothness.

The color-vector matrix $\mathbf{M} = [\mathbf{m}_1, \ldots, \mathbf{m}_{n_s}]$ is also unknown, because it depends on the staining procedures and microscopes. In [9], standard color-vectors for hematoxylin, eosin, and DAB stains were proposed. Although those standard color-vectors are not usually exact for each single image, they are very representative and have been frequently used. In this paper we incorporate the similarity to a representative color-vector matrix $\underline{\mathbf{M}} = [\underline{\mathbf{m}}_1, \ldots, \underline{\mathbf{m}}_{n_s}]$ into the Gaussian prior model

$$p(\mathbf{M}|\boldsymbol{\gamma}) = \prod_{s=1}^{n_s} p(\mathbf{m}_s|\gamma_s) \propto \prod_{s=1}^{n_s} \gamma_s^{\frac{3}{2}} \exp\left(-\frac{1}{2}\gamma_s \|\mathbf{m}_s - \underline{\mathbf{m}}_s\|^2\right). \tag{5}$$

where γ_s, $s = 1, \ldots, n_s$, controls our confidence on the accuracy of $\underline{\mathbf{m}}_s$.

The joint probability distribution for our problem is

$$p(\mathbf{Y}, \mathbf{C}, \mathbf{M}|\beta, \boldsymbol{\alpha}, \boldsymbol{\gamma}) = p(\mathbf{Y}|\mathbf{C}, \mathbf{M}, \beta)p(\mathbf{M}|\boldsymbol{\gamma})p(\mathbf{C}|\boldsymbol{\alpha}). \tag{6}$$

Following the Bayesian paradigm, inference will be based on the posterior distribution $p(\mathbf{C}, \mathbf{M}, \beta, \boldsymbol{\alpha}, \boldsymbol{\gamma}|\mathbf{y})$ which cannot be obtained in closed form, so a variational approach [2] is applied.

The hyperparameters $\{\beta, \boldsymbol{\alpha}, \boldsymbol{\gamma}\}$ have not been considered as variables for the variational method, but as model parameters for which a Maximum Likelihood Estimator (MLE) will be obtained and $p(\mathbf{C}, \mathbf{M}, \beta, \boldsymbol{\alpha}, \boldsymbol{\gamma}|\mathbf{y})$ is approximated by the distribution

$$q(\mathbf{C}, \mathbf{M}) = \prod_{s=1}^{n_s} q(\mathbf{m}_s) \prod_{s=1}^{n_s} q(\mathbf{c}_s). \tag{7}$$

It can then be shown [2] that for each unknown $\theta \in \Theta = \{\mathbf{m}_1, \ldots, \mathbf{m}_{n_s}, \mathbf{c}_1, \ldots, \mathbf{c}_{n_s}\}$, $q(\theta)$ will have the form

$$q(\theta) \propto \exp \langle \log p(\mathbf{y}, \mathbf{C}, \mathbf{M}|\beta, \boldsymbol{\alpha}, \boldsymbol{\gamma}) \rangle_{q(\Theta \setminus \theta)}, \tag{8}$$

where $\Theta \setminus \theta$ represents all the variables in Θ except θ and $\langle \cdot \rangle_{q(\Theta \setminus \theta)}$ denotes expected value calculated using the distribution $q(\Theta \setminus \theta)$. Estimates for the different variables can be obtained as $\hat{\theta} = \langle \theta \rangle_{q(\theta)}$. Let us now obtain the analytic expressions for each unknown estimate.

Concentration Update. Let us define

$$\mathbf{e}_{i,:}^{-s} = \mathbf{y}_{i,:} - \sum_{k \neq s} \langle c_{ik} \rangle \langle \mathbf{m}_k \rangle \quad \text{and} \quad z_i^{-s} = \langle \mathbf{m}_s \rangle^{\mathrm{T}} \mathbf{e}_{i,:}^{-s}, \quad \text{for } i = 1, \ldots, MN \tag{9}$$

From (6) and (8) we have

$$\langle \log p(\mathbf{y}, \mathbf{C}, \mathbf{M}|\beta, \boldsymbol{\alpha}, \boldsymbol{\gamma}) \rangle_{q(\Theta \setminus \mathbf{c}_s)} = -\frac{\beta}{2} \left(\|\mathbf{c}_s\|^2 \langle \|\mathbf{m}_s\|^2 \rangle - 2\mathbf{c}_s^{\mathrm{T}} \mathbf{z}^{-s} \right)$$
$$- \frac{1}{2}\alpha_s \mathbf{c}_s^{\mathrm{T}} \mathbf{F}^{\mathrm{T}} \mathbf{F} \mathbf{c}_s + \text{const} \tag{10}$$

which produces $q(\mathbf{c}_s) = \mathcal{N}(\mathbf{c}_s| \langle \mathbf{c}_s \rangle, \boldsymbol{\Sigma}_{\mathbf{c}_s})$, where

$$\boldsymbol{\Sigma}_{\mathbf{c}_s}^{-1} = \beta \langle \|\mathbf{m}_s\|^2 \rangle \mathbf{I}_{MN \times MN} + \alpha_s \mathbf{F}^t \mathbf{F} \quad \text{and} \quad \langle \mathbf{c}_s \rangle = \beta \boldsymbol{\Sigma}_{\mathbf{c}_s} \mathbf{z}^{-s}. \tag{11}$$

Algorithm 1. Variational Bayesian Blind Color Deconvolution

Require: Observed image $\mathbf{I}$, reference color-vector matrix $\underline{\mathbf{M}}$.

From $\mathbf{I}$, obtain the observed OD image, $\mathbf{Y}$, and set $\langle \mathbf{m}_s \rangle^{(0)} = \underline{\mathbf{m}}_s$, $\boldsymbol{\Sigma}_{\mathbf{m}_s}^{(0)} = \mathbf{0}$, $\boldsymbol{\Sigma}_{\mathbf{c}_s}^{(0)} = \mathbf{0}$, and $\langle \mathbf{c}_s \rangle^{(0)}$, $\forall s = 1, \dots, n_s$, from the matrix $\mathbf{C}$ obtained as $\mathbf{C}^\mathrm{T} = \underline{\mathbf{M}}^+ \mathbf{Y}^\mathrm{T}$, with $\underline{\mathbf{M}}^+$ the Moore-Penrose pseudo-inverse of $\underline{\mathbf{M}}$, and $n = 0$.

while convergence criterion is not met **do**

  1. Set $n = n + 1$.
  2. Using $\langle \mathbf{m}_s \rangle^{(n-1)}$, $\boldsymbol{\Sigma}_{\mathbf{m}_s}^{(n-1)}$, $\langle \mathbf{c}_s \rangle^{(n-1)}$ and $\boldsymbol{\Sigma}_{\mathbf{c}_s}^{(n-1)}$ obtain the new parameter estimations $\beta^{(n)}$, $\boldsymbol{\alpha}^{(n)}$ and $\boldsymbol{\gamma}^{(n)}$ from (14), (15) and (16), respectively.
  3. Using $\beta^{(n)}$, $\alpha_s^{(n)}$, $\langle \mathbf{m}_s \rangle^{(n-1)}$ and $\boldsymbol{\Sigma}_{\mathbf{m}_s}^{(n-1)}$ obtain the concentration updates $\boldsymbol{\Sigma}_{\mathbf{c}_s}^{(n)}$ and $\langle \mathbf{c}_s \rangle^{(n)}$ from (11).
  4. Using $\beta^{(n)}$, $\gamma_s^{(n)}$, $\langle \mathbf{c}_s \rangle^{(n)}$ and $\boldsymbol{\Sigma}_{\mathbf{c}_s}^{(n)}$ obtain the color-vector update $\boldsymbol{\Sigma}_{\mathbf{m}_s}^{(n)}$ and $\langle \mathbf{m}_s \rangle^{(n)}$ from (13).

end while

Output the color-vector $\hat{\mathbf{m}}_s = \langle \mathbf{m}_s \rangle^{(n)}$ and the concentrations $\hat{\mathbf{c}}_s = \langle \mathbf{c}_s \rangle^{(n)}$.

Color-Vector Update. In a similar way, using Eq. (9), from Eqs. (6) and (8) we now have

$$\langle \log \mathrm{p}(\mathbf{y}, \mathbf{C}, \mathbf{M} | \beta, \boldsymbol{\alpha}, \boldsymbol{\gamma}) \rangle_{\mathrm{q}(\Theta \backslash \mathbf{m}_s)} = -\frac{\beta}{2} \left(\parallel \mathbf{m}_s \parallel^2 \sum_i \langle c_{is}^2 \rangle - 2\mathbf{m}_s^\mathrm{T} \sum_i \langle c_{is} \rangle \, \mathbf{e}_{i,:}^{-s} \right)$$

$$- \frac{1}{2} \gamma_s \parallel \mathbf{m}_s - \underline{\mathbf{m}}_s \parallel^2 + \mathrm{const} \tag{12}$$

which produces $\mathrm{q}(\mathbf{m}_s) = \mathcal{N}(\mathbf{m}_s | \langle \mathbf{m}_s \rangle, \boldsymbol{\Sigma}_{\mathbf{m}_s})$, where

$$\boldsymbol{\Sigma}_{\mathbf{m}_s}^{-1} = (\beta \sum_i \langle c_{is}^2 \rangle + \gamma_s) \mathbf{I}_{3\times 3} \quad \text{and} \quad \langle \mathbf{m}_s \rangle = \boldsymbol{\Sigma}_{\mathbf{m}_s} (\beta \sum_i \langle c_{is} \rangle \, \mathbf{e}_{i,:}^{-s} + \gamma_s \underline{\mathbf{m}}_s). \tag{13}$$

Notice that $\langle \mathbf{m}_s \rangle$ may not be an unitary vector. We can always replace $\langle \mathbf{m}_s \rangle$ by $\langle \mathbf{m}_s \rangle / \parallel \langle \mathbf{m}_s \rangle \parallel$ and $\boldsymbol{\Sigma}_{\mathbf{m}_s}$ by $\boldsymbol{\Sigma}_{\mathbf{m}_s} / \parallel \langle \mathbf{m}_s \rangle \parallel^2$. Notice also that $\langle c_{is}^2 \rangle$ can be calculated using (11) and $\langle \parallel \mathbf{m}_s \parallel^2 \rangle$ can be easily calculated from (13).

Parameter Update. Finally, the MLE estimators of the noise, concentration, and color-vectors precisions are

$$\hat{\beta}^{-1} = \frac{\mathrm{tr} \left\langle (\mathbf{Y}^\mathrm{T} - \mathbf{M}\mathbf{C}^\mathrm{T})(\mathbf{Y}^\mathrm{T} - \mathbf{M}\mathbf{C}^\mathrm{T})^\mathrm{T} \right\rangle_{\mathrm{q}(\Theta)}}{3MN}, \tag{14}$$

$$\hat{\alpha}_s^{-1} = \frac{\mathrm{tr}(\mathbf{F}^\mathrm{T}\mathbf{F} \langle \mathbf{c}_s \mathbf{c}_s^\mathrm{T} \rangle)}{MN}, \tag{15}$$

$$\hat{\gamma}_s^{-1} = \frac{\mathrm{tr}(\langle (\mathbf{m}_s - \underline{\mathbf{m}}_s)(\mathbf{m}_s - \underline{\mathbf{m}}_s)^\mathrm{T} \rangle)}{3}. \tag{16}$$

respectively. Notice that the involved expected values can be easily calculated.

The proposed Variational Bayesian Blind Color Deconvolution method, summarized in Algorithm 1, allows to obtain the estimated concentrations $\hat{\mathbf{c}}_s$ and color-vector $\hat{\mathbf{m}}_s$ iterating on the concentration and color-vector updates until convergence. Finally, an RGB image of each separated stain, $\hat{\mathbf{i}}_s^{\text{sep}}$, can be obtained as $\hat{\mathbf{i}}_s^{\text{sep}} = \exp_{10}(-\hat{\mathbf{m}}_s \hat{\mathbf{c}}_s^{\text{T}})$.

4   Experiments

We compared the proposed fully automated approach with classical and state-of-the-art CD methods on the stain separation benchmark in [7]. This dataset is formed by three H&E images and their corresponding H-only and E-only images that can be used as ground truth images for the color deconvolution procedure. Each image in the dataset was obtained by eosin staining the tissue, imaging, destaining, staining with hematoxylin, imaging, staining also with eosin and imaging. An example of H&E stained image in the dataset is shown in Fig. 1(a) and its corresponding E-only and H-only images are shown in the left and right hand side of Fig. 1(b), respectively.

The election of a reference color-vector matrix depends on the used stains. For the H&E stains used in this paper, the value of $\underline{\mathbf{M}}$ was set to the H&E values proposed in [9]. We want to note that, for stains different from H&E, simply measuring the tissue response to a single stain might provide its corresponding reference color-vector. The convergence criterion $\| \langle \mathbf{c}_s \rangle^{(n)} - \langle \mathbf{c}_s \rangle^{(n-1)} \|^2 / \| \langle \mathbf{c}_s \rangle^{(n)} \|^2 < 10^{-5}$ for both stains, that is, $s = 1, 2$, was used. This is met in about 15 iterations of the algorithm. We compare against the classical method in [6] and the recent methods in [7,11]. For all the competing algorithms, parameters were selected following the recommendations on the original paper or the reference software freely available.

Figure 1(c)–(f) shows the separations with the proposed and competing methods. From the images, it is clear that the method in [7] and the proposed algorithm produce results closer to the ground truth (see Fig. 1(b)) than the methods in [6,11]. Although all methods effectively separate epithelial and stromal structures, ours seems closer to ground truth. Note, for instance, that the long structure in the center of the image (corresponding to bone tissue [7]) is not clearly shown in the hematoxylin estimations in Figs. 1(c) and (e). All eosin estimations present a higher contrast than the ground truth although, estimations obtained by the proposed method and the method in [7] are more similar to the ground truth. The eosin estimation from the method in [7] seems to be slightly less contrasted than ours.

Numerical results, using the *Peak Signal to Noise Ratio* (PSNR) and *Structural Similarity* (SSIM) [12] measures, are presented in Table 1. This table includes the results for the non-blind method in [9] as a reference. The figures-of-merit confirm the visual inspection results. The proposed method performs better than the competitors, except for the case of the eosin stain for the algorithm in [7]. This was expected since this algorithm selectively modifies the obtained values for the stain separations to better accommodate ground truth. More precisely, in [7] the eosin separation is corrected in contrast by adding

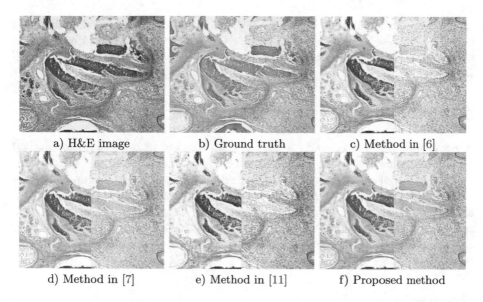

| a) H&E image | b) Ground truth | c) Method in [6] |
| d) Method in [7] | e) Method in [11] | f) Proposed method |

Fig. 1. Ground truth and separations for the proposed and the compared method.

a small part of the hematoxylin stain, and the hematoxylin stain is then computed again by taking into account interaction between the stains in those places where the contrast of the eosin coefficients is adjusted. Note that, in spite of these adjustments, our fully automated proposed method consistently provides better PSNR results for the hematoxylin stain than the method in [7]. Notice that the obtained PSNR and, especially, the SSIM values are quite low. This is due to the staining-destaining process that makes the tissue to move and deform. These deformations were partially corrected in [7] by geometrically registering the H-only and E-only to their corresponding estimations. Although we used the registered images from [7] as ground truth for all the tests, there still are misalignment between ground truth and estimations that deteriorate the figures-of-merit.

Table 1. PSNR and SSIM for the different methods and images in the dataset.

Image	Stain	Method in [9]		Method in [6]		Method in [7]		Method in [11]		Proposed	
		PSNR	SSIM	PSNR	SSIM	PSNR	SSIM	PSNR	SSIM	PSNR	SSIM
HE1	H	17.07	0.4275	17.35	0.4304	18.20	0.4614	16.56	0.3745	**18.33**	**0.4702**
	E	18.44	0.6675	18.70	0.6816	**20.04**	**0.6964**	18.17	0.6248	19.36	0.6922
HE2	H	16.21	0.4200	16.75	0.4578	17.52	**0.4662**	16.16	0.3945	**17.63**	0.4540
	E	17.15	0.6592	17.54	0.6850	**19.37**	**0.7008**	17.08	0.6593	18.16	0.6949
HE3	H	16.89	0.4660	17.33	0.4724	18.54	0.5241	16.53	0.4106	**18.58**	**0.5255**
	E	17.79	0.6905	18.12	0.7247	**20.29**	0.7158	17.57	0.6732	18.92	**0.7288**

The proposed method is faster than the recent method in [11], taking 14 s on a i7-5550U @ 2.40 GHz laptop with 16 GB RAM versus 50.2 s. However it is slower than the classical method in [6], that took 0.4 s, and the method in [7] that took 2.78 s.

5   Conclusions

A novel fully automated variational Bayesian blind color deconvolution method for histological images is proposed. The method estimates the color-vector matrix, the concentration of the stains and all the model parameters. The proposed model takes into account the spatial relations between pixels as well as the similarity to a standard color-vector matrix. Comparison with classical and recent methods demonstrated that the proposed method produces better results than the competitors, except for the eosin stain by the algorithm in [7] as already mentioned.

References

1. Alsubaie, N., Trahearn, N., et al.: Stain deconvolution using statistical analysis of multi-resolution stain colour representation. PLOS ONE **12**(1), e0169875 (2017)
2. Bishop, C.: Pattern Recognition and Machine Learning, pp. 454–455. Springer, New York (2006)
3. Carey, D., Wijayathunga, V.N., Bulpitt, A.J., Treanor, D.: A novel approach for the colour deconvolution of multiple histological stains. In: Proceedings of the 19th Conference of Medical Image Understanding and Analysis, pp. 156–162 (2015)
4. Gavrilovic, M., Azar, J.C., et al.: Blind color decomposition of histological images. IEEE Trans. Med. Imaging **32**(6), 983–994 (2013)
5. Khan, A.M., Rajpoot, N., Treanor, D., Magee, D.: A nonlinear mapping approach to stain normalization in digital histopathology images using image-specific color deconvolution. IEEE Trans. Biomed. Eng. **61**(6), 1729–1738 (2014)
6. Macenko, M., Niethammer, M., et al.: A method for normalizing histology slides for quantitative analysis. In: 2009 IEEE International Symposium on Biomedical Imaging: From Nano to Macro, pp. 1107–1110 (2009)
7. McCann, M.T., Majumdar, J., et al.: Algorithm and benchmark dataset for stain separation in histology images. In: IEEE International Conference on Image Processing (ICIP), pp. 3953–3957 (2014)
8. Rabinovich, A., Agarwal, S., Laris, C., Price, J.H., Belongie, S.J.: Unsupervised color decomposition of histologically stained tissue samples. In: Advances in Neural Information Processing Systems, pp. 667–674 (2004)
9. Ruifrok, A.C., Johnston, D.A.: Quantification of histochemical staining by color deconvolution. Anal. Quant. Cytol. Hist. **23**(4), 291–299 (2001)
10. Taylor, C.R., Levenson, R.M.: Quantification of immunohistochemistry-issues concerning methods, utility and semiquantitative assessment II. Histopathology **49**(4), 411–424 (2006)
11. Vahadane, A., Peng, T., et al.: Structure-preserving color normalization and sparse stain separation for histological images. IEEE Trans. Med. Imaging **35**(8), 1962–1971 (2016)

12. Wang, Z., Bovik, A.C., et al.: Image quality assessment: from error visibility to structural similarity. IEEE Trans. Image Proc. **13**, 600–612 (2004)
13. Xu, J., Xiang, L., Wang, G., et al.: Sparse Non-negative Matrix Factorization (SNMF) based color unmixing for breast histopathological image analysis. Comput. Med. Imaging Graph. **46**, 20–29 (2015)

Improving Whole Slide Segmentation Through Visual Context - A Systematic Study

Korsuk Sirinukunwattana[1(✉)], Nasullah Khalid Alham[1,2], Clare Verrill[2], and Jens Rittscher[1(✉)]

[1] Institute of Biomedical Engineering, Department of Engineering Science, University of Oxford, Oxford, UK
{korsuk.sirinukunwattana,jens.rittscher}@eng.ox.ac.uk
[2] Nuffield Department of Surgical Sciences and Oxford NIHR Biomedical Research Centre (BRC), University of Oxford, John Radcliffe Hospital, Oxford, UK

Abstract. While challenging, the dense segmentation of histology images is a necessary first step to assess changes in tissue architecture and cellular morphology. Although specific convolutional neural network architectures have been applied with great success to the problem, few effectively incorporate visual context information from multiple scales. With this paper, we present a systematic comparison of different architectures to assess how including multi-scale information affects segmentation performance. A publicly available breast cancer and a locally collected prostate cancer datasets are being utilised for this study. The results support our hypothesis that visual context and scale plays a crucial role in histology image classification problems.

Keywords: Digital pathology · Whole slide imaging
Dense segmentation · Deep learning

1 Introduction

Statistical learning approaches, primarily those embodied by deep learning, have demonstrated the potential for advancing our ability to extract information from histology images. The concept of end-to-end learning has been applied to predict cancer grade [1], genotype [2], and outcome [3] directly from the digitised haematoxylin and eosin (H&E) images. As opposed to summarising the vast amount of information in the form of a single number or category, we aim to capture potentially diagnostically relevant information and to support a more objective decision making process. Providing a dense segmentation of the entire image is a challenging and important first step towards achieving this goal.

Electronic supplementary material The online version of this chapter (https://doi.org/10.1007/978-3-030-00934-2_22) contains supplementary material, which is available to authorized users.

© Springer Nature Switzerland AG 2018
A. F. Frangi et al. (Eds.): MICCAI 2018, LNCS 11071, pp. 192–200, 2018.
https://doi.org/10.1007/978-3-030-00934-2_22

Tissue architecture is characterised by an organ-specific hierarchical assembly of various components (e.g. stroma, epithelium, glands, blood vessels), their shape and topology. Progressing disease can severely disrupt this multi-scale organisation. Examples like those shown in Fig. 1 illustrate how the increased amount of visual context improves the likelihood of correct identification. Classical medical imaging and computer vision research provides numerous examples on how information from multiple scales can be utilised. More recently, various deep learning approaches [4] have been introduced that effectively learn visual context directly from training data. With this paper we provide a more systematic comparison of these approaches and study how these effect the ability of differentiating between different tissue components. In addition, we introduce a computational model that utilises feature sharing across scales and learns dependencies between scales using long-short term memory (LSTM) unit [5].

An openly available collection of breast cancer samples [6] and a local collection of prostate cancer histology provide the necessary disease context. An overview of the relevant deep learning approaches is provided in Sect. 2. The set of architectures that are being used for a comparison and details of the datasets used in this study are being presented in Sect. 3. Our results in Sect. 4 give a strong indication that the modelling visual context impacts the quality of dense segmentation of histology images. While these results are extremely encouraging, we need to take shortcomings of the datasets into account. In our conclusions we outline what future studies are necessary to overcome the bias included in the present datasets.

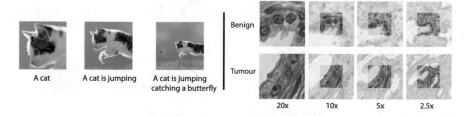

Fig. 1. Visual context. The different images of the scene containing a jumping cat effectively highlight that the correct interpretation of a scene depends on visual context. We content the accuracy of dense segmentation of histology images into different tissue types depends on our ability to make effective use of multiple scales.

2   Related Work

Two main approaches to medical image segmentations are semantic segmentation and patch-wise classification. For example, Ronneberger *et al.* [7] incorporate a dense prediction step in their U-Net convolutional neural network (CNN) architecture, which has been applied with great success to a range of biomedical applications. Zhang *et al.* [8] use a patch-based CNN approach to segment regions of infant MR brain images. In whole slide histology image segmentation, patch-based prediction models appear to dominate the landscape since the lack of comprehensive annotation ground-truth prohibits the use of semantic segmentation approach. Patch-based approaches have proven successful in various applications [9,10]. To detect cancer metastases in breast atypical lymph nodes at a fine-grained level, Wang and colleagues [9] divide large whole slide images into small patches and employ a CNN to assign a prediction score to every patch. The final decision is aggregated from the micro predictions. Nonetheless, processing each patch independently does not take contextual information and long range spatial dependencies into account. To address this shortcoming, Moeskops *et al.* [11] extract patches of different sizes centred at the same pixel location. Each patch is processed on a separated branch of a CNN, yielding multiple-scale features which are then combined for the final prediction. Instead of extracting multiple patches at different scales, Kong *et al.* [12] use a CNN with a 2-dimensional long-short term (LSTM) architecture [4] to learn spatial dependencies of image patches and their neighbours. Incorporating multi-scale and contextual information into a patch-wise classification scheme is still an open problem. A systematic comparison of different network architectures is necessary to establish how visual context should be utilised in whole slide image segmentation.

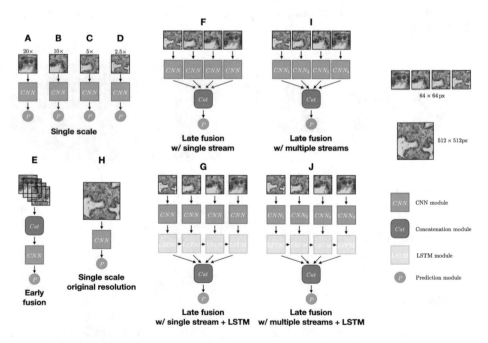

Fig. 2. Used architectures. Model complexity and run time are specified in Table 1.

3   Methods

Comparative Methods. The 10 different architectures that are being used in this study are presented in Fig. 2. These can be categorised into three groups: (1) those that operates at a particular image resolution (A, B, C, D, and H), (2) those that fuse information at multiple resolutions before passing through a neural network (also known as early fusion approach, E), and (3) those that combine multi-scale output features from the networks before prediction (late fusion; F, G, I, and J). Two different approaches to late fusion are being considered. Architectures G and J apply an LSTM unit for integrating the multi-scale information, while methods F and I fuse the features as is. By using the same CNN for all scales (F & G) we test if it is beneficial to share features. In contrast, separate CNNs are being learnt for each spatial scale (I & J).

With the exception of model H the same CNN architecture is used to compare how the different approaches utilise the multi-scale context. It consists of 4 layers, where each layer starts with convolution of size 4×4, followed by a batch normalisation and rectify linear unit activation before downsampling. In method H, there are instead 8 of these convolutional layers. After these layers, the feature responses are fed to 2 fully connected layers, each with 512 hidden neural units. Dropout is employed after each fully connected layer. A linear classifer is used in the final layer of the network. The spatial dimensions of an input images in all methods is 64×64, except method H which uses large high-resolution images (512×512) as input. The LSTM layer has a hidden state of size 512. See Supplementary Material for the detailed definition of each model.

The data are separated into 56% for training, 14% for validation, and 30% for testing at the patient level. The methods are trained using ADAM optimiser [13] with an initial learning rate of 0.0002. The training processed is stopped once the validation loss is no longer improving. Otherwise, the training is abort after 100 epochs.

Datasets. Two datasets are employed for quantitative evaluation. **Prostate:** the dataset consists of 4 tissue classes, including benign, lumen, stroma, and normal. Image patches are extracted from 28 whole slide images at 4 resolutions ($2.5\times$, $5\times$, $10\times$, and $20\times$). This implies that there are 4 images at an individual image location. There are no patches from the same whole slide image that appear in more than one of the training, validation, and test partitions. All annotations were provided by an expert prostate pathologist. In total, there are 41,442 patches at each scale before augmentation (lumen 8361, stroma 14547, benign 12,016, and tumour 6,518) **Breast:** this publically available dataset [6] consists of 4 tissue classes, namely normal, benign, in situ, and invasive. There are approximately 100 images in each classes. Training and test partitions are provided by the authors. Here, we extracted patches at 4 resolutions: $1.25\times$, $2.5\times$, $5\times$, and $10\times$. For each resolution, there are 27,060 patches before augmentation (normal 6,616, benign 7,050, in situ 8239, and invasive 5,155).

Performance Evaluation. Since the segmentation problem is treated as a patch-based classification in this study, we consider an F1-measure for the performance evaluation. F1-measure is mathematically equivalent to the Dice index, a standard measure for segmentation accuracy. Due to the stochastic nature in the training process of the algorithms, we trained each approach 3 times, and in the evaluation, we use the average value of true positives, false positives, and false negatives across the 3 runs.

Table 1. Classification accuracy as measured by the F1-measure. Bold indicates the best performance. Green, blue, yellow, and red colour codings indicate that the results are within 97.5%, 95%, 90%, and 85% of the best performance, respectively. This colour coding scheme can be used to rank the methods (bold = 1, green = 2, blue = 3, yellow = 4, red = 5, and no colour = 6). The overall ranking is summarised by the rank-sum. A total running time is measured on the test set of the prostate cancer data.

Dataset	Class	Method									
		A	B	C	D	E	F	G	H	I	J
Prostate	Lumen	0.728	0.663	0.705	0.716	0.739	0.738	0.748	0.713	0.722	**0.758**
	Stroma	0.797	0.855	0.849	0.790	0.875	0.869	0.884	**0.891**	0.862	0.883
	Benign	0.508	0.646	0.712	0.717	0.734	0.745	0.766	0.763	0.765	**0.782**
	Tumour	0.562	0.653	0.629	0.579	0.699	0.687	0.728	**0.746**	0.674	0.712
Breast	Normal	0.501	0.468	0.523	0.513	0.509	**0.603**	0.573	0.252	0.241	0.323
	Benign	0.453	0.468	0.482	0.444	0.410	0.369	0.423	**0.489**	0.333	0.437
	InSitu	0.468	0.476	0.486	0.533	**0.615**	0.614	0.581	0.286	0.311	0.452
	Invasive	0.401	0.477	0.430	0.540	0.557	0.548	0.576	0.520	0.446	**0.580**
Rank-sum (Prostate)		20	19	17	19	13	13	8	8	12	7
Rank-sum (Breast)		22	21	19	18	16	13	14	18	24	18
Total rank-sum		42	40	36	37	29	26	22	26	36	25
No. of parameters		7.2M	7.2M	7.2M	7.2M	7.3M	8.0M	10.1M	19.8M	28.9M	31.0M
Running time (s)		7.16	7.16	7.16	7.16	7.21	7.61	7.62	35.59	7.60	7.70

4 Results and Discussion

The results summarised in Table 1 provide some clear indication that including information from multiple different scales (E, F, G, I, and J) improves segmentation performance. When ranked with respect to performance, approaches that operate on a fixed resolution are clearly inferior. Rather than simply reporting out top performance with respect to each tissue category, we would like to highlight approaches that perform consistently well. A colour code is used in Table 1 to mark how each method relates to the top performer. In addition, we compute an accumulative rank.

While model H yields the top performance for selected classes, it also performs rather poorly on others. Given that this model performs extremely well on detecting stroma in prostate tissue, one could argue that it specialises on capturing certain texture patters extremly well. When comparing models G and J we can make some interesting observations. On the given data sets model G performs consistently well in all of the tissue classes and has the lowest accumulative rank. Only considering the prostate samples model J is clearly the best.

However, the performance of this model degrades on the breast cancer cases. Here, the interplay between model complexity and size of the data set needs to be taken into account. Later we discuss this issue in more detail. Overall, these results support our hypothesis that visual context and scale matters in histology image classification problems.

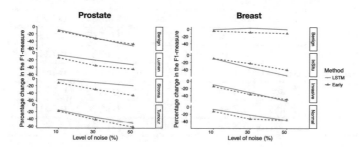

Fig. 3. Resilience to noise. The percentage change in the F1-measure at different noise levels of model E (in red) and model G (in green) is shown. The performance at the zero noise level is used as a reference. On each scale, an image is randomly replaced by a noisy image $(\sim \mathcal{N}(\cdot|\mu = 127, \sigma^2 = 1))$ with probability $p \in \{0.1, 0.3, 0.5\}$

Dataset Size and Makeup. It is crucial to mention that we observe a high degree of visual variation within each class in the breast cancer data. But each of these categories only contains a limited number of instances. This has two major consequences. When compared to the prostate experiments, all of the methods perform worse. More importantly, the breast cancer data set disadvantages more complex architectures. For example, consider method I and its counterpart with a significantly smaller number of parameters, method F. There is a dramatic drop in the performance of method I in relative to that of method F in most of the tissue classes. The same behaviour can be observed across a pair of methods J and G and a pair H and D in some of the tissue classes. This is why we need to interpret the results obtained on this breast data set with great caution.

Feature Integration. From Table 1, the models which utilise a LSTM unit (G and J) perform better than their counterparts with no LSTM (F and I) in most of the cases. Importantly, the LSTM unit also improves the resilience to noise. The direct comparison between models E and G shown in Fig. 3 shows the percentage change in the F1-measure when we contaminate the images with noise. As one would expect, G is more resilient to noise as the percentage of reduction in the performance is consistently smaller than that of strategy E across tissue classes in both datasets.

Computation Efficiency vs Accuracy. Especially when working on whole side images, computational efficiency needs to be taken into account. Here, memory usage and running time are important factors. In terms of the number of

Table 2. Effect of the order of image scales. F1-measures of the method with a single stream of CNN and LSTM (G) subjected to different sequences of the image scale orders.

Dataset	Class	Order			
		Low → High	High → Low	Random	Bidirectional
Prostate	Lumen	0.719	0.737	0.750	**0.756**
	Stroma	0.874	0.881	0.889	**0.891**
	Benign	**0.790**	0.779	0.787	0.776
	Tumour	**0.750**	0.706	0.724	0.734
Breast	Normal	0.573	0.588	0.590	**0.609**
	Benign	**0.423**	0.419	0.409	0.374
	InSitu	**0.581**	0.567	0.545	0.561
	Invasive	**0.576**	0.567	0.541	0.548

parameters, methods E, F and G and have a significantly lower number of parameters than H, I, and J. Based on the trend observed in the prostate dataset there is a possibility that when trained on more samples and longer methods I and J will yield an even better performance. On the other hand, methods E, F, G, I, and J run significantly faster than H (Table 1). In the medical context, the cost of running time has more weight than the cost of memory usage (number of parameters). As such, method H, which operates on the highest image resolution and full image dimensions, is considered very costly without offering significant improvement in the performance.

Sensitivity of Method G to the Order of Image Scales. To inspect whether the order of image scales affects the performance, we considered the following sequences of scale orders: (1) low to high, (2) high to low, (3) random ($5\times \rightarrow 2.5\times \rightarrow 20\times \rightarrow 10\times$ for the prostate and $2.5\times \rightarrow 1.25\times \rightarrow 10\times \rightarrow 5\times$

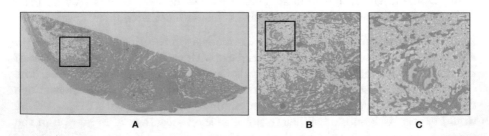

Fig. 4. Segmentation example. This whole slide segmentation was obtained with architecture G on one prostate cancer sample. Benign, tumour, lumen, and stroma regions are highlighted in orange, yellow, green, and purple. Note that the background white region is intentionally highlighted in green. Figures B and C correspond to the areas marked by rectangles in figure A and B.

for the breast dataset), and (4) bidirectional (low $\leftrightarrow$ high). From Table 2, there is no strong difference between F1-measures produced by different experimental conditions. This implies that the performance of the method G does not depend on the order of the image scales.

5   Conclusions

To address the lack of comprehensive annotations we cast the segmentation problem as a patch-based classification rather than semantic segmentation task. In summary we conclude:

– **Visual context:** Our results support the claim that incorporating larger context produces superior results.
– **Feature integration:** LSTM units effectively capture the dependencies between different scales and generally improves performance. LSTMs are resilient to noise and not sensitive to the order of inputs.
– **Dataset design:** Small datasets typically do not represent the true variation of the data. Real clinical samples should be used for validation.

In addition, we have introduced a computationally efficient model (G) which performs well on various different tissue categories. Visual inspection of the segmentation results on whole slide images of this approach also looks highly encouraging (Fig. 4). To overcome the problem of insufficient training data we aim at establish a standard dataset which includes data and annotation from multiple institutions. In addition to the manual annotation, immunohistochemistry staining will be considered to provide biological ground truth.

Acknowledgements. This research was funded by the National Institute for Health Research (NIHR) Oxford Biomedical Research Centre (BRC) and the EPSRC See-BiByte Programme Grant (EP/M013774/1). The views expressed are those of the authors and not necessarily those of the NHS, the NIHR or the Department of Health.

References

1. Shah, M., Rubadue, C., Suster, D., Wang, D.: Deep learning assessment of tumor proliferation in breast cancer histological images. arXiv preprint arXiv:1610.03467 (2016)
2. Schaumberg, A.J., Rubin, M.A., Fuchs, T.J.: H&E-stained whole slide deep learning predicts SPOP mutation state in prostate cancer. bioRxiv, page 064279 (2016)
3. Bychkov, D., et al.: Deep learning based tissue analysis predicts outcome in colorectal cancer. Sci. Rep. **8**(1), 3395 (2018)
4. Liang, X., Shen, X., Xiang, D., Feng, J., Lin, L., Yan, S.: Semantic object parsing with local-global long short-term memory. In: Proceedings of the IEEE Conference on Computer Vision and Pattern Recognition, pp. 3185–3193 (2016)
5. Hochreiter, S., Schmidhuber, J.: Long short-term memory. Neural Comput. **9**(8), 1735–1780 (1997)

6. Araújo, T., et al.: Classification of breast cancer histology images using convolutional neural networks. PloS one **12**(6), e0177544 (2017)
7. Ronneberger, O., Fischer, P., Brox, T.: U-Net: convolutional networks for biomedical image segmentation. In: Navab, N., Hornegger, J., Wells, W.M., Frangi, A.F. (eds.) MICCAI 2015. LNCS, vol. 9351, pp. 234–241. Springer, Cham (2015). https://doi.org/10.1007/978-3-319-24574-4_28
8. Zhang, W., et al.: Deep convolutional neural networks for multi-modality isointense infant brain image segmentation. NeuroImage **108**, 214–224 (2015)
9. Wang, D., Khosla, A., Gargeya, R., Irshad, H., Beck, A.H.: Deep learning for identifying metastatic breast cancer. arXiv preprint arXiv:1606.05718 (2016)
10. Hou, L., Samaras, D., Kurc, T.M., Gao, Y., Davis, J.E., Saltz, J.H.: Patch-based convolutional neural network for whole slide tissue image classification. In: Proceedings of the IEEE Conference on Computer Vision and Pattern Recognition, pp. 2424–2433 (2016)
11. Moeskops, P., Viergever, M.A., Mendrik, A.M., de Vries, L.S., Benders, M.J.N.L., Išgum, I.: Automatic segmentation of MR brain images with a convolutional neural network. IEEE Trans. Med. Imaging **35**(5), 1252–1261 (2016)
12. Kong, B., Wang, X., Li, Z., Song, Q., Zhang, S.: Cancer metastasis detection via spatially structured deep network. In: Niethammer, M., et al. (eds.) IPMI 2017. LNCS, vol. 10265, pp. 236–248. Springer, Cham (2017). https://doi.org/10.1007/978-3-319-59050-9_19
13. Kingma, D.P., Ba, J.: Adam: a method for stochastic optimization. CoRR, abs/1412.6980 (2014)

Adversarial Domain Adaptation for Classification of Prostate Histopathology Whole-Slide Images

Jian Ren[1]([⊠]), Ilker Hacihaliloglu[2], Eric A. Singer[3], David J. Foran[3], and Xin Qi[3]

[1] Department of Electrical and Computer Engineering, Rutgers University, Piscataway, USA
jian.ren0905@rutgers.edu
[2] Department of Biomedical Engineering, Rutgers University, Piscataway, USA
[3] Rutgers Cancer Institute of New Jersey, New Brunswick, USA

Abstract. Automatic and accurate Gleason grading of histopathology tissue slides is crucial for prostate cancer diagnosis, treatment, and prognosis. Usually, histopathology tissue slides from different institutions show heterogeneous appearances because of different tissue preparation and staining procedures, thus the predictable model learned from one domain may not be applicable to a new domain directly. Here we propose to adopt unsupervised domain adaptation to transfer the discriminative knowledge obtained from the source domain to the target domain without requiring labeling of images at the target domain. The adaptation is achieved through adversarial training to find an invariant feature space along with the proposed Siamese architecture on the target domain to add a regularization that is appropriate for the whole-slide images. We validate the method on two prostate cancer datasets and obtain significant classification improvement of Gleason scores as compared with the baseline models.

1 Introduction

Prostate cancer is the most common non-cutaneous malignancy and affects 1 in 7 men in the United States [1]. Gleason scores, graded from whole-slide images (WSIs), have been shown to serve as one of the best predictors for prostate cancer diagnosis [2]. Gleason grading is crucial for studying disease onset, progression and decision making for targeted therapy. However, Gleason grading is a time-consuming process due to the giga-pixel size of the WSIs. Furthermore, inter- and intra-observer variability errors often arise when pathologists make diagnosis based on WSIs. In order to provide an objective and quantitative Gleason grading score, computational methods have been applied for detection, extraction, and recognition of histopathological patterns. Methods based on convolutional neural networks (CNN) are considered state-of-the-art due to their high classication rates [3–5]. Most of these studies focus on the supervised

© Springer Nature Switzerland AG 2018
A. F. Frangi et al. (Eds.): MICCAI 2018, LNCS 11071, pp. 201–209, 2018.
https://doi.org/10.1007/978-3-030-00934-2_23

classification. Histopathology WSIs obtained from different institutions usually present distinct glandular region distributions due to differences in appearance that may be caused by using different microscope scanners and staining procedures. These differences may render the supervised classification model used for predicting the Gleason score for one annotated dataset (source domain) ineffective on another prostate dataset (target domain). A widely used approach to address the challenge is to label new images on the target domain and fine-tune the model trained on source domain [6]. Instead, methods that can learn from existing datasets and adapt to new target domains, without the need for additional labeling, are highly desirable.

Thus in this work, we aim to classify the newly given prostate datasets into low and high Gleason grade through unsupervised learning. To achieve this goal, we adopt the unsupervised domain adaptation paradigm to align the image distributions along the annotated source domain and the unlabeled target domain, where the two domains have the same number of high-level classes [7,8]. We apply adversarial training to minimize the distribution discrepancy at the feature space between the domains, with the loss function adopted from the Generative Adversarial Network (GAN) [9]. Furthermore, we developed a Siamese architecture for the target network to serve as a regularization of patches within the WSIs. The proposed method is validated on public prostate datasets and a newly collected local dataset. The experimental results show the approach significantly improves the classification accuracy of Gleason score as compared with the baseline model. To the best of our knowledge, this is the first study of domain adaptation for unsupervised prostate histopathology WSIs classification.

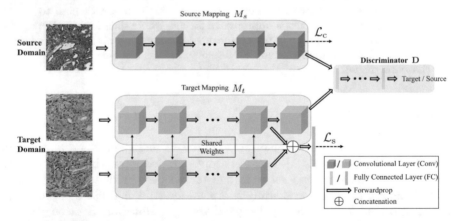

Fig. 1. The architecture of the networks for the unsupervised domain adaptation. The source network and the target network map the input samples into the feature space. The adaptation is accomplished by jointly training the discriminator and target network using the GAN loss to find the domain invariant feature. A Siamese network at target domain adds constrains for the WSIs.

2   Method

In this section, we present our approach on the unsupervised domain adaptation for the classification of prostate histopathology WSIs, as illustrated in Fig. 1 above.

Problem Formulation: Formally, we have a source domain distribution $\mathcal{S}$ that includes N_s labeled prostate histopathology images $\{(\mathbf{x}_i^s, \mathbf{y}_i^s)\}_{i=1}^{N_s}$ where $\mathbf{y}_i^s$ is one-hot vector denoting the Gleason score, and a target domain distribution $\mathcal{T}$ contains N_t unlabeled prostate histopathology images $\{(\mathbf{x}_i^t)\}_{i=1}^{N_t}$. We use the source domain to generate a feature space through the mapping function M_s, and seek to find the mapping M_t at the target domain to obtain a similar feature space with the one from source domain. Thus the Gleason score prediction for the target domain is easily achieved by using the M_t.

Learning at Source Domain: Since the Gleason scores for the prostate images from the source domain are available, we train the network on the source domain to get the discriminative feature space using the supervised learning. In order to feed the WSIs into the network, we crop them into patches and adopt the cross-entropy loss $\mathcal{L}_c$ to optimize the classifier $\mathbf{C}$, with weights as θ^S, to classify the images into low-grade (score as 6 and 7) and high-grade (score higher than 7) Gleason scores, which are highly related to clinical outcomes.

$$\mathcal{L}_c = \mathbb{E}_{\mathbf{x}_s \sim \mathcal{S}} \sum_{i=1}^{N_s} \mathbf{y}_i^s \cdot \log \mathbf{C}(M_s(\mathbf{x}_s; \theta^S)) \tag{1}$$

The majority vote is applied on the cropped patches within each WSI to obtain the final Gleason score for the WSIs.

Adversarial Adaptation for Target Domain: Due to lack of annotations for the training set on the target domain, the $\mathcal{L}_c$ is only applied on the source domain. To optimize the target network, we leverage the adversarial training to minimize the discrepancy between the feature space of the target domain and the one of the source domain. We perform an asymmetric adaptation where the network at the target domain is fine-tuned from the network of the source domain. Through optimization, the feature space of the target domain learns to mimic the distribution of the source feature space. Thus the target network is trained to extract the domain invariant features from input samples, which has the same distribution as the source domain.

Adversarial training is achieved by utilizing a GAN loss [9]. Two feature spaces generated from the source network and target network are fed into the discriminator $\mathbf{D}$. $\mathbf{D}$ is trained to map the input feature spaces into a binary domain label, where the true denotes the source domain and false denotes the target domain. Additionally, the target mapping M_t, is learned in an adversarial manner to purposely mislead the discriminator by reversing the domain label so that it cannot distinguish between the two feature spaces. Since the mapping parameterization of source model is determined before the adversarial training, we only optimize the target mapping. By using adversarial learning, we minimize the discrepancy between the two spaces. Therefore, estimating the Gleason scores for the images from target domain can be implemented by M_t. More specifically, the adversarial loss $\mathcal{L}_{\text{adv}_D}$ for optimizing the discriminator and the mapping loss $\mathcal{L}_{\text{adv}_M}$ for optimizing the target mapping are represented as:

$$\min_{D} \mathcal{L}_{\text{adv}_D} = -\mathbb{E}_{\mathbf{x}_s \sim \mathcal{S}} \log \mathbf{D}(M_s(\mathbf{x}_s; \theta^S); \theta^D) - \mathbb{E}_{\mathbf{x}_t \sim \mathcal{T}} \log(1 - \mathbf{D}(M_t(\mathbf{x}_t; \theta^T); \theta^D)) \quad (2)$$

$$\min_{M_t} \mathcal{L}_{\text{adv}_M} = -\mathbb{E}_{\mathbf{x}_t \sim \mathcal{T}} \log(\mathbf{D}(M_t(\mathbf{x}_t; \theta^T); \theta^D)) \quad (3)$$

For the adversarial training, we optimize the $\mathcal{L}_a$, where $\mathcal{L}_a = \mathcal{L}_{\text{adv}_D} + \mathcal{L}_{\text{adv}_M}$.

Algorithm 1: Learning Algorithm for the Network at Target Domain

Input: Initialized target network from source network with weights $\theta^T = \theta^S$

1 **for** *number of training iterations* **do**
2   sample two same number of mini-batches $\mathbf{x_s} \sim \mathcal{S}$, $\mathbf{x_t} \sim \mathcal{T}$;
3   obtain the estimation $\mathbf{y} = M_s(\mathbf{x_s}; \theta^S)$, $\mathbf{y}' = M_t(\mathbf{x_t}; \theta^T)$;
4       $\theta^D \leftarrow$ back propagate with stochastic gradient $\nabla \mathcal{L}_{\text{adv}_D}(\mathbf{y}, \mathbf{y}')$;
5       $\theta^T \leftarrow$ back propagate with stochastic gradient $\nabla \mathcal{L}_{\text{adv}_M}(\mathbf{y}')$;
6   sample mini-batches with paired of images $\mathbf{x_t^1}, \mathbf{x_t^2} \sim \mathcal{T}$;
7   obtain the estimation $\mathbf{y_f} = f(\mathbf{x_t^1}, \mathbf{x_t^2}; \theta^F)$;
8       $\theta^F \leftarrow$ back propagate with stochastic gradient $\nabla \mathcal{L}_s(\mathbf{y_f})$;

Siamese Architecture at Target Domain: Although there are no annotations for the prostate WSIs at the target domain, the cropped patches from the same WSI should still be predicted with the same Gleason score by the target network. While the adversarial loss forces the distribution across two domains to be similar, it can not constrain the target network to determine the similarity of the input patches. Therefore, we introduce a Siamese architecture at target domain to explicitly regularize patches from the same WSI to have the same Gleason score. As shown in Fig. 1, the two identical networks share the same weights with the input as a pair of images $(\mathbf{x}_t^1, \mathbf{x}_t^2) \subseteq \mathcal{T} \times \mathcal{T}$. The feature maps obtained from the second to the last layer of the two networks are concatenated to serve as the input for a one-layer perceptron to classify the features. Therefore, the input samples are classified by the function $f(\mathbf{x}_t^1, \mathbf{x}_t^2; \theta^F)$, that $f : \mathcal{T} \times \mathcal{T} \mapsto 0, 1$, where 1 indicates input patches belong to the same WSI while 0 denotes not. We learn the binary classifier f using cross-entropy loss $\mathcal{L}_s$.

To learn the network at target domain, we adopt a two-stage training process. For the first stage, we train the network at source domain. For the second stage, we optimize the Siamese network at target domain by applying $\mathcal{L}_t$ where $\mathcal{L}_t = \mathcal{L}_a + \mathcal{L}_s$. The learning algorithm for the target network is shown in Algorithm 1.

3   Experimental Validation and Results

Validation of the proposed method is performed in two datasets: (1) publicly available The Cancer Genome Atlas (TCGA) dataset [10], and (2) a local data set collected from Cancer Institute of New Jersey (CINJ) after obtaining the institutional review board (IRB) approval.

Table 1. The number of WSIs and patches for the prostate histopathology images from TCGA under different Gleason scores. The images from University of Pittsburgh (UP) are shown in parentheses.

	Gleason 6	Gleason 7	Gleason 8	Gleason 9	Gleason 10
# WSIs	115 (32)	395 (95)	94 (20)	128 (24)	4 (0)
# Patches	16293 (6517)	67162 (26583)	16204 (4968)	23978 (9606)	342 (0)

Dataset. In the first unsupervised domain adaptation experiment, we only use the TCGA dataset. The TCGA prostate cancer data includes histopathology WSIs uploaded from 32 institutions that have been acquired at 40× and 20× magnifications. We crop the WSIs into patches by the size of 2048 × 2048. We calculate the tissue area on the grayscale images and remove the images with tissue area less than the half of the patch size. The dataset includes the Gleason scores annotated by pathologists ranging from 6 to 10. As the University of Pittsburgh (UP) has contributed more images than other institutions, we treat the UP as the target domain where the annotations are withheld and the images from other institutions as the source domain, which we denote it as TCGA (w/o UP). We show the total number of WSIs and the cropped patches from TCGA in Table 1 and UP in the parentheses. We denote the adaptation as TCGA (w/o UP) → UP. For the second unsupervised domain adaptation experiment, we use all the images from TCGA as the source domain, and the images from CINJ as the target domain. The images from CINJ are acquired at 20× magnification. More details of the CINJ dataset is shown in Table 2. The dataset is labeled by one pathologist with the Gleason scores as 6 or 8. We denote the adaptation as TCGA → CINJ.

Implementation Details. For the two sets of experiments, we aim to optimize the network at target domain that could classify the WSIs into low and high Gleason scores. Thus we divide the TCGA dataset into low Gleason grade for the WSIs with score as 6 and 7, and high Gleason grade for the WSIs with score as 8, 9 and 10. For the CINJ dataset, the WSIs with Gleason score of 6 belong to the low Gleason grade and Gleason score of 8 belong to high Gleason grade. The training process is composed of two steps. We first train the binary classification network using the data from the source domain. We use a modified fully convolutional AlexNet [12], which only contains convolutional layers, as the network for the classification task. All the convolutional layers are followed by the Batch Normalization layer except the last one that gives the prediction. The data

Table 2. The number of WSIs and patches for the dataset from CINJ under different Gleason grades.

	Gleason 6	Gleason 8
# WSIs	57	26
# Patches	3933	666

Table 3. The network performance at the source domain. The two source networks both have better performance than [11].

	Accuracy (%)
Previous Study [11]	73.5
TCGA (w/o UP)	**76.9**
TCGA	**83.0**

from source domain is randomly divided into the training and the testing sets at a ratio of 80% (validation set is selected from the training set)/20%. The patients with more than one WSIs can only contribute the images to the training set or the testing set. During the training process, the images are resized as 256×256 and randomly cropped to 224×224 to feed into the network. And we train the network from scratch. The second step is to optimize the Siamese network at target domain. During the second step, we fix the parameters of the source network, and train the target network and the discriminator network at the same time. The feature vectors from the two domains are sent into the discriminator network that contains three fully connected layers. And the last layer gives the domain label estimation for the input feature samples. The prostate images at the target domain are randomly divided into the training and the testing sets at a ratio of 80%/20%.

Source Network Performance. As the training process contains two steps, we first show the performance of the network at the source domain. The comparison between the source network and the previous study [11] is shown in Table 3. From the results, we can see both of our models have better performance than [11]. However, the study at [11] uses less WSIs than ours and the network with the best performance reported in [11] is wider and deeper than our study. Although such differences lead to biased comparison, it still demonstrates the source domain network is well trained to classify the TCGA prostate images into low Gleason score and high Gleason score.

Adaptation of TCGA (w/o UP) $\rightarrow$ UP. In order to prove the effectiveness of the knowledge transfer from source domain to the target domain, we show the quantitative results for TCGA (w/o UP) $\rightarrow$ UP in Table 4. We can see that due to the different image distribution for the TCGA (w/o UP) and UP, the network learned from TCGA (w/o UP) is not working appropriately on UP. But through the unsupervised adaptation, we could effectively adapt the discriminative knowledge from TCGA (w/o UP) to the UP without requiring additional annotations. We further calculate the statistically significance of the accuracy improvement between the adapted network and the baseline network using McNemar Test [13] and demonstrates the improvement of classification accuracy is statistically significant with a p-value as 0.039. In addition, we show the result of the ablation study in Table 4 that using $\mathcal{L}_t$ achieves better classi-

Table 4. The unsupervised adaptation of TCGA (w/o UP) → UP.

	Accuracy (%)
Baseline	54.3
$\mathcal{L}_a$ only	71.4
$\mathcal{L}_t$	**77.1**

Table 5. The unsupervised adaptation of TCGA → CINJ.

	Accuracy (%)
Baseline	56.3
$\mathcal{L}_a$ only	62.5
$\mathcal{L}_t$	**75.0**

fication accuracy than $\mathcal{L}_a$ only. The confusion matrices for the adaptation are shown in Fig. 2a and b. After the adaptation, the classification accuracy for both WSIs of low and high Gleason scores are significantly improved.

Adaptation of TCGA → CINJ. The results showing in Table 5 also proves $\mathcal{L}_t$ could achieve the best adaptation performance. The confusion matrices are shown in Fig. 2c and d. We further show the qualitative results in Fig. 3. We use the probability predicted by the network on the patches to generate a Gaussian heatmap and overlay the heatmap on the original image. The red color indicates the high Gleason grade and blue color indicates the low Gleason grade. Figure 3a shows an example prostate WSI from CINJ with the high Gleason grade (Gleason score 8) and the ground-truth heatmap overlaid on it. The heatmap generated from the baseline network is shown in Fig. 3b. The heatmap indicates many low Gleason grade areas, which are misclassified. The heatmap obtained from the target network that optimized by $\mathcal{L}_a$ is shown in Fig. 3c, which presents less low Gleason grade areas. Using $\mathcal{L}_t$, the target network could correctly classify all the patches into high Gleason grade, as demonstrated in Fig. 3d.

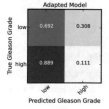 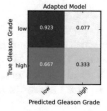 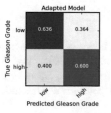 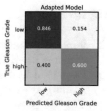

(a) The confusion matrix for UP before adaptation.

(b) The confusion matrix for UP after adaptation.

(c) The confusion matrix for CINJ before adaptation.

(d) The confusion matrix for CINJ after adaptation.

Fig. 2. The confusion matrix of the target network before and after the adaptation for TCGA (w/o UP) → UP and TCGA → CINJ.

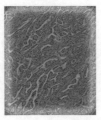 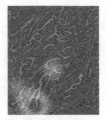 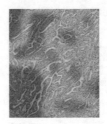 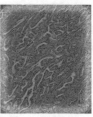

(a) Example image from CINJ with Gleason grade 8.

(b) Heatmap generated from the baseline model.

(c) Heatmap generated from the model optimized with $\mathcal{L}_a$.

(d) Heatmap generated from the model optimized with $\mathcal{L}_t$.

Fig. 3. We show an example image from CINJ with high Gleason grade and the heatmap generated from the prediction models.

4 Conclusion

In this work, we adopt an adversarial training and Siamese architecture to improve the classification performance of a target network in an unsupervised manner. We show that by using the proposed domain adaptation method statistically significant classification results can be achieved. Future work will include improvement of the method by using extensive datasets and extension to a wide range of histopathology image classification problems.

Acknowledgment. This research was funded, in part, by grants from NIH/NCI contracts 4R01LM009239-08, 7R01CA161375-05, 1UG3CA225021-01, and P30CA072720.

References

1. Ferlay, J.: Cancer incidence and mortality worldwide: sources, methods and major patterns in GLOBOCAN 2012. Int. J. Cancer **136**(5), E359–E386 (2015)
2. Epstein, J.I., Zelefsky, M.J., Sjoberg, D.D., et al.: A contemporary prostate cancer grading system: a validated alternative to the Gleason score. Eur. Urol. **69**(3), 428–435 (2016)
3. Hou, L., Samaras, D., Kurc, T.M., Gao, Y., Davis, J.E., Saltz, J.H.: Patch-based convolutional neural network for whole slide tissue image classification. In: CVPR, pp. 2424–2433 (2016)
4. Litjens, G., et al.: Deep learning as a tool for increased accuracy and efficiency of histopathological diagnosis. Sci. Rep. **6**, 26286 (2016)
5. Otálora, S., et al.: Combining unsupervised feature learning and Riesz Wavelets for histopathology image representation: application to identifying anaplastic Medulloblastoma. In: Navab, N., Hornegger, J., Wells, W.M., Frangi, A.F. (eds.) MICCAI 2015. LNCS, vol. 9349, pp. 581–588. Springer, Cham (2015). https://doi.org/10.1007/978-3-319-24553-9_71
6. Schmidhuber, J.: Deep learning in neural networks: an overview. Neural Netw. **61**, 85–117 (2015)

7. Tzeng, E., Hoffman, J., Saenko, K., Darrell, T.: Adversarial discriminative domain adaptation. In: CVPR, vol. 1, p. 4 (2017)
8. Ganin, Y., et al.: Domain-adversarial training of neural networks. J. Mach. Learn. Res. **17**(59), 1–35 (2016)
9. Goodfellow, I., et al.: Generative adversarial nets. In: NIPS, pp. 2672–2680 (2014)
10. Kandoth, C., et al.: Mutational landscape and significance across 12 major cancer types. Nature **502**(7471), 333 (2013)
11. Jimenez-del Toroab, O., et al.: Convolutional neural networks for an automatic classification of prostate tissue slides with high-grade Gleason score. In: Proceedings of SPIE, vol. 10140 (2017). 101400O–1
12. Krizhevsky, A., Sutskever, I., Hinton, G.E.: Imagenet classification with deep convolutional neural networks. In: NIPS, pp. 1097–1105 (2012)
13. Fagerland, M.W., Lydersen, S., Laake, P.: The McNemar test for binary matched-pairs data: mid-p and asymptotic are better than exact conditional. BMC Med. Res. Methodol. **13**(1), 91 (2013)

Rotation Equivariant CNNs
for Digital Pathology

Bastiaan S. Veeling[✉], Jasper Linmans, Jim Winkens, Taco Cohen,
and Max Welling

University of Amsterdam, Amsterdam, The Netherlands
basveeling@gmail.com

Abstract. We propose a new model for digital pathology segmentation,
based on the observation that histopathology images are inherently symmetric under rotation and reflection. Utilizing recent findings on rotation
equivariant CNNs, the proposed model leverages these symmetries in a
principled manner. We present a visual analysis showing improved stability on predictions, and demonstrate that exploiting rotation equivariance significantly improves tumor detection performance on a challenging lymph node metastases dataset. We further present a novel derived
dataset to enable principled comparison of machine learning models, in
combination with an initial benchmark. Through this dataset, the task of
histopathology diagnosis becomes accessible as a challenging benchmark
for fundamental machine learning research.

1 Introduction

The field of digital pathology is developing rapidly, following recent advancements in microscopic imaging hardware that allow digitizing glass slides into
whole-slide images (WSIs). This digitization has facilitated image analysis algorithms to assist and automate diagnostic tasks. A proven approach is to use
convolutional neural networks (CNNs), a type of deep learning model, trained
on patches extracted from whole-slide images. The aggregate of these patch-
based predictions serves as a slide-level representation used by models to identify metastases, stage cancer or diagnose complications. This approach has been
shown to outperform pathologists in a variety of tasks [1–3].

This performance is achieved using off-the-shelf CNN architectures originally
designed for natural images [2]. The effectiveness of these models can be largely
attributed to the efficient sharing of parameters in convolutional layers. As a
result, local patterns are encoded independently of their spatial location, and
shifting the input leads to a predictable shift in the output. This property,
known as translational equivariance, effectively exploits the translational symmetry inherent in natural images leading to strong generalization.

B.S. Veeling, J. Linmans and J. Winkens—Equal contribution.

© Springer Nature Switzerland AG 2018
A. F. Frangi et al. (Eds.): MICCAI 2018, LNCS 11071, pp. 210–218, 2018.
https://doi.org/10.1007/978-3-030-00934-2_24

In contrast to natural images, WSIs exhibit not only translational symmetry but rotation and reflection symmetry as well. CNNs do not exploit these symmetries, and as a result are found empirically to spend a large part of their parameter budget on multiple rotated and reflected copies of filters [4]. Additionally, we find that CNNs trained on histopathology data exhibit erratic fluctuations in predictions under input rotation and reflection. Enforcing equivariance in the model under these transformations is expected to reduce such instabilities, and lower the risk of overfitting by improving parameter sharing.

To encode these symmetries, we leverage recent findings in rotation equivariant CNNs [5–7], a current topic of interest in the machine learning community. These methods show strong generalization under limited dataset size and are more robust under adversarial perturbations in rotation, translation and local geometric distortions [8]. We propose a fully-convolutional patch-classification model that is equivariant to 90° rotations and reflection, using the method proposed by [5]. We evaluate the model on the Camelyon16 benchmark [9], showing significant improvement over a comparable CNN on slide level classification and tumor localization tasks.

As slide-level metrics potentially obscure the relative performance of patch-level models, we further validate on a patch-level task. In this regime, there is currently no benchmark that harbors the high volume, quality and variety of Camelyon16. Thus, we present *PatchCamelyon*(PCam), a large-scale patch-level dataset derived from Camelyon16 data. Through this dataset, we demonstrate that the proposed model is more accurate and more robust under input rotation and reflection, compared to an equivalent standard CNN.

The contributions of this work are as follows: **(1)** we propose a novel deep learning model that utilizes symmetries inherent to histopathology[1], **(2)** demonstrate that rotation equivariance improves model reliability and **(3)** present a new large-scale histopathology dataset that enables precise model evaluation.

Related Work. A common approach to improve orientation robustness is to train CNNs using extensive *data augmentation*, perturbing data with random transformations [1,2]. Although this may improve generalization, it fails to capture local symmetries and does not guarantee equivariance at every layer. As CNNs have to learn rotation equivariance from data, they require a larger model capacity to hold copies of identical filters. Even if rotation equivariance is achieved on training data, there is no guarantee that this generalizes to a test set. Orthogonally, [1,10] propose a test-time augmentation strategy that averages the predictions of 90°-rotated and mirrored versions to improve robustness to orientation-induced instability. As a downside, this comes at 8 times the computational cost and does not provide guarantees on equivariance [11].

Methods that enable equivariance under rotations and other transformations include Harmonic Networks [6], which constrain the set of filters to circular harmonics, allowing for full 360°-equivariance. [7] employs steerable filters and evenly samples a small number of rotations. In this work, we focus on the

---

[1] PCam details and data at https://github.com/basveeling/pcam. Implementations of equivariant layers available at https://github.com/basveeling/keras_gcnn.

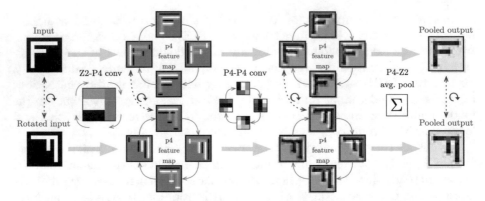

Fig. 1. Given a canonical input and a rotated duplicate, we demonstrate how a 2-layer G-CNN is equivariant in $p4$. Feature maps of one kernel per layer are shown, and the dashed blue arrows indicate how (intermediate) representations of the two inputs correspond. The $\mathbb{Z}^2 \to p4$ convolution correlates the input with 4 rotated versions of the same kernel. The $p4 \to p4$ convolution correlates the resulting feature map with the $p4$-kernel, cyclically-shifting and rotating the kernel for each orientation. The final layer demonstrates how average-pooling over the orientations produces a representation that is locally invariant and globally equivariant to rotation. *Global* average pooling over $p4$ would result in a representation globally invariant to both translation and rotation.

straight-forward G-CNN method from [5] applied on discrete rotation/reflection groups. Although these groups do not cover the full continuous rotational symmetry inherent in WSIs, the empirical evidence gathered so far shows that 90° rotation equivariance improves performance significantly [7].

2   Methods

2.1   Background

In the mathematical model of CNNs and G-CNNs introduced in [5], input images and output segmentation masks are considered to be functions $f : \mathbb{Z}^2 \to \mathbb{R}^K$, where K denotes the number of channels, and f is implicitly assumed to be zero outside of some rectangular domain.

A standard convolution[2] (denoted $*$) of an input f with filter ψ is defined as:

$$[f * \psi](x) = \sum_{y \in \mathbb{Z}^2} \sum_{k=1}^{K} f_k(y)\psi_k(x - y). \tag{1}$$

G-CNNs are a generalization of CNNs that are equivariant under more general symmetry groups, such as the group $G = p4$ of 90° rotations, or $G = p4m$ which additionally includes reflection. In a G-CNN, the feature maps are thought

---

[2] Technically, this is a cross-correlation.

of as functions on this group. For $p4$ and $p4m$, this simply means that feature channels come in groups of 4 or 8, corresponding to the 4 pure rotations in $p4$ or the 8 roto-reflections in $p4m$. In the first layer, these are produced using the $(\mathbb{Z}^2 \to G)$-convolution:

$$[f * \psi](g) = \sum_{y \in \mathbb{Z}^2} \sum_{k=1}^{K} f_k(y) \psi_k(g^{-1}y), \tag{2}$$

where $g = (r, t)$ is a roto-translation (in case $G = p4$) or roto-reflection-translation (in case $G = p4m$).

In further layers, both feature maps and filters are functions on G, and these are combined using the $(G \to G)$-convolution:

$$[f * \psi](g) = \sum_{h \in G} \sum_{k=1}^{K} f_k(h) \psi_k(g^{-1}h). \tag{3}$$

In the final layer, a group-pooling layer is used to ensure that the output is either invariant (for classification tasks) or equivariant as a function on the plane (for segmentation tasks, where the output is supposed to transform together with the input). In Fig. 1 we demonstrate how equivariance is achieved through this process. Non-linear activations and pooling operations are equivariant in $p4m$ [5], allowing layers to be freely stacked to enable deep architectures.

2.2   G-CNN DenseNet Architecture

The proposed patch-classification model is shown in Fig. 2 for $p4$ (the $p4m$-variant is a trivial extension). The architecture is based on the densely connected convolutional network (DenseNet) [12], which consist of dense blocks with layers that use the stack of all previous layers as input, alternated with transition blocks consisting of a 1×1 convolutional layer and 2×2 strided average pooling. We use one layer per dense block due to the limited receptive field of the model, with 5 dense-block/transition-block pairs. The model spatially-pools the input by a factor of 2^5, the output of which resembles the segmentation resolution used in [1].

Full-model group equivariance is achieved by replacing all convolution layers with group-equivariant versions [5]. Batch normalization layers [13] are made group-equivariant by aggregating moments per *group* feature map rather than spatial feature map (as proposed by [5]). Zero-padding is removed to prevent boundary-effects. The final layer consists of a group-pooling layer followed by a sigmoid activation, resulting in tumor-probability output on the plane $\mathbb{Z}^2$. As the model is fully convolutional, efficient inference can be achieved at test time by reusing computation of neighbouring patches, reducing segmentation time of a full WSI from hours to $\sim$2 min on a NVIDIA Titan XP.

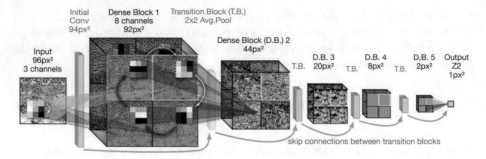

Fig. 2. The proposed equivariant DenseNet architecture for the $p4$ group, consisting of 5 Dense Blocks (D.B.) alternated with Transition Blocks (T.B.). The final layer of the model is a $p4 \rightarrow \mathbb{Z}^2$ group pooling layer followed by a sigmoid activation. The four orientations in $p4$ are illustrated through primary colors. A $\mathbb{Z}^2 \rightarrow p4$ kernel (*left*), $p4 \rightarrow p4$ kernel (*middle*) and $p4 \rightarrow \mathbb{Z}^2$ kernel (*right*) illustrate how equivariance arises in the model.

3   Experimental Results

3.1   Datasets and Evaluation

To evaluate the proposed model, we use Camelyon16 [9] and PCam. Additional testing is performed on BreakHis [14]. **(1)** The Camelyon16 dataset contains 400 H&E stained WSIs of sentinel lymph node sections split into 270 slides with pixel-level annotations for training and 130 unlabeled slides for testing. The slides were acquired and digitized at 2 different centers using a $40\times$ objective (resultant pixel resolution of 0.243 microns). In the Camelyon16 challenge, model performance is evaluated using the FROC curve for tumor localization. **(2)** The PCam dataset contains 327,680 patches extracted from Camelyon16 at a size of 96×96 pixels @ $10\times$ magnification, with a 75/12.5/12.5% train/validate/test split, selected using a hard-negative mining regime[1]. **(3)** The BreakHis dataset contains 7909 H&E stained microscopy images at a size of 700×460 pixels. The task is to classify the images into benign or malignant cases for multiple magnification factors. We limit our evaluation to the images at $4\times$ magnification, for which previous approaches [14,15] have reported the highest accuracy.

For the evaluation on the WSI-level Camelyon16 benchmarks, we largely follow the pipeline proposed in [1], uniformly sampling WSIs and drawing tumor/non-tumor patches with equal probability. To prevent overrepresentation of background and non-tissue patches, slides are converted to HSV, blurred, and rejected if the max. pixel saturation lies below 0.07 (range [0,1]) and value above 0.1. This was empirically verified to not drop tissue patches. For computing the FROC score, tumor location candidates are selected with an efficient square non-maximum suppression window rather than radial. The window-size is tuned per model on the validation set. FROC score confidence bounds are computed using 2000 bootstrap samples [1]. Train and validation splits are created by dividing the available WSIs randomly, maintaining equal tumor/normal ratio. We focus on the WSI data at $10\times$ magnification (4 times smaller than the original dataset, at 0.972 microns per pixel) to fit the compute budget available for this work. Following [1], we focus on the more-granular tumor-detection FROC metric in favor of slide-level AUC.

Training Details: Models are optimized using Adam [16] with batch size 64 and initial learning rate $1e-3$ (halved after 20 epochs of no improvement in validation loss). Epochs consists of 312 batches with a batch size of 64. Validation loss is computed using 40.000 sampled patches. Weights with lowest validation loss are selected for test evaluation.

3.2 Model Reliability

We evaluate stability of predictions under rotation of the input. We present a visual analysis in Fig. 3. For a comparable baseline we use an equivalent model with standard convolutions. For a fair model comparison, we keep the number of parameters consistent by multiplying the growth rate of the baseline model by the square root of the group size [5]. Bar the expected fluctuation around the tumor boundary (that arises due to the sub-sampled segmentation), the *p4m*-model is more robust to transformations even outside the group (sub-90° rotations). In addition, we observe a higher confidence for predictions inside the tumor regions for P4M-DenseNet as compared to the baseline.

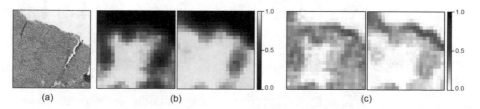

Fig. 3. (a) shows a large input region spanning multiple patches, with the tumor ground truth overlayed in green. The region is predicted under 32 evenly spaced sub-90° rotations, and prediction maps rotated back to original orientation. (b) shows the mean prediction and (c) shows the standard deviation of the predictions across all rotations, using DenseNet (*left*) and P4M-DenseNet (*right*). Both networks are trained on the 12.5% data regime.

3.3 P4M-DenseNet Performance

PatchCamelyon (PCam). We assess the performance of our main contribution, the P4M-DenseNet architecture, on the PCam dataset. Table 1 reports the performance. P4M-DenseNet outperforms other models, closely followed by the P4-DenseNet, indicating that both rotation and reflection are useful inductive biases, that can not be learned by data augmentation alone. Keeping the number of $\mathbb{Z}^2$ maps fixed in the baseline degrades performance further, demonstrating the sample-efficiency of the P4M model (Table 2).

Table 1. Performance on PCam, measured by negative log-likelihood, accuracy and AUC. Experiments with additional data augmentation with 90° rotations and reflections are marked by +. M indicates matching number of $\mathbb{Z}^2$ maps, $\#W$ number of weights, K number of $\mathbb{Z}^2$ maps per layer.

Network	K	$\#W$	NLL	Acc	AUC
P4M-DenseNet	64	119K	**0.260**	**89.8**	**96.3**
P4M-DenseNet M	24	19K	0.273	89.3	95.8
P4-DenseNet	48	125K	0.329	89.0	94.5
DenseNet+	24	128K	0.306	88.1	95.1
DenseNet+ M	64	902K	0.365	87.2	94.6
DenseNet	24	128K	0.315	87.6	95.5

Table 2. Performance on the Camelyon16 test set. The confidence bounds are obtained using a 2000-fold bootstrap regime. *Challenge winner [17] uses 40× resolution and is not directly comparable.

Model	Data	FROC
P4M-DenseNet 123k params	100%	84.0 (75.5, 91.5)
	50%	81.5 (72.2, 89.3)
	25%	72.6 (58.7, 84.6)
	12.5%	60.7 (46.0, 74.1)
DenseNet 126k params	100%	81.7 (72.1, 90.3)
	50%	80.0 (69.3, 89.1)
	25%	71.0 (57.7, 82.0)
	12.5%	55.4 (42.6, 68.5)
Liu et al. [1] 10×	100%	79.3 (74.2, 84.1)
Wang et al. [17]	100%	80.7*
Pathologist [9]	–	73.3

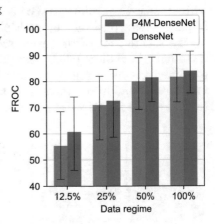

Fig. 4. Performance on the Camelyon16 test set. The confidence bounds are obtained using a 2000-fold bootstrap regime. *Challenge winner [17] uses 40× resolution and is not directly comparable.

Camelyon16. We evaluate our patch-based model on the slide-level tumor localization task of the Camelyon16 challenge. Figure 4 reports the performance on the FROC score, next to those of a pathologist [9] and the state-of-the-art approaches reported on this dataset, including [1,17]. For the baseline DenseNet, the training data is augmented with 90° rotations and reflection. We experiment with multiple data regimes, where the number of WSIs in the training set is incrementally reduced by a factor of two.

The results indicate that the proposed method performs consistently better than all compared methods in terms of the FROC metric. Comparing to the baseline DenseNet results, we see that the superiority of our proposed architecture is predominantly due to the increased parameter sharing by the $p4m$-equivariance, which frees up model capacity and reduces the redundancy of detecting the same histological patterns in different orientations.

We also observe that the performance gap between our model and the baseline increases when we limit the dataset size by removing WSIs. This seems to indicate that the performance in the small-data regime benefits significantly from the sample efficiency of P4M-DenseNet, with diminishing returns when the amount of data is sufficient for the baseline network to achieve (approximate) rotation equivariance. This performance gap remains for the full data set.

BreakHis. As an additional evaluation method, we assess the performance of the proposed model on the binary classification task of BreakHis as described in Sect. 3.1. As training the model from scratch is impractical given the small dataset, we pre-train on Camelyon16 at a similar pixel resolution. Similar to [14], we predict the malignancy of a test image by using the maximum activation of 1000 random crops. We obtain an accuracy of 96.1 ± 3.2 and 93.5 ± 4.7 for P4M-Densenet and the baseline respectively, outperforming previous approaches [14, 15].

4   Conclusion

We present a novel histopathology patch-classification model that outperforms a competitive traditional CNN by enforcing rotation and reflection equivariance. A derived patch-level dataset is presented, allowing straightforward and precise evaluation on a challenging histopathology task. We demonstrate that rotation equivariance improves reliability of the model, motivating the application and further research of rotation equivariant models in the medical image analysis domain.

Acknowledgements. We thank Geert Litjens, Jakub Tomczak, Dimitrios Mavroeidis and the anonymous reviewers especially for their insightful comments. This research was supported by Philips Research, the SURFSara Lisa cluster and the NVIDIA GPU Grant.

References

1. Liu, Y., et al.: Detecting cancer metastases on gigapixel pathology images (2017)
2. Litjens, G., et al.: A survey on deep learning in medical image analysis (2017)
3. Bejnordi, B.E.: Stain specific standardization of Whole-Slide histopathological images. IEEE Trans. Med. Imaging **35**(2), 404–415 (2016)
4. Zeiler, M.D., Fergus, R.: Visualizing and understanding convolutional networks. In: Fleet, D., Pajdla, T., Schiele, B., Tuytelaars, T. (eds.) ECCV 2014. LNCS, vol. 8689, pp. 818–833. Springer, Cham (2014). https://doi.org/10.1007/978-3-319-10590-1_53

5. Cohen, T.S., et al.: Group equivariant convolutional networks (2016)
6. Worrall, D.E., et al.: Harmonic networks: deep translation and rotation equivariance. In: Proceedings of IEEE CVPR, vol. 2 (2017). openaccess.thecvf.com
7. Weiler, M., et al.: Learning steerable filters for rotation equivariant CNNs (2017)
8. Dumont, B., et al.: Robustness of Rotation-Equivariant networks to adversarial perturbations (2018)
9. Ehteshami, B.B.: Diagnostic assessment of deep learning algorithms for detection of lymph node metastases in women with breast cancer. JAMA **318**(22), 2199–2210 (2017)
10. Cireşan, D.C.: Mitosis detection in breast cancer histology images with deep neural networks. MICCAI **16**(Pt 2), 411–418 (2013)
11. Lenc, K., et al.: Understanding image representations by measuring their equivariance and equivalence. In: 2015 IEEE CVPR, pp. 991–999 (2015)
12. Huang, G., et al.: Densely connected convolutional networks (2016)
13. Ioffe, S., et al.: Batch normalization: accelerating deep network training by reducing internal covariate shift. In: ICML, pp. 448–456 (2015)
14. Spanhol, F.A.: A dataset for breast cancer histopathological image classification. IEEE Trans. Biomed. Eng. **63**(7), 1455–1462 (2016)
15. Song, Y., Chang, H., Huang, H., Cai, W.: Supervised intra-embedding of fisher vectors for histopathology image classification. In: Descoteaux, M., Maier-Hein, L., Franz, A., Jannin, P., Collins, D.L., Duchesne, S. (eds.) MICCAI 2017. LNCS, vol. 10435, pp. 99–106. Springer, Cham (2017). https://doi.org/10.1007/978-3-319-66179-7_12
16. Kingma, D.P., et al.: Adam: a method for stochastic optimization (2014)
17. Wang, D., et al.: Deep learning for identifying metastatic breast cancer (2016)

A Probabilistic Model Combining Deep Learning and Multi-atlas Segmentation for Semi-automated Labelling of Histology

Alessia Atzeni[1]([⊠]), Marnix Jansen[2], Sébastien Ourselin[3,4P],
and Juan Eugenio Iglesias[1]

[1] Medical Physics and Biomedical Engineering,
University College London, London, UK
alessia.atzeni.14@ucl.ac.uk
[2] University College London Hospital, London, UK
[3] Wellcome EPSRC Centre for Interventional and Surgical Sciences (WEISS),
University College London, London, UK
[4] The School of Biomedical Engineering and Imaging Science, King's College
London, London, UK

Abstract. Thanks to their high resolution and contrast enhanced by different stains, histological images are becoming increasingly widespread in atlas construction. Building atlases with histology requires manual delineation of a set of regions of interest on a large amount of sections. This process is tedious, time-consuming, and rather inefficient due to the high similarity of adjacent sections. Here we propose a probabilistic model for semi-automated segmentation of stacks of histological sections, in which the user manually labels a sparse set of sections (e.g., one every n), and lets the algorithm complete the segmentation for other sections automatically. The proposed model integrates in a principled manner two families of segmentation techniques that have been very successful in brain imaging: multi-atlas segmentation (MAS) and convolutional neural networks (CNNs). Within this model, we derive a Generalised Expectation Maximisation algorithm to compute the most likely segmentation. Experiments on the Allen dataset show that the model successfully combines the strengths of both techniques (effective label propagation of MAS, and robustness to misregistration of CNNs), and produces significantly more accurate results than using either of them independently.

1 Introduction

Histological sections, which can be digitised at sub-micron resolution, allow to differentiate and characterise brain substructures that are not visible with mm-scale imaging (e.g., MRI), and are becoming increasingly popular for building high resolution brain atlases, e.g., BigBrain [1] or Allen [2]. An important component of many of these atlases is a set of associated manual delineations of regions

© Springer Nature Switzerland AG 2018
A. F. Frangi et al. (Eds.): MICCAI 2018, LNCS 11071, pp. 219–227, 2018.
https://doi.org/10.1007/978-3-030-00934-2_25

of interest. Manual segmentation is however tedious and time-consuming – and thus expensive. In histological datasets, where stacks of 2D sections are labelled to create a 3D segmentation, manually delineating adjacent sections is very inefficient due to their similarity. A possible solution is the use of semi-automated algorithms, which allow labelling one slice every n, letting the method complete the segmentation task automatically, with the possibility of final user refinement.

Many semi-automated algorithms rely on the introduction of user defined scribbles or boundary points, which are treated as prior information by the algorithm to produce a dense segmentation of the whole image. If the computational complexity of the method is low enough, the user can interactively review the output and add or remove scribbles/points to correct mistakes, refining the segmentation until it is satisfactory. Popular semi-automated segmentation techniques include Random walker [3] or GeoS [4]. For 3D modalities like MR or CT, one can label a subset of slices and use them as input for these algorithms to complete the segmentation for the whole volume. However, for stacks of histological images, these techniques cannot be used due to the absence of 3D continuity between sections.

An alternative approach is to treat the labelled sections as training data, and use supervised segmentation techniques to segment the unlabelled sections in between. A very successful family of techniques in brain image segmentation are multi-atlas based [5,6]. Multi-atlas segmentation (MAS) relies on non-rigid registration between a set of atlases and a test image. The deformations resulting from the registration are used to propagate the atlas labels to the novel image coordinates, where the segmentation of each pixel is decided through a label fusion approach. These techniques are well suited for inter-slice labelling as long as the registered sections are not too far apart, such that the registration can be expected to be good.

Meanwhile, deep learning techniques, best represented by convolutional neural networks (CCNs), have become increasingly popular in medical image segmentation. Deep learning can be directly applied to semi-automated segmentation of medical images. For example, a 3D U-net was trained on few manually annotated orthogonal slices in [7], in order to produce a segmentation for the whole volume. The negative effects of the limited training data were ameliorated with aggressive data augmentation.

The present paper integrates deep learning and label fusion into a joint probabilistic model in a principled way. Along with the model, we present an inference method – based on the Generalised Expectation Maximisation (GEM) algorithm – to compute the most likely segmentation for an input histological image, given the labelled neighbouring sections. The proposed algorithm successfully combines the advantages of the two techniques, inheriting: 1. from CNNs, the robustness to registration errors, which might happen due to artefacts or large separation between the sections to register; and 2. from MAS, the ability to preserve anatomical shape, including faint or invisible boundaries that rely on prior knowledge, e.g., between brain substructures or cortical regions.

2   Methods

2.1   Probabilistic Model

The graphical model of the proposed probabilistic framework is shown in Fig. 1. Let $\{I_n(\boldsymbol{x})\}_{n=1,\dots,N}$ be N histological sections defined on discrete coordinates $\boldsymbol{x}$ over an image domain $\Omega \subset \mathbb{R}^2$, for which a manual segmentation is available. In a similar manner, let $\{L_n(\boldsymbol{x})\}_{n=1,\dots,N}$ be the corresponding (manual) segmentations. $\{I_n(\boldsymbol{x})\}$ and $\{L_n(\boldsymbol{x})\}$ define thus a training dataset of atlases. We assume that these atlases have been pre-registered to a test image $I(\boldsymbol{x})$, whose labels $L(\boldsymbol{x})$ are unknown. A label fusion approach aims to estimate the label map $\boldsymbol{L}$ associated with $\boldsymbol{I}$, given the registered atlases. Here we assume the availability of a probabilistic fusion algorithm that produces a posterior probability of the segmentation p^f that factorises over voxels:

$$p^f(\boldsymbol{L}|\{\boldsymbol{I_n}\}, \{\boldsymbol{L_n}\}, \boldsymbol{I}) = \prod_{\boldsymbol{x} \in \Omega} p_{\boldsymbol{x}}^f(L(\boldsymbol{x})|\ \{\boldsymbol{I_n}\}, \{\boldsymbol{L_n}\}, \boldsymbol{I}).$$

Let $\boldsymbol{\theta}$ be the parameters of a semantic segmentation neural network trained on all images and corresponding segmentations within our framework – both the atlases and the test image. We can then derive a discriminative probability density function on $\boldsymbol{\theta}$, conditioned on the training data:

$$p(\boldsymbol{\theta}|\ \boldsymbol{I}, \{\boldsymbol{I_n}\}, \boldsymbol{L}, \{\boldsymbol{L_n}\})$$
$$\propto p(\boldsymbol{\theta}) \exp\left[\lambda\left(\sum_{\boldsymbol{x}} H\Big[L(\boldsymbol{x})|\ p_{\boldsymbol{x}}^d(L(\boldsymbol{x})|\ \boldsymbol{I}; \theta)\Big] + \sum_{n=1}^{N} H\Big[L_n(\boldsymbol{x})|\ p_{\boldsymbol{x}}^d(L_n(\boldsymbol{x})|\ \boldsymbol{I_n}; \theta)\Big]\right)\right],$$

where $p(\boldsymbol{\theta})$ is the prior on $\boldsymbol{\theta}$ (e.g., penalty on parameters), H is the cross-entropy function, λ is a constant that weights the importance of the cross entropy, and $p_{\boldsymbol{x}}^d(l|\ \boldsymbol{I}; \boldsymbol{\theta})$ is the soft prediction of the network for label l and image $\boldsymbol{I}$ at location $\boldsymbol{x}$, when the network parameters are equal to $\boldsymbol{\theta}$.

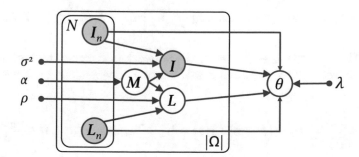

Fig. 1. Graphical model representing the relationship between the model variables. Replications are illustrated with plates. Shaded variables are observed.

2.2   Inference: Proposed Method

The goal of the proposed method is to compute the most likely segmentation $\boldsymbol{L}$ of the test image, given the observed variables $\boldsymbol{I}, \{\boldsymbol{L}_n\}, \{\boldsymbol{I}_n\}$. In a fully Bayesian approach, we would marginalise over the neural network weights $\boldsymbol{\theta}$ when computing the posterior distribution of $\boldsymbol{L}$ that we aim to maximise. However, this leads to an intractable integral over $\boldsymbol{\theta}$. Instead, we make the standard assumption that the posterior distribution of the parameters $\boldsymbol{\theta}$ is heavily peaked, and therefore we can approximate:

$$\hat{\boldsymbol{L}} = \underset{L}{\arg\max}\, p(\boldsymbol{L}|\ \boldsymbol{I}, \{\boldsymbol{I}_n\}, \{\boldsymbol{L}_n\}, \hat{\boldsymbol{\theta}}), \quad \text{with} \quad \hat{\boldsymbol{\theta}} = \underset{\theta}{\arg\max}\, p(\boldsymbol{\theta}|\ \boldsymbol{I}, \{\boldsymbol{I}_n\}, \{\boldsymbol{L}_n\}),$$

which we can rewrite as:

$$\hat{\boldsymbol{\theta}} = \underset{\theta}{\arg\max}\, \sum_L p(\boldsymbol{\theta}|\ \boldsymbol{L}, \{\boldsymbol{L}_n\}, \boldsymbol{I}, \{\boldsymbol{I}_n\}) p(\boldsymbol{L}|\ \boldsymbol{I}, \{\boldsymbol{I}_n\}, \{\boldsymbol{L}_n\})$$

$$= \underset{\theta}{\arg\max}\, \prod_{x \in \Omega} \prod_{n'=1}^{N} \left[p_x^d\left(L_{n'}(\boldsymbol{x})|\ \boldsymbol{I}_{n'}; \boldsymbol{\theta} \right) \right]^\lambda \sum_l \left[p_x^d\left(l|\boldsymbol{I}; \boldsymbol{\theta} \right) \right]^\lambda p_x^f\left(l|\ \boldsymbol{I}, \{\boldsymbol{L}_n\}, \{\boldsymbol{I}_n\} \right) p(\boldsymbol{\theta}).$$

Taking logarithm, we obtain the following objective function:

$$\mathcal{L}(\boldsymbol{\theta}) = \log p(\boldsymbol{\theta}) + \lambda \sum_{x \in \Omega} \sum_{n'=1}^{N} \log p_x^d\left(L_{n'}(\boldsymbol{x})|\boldsymbol{I}_{n'}; \boldsymbol{\theta} \right)$$

$$+ \sum_{x \in \Omega} \log \left\{ \sum_l \left[p_x^d\left(l|\ \boldsymbol{I}; \boldsymbol{\theta} \right) \right]^\lambda p_x^f\left(l|\ \boldsymbol{I}, \boldsymbol{L}_n, \boldsymbol{I}_n \right) \right\}. \tag{1}$$

The objective function in Eq. 1 can be optimised with GEM [8]:

E-step. We build a lower bound to the objective function $\mathcal{L}(\boldsymbol{\theta})$ that touches it at the current estimate of the parameters. This involves computing a soft segmentation $w_l(\boldsymbol{x})$ at each pixel of the test image $\boldsymbol{I}$:

$$w_l(\boldsymbol{x}) = \left[p_x^d(l|\ \boldsymbol{I}, \boldsymbol{\theta}) \right]^\lambda p_x^f(l|\ \boldsymbol{I}, \boldsymbol{L}_n, \boldsymbol{I}_n) \bigg/ \sum_{l'} \left[p_x^d(l'|\ \boldsymbol{I}, \boldsymbol{\theta}) \right]^\lambda p_x^f(l'|\ \boldsymbol{I}, \boldsymbol{L}_n, \boldsymbol{I}_n). \tag{2}$$

M-step. We update the estimates of the network parameters by optimising the bound with respect to $\boldsymbol{\theta}$. Leaving aside terms independent of $\boldsymbol{\theta}$, we seek to maximise:

$$\underset{\theta}{\arg\max}\, \sum_{x \in \Omega} \sum_{n'=1}^{N} \log p_x^d\left(L_{n'}(\boldsymbol{x})|\ \boldsymbol{I}_{n'}; \boldsymbol{\theta} \right) + \sum_{x \in \Omega} \sum_l w_l(\boldsymbol{x}) \log p_x^d(l|\ \boldsymbol{I}, \boldsymbol{\theta}) + \frac{\log p(\boldsymbol{\theta})}{\lambda}. \tag{3}$$

Maximising Eq. 3 amounts to training a neural network with regulariser $\lambda^{-1} \log p(\boldsymbol{\theta})$, using the standard cross entropy loss – and including not only the atlases in the training dataset, but also the target image with its soft segmentation $w_l(\boldsymbol{x})$. This can be achieved with standard numerical techniques, e.g., based on stochastic gradient descent. We note that a standard EM algorithm would require exact maximisation of Eq. 3, whereas numerical methods will only improve the bound. However, improving the bound also leads to an improvement in the original objective function; hence "generalised EM".

The GEM algorithm alternates between the E and M steps until convergence. At that point, it is straightforward to show that:

$$p(\boldsymbol{L}|\ \boldsymbol{I}, \{\boldsymbol{I}_n\}, \{\boldsymbol{L}_n\}, \hat{\boldsymbol{\theta}}) = \prod_{\boldsymbol{x} \in \Omega} w_{L(\boldsymbol{x})}(\boldsymbol{x}),$$

and the final segmentation is given by: $\hat{L}(\boldsymbol{x}) = \mathrm{argmax}_l\, w_l(\boldsymbol{x})$.

2.3   Model Instantiation

In our semi-automated histology segmentation problem, labelled sections play the role of atlases, whereas $\boldsymbol{I}$ is an unlabelled section. To model $p_{\boldsymbol{x}}^f$, we choose the local label fusion model from [9], which relies on a latent discrete field $M(\boldsymbol{x})$ that indexes what atlas generates the test image and its segmentation at each location. The model further assumes that the image intensities $\boldsymbol{I}$ and labels $\boldsymbol{L}$ are conditionally independent given the field $\boldsymbol{M}$. As in [9], we use a Gaussian likelihood term for the image intensities and a LogOdds model based on the signed distance transform for the labels. In addition, we use a prior for the field $\boldsymbol{M}$ that reflects lower reliability of the registration for sections at larger distances from one another, independently from the 2D location $\boldsymbol{x}$: $p(M(\boldsymbol{x}) = n) \propto \exp(-\alpha|z - z_n|)$, where z and z_n be section indices for the test image and atlas n, respectively, and α is a parameter controlling the sharpness of the prior. Following [9], the posterior probability for the labels is then:

$$p_{\boldsymbol{x}}^f(L(\boldsymbol{x})|\ \{\boldsymbol{I}_n\}, \{\boldsymbol{L}_n\}, \boldsymbol{I}) = \frac{\sum_{n=1}^{N} \mathcal{N}[I(\boldsymbol{x}); I_n(\boldsymbol{x}), \sigma^2] e^{\rho D_{\boldsymbol{x}}[L(\boldsymbol{x}); \boldsymbol{L}_n]} e^{-\alpha|z - z_n|}}{\sum_{n=1}^{N} e^{-\alpha|z - z_n|} \mathcal{N}[I(\boldsymbol{x}); I_n(\boldsymbol{x}), \sigma^2] \sum_l e^{\rho D_{\boldsymbol{x}}[l; \boldsymbol{L}_n]}} \quad (4)$$

where $\mathcal{N}$ is the Gaussian distribution; $D_{\boldsymbol{x}}$ is the signed distance transform evaluated at location $\boldsymbol{x}$; and σ^2 and ρ are the likelihood parameters.

For the deep learning framework we use a fully convolutional network (FCN) [10]. We built a FCN on top of a VGG-16 architecture [11], with publicly available weights pre-trained on ImageNet [12]. This architecture was modified by removing the classification layer, and converting fully connected layers to convolutions. A 1×1 convolution layer, with as many channels as output classes, was added at each of the coarse output locations, followed by deconvolution layers to upsample the coarse outputs to fine-grain outputs. Skip connections were added between lower and higher layers, enabling prediction at input resolution. Finally, we used an L2 norm penalty on the network weights, i.e., as $-\log p(\boldsymbol{\theta})$.

3   Experiments and Results

3.1   Data

We used the publicly available Allen atlas [2], which includes 106 (unevenly spaced) Nissl-stained histological sections of a human hemisphere with associated manual segmentations for 862 brain structures. The sections are $50\,\mu$m thick and digitised at $1\,\mu$m resolution, but we downsampled them to $250\,\mu$m – as a compromise between detail and computational requirements. Using the label ontology from the Allen Institute, we created two simplified sets of labels: one at the tissue type level (white matter, grey matter, cerebrospinal fluid), and another at the whole structure level, including: cerebral WM, cerebral cortex, lateral ventricle, cerebellar WM, cerebellar cortex, thalamus, caudate, putamen, pallidum, brainstem, hippocampus and amygdala. The tissue level labels are useful for coarse fine-tuning, and the structure level labels will be used in evaluation: using the full Allen ontology introduces excessive noise in the results, due to large differences in the sets of structures appearing in consecutive sections.

3.2   Experimental Setup

We perform a cross-validation on the 106 labelled sections using two folds: one in which even sections are used to predict the segmentation of the odds sections, and vice versa. We compared our proposed method with three competing approaches: the local label fusion method, the CNN alone (with global and local fine-tuning), and an *ad hoc* combination of the two using the product rule, i.e., $p(L) \propto p^d(L)p^f(L)$. As metric of performance, we used the percentage of correctly classified pixels based on the labelling at the structure level.

Each fold was processed as follows. First we globally fine-tuned the network using all available labelled sections of the training fold and the tissue type labels. This enabled a fast transition from the ImageNet weights, effectively adapting the features to the histological images. The learning rates of the final

Table 1. Minimum and median pixel classification accuracy. The p values are for a non-parametric, paired, two-sided Wilcoxon statistical test comparing medians.

Method	Min. acc. (%)	Med. acc. (%)	p-val vs. CNN	p-val vs. LF	p-val vs. *ad hoc*
CNN	75.35	90.55	N/A	N/A	N/A
Lab. Fus.	73.61	91.81	0.03	N/A	N/A
Ad hoc	85.30	92.62	5×10^{-15}	9×10^{-6}	N/A
Proposed	85.83	92.91	3×10^{-15}	5×10^{-8}	4×10^{-8}

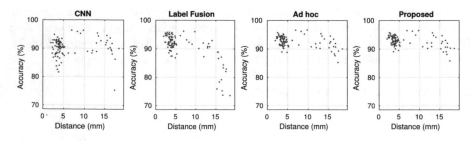

Fig. 2. Pixel classification accuracy vs. average distance between atlas and test sections.

four convolutional layers were increased by a factor of 20 for fine-tuning. We used rotation, translation, scaling and contrast/brightness changes for data augmentation. Then, we visit one unlabelled section at the time, and go over the following three steps: label fusion, local fine-tuning and GEM. For the label fusion, we used the preceding and succeeding labelled sections as atlases. We used NiftyReg with stationary velocity field parameterisation [13] for the registration (default parameters with local correlation metric), and computed soft predictions for the structure level labels with Eq. 4. The local fine-tuning used the same two sections as training data. We replaced the final layers from the globally fine-tuned network, and further fine-tuned to the structure level labels, with the same augmentation scheme. Finally, we iterated between the E and M steps of the GEM algorithm (Eqs. 2 and 3) to produce the final output. The parameters were kept constant for all experiments: $\sigma^2 = 400$, $\rho = 21\text{mm}^{-1}$, $\alpha = 1\text{mm}^{-1}$, $\lambda = 2$.

3.3   Results

Table 1 shows the median pixel classification accuracy for the competing methods, computed inside a mask obtained by dilating 2 mm the union of the ground truth segmentations. The table also shows p-values for paired, non-parametric tests comparing the medians achieved by the different methods, as well as the minimal accuracy across the dataset – which is a measure of robustness.

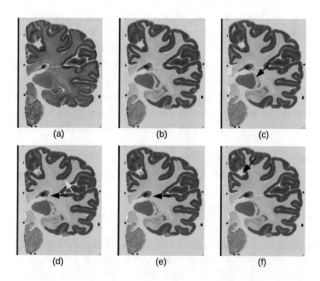

Fig. 3. Sample section from the Allen dataset with segmentation results overlaid. (a) Histological section. (b) Manual segmentation. (c) Label fusion. (d) CNN. (e) *Ad hoc* combination with product rule. (f) Proposed method.

Figure 2 plots accuracy against the mean separation between the atlas and test sections $(1/2)(|z - z_1| + |z - z_2|)$. The CNN provides consistent performance across distances, remaining robust even at large separations. Label fusion alone, in contrast, yields higher scores at low separations (when registration is generally more accurate) but falters at larger distances. Combining the algorithms enables us to take advantage of the strengths of both: the *ad hoc* method outperforms CNN and label fusion, and a further improvement is obtained when integrating the two approaches into a unified model in a principled way. Albeit small (0.3% accuracy), this improvement is consistent ($p < 10^{-7}$) and visually noticeable.

The differences between the methods are illustrated in Fig. 3. Label fusion fails to segment the retrosplenial cortex (Fig. 3c, yellow arrow) and to recover the reticular nucleus of the thalamus (black arrow). The CNN (Fig. 3d) ameliorates these issues, but introduces new errors, e.g., voxels labeled as ventricle due to tears (yellow arrow), or completely missing the caudate due to insufficient contrast (black arrow). The *ad hoc* method (Fig. 3e) solves some of these problems, but still fails to recover the caudate (black arrow). Our approach not only manages to segment the caudate, but also cleans up some other segmentation errors, e.g., the false positives in cortical areas (black arrow in Fig. 3f).

4   Discussion and Conclusion

We have presented a probabilistic model for semi-automated segmentation of stacks of 2D histological sections, which allows to incorporate label fusion techniques with deep learning. The model is flexible both in terms of CNN architecture and label fusion methods – as long as the posterior distribution of the segmentation factorises over voxels, which is the case for most available algorithms. Since each iteration requires fine-tuning the network in the M-step (which takes ca. 4 min on a Titan Xp GPU), the method is computationally expensive. However, this is seldom a problem in practice because the algorithm can be run offline. Future work will focus on integrating the registration with the segmentation in the framework, such that the registration of atlas sections further away from the test image can benefit from the more robust CNN classification.

Acknowledgement. supported by the EPSRC (CDT in Medical Imaging, EP/ L016478/1), ERC (Starting Grant 677697) and NVIDIA (donation of GPU).

References

1. Amunts, K., Lepage, C., Borgeat, L., Mohlberg, H., Dickscheid, T., et al.: BigBrain: an ultrahigh-resolution 3D human brain model. Science **340**, 1472–1475 (2013)
2. Ding, S.L., Royall, J.J., Sunkin, S.M., Ng, L., Facer, B.A., et al.: Comprehensive cellular-resolution atlas of the adult human brain. J. Comp. Neurol. **524**(16), 3127–3481 (2016)
3. Grady, L.: Random walks for image segmentation. IEEE Trans. Pattern Anal. Mach. Intell. **28**(11), 1768–1783 (2006)
4. Criminisi, A., Sharp, T., Blake, A.: GeoS: Geodesic image segmentation. In: Forsyth, D., Torr, P., Zisserman, A. (eds.) ECCV 2008. LNCS, vol. 5302, pp. 99–112. Springer, Heidelberg (2008). https://doi.org/10.1007/978-3-540-88682-2_9

5. Rohlfing, T., Brandt, R., Menzel, R., Maurer Jr., C.R.: Evaluation of atlas selection strategies for atlas-based image segmentation with application to confocal microscopy images of bee brains. NeuroImage **21**(4), 1428–1442 (2004)
6. Iglesias, J.E., Sabuncu, M.R.: Multi-atlas segmentation of biomedical images: a survey. Med. Image Anal. **24**(1), 205–219 (2015)
7. Çiçek, Ö., Abdulkadir, A., Lienkamp, S.S., Brox, T., Ronneberger, O.: 3D U-Net: learning dense volumetric segmentation from sparse annotation. In: Ourselin, S., Joskowicz, L., Sabuncu, M.R., Unal, G., Wells, W. (eds.) MICCAI 2016. LNCS, vol. 9901, pp. 424–432. Springer, Cham (2016). https://doi.org/10.1007/978-3-319-46723-8_49
8. Dempster, A.P., Laird, N.M., Rubin, D.B.: Maximum likelihood from incomplete data via the EM algorithm. J. R. Stat. Soc., 1–38 (1977)
9. Sabuncu, M.R., Yeo, B.T., Van Leemput, K., Fischl, B., Golland, P.: A generative model for image segmentation based on label fusion. IEEE Trans. Med. Imaging **29**(10), 1714–1729 (2010)
10. Long, J., Shelhamer, E., Darrell, T.: Fully convolutional networks for semantic segmentation. In: CVPR, pp. 3431–3440 (2015)
11. Simonyan, K., Zisserman, A.: Very deep convolutional networks for large-scale image recognition. arXiv:1409.1556 (2014)
12. Deng, J., Dong, W., Socher, R., Li, L.J., Li, K., Fei-Fei, L.: Imagenet: a large-scale hierarchical image database. In: CVPR, pp. 248–255 (2009)
13. Modat, M., Daga, P., Cardoso, M.J., Ourselin, S., Ridgway, G.R., Ashburner, J.: Parametric non-rigid registration using a stationary velocity field. In: Mathematical Methods in Biomedical Image Analysis, pp. 145–150 (2012)

BESNet: Boundary-Enhanced Segmentation of Cells in Histopathological Images

Hirohisa Oda[1(✉)], Holger R. Roth[2], Kosuke Chiba[3], Jure Sokolić[4],
Takayuki Kitasaka[5], Masahiro Oda[3], Akinari Hinoki[3], Hiroo Uchida[3],
Julia A. Schnabel[4], and Kensaku Mori[2,6,7]

[1] Graduate School of Information Science, Nagoya University, Nagoya, Japan
hoda@mori.m.is.nagoya-u.ac.jp
[2] Graduate School of Informatics, Nagoya University, Nagoya, Japan
[3] Nagoya University Graduate School of Medicine, Nagoya, Japan
[4] Division of Imaging Sciences and Biomedical Engineering, King's College London,
London, UK
[5] School of Information Science, Aichi Institute of Technology, Toyota, Japan
[6] Information Technology Center, Nagoya University, Nagoya, Japan
[7] Research Center for Medical Bigdata, National Institute of Informatics,
Tokyo, Japan

Abstract. We propose a novel deep learning method called Boundary-Enhanced Segmentation Network (BESNet) for the detection and semantic segmentation of cells on histopathological images. The semantic segmentation of small regions using fully convolutional networks typically suffers from inaccuracies around the boundaries of small structures, like cells, because the probabilities often become blurred. In this work, we propose a new network structure that encodes input images to feature maps similar to U-net but utilizes two decoding paths that restore the original image resolution. One decoding path enhances the boundaries of cells, which can be used to improve the quality of the entire cell segmentation achieved in the other decoding path. We explore two strategies for enhancing the boundaries of cells: (1) skip connections of feature maps, and (2) adaptive weighting of loss functions. In (1), the feature maps from the boundary decoding path are concatenated with the decoding path for entire cell segmentation. In (2), an adaptive weighting of the loss for entire cell segmentation is performed when boundaries are not enhanced strongly, because detecting such parts is difficult. The detection rate of ganglion cells was 80.0% with 1.0 false positives per histopathology slice. The mean Dice index representing segmentation accuracy was 74.0%. BESNet produced a similar detection performance and higher segmentation accuracy than comparable U-net architectures without our modifications.

© Springer Nature Switzerland AG 2018
A. F. Frangi et al. (Eds.): MICCAI 2018, LNCS 11071, pp. 228–236, 2018.
https://doi.org/10.1007/978-3-030-00934-2_26

1   Introduction

The detection or the semantic segmentation of cells in histopathological images using fully convolutional networks has been explored [1,2] for many diagnostic or medical research purposes. Our focus in this work is the ganglion cell detection of the HE-stained images of pediatric intestine specimens of Hirschsprung's disease [3]. To quicken and increase the accuracy of its pathologic diagnosis during surgery, an automatic segmentation method of ganglion cells is required. There may be several ganglion cells on HE-stained images, which have variations of color, size, shape, and contrast. Many cells or tissues also resemble ganglion cells on HE-stained images.

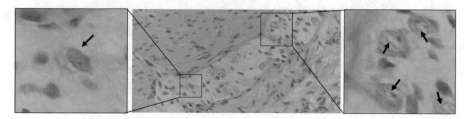

Fig. 1. Ganglion cells on HE-stained images: Green circles or black arrows represent ganglion cells, which have variations of color, shape, and contrast. Cells or tissues also exist that resemble ganglion cells.

U-net [1] is one of the most popular and widely used fully convolutional architectures, which segment biomedical images well. However, for small objects in large images, blurring of the probability response maps occurs around the boundaries of these small objects. This problem is caused by lack of consideration of difficulties around the target object borders. Hand-crafted weighting schemes of the loss for outside objects have been introduced for improving the prediction in these regions [1,2]. However, adaptive weighting schemes for improving the responses around the border based on the difficulty of training have not yet been considered. We tackle these problems by proposing a (1) new network architecture called Boundary-Enhanced Segmentation Network (BESNet) and a (2) Boundary-Enhanced Cross Entropy (BECE) loss. BESNet consists of a network with two decoding paths. One is trained for boundary prediction but suffers from inaccuracies because detecting the boundaries is difficult. This information on the degree of difficulty of detecting a network's boundaries can be fused with the decoder path for entire cell segmentation by skip connections and (2) Boundary-Enhanced Cross Entropy loss. Accessing and modifying feature maps in the layers that haven't been decoded yet is inspired by deep supervision, which is especially useful for edge enhancement [4]. In this work, we enhance the segmentation of the entire cell by utilizing the feature maps of boundaries.

The BESNet performance is shown by the detection and the segmentation of ganglion cells from the HE-stained images of the histopathological samples of pediatric intestine. As shown in Fig. 1, ganglion cells are scattered on HE-stained images, and many similar regions surround them. A computer-aided diagnosis system that detects and measures the size of the ganglion cells is required for assisting the rapid pathologic diagnosis during surgery, which finds ganglion cells from HE-stained images. To the best of our knowledge, no other work has addressed the detection or segmentation of ganglion cells apart from our preliminary work [5].

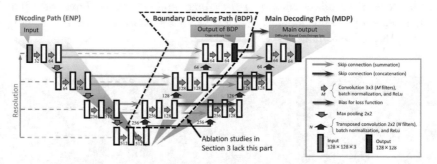

Fig. 2. Network structure of BESNet: While encoding part resembles standard U-net, BESNet has two decoding parts, Boundary Decoding Path (BDP) and Main Decoding Path (MDP). Feature maps in BDP are concatenated with MDP. Loss function for MDP is weighted by BDP output.

2   Method

2.1   Boundary-Enhanced Segmentation Network (BESNet)

BESNet is a novel, fully convolutional network for semantic segmentation. Its concept is to train the boundaries of the targeted cells and use their responses to adaptively weight the training loss for entire cell segmentation. This allows us to apply a stronger weight in the more difficult part of the targeted cell during training. Our proposed network structure is shown in Fig. 2. Any input patch is encoded into feature maps in a similar way to U-net [1] on the ENcoding Path (ENP). Unlike U-net, BESNet has two decoding paths. A Boundary Decoding Path (BDP) is trained using the boundary labels of the annotated cells. Feature maps in this path are concatenated with Main Decoding Path (MDP), which is trained on all of the cell labels. After two layers of 3×3 convolution (CV), batch normalization (BN), and ReLU activation functions (RA), 2×2 max pooling (MP) decreases the resolution at each level of the ENP. After repeating these layers (CV, BN, RA, CV, BN, RA, and MP) three times and this sequence twice (CV, BN, RA), we obtain feature maps whose resolution is the lowest but has the highest level of abstraction for effective semantic segmentation. Here, the network is branched into BDP and MDP. The resolution is restored by 2×2 transposed convolutions (TC) at each resolution level. Both BDP and MDP have three times of the sequence (RA, TC, CV, BN) with a final CV layer with 1×1

convolution kernels and *sigmoid* activations. For each TC on BDP and MDP, feature maps after the last RA in the same resolution in ENP are summed by skip connections. Moreover, for each RA on MDP, feature maps after the last RA in the same resolution in BDP is concatenated using skip connections.

2.2 Boundary-Enhanced Cross-Entropy (BECE) Loss

The basic idea of cross-entropy, which is one of the most commonly used loss functions, is to penalize the loss more when the network's output is more different than the ground-truth. We utilize cross-entropy loss $\mathcal{L}_C$ for BDP. Since this is a binary problem but we are only interested in how difficult it is to learn the foreground pixels of the boundary, $\mathcal{L}_C$ is defined by

$$\mathcal{L}_C = - \sum_{x \in M} B(x) \log\big(p_B(x)\big) \tag{1}$$

where x represents a pixel in mini-batch M, $B(x) \in \{0, 1\}$ represents the boundary label of the ground-truth at x, and $p_B(x) \in \{0, \cdots, 1\}^{\mathbb{R}}$ represents the BDP output at x.

BDP output $p_B(x)$ usually performs well at the boundaries, but it may become low at the boundary parts that are less clear or have rare types of appearances. This means that the features of the boundaries with low output of BDP probability are difficult to train by the network. Therefore, these parts should be trained more strongly by MDP by adaptively weighting the loss function for the MDP branch. For MDP, we newly define a Boundary-Enhanced Cross-Entropy (BECE) loss:

$$\mathcal{L}_D = - \sum_{x \in M} \big\{ [1 + b(x)] G(x) \log\big(p_M(x)\big) + w[1 - G(x)] \log\big(1 - p_M(x)\big) \big\} \tag{2}$$

$$b(x) = \alpha \, \max\big(\beta - p_G(x), 0\big) \tag{3}$$

where $G(x) \in \{0, 1\}$ and $p_M(x) \in \{0, \cdots, 1\}^{\mathbb{R}}$ represent the ground-truth label and the MDP output at x, respectively. $b(x)$ is a function that represents the training difficulty of the boundary at x. $\alpha \in \{0, \cdots, 1\}^{\mathbb{R}}$ and $\beta \in \{0, \cdots, 1\}^{\mathbb{R}}$ are coefficients for the strength of boundary-enhanced weighting and minimum value of p_B that are enhanced well, respectively. w is weight for background pixels, which is the ratio between numbers of positive and negative pixels. This loss definition is partly inspired by Focal Loss [6], but it adjusts the weighting just from the probabilities of the same output of the network.

2.3 Training and Testing

Input and Output: Our method detects and segments cells from histopathological images. For training, a set of images and their ground-truth labels G_n

are required. Detection and segmentation of cells are performed on the images for testing. The output is a set of ganglion cell regions.

Training: Histopathological images, which are usually scanned in high resolution, are much bigger (e.g., 1636×1088 pixels) than what we can fit on GPU memory as input to BESNet, (see Sect. 2.1 for more details). Hence, we first perform d-times downsampling of the images and the ground-truth. Then patches ($s_x \times s_y$ pixels) are cropped randomly, but at least one positive pixel must exist in the ground-truth. We employ a data augmentation process during training that consists of random rotation, translation, and elastic deformations by B-spline splitting. We collect m images as a mini-batch for training at each iteration.

Testing: BESNet is reshaped so that the input and output sizes cover larger region $s_{rx} \times s_{ry}$ pixels. The testing image is divided into patches in a grid pattern with v-voxel overlap to the neighboring patches. The MDP output is computed for each patch, and the output for every histopathological image is combined from all the patch predictions. The average responses are computed on the overlapping parts of multiple patches to allow smooth transitions of the responses across patches.

3   Experiments

Overview: To evaluate the segmentation accuracy of our proposed model without decreasing the detection performance of the cells, we conducted detection and segmentation of the ganglion cells on the HE-stained images of histopathological samples. The detection performance was evaluated by the detection rate and the number of false positives (FPs) per image (FPs/image). Segmentation accuracy was evaluated by Dice index, precision, and recall. Probability threshold t was set to $0.05, 0.10, \cdots, 0.95$ for FROC evaluation.

Dataset: The HE-stained images of the intestine parts whose peristaltic movement is functioning properly were obtained from 25 patients suffering from Hirschsprung disease from whom we received ethical approval from Nagoya University Hospital (Japan). They include 741 ganglion cells from 224 images. Each specimen was imaged with an ECLIPSE Ni-U (Nikon) microscope and scanned by a DS-Ri2 (Nikon) camera as RGB-color images consisting of 1636×1088 pixels. Resolution is $250 \times 250 \, \text{nm}^2$. The ground-truth labels were manually created by an expert pediatric surgeon.

Condition: Three-fold cross validation was conducted by dividing the patients into three groups. The network was implemented on Keras with a TensorFlow backend. The parameters were empirically set to $d = 2, s_x \times s_y = 256 \times 256$, $s'_x \times s'_y = 768 \times 256$, $\alpha = 0.5$ and $\beta = 0.1$. DeepLearningBOX (GDEP Advance) workstations with GTX 1080 Ti (NVIDIA) GPUs, CUDA 8.0, and cuDNN 6.0 was used for the computation. We fixed the random number of seeds of NumPy and TensorFlow for reproducibility. Other training conditions were set as follows: mini-batch size to 8, iterations to 30000, and optimizer to Adam.

Ablation Studies: For a comparison with the proposed method, we conducted two ablation studies: "U-net & Cross-entropy" and "U-net & Dice", using cross-entropy loss or Dice loss, respectively. As annotated in Fig. 2, removing BDP from BESNet allows us to get a U-net-like structure. It contains BN layers, and have four levels of resolution (original one [1] has five).

4   Results and Discussions

Detection: The partial FROC curves of the three methods that were obtained by changing threshold t are shown in Fig. 3. Table 1 shows the detection performance when t is 0.20, 0.50, or 0.80. The proposed method's performance was 89.5% of the detection rate with 2.5 ± 7.1 FPs/slice with $t = 0.50$, and an example slice of the results is shown in Fig. 4. All three methods produced similar results. One difference between (c) Dice and the others is the change of the balance between the detection rate and the FPs/slice.

Table 1. Performances of three methods: Partial FROC curves were linearly interpolated and FPs/slice were estimated at 80.0%, 85.0%, and 90.0% of detection rates. Bold FPs/slice represent smallest average. FPs/slice of U-net & Dice at 90.0% of detection rate could not be estimated since no threshold produced detection rate of 90.0% or above.

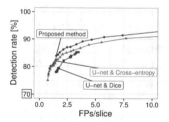

Fig. 3. Partial FROC curves: Proposed method, U-net & Cross-entropy, and U-net & Dice produced similar detection performances.

	Detection rate	FPs/slice
Proposed method	80.0%	**1.0 ± 1.7**
U-net & Cross-entropy		1.1 ± 2.0
U-net & Dice		1.8 ± 2.9
Proposed method	85.0%	**1.8 ± 2.6**
U-net & Cross-entropy		2.4 ± 3.5
U-net & Dice		3.3 ± 4.8
Proposed method	90.0%	**4.8 ± 5.4**
U-net & Cross-entropy		7.1 ± 7.6
U-net & Dice	N/A	

Segmentation: Segmentation accuracies are shown in Table 2 and Figs. 6(a)–(c). The Dice index, precision, and recall of the proposed method were 71.4±31.9, 81.2 ± 32.9, and 67.2 ± 31.7 (mean ± std. dev.), respectively, when threshold t was 0.50. The scores of the true positives (TPs) were computed for the highest regions obtained by the methods, and the scores of all the false negatives are zero. Our proposed method produced the highest Dice index and precision. Using the Wilcoxon rank sum test, most results between the proposed method and others showed significant differences (Table 2).

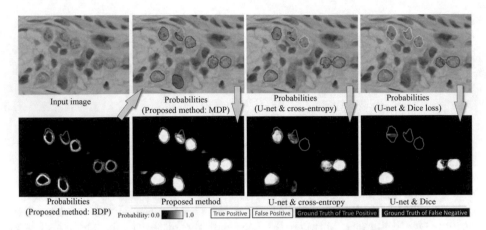

Fig. 4. Probabilities and outputs of three methods.

Table 2. Segmentation accuracy of three methods when t is 0.20, 0.50, or 0.80. Mean $\pm$ standard deviation of each measure is shown. Bold numbers show best mean of all scores among three methods with common t. (*) and (**) represent significant differences between proposed method, which has $p < 0.05$ and $p < 0.01$, respectively.

t	Method	Dice index	Precision	Recall
0.20	Proposed method	**74.0 ± 31.8**	**81.8 ± 29.9**	72.3 ± 32.8
	U-net & Cross-entropy	70.9 ± 33.6 (**)	75.7 ± 31.3 (**)	**72.6 ± 35.8** (**)
	U-net & Dice	69.7 ± 35.1 (**)	74.1 ± 34.3 (**)	70.7 ± 36.8 (**)
0.50	Proposed method	**69.1 ± 34.8**	**79.9 ± 35.2**	64.7 ± 34.1
	U-net & Cross-entropy	66.8 ± 36.7 (*)	75.8 ± 35.9 (**)	65.1 ± 37.3 (**)
	U-net & Dice	67.5 ± 36.9 (*)	73.9 ± 36.2 (**)	**67.0 ± 38.0** (**)
0.80	Proposed method	**63.5 ± 35.9**	**77.7 ± 38.9**	56.9 ± 33.8
	U-net & Cross-entropy	61.6 ± 37.9 (**)	74.2 ± 39.7 (**)	56.8 ± 36.8 (**)
	U-net & Dice	63.3 ± 38.3 (**)	71.3 ± 38.9 (**)	**61.1 ± 38.8** (**)

Three cells on a slice are magnified in Fig. 5. Cell A had blurred probabilities around the boundaries from the U-net & Cross-entropy, as shown in dotted cyan squares. Predicting this part is also difficult by the BDP of our proposed method. Due to the adaptive weighting of such boundaries during training, a clearer and more accurate region segmentation was obtained by MDP. Cell B and C also had weak boundary probabilities from BDP in almost the entire cell. The MDP of our proposed method accurately produced high probabilities on entire of each cell regions, and two cells were divided well. U-net & Cross-entropy produced higher probabilities even gap between two cells, and segmentation results of two cells were connected. This is why Dice index of Cell B was only 57.4% with U-net & Cross-entropy. U-net & Dice produced high probabilities only on Cell B, and Cell C was a false negative. While just dividing two neighboring cells gives the same advantage as other works [1] including methods specific to instance segmentation [2], BESNet also can achieve better segmentation accuracy inside cells.

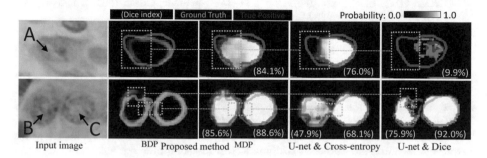

Fig. 5. Probabilities on three cells: Yellow numbers show Dice index of segmentation results where $t = 0.50$. Green circles show ground-truth. In dotted cyan squares of each cell, BDP output does not clearly show boundaries. In such regions, our proposed method produced higher probabilities inside cell and low at ones outside it, compared to U-net.

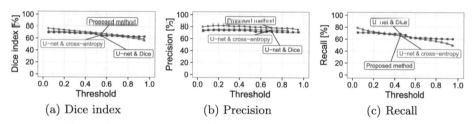

Fig. 6. Segmentation accuracy of three methods. Proposed method had higher Dice index and precision than others.

5   Conclusions

We proposed a novel deep learning method called Boundary-Enhanced Segmentation Network (BESNet) for the detection and semantic segmentation of cells on pathological images. Experimental results on ganglion cells show similar detection performances but significantly better segmentation results. One limitation is computational complexity. Ablation studies with U-net required only about 6 GB GPU memory, but BESNet required about 10 GB. More comparisons to related works are left for future work.

Acknowledgements. Parts of this research were supported by JSPS KAKENHI (26108006, 17H00867, 17K20099) and JSPS Bilateral Joint Research Project.

References

1. Ronneberger, O., Fischer, P., Brox, T.: U-Net: convolutional networks for biomedical image segmentation. In: Navab, N., Hornegger, J., Wells, W.M., Frangi, A.F. (eds.) MICCAI 2015. LNCS, vol. 9351, pp. 234–241. Springer, Cham (2015). https://doi.org/10.1007/978-3-319-24574-4_28
2. Chen, H., Qi, X., Yu, L., Heng, P.A.: DCAN: deep contour-aware networks for accurate gland segmentation. In: Proceedings of the IEEE conference on Computer Vision and Pattern Recognition, pp. 2487–2496 (2016)
3. Amiel, J., Lyonnet, S.: Hirschsprung disease, associated syndromes, and genetics: a review. J. Med. Genet. **38**(11), 729–739 (2001)
4. Xie, S., Tu, Z.: Holistically-nested edge detection. In: Proceedings of the IEEE International Conference on Computer Vision, pp. 1395–1403 (2015)
5. Oda, H., et al.: Automated ganglion cell detection using fully convolutional networks and evaluation under different training losses. In: Computer Assisted Radiology and Surgery (CARS) 2018 (2018)
6. Lin, T.Y., Goyal, P., Girshick, R., He, K., Dollar, P.: Focal loss for dense object detection. In: The IEEE International Conference on Computer Vision (ICCV) (2017)

Panoptic Segmentation with an End-to-End Cell R-CNN for Pathology Image Analysis

Donghao Zhang[1(✉)], Yang Song[1], Dongnan Liu[1], Haozhe Jia[2], Siqi Liu[1], Yong Xia[2], Heng Huang[3], and Weidong Cai[1]

[1] School of Information Technologies, University of Sydney, Sydney, NSW 2006, Australia
dzha9516@uni.sydney.edu.au

[2] School of Computer Science and Engineering, Northwestern Polytechnical University, Xi'an 710072, China

[3] Department of Electrical and Computer Engineering, University of Pittsburgh, Pittsburgh, USA

Abstract. The morphological clues of various cancer cells are essential for pathologists to determine the stages of cancers. In order to obtain the quantitative morphological information, we present an end-to-end network for panoptic segmentation of pathology images. Recently, many methods have been proposed, focusing on the semantic-level or instance-level cell segmentation. Unlike existing cell segmentation methods, the proposed network unifies detecting, localizing objects and assigning pixel-level class information to regions with large overlaps such as the background. This unifier is obtained by optimizing the novel semantic loss, the bounding box loss of Region Proposal Network (RPN), the classifier loss of RPN, the background-foreground classifier loss of segmentation Head instead of class-specific loss, the bounding box loss of proposed cell object, and the mask loss of cell object. The results demonstrate that the proposed method not only outperforms state-of-the-art approaches to the 2017 MICCAI Digital Pathology Challenge dataset, but also proposes an effective and end-to-end solution for the panoptic segmentation challenge.

1 Introduction

Cancer diagnosis by pathologists mainly relies on the visual inspection of tissue sample images captured by microscopy. The morphological features of cells such as the shape and nuclei size are significant to the diagnosis of the cancer stages (benign and malignant). It is impractical and labour-intensive for pathologists to produce manual morphological annotations for the whole slide image.

The general semantic scene understanding can be categorized into semantic segmentation, object detection, instance segmentation, and panoptic segmentation, as shown in Fig. 1. The instance segmentation assigns pixel-level segmentation masks to each individual object. The semantic segmentation obtains pixel-level whole image classification without differentiating different objects belong

© Springer Nature Switzerland AG 2018
A. F. Frangi et al. (Eds.): MICCAI 2018, LNCS 11071, pp. 237–244, 2018.
https://doi.org/10.1007/978-3-030-00934-2_27

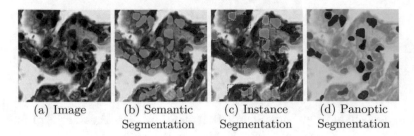

(a) Image   (b) Semantic   (c) Instance   (d) Panoptic
             Segmentation   Segmentation   Segmentation

Fig. 1. An example of illustrating the difference between semantic segmentation, instance segmentation and panoptic segmentation.

to the same class, but panoptic segmentation produces its semantic label (class) and its instance id. Recently in general computer vision, semantic segmentation has drawn a lot of attention, and many methods [1,10,16] based on convolutional neural network architectures are proposed. A U-shaped neural network [12] further includes more feature channels in the upsampling layer, which is proven to generate reasonable segmentation from limited training data such as neuronal structure segmentation of electron microscopy images. LinkNet [1] accelerates the processing time and reduces the network parameters by utilizing addition of feature channels instead of concatenation. Besides semantic segmentation, breakthroughs of object detection and instance segmentation happen due to the region proposal strategy by Faster R-CNN [11] and mask head segmentation by Mask R-CNN [5,6]. The recently introduced panoptic segmentation [9] defines its meaning by unifying semantic segmentation and instance segmentation.

In addition to recent developments of semantic scene understanding in general computer vision, there have been attempts [2,13–15] particularly targeting cell segmentation. The major difference between bio-medical related segmentation and general computer vision is the limited training data due to the difficulty of manual labelling requiring the prior knowledge of the specialists. Some proposed to use unannoted images with adversarial network [15] and others attempt to include contour-aware loss [2] and suggestive annotation [13] to solve these bio-medical segmentation problems. Cell segmentation requires a unique id for each cell so only semantic segmentation is not enough to produce individual object segmentation masks. Although instance segmentation can produce unique ids for each cell object, it only relies on image features of intracellular materials. Moreover, the panoptic segmentation not only produces instance cell masks but also fully utilizes the potential information relation between intercellular and intracellular materials.

Inspired by the related work mentioned above, we propose an end-to-end panoptic segmentation method, named Cell R-CNN, to perform morphological analysis of pathology images. Our contribution is three-fold. First, we propose a unified solution of combining semantic segmentation and instance segmentation by introducing the novel semantic segmentation branch. Second, the proposed branch is capable of detecting regions having large overlaps with objects.

Third, we propose to use upsampling layers to replace deconvolution layers in GCN [10] to reduce the required parameters. Evaluated on the 2017 MICCAI Digital Pathology Challenge dataset, results indicate that the proposed Cell R-CNN outperforms state-of-the-art methods in terms of segmentation metrics including F1-score, Dice, and Hausdorff distance.

2   Methods

The main idea of the proposed framework is to unify semantic segmentation and instance segmentation. The convolutional features like ResNet [4] are used by the RPN [11] in object detection to reduce the computation time of the proposal. Similarly, some recent advances in semantic segmentation also demonstrate that the accuracy of semantic segmentation is improved by applying ResNet as its encoder. Is that possible to share these convolutional features between semantic segmentation and instance segmentation? In this paper, we simply and intuitively choose the global convolutional network (GCN) [10] as our base of semantic segmentation branch. The proposed Cell R-CNN firstly generates the convolutional features using the backbone ResNet, which are shared by the novel and intuitive semantic segmentation branch and feature map branch. This sharing operation improves the potential feature representation ability of backbone network (ResNet). The outputs of feature map branch are then fed into RPN to generate proposals. The region of interest proposals are the inputs of the instance segmentation branches [5]. Finally, the multi-task losses are optimized together to obtain the panoptic segmentation result.

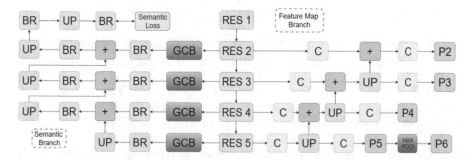

Fig. 2. The network architecture of semantic segmentation branch and feature map branch. C, BR, UP, GCB and RES X represent convolutional layer, boundary refine block, upsampling layer, global convolution block and specific ResNet layer respectively.

2.1   Semantic Segmentation Branch and Feature Map Branch

The overview of the semantic segmentation branch and the feature map branch is shown in Fig. 2. The semantic segmentation branch generates segmentation by assigning pixel-level object class information and the feature map branch prepares the features shared by RPN and instance branches (Sect. 2.2). GCN is chosen for the semantic segmentation branch because it is highly efficient and has global receptive field. ResNet101 is used as the backbone of GCN. The GCB employs convolutional kernels with the size $1 \times k + k \times 1$ and $k \times 1 + 1 \times k$ to ensure that there is enough valid receptive field. Instead of directly using the convolutional kernels with $k \times k$, the GCB is designed to greatly reduce the required training parameters for the network. BR consists of a *conv+relu+conv* block and a residual design: $x = F(x) + x$. BR aims to replace non-trainable conditional random field or other post-processing techniques. In simple words, everything is learnable. Besides the semantic segmentation branch, the features generated by ResNet are also shared by the feature map branch. This design not only maximizes the potential feature representation ability of ResNet but also greatly reduces the required parameters. The feature map branch targets at sharing features $(P2, P3, P4, P5, P6)$ between RPN and the Instance Branch (Sect. 2.2). The first and second the convolutional kernel sizes of feature map branch after ResNet X are 1×1 and 3×3, respectively.

2.2 Region Proposal Network and Instance Branch

The inputs of RPN are the feature maps (P2, P3, P4, P5, P6) and its outputs are bounding box proposals with a score showing the possibility of being an object. The anchors (rectangular bounding boxes) are initially generated by sliding window strategy. At each sampling point, anchors with different ratios and sizes are generated. Each anchor is assigned a score and box delta $(t_x^*, t_y^*, log(w/w_a), log(h/h_a))$ by the RPN shown in Fig. 3. The bounding box regression [3] is defined with the following equations:

$$
\begin{aligned}
t_x = (x - x_a)/w_a, \; t_y = (y - y_a)/h_a, \; t_w = log(w/w_a), \; t_h = log(h/h_a) \\
t_x^* = (x^* - x_a)/w_a, \; t_y^* = (y^* - y_a)/h_a, \; t_w^* = log(w^*/w_a), \; t_h^* = log(h^*/h_a)
\end{aligned}
\tag{1}
$$

where x, y, w and h represent the coordinates of the center sampling points, the width and height of the predicted bounding box (ROIs). Similarly, x_a, y_a, w_a and h_a denote corresponding variables of the anchor box. The other variables are for the ground truth. The outputs of RPN are further refined by the proposal layer. The proposal layer sorts anchors by scores decreasingly. The box delta refinement is then applied and non-max suppression removes candidates of refined bounding boxes with strong overlaps with each other. For optimization of boxes and scores loss, only the positive anchors contribute to the loss calculation. In order to successfully train RPN, the ratio of positive anchors to negative anchors is maintained within a certain range. The kernel sizes of first and last RPN convolution layers are 3×3 and 1×1, respectively.

The instance branches consist of instance location and discriminator branch and instance mask branch. The instance location and discriminator branch further refine bounding box location and evaluate the possibility of each object category (foreground or background), which is a two-stage detector. The instance

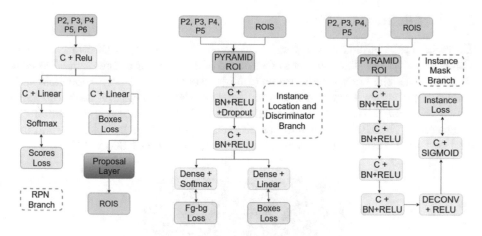

Fig. 3. Region proposal network and instance branch. ROIS, PYRAMID ROI, and DECONV indicate regions of interest, pyramid ROI aligning layer and deconvolutional layer, respectively.

branches use refined ROIs generated by the proposal layer as part of its input, and the other inputs are the feature maps (P2, P3, P4, P5). The pyramid ROI aligning layer selects the corresponding level of feature map based on the size of ROI. Here, instead of class specific loss, we use foreground-background loss. This particular design attempts to segment cells from different classes using the same network inspired by the segment everything work [6]. The instance mask branch is to generate an instance object segmentation when an ROI is given. For kernel sizes of convolutional layer for instance mask branch, all of them are 3×3 except the last convolutional layer is 3×3. The kernel size of deconvolutional layer is 2×2 with stride 2. For the computation of instance loss, the ground truth of object mask is resized into 28×28. This design is to preserve the spatial relation information. Due to pixel-to-pixel correspondence of pyramid ROI aligning layer, the prediction result of instance mask branch can be accurate.

The final loss is defined with the following equation:

$$
\begin{aligned}
L_{total} = L_{semantic} + L_{score} + L_{boxes}(RPN) \\
+ L_{(fg-bg)} + L_{boxes}(Instance) + L_{instance}
\end{aligned}
\tag{2}
$$

where L_{total}, $L_{semantic}$, L_{score}, $L_{boxes}(RPN)$, $L_{(fg-bg)}$, $L_{boxes}(Instance)$, and $L_{instance}$ represent the total loss of Cell R-CNN, semantic segmentation loss, classifier loss of RPN, bounding box regression loss of RPN, foreground-background loss of instance branch, bounding box regression loss of instance branch, and mask segmentation loss of each object respectively as shown in Figs. 2 and 3; $L_{semantic}$ and $L_{instance}$ are categorical cross-entropy loss and binary cross-entropy loss respectively; $L_{boxes}(RPN)$ and $L_{boxes}(Instance)$ are the smoothed $L1$ regression losses, $L1(t - t^*)$. L_{score} and $L_{(fg-bg)}$ are simple log losses between different classes.

3   Experiment

Experimental evaluation was performed on the 2017 MICCAI Digital Pathology Challenge dataset. The dataset is composed of 32 training images and 32 testing images. Both the training and testing images were sampled from the whole slide image of patients with glioblastoma multiforme (GBM), head and neck squamous cell carcinoma (HNSCC), lower grade glioma (LGG) tumors or non small cell lung cancer (NSCLC). The number of each category is 8 in both the training and testing datasets. The image size is either 500×500 or 600×600.

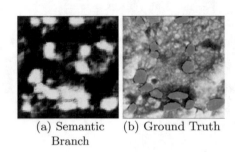

(a) Semantic   (b) Ground Truth
Branch

Fig. 4. An example of semantic segmentation branch result.

The data augmentation technique was applied to both the proposed method and comparison methods. The proposed method is implemented using keras and tensorflow. The convolutional kernel size for GCN block of semantic segmentation branch is constant as 5. The upsampling size along x, y dimension of semantic segmentation branch is 2. Since the maximum number of cells is less than 100, the number of training regions of interest is set to 400 to increase potential candidates. The pixel-size of the anchors are $\{8, 16, 32, 64, 128\}$. The stride of the anchors is 2. The optimizer is stochastic gradient descent (SGD) whose initial learning rate, momentum and weight decay are $2e^{-3}$, 0.9 and $1e^{-4}$, respectively. The non-maximum suppression threshold is set to 0.3 to ensure the successful detection of boundary-touching cells. The minimum detection confidence is set to 0.5.

An example of semantic branch result is shown in Fig. 4. The semantic branch is able to learn the region with large overlaps with other objects. In this particular example, the non-cell background region overlaps with individual cell objects but successfully distinguished by the semantic segmentation branch. One challenging condition is that only limited training data was provided while various cancer categories lead to different imaging conditions shown in Fig. 5. Overall, the proposed method is capable of producing accurate and reliable panoptic segmentation of different cancer images. According to the segmentation results, there are still incomplete cell segmentation of prediction result such as top left of prediction result on NSCLC image in Fig. 5. For quantitative evaluation, F1 score, object-level Dice, and Hausdorff distance are computed. The detailed definitions of F1 score, object-level Dice, and Hausdorff distance are referred to [2].

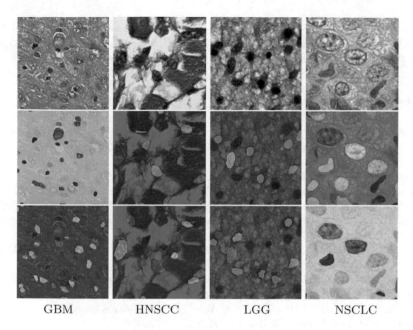

GBM   HNSCC   LGG   NSCLC

Fig. 5. Panoptic-level cell segmentation results of various cancer categories (from top to bottom): testing image, prediction, ground truth.

Table 1. The quantitative cell segmentation results.

Network	F1-score	Dice	Hausdorff
UNet [12]	0.4059 ± 0.2311	0.4942 ± 0.1872	54.1130 ± 73.4936
Pix2Pix [7]	0.6208 ± 0.1126	0.6351 ± 0.0706	19.1441 ± 6.0933
LinkNet [1]	0.4117 ± 0.1852	0.5611 ± 0.0899	19.7294 ± 9.0798
FnsNet [8]	0.7413 ± 0.0668	0.6165 ± 0.0839	25.9102 ± 9.5834
Ours w/o Semantic branch	0.8004 ± 0.0722	0.7070 ± 0.0598	12.6723 ± 3.4591
Ours	0.8216 ± 0.0625	0.7088 ± 0.0564	11.3141 ± 2.6917

It can be seen from Table 1 that the proposed method ranked first in terms of F1-score with 0.8216, Dice with 0.7088, and minimum Hausdorff distance with 11.3141. Based on the average and standard deviation of the evaluation metrics, the proposed framework is most robust and stable among all compared methods.

4 Conclusions

In this paper, we propose a novel and end-end Cell R-CNN framework to generate panoptic segmentation. The proposed method unifies individual semantic and instance segmentation tasks with a novel semantic segmentation branch. The semantic segmentation branch is capable of learning features from regions with large overlaps with other objects. Evaluated on the 2017 MICCAI Digital Pathology Challenge dataset, the proposed method outperforms compared methods in terms of F1 score, cell-object Dice, and Hausdorff distance.

References

1. Chaurasia, A., Culurciello, E.: Linknet: exploiting encoder representations for efficient semantic segmentation. arXiv preprint arXiv:1707.03718 (2017)
2. Chen, H., Qi, X., Yu, L., Heng, P.: DCAN: deep contour-aware networks for accurate gland segmentation. In: CVPR, pp. 2487–2496 (2016)
3. Girshick, R., Donahue, J., Darrell, T., Malik, J.: Rich feature hierarchies for accurate object detection and semantic segmentation. In: CVPR, pp. 580–587 (2014)
4. He, K., Zhang, X., Ren, S., Sun, J.: Deep residual learning for image recognition. In: CVPR, pp. 770–778 (2016)
5. He, K., Gkioxari, G., Dollár, P., Girshick, R.: Mask r-cnn. In: ICCV, pp. 2980–2988 (2017)
6. Hu, R., Dollár, P., He, K., Darrell, T., Girshick, R.: Learning to segment every thing. In: CVPR (2018)
7. Isola, P., Zhu, J.Y., Zhou, T., Efros, A.A.: Image-to-image translation with conditional adversarial networks. In: CVPR, pp. 5967–5976 (2017)
8. Johnson, J., Alahi, A., Fei-Fei, L.: Perceptual losses for real-time style transfer and super-resolution. In: Leibe, B., Matas, J., Sebe, N., Welling, M. (eds.) ECCV 2016. LNCS, vol. 9906, pp. 694–711. Springer, Cham (2016). https://doi.org/10.1007/978-3-319-46475-6_43
9. Kirillov, A., He, K., Girshick, R., Rother, C., Dollár, P.: Panoptic segmentation. arXiv preprint arXiv:1801.00868 (2018)
10. Peng, C., Zhang, X., Yu, G., Luo, G., Sun, J.: Large kernel matters-improve semantic segmentation by global convolutional network. In: CVPR, pp. 1743–1751 (2017)
11. Ren, S., He, K., Girshick, R., Sun, J.: Faster r-cnn: towards real-time object detection with region proposal networks. In: NIPS, pp. 91–99 (2015)
12. Ronneberger, O., Fischer, P., Brox, T.: U-Net: convolutional networks for biomedical image segmentation. In: Navab, N., Hornegger, J., Wells, W.M., Frangi, A.F. (eds.) MICCAI 2015. LNCS, vol. 9351, pp. 234–241. Springer, Cham (2015). https://doi.org/10.1007/978-3-319-24574-4_28
13. Yang, L., Zhang, Y., Chen, J., Zhang, S., Chen, D.Z.: Suggestive annotation: a deep active learning framework for biomedical image segmentation. In: Descoteaux, M., Maier-Hein, L., Franz, A., Jannin, P., Collins, D.L., Duchesne, S. (eds.) MICCAI 2017. LNCS, vol. 10435, pp. 399–407. Springer, Cham (2017). https://doi.org/10.1007/978-3-319-66179-7_46
14. Zhang, D., Song, Y., Liu, S., Feng, D., Wang, Y., Cai, W.: Nuclei instance segmentation with dual contour-enhanced adversarial network. In: ISBI (2018)
15. Zhang, Y., Yang, L., Chen, J., Fredericksen, M., Hughes, D.P., Chen, D.Z.: Deep adversarial networks for biomedical image segmentation utilizing unannotated images. In: Descoteaux, M., Maier-Hein, L., Franz, A., Jannin, P., Collins, D.L., Duchesne, S. (eds.) MICCAI 2017. LNCS, vol. 10435, pp. 408–416. Springer, Cham (2017). https://doi.org/10.1007/978-3-319-66179-7_47
16. Zhao, H., Shi, J., Qi, X., Wang, X., Jia, J.: Pyramid scene parsing network. In: CVPR, pp. 6230–6239 (2017)

Integration of Spatial Distribution in Imaging-Genetics

Vaishnavi Subramanian[1]([✉]), Weizhao Tang[1], Benjamin Chidester[2], Jian Ma[2], and Minh N. Do[1]

[1] Department of Electrical and Computer Engineering, University of Illinois at Urbana-Champaign, Urbana, IL, USA
vs5@illinois.edu
[2] School of Computer Science, Carnegie Mellon University, Pittsburgh, PA, USA

Abstract. To better understand diseases such as cancer, it is crucial for computational inference to quantify the spatial distribution of various cell types within a tumor. To this end, we used Ripley's K-statistic, which captures the spatial distribution patterns at different scales of both individual point sets and interactions between multiple point sets. We propose to improve the expressivity of histopathology image features by incorporating this descriptor to capture potential cellular interactions, especially interactions between lymphocytes and epithelial cells. We demonstrate the utility of the Ripley's K-statistic by analyzing digital slides from 710 TCGA breast invasive carcinoma (BRCA) patients. In particular, we consider its use in the context of imaging-genetics to understand correlations between gene expression and image features using canonical correlation analysis (CCA). Our analysis shows that including these spatial features leads to more significant associations between image features and gene expression.

1 Introduction

An important factor in cancer diagnosis is the distribution of heterogeneous cells within the tumor microenvironment. A scenario where the lymphocytes are well mixed with the cancerous epithelial cells (high lymphocyte infiltration) is significantly different from when the two are well-separated spatially (low lymphocyte infiltration), which has been shown to be linked to clinical outcome [1]. While advanced deep learning based techniques have been employed to accurately segment the nuclei from histopathology images [2,3], there is still a need in computational pathology for subsequent analysis of the spatial interaction of cells. Traditional methods to capture the distribution of cells in the tissue include plane partitioning techniques, such as Delaunay triangulation and Voronoi diagrams. These methods, however, only look at the local neighborhood (of a few adjacent nuclei), and do not account for the overall distribution of cells at different scales, or the interactions between different types of cells.

A similar problem arises in the area of geography to quantify the distribution of population across a region, for example. Classical tools used to identify the

© Springer Nature Switzerland AG 2018
A. F. Frangi et al. (Eds.): MICCAI 2018, LNCS 11071, pp. 245–253, 2018.
https://doi.org/10.1007/978-3-030-00934-2_28

level of randomness of spatial point process include nearest-neighbour statistics, spectral analysis of point processes, and location-based functions. These tools can be readily applied to the tissue setting to describe spatial statistics of cells, and even cells of differing types, as demonstrated recently [4,5]. In this work, we employ Ripley's K-function [6], a location based function, to capture the second order statistics of the point sets in the context of histopathology images.

In addition to the spatial distribution, understanding tissue environment from different viewpoints can provide key information for use in diagnosis and understanding of diseases. With an increase of multimodal datasets, such as The Cancer Genomic Atlas (TCGA) [7], we now have access to both imaging and genomic data from patients. To integrate multimodal data, different linear techniques such as partial least squares, canonical correlation analysis (CCA), and deep learning techniques (e.g., deep multimodal autoencoders and deep multimodal Boltzmann machines) have been developed.

Recent works analyzing multimodal data using spatial information of cell distribution [4,5] have considered its value for prediction of patient outlook. In contrast, the focus of our study is to enable the discovery of novel biological connections between image features and genes, through CCA and sparse-CCA (SCCA), to improve the understanding of diseases, as demonstrated recently [8]. We hope that the discovery of such connections will help not only to predict cancer subtype or survival but also to learn more about the fundamental biological connection between genotype and phenotype.

We applied our new method to 710 breast invasive carcinoma (BRCA) patients from TCGA and observed an increased correlation between the resulting image features and gene expressions, suggesting a more informative image feature vector in terms of its connection with molecular signatures. Further, after identifying the highly correlated genes, we investigated their association with specific pathways and found several significantly associated pathways that are known to be related to cancer. This analysis demonstrates a proof-of-concept workflow which, we believe, will be important for future unsupervised discovery of genotype-phenotype connections in disease as more imaging-genomic data becomes available and techniques for cell segmentation and feature extraction become more refined.

2   Method

To work with a multimodal dataset comprising histopathology images and their gene expression measurements from the tumors of cancer patients, we use the overall workflow shown in Fig. 1a consisting of image feature extraction, spatial feature computation, and CCA (or SCCA) between the gene expressions and image features to reveal important connections between the two different modalities.

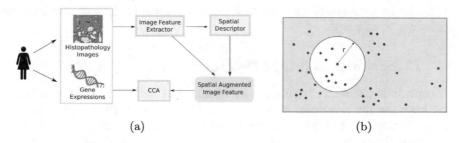

(a)   (b)

Fig. 1. (a) Our work-flow comprising CNN-based image feature extraction, spatial feature descriptor, and CCA between the features. (b) Pictorial representation of the K-function evaluated at radius r for the blue process, by counting blue points (self K-function) and red stars (cross K-function) within radius r.

2.1   Extraction of Image Features

For cancer patients, hematoxylin and eosin (H&E) histopathology images are routinely obtained for diagnosis, and we use these images to acquire quantitative measures of relevant nuclear and cellular characteristics, including morphology, granularity, and spatial distribution. This process of image feature extraction is described in our earlier work [2], which we summarize briefly here. First, we segment nuclei using a patch-based convolutional neural network (CNN) approach, which outputs a binary label indicating if the center of the patch is within nucleus or not. The entire image is scanned by our CNN, producing a binary label at each pixel. CellProfiler [9], a cell analysis tool, is used with the binary segmentation mask to extract quantitative features of the texture, morphology, and color of nuclei and cells. To obtain a single feature vector for the patient, each of the nuclear and cellular features are summarized across all the cells in the image by their mean, standard deviation, and percentiles (with 10% increments), yielding ~2400 unique features for each patient. In our analysis, since we analyzed whole-slide images (WSIs) provided by TCGA, we processed only a few representative patches per slide for computational feasibility.

In order to distinguish lymphocytes from epithelial cells for subsequent spatial analysis, a simple thresholding based on the area and intensity of the cell is used. Let c denote a cell detected by the CNN. Then,

if Area$(c) < \tau_1$ **and** Average-Intensity$(c) > \tau_2$, mark c as a lymphocyte,

where τ_1 and τ_2 are thresholds chosen to manually. Some sample results are shown in Fig. 2. This yields nuclei of two different types: *epithelial* – potentially cancerous in nature, and *lymphocytes* – white blood cells indicating immune activity. It is possible that some false positives (such as small epithelial or stromal cells) may be incorrectly detected as lymphocytes by this method, but we believe the relative frequency of such will be small since lymphocytes are well-discriminated by their small size and dark color. This threshold could be replaced in the future by a neural network that both segments nuclei and classifies them according to cell type.

2.2 Computation of Spatial Descriptor

To capture the spatial distribution information of individual cells, and interaction between the two types of cells (i.e., ephithelial and lymphocyte), we make use of Ripley's K-function [6]. For two sets random points $\mathcal{A}$ and $\mathcal{B}$ in a d-dimensional space, with $d \geq 2$ and respective point densities λ_1, λ_2, the self K-function ($K_\mathcal{A}(r)$ for $\mathcal{A}$) and cross K-function ($K_{\mathcal{A},\mathcal{B}}(r)$ between $\mathcal{A}$ and $\mathcal{B}$) are

$$K_\mathcal{A}(r) = \frac{1}{\lambda_1}\mathbb{E}\{f_\mathcal{A}(\mathcal{A}, r)\}, \tag{1}$$

$$K_{\mathcal{A},\mathcal{B}}(r) = \frac{1}{2}\Big(\frac{1}{\lambda_1}\mathbb{E}\{f_\mathcal{A}(\mathcal{B}, r)\} + \frac{1}{\lambda_2}\mathbb{E}\{f_\mathcal{B}(\mathcal{A}, r)\}\Big), \tag{2}$$

where $f_{\mathcal{P}_1}(\mathcal{P}_2, r)$ is the number of points from point set $\mathcal{P}_2$ within a distance r of a randomly chosen point from $\mathcal{P}_1$, and $\mathbb{E}$ denotes expected value. Note that by way of definition, the K-function is an increasing curve with respect to radius r. A pictorial representation of the evaluation is shown in Fig. 1b.

In practice, the average value is computed to estimate the K-function in place of the expectation. The resulting function, sampled at a range of different radii, represents the spatial feature vector of the patient, which is then combined with the previously obtained nuclear and cellular features to obtain the overall image feature vector of each patient.

2.3 Canonical Correlation Analysis

To assess the relationship between the image features and gene expression extracted from tumors, we make use of canonical correlation analysis. CCA [10] is a linear method to identify the correlation between two sets of variables. Mathematically, given $\mathbf{X} \in \mathbb{R}^{p \times n}$ and $\mathbf{Y} \in \mathbb{R}^{q \times n}$ normalized to zero mean and unit variance, CCA looks for $\alpha \in \mathbb{R}^p$ and $\beta \in \mathbb{R}^q$ to maximize the Pearson's correlation coefficient ρ based on the optimization problem in Eq. 3.

$$\max_{\alpha,\beta} \rho(\alpha, \beta) = \alpha^T \mathbf{X}^T \mathbf{Y} \beta \text{ such that } \alpha^T \mathbf{X}^T \mathbf{X} \alpha = \beta^T \mathbf{Y}^T \mathbf{Y} \beta = 1. \tag{3}$$

To obtain more than one linear combination, or *variate*, the above process can be repeated, imposing orthogonality constraints.

The setup of CCA requires $n \geq \max(p, q)$, which often does not hold for imaging-genetic data, since there are thousands of genes, and potentially thousands of image features, and possibly only a few hundred samples, or patients. Thus, to deal with high dimensional data, the SCCA formulation by Witten *et al.* [11], which optimizes the same objective function over convex sparsity constraints, is used. The algorithm is iterated to obtain multiple variates.

3   Experiments and Results

The framework was applied to WSIs of 710 TCGA-BRCA patients. To make the processing of WSIs feasible, up to 15 manually chosen 1000×1000 representative patches in the tumor regions were used for feature extraction. The gene expression data was obtained from cBioPortal [12].

3.1   Ripley's K-Function on Real Data

The variation in K-functions can be seen by computing the self K and cross K-functions for a couple of point sets (Fig. 2a and b) obtained after processing the TCGA-BRCA histopathology images. Configuration 1 is denoted by dashed lines and configuration 2 by solid lines in Fig. 2c. Firstly, all the identified cells obtained from the CNN are utilized together to obtain the self K-functions $K_{all,1}$ and $K_{all,2}$ shown in black. We observe that there is slight difference in these self K-functions, though the distinction is not prominent.

Next, the identified cells were differentiated into epithelial and lymphocytes, shown in Fig. 2 in cyan and red, respectively, as described previously. The self K - functions computed for the resulting epithelial cells ($K_{epi,1}$, $K_{epi,2}$) are not very different. In contrast, the self K-functions of the lymphocytes ($K_{lym,1}$, $K_{lym,2}$) show considerable difference with $K_{lym,1}$ lying below $K_{lym,2}$ for smaller values of radius r and thereby capturing the clustered nature of lymphocytes in configuration 2. The cross K-functions between the epithelial cells and lymphocytes ($K_{cross,1}$, $K_{cross,2}$) are such that $K_{cross,2}$ lies well below $K_{cross,1}$ indicating the absence of considerable interaction between the points sets in configuration 2.

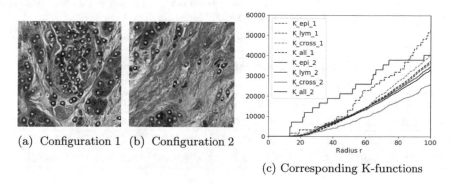

(a) Configuration 1   (b) Configuration 2

(c) Corresponding K-functions

Fig. 2. The variation in self K and cross K-function (c) for two configurations (a) and (b) where epithelial cells are shown in cyan, and lymphocytes in red.

3.2   CCA with Image and Spatial Features

To apply CCA, a subset of both image features and genes need to be chosen. For the nuclei-based image features, those corresponding to the mean and standard deviation of fundamental cellular and nuclear properties such as the color, texture and shape features are chosen, yielding a restricted set of 84 features. For the spatial features, we considered two different settings: (1) the self K-function evaluated on all detected cells, without differentiation of epithelial cells and lymphocytes (corresponding to the black curves in Fig. 2c), and (2) the cross K-function between the lymphocytes and epithelial cells (green curves in Fig. 2c) based on thresholding, as described earlier. In both settings, the K-function is evaluated for several different ranges of radii, sampled evenly at 100 values. The resulting spatial feature is augmented with the nuclei-based 84-dimensional feature vector to yield an overall 184-dimensional feature vector per patient. For the genes, the PAM50 subset of genes, which have been shown to be informative in breast cancer subtyping, is chosen.

The resulting correlation coefficients (ρ) and associated p-values for the correlations (computed using Wilk's lambda statistic) identified by CCA are presented in Table 1 for both settings. The spatial feature is modified in each setting by varying the maximum radius for computation of the K-functions as shown in the first column. It is observed that the augmentation of spatial features significantly improves the correlation for the first 3 variates in both the settings. The correlation achieved by the first variate increases by a factor of around 5%, while both second and third variates show an improvement in correlation by a factor of 10% for both settings. This increase in correlation implies a stronger and, therefore, more meaningful, association between the representations of image and genomic features. Beyond the 3 variates, the combined spatial image features did not yield statistically significant results.

Table 1. Correlation coefficient (ρ) and associated p-values of self K-function and cross K-function based image features with PAM50 Genes for top 3 variates

Radii	Self K						Cross K					
	1st variate		2nd variate		3rd variate		1st variate		2nd variate		3rd variate	
	ρ	p-value	ρ	p-value	ρ	p-value	ρ	p-value	ρ	p-value	ρ	p-value
None	0.74	$1e^{-15}$	0.63	$4.6e^{-14}$	0.60	$7.7e^{-09}$	0.74	$1e^{-15}$	0.62	$4.6e^{-14}$	0.60	$7.7e^{-09}$
$r < 100$	0.81	$1.8e^{-13}$	0.74	$1.3e^{-05}$	0.70	$1.2e^{-02}$	0.79	$1.9e^{-15}$	0.74	$1.3e^{-08}$	0.71	$1.1e^{-03}$
$r < 300$	0.81	$1.4e^{-14}$	0.75	$2.2e^{-06}$	0.71	$2.9e^{-03}$	0.79	$7.6e^{-09}$	0.75	$1.7e^{-03}$	0.71	$1.9e^{-03}$
$r < 500$	0.80	$2.4e^{-13}$	0.74	$3.4e^{-06}$	0.72	$4.0e^{-03}$	0.78	$9.4e^{-09}$	0.75	$1.2e^{-03}$	0.73	$1.5e^{-03}$

3.3   Sparse CCA with Image and Spatial Features

As mentioned, SCCA avoids the need to prune the gene and image feature set *a priori* and instead discovers which features of both modalities lead to the highest correlation and, therefore, the most meaningful association. We ran SCCA iteratively until we obtained five variates. Beyond the first five variates, we obtained variates similar to the first five due to the lack of orthogonality enforcement in

SCCA. The L_1 penalty factor was determined automatically by the algorithm to obtain the result with the highest statistical significance. We used the set of 3400 genes with the highest variance of expression and 3400 image features comprising the 2400 dimensional nuclear and cellular features augmented with the cross K-function between detected lymphocytes and epithelial cells evaluated at 1000 equally-spaced radii in different ranges. The other setting of using the self K-function treating all cells as the same type did not yield statistically significant results, so we do not report the results here. The resulting correlations discovered by SCCA are shown in Table 2. We observe that the inclusion of the spatial features increases the correlation for variates numbered three through five, while having little effect on the first two variates.

Table 2. Correlation coefficient of spatially-augmented image features with gene expression based on SCCA for the first five variates

Radii	L1 penalty	1st variate	2nd variate	3rd variate	4th variate	5th variate
None	0.05	0.490	0.404	0.321	0.424	0.399
$r \leq 100$	0.05	0.489	0.403	0.466	0.424	0.382
$r \leq 300$	0.52	0.470	0.345	0.457	0.478	**0.460**
$r \leq 500$	0.05	0.489	0.403	**0.466**	**0.535**	0.424

We next identified the genes and image features which are highly correlated with the variates for the setting that yields the highest correlation coefficient ($r \leq 500$). For the image features, we observe that the 4th variate is dominated by spatial features, while being uncorrelated with the nuclei-based features (Fig. 3a). We refer to this variate as the *spatial* variate. The presence of such a variate highlights the importance of spatial features in correlations with genes by implying that these features capture important properties of gene expression variation.

The correlation of all genes with the corresponding spatial variate, ordered decreasingly, is shown in Fig. 3b. To interpret the function of the genes chosen by the spatial variate of SCCA, we used the online functional annotation tool DAVID [13] to determine the Kyoto Encyclopedia of Genes and Genomes (KEGG) pathways associated with genes with a correlation of more than 0.4, a threshold chosen by studying Fig. 3b. Of the different pathways we obtained, the most significant ones are shown in Table 3. These belong to categories important in cancer in the different properties of cells' growth, death and interaction.

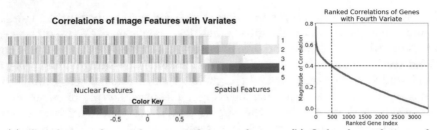

(a) Correlation of spatial-augmented image features with variates (K-function evaluated for $r \leq 500$).

(b) Ordered correlations of gene with spatial variate.

Fig. 3. SCCA for gene expression and image features, with spatial features added. (a) The fourth variate has a strong negative correlation with most spatial features. (b) The correlation of gene expression with this variate showed very high correlation with a few genes and then a linear decay in correlation. We chose the transition at the 480th gene, corresponding to a correlation threshold of 0.4, for use in pathway analysis.

Table 3. Pathways involved, number of overlapping genes, percentage of pathway genes identified, p-value and Benjamini-Hochberg corrected p-value of the top 480 correlated genes for the fourth variate from SCCA

KEGG pathway	Gene count	%	p-value	Benjamini
Cell cycle	12	2.7	$7.5e^{-4}$	0.034
p53 signaling pathway	9	2.0	$6.0e^{-4}$	0.041
Pathways in cancer	17	3.8	$2.2e^{-2}$	0.300

4   Discussion and Conclusions

We have demonstrated the use of Ripley's K-function in the histopathology setting to encode spatial information. We showed that incorporating spatial features increases correlation with PAM50 genes expression by factors of 10%. Additionally, by employing SCCA, we verified that the spatial features are able to capture significant association with genes independent of other image features. We demonstrated how this discovered association could be used to implicate associated pathways in the spatial distribution of cells in a tumor. We believe such analysis will be significant for future research in understanding the connections of genes to the heterogeneity of the tumor microenvironment in diseases.

References

1. Stanton, S.E., Disis, M.L.: Clinical significance of tumor-infiltrating lymphocytes in breast cancer. J. Immunother. Cancer **4**(1), 59 (2016)
2. Chidester, B., Do, M., Ma, J.: Discriminative bag-of-cells for imaging-genomics. In: Pacific Symposium on Biocomputing (2018)
3. Janowczyk, A., et al.: Deep learning for digital pathology image analysis: a comprehensive tutorial with selected use cases. J. Pathol. Inf. (2016)
4. Chang, Y.H., et al.: Quantitative analysis of histological tissue image based on cytological profiles and spatial statistics. In: Engineering in Medicine and Biology Society (EMBC). pp. 1175–1178. IEEE (2016)
5. Yuan, Y., et al.: Quantitative image analysis of cellular heterogeneity in breast tumors complements genomic profiling. Sci. Transl. Med. **4**(157), 157ra143 (2012)
6. Dixon, P.M.: Ripley's K function. In: Encyclopedia of Environmetrics (2002)
7. Cancer Genome Atlas Network: Comprehensive molecular portraits of human breast tumours. Nature **490**(7418), 61 (2012)
8. Subramanian, V., et al.: Correlating cellular features with gene expression using CCA. In: IEEE International Symposium on Biomedical Imaging, p. 805 (2018)
9. Carpenter, A., et al.: CellProfiler: image analysis software for identifying and quantifying cell phenotypes. Genome Biol. **7**(10), R100 (2006)
10. Hotelling, H.: Relations between two sets of variates. Biometrika **28**, 321–377 (1936)
11. Witten, D.M., et al.: A penalized matrix decomposition, with applications to sparse principal components and canonical correlation analysis. Biostatistics **10**(3), 515–534 (2009)
12. Cerami, E., et al.: The cBio cancer genomics portal: an open platform for exploring multidimensional cancer genomics data. Cancer Discov. **2**(5) (2012)
13. Huang, D.W., et al.: Systematic and integrative analysis of large gene lists using DAVID bioinformatics resources. Nat. Protoc. **4**(1), 44 (2008)

Multiple Instance Learning for Heterogeneous Images: Training a CNN for Histopathology

Heather D. Couture[1]([✉]), J. S. Marron[2,3], Charles M. Perou[2,4], Melissa A. Troester[2,5], and Marc Niethammer[1,6]

[1] Department of Computer Science, University of North Carolina, Chapel Hill, NC, USA
heather@cs.unc.edu
[2] Lineberger Comprehensive Cancer Center, University of North Carolina, Chapel Hill, NC, USA
[3] Department of Statistics and Operations Research, University of North Carolina, Chapel Hill, NC, USA
[4] Department of Genetics, University of North Carolina, Chapel Hill, NC, USA
[5] Department of Epidemiology, University of North Carolina, Chapel Hill, NC, USA
[6] Biomedical Research Imaging Center, University of North Carolina, Chapel Hill, NC, USA

Abstract. Multiple instance (MI) learning with a convolutional neural network enables end-to-end training in the presence of weak image-level labels. We propose a new method for aggregating predictions from smaller regions of the image into an image-level classification by using the quantile function. The quantile function provides a more complete description of the heterogeneity within each image, improving image-level classification. We also adapt image augmentation to the MI framework by randomly selecting cropped regions on which to apply MI aggregation during each epoch of training. This provides a mechanism to study the importance of MI learning. We validate our method on five different classification tasks for breast tumor histology and provide a visualization method for interpreting local image classifications that could lead to future insights into tumor heterogeneity.

1 Introduction

Deep learning has become the standard solution for classification when a large set of images with detailed annotations is available for training. When the annotations are weaker, such as with large, heterogeneous images, we turn to multiple instance (MI) learning. The image (called a bag) is broken into smaller regions (called instances). We are given a label for each bag, but the instance labels are unknown. Some form of pooling aggregates instances into a bag-level classification. By integrating MI learning into a convolutional neural network (CNN), we can learn an instance classifier and aggregate the predictions so the entire system is trained end-to-end [5,7,12].

© Springer Nature Switzerland AG 2018
A. F. Frangi et al. (Eds.): MICCAI 2018, LNCS 11071, pp. 254–262, 2018.
https://doi.org/10.1007/978-3-030-00934-2_29

We propose a more general approach for aggregating instance predictions that looks at the full distribution by pooling with the quantile function (QF) and learning how much heterogeneity to expect for each class. As data augmentation is especially critical in training large CNNs, we also created an augmentation technique for training MI methods with a CNN (Fig. 1). Through MI augmentation, we study the importance of the MI formulation during training.

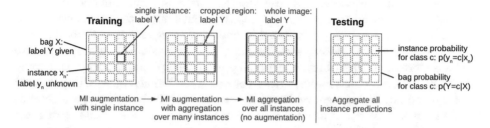

Fig. 1. In MI learning, each bag contains one or more instances. Labels are given for the bag, but not the instances. MI augmentation is a technique to provide additional training samples by randomly selecting a cropped image region and the instances within it. When the bag label is applied to a small number of instances, it is weak because this small region may not be representative of the bag class. Applying the bag label to larger cropped regions provides a stronger label, while still providing benefit from image augmentation. Training with the whole image maximizes the opportunity for MI learning, but restricts the benefits of image augmentation. *At test time, the whole image is processed and the predictions from all instances are aggregated into a bag prediction.*

Using MI learning to make class predictions over smaller regions of the image provides insight into how different parts of the image contribute to the classification. Visualizing the instance predictions provides a method of interpretability that we demonstrate on a data set of breast tumor tissue microarray (TMA) images stained with hematoxylin and eosin (H&E) by predicting grade, receptor status, and subtype. Some of these tasks are not previously known to be achievable from H&E alone. Our quantitative results conclude that the MI component is critical to successful classification, demonstrating the importance of accounting for heterogeneity. This method could provide future insights into tumor heterogeneity and its connection with cancer progression [3,9].

Contributions. (1) A more general MI aggregation method that uses the quantile function for pooling and learns how to aggregate instance predictions. (2) An MI augmentation technique for training MI methods. (3) Exploration of single instance and MI learning on a continuous spectrum, demonstrating the importance of MI learning on heterogeneous images. (4) Evaluation on a large data set of 1713 patient samples (5970 images), showing significant gains in classifying breast cancer TMAs. (5) A method for visualizing the predictions of each instance, providing interpretability to the method.

2   Background

Aggregating Instance Predictions. A *permutation invariant* pooling of instances is needed to accommodate images of different sizes, whereas a fully connected neural network cannot. Existing pooling approaches are very aggressive; they compute a single number rather than looking at the distribution of instance predictions. Most MI applications use the maximum, which works well for problems such as cancer diagnosis where, if there is a small amount of tumor, the sample is labeled as cancerous [6,16]. A smooth approximation, such as the generalized mean or noisy-OR, provide better convergence in a CNN [5,7,12]. For other tasks, a majority vote, median, or mean is more appropriate. We include more of the distribution by pooling with the QF and learning a mapping to the bag class prediction, improving the classification accuracy. Our proposed method of quantile aggregation learns how to predict the bag class from instance predictions and so could provide a solution when the most suitable aggregator is unknown. The QF is a new general type of feature pooling that could provide an alternative to max pooling in a CNN.

Training MI Methods with a CNN. Image augmentation is commonly applied in training a CNN by randomly cropping large portions of each image during each epoch. At test time, the whole image is used. We propose MI augmentation, in which a subset of instances is randomly selected from each bag during each epoch. Instances are always the same size, but we choose how many instances to aggregate over. In selecting the number of instances, there are two extremes: a single instance vs. the whole bag. In the former, the bag label is assigned to each instance and is often called single instance learning. In the latter, MI aggregation is incorporated while training the bag classifier as in other MI methods [1,4]. Comparison studies have found little or no improvement from these MI methods on some data sets [14,15]. We found MI learning to be very beneficial and show that it is critical in dealing with heterogeneous data.

3   Multiple Instance Learning with a CNN

We denote a bag by X, its label by $Y \epsilon \{1, 2, ..., C\}$, and the instances it contains by x_n for $n = 1, ..., N$. The instance labels y_n are unknown. On a novel sample, an instance classifier f_{inst}^c predicts the probability of each class c and a function f_{agg}^c aggregates these instance probabilities into a bag probability:

$$s_{n,c} = f_{inst}^c(x_n) = \Pr(y_n = c|x_n) \qquad S_c = f_{agg}^c(s_{1,1}, ..., s_{N,C}) = \Pr(Y = c|X).$$

MI learning can be implemented with many different types of classifiers [1,6,14]. When implemented as a CNN, a fully convolutional network (FCN) forms the instance classifier f_{inst}, followed by a global MI layer for instance aggregation f_{agg}. The FCN consists of convolutional and pooling layers that downsize the representation, followed by a softmax operation to predict the probability for each class. For an input image of size $w \times w \times 3$, the FCN output is $w_d \times w_d \times C$. An instance is defined as the receptive field from the original image used in creating a point in this $w_d \times w_d$ grid; the instances are overlapping. The MI aggregation layer takes the instance probabilities and the foreground mask for the input image (downscaled to $w_d \times w_d$), thereby aggregating over only the foreground instances. Figure 2 provides an overview.

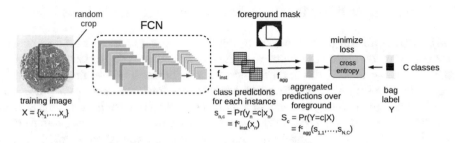

Fig. 2. During training, a cropped region of a given size is randomly selected. An FCN is applied to predict the class, producing a grid of instance predictions. The instance predictions are aggregated over the foreground of the image (as indicated by the foreground mask) using quantile aggregation to predict the class of the cropped image region. With a cross entropy loss applied, backpropagation then learns the FCN and aggregation function weights. At test time, the whole image is used.

4   Multiple Instance Aggregation

Instance predictions can be used to form a bag prediction in different ways. The bag prediction function should be invariant to the number and spatial arrangement of instances, so some pooling of predictions is needed. Mean aggregation is well suited for global pooling as it is permutation invariant and can incorporate a foreground mask for the input image. Denoting the mask as M and its value for each instance as $m_n \epsilon \{0, 1\}$, the mean aggregation function is

$$S_c = f^c_{\text{mean agg}}(s_{1,1}, ..., s_{N,C}) = \frac{\sum_{n=1}^{N} m_n s_{n,c}}{\sum_{n=1}^{N} m_n}.$$

Mean pooling incorporates predictions from all instances, but a lot of information is lost in compressing to a single number. A histogram is a more complete description of the probability distribution, but is dependent upon a suitable bin width. Alternatively, the QF (inverse cumulative distribution) represents the boundary points between fractions of the population, providing a better discretization [2]. We propose quantile aggregation to provide a more complete description of the instance predictions in a bag. If the instance predictions for class c are represented by $S_c = \{s_{1,c}, ..., s_{N,c}\}$, then the q-th Q-quantile is the value z such that $\Pr(S_c \leq z) = (q - 0.5)/Q$. To pool with the QF, we first sort S_c and exclude instances not in the foreground, leaving the set $\tilde{S}_c = \{\tilde{s}_{1,c}, ..., \tilde{s}_{\tilde{N},c}\}$.

The sorted values in $\tilde{S}_c$ are used to extract the QF vector for each class c as $z_c = [z_{1,c}, ..., z_{Q,c}]$ where $z_{q,c} = \tilde{s}_{\lceil \tilde{N}(q-0.5)/Q \rceil, c}$. The QF vectors for all classes are concatenated as $Z = [z_1, ..., z_C]$. We then use a softmax function operating on Z to predict the bag class. The QF from all classes is used in order to learn the interaction of different subtypes in a bag. Backpropagtion through the QF operates in a similar manner to max pooling by passing the gradient back to the instance that achieved each quantile.

5   Training with Multiple Instance Augmentation

Image augmentation by random cropping is an important technique for creating extra training samples that helps to reduce over-fitting. We propose an augmentation strategy for MI methods to increase the number of training samples by randomly selecting a different subset of instances for each epoch. We randomly crop the image to select the set of instances, such that each crop contains at least 75% foreground according to the foreground mask. It is important to note that the image is never resized and the instance size remains constant. For each crop size chosen, the FCN is applied to the cropped image at full resolution. MI augmentation is a strategy used during training. *As the MI aggregation layer is invariant to input size, the entire image and all its instances are always used at test time.*

6   Experiments

Data Set. Our data set consists of 1713 patient samples from the Carolina Breast Cancer Study, Phase 3 [13]. There are typically four 1.0 mm cores per patient in the TMA, with a total of 5970 cores. Each core is selected from the H&E-stained whole slide by a pathologist such that it contains a substantial amount of tumor tissue. Each image has a diameter of around 2400 pixels and a maximum of 3500 pixels. One sample core is shown in Fig. 2. We use a random subset of half the patients for training and the other half for testing. Classification accuracy is measured for five different tasks, some of them multi-class: (1) histologic subtype (ductal or lobular), (2) estrogen receptor (ER) status (positive or negative), (3) grade (1, 2, or 3), (4) risk of recurrence score (ROR) (low, intermediate, or high), (5) genetic subtype (basal, luminal A, luminal B, HER2, or normal-like). Ground truth for histologic subtype and grade are from a pathologist looking at the original whole slide. ER status is determined from immunohistochemistry, genetic subtype from the PAM50 array [11], and ROR from the ROR-PT score-based method [11].

Implementation Details. The TMA images are intensity normalized to standardize the appearance across slides [10]. The hematoxylin, eosin, and residual channels are extracted from the normalization process and used as the three-channel input for the rest of our algorithm. A binary mask distinguishing tissue from background is also provided as input.

We use the pre-trained CNN AlexNet [8] and fine-tune with the MI architecture shown in Fig. 2. All five tasks are equally weighted in a multi-task CNN as shared features help to reduce over-fitting. For each patient, ground truth labels are available for most tasks. The cross entropy loss is adjusted to ignore patients missing a label for a particular task.

In addition to MI augmentation, we randomly mirror and rotate each training image. To accommodate the larger cropped image sizes in GPU memory, we reduce the batch size. A typical image with tissue of diameter 2400 pixels produces a 68×68 grid of instances. After applying the foreground mask, there are roughly 3600 instances. $Q = 15$ quantiles are used in all experiments. There are typically four core images per patient; we assign the patient label to each during training and, at test time, take the mean prediction across the images. Further MI learning could be done to address the multiple core images per patient, however our current focus is only on MI learning within each image.

MI Augmentation and the Importance of MI Learning. We study the effect of MI learning on large images by selecting the cropped image size for training. The smallest possible size is 227×227 (the input size for AlexNet), consisting of a single instance. When the bag label is applied to each instance during training, this is called single instance learning. Alternatively, a larger cropped region of size $w \times w$ can be selected; we test multiples of 500 up to 3500 and use mean aggregation in this experiment. By assigning the bag label to this larger cropped region during training and keeping the instance size constant, we perform MI learning. Multiple random crops are obtained from each training image such that roughly the same number of pixels is sampled for each crop size (i.e., the whole image for the largest crop size of 3500, $\frac{3500^2}{w^2}$ random crops for a training crop of size w). For the largest crop size, the whole image is used without MI augmentation. Random mirroring and rotations are used for augmentation at all crop sizes. At test time, the whole image is always used, with the bag prediction formed by aggregating across all instances.

Figure 3 shows that larger crop sizes *for training* significantly increases classification accuracy ($p < 10^{-3}$ with McNemar's test for $w = 500$ vs. $w = 1500$ on all tasks). The benefits level off for larger crops. As GPU memory requirements increase for larger crop sizes, selecting an intermediate crop size provides most of the benefits of MI augmentation.

Although it should not be surprising that a larger crop size at training works better, the magnitude of improvement is very significant. If

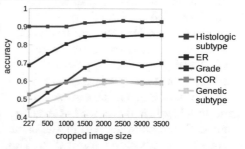

Fig. 3. Classification accuracy using mean aggregation as the number of instances (cropped image size) used for training is increased, while keeping instance size constant.

the images were homogeneous (at the scale of a single instance, $w = 227$), then applying the bag label to each instance should produce a classification accuracy similar to when MI aggregation over the whole image is used during training. This is clearly not the case in Fig. 3. For example, ER status increases from 68.6% to 85.6% when applying MI learning over the whole image. *This demonstrates the importance of MI learning and the effect of heterogeneity.* Our data set consists of cores selected from a whole slide by a pathologist. MI learning may be even more crucial when classifying larger and more heterogeneous images like whole slides.

MI Aggregation. We compared aggregation methods by training our model on a crop size $w = 2000$ and taking the average classification accuracy over four runs. Table 1 shows that mean and quantile aggregation both significantly outperform max ($p < 10^{-8}$ with McNemar's test). While quan-

Table 1. Average classification accuracy for different types of MI aggregation. The standard error is in brackets.

Task	Max	Mean	Quantile
Histologic subtype	.898 (.004)	.931 (.004)	.952 (.003)
ER	.683 (.006)	.833 (.008)	.841 (.006)
Grade	.408 (.019)	.680 (.003)	.676 (.006)
ROR	.542 (.010)	.595 (.003)	.582 (.008)
Genetic subtype	.321 (.032)	.548 (.006)	.544 (.003)

tile aggregation performance is similar to mean for some tasks, a significant increase in performance (93.1% to 95.2%) is observed for predicting the histologic subtype of ductal vs. lobular ($p < 10^{-10}$ with McNemar's test). This improvement is due to quantile aggregation predicting the bag class from a more complete view of the instance predictions using QF pooling, thereby capturing the heterogeneity.

Heterogeneity. By computing the class predictions for each instance, we get an idea of each region's contribution to the classification. Figure 4 provides a visualization for a sample image where the instance predictions are colored for each class. The $w = 2000$ crop size was used for this example. With the same computation performed over the whole test set, we calculated the proportion of instances predicted to belong to each class. Figure 5 plots the results for grade 1 vs. 3 and genetic subtype basal vs. luminal A. Heterogeneity is expected for grade, as the three tumor grades are not discrete, but a continuous spectrum from low to high. On the other hand, the level of heterogeneity to expect for genetic subtype is unknown because no studies have yet assessed genetic subtype from multiple samples within the same tumor. The graph shows a continuous spectrum from basal to luminal A. The luminal B, HER2, and normal samples lie mostly on the luminal A side, but with some mixing into the basal side.

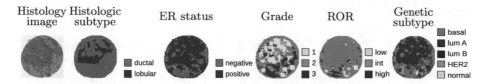

Fig. 4. Visualization of instance predictions for a sample with ground truth labels of ductal, ER positive, grade 1, low ROR, and luminal A.

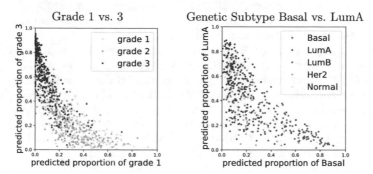

Fig. 5. Predicted heterogeneity for grade 1 vs. 3 and genetic subtype basal vs luminal A. The predicted proportion for each class is calculated as the proportion of instances in the sample predicted to be from each class. Test samples for all classes are plotted.

7   Discussion

We have shown that MI learning while training a CNN is critical in achieving high classification accuracy on large, heterogeneous images. Even with a small number of labeled samples, our model was successful in fine-tuning the AlexNet CNN because of the large size of the images providing plenty of opportunity for MI augmentation. The impact of MI learning indicates that accommodating image heterogeneity is essential. While aggregating instance predictions with the mean is sufficient for some tasks, quantile aggregation produces a significant improvement for others. Instance-level predictions will enable future work studying tumor heterogeneity, perhaps leading to biological insights of tumor progression.

Acknowledgments. This work was supported by a grant from the UNC Lineberger Comprehensive Cancer Center funded by the University Cancer Research Fund (LCCC2017T204), NCI Breast SPORE program (P50-CA58223), and the Breast Cancer Research Foundation.

References

1. Andrews, S., Tsochantaridis, I., Hofmann, T.: Support vector machines for multiple-instance learning. In: NIPS, pp. 561–568 (2002)
2. Broadhurst, R.E.: Compact appearance in object populations using quantile function based distribution families. Ph.D. thesis, The University of North Carolina at Chapel Hill (2008)
3. Hiley, C.T., Swanton, C.: Spatial and temporal cancer evolution: causes and consequences of tumour diversity. Clin. Med. **14**(Suppl-6), s33–s37 (2014)
4. Hou, L., Samaras, D., et al.: Patch-based convolutional neural network for whole slide tissue image classification. In: CVPR (2016)
5. Jia, Z., Huang, X., Chang, E.I.C., Xu, Y.: Constrained deep weak supervision for histopathology image segmentation. arXiv preprint: 1701.00794 (2017)
6. Kandemir, M., Hamprecht, F.A.F.: Computer-aided diagnosis from weak supervision: a benchmarking study. Comput. Med. Imaging Graph. **42**, 44–50 (2014)
7. Kraus, O.Z., Ba, J.L., Frey, B.J.: Classifying and segmenting microscopy images with deep multiple instance learning. Bioinformatics **32**(12), i52–i59 (2016)
8. Krizhevsky, A., Sutskever, I., Hinton, G.: Imagenet classification with deep convolutional neural networks. In: NIPS, pp. 1106–1114 (2012)
9. McGranahan, N., Swanton, C.: Biological and therapeutic impact of intratumor heterogeneity in cancer evolution. Cancer Cell **27**(1), 15–26 (2015)
10. Niethammer, M., Borland, D., Marron, J.S., Woosley, J., Thomas, N.E.: Appearance normalization of histology slides. In: Wang, F., Yan, P., Suzuki, K., Shen, D. (eds.) MLMI 2010. LNCS, vol. 6357, pp. 58–66. Springer, Heidelberg (2010). https://doi.org/10.1007/978-3-642-15948-0_8
11. Parker, J.S., Mullins, M.: Supervised risk predictor of breast cancer based on intrinsic subtypes. J. Clin. Oncol. **27**(8), 1160–1167 (2009)
12. Sun, M., Han, T.X., Liu, M.C., Khodayari-Rostamabad, A.: Multiple instance learning convolutional neural networks for object recognition. In: ICPR (2016)
13. Troester, M., Sun, X., et al.: Racial differences in PAM50 subtypes in the Carolina breast cancer study. J. Natl. Cancer Inst. **110**(2), 176–182 (2018)
14. Vanwinckelen, G., do Tragante, O.V., Fierens, D., Blockeel, H.: Instance-level accuracy versus bag-level accuracy in multi-instance learning. Data Min. Knowl. Discov. **30**(2), 313–341 (2016)
15. Wang, X., Yan, Y., Tang, P., Bai, X., Liu, W.: Revisiting Multiple Instance Neural Networks. Pattern Recognit. **74**, 15–24 (2018)
16. Xu, Y., Zhu, J.Y.: Weakly supervised histopathology cancer image segmentation and classification. Med. Image Anal. **18**(3), 591–604 (2014)

Optical and Histology Applications: Microscopy Applications

Cell Detection with Star-Convex Polygons

Uwe Schmidt[1,2(✉)], Martin Weigert[1,2(✉)], Coleman Broaddus[1,2],
and Gene Myers[1,2,3]

[1] Max Planck Institute of Molecular Cell Biology and Genetics, Dresden, Germany
{uschmidt,mweigert}@mpi-cbg.de
[2] Center for Systems Biology Dresden, Dresden, Germany
[3] Faculty of Computer Science, Technical University Dresden, Dresden, Germany

Abstract. Automatic detection and segmentation of cells and nuclei in microscopy images is important for many biological applications. Recent successful learning-based approaches include per-pixel cell segmentation with subsequent pixel grouping, or localization of bounding boxes with subsequent shape refinement. In situations of crowded cells, these can be prone to segmentation errors, such as falsely merging bordering cells or suppressing valid cell instances due to the poor approximation with bounding boxes. To overcome these issues, we propose to localize cell nuclei via *star-convex polygons*, which are a much better shape representation as compared to bounding boxes and thus do not need shape refinement. To that end, we train a convolutional neural network that predicts for every pixel a polygon for the cell instance at that position. We demonstrate the merits of our approach on two synthetic datasets and one challenging dataset of diverse fluorescence microscopy images.

1 Introduction

Many biological tasks rely on the accurate detection and segmentation of cells and nuclei from microscopy images [11]. Examples include high-content screens of variations in cell phenotypes [2], or the identification of developmental lineages of dividing cells [1,17]. In many cases, the goal is to obtain an *instance segmentation*, which is the assignment of a cell instance identity to every pixel of the image. To that end, a prevalent *bottom-up* approach is to first classify every pixel into semantic classes (such as *cell* or *background*) and then group pixels of the same class into individual instances. The first step is typically done with learned classifiers, such as random forests [16] or neural networks [4,5,15]. Pixel grouping can for example be done by finding connected components [4]. While this approach often gives good results, it is problematic for images of very crowded cell nuclei, since only a few mis-classified pixels can cause bordering but distinct cell instances to be fused [3,19].

U. Schmidt and M. Weigert—Equal contribution.

© Springer Nature Switzerland AG 2018
A. F. Frangi et al. (Eds.): MICCAI 2018, LNCS 11071, pp. 265–273, 2018.
https://doi.org/10.1007/978-3-030-00934-2_30

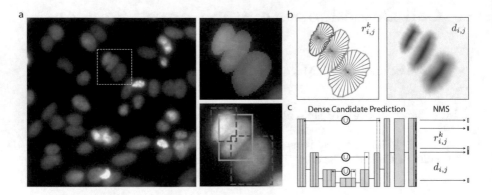

Fig. 1. *(a)* Potential segmentation errors for images with crowded nuclei: Merging of touching cells (upper right) or suppression of valid cell instances due to large overlap of bounding box localization (lower right). *(b)* The proposed STARDIST method predicts object probabilities $d_{i,j}$ and star-convex polygons parameterized by the radial distances $r_{i,j}^k$. *(c)* We densely predict $r_{i,j}^k$ and $d_{i,j}$ using a simple U-Net architecture [15] and then select the final instances via non-maximum suppression (NMS).

An alternative *top-down* approach is to first localize individual cell instances with a rough shape representation and then *refine* the shape in an additional step. To that end, state-of-the-art object detection methods [9,12,14] predominately predict axis-aligned bounding boxes, which can be refined to obtain an instance segmentation by classifying the pixels within each box (*e.g., Mask R-CNN* [6]). Most of these methods have in common that they avoid detecting the same object multiple times by performing a *non-maximum suppression* (NMS) step where boxes with lower confidence are suppressed by boxes with higher confidence if they substantially overlap. NMS can be problematic if the objects of interest are poorly represented by their axis-aligned bounding boxes, which can be the case for cell nuclei (Fig. 1a). While this can be mitigated by using *rotated* bounding boxes [10], it is still necessary to refine the box shape to accurately describe objects such as cell nuclei.

To alleviate the aforementioned problems, we propose STARDIST, a cell detection method that predicts a shape representation which is flexible enough such that – without refinement – the accuracy of the localization can compete with that of instance segmentation methods. To that end, we use *star-convex polygons* that we find well-suited to approximate the typically roundish shapes of cell nuclei in microscopy images. While Jetley et al. [7] already investigated star-convex polygons for object detection in natural images, they found them to be inferior to more suitable shape representations for typical object classes in natural images, like people or bicycles.

In our experimental evaluation, we first show that methods based on axis-aligned bounding boxes (we choose Mask R-CNN as a popular example) cannot cope with certain shapes. Secondly, we demonstrate that our method performs well on images with very crowded nuclei and does not suffer from merging bordering cell instances. Finally, we show that our method exceeds the performance of strong competing methods on a challenging dataset of fluorescence microscopy images. STARDIST uses a light-weight neural network based on *U-Net* [15] and is easy to train and use, yet is competitive with state-of-art methods.

2   Method

Our approach is similar to object detection methods [7,9,12] that directly predict shapes for each object of interest. Unlike most of them, we do not use axis-aligned bounding boxes as the shape representation ([7,10] being notable exceptions). Instead, our model predicts a *star-convex polygon* for every pixel[1]. Specifically, for each pixel with index i,j we regress the distances $\{r_{i,j}^k\}_{k=1}^n$ to the boundary of the object to which the pixel belongs, along a set of n predefined radial directions with equidistant angles (Fig. 1b). Obviously, this is only well-defined for (non-background) pixels that are contained within an object. Hence, our model also separately predicts for every pixel whether it is part of an object, so that we only consider polygon proposals from pixels with sufficiently high object probability $d_{i,j}$. Given such polygon candidates with their associated object probabilities, we perform non-maximum suppression (NMS) to arrive at the final set of polygons, each representing an individual object instance.

Object probabilities. While we could simply classify each pixel as either object or background based on binary masks, we instead define its object probability $d_{i,j}$ as the (normalized) Euclidean distance to the nearest background pixel (Fig. 1b). By doing this, NMS will favor polygons associated to pixels near the cell center (*cf.* Fig. 5b), which typically represent objects more accurately.

Star-convex polygon distances. For every pixel belonging to an object, the Euclidean distances $r_{i,j}^k$ to the object boundary can be computed by simply following each radial direction k until a pixel with a different object identity is encountered. We use a simple GPU implementation that is fast enough that we can compute the required distances on demand during model training.

2.1   Implementation

Although our general approach is not tied to a particular regression or classification approach, we choose the popular U-Net [15] network as the basis of our model. After the final U-Net feature layer, we cautiously add an additional 3×3 convolutional layer with 128 channels (and *relu* activations) to avoid that the subsequent two output layers have to "fight over features". Specifically, we use a single-channel convolutional layer with *sigmoid* activation for the object probability output. The polygon distance output layer has as many channels as there are radial directions n and does not use an additional activation function.

---

[1] Although we only consider the single object class *cell nuclei* in our experiments, note that we are not limited to that and thus use the generic term *object* in the following.

Training. We minimize a standard *binary cross-entropy* loss for the predicted object probabilities. For the polygon distances, we use a *mean absolute error* loss weighted by the ground truth object probabilities, *i.e.* the pixel-wise errors are multiplied by the object probabilities before averaging. Consequently, background pixels will not contribute to the loss, since their object probability is zero. Furthermore, predictions for pixels closer to the center of each object are weighted more, which is appropriate since these will be favored during non-maximum suppression. The code is publicly available[2].

Non-maximum Suppression. We perform common, greedy non-maximum suppression (NMS, *cf.* [9,12,14]) to only retain those polygons in a certain region with the highest object probabilities. We only consider polygons associated with pixels above an object probability threshold as candidates, and compute their intersections with a standard polygon clipping method.

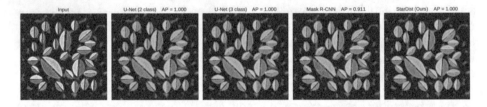

Fig. 2. Segmentation result ($\tau = 0.5$) for TOY image. Predicted cell instances are depicted in green if correctly matched (*TP*), otherwise highlighted in red (*FP*). Ground truth cells are always shown by their blue outlines in the input image (left), and in all other images only when they are not matched by any predicted cell instance (*FN*).

3   Experiments

3.1   Datasets

We use three datasets that pose different challenges for cell detection:

Dataset TOY: Synthetically created images that contain pairs of touching half-ellipses with blur and background noise (*cf.* Fig. 2). Each pair is oriented in such a way that the overlap of both enclosing bounding boxes is either very small (along an axis-aligned direction) or very large (when the ellipses touch at an oblique angle). This dataset contains 1000 images of size 256×256 with associated ground truth labels. We specifically created this dataset to highlight the limitations of methods that predict axis-aligned bounding boxes.

Dataset TRAGEN: Synthetically generated images of an evolving cell population from [18] (*cf.* Fig. 3). The generative model includes cell divisions, shape

---

[2] https://github.com/mpicbg-csbd/stardist.

deformations, camera noise and microscope blur and is able to simulate realistic images of extremely crowded cell configurations. This dataset contains 200 images of size 792×792 along with their ground truth labels.

Dataset DSB2018: Manually annotated real microscopy images of cell nuclei from the 2018 Data Science Bowl[3]. From the original dataset (670 images from diverse modalities) we selected a subset of fluorescence microscopy images and removed images with labeling errors, yielding a total of 497 images (*cf.* Fig. 4).

For each dataset, we use 90% of the images for training and 10% for testing. We train all methods (Sect. 3.3) with the same random crops of size 256×256 from the training images (augmented via axis-aligned rotations and flips).

3.2 Evaluation Metric

We adopt a typical metric for object detection: A detected object I_{pred} is considered a match (*true positive* TP_τ) if a ground truth object I_{gt} exists whose *intersection over union* $IoU = \frac{I_{pred} \cap I_{gt}}{I_{pred} \cup I_{gt}}$ is greater than a given threshold $\tau \in [0,1]$. Unmatched predicted objects are counted as *false positives* (FP_τ), unmatched ground truth objects as *false negatives* (FN_τ). We use the *average precision* $AP_\tau = \frac{TP_\tau}{TP_\tau + FN_\tau + FP_\tau}$ evaluated across all images as the final score.

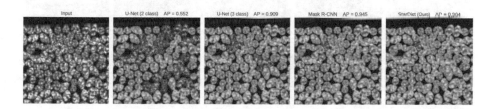

Fig. 3. Segmentation result ($\tau = 0.5$) for TRAGEN image. See Fig. 2 caption for legend.

3.3 Compared Methods

U-Net (2 class): We use the popular U-Net architecture [15] as a baseline to predict 2 output classes (cell, background). We use 3 down/up-sampling blocks, each consisting of 2 convolutional layers with $32 \cdot 2^k (k = 0,1,2)$ filters of size 3×3 (approx. 1.4 million parameters in total). We apply a threshold σ on the cell probability map and retain the connected components as final result (σ is optimized on the validation set for every dataset).

U-Net (3 class): Like U-Net (2 class), but we additionally predict the *boundary pixels* of cells as an extra class. The purpose of this is to differentiate crowded cells with touching borders (similar to [4,5]). We again use the connected components of the thresholded cell class as final result.

---

[3] https://www.kaggle.com/c/data-science-bowl-2018.

Mask R-CNN: A state-of-the-art instance segmentation method combining a bounding-box based region proposal network, non-maximum-suppression (NMS), and a final mask segmentation (approx. 45 million parameters in total). We use a popular open-source implementation[4]. For each dataset, we perform a grid-search over common hyper-parameters, such as detection NMS threshold, region proposal NMS threshold, and number of anchors.

STARDIST: Our proposed method as described in Sect. 2. We always use $n = 32$ radial directions (*cf.* Fig. 1b) and employ the same U-Net backbone as for the first two baselines described above.

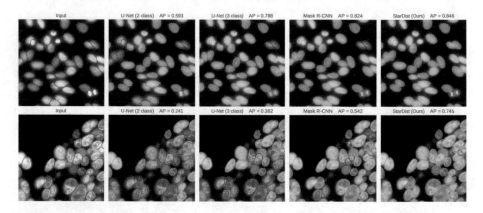

Fig. 4. Two segmentation results ($\tau = 0.5$) for DSB2018. See Fig. 2 caption for legend.

3.4   Results

We first test our approach on dataset TOY, which was intentionally designed to contain objects with many overlapping bounding boxes. The results in Table 1 and Fig. 2 show that for moderate IoU thresholds ($\tau < 0.7$), STARDIST and both U-Net baselines yield essentially perfect results. Mask R-CNN performs substantially worse due to the presence of many slanted and touching pairs of objects (which have almost identical bounding boxes, hence one is suppressed). This experiment highlights a fundamental limitation of object detection methods that predict axis-aligned bounding boxes.

On dataset TRAGEN, U-Net (2 class) shows the lowest accuracy mainly due to the abundance of touching cells which are erroneously fused. Table 1 shows that all other methods attain almost perfect accuracy for many IoU thresholds even on very crowded images, which might be due to the stereotypical size and texture of the simulated cells. We show the most difficult test image in Fig. 3.

---

[4] https://github.com/matterport/Mask_RCNN.

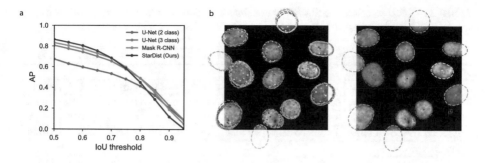

Fig. 5. *(a)* Detection scores on dataset DSB2018 (*cf.* Table 1, bottom). *(b)* Example of STARDIST polygon predictions for 200 random pixels (left) and for all pixels after non-maximum suppression (right); pixels and associated polygons are color-matched.

Finally, we turn to the real dataset DSB2018 where we find STARDIST to outperform all other methods for IoU thresholds $\tau < 0.75$, followed by the next best method Mask R-CNN (*cf.* Table 1 and Fig. 5a). Figure 4 shows the results and errors for two different types of cells. Common segmentation errors include merged cells (mostly for the 2 class U-Net), bounding box artifacts (Mask R-CNN) and missing cells (all methods). The bottom example of Fig. 4 is particularly challenging, where out-of-focus signal results in densely packed and partially overlapping cell shapes. Here, merging mistakes are pronounced for both U-Net baselines. All false positives predicted by STARDIST retain a reasonable shape, whereas those predicted by Mask R-CNN sometimes exhibit obvious artifacts.

We observe that STARDIST yields inferior results for the largest IoU thresholds τ for our synthetic datasets. This is not surprising, since we predict a parametric shape model based on only 32 radial directions, instead of a per-pixel segmentation as all other methods. However, an advantage of a parametric shape model is that it can be used to predict reasonable complete shape hypotheses from nuclei that are only partially visible at the image boundary (*cf.* Fig. 5b, also see [20]).

4   Discussion

We demonstrated that star-convex polygons are a good shape representation to accurately localize cell nuclei even under challenging conditions. Our approach is especially appealing for images of very crowded cells. When our STARDIST model makes a mistake, it does so gracefully by either simply omitting a cell or by predicting at least a plausible cell shape. The same cannot by said for the methods that we compared to, whose predicted shapes are sometimes obviously implausible (*e.g.*, containing holes or ridges). While STARDIST is competitive to the state-of-the-art Mask R-CNN method, a key advantage is that it has an order of magnitude fewer parameters and is much simpler to train and use. In contrast to Mask R-CNN, STARDIST has only few hyper-parameters that do not need careful tuning to achieve good results.

Table 1. Cell detection results for three datasets and four methods, showing *average precision* (AP) for several *intersection over union* (IoU) thresholds τ.

Threshold τ	0.50	0.55	0.60	0.65	0.70	0.75	0.80	0.85	0.90
Toy									
U-Net (2 class)	0.9994	0.9990	0.9977	0.9931	0.9641	0.8659	0.6229	0.2939	0.0667
U-Net (3 class)	**0.9998**	**0.9998**	**0.9998**	**0.9998**	**0.9998**	**0.9998**	**0.9990**	**0.9874**	**0.9243**
Mask R-CNN	0.9104	0.9061	0.9014	0.8944	0.8729	0.8471	0.7728	0.6075	0.3717
StarDist (Ours)	**0.9998**	**0.9998**	**0.9998**	**0.9998**	0.9994	0.9890	0.8695	0.4630	0.0748
TrAGen									
U-Net (2 class)	0.9030	0.8908	0.8852	0.8815	0.8811	0.8783	0.8566	0.6937	0.4056
U-Net (3 class)	0.9918	0.9904	0.9899	0.9897	0.9890	0.9883	**0.9848**	**0.9679**	**0.8995**
Mask R-CNN	0.9924	0.9919	0.9912	0.9898	0.9863	0.9777	0.9594	0.8948	0.5280
StarDist (Ours)	**0.9984**	**0.9981**	**0.9976**	**0.9967**	**0.9953**	**0.9934**	0.9841	0.9465	0.4259
DSB2018									
U-Net (2 class)	0.6739	0.6295	0.5975	0.5650	0.5339	0.4819	0.4151	0.3248	0.2032
U-Net (3 class)	0.8060	0.7753	0.7431	0.7011	0.6543	0.5777	**0.4910**	**0.3738**	**0.2258**
Mask R-CNN	0.8323	0.8051	0.7728	0.7299	0.6838	**0.5974**	0.4893	0.3525	0.1891
StarDist (Ours)	**0.8641**	**0.8361**	**0.8043**	**0.7545**	**0.6850**	0.5862	0.4495	0.2865	0.1191

Our approach could be particularly beneficial in the context of cell tracking. There, it is often desirable to have multiple diverse segmentation hypotheses [8,13], which could be achieved by suppressing fewer candidate polygons. Furthermore, StarDist can plausibly complete shapes for partially visible cells at the image boundary, which could make it easier to track cells that enter and leave the field of view over time.

References

1. Amat, F., Lemon, W., Mossing, D.P., McDole, K., Wan, Y., Branson, K., Myers, E.W., Keller, P.J.: Fast, accurate reconstruction of cell lineages from large-scale fluorescence microscopy data. Nat. Methods **11**(9), 951 (2014)
2. Boutros, M., Heigwer, F., Laufer, C.: Microscopy-based high-content screening. Cell **163**(6), 1314–1325 (2015)
3. Caicedo, J.C., et al.: Evaluation of deep learning strategies for nucleus segmentation in fluorescence images. bioRxiv (2018)
4. Chen, H., Qi, X., Yu, L., Heng, P.A.: DCAN: deep contour-aware networks for accurate gland segmentation. In: CVPR (2016)
5. Guerrero-Pena, F.A., Marrero Fernandez, P.D., Ren, T.I., Yui, M., Rothenberg, E., Cunha, A.: Multiclass weighted loss for instance segmentation of cluttered cells. arXiv (2018)
6. He, K., Gkioxari, G., Dollár, P., Girshick, R.: Mask R-CNN. In: ICCV (2017)
7. Jetley, S., Sapienza, M., Golodetz, S., Torr, P.H.: Straight to shapes: real-time detection of encoded shapes. In: CVPR (2017)
8. Jug, F., Levinkov, E., Blasse, C., Myers, E.W., Andres, B.: Moral lineage tracing. In: CVPR (2016)
9. Liu, W., et al.: SSD: single shot multibox detector. In: ECCV (2016)

10. Ma, J., et al.: Arbitrary-oriented scene text detection via rotation proposals. IEEE Trans. Multimed. (2018)
11. Meijering, E.: Cell segmentation: 50 years down the road. IEEE Signal Process. Mag. **29**(5), 140–145 (2012)
12. Redmon, J., Divvala, S., Girshick, R., Farhadi, A.: You only look once: unified, real-time object detection. In: CVPR (2016)
13. Rempfler, M., Kumar, S., Stierle, V., Paulitschke, P., Andres, B., Menze, B.H.: Cell lineage tracing in lens-free microscopy videos. In: Descoteaux, M., Maier-Hein, L., Franz, A., Jannin, P., Collins, D.L., Duchesne, S. (eds.) MICCAI 2017. LNCS, vol. 10434, pp. 3–11. Springer, Cham (2017). https://doi.org/10.1007/978-3-319-66185-8_1
14. Ren, S., He, K., Girshick, R., Sun, J.: Faster R-CNN: towards real-time object detection with region proposal networks. In: NIPS (2015)
15. Ronneberger, O., Fischer, P., Brox, T.: U-Net: convolutional networks for biomedical image segmentation. In: Navab, N., Hornegger, J., Wells, W.M., Frangi, A.F. (eds.) MICCAI 2015. LNCS, vol. 9351, pp. 234–241. Springer, Cham (2015). https://doi.org/10.1007/978-3-319-24574-4_28
16. Sommer, C., Straehle, C., Koethe, U., Hamprecht, F.A.: Ilastik: interactive learning and segmentation toolkit. In: International Symposium on Biomedical Imaging (2011)
17. Ulman, V., et al.: An objective comparison of cell-tracking algorithms. Nat. Methods **14**(12), 1141 (2017)
18. Ulman, V., Orémuš, Z., Svoboda, D.: TRAgen: a tool for generation of synthetic time-lapse image sequences of living cells. In: Murino, V., Puppo, E. (eds.) ICIAP 2015. LNCS, vol. 9279, pp. 623–634. Springer, Cham (2015). https://doi.org/10.1007/978-3-319-23231-7_56
19. Xie, W., Noble, J.A., Zisserman, A.: Microscopy cell counting and detection with fully convolutional regression networks. Comput. Methods Biomech. Biomed. Eng. Imaging Vis. **6**(3), 283–292 (2018)
20. Yurchenko, V., Lempitsky, V.: Parsing images of overlapping organisms with deep singling-out networks. In: CVPR (2017)

Deep Convolutional Gaussian Mixture Model for Stain-Color Normalization of Histopathological Images

Farhad Ghazvinian Zanjani[✉], Svitlana Zinger, and Peter H. N. de With

Eindhoven University of Technology, 5612 AJ Eindhoven, The Netherlands
f.ghazvinian.zanjani@tue.nl

Abstract. Automated microscopic analysis of stained histopathological images is degraded by the amount of color and intensity variations in data. This paper presents a novel unsupervised probabilistic approach by integrating a convolutional neural network (CNN) and the Gaussian mixture model (GMM) in a unified framework, which jointly optimizes the modeling and normalizing the color and intensity of hematoxylin-and eosin-stained (H&E) histological images. In contrast to conventional GMM-based methods that are applied only on the color distribution of data for stain color normalization, our proposal learns how to cluster the tissue structures according to their shape and appearance and simultaneously fits a multivariate GMM to the data. This approach is more robust than standard GMM in the presence of strong staining variations because fitting the GMM is conditioned on the appearance of tissue structures in the density channel of an image. Performing a gradient descent optimization in an end-to-end learning, the network learns to maximize the log-likelihood of data given estimated parameters of multivariate Gaussian distributions. Our method does not need ground truth, shape and color assumptions of image contents or manual tuning of parameters and thresholds which makes it applicable to a wide range of histopathological images. Experiments show that our proposed method outperforms the state-of-the-art algorithms in terms of achieving a higher color constancy.

Keywords: Computational pathology · Stain-color normalization
Gaussian mixture model (GMM)
Convolutional neural network (CNN)

1 Introduction

Computational histopathology involves computer-aided diagnosis (CAD) for microscopic analysis of stained histopathological slides to study presence, localization or grading of disease. Manual staining by adding contrasting dyes prior to microscopic imaging is a common clinical practice. Such a non-quantified manual procedure causes significant variations in tissue intensity and color, which also

© Springer Nature Switzerland AG 2018
A. F. Frangi et al. (Eds.): MICCAI 2018, LNCS 11071, pp. 274–282, 2018.
https://doi.org/10.1007/978-3-030-00934-2_31

originate from other factors such as imaging device characteristics. Such undesirable effects become more problematic when different laboratories share digital
images [1]. A well-known approach for compensating the color variations is applying color normalization techniques. Recent studies show that color normalization
as preprocessing stage leads to a higher performance in a CAD system [2]. To do so,
several methods are investigated [1,3–9]. The proposed approaches can be divided
into two categories:*stain-color deconvolution* and *template color matching*, which
are first briefly explained below, and then we describe our contributions.

Stain-color deconvolution [10] methods are considering prior knowledge of
the reference stain vector for every dye and split an input RGB image into three
stain channels, each representing the actual stain color. Ruifrok *et al.* [10] introduce this prior knowledge by manually selecting pixels that represent a specific
stain class and then compute the color deconvolution vector. Because of the semi-
automatic nature, several studies are performed later for automated extraction
of stains by e.g. using the singular value decomposition (SVD) technique [6],
probabilistic Gaussian mixture model (GMM) [8], using a prior for stain matrix
estimation [3] and stain color descriptions along with training a supervised relevance vector machine [4]. Although these solutions lead to a better stain estimation, they solely limited to image color information, while the spatial dependency
among tissue structures has been ignored [1]. This causes shortcomings for stain
deconvolution approaches when severe staining variations occur in the data.

Template color matching methods proposed by Reinhard *et al.* [5] rely on
aligning the statistical color distribution (e.g. mean and standard deviation) of
a *source* image with a *template* image. The authors used a set of linear transformations for assigning a unimodal distribution to each channel of the CIELAB
color model. Afterwards, each channel was treated independently for alignment.
Since there is a dependency between the color channels due to dye contribution,
this approach has drawbacks which have been addressed in [1,4]. For solving
this problem, separate transformations are performed on stain classes [8], or on
tissue classes [1,9]. For avoiding artifacts at the border of different classes under
different transformations, a weighted contribution of these transformations in
the final color image is considered. Two proposed solutions consist of estimating
weights of the GMM [8] and training a naive Bayesian classifier [1]. This solution
introduce multiple parameters and thresholds which cannot be optimally applied
to a new dataset or even fail if the tissue type changes.

Regarding to [8,9], we propose a stain-color normalization method based on
GMM but with a different approach. Our contribution is threefold. First, we introduce a new unsupervised stain-color normalization method based on deep convolutional Gaussian mixture models (DCGMM). Our proposal benefits from a
convolutional neural network (CNN) for performing soft-assignment clustering
of tissue structures in an unsupervised manner. Second, in contrast to the previous GMM-based color normalization methods that work on color point-clouds
by considering each pixel independently in input space, our method fits a GMM
to an input color image with processing and involving the visual contents, such as
the appearance and shape of regions in the image intensity (density) channel by

means of the CNN. Such an approach outperforms the previous methods specifically when strong staining variations appear in the data (see Fig. 1). This outcome occurs because our method is independent from the chromatic information for tissue class assignment and consequent distribution modeling. Finally, instead of using a common expectation-maximization (EM) algorithm for optimizing the GMM, we introduce an end-to-end learning procedure for optimizing the parameters of the CNN and the GMM together. To our knowledge, it is the first time that this approach is used for training a DCGMM.

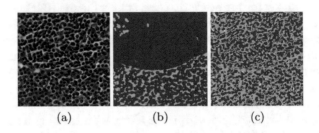

(a)   (b)   (c)

Fig. 1. Example of standard GMM failure in tissue clustering using HSD color space; (a) RGB H&E image; (b) 3-class standard GMM; (c) 3-class DCGMM.

2   Methods

We first provide a brief overview of the standard GMM method and introduce the notation used in the paper. Afterwards, we introduce our DCGMM method.

Gaussian Mixture Model of data ($\mathbf{x}$), can be presented as a linear superposition of K Gaussian mixtures in terms of discrete *latent* variables ($\mathbf{z}$), in the form of

$$p(\mathbf{x}) = \Sigma_{k=1}^{K} \pi_k \mathcal{N}(\mathbf{x}|\boldsymbol{\mu}_k, \boldsymbol{\Sigma}_k). \tag{1}$$

The K-dimensional binary random variable $\mathbf{z}$ has one-hot encoding ($z_k \in \{0,1\}$; $\Sigma_{k=1}^{K} z_k = 1$), which represents the tissue class in our study. In Eq. (1), the mixing coefficients π_k must satisfy $0 \leq \pi_k \leq 1$ together with $\Sigma_{k=1}^{K} \pi_k = 1$, in order to fulfill a valid probability definition [11]. Here, $\mathcal{N}$ stands for a multivariate normal distribution with mean $\boldsymbol{\mu}_k$ and covariance matrix $\boldsymbol{\Sigma}_k$. If we consider π_k as prior probability of class z_k, its posterior probability called *responsibility* can be written as follows [11]:

$$\gamma(z_k) = p(z_k = 1|\mathbf{x}) = \frac{\pi_k \mathcal{N}(\mathbf{x}|\boldsymbol{\mu}_k, \boldsymbol{\Sigma}_k)}{\Sigma_{j=1}^{K} \pi_j \mathcal{N}(\mathbf{x}|\boldsymbol{\mu}_j, \boldsymbol{\Sigma}_j)}. \tag{2}$$

According to Eq. (1), the (natural) log-likelihood function for an image ($\mathbf{X} = \{\mathbf{x}_1, \mathbf{x}_2, ..., \mathbf{x}_N\}$) with total number of pixels (observations) equal to N is

$$\ln p(\mathbf{X}|\boldsymbol{\pi}, \boldsymbol{\mu}, \boldsymbol{\Sigma}) = \Sigma_{n=1}^{N} \ln\{\Sigma_{k=1}^{K} \pi_k \mathcal{N}(\mathbf{x}|\boldsymbol{\mu}_k, \boldsymbol{\Sigma}_k)\}. \tag{3}$$

Given the GMM, the goal is to maximize the likelihood function (Eq. (3)) with respect to the parameters (μ_k, Σ_k, π_k). The common approach for this is using the EM algorithm by iteratively evaluating the responsibilities (Eq. (2)) and re-estimating the parameters.

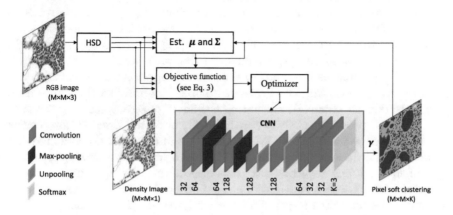

Fig. 2. Block diagram of DCGMM in training phase.

Deep Convolutional GMM (DCGMM): The recent development of deep generative models has invoked some extensions to the standard GMM [12,13]. Two proposed approaches are (1) constructing a stack of multiple GMM layers on top of each other in a hierarchical architecture [13] that is optimized by EM-based algorithm and (2) using auto-encoder neural networks while applying the GMM on their low-dimensional representations [12] that has been studied for unsupervised anomaly detection. This paper presents a different extension to the standard GMM by introducing the DCGMM that is a fully-convolutional CNN of which the parameters are optimized to fit a GMM to the input image, in an end-to-end learning, using gradient descent and back-propagation algorithms.

We aim to fit a GMM to the pixel-color distribution conditioned on tissue classes. For processing the image and detecting the tissue classes, the high capability of the CNN has been exploited. To do so, estimating the responsibility coefficients (Eq. (2)) is performed by a CNN. For a better understanding, one can consider that the E-step in an EM-based optimization is replaced by a CNN. However, all parameters of the GMM and CNN are jointly optimized by the gradient descent algorithm. In the DCGMM, the negative log-likelihood (maximizing Eq. (3)) is used as the loss function.

Our color normalization algorithm can be split into two phases, training the DCGMM and the color transformation (inference). In the training phase, we fit a GMM to the data. After the training stage is finished and in inference mode, the template image and source image are separately supplied to the model. Consequently, the parameters of the fitted Gaussian distributions and their mixture coefficients (π) are computed in those two images. Afterwards, the multivariate

Gaussian distributions of the source image are transformed (aligned) to have similar parameters of distributions as the template image, while $\boldsymbol{\pi}$ is kept unchanged. In the rest of this section, we explain these two phases in detail.

Fitting Gaussian Distribution to Data: First the RGB color values are transferred to the hue-saturation-density (HSD) color system [14]. In a HSD model of histopathological images, the density channel (D) is linearly related to the amount of stain while the other two chromatic channels are independent. This property suits well to the analysis of transmitted light microscopy, compared to the alternative color spaces [1]. We only use the normalized to zero-mean (centered) density channel as the input to the network. Ignoring the chromatic information and only clustering the tissue structures according to their appearance (normalized density channel), alleviating the effect of strong staining variations in images. The proposed CNN has a fully-convolutional architecture, consisting of several convolutional layers, rectified linear units (ReLU) as nonlinearity functions and (un)pooling operators. The reduced image size after applying two stages of max-pooling returns back to it original size by applying un-pooling operations. After the last convolutional layer, there is a softmax layer. The network aims to estimate the responsibility values (see Eq. (2)) for each pixel in the input image. Using the softmax layer at the output of the network guarantees the constraint of $\Sigma_{k=1}^{K}\gamma_k = 1$. Since we are working on H&E histopathological images, each pixel in the image mostly belongs to one out of three clusters ($K = 3$): hematoxylin, eosin and background (not stained). Because the biological composition of tissue related to each pixel in the image leads to a varying stain absorption ratio between pixels, the color of each pixel can be presented by a weighted sum of the different stains used. This property can be reflected in the responsibility coefficient ($\boldsymbol{\gamma}$) of a GMM, which is estimated in the softmax layer of the network in our proposed model. The calculation of the required partial derivatives of negative log-likelihood (loss function) with respect to its parameters ($\boldsymbol{\pi}, \boldsymbol{\mu}$ and $\boldsymbol{\Sigma}$) for performing a gradient descent algorithm can be found in [15, p. 45].

Algorithm 1. DCGMM training (left) and inference (right) algorithm

$\theta_{net} \leftarrow$ random CNN parameters	$\mathbf{X}^t_{h,s,d} \leftarrow$ HSD Template image
repeat	$\gamma^t, \mu^t, \Sigma^t, \pi^t \leftarrow$ Ops. (1-5)
$\mathbf{X} \leftarrow$ input image	$\mathbf{X}^s_{h,s,d} \leftarrow$ HSD Source image
$\mathbf{X}_h, \mathbf{X}_s, \mathbf{X}_d \leftarrow \mathrm{HSD}(\mathbf{X})$	$\gamma^s, \mu^s, \Sigma^s, \pi^s \leftarrow$ Ops. (1-5)
$\gamma \leftarrow f_{net}(\bar{\mathbf{X}}_d, \theta_{net})$ $\triangleright$ (1)	**for** k:=1 to K step 1 **do**
$N_k \leftarrow \Sigma_{n=1}^N \gamma(z_{nk})$ $\triangleright$ (2)	$\mathbf{Y} \leftarrow \mathbf{X}^s_k - \mu^s_k$ $\triangleright$ Centering
$\mu_k \leftarrow \frac{1}{N_k}\Sigma_{n=1}^N \gamma(z_{nk})\mathbf{x}_n$ $\triangleright$ (3)	$\Phi^s \Lambda^s \Phi^{s-1} \leftarrow \Sigma^s_k$ $\triangleright$ SVD
$\Sigma_k \leftarrow \frac{1}{N_k}\Sigma_{n=1}^N \gamma(z_{nk})(\mathbf{x}_n - \mu_k)(\mathbf{x}_n - \mu_k)^T \triangleright$ (4)	$\mathbf{Z} \leftarrow \Lambda^{s-\frac{1}{2}}\Phi^{sT}\mathbf{Y}$ $\triangleright$ Whitening
$\pi_k \leftarrow \frac{N_k}{N}$ $\triangleright$ (5)	$\Phi^t \Lambda^t \Phi^{t-1} \leftarrow \Sigma^t_k$ $\triangleright$ SVD
$\mathcal{L} \leftarrow -\Sigma_{n=1}^N \ln\{\Sigma_{k=1}^K \pi_k \mathcal{N}(\mathbf{x}|\mu_k, \Sigma_k)\}$ $\triangleright$ loss	$\mathbf{X}^{new}_k \leftarrow \Phi^t \Lambda^{t\frac{1}{2}}\mathbf{Z} + \mu^t_k$
$\theta_{net} \overset{+}{\leftarrow} -\nabla_{\theta_{net}}(\mathcal{L})$	**end for**
until stopping criterion	$\mathbf{X}^{new} \leftarrow \Sigma_{k=1}^K [\gamma^s_k \circ \mathbf{X}^{new}_k]$

Table 1. Standard Deviation (SD) and Coefficient of Variation (CV) of NMI for all five laboratories for hematoxylin and eosin dyes.

Method	Hematoxylin												Eosin	
	Lab 1		Lab 2		Lab 3		Lab 4		Lab 5		Average			
	SD	CV	SD	CV	SD	CV	SD	CV	SD	CV	SD	CV	SD	CV
Original	0.033	0.065	0.031	0.060	0.037	0.078	0.029	0.049	0.028	0.051	0.032	0.060	0.0563	0.0748
Macenko [6]	0.029	0.052	0.026	0.046	0.020	0.037	0.025	0.044	0.020	0.035	0.024	0.043	0.0362	0.0439
Reinhard [5]	0.032	0.058	0.025	0.044	0.020	0.035	0.030	0.052	0.029	0.049	0.027	0.047	0.0386	0.0494
Khan [4]	0.066	0.156	0.067	0.155	0.085	0.158	0.054	0.110	0.049	0.093	0.064	0.135	0.0434	0.0555
Vahadane [7]	0.036	0.065	0.032	0.058	0.024	0.046	0.023	0.042	0.020	0.038	0.027	0.050	0.034	0.041
Bejnordi [1]	**0.016**	**0.029**	**0.015**	0.027	0.018	0.034	0.029	0.055	0.024	0.044	0.021	0.038	0.0191	0.0220
Ours	0.022	0.045	0.017	0.034	**0.017**	0.036	**0.014**	0.030	**0.017**	0.035	**0.017**	**0.036**	**0.0188**	**0.0209**

Although the responsibility term is estimated by the CNN from only the density channel of the image, the mean and covariance matrices (μ_k and Σ_k) are estimated from all three channels of the HSD color image. The randomly initialized parameters of the CNN are updated by ADAM gradient-based optimization with a fixed learning rate of 10^{-3}. The scheme of our model is depicted in Fig. 2.

Transformation of Multivariate Gaussian Distributions: By training the model in the color normalization task, two GMMs are fitted to the source and template images, individually. Afterwards, a set of transformations are applied to align the multivariate Gaussian distributions between the source and the template. These transformations consist of three operations: *mean centering, whitening* and *coloring* transformation. Let us assume that (μ^s, Σ^s) and (μ^t, Σ^t) are the estimated parameters of the two distributions in source and template image, respectively. By shifting the mean of source image to the origin (*centering*) and then whitening which involves the SVD algorithm, the source image will have a zero mean and an identity covariance matrix. Consequently, by applying a coloring transformation which is the inverse of whitening but after replacing the eigenvalues (Λ) and eigenvectors (Φ) of source distribution with the template distribution, the whitened Gaussian distribution of source image scales and rotates to have the same covariance matrix as the template image (Σ^t). Finally, the distribution is shifted to obtain the same mean as the template distribution. For clarifying this procedure, pseudocode in Algorithm 1 shows these steps in detail.

3   Experimental Results

Histopathology Image Dataset: We focus on inter-laboratory variations of the H&E staining, as it is a major concern in large-scale application of CAD in pathology. For better comparison with recent studies, we use the same dataset as has been introduced in [1]. The dataset contains 625 images (each 1388×1040 pixels) from 125 digitized H&E stained WSIs of lymph nodes from 3 patients and was collected from five Dutch pathology laboratories, each using their own routine staining protocols (more details can be found in [1]). Our model is trained on randomly cropped patches (576 × 576 pixels) and evaluated on full-sized images by using leave-one-out cross-validation based on the above laboratories.

Results: We trained the DCGMM on the dataset. The model easily converges in a few minutes. The inference computation time for each image in its original size (1388 × 1040 pixels) is about 0.6 s, implemented in the TensorFlow library and running on a TITAN Xp GPU. The performance of our method is compared to that of five competing state-of-the-art algorithms: linear appearance normalization by Macenko *et al.* [6], statistical color properties alignment by Reinhard *et al.* [5], nonlinear mapping for stain normalization by Khan *et al.* [4], sparse non-negative matrix factorization by Vahadane*et al.* [7] and WSI color standardizer by Bejnordi *et al.* [1]. The normalized median intensity (NMI) measure [1,9] is used to evaluate color constancy of normalized images. Quantitative analysis is based on independently evaluating the color constancy in the regions that show mostly absorbed hematoxylin or eosin. Since nuclei mostly absorb hematoxylin, they first are detected automatically by using a fast radial symmetry transform and a marker-controlled watershed algorithm [1]. Since our generated hematoxylin masks slightly differ from what were used in [1], the obtained NMI scores in our benchmark are not exactly the same as [1]. However, the results are in agreement with [1]. For evaluation of the eosin analysis, several regions are manually annotated for 25 images. The evaluation results of different methods for assessing hematoxylin and eosin regions are shown in Table 1. The results clearly indicate that our proposed method results in the lowest variation in color after normalization of the images and it outperforms competing state-of-the-art methods. Figure 3 illustrates an example of the template image, a source image and the outcomes of color normalization by the different methods.

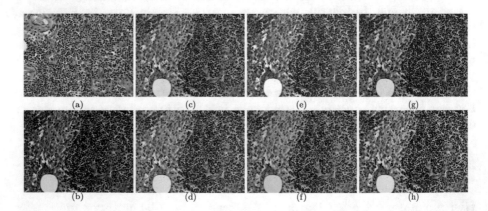

Fig. 3. Performance of different stain color-normalization methods on an *H&E* image. (a) template image (b) original images, (c) Macenko *et al.*[6], (d) Vahadane *et al.*[7], (e) Reinhard *et al.*[5], (f) Bejnordi *et al.*[1], (g) Khan *et al.* [4], (h) DCGMM.

4 Conclusions

We have introduced a framework for modeling and normalizing the colors in H&E histopathological images. Our model jointly optimizes the parameters of a CNN and the parameters of multivariate GMM in an end-to-end learning framework. By minimizing the negative log-likelihood loss function, the CNN learns how to cluster the image structures for optimally fitting the GMM on the data. Our proposal takes only one assumption on the number of clusters that is evidently chosen to three ($K = 3$) for H&E images. It does not need manual tuning of parameters and thresholds which makes it applicable to a wide range of histopathological images collected from different organs. Since our method processes and fits the GMM conditioned on the tissue classes, in comparison with previous methods, it is more robust in presence of strong stain variations.

References

1. Bejnordi, B., et al.: Stain specific standardization of whole-slide histopathological images. IEEE Trans. Med. Imaging **35**(2), 404–415 (2016)
2. Ciompi, F., Geessink, O., Bejnordi, B.E., et al.: The importance of stain normalization in colorectal tissue classification with convolutional networks. In: 2017 IEEE 14th International Symposium on Biomedical Imaging (ISBI 2017), pp. 160–163. IEEE (2017)
3. Niethammer, M., Borland, D., Marron, J.S., Woosley, J., Thomas, N.E.: Appearance normalization of histology slides. In: Wang, F., Yan, P., Suzuki, K., Shen, D. (eds.) MLMI 2010. LNCS, vol. 6357, pp. 58–66. Springer, Heidelberg (2010). https://doi.org/10.1007/978-3-642-15948-0_8
4. Khan, A., Rajpoot, N., Treanor, D., Magee, D.: A nonlinear mapping approach to stain normalization in digital histopathology images using image-specific color deconvolution. IEEE Trans. Biomed. Eng. **61**(6), 1729–1738 (2014)
5. Reinhard, E., Adhikhmin, M., Gooch, B., Shirley, P.: Color transfer between images. IEEE Comput. Graph. Appl. **21**(5), 34–41 (2001)
6. Macenko, M., et al.: A method for normalizing histology slides for quantitative analysis. In: Proceedings of IEEE International Symposium on Biomedical Imaging Nano Macro, pp. 1107–1110 (2009)
7. Vahadane, A., et al.: Structure-preserving color normalization and sparse stain separation for histological images. IEEE Trans. Med. Imaging **35**(8), 1962–1971 (2016)
8. Magee, D., et al.: Color normalization in digital histopathology images. In: Proceedings of Optical Tissue Image Analysis Microscopy, Histopathology Endoscopy, pp. 100–111 (2009)
9. Ajay Basavanhally, A.M.: Em-based segmentation-driven color standardization of digitized histopathology. Proc. SPIE **12**, 8676–8676-12 (2013)
10. Ruifrok, A.C., Johnston, D.A.: Quantification of histochemical staining by color deconvolution. Analyt. Quant. Cytol. Histol. Int. Acad. Cytol. Am. Soc. Cytol. **23**(4), 291–299 (2001)
11. Christopher, M.B.: Pattern Recognition and Machine learning. Springer, New York (2016)

12. Zong, B., et al.: Deep autoencoding gaussian mixture model for unsupervised anomaly detection. In: International Conference on Learning Representations (2018)
13. van den Oord, A., Schrauwen, B.: Factoring variations in natural images with deep gaussian mixture models. In: Advances in Neural Information Processing Systems, vol. 27, pp. 3518–3526. Curran Associates, Inc. (2014)
14. van der Laak, J.A., Pahlplatz, M.M., Hanselaar, A.G., de Wilde, P.C.: Hue-saturation-density (hsd) model for stain recognition in digital images from transmitted light microscopy. Cytometry **39**(4), 275–284 (2000)
15. Petersen, K.B., Pedersen, M.S.: The Matrix Cookbook. Technical University of Denmark, version 20121115, November 2012

Learning to Segment 3D Linear Structures Using Only 2D Annotations

Mateusz Koziński(✉), Agata Mosinska, Mathieu Salzmann, and Pascal Fua

Computer Vision Laboratory, École Polytechnique Fédérale de Lausanne,
Lausanne, Switzerland
{mateusz.kozinski,agata.mosinska,mathieu.salzmann,pascal.fua}@epfl.ch

Abstract. We propose a loss function for training a Deep Neural Network (DNN) to segment volumetric data, that accommodates ground truth annotations of 2D projections of the training volumes, instead of annotations of the 3D volumes themselves. In consequence, we significantly decrease the amount of annotations needed for a given training set. We apply the proposed loss to train DNNs for segmentation of vascular and neural networks in microscopy images and demonstrate only a marginal accuracy loss associated to the significant reduction of the annotation effort. The lower labor cost of deploying DNNs, brought in by our method, can contribute to a wide adoption of these techniques for analysis of 3D images of linear structures.

1 Introduction

Linear structures such as blood vessels, bronchi and dendritic trees are pervasive in medical imagery. Automatically recovering their topology has therefore become critically important to fully exploit the vast amounts of data that modern imaging devices can now produce. Machine Leaning based techniques have demonstrated their effectiveness for this purpose, but usually require substantial amounts of annotated training data to reach their full potential.

Unfortunately, annotating complex topologies in 3D volumes by means of an inherently 2D computer interface is slow and tedious. The annotator must frequently rotate and move the volume to verify the correct placement of control points and to reveal occluded details. Not only is this inherently slow, but such interactions require continuously re-displaying large amounts of data, which often exceeds the capacity of a workstation, thus introducing further delays.

In this paper, we show that we can train a Deep Net to perform 3D volumetric delineation given *only* 2D annotations in Maximum Intensity Projections (MIP), such as those shown on the right side of Fig. 1. This is a major time-saver because

---

M. Koziński—The author was supported by the FastProof ERC Proof of Concept Grant.

A. Mosinska—The author was supported by the Swiss National Science Foundation.

© Springer Nature Switzerland AG 2018
A. F. Frangi et al. (Eds.): MICCAI 2018, LNCS 11071, pp. 283–291, 2018.
https://doi.org/10.1007/978-3-030-00934-2_32

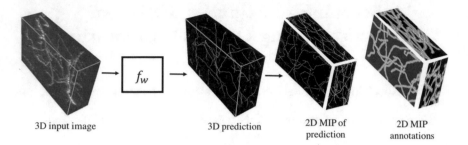

3D input image   3D prediction   2D MIP of   2D MIP
                                           prediction   annotations

Fig. 1. 3D training using 2D annotations only. We first annotate the 2D Maximum Intensity Projections (MIP) of the training image stacks. Then, we minimize a cross entropy loss between the annotated 2D MIPs and the corresponding projections of the 3D prediction made by the network f_w we are training.

delineating linear structures in 2D images is much easier than in 3D volumes and involves none of the difficulties mentioned above. Furthermore, semi-automated annotation tools work more smoothly on 2D than on 3D data. In short, limiting the annotation effort to the projections leads to a considerable labor saving without compromising the performance of the trained network.

More specifically, we introduce a loss function that penalizes discrepancies between the maximum intensity projection of the predictions and the 2D annotations. We show that it yields a network that performs as well as if it had been trained using full 3D annotations. The loss is inspired by *space carving*, a classical approach to reconstructing complex 3D shapes from arbitrarily-positioned cameras [1]. Space carving exploits the fact that visual rays corresponding to background pixels in 2D images cannot cross any foreground voxel when passing through the volume. Conversely, rays emanating from foreground pixels have to cross at least one foreground voxel. In our case, the rays are parallel to the projection axes. The network is trained to minimize the cross-entropy between the 2D annotations and the maximum values along the rays.

Our contribution is therefore a principled approach to reducing the annotators' burden when training a Deep Net by enabling them to trace in 2D instead of 3D, while still capturing the full 3D topology of complex linear structures. We demonstrate this on 3D light microscopy images of neurons and retinal blood vessels and on Magnetic Resonance Angiography (MRA) brain scans.

2   Related Work

Early approaches to delineation of 3D curvilinear structures relied on filters manually designed to respond strongly to tubular segments [2–4]. They do not require to be trained, but their performance degrades when the structures become irregular and the images noisy. This has led to the emergence of machine learning based methods that can cope with such difficulties, given enough annotated data [5–8]. The most recent one of these [8] relies on Deep Learning for neuron tracing by adaptive exploration of 3D light microscopy images.

However, using Machine Learning, and Deep Learning in particular, requires large amounts of annotated training data. Furthermore, annotating 3D stacks is much more labor-intensive than annotating 2D images. Only true experts, whose time is precious, are able to orient themselves and follow complex structures in large volumes [9]. Until now, this problem has been handled by developing better ways to visualize and interact with image stacks [8,10]. In [11], only a few slices of a volume are annotated and the loss is computed using only them. The technique of [9], like ours, allows the annotator to trace a linear structure in a maximum intensity projection and then attempts to guess the value of the third coordinate using a simple heuristic. While effective when the structures are relatively sparse, this can easily get confused as the scene becomes more cluttered.

The originality of our approach is to introduce a method that relies solely on 2D annotations in Maximum Intensity Projections and, yet, captures the 3D structure of complex linear structures when the projections are used jointly.

3 Method

3.1 From 3D to 2D Annotations

Let us first consider the problem of training a neural network f_w, parameterized by weights w, to segment linear structures within 3D image stacks, given a training set T of pairs $(\mathbf{x}, \tilde{\mathbf{y}})$, where each 3D image $\mathbf{x}$ is accompanied by the corresponding volumetric ground-truth annotations $\tilde{\mathbf{y}}$. We denote the elements of $\mathbf{x}$ and $\tilde{\mathbf{y}}$ by x_{ijk} and $\tilde{y}_{ijk}$, where i, j, k index the positions of the elements within the volumes. The ground-truth labels take a value in the set $\{1, 0, \varnothing\}$, which indicate the presence of a linear structure in voxel i, j, k if $\tilde{y}_{ijk} = 1$, the absence of a linear structure if $\tilde{y}_{ijk} = 0$, and uncertainty of the annotator if $\tilde{y}_{ijk} = \varnothing$. Delineation can then be cast as a binary segmentation problem by simply ignoring the voxels labeled as $\varnothing$ during training. The network output $\mathbf{y} = f_w(\mathbf{x})$ has the same size as the input and contains probabilities of presence of a linear structure in each voxel. To train the network, we find

$$\arg \min_w \sum_{(\mathbf{x}, \tilde{\mathbf{y}}) \in T} \sum_{i,j,k} L(f_w(\mathbf{x})_{ijk}, \tilde{y}_{ijk}), \qquad (1)$$

where $f_w()_{ijk}$ denotes voxel i, j, k of the prediction, and the loss $L(y, \tilde{y})$ is taken to be the cross entropy $C(y, \tilde{y}) = [\tilde{y} = 1] \log y + [\tilde{y} = 0] \log(1 - y)$, where $[\cdot]$ is the Iverson bracket. As discussed in the introduction, the drawback of this approach is that generating the ground-truth labels $\tilde{\mathbf{y}}$ in sufficient numbers to train a deep network is tedious and expensive when operating on large volumes.

To alleviate this problem, we reformulate the loss function of Eq. 1 so that it can exploit annotated Maximum Intensity Projections (MIPs) of the input volumes. A MIP of volume $\mathbf{x}$ along direction i, which we denote as $\mathbf{x}^i$, is a 2D image with elements $x_{jk}^i = \max_i x_{ijk}$. Annotating MIPs is easy when the structures of interest have high intensity and are clearly visible in the projections. A MIP annotation $\tilde{\mathbf{y}}^i$ comprises elements $\tilde{y}_{jk}^i \in \{1, 0, \varnothing\}$, which can also be

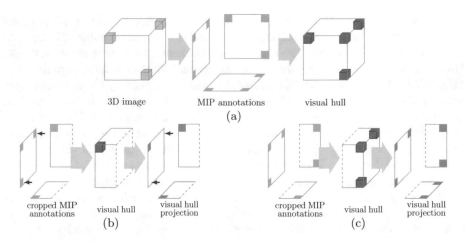

3D image   MIP annotations   visual hull
(a)

cropped MIP   visual hull   visual hull   cropped MIP   visual hull   visual hull
annotations   projection   annotations   projection
(b)   (c)

Fig. 2. Handling cropped volumes. *(a)* A 3D volume with three foreground voxels, the annotations of its MIPs in green, and the visual hull computed from these in blue. *(b)* The volume has been cropped so that only the left half remains. The annotations have been cropped to match, leaving a single blue voxel in the visual hull. Reprojecting it into the MIPs lets us eliminate the extraneous annotations, indicated with red arrows. *(c)* However, there are situations such as the one depicted here, where some will survive.

thought of as $\tilde{y}^i_{jk} = \max_i \tilde{y}_{ijk}$. MIPs of the volume along the directions j and k, and their annotations, are defined similarly.

Since $\tilde{y}^i_{jk} = 0$ tells us that *all* voxels of the input column jk contain background while $\tilde{y}^i_{jk} = 1$ tells us that at least one voxel in the input column contains a linear structure, we define the max-projection $f^i_w(\mathbf{x})$ along direction i of the network output as the image with elements $f^i_w(\mathbf{x})_{jk} = \max_i f_w(\mathbf{x})_{ijk}$. We proceed similarly for directions j and k. We then rewrite our training loss as

$$\sum_{(\mathbf{x},\tilde{\mathbf{y}})\in T} \left(\sum_{jk} L\big(f^i_w(\mathbf{x})_{jk}, \tilde{y}^i_{jk}\big) + \sum_{ik} L\big(f^j_w(\mathbf{x})_{ik}, \tilde{y}^j_{ik}\big) + \sum_{ij} L\big(f^k_w(\mathbf{x})_{ij}, \tilde{y}^k_{ij}\big) \right). \quad (2)$$

Note that $f^i_w(\mathbf{x})_{jk}$ upper bounds the probability of presence of a linear structure in column jk. Equation 2 penalizes large values of this upper bound whenever $\tilde{y}^i_{jk} = 0$, thus mimicking space carving. When $\tilde{y}^i_{jk} = 1$, minimizing the loss increases the largest prediction in the column.

3.2   Visual Hull for Training on Cropped Volumes

Due to memory limitations, the annotated training volumes are typically cropped into sub-volumes and the MIP can be cropped to match. However, the cropped annotations may then contain labels for structures located outside the volume crop, as illustrated by Fig. 2. To reduce the influence of these extraneous annotations, we use another element of the space carving theory, the visual hull **h**. **h** is a volume containing the original one, and constructed from its projections [1].

By construction, an element of the hull $h_{ijk} = 1$ if and only if *all* of its projections are labelled as foreground. In our context, a foreground voxel outside a crop only produces an incorrect annotation in *a single* projection. Therefore, as shown in Fig. 2, we can very often eliminate it by projecting the visual hull back to the 2D annotations and discarding those that fall outside.

3.3   Implementation

In practice, we use a U-Net style architecture [12] to implement f_w. Specifically, we made the original convolution-ReLU-convolution-ReLU blocks residual, and rely on only two max-pooling operations instead of the usual four ones, which resulted in a more compact network that fits in memory even with larger volume crops. In all our experiments, we trained the network for two hundred thousand iterations, using the ADAM update scheme [13] with momentum of 0.9, weight decay 10^{-4} and step size 10^{-5}.

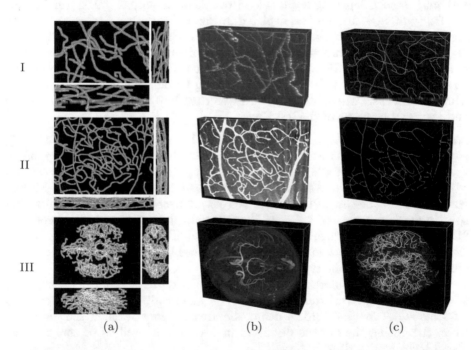

Fig. 3. Results on our three datasets, from top to bottom, axons, retinal blood vessels, and brain vasculature in MRA scans. (a) 2D annotations in 3 MIPs of a training volume. The foreground centerline annotations are marked in white and the regions to be ignored around them in gray. (b) Input test image volume. (c) Output segmentation.

4   Experimental Evaluation

4.1   Data and Annotations

We tested our approach on three data sets that differ in terms of the imaged tissue, the acquisition modality and the image resolution. As a result, there are substantial variations with respect to the density of the structures of interest, their appearance and the amount of clutter originating from extraneous objects.

Axons. The dataset comprises 16 stacks of 2-photon microscopy images of neural tissue in mouse brain, with sizes ranging from $40 \times 200 \times 200$ to $136 \times 322 \times 500$ voxels and a resolution of $0.8 \times 0.26 \times 0.26$ μm. We split the data into a test set of two volumes, both of size $136 \times 233 \times 500$, and a training set of 14 smaller volumes. Figure 1 depicts one of the training sets and the top row of Fig. 3 one of the testing ones.

Retina. The dataset is made of two stacks of confocal microscopy $1024 \times 1024 \times 110$ image stacks depicting retinal blood vessels of resolution of 0.62 μm. We use one for training and the other, depicted in Fig. 3, for testing. Since most vessels are located within a 50-pixel high XY slice, MIPs in the X and Y directions are very cluttered. Therefore, we split the volume into 16 $256 \times 256 \times 110$ subvolumes and their annotated MIPs. In other words, we also traced the vertical faces of the smaller volumes. This only requires annotating 6 additional 1024×110 images, which is still fast. The middle row of Fig. 3 describes both our 2D annotations and the results on one of the test sets.

Angiography. This set of MRI brain scans [14], one of which is shown in Fig. 3, is publicly available. It consists of 42 annotated stacks, which we cropped to a size of $416 \times 320 \times 128$ voxels by removing the margins. Their resolution is $0.5 \times 0.5 \times 0.6$ mm. We partitioned the data into 31 training and 11 test volumes. As in the case of the retinal vessels, we decreased the visual clutter by splitting each volume into 4 $208 \times 160 \times 128$ subvolumes for which we produced 2D annotations. This requires annotating an additional 416×128 image and a 320×128 one. The bottom row of Fig. 3 describes both our 2D annotations and our results on one of the test sets.

All the manual annotations are expressed in terms 2D and 3D centerlines of the underlying structures. We then use a pixel-width of 11 for the first two datasets and 7 for the third to define the area to ignore around the centerline when computing the loss, as discussed in Sect. 3.1, as well as to compute the visual hulls, as described in Sect. 3.2.

4.2   User Study

The usefulness of our approach is predicated on the claim that tracing in 2D is much easier than in 3D. To substantiate it, we conducted a small user study involving 5 PhD students used to performing such delineation tasks for research purposes. We asked them to annotate three volumes from the axon dataset using the Fiji Simple Neurite Tracer plugin [2], both in 2D and in 3D, and recorded

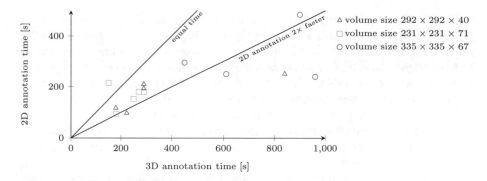

Fig. 4. Annotation times captured during the user study. Each user annotated volumes both in 3D and in 2D, and a pair of annotation times is represented as a single point in the plot. Different colors denote different volumes.

how long it took them to complete these two tasks. We report the results in Fig. 4. For the two smaller volumes—$292 \times 292 \times 40$ and $231 \times 231 \times 71$—it took people 3 to 4 min to create the 3D annotations and about 25% to 50% less in 2D. For the larger $335 \times 335 \times 67$ volume, the 3D annotation time grew substantially but, it took about half as long to annotate in 2D.

While this study is too small to be statistically significant, it shows a clear trend. The larger the volume to be annotated, the more tedious the 3D annotation process, and the more attractive it becomes to annotate solely in 2D.

4.3   3D vs 2D Annotations

The 2D annotations are faster and easier but are *a priori* less informative than the 3D ones, and we could expect a drop in performance when using the former. We now show that our reconstruction framework *prevents* this drop from materializing.

Table 1. F1 score performance and corresponding time savings.

	F1 score			Time saving [%]
	Axons	Retina	Angiography	
UNet/3D annot	75.4	**81.5**	**77.6**	0
UNet/3 MIP annot./volume	**78.1**	78.2	75.9	50
UNet/2 MIP annot./volume	75.0	77.8	74.8	60
UNet/1 MIP annot./volume	72.3	39.0	57.7	70
Slice annot. [11]	70.8	75.8	74.1	50
Tubularity Score [4]	58.8	77.1	22.7	100
Centerline Detection [7]	68.5	62.6	50.3	0

In Table 1, we compare results obtained by training either on 2D or on 3D annotations in terms of the F1 score—the harmonic mean of precision and recall, which is a standard measure of binary segmentation performance—computed in 3D with respect to the 3D annotations. To ensure that the scores are comparable in both scenarios, we use here the projections of the 3D annotations in all three directions as our 2D annotations. In the rightmost column, we give an estimate of the time saved by generating the 2D annotations instead of the 3D ones on the basis of the above user study. In short, we obtain roughly the same results— slightly better for the axons, slightly worse for the retina and brain scans—at half the annotation cost.

We can further reduce the amount of annotations used by training our app- roach using only 2 or even 1 single projection. The performance remains com- petitive when two projections are used, but decreases for a single one.

Whether using 3D or 2D annotations, these results rely on the modified U-Net architecture discussed in Sect. 3.3. For completeness, we also list in Table 1 the performance of an earlier Deep Net approach that relies on annotating a subset of slices [11]—and requires about the same amount of annotation as ours— and on techniques that do not use Deep Learning [4,7], which our approach also outperforms.

5   Conclusion

We have proposed a method for training DNNs to segment 3D images of linear structures using only annotations of 2D maximum intensity projections of the training data instead of full 3D annotations. We demonstrated that this results in decreased annotation requirements without loss of performance. To this end, we have exploited properties of visual hulls that are not specific to linear structures. In future work, we therefore intend to show that the scope of this technique is in fact much broader, for example by applying it to 3D membrane extraction.

References

1. Kutulakos, K., Seitz, S.: A theory of shape by space carving. IJCV **38**(3), 197–216 (2000)
2. Frangi, A.F., Niessen, W.J., Vincken, K.L., Viergever, M.A.: Multiscale vessel enhancement filtering. In: Wells, W.M., Colchester, A., Delp, S. (eds.) MICCAI 1998. LNCS, vol. 1496, pp. 130–137. Springer, Heidelberg (1998). https://doi.org/10.1007/BFb0056195
3. Law, M.W.K., Chung, A.C.S.: Three dimensional curvilinear structure detection using optimally oriented flux. In: Forsyth, D., Torr, P., Zisserman, A. (eds.) ECCV 2008. LNCS, vol. 5305, pp. 368–382. Springer, Heidelberg (2008). https://doi.org/10.1007/978-3-540-88693-8_27
4. Turetken, E., Becker, C., Glowacki, P., Benmansour, F., Fua, P.: Detecting irreg- ular curvilinear structures in gray scale and color imagery using multi-directional oriented Flux. In: ICCV, December 2013

5. Becker, C., Rigamonti, R., Lepetit, V., Fua, P.: Supervised feature learning for curvilinear structure segmentation. In: Mori, K., Sakuma, I., Sato, Y., Barillot, C., Navab, N. (eds.) MICCAI 2013. LNCS, vol. 8149, pp. 526–533. Springer, Heidelberg (2013). https://doi.org/10.1007/978-3-642-40811-3_66
6. Breitenreicher, D., Sofka, M., Britzen, S., Zhou, S.K.: Hierarchical discriminative framework for detecting tubular structures in 3D images. In: Gee, J.C., Joshi, S., Pohl, K.M., Wells, W.M., Zöllei, L. (eds.) IPMI 2013. LNCS, vol. 7917, pp. 328–339. Springer, Heidelberg (2013). https://doi.org/10.1007/978-3-642-38868-2_28
7. Sironi, A., Turetken, E., Lepetit, V., Fua, P.: Multiscale centerline detection. PAMI **38**(7), 1327–1341 (2016)
8. Peng, H., Zhou, Z., Meijering, E., et al.: Automatic tracing of ultra-volumes of neuronal images. Nat. Methods **14**, 332–333 (2017)
9. Peng, H., Tang, J., Xiao, H.: Virtual finger boosts three-dimensional imaging and microsurgery as well as terabyte volume image visualization and analysis. Nat. Commun. **5**, 4342 (2014)
10. Vitanovski, D., Schaller, C., Hahn, D., Daum, V., Hornegger, J.: 3D annotation and manipulation of medical anatomical structures. In: Proceedings of SPIE on Medical Imaging, vol. 7261 (2009)
11. Çiçek, Ö., Abdulkadir, A., Lienkamp, S.S., Brox, T., Ronneberger, O.: 3D U-Net: learning dense volumetric segmentation from sparse annotation. In: Ourselin, S., Joskowicz, L., Sabuncu, M.R., Unal, G., Wells, W. (eds.) MICCAI 2016. LNCS, vol. 9901, pp. 424–432. Springer, Cham (2016). https://doi.org/10.1007/978-3-319-46723-8_49
12. Ronneberger, O., Fischer, P., Brox, T.: U-Net: convolutional networks for biomedical image segmentation. In: Navab, N., Hornegger, J., Wells, W.M., Frangi, A.F. (eds.) MICCAI 2015. LNCS, vol. 9351, pp. 234–241. Springer, Cham (2015). https://doi.org/10.1007/978-3-319-24574-4_28
13. Kingma, D.P., Ba, J.: Adam: A Method for Stochastic Optimization. arXiv Preprint (2014)
14. Bullitt, E., Zeng, D., Gerig, G.: Vessel tortuosity and brain tumor malignancy: a blinded study. Acad. Radiol. **12**(10), 1232–1240 (2005)

A Multiresolution Convolutional Neural Network with Partial Label Training for Annotating Reflectance Confocal Microscopy Images of Skin

Alican Bozkurt[1]([✉]), Kivanc Kose[2], Christi Alessi-Fox[3], Melissa Gill[4,5],
Jennifer Dy[1], Dana Brooks[1], and Milind Rajadhyaksha[2]

[1] Northeastern University, Boston, MA, USA
alican@ece.neu.edu
[2] Memorial Sloan Kettering Cancer Center, New York, NY, USA
[3] Caliber I.D. Inc, Rochester, NY, USA
[4] SkinMedical Research and Diagnostics, P.L.L.C., Dobbs Ferry, NY, USA
[5] Department of Pathology, SUNY Downstate Medical Center, Brooklyn, NY, USA

Abstract. We describe a new multiresolution "nested encoder-decoder" convolutional network architecture and use it to annotate morphological patterns in reflectance confocal microscopy (RCM) images of human skin for aiding cancer diagnosis. Skin cancers are the most common types of cancers, melanoma being the most deadly among them. RCM is an effective, non-invasive pre-screening tool for skin cancer diagnosis, with the required cellular resolution. However, images are complex, low-contrast, and highly variable, so that it requires months to years of expert-level training for clinicians to be able to make accurate assessments. In this paper we address classifying 4 key clinically important structural/textural patterns in RCM images. The occurrence and morphology of these patterns are used by clinicians for diagnosis of melanomas. The large size of RCM images, the large variance of pattern size, the large scale range over which patterns appear, the class imbalance in collected images, and the lack of fully-labelled images all make this a challenging problem to address, even with automated machine learning tools. We designed a novel nested U-net architecture to cope with these challenges, and a selective loss function to handle partial labeling. Trained and tested on 56 melanoma-suspicious, partially labelled, 12k × 12k pixel images, our network automatically annotated RCM images for these diagnostic patterns with high sensitivity and specificity, providing consistent labels for unlabelled sections of the test images. We believe that providing such annotation in a fast manner will aid clinicians in achieving diagnostic accuracy, and perhaps more important, dramatically facilitate clinical training, thus enabling much more rapid adoption of RCM into widespread clinical use process. In addition our adaptation

A. Bozkurt and K. Kose—Authors contributed equally to this work.
This project was supported by NIH grant R01CA199673 from NCI and MSKCC's Cancer Center core support NIH grant P30CA008748 from NCI.

© Springer Nature Switzerland AG 2018
A. F. Frangi et al. (Eds.): MICCAI 2018, LNCS 11071, pp. 292–299, 2018.
https://doi.org/10.1007/978-3-030-00934-2_33

of U-net architecture provides an intrinsically multiresolution deep network that may be useful in other challenging biomedical image analysis applications.

Keywords: Reflectance confocal microscopy
Melanoma · Segmentation

1   Introduction

Approximately 3.6 million new cases of skin cancer are diagnosed in the USA every year, and another million worldwide [12]. The current gold standard in diagnosis is invasive, costly and laborious biopsy followed histology, with associated morbidity, cost, and patient anxiety. Moreover, a biopsy-based workflow is inefficient: the benign-to-malignant biopsy ratios still range from as low as 2-to-1 to as high as 600-to-1 depending on the clinical setting and the experience level of the clinician, even after "preselection" using clinical imaging and dermoscopy [13]. Recent advances in in-vivo microscopy offer non-invasive, cost-effective and efficient ways of examining tissue morphology and cytology. Among several available methods, reflectance confocal microscopy (RCM) stands out because it offers resolution and sectioning comparable to histology. Diagnostic information in RCM images, similar to histology, is based on the morphological and cytological appearance of the tissue under the microscope. However, whereas histology images contain color contrast due to staining agents, RCM images are scalar-valued (grayscale) with the difference between reflective properties of the tissue components the only source of contrast. Lack of tissue-specific color contrast makes RCM images harder to analyze compared to histology. Even though users who have been sufficiently trained can read these with high sensitivity and specificity, "novice" users struggle to achieve the same level of diagnostic confidence in their analysis; they need months to years of training and guidance in order to reach the level of the early adopters.

Unlike traditional black box approaches that simply classify a lesion as malignant vs. benign, here we offer a framework that can segment different morphological patterns that are encountered in RCM images collected at dermal epidermal junction (DEJ) level of melanocytic lesions. Thus, rather than giving a blind diagnostic support to the clinicians, we aim to help them to detect, and learn to recognize, these morphological patterns and thus increase clinician confidence about their diagnoses. By highlighting different morphological patterns, together with potential suspicious regions for further examination, the framework can serve as both a training tool and diagnostic support system. Ultimately, this platform will help (i) the novice clinicians to adopt RCM imaging technology in their clinical practice more easily and (ii) the general cohort of users to make RCM imaging based clinical practice more efficient by limiting the tissue regions to be analyzed.

We assessed and labeled mosaics of melanocytic lesions captured at the dermal-epidermal junction (DEJ), for 6 morphological patterns (Fig. 1). The

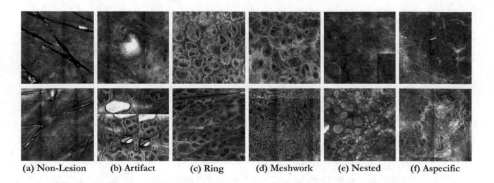

(a) Non-Lesion　　(b) Artifact　　(c) Ring　　(d) Meshwork　　(e) Nested　　(f) Aspecific

Fig. 1. Skin structures under reflectance confocal microscopy

presence of these patterns, their locations within the lesion, and the percentage of the lesion where the pattern appears, all can have diagnostic significance. *Background* describes the "normal" skin surrounding the lesion and allows for delineation of the lesion. *Artifact* pixels are non-skin regions in image, such as oil droplets, hair, or wrinkles. *Meshwork* pattern is characterized by thickening of the interpapillary spaces at the DEJ due to nesting of melanocytes, creating a "basket weave" appearance. *Ring* or "ringed" pattern is characterized by bright cells demarcating dermal papillae giving it the appearance of "beaded bracelets", or bright rings. Ring is often associated with lesions that have a lentiginous component and is frequently observed at the periphery of melanocytic lesions. *Clod* or "nested" pattern is represented by dense nests of melanocytes that can be attached to the DEJ or separated from it, indicating a dermal lesion. The final pattern, *aspecific*, is most commonly associated with features of concern or suspicion for malignancy. An aspecific pattern indicates that, although image resolution is not compromised and cells and vessels are clearly observed, part or all the lesion pattern is completely disorganized, a hallmark of dysplasia or malignancy. This feature is most commonly associated with disruption of the DEJ. A single pattern can predominate a lesion, but typically multiple patterns are present. For example, in benign compound nevi, the center of the lesion may have a nested pattern with clods and meshwork, while the periphery of the lesion may be predominantly ringed.

2 Related Work

Automatically annotating RCM images has seldom been reported, presumably due to lack of labeled data. The only prior work in the literature that we are aware of is [7], where authors use "bag of finetuned CNN features" and support vector machines. Their dataset consists of 20 fully labeled mosaics.

Using multiscale information for semantic segmentation of medical images, or semantic segmentation in general, is an active area of research. There are two main paradigms: using input images at a several scales and corresponding deep feature extraction networks, and (ii) merging features from different layers of a single deep architecture, with several recent works combining these two approaches [1,2,5,9,10,14]. Our work also combines the two ends of the spectrum: We are using input images at a several scales, and merging features from different layers of a single deep architecture. Whereas most prior work fuses intermediate features between different layers, we fuse input images and segmentation maps at different scales.

Augmenting the loss function with auxiliary losses calculated at intermediate layers of a network, which is known as deep supervision [8], has been shown to be helpful during training deep architectures, and was used in several segmentation works [11,15]. In our case, this auxiliary loss is directly the Dice loss between ground truth and segmentation map at lower resolutions.

3   Proposed Model

A typical RCM mosaic is 12000×12000 pixels, covering an area of 36 mm^2 (1μ m/px resolution). We chose not to process these images at this scale, but to use a version downsampled to $1/4$ of their size in each dimension (3000×3000 with 4 mm/px resolution). The model is a fully convolutional encoder-decoder type of network, which can technically take an images with any size (limited by the memory size) as input and generate a segmentation map for it. However, due to use of strides (max 4 level of strides in the presented architecture) in our model, the size of the input images should be at least a multiple of 2^4. We use a 256×256 pixel sliding window with %75 overlap and pass each window through a convolutional neural network as detailed in the following section. Our network is therefore generating probability maps over a ~ 1.25 mm^2 area. To get a segmentation map for whole image, we take the average of overlapping probability maps and choose the class with highest average probability for each pixel.

3.1   Architecture

Our proposed network, named MUNet, is composed of M U-Net [14] subnetworks nested together, with variable depths depending on need and computational capabilities. For $M = 1$, our architecture is equivalent to the original U-Net, whereas for this study we chose $M = 3$. For $M > 1$, let I_0 and L_0 be original image and corresponding ground truth labels, and I_m and L_m be $2m$-downsampled versions, $m = 1, \ldots, M - 1$. The U-Net at the deepest layer ($UNet_{M-1}$) takes only I_{M-1} as input and produces a probability map $\hat{L}_{M-1}$. For all other U-Nets $UNet_k$, we upsample and concatenate $\hat{L}_{k+1}$ with $\hat{I}_k$ to get the input. $\hat{L}_0$ is the final probability map at full resolution. At each level, we calculate a loss between $\hat{L}_m$ and L_m (see Fig. 2).

By feeding the coarser level segmentation output to the next level, we actually introduce a prior subnetwork segmentation (except at the deepest level) and allow the overall model to improve the results of the coarser estimates. Moreover, we observed that this topology helped in obtaining more coherent segmentation, which prevents over-segmentation and formation of very small, isolated label clusters. In order to increase the detail level of the segmentation, we increase the depth of the U-Net subnetworks at each level by one. The resulting 3-level network is composed of ~50 layers and ~6M learnable parameters.

In order to facilitate better-behaved training, we calculate and back-propagate the error between intermediate segmentation results and the down-sampled version of the ground truth segmentation. In this way, we (i) obtain direct access and update deeper level coefficients of the network as well as, (ii) we control the behavior of the network at the earlier stages and help it to obtain better priors for the later stages of the topology.

3.2   Loss Function

Our loss function should (i) be appropriate for segmentation, (ii) be multi-class, (iii) handle unlabeled pixels in ground truth. Dice coefficient [4] is a very common statistic used for binary segmentation: $DSC(A, B) = 2|A \wedge B| / (|A| + |B|)$. Modifying Dice coefficient for our case, suppose we have $W \times H \times K$ sized tensors A and B, where A is one-hot encoded ground truth $A_{ij} = \mathbf{e}_k$ if pixel (i, j) contains class k. ($\mathbf{e}_k$ is K-length one-hot vector with 1 in kth entry and 0 everywhere else). B is the output of neural network $B_{ijk} = [0, 1]$, $\sum_k B_{ijk} = 1$. Our modified statistic is:

$$DSC(A, B) = \sum_{k=0}^{K-1} \frac{\alpha_k \sum_{i,j} \mathbf{1}_{ij} A_{ijk} B_{ijk}}{\epsilon + \sum_{i,j} \mathbf{1}_{ij} (A_{ijk} + B_{ijk})}$$

where α_k are coefficients inversely proportional to abundance of class k in training dataset (see Fig. 3), $\mathbf{1}_{ij}$ indicating whether pixel (i, j) is labeled or not, and ϵ is added for numerical stability. In our multi-level architecture, we calculate the loss at each level. Using the notation in Sect. 3.1, the overall loss function becomes

$$\mathcal{L} = 1 - \sum_{m=0}^{M-1} \beta_m DSC(L_m, \hat{L}_m),$$

where we introduce β_m, to assign relative importance to particular level. Empirically, we choose $\beta_0 = 0.8$, $\beta_1 = 0.16$, $\beta_3 = 0.04$ (It is important that $\sum_m \beta_m = 1$ to keep $\mathcal{L}$ in reasonable bounds).

4   Dataset and Experiments

Our dataset is composed of 56 RCM mosaics (each covering 36 mm^2 area), collected from "melanoma suspicious" lesions. The mosaics are consensus labeled by 2 expert readers for 6 different labels: Non-Lesion, Artifact, Meshwork Pattern, Ring Pattern, Nested Pattern, and Aspecific/Patternless. We randomly select 10 mosaics for test and use the rest for training. Mosaics are too large (24MP) to be processed as a whole, so at every epoch, we extract random patches from

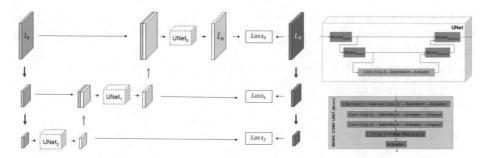

Fig. 2. Our architecture (a) is composed of 3 nested U-Net networks, that generate semantic segmentation at different resolutions. Red arrows denote 2x downsampling, and green arrows denote 2x upsampling. The topology $UNet_2$ and basic convolutional layer (BConv) are presented on the right.

the mosaics and input them to the segmentation network. We cover the whole mosaic area, extracting 0.5 mm × 0.5 mm sized patches from every 1 mm × 1 mm with 50% overlap in a sliding window fashion. In this way, we aim to homogeneously sample from all spatial neighborhoods in the mosaic. In order to further improve the training efficiency, we also increase the training data amount using data augmentation (random rotation, flipping, shearing and mean intensity level change). We trained the described model end-to-end using Keras [3,6].

In Table 1, we present the segmentation performance of MUNet in terms of sensitivity, specificity, Dice coefficient and precision. We also compare MUNet against other SOTA semantic segmentation models available in the literature. For the comparisons, we implemented and trained all the models in Keras, with following modifications: For SegNet, we are using "SegNet-basic" variant, for FCN, we are using ResNet-32, for DeepLab, we are omitting CRF layer at the end. For most of the patterns and metrics, the MUNet model outperformed the other models, achieving an overall accuracy of 73%, which is almost 4% better than its closest competitor. An exemplar segmentation result for all the methods is given Fig. 4.

Overall, MUNet performs quite well in automatically annotating the diagnostic labels except for the meshwork pattern. Further comparison of the model outputs with the ground truth labels show that the model confuses meshwork

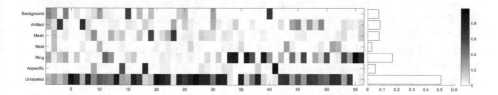

Fig. 3. Class distribution per image and marginal class distribution in our dataset.

Table 1. Sensitivity, specificity, dice coefficient, and precision values of the proposed algorithm (MUNet) on the test set, compared with DeepLab [2], SegNet [1], FCN [10], and UNet [14].

	Sensitivity					Specificity				
	MUNet	DeepLab	Segnet	FCN	Unet	MUNet	DeepLab	Segnet	FCN	Unet
Background	**72.89**	58.01	51.75	47.57	37.19	95.26	96.00	96.15	92.17	**96.40**
Artifact	79.16	78.37	**83.56**	78.97	75.96	**97.44**	95.36	95.92	95.30	96.22
Mesh	50.52	47.79	**66.99**	24.72	46.82	97.88	95.07	91.01	**98.30**	97.80
Nest	77.39	**91.15**	73.70	57.80	60.94	**96.11**	82.45	96.09	89.74	96.09
Ring	93.86	82.25	91.53	88.74	**94.11**	90.38	**94.70**	84.61	86.66	71.07
Aspecific	**87.26**	59.34	45.31	55.01	65.00	91.20	95.73	**97.50**	85.41	93.67
	Dice					Precision				
Background	**78.36**	68.60	63.72	56.18	50.53	**84.71**	83.91	82.88	68.61	78.78
Artifact	**80.61**	74.78	79.21	74.99	75.43	**82.12**	71.51	75.29	71.39	74.90
Mesh	64.71	59.41	**70.19**	38.26	61.34	**89.97**	78.49	73.72	84.57	88.91
Nest	**59.08**	31.82	56.98	30.33	49.55	**47.77**	19.28	46.45	20.56	41.74
Ring	**81.71**	81.44	73.56	74.43	62.33	72.35	**80.64**	61.48	64.09	46.60
Aspecific	**59.59**	56.34	51.70	33.32	53.95	45.24	53.62	**60.17**	23.89	46.11

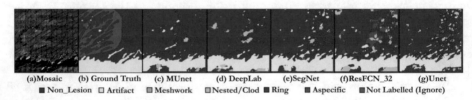

(a)Mosaic   (b) Ground Truth   (c) MUnet   (d) DeepLab   (e)SegNet   (f)ResFCN_32   (g)Unet
■ Non_Lesion □ Artifact ■ Meshwork □ Nested/Clod ■ Ring ■ Aspecific ■ Not Labelled (Ignore)

Fig. 4. Example segmentation results

pattern with ring pattern and aspecific classes. This result is interesting because novice clinicians also suffer from the same problem due to the wide range of variations in the appearance of the meshwork pattern. Moreover, visual examination of the results also confirms that most of the falsely classified meshwork pattern samples contain deformed variations of the pattern, which can also be misclassified by novice readers. We believe that it is possible to overcome this problem by using more training data of meshwork pattern that contain such deformations.

For a qualitative assessment, we have presented the output segmentation map of the MUNet model to the experts, who initially labelled the RCM mosaics for this study. We asked them to review the automated annotation of the algorithm over the originally unlabelled areas. They responded very positively about the results and confirmed that in most of the not-labelled areas, model performed very well in annotating the mosaics. Currently, we are working on, how this secondary assessment of the expert readers can be translated into a performance metric in order to measure the success of the algorithm over these areas in a quantitative manner and also utilize this assessment to fine-tune the model.

References

1. Badrinarayanan, V., Kendall, A., Cipolla, R.: SegNet: a deep convolutional encoder-decoder architecture for image segmentation. IEEE Trans. Patt. Anal. Mach. Intell. **39**(12), 2481–2495 (2017)
2. Chen, L.-C., Papandreou, G., Kokkinos, I., Murphy, K., Yuille, A.L.: DeepLab: semantic image segmentation with deep convolutional nets, atrous convolution, and fully connected CRFs. arXiv preprint arXiv:1606.00915 (2016)
3. Chollet, F.: Keras (2015). https://github.com/fchollet/keras
4. Dice, L.R.: Measures of the amount of ecologic association between species. Ecology **26**(3), 297–302 (1945)
5. Harrison, A.P., Xu, Z., George, K., Lu, L., Summers, R.M., Mollura, D.J.: Progressive and multi-path holistically nested neural networks for pathological lung segmentation from CT images. In: Descoteaux, M., Maier-Hein, L., Franz, A., Jannin, P., Collins, D.L., Duchesne, S. (eds.) MICCAI 2017. LNCS, vol. 10435, pp. 621–629. Springer, Cham (2017). https://doi.org/10.1007/978-3-319-66179-7_71
6. Hundt, A.: Keras-FCN. https://github.com/ahundt/Keras-FCN
7. Kose, K., et al.: Deep learning based classification of morphological patterns in RCM to guide noninvasive diagnosis of melanocytic lesions. In: Photonics in Dermatology and Plastic Surgery, vol. 10037, p. 100370C. International Society for Optics and Photonics (2017)
8. Lee, C.-Y., Xie, S., Gallagher, P., Zhang, Z., Tu, Z.: Deeply-supervised nets. In: Artificial Intelligence and Statistics, pp. 562–570 (2015)
9. Lin, G., Milan, A., Shen, C., Reid, I.: RefineNet: multi-path refinement networks for high-resolution semantic segmentation. In: IEEE Conference on Computer Vision and Pattern Recognition (CVPR) (2017)
10. Long, J., Shelhamer, E., Darrell, T.: Fully convolutional networks for semantic segmentation. In: Proceedings of the IEEE Conference on Computer Vision and Pattern Recognition, pp. 3431–3440 (2015)
11. Mo, J., Zhang, L.: Multi-level deep supervised networks for retinal vessel segmentation. Int. J. Comput. Assist. Radiol. Surgery **12**(12), 2181–2193 (2017)
12. Nikolaou, V., Stratigos, A.J.: Emerging trends in the epidemiology of melanoma. Br. J. Dermatol. **170**(1), 11–19 (2014)
13. Rajadhyaksha, M., Marghoob, A., Rossi, A., Halpern, A.C., Nehal, K.S.: Reflectance confocal microscopy of skin in vivo: from bench to bedside. Lasers Surg. Med. **49**(1), 7–19 (2017)
14. Ronneberger, O., Fischer, P., Brox, T.: U-Net: convolutional networks for biomedical image segmentation. In: Navab, N., Hornegger, J., Wells, W.M., Frangi, A.F. (eds.) MICCAI 2015. LNCS, vol. 9351, pp. 234–241. Springer, Cham (2015). https://doi.org/10.1007/978-3-319-24574-4_28
15. Zhu, Q., Du, B., Turkbey, B., Choyke, P.L., Yan, P.: Deeply-supervised CNN for prostate segmentation. In: 2017 International Joint Conference on Neural Networks (IJCNN), pp. 178–184. IEEE (2017)

Weakly-Supervised Learning-Based Feature Localization for Confocal Laser Endomicroscopy Glioma Images

Mohammadhassan Izadyyazdanabadi[1,2], Evgenii Belykh[2,3],
Claudio Cavallo[2], Xiaochun Zhao[2], Sirin Gandhi[2],
Leandro Borba Moreira[2], Jennifer Eschbacher[2], Peter Nakaji[2],
Mark C. Preul[2], and Yezhou Yang[1(✉)]

[1] School of Computing, Informatics, and Decision System Engineering,
Arizona State University, Tempe, AZ 85281, USA
yz.yang@asu.edu
[2] Department of Neurosurgery, Barrow Neurological Institute,
Phoenix, AZ 85013, USA
[3] Department of Neurosurgery, Irkutsk State Medical University,
Irkutsk 664003, Russia

Abstract. Confocal Laser Endomicroscopy (CLE) is novel handheld fluorescence imaging technology that has shown promise for rapid intraoperative diagnosis of brain tumor tissue. Currently CLE is capable of image display only and lacks an automatic system to aid the surgeon in diagnostically analyzing the images. The goal of this project was to develop a computer-aided diagnostic approach for CLE imaging of human glioma with feature localization function. Despite the tremendous progress in object detection and image segmentation methods in recent years, most of such methods require large annotated datasets for training. However, manual annotation of thousands of histopathology images by physicians is costly and time consuming. To overcome this problem, we constructed a Weakly-Supervised Learning (WSL)-based model for feature localization that trains on image-level annotations, and then localizes incidences of a class-of-interest in the test image. We developed a novel convolutional neural network for diagnostic features localization from CLE images by employing a novel multiscale activation map that is laterally inhibited and collaterally integrated. To validate our method, we compared the model output to the manual annotation performed by four neurosurgeons on test images. The model achieved 88% mean accuracy and 86% mean intersection over union on intermediate features and 87% mean accuracy and 88% mean intersection over union on restrictive fine features, while outperforming other state of the art methods tested. This system can improve accuracy and efficiency in characterization of CLE images of glioma tissue during surgery, and may augment intraoperative decision-making regarding the tumor margin and improve brain tumor resection.

Keywords: Deep learning · Convolutional neural networks
Weakly-supervised localization · Endomicroscopy · Glioma
Brain tumor diagnosis · Digital pathology

© Springer Nature Switzerland AG 2018
A. F. Frangi et al. (Eds.): MICCAI 2018, LNCS 11071, pp. 300–308, 2018.
https://doi.org/10.1007/978-3-030-00934-2_34

1   Introduction

Rapid intraoperative interpretation of suspected brain tumor tissue is of paramount importance for planning the treatment and guiding the neurosurgeon towards the optimal extent of tumor resection. Handheld, portable Confocal Laser Endomicroscopy (CLE) is being explored as a fluorescence imaging technique for its ability to image histopathological features of tissue at cellular resolution in real time during brain tumor surgery [1–4]. CLE systems can acquire up to 20 images per second, with areas in the tumor resection bed interrogated as an "optical biopsy". Hundreds of images may be acquired showing thousands of cells, but the images may be affected with artifacts such as red blood cells (for CLE systems operating in the blue laser range) and motion distortion, making them complicated to analyze. Although images may be interpreted as largely artefactual, detailed inspection often reveals image areas that may be diagnostic. CLE images present a new fluorescent image environment for the pathologist. Augmenting CLE technology with a computer aided system that can rapidly highlight image regions that may reveal malignant or spreading tumor would have great impact on intraoperative diagnosis. This is relevant for tumors such as gliomas where discrimination of margin regions is key to achieve maximal safe resection, which has been correlated with increased patient survival duration [5, 6].

Recent studies have shown that off-the-shelf Convolutional Neural Networks (CNNs) can be used effectively for classifying CLE images based on their diagnostic value [7, 8] and tumor type [9]. However, feature localization models have not been previously applied to CLE images. Feature localization models based on fully supervised learning require large number of images for object-level annotation of the features, which is expensive and time consuming. To overcome this limitation, we used a weakly-supervised localization (WSL) approach. A WSL approach allowed the model to learn and localize the class-specific features from image-level labels.

A few groups have recently applied WSL approaches to medical images, including placenta scans [10], whole-slide images of colorectal cancer [11], diabetic retinopathy [12], microscopic cellular images [13], and lung computed tomography scans [14]. Here, we present a novel model for detection of histological features of glioma on CLE images trained on a dataset of CLE images acquired during brain surgery for this invasive tumor. The architecture included end-to-end Multi-Layer Class Activation Map (MLCAM) with Lateral Inhibition (LI) and Collateral Integration (CI) of the glioma feature localizer neurons. The model was able to segment the CLE images semantically by disentangling class-specific discriminative features that can complement interpretation by the physicians. Performance of the model was assessed by comparing its output to CLE image segmentations performed by neurosurgeons and other deep learning models. Additionally, we validated the significance of the MLCAM, LI and CI architecture components on the overall performance of the model. The model localized known diagnostic CLE features and revealed new CLE features that correlated with the final classification and were not previously recognized by the reviewers.

Unlike previous models that require patch labeling [11] or an extra step for creating the activation maps during testing [15], our model is solely trained based on the whole image-level labels. Furthermore, we did not limit the network to localize features that are already known phenotypes to the physicians [13, 14]. CLE images are relatively novel to the pathology tissue diagnosis workflow. Although the tissue architecture suggestive for a certain tumor type can be identified on CLE images [1–4], detailed characteristic brain tumor patterns for CLE images are not yet well described. There-fore, we used a more general concept (glioma diagnostic vs. nondiagnostic) that includes a range of known histological diagnostic elements (i.e., large nucleus, mitotic figures, hypercellularity, etc.) and allows for discovery of previously unrecognized features that may correlate with final image classification. Further investigation of detected features may deepen the understanding of glioma histopathological pheno-types in CLE images, consequently improving their theranostic implications.

2   Methods

We constructed a WSL-based model to generate glioma Diagnostic Feature Maps (DFM) from CLE images, which includes three main components (see Fig. 1): (1) Customized CNN architecture with new design of CAM at different CNN layers. (2) Lateral inhibition (LI) mechanism that suppresses the activation of DFM at loca-tions where its competitor, nondiagnostic feature map (NFM), also exhibit high acti-vation. (3) Collateral integration (CI) mechanism that amplifies activation of DFM at locations where its allies at other layers also have high activations.

For an input image I_m supplied to the CNN, the class scores (S_D for diagnostic and S_N for nondiagnostic) are defined from three layers via global pooling of discriminative regions estimated in each activation map (DFM, NFM). The class scores achieved from each layer, are then passed to independent softmax layers. The three predictions (probability of I_m being diagnostic (D) and nondiagnostic (ND)) achieved from the softmax layers are streamed into three multinomial logistic loss layers and inject the weight update into the CNN during backpropagation. The total loss is calculated by summing the three loss values.

2.1   New Design of Class Activation Map (CAM)

To produce the CAM from each layer, a new convolutional layer is stacked to sum its weighted feature planes. Formally, the DFM and NFM at location (x, y) achieved from layer z^j, are defined as:

$$DFM(x, y, z^j) = \sum_l w_{k1}^{z^j} f_l(x, y, z^j), \tag{1}$$

$$NFM(x, y, z^j) = \sum_l w_{k0}^{z^j} f_l(x, y, z^j), \tag{2}$$

where $f_l(x, y, z^j)$ is the activation of lth feature plane of layer z^j at location (x, y) and $w_{k1}^{z^j}$ and $w_{k0}^{z^j}$ are the weights to produce the DFM and NFM, respectively. By applying GAP and then softmax function on DFM and NFM, the classification scores for different classes are calculated at each layer. Therefore, the softmax input for diagnostic (S_D) and nondiagnostic (S_N) class at layer z^j can be formulated as:

$$S_D = \frac{1}{W^{z^j} \times H^{z^j}} \sum_{x,y} \text{DFM}(x, y, z^j) = \frac{1}{W^{z^j} \times H^{z^j}} \sum_{x,y} \sum_l w^{z^j}_{k_1} f_l(x, y, z^j), \quad (3)$$

$$S_N = \frac{1}{W^{z^j} \times H^{z^j}} \sum_{x,y} \text{NFM}(x, y, z^j) = \frac{1}{W^{z^j} \times H^{z^j}} \sum_{x,y} \sum_l w^{z^j}_{k_0} f_l(x, y, z^j), \quad (4)$$

where W^{z^j} and H^{z^j} are the width and height of DFM and NFM at layer z^j. With the novel design of MLCAM, DFM, and NFM are produced in every forward pass and are updated through backpropagation. Furthermore, producing DFM from deeper layers empowers the overall predictive power of the model (i.e. labeling the detected region as diagnostic or nondiagnostic), while DFM from shallower layers allows larger spatial resolution and more precise detection of fine regions.

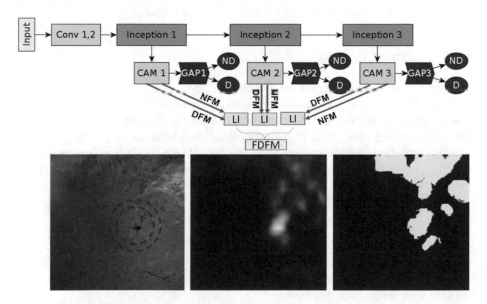

Fig. 1. Network architecture with Lateral Inhibition (LI) and Collateral Integration (CI) components for weakly supervised localization of glioma diagnostic features. Bottom image shows a CLE image along with the final diagnostic feature map generated by the model.

2.2 Lateral Inhibition and Collateral Integration of Localizer Neurons

During the computation of DFM and NFM, some locations might be activated in both feature maps, which indicates the model's confusion about the diagnostic value of those regions. The activation of DFM is downregulated in these regions, using NFM activations. This mechanism is known as neuronal lateral inhibition in neurobiology [16]. Furthermore, we upregulate the activation of regions which had higher recurrence of activation by integrating DFMs achieved from different layers. To combine these two neural interactions, we compose the following equation to produce the Final DFM (FDFM):

$$FDFM(x,y) = \sum_{z^i, z^j(i \neq j)} \left[DFM'(x,y,z^i) \right.$$
$$- DFM'(x,y,z^i).NFM'(x,y,z^i) \left. \right]. \tag{5}$$
$$\left[DFM'(x,y,z^j) - DFM'(x,y,z^i).NFM'(x,y,z^j) \right],$$

where $DFM'(x,y,z^i)$ and $NFM'(x,y,z^i)$ are the value of normalized diagnostic and nodiagnostic feature maps achieved from layer z^i, after up-sampling to the original input image size. As shown in Eq. (5), the downregulation for layer z^i is implemented by subtracting the $DFM(x,y,z^i).NFM(x,y,z^i)$ term, which represents the confusing regions at this layer, from $DFM(x,y,z^i)$. Lastly, $FDFM(x,y)$ is also normalized. Figure 1 presents the developed network's architecture. The three inception modules have the same architecture, each combines filters of size $1 \times 1, 3 \times 3, 5 \times 5$ in parallel, and concatenates the outputs from each filter into a single tensor [17].

3   Experimental Setup and Results

To train our model on image-level annotations, first, a "classification dataset" was created. The CLE images were acquired with an Optiscan 5.1 CLE as described previously [1]. The classification dataset included 6,287 CLE images (3,126 diagnostic and 3,161 nondiagnostic) from 20 patients with glioma brain tumors. If the CLE image depicted any distinguishable diagnostic features, it was labeled as diagnostic and otherwise as nondiagnostic. Table 1 shows the composition of the classification dataset and the number of images used in each stage (Fig. 2).

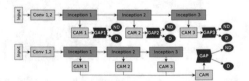

Table 1. Number of Diagnostic (D) and Nondiagnostic (ND) images used for training, validation (Val), and test stage is presented.

	D	ND	All
Train	1714	1729	3443
Val	487	511	998
Test	925	921	1846
Total	3126	3161	6287

Fig. 2. Network architectures used for the ablation study. Top network shows the developed architecture without the LI and CI components. Bottom network shows the MLGAP architecture [14] which combines the three CAMs and then uses a GAP layer for classification.

The classification dataset was divided on a patient level for model development and test (12 cases for training, 4 cases for validation and 4 cases isolated for testing). Stochastic Gradient Descent (SGD) with an initial learning rate of 0.001 and momentum of 0.9 was used to optimize the model's parameters. Learning rate decay policy was set to step function with a gamma of 0.9 and step size of 500 iterations. Image cropping and rotation were not used for augmentation because these might harm the validity of images. Since the diagnostic features could be very small, not every crop of a diagnostic image would be diagnostic. Also, there is no guarantee that the acquired CLE images are rotation invariant (e.g. the surgeons' preference for holding the CLE probe). Training batch size was set to 15 images and it took 22,000 iterations to achieve the model with the minimum loss on classification of validation images. All the experiments were performed in Caffe [18] deep learning framework, using a GeForce GTX 980 Ti GPU (6 GB memory).

The classification accuracy of the model was 84% on the test set (sensitivity = 83.8%, specificity = 84.1%). To validate the efficacy of the WSL model, we tested the following three hypotheses. *First*, the model can correctly segment the image regions which have features that are indicative of glioma, confirmed by physicians at different scales (i.e., medium-sized intermediate and small-sized restrictive scales) and without much reliance on previous exposure (i.e., images from training, validation and test stages). *Second*, the new components utilized (MLCAM, LI, and CI) increase the performance of the model in detecting the features (especially restrictive features) compared to the other state of the art WSL methods that lack them and removing any of these would affect the model performance negatively. *Third*, the developed method can detect novel features in CLE images that were not previously recognized by the physicians. The three hypotheses were tested empirically, using image semantic segmentation task with the following evaluation metrics: mean accuracy (mean_acc), mean intersection over union (mean_IU), and frequency-weighted intersection over union (fw_IU).

A segmentation dataset including 310 CLE images was acquired from images annotated by four neurosurgeons. Each observer highlighted the diagnostic glioma features of each CLE images, independently. We used majority voting to process the annotation variations from the neurosurgeons. For rigorous assessment of the first hypothesis, the segmentation dataset included diagnostic regions at different scales. (145 images were annotated for both Intermediate (Set2-I) and Restrictive (Set2-R) features). Also, to study the effect of previous exposure of CLE image to the model, we used images from all three stages: 30 images from training (Set1), 145 images form validation (Set2), and 135 images from test set (Set3 and Set4)). To appraise the second hypothesis, we sequentially altered components of the designed architecture and assessed the resulting performance of the model ("ablation study"). All models were trained and tested on the same data with the same parameters to avoid any bias. Finally, to test the third hypothesis, our dataset included 55 CLE images that were known to be from glioma tumors but were initially classified as nondiagnostic (Set4). The model generated the segmentation mask by creating the FDFM of the input image with one forward pass and then thresholding (threshold value of 0.03 for intermediate and 0.2 for restrictive features).

Table 2 shows experimental results of segmentation performance by ten different models with respect to the annotators. Each model constructs a DFM to create a segmentation map: M1, similar to [14]; M2 – DFM and NFM of CAM 1,2, and 3 are first laterally inhibited and then collaterally integrated; M3 – CAM 1,2, and 3 are collaterally integrated; M4, M5, M6 – by laterally inhibiting the DFM and NFM of CAM 1, 2, and 3, respectively; M7, M8, M9 – by using the DFMs from CAM 1, 2, and 3 without any further processing; M10, similar to [15]. The first hypothesis proved to be true, since our developed model, M2, produced high mean_acc, mean_IU, and fw_IU for all the intermediate features from diagnostic images (Set1, Set2-I, and Set3). Moreover, it could segment the images from Set3 without significant change in mean_acc, while producing better fw_IU and mean_IU values on images that were previously revealed to it (Set1). Results from Set2-I and Set2-R images showed that all models generated much lower mean_IU and fw_IU on restrictive features compared to intermediate features, except for M1 and M2 models, both of which utilize shallower layers for enhancing the DFM's spatial resolution. In all experiments, M2 made the best performance for three measures (except in mean_acc for Set2-R), supporting the second hypothesis about the significance of the utilized components (MLCAM, LI, and CI). Specifically, M4-M6 models outperformed other ablated models (M7-M9), highlighting the significant value of LI. The higher mean_IU value of M6 and M9 compared to M4,5 and M7,8, respectively, indicates that more abstract features were learned by inception 3 than by inception 1,2. In the first round of review, clinicians labeled Set4 images as nondiagnostic, however, after features were highlighted by the developed model, the clinicians re-classified Set4 images as diagnostic. The highest performance in Set4 belonged to M2 (mean_acc = 88% and mean_IU = 89%). High mean_IU value achieved by the model and clinical feedback emphasize significance and novelty of the features.

Table 2. Segmentation performance by different models. M2* is the developed model.

	Set	M1	M2*	M3	M4	M5	M6	M7	M8	M9	M10
mean_acc	Set1	0.71	**0.88**	0.71	0.75	0.75	0.77	0.71	0.71	0.71	0.7
	Set2-I	0.76	**0.85**	0.74	0.76	0.76	0.77	0.74	0.74	0.74	0.74
	Set3	0.72	**0.86**	0.72	0.75	0.75	0.76	0.72	0.72	0.72	0.72
	Set2-R	0.78	0.87	0.79	**0.88**	**0.88**	0.85	0.78	0.79	0.81	0.78
	Set4	0.74	**0.88**	0.74	0.76	0.76	0.78	0.74	0.74	0.74	0.72
mean_IU	Set1	0.65	**0.9**	0.61	0.69	0.69	0.72	0.61	0.61	0.61	0.63
	Set2-I	0.69	**0.86**	0.67	0.69	0.71	0.73	0.65	0.67	0.67	0.69
	Set3	0.57	**0.82**	0.56	0.59	0.61	0.63	0.56	0.56	0.56	0.59
	Set2-R	0.77	**0.88**	0.29	0.57	0.63	0.59	0.27	0.29	0.31	0.63
	Set4	0.48	**0.89**	0.48	0.52	0.55	0.57	0.48	0.48	0.48	0.5
fw_IU	Set1	0.8	**0.99**	0.8	0.83	0.85	0.87	0.8	0.8	0.8	0.8
	Set2-I	0.88	**0.98**	0.86	0.88	0.9	0.92	0.86	0.86	0.86	0.86
	Set3	0.65	**0.88**	0.65	0.69	0.71	0.73	0.65	0.65	0.65	0.67
	Set2-R	0.9	**0.97**	0.18	0.5	0.61	0.58	0.14	0.16	0.2	0.67
	Set4	0.38	**0.79**	0.35	0.42	0.44	0.46	0.35	0.35	0.35	0.4

4   Conclusions

In this study, a WSL model was developed to localize the diagnostic features of gliomas in CLE images. It utilizes three fundamental components for creating the final glioma DFM: multi-scale DFM, LI for removing confusing regions, and CI to spatially infuse diagnostic areas from DFMs with different spatial resolutions. The model could detect the diagnostic regions with high agreement compared with annotation by neurosurgeon, from both diagnostic and nondiagnostic images (i.e., images that were initially designated as lacking diagnostic features) in intermediate and restrictive features, while outperforming other methods. Such an approach should be tested on larger datasets. Initial testing demonstrated that WSL has the potential to identify not only relevant, but novel or unrecognized diagnostic features in CLE images that were not previously discriminated by human inspection, requiring further investigation. This approach can be augmented with active learning and patch clustering to create an atlas of glioma phenotypes in CLE images. Further detailed studies correlating regular histology and CLE images are necessary for better understanding of glioma histopathological features on CLE images.

Acknowledgement.   YY is partially supported by NSF grant #1750802. This work was supported by the Newsome Chair in Neurosurgery Research held by MCP and by funds from the Barrow Neurological Foundation. EB acknowledges SP-2044.2018.4.

References

1. Martirosyan, N.L., et al.: Prospective evaluation of the utility of intraoperative confocal laser endomicroscopy in patients with brain neoplasms using fluorescein sodium: experience with 74 cases. Neurosurg. Focus **40**, E11 (2016)
2. Foersch, S., et al.: Confocal laser endomicroscopy for diagnosis and histomorphologic imaging of brain tumors in vivo. PLoS ONE **7**, e41760 (2012)
3. Belykh, E., et al.: Intraoperative fluorescence imaging for personalized brain tumor resection: current state and future directions. Front. Surg. **3**, 55 (2016)
4. Eschbacher, J., et al.: In vivo intraoperative confocal microscopy for real-time histopathological imaging of brain tumors: clinical article. J. Neurosurg. **116**, 854–860 (2012)
5. Almeida, J.P., Chaichana, K.L., Rincon-Torroella, J., Quinones-Hinojosa, A.: The Value of Extent of Resection of Glioblastomas: Clinical Evidence and Current Approach (2015)
6. Sanai, N., Polley, M.-Y., McDermott, M.W., Parsa, A.T., Berger, M.S.: An extent of resection threshold for newly diagnosed glioblastomas: clinical article. J. Neurosurg. **115**, 3–8 (2011)
7. Izadyyazdanabadi, M., et al.: Convolutional neural networks: ensemble modeling, fine-tuning and unsupervised semantic localization for neurosurgical CLE images. J. Vis. Commun. Image Represent. **54**, 10–20 (2018)
8. Izadyyazdanabadi, M., et al.: Improving utility of brain tumor confocal laser endomicroscopy: objective value assessment and diagnostic frame detection with convolutional neural networks. In: Progress in Biomedical Optics and Imaging - Proceedings of SPIE (2017)

9. Murthy, N.V., Singh, V., Sun, S., Bhattacharya, S., Chen, T., Comaniciu, D.: Cascaded deep decision networks for classification of endoscopic images. In: Styner, M.A., Angelini, E.D. (eds.) Medical Imaging 2017: Image Processing, p. 101332B (2017)

10. Qi, H., Collins, S., Noble, A.: Weakly supervised learning of placental ultrasound images with residual networks. In: Annual Conference on Medical Image Understanding and Analysis, pp. 98–108 (2017)

11. Korbar, B., et al.: Looking under the hood: deep neural network visualization to interpret whole-slide image analysis outcomes for colorectal polyps. In: 2017 IEEE Conference on Computer Vision and Pattern Recognition Workshops (CVPRW), pp. 821–827 (2017)

12. Gondal, W.M., Köhler, J.M., Grzeszick, R., Fink, G.A., Hirsch, M.: Weakly-supervised localization of diabetic retinopathy lesions in retinal fundus images. arXiv Prepr. arXiv1706.09634. (2017)

13. Sailem, H., Arias–Garcia, M., Bakal, C., Zisserman, A., Rittscher, J.: Discovery of rare phenotypes in cellular images using weakly supervised deep learning. In: Proceedings of the IEEE Conference on Computer Vision and Pattern Recognition. pp. 49–55 (2017)

14. Feng, X., Yang, J., Laine, A.F., Angelini, E.D.: Discriminative localization in CNNs for weakly-supervised segmentation of pulmonary nodules. In: International Conference on Medical Image Computing and Computer-Assisted Intervention. pp. 568–576 (2017)

15. Zhou, B., Khosla, A., Lapedriza, A., Oliva, A., Torralba, A.: Learning deep features for discriminative localization. In: Proceedings of the IEEE Conference on Computer Vision and Pattern Recognition. pp. 2921–2929 (2016)

16. Baars, B.J., Gage, N.M.: Cognition, Brain and Consciousness (2010)

17. Szegedy, C., et al.: Going deeper with convolutions. In: Proceedings of the IEEE Conference on Computer Vision and Pattern Recognition, pp. 1–9 (2015)

18. Jia, Y., et al.: Caffe: Convolutional Architecture for Fast Feature Embedding. arXiv Prepr. arXiv1408.5093 (2014)

Synaptic Partner Prediction from Point Annotations in Insect Brains

Julia Buhmann[1](✉), Renate Krause[1,2](✉), Rodrigo Ceballos Lentini[1],
Nils Eckstein[1], Matthew Cook[1], Srinivas Turaga[2], and Jan Funke[2,3]

[1] Institute of Neuroinformatics UZH/ETHZ, Zurich, Switzerland
{juliab,rekrau}@ini.uzh.ch
[2] HHMI Janelia Research Campus, Ashburn, USA
[3] Institut de Robotica i Informatica Industrial, UPC, Barcelona, Spain

Abstract. High-throughput electron microscopy allows recording of large stacks of neural tissue with sufficient resolution to extract the wiring diagram of the underlying neural network. Current efforts to automate this process focus mainly on the segmentation of neurons. However, in order to recover a wiring diagram, synaptic partners need to be identified as well. This is especially challenging in insect brains like *Drosophila melanogaster*, where one presynaptic site is associated with multiple postsynaptic elements. Here we propose a 3D U-Net architecture to directly identify pairs of voxels that are pre- and postsynaptic to each other. To that end, we formulate the problem of synaptic partner identification as a classification problem on long-range edges between voxels to encode both the presence of a synaptic pair and its direction. This formulation allows us to directly learn from synaptic point annotations instead of more expensive voxel-based synaptic cleft or vesicle annotations. We evaluate our method on the MICCAI 2016 CREMI challenge and improve over the current state of the art, producing 3% fewer errors than the next best method (Code at: https://github.com/juliabuhmann/syntist).

1 Introduction

The field of Connectomics studies the reconstruction and connectivity of neurons. So far, only electron microscopy (EM) methods are able to image neural tissue with a resolution high enough to resolve connectivity at a synaptic level. This results in large amounts of data, requiring automated methods in order to be processed in a reasonable amount of time. In order to acquire a full connectivity diagram we need to solve two main problems: First, the neurons have to be segmented to reconstruct their morphology. Second, synaptic connections between neurons have to be identified, since neuron morphology does not provide enough information to estimate connectivity [7].

The segmentation of neurons has received considerable attention by the computer vision community, for recent methods see [3,6]. Automated synapse detection methods have also seen progress, for instance in [2], where automatically

---

J. Buhmann and R. Krause—Equal contribution.

© Springer Nature Switzerland AG 2018
A. F. Frangi et al. (Eds.): MICCAI 2018, LNCS 11071, pp. 309–316, 2018.
https://doi.org/10.1007/978-3-030-00934-2_35

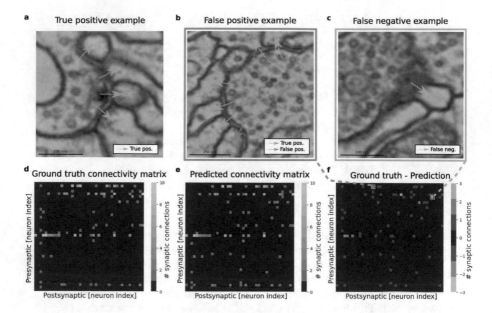

Fig. 1. Qualitative results on the validation set. First row: examples of **(a)** True Positive (TP), **(b)** False Positive (FP) and **(c)** False Negative (FN) in 2D sections. Note that in (b) the predicted partner is likely correct and was overlooked during ground truth annotation while (c) represents an ambiguous case. Second row: Connectivity matrices of **(d)** ground truth and **(e)** predicted connectome. Each row and each column in a connectivity matrix corresponds to one neuron. A positive entry in the matrix stands for the number of connections/synapses that exist between the two neurons. In **(f)** the ground truth matrix is subtracted from the prediction matrix (blue: FP, red: FN). Results shown for the validation set (f-score 0.75) and ground truth segmentation based synaptic partner extraction.

identified synapses allow the analysis of different neuron cell types. Most of the proposed methods identify synaptic *sites* [1,5,10–12]. For the overall goal of reconstructing the connectome, however, it is necessary to additionally identify the pre- and postsynaptic *partners*. In mouse, zebrafish, or zebra finch, a synaptic site usually has only one pre- and one postsynaptic partner, whereas in insects such as *Drosophila melanogaster*, synapses form one-to-many connections which are called polyadic synapses (for an example, see Fig. 1a and b).

To identify partners in one-to-one synapses, a common strategy is to first identify contact sites of neuronal segments to extract a set of potential synaptic partners, and second to collect features for them which are then handed over to a classifier to decide if a given candidate is valid [2,14].

In [4], a similar strategy is used to detect synaptic partners in polyadic synapses found in insects. Specific changes are required to make the method applicable. For instance, while a vesicle cloud is quite indicative for a presynaptic site in songbird [2], the *Drosophila melanogaster* presynaptic site includes a characteristic T-shaped appearance (called T-bar). In a first step, a convolutional neural network is trained to detect T-bars. Subsequent partner prediction is constrained to those identified locations. This method was shown to perform well on isotropic data.

However, for anisotropic datasets, the task of automatically detecting presynaptic locations is potentially harder.

The only currently proposed method to detect synaptic partners in anisotropic datasets with polyadic synapses by [9] requires the neuron segmentation as well as predicted synapse locations. Based on these, the method identifies a set of potential synaptic partners. Then unary and pairwise factors are assigned to all candidate pairs and an Integer Linear Program (ILP) is solved to select correct synaptic partners.

2   Method

A common approach for synaptic partner detection is to first identify potential pre- and postsynaptic point locations while the correct pairing of candidate sites is performed in a second, separate step [2,9,14]. Here we propose a method for synaptic partner prediction that fuses these two, formerly independent steps, into one. We achieve this reduction by formulating the problem as a classification task on the space of directed edges between voxels. An advantage of this approach is that potential pre- or postsynaptic sites are only classified as such if there is evidence for a corresponding partner. The proposed representation also allows us to learn from synaptic point annotations only, since we do not rely on labeled synaptic features, such as synaptic clefts or vesicle clouds.

In the following subsections, we describe how we (1) represent neuron connectivity by directed long-range edges, (2) train a U-Net to classify those edges, and (3) post-process the U-Net output to directly obtain synaptic partners.

2.1   Directed edges for synaptic partner representation

In order to constrain the learning problem we fuse synaptic site detection and partner identification in a single step. To this end we consider a directed graph $G(V, E)$, where each voxel is represented as a vertex $v \in V$ and we encode relations between voxels as directed edges $e_{i \to j} = (v_i, v_j) \in E$.

If we were to connect each voxel v_i in a given volume with each other voxel $v_{j \neq i}$, we could identify synaptic partners by selecting the subset of those edges $e_{i \to j} = (v_i, v_j)$ whose vertices v_i and v_j lie inside a pre- and corresponding postsynaptic region respectively, pointing from one site to the other. However, in such a scheme the number of candidate edges we would need to consider scales as $|V|^2$, which is infeasible and not necessary.

We thus limit the space of candidate edges to lie within a biologically plausible range using the prior that pre- and postsynaptic sites are separated from each other by a certain distance. That is, for each voxel v_i, we only consider n_e edges with associated relative offsets $r_j \in \mathbb{Z}^3$, $j = 1, \ldots, n_e$. The number of edges n_e trades off the coverage rate of synaptic partners. For example, if we use too few edges, there might be synaptic partners that are missed by our representation. In order to select a minimal set of sufficient edges, we perform a grid search on a training and validation set over the number of candidate edges n_e, the length of the vectors $|r_j|$, and radius of pre- and postsynaptic region r_{syn} such that we obtain a coverage rate of 100% of synaptic partners. We denote the set of edges that we find with the proposed method E^{syn}.

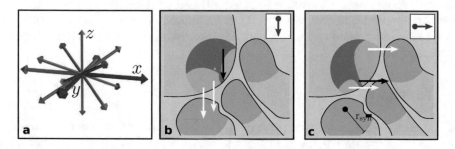

Fig. 2. Illustration of synaptic partner representation. **(a)** 3D rendering of the 14 offset vectors r_j found with grid search on the CREMI dataset. **(b, c)** One presynaptic neuron with its 3 postsynaptic partners. An example is shown for two offset vectors **(b)** $r_1 = (0, 120, 0)$, **(c)** $r_2 = (120, 0, 0)$ in the x-y plane, their direction shown in the upper right corner and marked in (a) in blue and red. Green dots represent synaptic point annotations, with their pre- (brown) and post- (green) synaptic location area. White arrow: selected edge $s(e_{i \rightarrow j} = 1)$, black arrow: unselected edge $s(e_{i \rightarrow j} = 0)$. Teal colored regions correspond to the resulting activation map: each voxel v_i is colored teal if the corresponding edge $e_{i \rightarrow j}$ is selected, i.e., voxel v_j lies inside the postsynaptic area.

2.2   Edge classification

We train a 3D U-Net to classify for each voxel v_i which of its directed edges $e_{i \rightarrow j} \in E^{syn}$ is synaptic or non-synaptic. That is, we predict an n_e dimensional vector y^i for each voxel in the input volume. Each entry y^i_j then represents the score $s(e_{i \rightarrow j} = 1)$ that edge $e_{i \rightarrow j}$ is synaptic. Consistent with the search for E^{syn}, we annotate synaptic regions for training by expanding the ground truth point annotation of pre- and postsynaptic sites into a ball of radius r_{syn}, shown in brown/green in Fig. 2. Note that we constrain each synaptic region to lie within its corresponding neuron. An illustration of pre- and postsynaptic regions, selected and unselected edges for two offset vectors r_1 and r_2 in the x-y plane is shown in Fig. 2.

2.3   Synaptic partner extraction

We formalize the notion of a connectome by introducing a directed connectome graph $G_c = (S, A)$, with vertices $s \in S \subset P(V)$ representing neuron segments as subsets of voxels $v \in V$ and candidate synapses between neurons $a \in A \subset P(E)$ as subsets of edges $e \in E$, where $P(\cdot)$ is the power set. We extract candidate synapses $a_{k \to l}$ from the edge predictions in the following way: we use an underlying neuron segmentation (this can be either ground truth or automatically generated) to collect all edges e that start in segment s_k and end in another segment $s_{l \neq k}$. We only consider edges as evidence for a synapse a if the predicted edge score $s(e = 1)$ is above a certain threshold t_1. In order to account for neuron pairs that have multiple synapses at different locations, we introduce a separate candidate synapse $a_{l \to k}^m \subset a_{l \to k}$ for each set of edges whose target voxels form a connected component in segment s_k. A confidence score for candidate synapses $a_{l \to k}^m$ is obtained by calculating the sum over all edge scores per synapse:

$$\text{confidence}(a_{l \to k}^m) = \sum_{e \in a_{l \to k}^m} s(e) \tag{1}$$

A candidate synapse $a_{l \to k}^m$ is finally selected if $\text{confidence}(a_{l \to k}^m) > t_2$. The parameters t_1 and t_2 are used to control precision and recall of the method. Finally we extract single locations for the identified partners by calculating the center of mass of the start and end points of synapses $a_{l \to k}^m$. Synaptic partners are thus represented by a single pre- and a single postsynaptic location. In cases of reciprocal synapses, we remove the synapse with lower predicted evidence.

Error Metric. We evaluate our method using the synaptic partner identification metric proposed by the MICCAI 2016 CREMI challenge[1]. First it uses Hungarian Matching to match each predicted synaptic pair $a_{l \to k}^m$ to a ground truth pair within a tolerance distance d. It further requires that the underlying segment IDs of ground-truth and predicted pair match. This means that a slight shift of the location is only tolerated if the underlying voxel still corresponds to the correct segment.

3   Results

CREMI Dataset. We tested our method on the publicly available serial section EM dataset from the MICCAI 2016 CREMI challenge[1]. The dataset consists of six cutouts from an adult *Drosophila melanogaster* brain, divided into three training volumes (A, B and C) and three test volumes (A+, B+ and C+), with a size of $1250 \times 1250 \times 125$ voxels each and a highly anisotropic resolution of $4 \times 4 \times 40$ nm. We split the three training volumes into a training set (A, B and half C) and a validation set (the other half of C). The validation set is used for model optimization and qualitative analysis of the results. The ground truth for the training set includes volumetric neuron labels and synaptic partner annotations. Each partner is represented with a pre- and postsynaptic location (as shown in Fig. 1a). We use the training volumes to carry out a grid search in order to obtain parameters for our synaptic representation (discussed in 2.1).

---

[1] https://cremi.org.

We find $r_{\text{syn}} = 100$ nm and 14 edges $e_{i \to j}$ per voxel and the following offset vectors: $\boldsymbol{r}_1, \ldots, \boldsymbol{r}_{14} = (0, 0, \pm 80)$, $(\pm 120, 0, 0)$, $(0, \pm 120, 0)$, $(\pm 40, \pm 60, \pm 40)$ (shown in Fig. 2a).

Architecture. Our architecture is based on the U-Net architecture proposed by [13]. It has been shown to be well suited to a number of applications in biomedical imaging and neuron segmentation in particular (e.g. [3]). We use the same U-Net architecture as in [3] and we do not carry out any further experiments with regards to the hyperparameters of the network. We use three down- and three up-sampling layers where each layer consists of two convolutions with kernel size $(3 \times 3 \times 3)$. We downsample via max-pooling operations of size $(3 \times 3 \times 1)$ and upsample via transposed convolutions of the same size. Lastly, we apply a convolutional layer with kernel size 1 and a sigmoid activation function. Here, each output voxel has a context of x $= 212$, y $= 212$, z $= 28$ voxel (848, 848, 1120 nm). We use the Adam optimizer [8] with a learning rate of $\alpha = 5 \cdot 10^{-6}$ for all our experiments.

CREMI: Challenge Results. We include in our training the whole samples A, B, and C in order to make use of all available training data. We carry out a grid search on the same training data to find $t_1 = 0.5$ and $t_2 = 2500$ as the parameters maximizing the f-score. For the synaptic partner extraction we use an automatically generated neuron segmentation (provided by the authors of [3]), in which we manually mask missing sections and sections with artifacts to exclude them from the synaptic partner extraction. Results for the CREMI challenge are summarized in Table 1. We obtain a 3% gain in the f-score over the previous challenge leader. Looking at the total number of FN and FP this translates to a clear improvement in accuracy of ~19%. Note that the f-score is averaged over all three samples equally, although sample A+, B+ contain presumably fewer synapses (the actual TP numbers are not revealed in the challenge). This explains the discrepancy of the ~3% gain in accuracy for the f-score and the 19% gain in accuracy for the absolute numbers.

Table 1. Results on the CREMI challenge for our method (lr U-Net) compared to the next best method (PSP unar). Highlighted in bold are our method and best values per column. Reported measures are (1) f-score, (2) FP and FN averaged over the three test datasets and (3) FN and FP summed over the three test datasets. For a detailed description of the used error metric, see Section 2.3

Method	f-score	avg. FP/FN	abs. FP/FN
PSP unar	0.539	266/**281**	800/**843**
lr U-Net	**0.553**	**175**/314	**526**/942
lr U-Net training	0.669	223/185	668/554

Qualitative Results. Since the ground truth is not public we cannot qualitatively analyze our results on the test set. Instead we summarize our observations for the validation set (f-score $= 0.75$). We find some errors in the ground truth annotations, where some synapses have not been annotated (FP) or at least are of ambiguous nature (see Fig. 1b and c). Furthermore we observe that our method has problems with very small postsynaptic neurons or synapses that lie in the cutting plane (not shown). Figure 1(d-f) show a visualization of our results in form of a connectivity matrix. Note that the overall appearance of the predicted matrix and the ground truth is surprisingly similar despite the comparably low precision and recall (0.78, 0.73).

4   Discussion

The main advantage of our method is the ability to directly predict synaptic partners. Using a state-of-the-art deep learning architecture, we currently lead the CREMI challenge. Nevertheless, the comparably low overall performance (f-score: 0.55) demonstrates how challenging the task remains. Although we can confidently attribute some "errors" to incorrect labels or ambiguous cases, there are many observed cases that are truly incorrect.

Our current synapse representation has the shortcoming of using a discretized approach: sparse, long range edges. Although we guarantee that all synapses in training and validation set are captured, synapse statistics of other parts of the dataset potentially vary. Our method might thus benefit from a continuous formulation, in which we predict x, y, z values for the direction of the postsynaptic partner. We thus propose to rephrase the classification task as a regression task in future work.

Acknowledgements. This work was funded by the SNF grants P2EZP2_165241 and 205321L_160133.

References

1. Becker, C., Ali, K., Knott, G., Fua, P.: Learning context cues for synapse segmentation. IEEE Trans. Med. Imaging **32**(10), 1864–1877 (2013)
2. Dorkenwald, S., et al.: Automated synaptic connectivity inference for volume electron microscopy. Nat. Methods **14**(4), 435 (2017)
3. Funke, J., et al.: Large scale image segmentation with structured loss based deep learning for connectome reconstruction. IEEE Trans. Pattern Anal. Mach. Intell. (early access). https://doi.org/10.1109/TPAMI.2018.2835450
4. Huang, G.B., Scheffer, L.K., Plaza, S.M.: Fully-automatic synapse prediction and validation on a large data set. arXiv preprint arXiv:1604.03075 (2016)
5. Jagadeesh, V., Anderson, J., Jones, B., Marc, R., Fisher, S., Manjunath, B.: Synapse classification and localization in electron micrographs. Pattern Recognit. Lett. **43**, 17–24 (2014)
6. Januszewski, M., Maitin-Shepard, J., Li, P., Kornfeld, J., Denk, W., Jain, V.: Flood-filling networks. arXiv preprint arXiv:1611.00421 (2016)
7. Kasthuri, N., et al.: Saturated reconstruction of a volume of neocortex. Cell **162**(3), 648–661 (2015)
8. Kingma, D.P., Ba, J.: Adam: A method for stochastic optimization. CoRR abs/1412.6980 (2014). http://arxiv.org/abs/1412.6980

9. Kreshuk, A., Funke, J., Cardona, A., Hamprecht, F.A.: Who is talking to whom: synaptic partner detection in anisotropic volumes of insect brain. In: Navab, N., Hornegger, J., Wells, W.M., Frangi, A.F. (eds.) MICCAI 2015. LNCS, vol. 9349, pp. 661–668. Springer, Cham (2015). https://doi.org/10.1007/978-3-319-24553-9_81
10. Kreshuk, A., Koethe, U., Pax, E., Bock, D.D., Hamprecht, F.A.: Automated detection of synapses in serial section transmission electron microscopy image stacks. PloS One **9**(2), e87351 (2014)
11. Kreshuk, A.: Automated detection and segmentation of synaptic contacts in nearly isotropic serial electron microscopy images. PloS One **6**(10), e24899 (2011)
12. Roncal, W.G., et al.: Vesicle: volumetric evaluation of synaptic interfaces using computer vision at large scale. arXiv preprint arXiv:1403.3724 (2014)
13. Ronneberger, O., Fischer, P., Brox, T.: U-Net: convolutional networks for biomedical image segmentation. In: Navab, N., Hornegger, J., Wells, W.M., Frangi, A.F. (eds.) MICCAI 2015. LNCS, vol. 9351, pp. 234–241. Springer, Cham (2015). https://doi.org/10.1007/978-3-319-24574-4_28
14. Staffler, B., Berning, M., Boergens, K.M., Gour, A., van der Smagt, P., Helmstaedter, M.: Synem, automated synapse detection for connectomics. eLife **6**, e26414 (2017)

Synaptic Cleft Segmentation in Non-isotropic Volume Electron Microscopy of the Complete *Drosophila* Brain

Larissa Heinrich[1], Jan Funke[1,2], Constantin Pape[1,3], Juan Nunez-Iglesias[1], and Stephan Saalfeld[1(✉)]

[1] HHMI Janelia Research Campus, Ashburn, USA
saalfelds@janelia.hhmi.org
[2] Institut de Robòtica i Informàtica Industrial, Barcelona, Spain
[3] University of Heidelberg, Heidelberg, Germany

Abstract. Neural circuit reconstruction at single synapse resolution is increasingly recognized as crucially important to decipher the function of biological nervous systems. Volume electron microscopy in serial transmission or scanning mode has been demonstrated to provide the necessary resolution to segment or trace all neurites and to annotate all synaptic connections.

Automatic annotation of synaptic connections has been done successfully in near isotropic electron microscopy of vertebrate model organisms. Results on non-isotropic data in insect models, however, are not yet on par with human annotation.

We designed a new 3D-U-Net architecture to optimally represent isotropic fields of view in non-isotropic data. We used regression on a signed distance transform of manually annotated synaptic clefts of the CREMI challenge dataset to train this model and observed significant improvement over the state of the art.

We developed open source software for optimized parallel prediction on very large volumetric datasets and applied our model to predict synaptic clefts in a 50 tera-voxels dataset of the complete *Drosophila* brain. Our model generalizes well to areas far away from where training data was available.

1 Introduction

Today, the neuroscience community widely agrees that the synaptic microcircuitry of biological nervous systems is important to understand what functions they implement. The only currently available method to densely reconstruct all axons, dendrites, and synapses is volume electron microscopy (EM) as it provides a resolution sufficient to unambiguously separate them (<15 nm per voxel, [19]). For EM *connectomics*, several flavors of volume EM have been used [3]: Serial block face scanning EM (SBFSEM), in combination with focused ion beam milling (FIB-SEM), provides the highest isotropic resolution of $\sim5^3$ nm per voxel

© Springer Nature Switzerland AG 2018
A. F. Frangi et al. (Eds.): MICCAI 2018, LNCS 11071, pp. 317–325, 2018.
https://doi.org/10.1007/978-3-030-00934-2_36

and excellent signal to noise ratio but is relatively slow. On the other end of the spectrum, serial section transmission EM (ssTEM) offers excellent lateral resolution, imaging speed, and signal to noise ratio but generates highly non-isotropic data with comparably poor axial resolution (>35 nm per voxel).

A remarkable number of projects are currently under way to reconstruct the connectomes of various model organisms [23], ranging from small invertebrate nervous systems like the larvae of *Drosophila melanogaster* [6,24] or *Platynereis dumerilii* [20], the adult *Drosophila* [27,28], to vertebrate models like the zebrafish larva [9], the retina of a mouse [8], or the zebra finch HVC [13].

2   Related Work

While many ongoing connectome reconstruction efforts still rely on manual annotation of synaptic contacts [24,28], automatic annotation of synaptic clefts from volume electron microscopy has been explored in recent years. On vertebrate model systems, existing solutions perform comparably to trained human annotators on both isotropic [2,5,14,15,26] and non-isotropic data [5,16]. Synapses in the insect brain, however, are more complicated, and typically smaller than in vertebrates. Accordingly, the performance on isotropic data is good [10,14,18], but not yet satisfying on non-isotropic data (see CREMI leaderboard).[1]

The methods follow the general trend in computer vision. Earlier approaches [2,14–16,18] use carefully designed image features and train pixel classifiers using random forests or gradient boosting. More recent approaches [5,10,26] train deep learning models to classify pixels or regions of interest as synapse candidates. All approaches rely on sensible post-processing to filter false detections.

The CREMI challenge provides three volumes with ground truth for neuron segmentation, synaptic clefts, and synaptic partner annotations in diverse regions of ssTEM of the adult *Drosophila* brain at 40×4^2 nm per voxel. The challenge data includes typical artifacts for ssTEM preparations such as missing sections, staining precipitate, or incorrect alignment. To our knowledge, it is the only existing challenge with secret test data that enables unbiased comparison of synapse detection in non-isotropic EM of the insect brain. The evaluation metric for synaptic cleft detection (CREMI score) is the average of the average false positive distance (FPD) and the average false negative distance (FND). The FPD is the distance of a predicted label to the nearest true label, the FND is the distance of a true label to the nearest predicted label.

3   Methods

3.1   Training Setup

We corrected the serial section alignment errors present in the CREMI volumes using elastic alignment with TrakEM2 [22] and split each volume into a training (75%) and validation (25%) subset, such that the statistics of each subset

---

[1] MICCAI Challenge on Circuit Reconstruction from Electron Microscopy Images (CREMI): https://cremi.org.

are visually similar to the whole block. We trained 3D-U-Nets [4] to predict a signed distance transform of binary synapse labels using TensorFlow [1]. We used Gunpowder[2] for batch loading, preprocessing, and training. We made heavy use of Gunpowder's support for data augmentations auch as transposing, intensity variation, elastic deformations, and ssTEM-specific artifacts like missing or noisy sections. We believe that these augmentations are crucial for our network to generalize well on large datasets without substantial engineering efforts.

As synaptic clefts are very sparse, we sample batches that contain synapses more frequently by rejecting batches without synapses with 95% probability. Additionally, we rebalance the loss with the frequency of positively annotated voxels to heavily penalize false negative predictions (unless otherwise stated).

We used Adam to minimize the L2 loss w.r.t. a signed Euclidean distance transform (SEDT) of the binary labels. As the SEDT is not meaningful far away from synapses, we scaled it and applied a tanh nonlinearity that saturates between $[-1, 1]$: $STDT = \tanh(SEDT/s)$. Our experiments indicated that the scaling factor has little effect on performance (data not shown), we chose $s = 50$. Simple thresholding converts the predicted $STDT$ into binary labels.

3.2   Experiments

3D-U-Nets Benefit from Isotropic Fields of View (FOV). The DTU-1 (distance transform U-Net) architecture is based on a design for neuron segmentation in non-isotropic ssTEM [7] (Fig. 1). The FOV of this architecture is highly non-isotropic across a large number of layers. Hypothesizing that an isotropic FOV would be beneficial to learn meaningful physical features, we tweaked the kernel sizes while retaining the overall design. The 'isotropic' network (DTU-2, Fig. 1) is restricted to 2D convolutions in the first few levels and has isotropic kernels once the voxel size is nearly isotropic. The encoding and decoding side are symmetric. Figure 2 shows that DTU-2 consistently outperforms DTU-1.

DTU-2 has significantly fewer parameters than DTU-1. This allows for a larger patch size (output size $23 \times 218 \times 218$ as opposed to $56 \times 56 \times 56$) which translates into a better estimate of the true gradient during stochastic gradient descent. While this constitutes an additional advantage of DTU-2, we showed that it is not sufficient to explain its superior performance. A smaller version of DTU-2, with output size $20 \times 191 \times 191$, still outperforms DTU-1 (Fig. 2a).

At the time of writing, DTU-2 is first on the CREMI synaptic cleft detection challenge, followed by DTU-1 in second place. Unlike the experiments shown in Fig. 2, those networks were trained for more iterations, on a curated version of the full CREMI ground truth.

Regression Outperforms Classification. Most deep-learning approaches for object detection in general, and synapse detection specifically [5], use a sigmoid nonlinearity and cross-entropy loss to predict a probability map for the object. Inspired by the recent success of long-range affinities as an auxiliary loss for

---

[2] Gunpowder: https://github.com/funkey/gunpowder.

boundary detection [17], we suspected that networks might generally benefit from being explicitly forced to gather information from a larger context. With this assumption in mind, we trained the network to predict a distance rather than a probability map. This approach turns the voxel-wise classification into a voxel-wise regression problem [12].

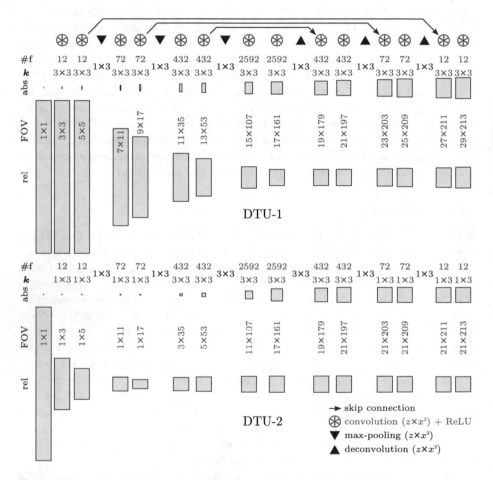

Fig. 1. Comparison of the physical FOV in each layer of the 3D-U-Net architectures DTU-1 and DTU-2. The top row shows a graphical representation of the general U-Net architecture. The network consists of modules of two convolutions and rectlinear units followed by max-pooling on the encoding side, and deconvolution followed by two convolutions and rectlinear units on the decoding side. Kernel sizes (k) are denoted as $z \times x$ as the x and y axes are isotropic. The number of features per convolutional layer (#f) is increased by a factor of six after max-pooling and decreased by a factor of six after deconvolution. In DTU-2, 3D-convolutions are replaced by 2D-convolutions where the resolution is highly non-isotropic, and 2D-max-pooling and deconvolution are replaced by 3D-max-pooling and deconvolution where the resolution is near-isotropic. The physical FOV in each layer, depicted as absolute (abs) and relative (rel) size boxes, is therefore closer to isotropic than in DTU-1.

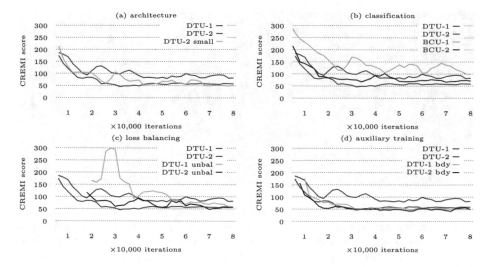

Fig. 2. Validation experiments. All plots show mildly smoothed validation results sampled in intervals of 2,000 iterations using the CREMI score averaged over the validation set. (a) shows that DTU-2 outperforms DTU-1, even if training blocks of the same size as for DTU-1 are used. (b) shows that DTU-1 and DTU-2 trained for regression on the distance transform outperform the same architectures trained for binary classification. (c) shows that loss balancing makes training more robust. (d) shows that auxiliary training for boundary distances improves performance on synaptic cleft detection.

In Fig. 2b, we compare the performance of probability map prediction using a sigmoid nonlinearity with binary cross entropy loss and the STDT prediction as shown before. All other hyperparameters are the same and the maps are converted into binary labels with a non-tweaked threshold (i.e. 0.5 and 0, respectively). For both network architectures, the CREMI score on the validation set improves when predicting the STDT.

Loss Balancing Is Important. Rebalancing the loss is an important feature of the training pipeline (Fig. 2c). In early iterations, the CREMI score cannot be properly evaluated as no voxel in the validation set is predicted to be above threshold, i.e. no synapses were detected.

Auxiliary Training Improves Performance. As synaptic clefts are, by definition, located at cell boundaries, we conducted experiments to determine whether an auxiliary loss from predicting a distance map of cell boundaries boosts performance. We added a second output channel to both DTU-1 and DTU-2 with an (unbalanced) L2 loss with respect to the STDT, now computed on the neuron labels. The two losses are weighed equally. Batch sampling is still done with respect to synaptic clefts.

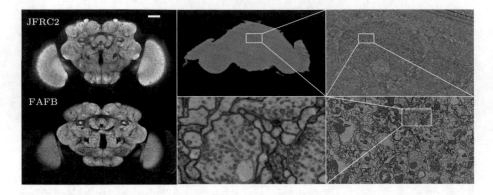

Fig. 3. Synaptic cleft prediction on the complete adult *Drosophila* brain. Left: Convolution of our predictions (FAFB) with a smooth PSF reproduces synaptic densities as visualized by fluorescent microscopy with the the nc82 antibody (JFRC2 template brain [11]), scale bar 50 μm. Right: Examplary zoom-series into our DTU-2 synaptic cleft predictions overlayed over the FAFB volume.

Figure 2d shows that both networks benefit from the auxiliary loss signal. Interestingly, the effect is more significant for DTU-1. A careful evaluation of the boundary detection is beyond the scope of this work.

3.3 Synaptic Cleft Prediction on the Complete *Drosophila* Brain

Prediction on large volumes can be performed in parallel on adjacent blocks. Since our network was trained on valid input, the input block-size needs to be padded by the FOV of the network, i.e. while output blocks are adjacent and non-overlapping, input blocks overlap.

We converted the full adult fly brain (FAFB) volume [28][3] into a scale-pyramid using the the N5 data format[4] on a shared filesystem. We used N5 for both input and output because it enables parallel reading and writing of compressed volumetric blocks. Prediction requires less memory than training because gradients do not need to be computed. We found $71 \times 650 \times 650$ voxels to be the maximum valid output block-size for the DTU-2 network that we could process on our NVIDIA Quadro M6000 GPUs with 12 GB of RAM. Using this increased block-size accelerated prediction by a factor of ∼2.5 compared to the block-size used for training.

The relevant biological sample covers only 20% of the FAFB volume. We used ilastik [25] to train a random forest classifier on scale-level 7 (downscaled by $13 \times 128 \times 128$, i.e. ∼0.5^3 μm per voxel) that separates relevant biological sample from background. Only output blocks that intersect with this mask were considered for prediction. This valid set of blocks has a volume of ∼50 tera-voxels, the entire FAFB volume including background contains ∼213 tera-voxels.

---

[3] Available for download at http://temca2data.org/.
[4] N5 specification: https://github.com/saalfeldlab/n5.

We distributed the list of output blocks over 48 GPUs. For each GPU, we used Dask [21] to load, preprocess, and store image blocks while the GPU performed prediction, achieving greater than 90% GPU utilization[5]. Our average prediction speed was ~3 mega-voxels per second and GPU, i.e. prediction of the complete volume was finished in less than five days.

The quality of predictions across the entire volume was consistent with our results on CREMI (see Fig. 3). Even in areas with different characteristics than the CREMI training volumes (such as the lamina), synaptic cleft predictions are mostly correct and consistent with our expectations. Predictions are correctly missing in axonal tracts and in the cortex. We produced a simulation of an nc82 labeled confocal image by applying a large non-isotropic Gaussian PSF to our predictions and visually compared the result with the JFRC2 template brain [11] (Fig. 3). Accounting for that the two volumes stem from different individuals and have not been registered, our predictions convincingly reproduce the synaptic density distribution as visualized with the nc82 antibody.

4   Conclusion

We achieved a significant improvement over the state of the art in detection and segmentation of synaptic clefts in non-isotropic ssTEM of the insect nervous system. We designed a 3D-U-Net architecture and training scheme that is particularly well suited to account for the non-isotropy in ssTEM data and the sparsity of synapses. We trained this architecture by regression on a signed distance transform of manually annotated synaptic clefts of the publicly available CREMI challenge. We showed that our new architecture compares favorably to a previously described architecture for the same data despite exposing fewer training parameters. We developed an optimized framework for parallel prediction on very large volumetric data and achieved a prediction throughput of ~3 mega-voxels per second and GPU. This efficiency enabled us to predict all synaptic clefts in the 50 tera-voxels full adult *Drosophila* brain [28] in less than five days. We made our code available as open source under a permissive license[6].

References

1. Abadi, M., Agarwal, A., Barham, P., Brevdo, E., et al.: TensorFlow: large-scale machine learning on heterogeneous systems (2015)
2. Becker, C., Ali, K., Knott, G., Fua, P.: Learning context cues for synapse segmentation in EM volumes. In: Ayache, N., Delingette, H., Golland, P., Mori, K. (eds.) MICCAI 2012. LNCS, vol. 7510, pp. 585–592. Springer, Heidelberg (2012). https://doi.org/10.1007/978-3-642-33415-3_72
3. Briggman, K.L., Bock, D.D.: Volume electron microscopy for neuronal circuit reconstruction. Curr. Opin. Neurobiol. **22**(1), 154–161 (2012)

---

[5] Parallel prediction framework: https://github.com/saalfeldlab/simpleference.

[6] CNNectome: https://github.com/saalfeldlab/cnnectome.

4. Çiçek, Ö., Abdulkadir, A., Lienkamp, S.S., Brox, T., Ronneberger, O.: 3D U-Net: learning dense volumetric segmentation from sparse annotation. In: Ourselin, S., Joskowicz, L., Sabuncu, M.R., Unal, G., Wells, W. (eds.) MICCAI 2016. LNCS, vol. 9901, pp. 424–432. Springer, Cham (2016). https://doi.org/10.1007/978-3-319-46723-8_49

5. Dorkenwald, S., Schubert, P.J., Killinger, M.F., Urban, G.: Automated synaptic connectivity inference for volume electron microscopy. Nat. Methods 14, 435–442 (2017)

6. Eichler, K., Li, F., Litwin-Kumar, A., Park, Y., et al.: The complete connectome of a learning and memory centre in an insect brain. Nature 548, 175–182 (2017)

7. Funke, J., Tschopp, F., Grisaitis, W., Sheridan, A., et al.: Large scale image segmentation with structured loss based deep learning for connectome reconstruction. IEEE Trans. Pattern Anal. Mach. Intell. (early access). https://doi.org/10.1109/TPAMI.2018.2835450

8. Helmstaedter, M., Briggman, K.L., Turaga, S.C., Jain, V., et al.: Connectomic reconstruction of the inner plexiform layer in the mouse retina. Nature 500, 168–174 (2013)

9. Hildebrand, D.G.C., Cicconet, M., Torres, R.M., Choi, W., et al.: Whole-brain serial-section electron microscopy in larval zebrafish. Nature 545, 345–349 (2017)

10. Huang, G.B., Plaza, S.: Identifying synapses using deep and wide multiscale recursive networks. arXiv:1409.1789 [cs.CV] (2014)

11. Jenett, A., Rubin, G., Ngo, T.T., Shepherd, D., et al.: A GAL4-driver line resource for Drosophila neurobiology. Cell Rep. 2(4), 991–1001 (2012)

12. Kainz, P., Urschler, M., Schulter, S., Wohlhart, P., Lepetit, V.: You should use regression to detect cells. In: Navab, N., Hornegger, J., Wells, W.M., Frangi, A.F. (eds.) MICCAI 2015. LNCS, vol. 9351, pp. 276–283. Springer, Cham (2015). https://doi.org/10.1007/978-3-319-24574-4_33

13. Kornfeld, J., Benezra, S.E., Narayanan, R.T., Svara, F., et al.: EM connectomics reveals axonal target variation in a sequence-generating network. eLife 6, e24364 (2017)

14. Kreshuk, A., Straehle, C., Sommer, C., Koethe, U., et al.: Automated detection and segmentation of synaptic contacts in nearly isotropic serial electron microscopy images. PloS One 6(10), e24899 (2011)

15. Kreshuk, A., Funke, J., Cardona, A., Hamprecht, F.A.: Who is talking to whom: synaptic partner detection in anisotropic volumes of insect brain. In: Navab, N., Hornegger, J., Wells, W.M., Frangi, A.F. (eds.) MICCAI 2015. LNCS, vol. 9349, pp. 661–668. Springer, Cham (2015). https://doi.org/10.1007/978-3-319-24553-9_81

16. Kreshuk, A., Koethe, U., Pax, E., Bock, D.D., Hamprecht, F.A.: Automated detection of synapses in serial section transmission electron microscopy image stacks. PLOS ONE 9(2), 1–11 (2014)

17. Lee, K., Zung, J., Li, P., Jain, V., Seung, H.S.: Superhuman accuracy on the SNEMI3D connectomics challenge. arXiv:1706.00120 [cs.CV] (2017)

18. Plaza, S., Parag, T., Huang, G., Olbris, D., et al.: Annotating synapses in large EM datasets. arXiv:1409.1801v2 (2014)

19. Plaza, S.M., Scheffer, L.K., Chklovskii, D.B.: Toward large-scale connectome reconstructions. Curr. Opin. Neurobiol. 25, 201–210 (2014)

20. Randel, N., Shahidi, R., Verasztó, C., Bezares-Calderón, L.A., et al.: Inter-individual stereotypy of the Platynereis larval visual connectome. eLife 4, e08069 (2015)

21. Rocklin, M.: Dask: parallel computation with blocked algorithms and task scheduling. In: Python in Science, pp. 130–136 (2015)

22. Saalfeld, S., Fetter, R., Cardona, A., Tomancak, P.: Elastic volume reconstruction from series of ultra-thin microscopy sections. Nat. Methods **9**(7), 717–720 (2012)
23. Schlegel, P., Costa, M., Jefferis, G.S.: Learning from connectomics on the fly. Curr. Opin. Insect Sci. **24**, 96–105 (2017)
24. Schneider-Mizell, C.M., Gerhard, S., Longair, M., Kazimiers, T., et al.: Quantitative neuroanatomy for connectomics in Drosophila. eLife **5**, e12059 (2016)
25. Sommer, C., Straehle, C., Köthe, U., Hamprecht, F.A.: Ilastik: interactive learning and segmentation toolkit. In: ISBI, pp. 230–233 (2011)
26. Staffler, B., Berning, M., Boergens, K.M., Gour, A.: SynEM, automated synapse detection for connectomics. eLife **6**, e26414 (2017)
27. Takemura, S.Y., Aso, Y., Hige, T., Wong, A.: A connectome of a learning and memory center in the adult Drosophila brain. eLife **6**, e26975 (2017)
28. Zheng, Z., Lauritzen, J.S., Perlman, E., Robinson, C.G., et al.: A complete electron microscopy volume of the brain of adult Drosophila melanogaster. Cell **174**(3), 730–743.e22 (2018). https://doi.org/10.1016/j.cell.2018.06.019

Weakly Supervised Representation Learning for Endomicroscopy Image Analysis

Yun Gu[1,2], Khushi Vyas[2], Jie Yang[1(✉)], and Guang-Zhong Yang[2]

[1] Institute of Image Processing and Pattern Recognition,
Shanghai Jiao Tong University, Shanghai, China
`jieyang@sjtu.edu.cn`
[2] Hamlyn Centre for Robotic Surgery, Imperial College London, London, UK

Abstract. This paper proposes a weakly-supervised representation learning framework for probe-based confocal laser endomicroscopy (pCLE). Unlike previous frame-based and mosaic-based methods, the proposed framework adopts deep convolutional neural networks and integrates frame-based feature learning, global diagnosis prediction and local tumor detection into a unified end-to-end model. The latent objects in pCLE mosaics are inferred via semantic label propagation and the deep convolutional neural networks are trained with a composite loss function. Experiments on 700 pCLE samples demonstrate that the proposed method trained with only global supervisions is able to achieve higher accuracy on global and local diagnosis prediction.

Keywords: Probe-based Confocal Laser Endomicroscopy
Feature learning · Semantic exclusivity

1 Introduction

Probe-based confocal laser endomicroscopy (pCLE) is a novel optical biopsy technique for real-time tissue characterization *in vivo*. Flexible coherent fiber-bundle probes, typically of the size of 1.0 mm in outer diameter, integrating confocal optics in the proximal end, are used to provide fluorescence imaging of the biological tissue. Furthermore, these miniaturized probes can be integrated into standard video endoscopes, making pCLE a popular choice for minimally invasive endoscopic procedures. Current applications include breast, gastro-intestinal and lung diseases.

Although pCLE enables the acquisition of *in-vivo* microscopic images that resemble the gold-standard (H&E) stained histology images, many challenges associated with disease characterization still remain. A major challenge being that the field of view (FOV), limited by the size of the fiber bundle, is typically less than 1 mm². A high resolution Cellvizio probe for example offers a lateral resolution of 1.4 μm but a FOV of just 240 μm. With such a small FOV, particularly when compared to histology slides, means that only a small number

© Springer Nature Switzerland AG 2018
A. F. Frangi et al. (Eds.): MICCAI 2018, LNCS 11071, pp. 326–334, 2018.
https://doi.org/10.1007/978-3-030-00934-2_37

of morphological features can be visualized in each image. Furthermore, conventionally histology images are examined by trained pathologists, which is different from the surgical setting where live pCLE images need to be assessed in real-time by surgeons who may have limited training on histopathology.

For these reasons, there has been extensive interests in developing computer-aided diagnosis for automated pCLE image classification in the recent years [1–5]. These methods can be broadly categorized into frame-based methods [2,3,5] and mosaic-based methods [1,4]. As shown in Fig. 1(a), the frame-based methods adopt the visual information of single frame based on Dense-SIFT [2], deep convolutional neural networks (CNN) [5] or transfer learning from histopathological images [3]. Although these methods provide diagnosis result for each pCLE frame, the FoV of each frame is relatively small leading to low confidence for final diagnosis. Moreover, the frame-based methods require massive annotations of training data which is often expensive and time-consuming. On the other hand, the mosaic-based methods [1,4], as shown in Fig. 1(b), help to increase the effective FoV along with direction of probe motion by stitching consecutive image frames. Even with this enlarged FoV, the pCLE diagnostic accuracy depends on the quality of reconstructed mosaics, which in turn is affected by several factors including the speed by which the operator can translate the probe across the tissue, as well as probe-tissue contact and tissue deformation. In addition, mosaic-based methods can only provide a global diagnosis for the large pCLE mosaic but not for the specific regions of the mosaic (e.g. for the regions that correspond to neoplastic tissue as shown in Fig. 1(c)). This would affect the overall diagnostic performance. To provide an objective support for pCLE diagnosis, it is critical to develop a learning framework that can provide both **global diagnosis** as well as **local tumour detection** for pCLE images.

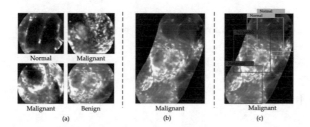

Fig. 1. Illustration of different types of methods: (a) Frame-based methods (e.g. MVMME [3] and Patch-CNN [5]); (b) Mosaic-based methods (e.g. DenseSIFT [6] and UMGM [4]; (c) The proposed method.

Given only the global diagnosis of the pCLE data[1], the task of local tumour detection is related to the weakly-supervised object detection (WSOD) that discovers the latent region of interests (ROIs) by only image-level labels. Unlike

---

[1] *pCLE videos* refer to a set of consecutive frames of pCLE images; *pCLE mosaics* refer to the image with large field of view which are generated by stitching the frames.

the WSOD tasks in general computer vision, the global labels of medical data may not cover all latent objects in the image. As shown in Fig. 1(c), the final diagnosis is 'malignant', which is determined by a small portion of the local regions while the rest are 'normal' tissues that are not included in the global label. In this paper, this observation is called 'semantic exclusivity' which leads to another critical task of discriminative feature learning for pCLE data to discover all latent objects in the pCLE video.

To this end, a weakly-supervised feature learning framework (WSFL) is proposed. The architecture of WSFL is illustrated in Fig. 2. Given a set of consecutive pCLE frames, WSFL firstly passes the frames through several convolutional layers which are then processed by fully connected layers to output fixed-size frame-based features. These frame-based features are branched into two different streams: one jointly learns the global-image representation and global diagnosis and the other further learns the frame-based annotations by label propagation. Only global diagnosis labels are used as supervisions to train the two streams based on composite loss. We validate the performance of the representation on dataset with 45 patient cases consisting of 700 pCLE videos. The experiments demonstrate that the proposed method is effective for both global diagnosis and local tumour detection compared to frame-based methods [3,5] and mosaic-based methods [1,4].

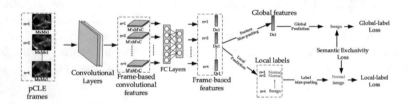

Fig. 2. The main framework of the proposed method.

2   Methodology

2.1   Frame-Based Feature Representation

In this paper, the pCLE data are denoted by $\{X_i\}, i = 1, \ldots, n$ where n is the number of pCLE videos. Each data sample X_i is composed with m_i frames $\{X_{i,j}\}$ where $j = 1, \ldots, m_i$. The goal of this paper is to learn global prediction function $H^g(\cdot)$ for global diagnosis Y_i^g and local prediction function $H^l(\cdot)$ for local labels $Y_{i,j}^l$ only with the global supervision. Given a pCLE video $X_i = \{X_{i,j}\}, j = 1, \ldots, m_i$, we firstly extract the frame-based features by convolutional neural networks. As shown in Fig. 2, the j-th pCLE frame $X_{i,j}$ is fed into the convolutional layers and then transformed into a D-dimensional representation $f_{i,j}^l$.

2.2   Local Label Classification

Unlike the frame-based approach, the frame-wise labels are not available during the training procedure in our work. Therefore, one challenge of the proposed method is to infer the labels of all frames based on global diagnosis results. However, it is common that the global label may not cover all regions of the image. This is called 'semantic exclusivity' in this paper. As shown in Fig. 1, if the pCLE video/mosaic is annotated with 'normal', all its frames should be labeled as 'normal'. For the 'benign' videos, the only confirmed issue is that the video includes at least one frame that indicates the existence of benign regions. Therefore, the status of frames can be either 'normal' or 'benign'. Similarly, the malignant videos are also likely to include benign and normal frames.

In order to infer the labels of all image frames, we built a frame-link graph and propagate the labels between the samples. For all frames $X_{i,j}$ from the training dataset, the frame-link graph $G = \{V, E\}$ is constructed where the nodes V are composed with pCLE frames and the edges E with the weight matrix W indicate the similarity between pCLE frames. In this paper, we use the k-NN graph based on RBF-Kernel where the similarity between $X_{i,j}$ and $X_{i',j'}$ is calculated by $\exp(-\|f_{i,j}^l - f_{i',j'}^l\|_2^2/\sigma)$ where $f_{i,j}^l$ and $f_{i',j'}^l$ are the frame-based features. In order to recover the latent 'normal' frames in 'benign' and 'malignant' videos, the labels of frames from normal videos are propagated via the frame-link graph as follows:

$$\min_Y Q_Y = Y^T L Y + \lambda \|Y_{normal} - Y_{normal}^*\|_2^2 \tag{1}$$

where L is the graph Laplacian of the similarity matrix W. Y is the set of labels of all frames after propagation. $\|Y_{normal} - Y_{normal}^*\|_2^2$ indicates the frames from normal videos should always labeled with 'normal'. The probability of a specific frame belongs to the normal class can be obtained via the label propagation from normal frames. However, the propagation scheme in Eq. (1) has no constraints on global labels. For a benign video, there is at least one frame belonging to the benign class. Therefore, we add the constraints to Eq. (1) as follows:

$$\min_Y Q_Y = Y^T L Y + \lambda \|Y_{normal} - Y_{normal}^*\|_2^2$$
$$s.t. \quad m_i \geq (1 - Y_i^l)^T \mathbf{1} \geq 1, \forall Y_i^g \neq 1 \tag{2}$$

where $Y_i^l = \{Y_{i,1}^l, \ldots, Y_{i,m_i}^l\}$ is the vector of labels of pCLE video X_i and $\mathbf{1}$ is a all-one vector which has the same number of element with Y_i^l; By adding this constraint, the frames which are not likely to be normal are assigned with low confidence for normal class. If the probability is lower than a pre-defined θ, it can be considered as a benign frame. Similarly, the label propagation is also conducted from the benign videos to malignant videos to recover the latent benign regions. The problem in Eq. (2) can be solved by Augmented Lagrangian method (ALM) [7]. After the label propagation, all frames $X_{i,j}$ are assigned with the pseudo labels $\bar{Y}_{i,j}^l$. The frame-based classification layers H^l are then trained by minimizing the cross-entropy loss as follows:

$$\min L_{local} = \sum H^l(f_{i,j}^l) \log Y_{i,j}^l \tag{3}$$

2.3   Global Label Classification

The mosaic-based methods take the holistic image as input to generate the global diagnosis result. However, the freehand capture of pCLE data can introduce irregular background in the mosaic image, thus leading to overfitting. Instead of using holistic features of the whole pCLE mosaics, we extract the features for all pCLE frames $f_{i,j}$ to generate the global features as follows:

$$f_i^g = \mathcal{F}(\{f_{i,j}^l\}), \quad f^g(d) = \max\left(\{f_{i,j}^l(d)\}\right) \tag{4}$$

where $\mathcal{F}$ is the max-pooling function. Therefore, the mosaic-based classification layers H^g are trained by minimizing the loss defined as follows:

$$\min L_{global} = \sum H^g(f_i^g) \log \bar{Y}_i^g \tag{5}$$

2.4   Semantic Exclusivity Loss

Although Eqs. (3) and (5) are introduced for global and local classification, the learning of two streams is still separated where only the lower feature extraction layers are shared. In order to preserve the consistency between the global and local results, we introduce the semantic exclusivity loss based on the exclusivity relationship between labels: If the global label is 'normal', the 'benign' and 'malignant' labels are not likely to co-exist in local label sets; If the global label is 'benign', there will be no 'malignant' local frames. Therefore, the semantic exclusivity loss is defined as follows:

$$L_{ex}(Y_{i,j}^l, Y_i^g, Y_i^{g*}) = \begin{cases} -Y_{i,n}^g(\log \bar{Y}_{i,n}^l - \log \bar{Y}_{i,b}^l - \log \bar{Y}_{i,m}^l) & \text{if } Y_{i,n}^{g*} = 1, \\ -Y_{i,b}^g(\log \bar{Y}_{i,b}^l - \log \bar{Y}_{i,m}^l) & \text{if } Y_{i,b}^{g*} = 1, \\ -Y_{i,m}^g \log \bar{Y}_{i,m}^l & \text{if } Y_{i,m}^{g*} = 1. \end{cases} \tag{6}$$

where $\bar{Y}^l$ is the max-pooled label over all frames; Y^{g*} is the ground-truth of global label where $Y_{i,n}^{g*}$, $Y_{i,b}^{g*}$ and $Y_{i,m}^{g*}$ are the probability of 'normal', 'benign' and 'malignant' respectively. The semantic exclusivity loss can be regarded as an alternative of the standard cross-entropy loss with additional penalizations on the impossible co-existence of local labels.

2.5   Final Objective and Alternative Learning

The final objective is a combination of global classification, local detection and semantic exclusivity loss as follows:

$$\min L_{final} = \lambda_{global} L_{global} + \lambda_{local} L_{local} + \lambda_{ex} L_{ex} \tag{7}$$

where λ_{global}, λ_{local} and λ_{ex} are balance weights of each terms. We set $\lambda_{global} = 1$, $\lambda_{local} = \lambda_{ex} = 0.001$ in this paper. It is worth nothing the label propagation process cannot be directly solved via back-propagation. In each epoch, the label propagation is firstly conducted to obtain the pseudo labels for each frame. Then the deep neural networks are trained via back propagation.

3   Experiments

Dataset and Experimental Settings: The dataset is collected by a pre-clinical pCLE system (Cellvizio, Mauna Kea Technologies, Paris, France) as described in [8]. Breast tissue samples are obtained from 45 patients that are diagnosed with three classes including normal, benign and malignant. We finally obtained 700 pCLE mosaics which consist of 8000 frames in total. Among them, 500 pCLE mosaics are used for training and the rest are for testing. For data annotation, each frame is manually labeled with the corresponding class by experts and the mosaics are also labeled with the final diagnosis.

The feature extraction layers in Fig. 2 is based on the residual architecture proposed in [9]. We use the Adam solver [10] with a batch size of 1. The Pytorch[2] framework is adopted to implement the deep convolution neural networks and the experiment platform is a workstation with Xeon E5-2630 and NVIDIA GeForce Titan Xp.

Qualitative Performance Evaluation. We firstly present two typical cases in Fig. 3. The first column is the original pCLE video[3]; The second column selects local prediction for the representative frames where the green rectangles indicates the normal frames while the red rectangle indicates the malignant frames. Given a new pCLE video, the local and global prediction are updated along with the time frames. For cases 1, several frames at the beginning include the stroma tissues which are similar to the malignant cases. Therefore, the probability of malignant class on both local and global prediction are over 0.1. After receiving sufficient numbers of pCLE frames, the prediction tends to be stable. For case 2, the pCLE starts with normal frames which supports both local and global prediction to 'normal'. However, the malignant frames exist from frame # 10 to #20 which leads to the global prediction to be 'malignant'. Although several frames are likely to be normal after frame #20, the global prediction is not changed which demonstrates the proposed method is able to handle the pCLE video with different classes of local cases. More examples can be found in supplementary materials.

Quantitative Performance Evaluation. We also present the quantitative results of global and local prediction on pCLE dataset. The average precision of each class and the mean average precision over all classes are reported to measure the accuracy of classification. Several baselines are implemented in this

---

[2] https://github.com/pytorch/pytorch.
[3] For better visualization, we present the pCLE mosaics in the experiment. However, the proposed method takes frames as input without mosaicking.

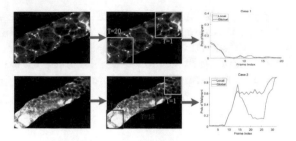

Fig. 3. Examples of global and local prediction.

Table 1. Performance of global and local prediction. WSFL-S refers to the proposed method without semantic exclusivity loss in Eq.(6). The best result is in **bold** and the second best result is <u>underlined</u>.

Global-Prediction	Normal	Benign	Malignant	Average
DenseSIFT [11]	0.805	0.754	0.842	0.816
MVMME [3]	0.823	0.762	0.829	0.827
UMGM [4]	0.834	0.781	0.855	0.834
CNN [9]	0.811	0.723	0.835	0.819
Patch-CNN [5]	**0.846**	0.802	0.867	0.833
WSFL-S	0.831	<u>0.829</u>	<u>0.855</u>	<u>0.832</u>
WSFL	<u>0.845</u>	**0.828**	**0.872**	**0.844**
Local-Prediction	Normal	Benign	Malignant	Average
DenseSIFT [11]	0.857	0.822	0.863	0.851
MVMME [3]	0.859	0.831	0.884	0.862
UMGM [4]	0.882	0.846	0.913	0.884
CNN [9]	0.901	0.885	0.914	0.903
Patch-CNN [5]	**0.922**	**0.905**	**0.943**	**0.921**
WSFL-S	0.897	0.882	0.926	0.903
WSFL	<u>0.903</u>	<u>0.894</u>	<u>0.938</u>	<u>0.914</u>

paper for comparison including dense-SIFT in [11], MVMME in [3], UMGM in [4], Residual CNN [9] and Patch-CNN in [5]. During the model training, all global and local labels are available for baselines while the proposed method is trained with only global supervision. Table 1 shows the classification performance of multiple baseline methods and the proposed WSFL. In overall view, the proposed WSFL achieves the competitive accuracy on both global and local prediction compared to all baselines. For global prediction task, the proposed method outperforms the methods with hand-crafted features even MVMME and UMGM adapt the knowledge from histopathological slides which demonstrated the good feature extraction of convolutional neural networks. However, the CNN model which directly takes the whole mosaic as input does not perform well on global prediction tasks. The main reason is that the pCLE mosaics are resized into the same sizes which are different from the original scales. Compared to the Patch-CNN method, the proposed method recovers the local label based on semantic propagation that helps to learn class-specific features. Moreover, the semantic exclusivity loss further improves the proposed method. For local prediction tasks, the proposed method outperforms most of the baselines even with only global supervision which is also closed to the Patch-CNN trained with frame labels.

4 Conclusion

In this paper, we have proposed a weakly-supervised feature learning (WSFL) framework to learn discriminative features for endomicroscopy analysis. A two-stream convolutional neural networks is adopted to jointly learn global and local prediction based on label propagation and semantic exclusivity loss. Compared to previous frame-based and mosaic-based methods, the proposed framework is trained under the global supervision only while the classification accuracy on both local and global tasks is promising on the breast tissue dataset with 700 pCLE samples. Our future work will focus on reformulating the label propagation process as forward/background operations in neural networks for end-to-end discriminative feature learning.

Acknowledgement. This research is partly supported by Committee of Science and Technology, Shanghai, China (No. 17JC1403000) and 973 Plan, China (No. 2015CB856004). Yun Gu is supported by Chinese Scholarship Council (CSC). We also thank NVIDIA to provide the device for our work. The tissue specimens were obtained using the Imperial tissue bank ethical protocol following the R-12047 project.

References

1. André, B., Vercauteren, T., Buchner, A.M., Wallace, M.B., Ayache, N.: A smart atlas for endomicroscopy using automated video retrieval. MedIA **15**(4), 460–476 (2011)
2. Kamen, A., et al.: Automatic tissue differentiation based on confocal endomicroscopic images for intraoperative guidance in neurosurgery. In: BioMed Research International 2016 (2016)
3. Gu, Y., Yang, J., Yang, G.Z.: Multi-view multi-modal feature embedding for endomicroscopy mosaic classification. In: CVPR, pp. 11–19 (2016)
4. Gu, Y., Vyas, K., Yang, J., Yang, G.-Z.: Unsupervised feature learning for endomicroscopy image retrieval. In: Descoteaux, M., Maier-Hein, L., Franz, A., Jannin, P., Collins, D.L., Duchesne, S. (eds.) MICCAI 2017. LNCS, vol. 10435, pp. 64–71. Springer, Cham (2017). https://doi.org/10.1007/978-3-319-66179-7_8
5. Aubreville, M., et al.: Automatic classification of cancerous tissue in laserendomicroscopy images of the oral cavity using deep learning. Sci. Rep. **7**(1), 11979 (2017)

6. André, B., Vercauteren, T., Buchner, A.M., Wallace, M.B., Ayache, N.: Endomicroscopic video retrieval using mosaicing and visual words. In: IEEE ISBI 2010, pp. 1419–1422. IEEE (2010)
7. Fortin, M., Glowinski, R.: Augmented Lagrangian Methods: Applications to the Numerical Solution of Boundary-Value Problems, vol. 15. Elsevier, New York (2000)
8. Chang, T.P., et al.: Imaging breast cancer morphology using probe-based confocal laser endomicroscopy: towards a real-time intraoperative imaging tool for cavity scanning. Breast Cancer Res. Treat. **153**(2), 299–310 (2015)
9. He, K., Zhang, X., Ren, S., Sun, J.: Deep residual learning for image recognition. In: CVPR, pp. 770–778 (2016)
10. Kingma, D.P., Ba, J.: Adam: a method for stochastic optimization. arXiv preprint arXiv:1412.6980 (2014)
11. André, B., Vercauteren, T., Perchant, A., Buchner, A.M., Wallace, M.B., Ayache, N.: Endomicroscopic image retrieval and classification using invariant visual features. In: IEEE ISBI 2009, pp. 346–349. IEEE (2009)

DeepHCS: Bright-Field to Fluorescence Microscopy Image Conversion Using Deep Learning for Label-Free High-Content Screening

Gyuhyun Lee[1], Jeong-Woo Oh[2], Mi-Sun Kang[4], Nam-Gu Her[3], Myoung-Hee Kim[4], and Won-Ki Jeong[1(✉)]

[1] School of Electrical and Computer Engineering, Ulsan National Institute of Science and Technology (UNIST), Ulsan, Korea
wkjeong@unist.ac.kr
[2] Department of Health Sciences and Technology, Samsung Advanced Institute for Health Science and Technology, Sungkyunkwan University, Seoul, Korea
[3] Samsung Medical Center (SMC), Seoul, Korea
[4] Department of Computer Science and Engineering, Ewha Womans University, Seoul, Korea

Abstract. In this paper, we propose a novel image processing method, *DeepHCS*, to transform bright-field microscopy images into synthetic fluorescence images of cell nuclei biomarkers commonly used in high-content drug screening. The main motivation of the proposed work is to automatically generate virtual biomarker images from conventional bright-field images, which can greatly reduce time-consuming and laborious tissue preparation efforts and improve the throughput of the screening process. DeepHCS uses bright-field images and their corresponding cell nuclei staining (DAPI) fluorescence images as a set of image pairs to train a series of end-to-end deep convolutional neural networks. By leveraging a state-of-the-art deep learning method, the proposed method can produce synthetic fluorescence images comparable to real DAPI images with high accuracy. We demonstrate the efficacy of this method using a real glioblastoma drug screening dataset with various quality metrics, including PSNR, SSIM, cell viability correlation (CVC), the area under the curve (AUC), and the IC50.

1 Introduction

A glioblastoma (GBM) is a brain tumor that is commonly found in the cerebral hemisphere of the brain. GBM is considered an obstinate brain tumor because even after medical advances in the past few decades, no effective treatment has been discovered that greatly improves life expectancy in patients. When patients are diagnosed with a GBM, in most cases, the best treatment option is surgery to eliminate as many tumor cells as possible. In addition to surgical treatments, patient-specific chemotherapy by analyzing patient-driven GBM tumor cells to

© Springer Nature Switzerland AG 2018
A. F. Frangi et al. (Eds.): MICCAI 2018, LNCS 11071, pp. 335–343, 2018.
https://doi.org/10.1007/978-3-030-00934-2_38

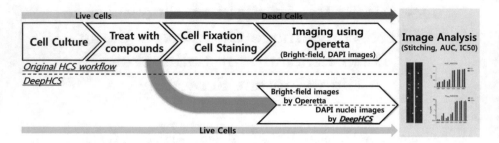

Fig. 1. DeepHCS eliminates the cell fixation and staining progress in the original HCS workflow and generates corresponding fluorescence image based bright-field image by Operetta. DeepHCS can keep the cells alive during the entire progress.

find the most effective drug for the target patient, called *precision medicine*, has become popular. High-throughput screening (HTS) and high-content screening (HCS) have demonstrated their effectiveness in precision medicine in recent studies [2,8]. Both approaches for precision medicine involve readouts of various drug responses to patient-derived cell cultures. Among them, HCS uses high-throughput imaging and automatic image analysis to evaluate changes in the phenotype of the whole cells, such as counting the number of living cells versus dead cells, measuring the size of the cells, comparing the shape of the cells, etc. In HCS, multiple imaging modalities are commonly used together to image various aspects of the cell phenotypes (Fig. 1). Such imaging modalities include bright-field and fluorescence microscopy, in which the former can capture the overall morphology of the cells, while the latter can image various fluorescent biomarkers. One advantage of using bright-field images in HCS is its ability to acquire a photographic record of cells without any extra preparation while fluorescence images require time-consuming cell fixation and staining procedures. Another advantage of the bright-field image method is its ability to capture the dynamics of cells because cell fixation and cell staining are not required (Fig. 1 lower row). However, fluorescence imaging can capture only a snapshot of the cells at any given point in time because cells die during fixation and staining (Fig. 1 upper row).

There have been many research efforts to develop image processing techniques for bright-field imaging to extract cell phenotypes without fluorescence imaging. Selinummi et al. [9] used multi-focal bright-field images to extract the shape of cells without whole cell fluorescence images. Their method calculates the intensity variation along the z-stack of multi-focal bright-field images to robustly detect cell boundaries. Ali et al. [1] proposed detection and segmentation of adherent HT1080 and HeLa cells from bright-field images. This method extracts local phase and local orientation from multi-focal bright-field images using the monogenic single framework to guide the evolution of the active contour. Tikkanen et al. [10] employed a machine learning approach using the histogram of oriented gradient (HOG) [3] feature for detecting cells in 25 focal images. The extracted features and their neighboring intensity histograms are combined for classification using a support vector machine (SVM). Liimatainen et al. [6] employed a logistic regression with a ℓ_1 penalty to classify the location of cells and non-cells using the intensity values from 25 focal images as features. However, most previous work focused only on cell segmentation and detection directly from bright-field images, and no state-of-the-art deep learning methods are leveraged. In addition, in spite of ongoing research efforts in bright-field image analysis, the standard HCS workflow still relies on detecting and analyzing biomarkers presented in fluorescence images.

Based on these observations, we propose *DeepHCS*, a novel data-driven image conversion technique for high-content screening. Unlike most existing methods that directly analyze bright-field images, DeepHCS converts bright-field images to fluorescence images as accurately as possible using end-to-end convolutional neural networks. By doing this, DeepHCS effectively avoids the time-consuming and laborious cell preparation process for generating biomarkers while providing accurate image analysis results by using the well-established conventional HCS workflow (Fig. 1 bottom row). We evaluate the accuracy of DeepHCS using widely used image quality metrics (e.g., PSNR and SSIM). In addition, we compare cell viability [4], the area under curve (AUC) and the IC50 of the results and real DAPI images to demonstrate that DeepHCS can replace the tissue preparation and fluorescence imaging process in the conventional HCS workflow with the software-based image conversion process.

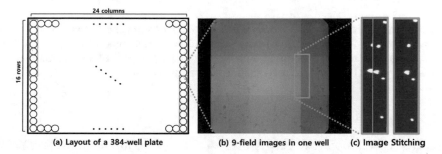

(a) Layout of a 384-well plate   (b) 9-field images in one well   (c) Image Stitching

Fig. 2. Overview of data acquisition and preprocessing: (a) layout of a 384-well plate, (b) nine overlapped images for a single well, (c) before and after stitching images (yellow line on the left is the border between adjacent images)

2 Method

2.1 Data

We acquired the image data from patients who had been diagnosed with a GBM brain tumor. The GBM tumor cells were divided evenly into a 384-well plate organized into a 24×16 grid (Fig. 2a) and stained with Hoechst 33342 solution. For drug screening, biologists added various FDA-approved drugs into the wells. Each drug was administered to a 1×8 column, starting with a $20\,\mu/\text{mol}$ dosage and tripling the dosage in each subsequent well (green box of Fig. 2a). The last wells in the 1×8 column contained no drugs and were used as a control (blue box of Fig. 2a). Each well was imaged with the Operetta CLS^{TM} high-content analysis system equipped with an high resolution 14bit CCD camera for cell imaging and the Harmony 3.5 software. Nine-field image montage per well (Fig. 2b) is generated by using an image stitching algorithm (Fig. 2c). The resolution of each image is 1360×1024 pixels. We took images from various locations with different drug dosages and evenly distributed cells, and made pairs for training set in which each pair consists of a bright-field image and its fluorescence nuclei image.

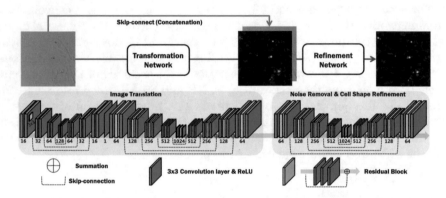

Fig. 3. DeepHCS consists of two sub-networks: a Transformation Network (green box); and a Refinement Network (pink box). Convolution layers (blue layer) include ReLU as a non-linear function. Residual blocks (purple layer) consist of three identical convolution layers. All filter sizes used in this system are 3×3.

2.2 Proposed Method: DeepHCS

DeepHCS is built upon two deep neural networks, *Transformation Network (TN)* and *Refinement Network (RN)* (see Fig. 3).

Transformation Network is the first part of DeepHCS, consisting of two sets of FusionNet variant networks [7]. The first network in the TN is used to gradu-ally transform the input bright-field image into the intermediate feature image, and the second network in the TN is used to actually perform the translation into the DAPI fluorescence image. The first network in the TN can effectively expand the depth of the network when the size of the input is relatively small, and adequately performs drop-out in which 16 feature maps are merged into one feature map at the end. The second network in the TN has more neuron weights by using residual blocks and actually translates the input image into DAPI flu-orescence images. The number of filters in the entire network is expressed under each layer in Fig. 3.

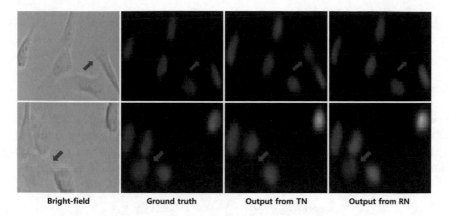

| Bright-field | Ground truth | Output from TN | Output from RN |

Fig. 4. Refinement Network improves the cell shapes and restores missing cells. A false positive (top row) and a false negative (bottom row) from the TN are corrected by the RN.

Refinement Network is the second part of DeepHCS and is designed to improve the image quality of the translated result from the TN in terms of the noise and the cell shape. In contrast to the TN, the RN takes a concatenation of the translated TN result and the input bright-field image of the TN, which provides a clue to rectify errors in the translated image generated by the TN. For example, as shown in Fig. 4, the RN can improve the cell shapes and restore falsely removed cells. Another benefit of using the concatenated input image is to help reducing the gradient-vanishing problem caused by the black background in the translated result by the TN.

Loss Function. For the TN, the mean-square error (MSE) is used to define the loss function to measure the pixel-wise error between the ground truth and the output image of the TN, as follows:

$$L_{TN}(x) = \frac{1}{n} \sum_{i=1}^{n} (\hat{y}_i - y_i)^2 \qquad (1)$$

where x is the input bright-field image, y_i is the real fluorescence image, and $\hat{y}_i$ is the output of the TN. For the RN, the mean-absolute error (MAE) and the SSIM are used as the loss function to deal with the shape of cells and the pixel intensity at the same time. The MAE is define as follows:

$$L_{MAE}(\hat{x}, y) = \frac{1}{n} \sum_{i=1}^{n} |r_i - y_i| \qquad (2)$$

where $\hat{x}$ is the concatenation of the translated result of the TN and the input bright-field image, and r_i is the output of the RN. In contrast to the TN, we employed the MAE to handle the translated result of the TN because the MSE penalizes larger errors and is more tolerant to smaller errors. The SSIM is defined as follows:

$$SSIM(x,y) = \frac{(2\mu_x\mu_y + c_1)(2\sigma_{xy} + c_2)}{(\mu_x^2 + \mu_y^2 + c_1)(\sigma_x^2 + \sigma_y^2 + c_2)} \tag{3}$$

where μ_x and σ_x represent the mean and the variance of image x, respectively; σ_{xy} represents the covariance of image x and y, and c_1 and c_2 are two constant variables for division stability. Based on Eq. 3, we can measure the degree of structural change in the image and additionally recognize the difference between the two images based on luminance and contrast. The SSIM values range between 0 and 1; therefore, we defined the loss function using the SSIM as follows:

$$L_{SSIM}(\hat{x},y) = \frac{1}{n}\sum_{i=1}^{n} 1 - SSIM(r_i, y_i) \tag{4}$$

By combining the two error measures, we can define the loss function for the RN as follows (α is empirically set to 0.8):

$$L_{RN}(\hat{x}) = (1-\alpha) \cdot L_{MAE}(\hat{x},y) + \alpha \cdot L_{SSIM}(\hat{x},y) \tag{5}$$

3   Results

We used the training set consisting of 2,860 pairs of bright-field images and their corresponding fluorescence images, each measuring 256×256 pixels (we cropped the center of each image to reduce boundary effects). To validate DeepHCS, we used eight cases (C1 to C8), including either 1,386 or 2,646 images.

Table 1. Accuracy of the proposed method for eight test cases.

	C1	C2	C3	C4	C5	C6	C7	C8
PSNR	33.91	33.90	33.79	33.93	38.52	39.04	38.65	38.46
SSIM	0.75	0.75	0.74	0.75	0.87	0.88	0.87	0.87
CVC	0.8663	0.9064	0.8794	0.8865	0.9583	0.9625	0.9673	0.9702

To assess the quality of the images generated by DeepHCS, we used two image error metrics (PSNR and SSIM) and cell viability correlation (CVC) that measures the similarity between the actual and generated DAPI fluorescence images using R^2 correlation, as shown in Table 1. In the experiment, we achieved an average of 0.9092 and a maximum of 0.9702 correlation with the ground truth. In addition, the shape of the cells and the status of the cells (living or dead) are clearly distinguished as shown in Fig. 5.

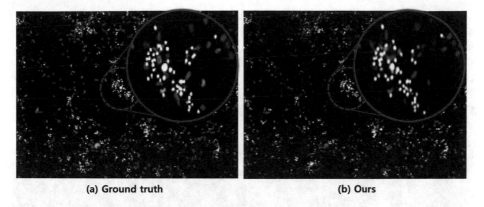

(a) Ground truth **(b) Ours**

Fig. 5. (a) Ground truth fluorescence image, (b) the result of our method. Zoom-in shows the similarity of the cell shapes between the ground truth and ours.

To further demonstrate the feasibility of DeepHCS for replacing biomarker generation in the conventional HCS workflow, we used seven other cases for the validation test. Figure 6 shows the correlation of real DAPI images and our synthetic fluorescence images in terms of AUC and IC50, respectively. In addition, the responses of two anti-cancer drugs (AMG232 and RG7112) measured by AUC and IC50 are also shown using heatmaps; clear separation of two groups in drug responses are identically shown in DAPI images and ours. These results confirm that the images generated by DeepHCS can be used to compute AUC and IC50 for the estimation of drug responses, which shows potential to replace the conventional fluorescence imaging process in the HSC workflow.

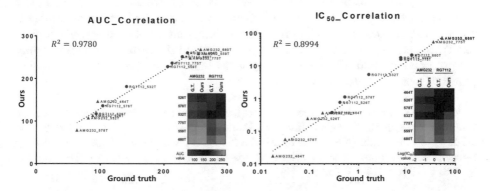

Fig. 6. Comparison of AUC and IC50 values from the real DAPI images (ground truth) and our results from the seven patients' data. The heat maps show the drug response (green is low, and red is high).

Finally, we compared DeepHCS with the latest GAN-based image translation method used in the Pix2Pix network [5]. As shown in Fig. 7, DeepHCS reproduces cell images close to real DAPI images while Pix2Pix fails to accurately generate cell shapes in some cases. The GAN attempts to approximate the data distribution of the training set as much as possible; therefore, the reconstructed images look like cell images. However, this does not imply that the reconstructed image satisfies the accuracy up to the HCS analysis. Even though Pix2Pix learns the morphological characteristics in the cell image by minimizing the ℓ_1 distance from the ground truth, it is not enough to satisfy this problem.

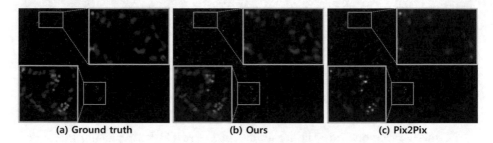

(a) Ground truth   (b) Ours   (c) Pix2Pix

Fig. 7. (a) Ground truth fluorescence image, (b) the results of the proposed method, (c) the results of the Pix2Pix network [5]. The results are generated after 300 training epochs. Our method can generate most of cell structures close to the ground truth.

4   Conclusion

In this paper, we introduced DeepHCS, a novel deep end-to-end convolution neural network for generating DAPI fluorescence images directly from bright-field images. We showed that the DeepHCS can generate results similar to real DAPI images and outperforms state-of-the-art image translation methods. The proposed method demonstrates the potential to reduce the laborious biomarker preparation process and to improve the throughput of the large-scale image-based drug screening process using deep learning. In the future, we plan to apply the proposed method to time-lapse bright-field images, and assess the efficacy of generating other biomarker images.

Acknowledgements. This work was partially supported by Basic Science Research Program through the National Research Foundation of Korea (NRF) funded by the Ministry of Education (NRF-2017R1D1A1A09000841) and Bio & Medical Technology Development Program of the National Research Foundation of Korea (NRF) funded by MSIT (NRF-2015M3A9A7029725).

References

1. Ali, R., Gooding, M., Szilágyi, T., Vojnovic, B., Christlieb, M., Brady, M.: Automatic segmentation of adherent biological cell boundaries and nuclei from bright-field microscopy images. Mach. Vis. Appl. **23**(4), 607–621 (2012)
2. Boutros, M., Heigwer, F., Laufer, C.: Microscopy-based high-content screening. Cell **163**(6), 1314–1325 (2015)

3. Dalal, N., Triggs, B.: Histograms of oriented gradients for human detection. In: 2005 IEEE Computer Society Conference on Computer Vision and Pattern Recognition (CVPR 2005), vol. 1, pp. 886–893. IEEE (2005)
4. Darzynkiewicz, Z., Li, X., Gong, J.: Assays of cell viability: discrimination of cells dying by apoptosis. Methods Cell Biol. **41**, 15–38 (1994)
5. Isola, P., Zhu, J.Y., Zhou, T., Efros, A.A.: Image-to-image translation with conditional adversarial networks. arXiv preprint arXiv:1611.07004 (2016)
6. Liimatainen, K., Ruusuvuori, P., Latonen, L., Huttunen, H.: Supervised method for cell counting from bright field focus stacks. In: 2016 IEEE 13th International Symposium on Biomedical Imaging (ISBI), pp. 391–394. IEEE (2016)
7. Quan, T.M., Hilderbrand, D.G., Jeong, W.K.: FusionNet: a deep fully residual convolutional neural network for image segmentation in connectomics. arXiv preprint arXiv:1612.05360 (2016)
8. Quartararo, C.E., Reznik, E., DeCarvalho, A.C., Mikkelsen, T., Stockwell, B.R.: High-throughput screening of patient-derived cultures reveals potential for precision medicine in glioblastoma. ACS Med. Chem. Lett. **6**(8), 948–952 (2015)
9. Selinummi, J., et al.: Bright field microscopy as an alternative to whole cell fluorescence in automated analysis of macrophage images. PloS One **4**(10), e7497 (2009)
10. Tikkanen, T., Ruusuvuori, P., Latonen, L., Huttunen, H.: Training based cell detection from bright-field microscope images. In: 2015 9th International Symposium on Image and Signal Processing and Analysis (ISPA), pp. 160–164. IEEE (2015)

Optical and Histology Applications: Optical Coherence Tomography and Other Optical Imaging Applications

A Cascaded Refinement GAN for Phase Contrast Microscopy Image Super Resolution

Liang Han and Zhaozheng Yin[✉]

Department of Computer Science, Missouri University of Science and Technology,
Rolla, USA
{lh248,yinz}@mst.edu

Abstract. Phase contrast microscopy is a widely-used non-invasive technique for monitoring live cells over time. High-throughput biological experiments expect a wide-view (i.e., a low microscope magnification) to monitor the entire cell population and a high magnification on individual cell's details, which is hard to achieve simultaneously. In this paper, we propose a cascaded refinement Generative Adversarial Network (GAN) for phase contrast microscopy image super-resolution. Our algorithm uses an optic-related data enhancement and super-resolves a phase contrast microscopy image in a coarse-to-fine fashion, with a new loss function consisting of a content loss and an adversarial loss. The proposed algorithm is both qualitatively and quantitatively evaluated on a dataset of 500 phase contrast microscopy images, showing its superior performance for super-resolving phase contrast microscopy images. The proposed algorithm provides a computational solution on achieving a high magnification on individual cell's details and a wide-view on cell populations at the same time, which will benefit the microscopy community.

1 Introduction

Phase Contrast Microscopy [19] allows researchers to acquire images on hundreds of live cells from different treatments over days or weeks without invasively staining them (Fig. 1(a)). The high-throughput experiments need a wide-view to monitor the entire cell population, so the magnification of phase contrast microscope is set low. But, the low magnification loses cell details and provides low-resolution (**LR**) images on individual cells (Fig. 1(b)). To obtain high-resolution (**HR**) images with cell details, we have to increase the magnification with a limited view on a small number of cells (Fig. 1(c)), which is not suitable for monitoring large-scale cell populations.

To simultaneously achieve a high magnification and wide-view, we propose a novel super-resolution approach to increase the image resolution on cell details while maintaining the wide-view on cell populations.

© Springer Nature Switzerland AG 2018
A. F. Frangi et al. (Eds.): MICCAI 2018, LNCS 11071, pp. 347–355, 2018.
https://doi.org/10.1007/978-3-030-00934-2_39

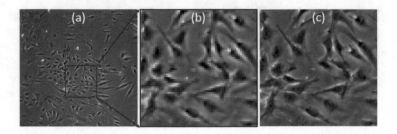

Fig. 1. (a) Monitoring cell populations with a low magnification; (b) A zoomed-in image shows the low resolution on individual cells; (c) A high magnification visualizes cell details but with a limited view.

2   Related Work and Our Proposal

The single image super-resolution problem is first tackled by some filtering approaches such as linear, bicubic [8] and Lanczos [4]. However, these filtering methods produce overly smoothed textures in the recovered HR images.

To preserve the edges in the recovered HR images, example-based approaches [17,18] aiming at learning a mapping between low- and high-resolution image patches are proposed. The example-based methods (or patch-based methods) exploit the self-similarity property and construct high-resolution image patches from the input image [5]. However, the example-based methods suffer from the heavy computational cost of patch search. Moreover, the found low- and high-resolution image patch pairs may not be sufficient to represent the large textural variations in the testing images.

In order to overcome the drawbacks of the example-based approaches, deep learning algorithms [3,9] are proposed to super-resolve an image. Instead of modeling the low- and high-resolution mapping in the patch space, these algorithms learn the nonlinear mapping in the image space. Dong *et al.* upscale an input LR image and train a three layer deep convolutional network to learn an end-to-end mapping between low- and high-resolution images [3]. Ledig *et al.* present a Generative Adversarial Network (GAN) for image super-resolution, which is capable of inferring photo-realistic natural images for 4× upscaling factors [12]. Lai *et al.* propose a Laplacian Pyramid Super-Resolution Network to progressively reconstruct the sub-band residuals of the high-resolution images [11]. However, these deep learning algorithms mainly focus on the natural image super-resolution, and may not be suitable for super-resolving microscopy images as no optical properties of the microscopy imaging are taken into account.

In this paper, we propose a cascaded refinement GAN for phase contrast microscopy image super-resolution. The contributions of this study are mainly in three aspects. *First*, to our best knowledge, this is the first framework capable of super-resolving phase contrast microscopy images for 8× upscaling factors. *Second*, we design a perceptual loss consisting of an adversarial loss and a content loss for our algorithm and achieve the best performance on phase contrast microscopy image super-resolution. *Third*, an optics-related data enhancement is developed to improve the performance of our algorithm on phase contrast microscopy image super-resolution.

3   Preliminaries

3.1   Generative Adversarial Networks

There are one generator network G and one discriminator network D in the Generative Adversarial Networks (GANs) [6]. These two networks are trained alternatively to compete in a two-player min-max game. The generator G is optimized to simulate the true data distribution by synthesizing images that are challenging for the discriminator D to tell from the real ones. The discriminator D is optimized to try not to be fooled by the generator G by correctly distinguishing the real images from the synthetic images. These two networks play the min-max game with the following objective function

$$\min_{G} \max_{D} V(D,G) = \mathbb{E}_{x \sim p_{data}}[logD(x)] + \mathbb{E}_{z \sim p_z(z)}[log(1 - D(G(z)))], \quad (1)$$

where x is a real image sampled from the real data distribution p_{data}, z is a noise vector drawn from distribution p_z (e.g., Gaussian or uniform distribution).

3.2   Optics-Related Data Enhancement

The properties of phase contrast microscopy images (e.g., halo artifact and low image contrast) motivated researchers to derive optics-related imaging models for microscopy image restoration [16], which include a series of Diffraction Pattern Filters (DPFs, Fig. 2(a1–a6)). Rather than solving the inverse problem of image restoration, we leverage the DPFs to enrich phase contrast microscopy images (Fig. 2(b0)) by convolving it with DPFs. As shown in Fig. 2(b1–b6), the convolution generates a set of images sensitive to different types of cell regions, which is an optics-related data enhancement to the original input.

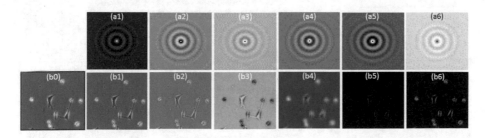

Fig. 2. DPFs and the enriched phase contrast microscopy images.

4 A Cascaded Refinement GAN for Super Resolution

In this section, we describe the network structure of the proposed cascaded refinement generative adversarial network (GAN) for phase contrast microscopy image super resolution, the loss function for network optimization, and the network implementation and training details.

4.1 Network Architecture

Generator Architecture: As shown in Fig. 3, the LR phase contrast image is first enhanced by convolving with some DPFs. The proposed generator takes the enhanced image stacks as input and then refines them with cascaded refinement modules. Each module operates at a certain resolution and the resolution is doubled between two consecutive modules.

All the modules $M_s(s \in \{1, 2, 3\})$ are structurally identical and consist of three layers: the input layer, the upsampling layer, and the convolutional layer (Fig. 3). The input layer of the first module is the enriched image stack of the LR image, while the input layers of the other modules are identical to the convolutional layers of the previous modules. The upsampling layer is obtained by bilinearly upsampling the input layer. As the upconvolutions is prone to introduce characteristic artifacts to the output image [2,14], we discard the upconvolution and use bilinear upsampling. The convolutional layer is obtained by implementing 3×3 convolutions, layer normalization [1], and Leaky ReLu nonlinearlity [13] operations on the upsampling layer. A linear projection (1×1 convolution) is applied on the convolutional layer to project the feature tensor to the output image. Note that the output image at each upsampling level is not used as the input of the next module.

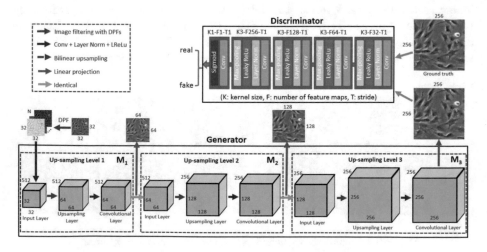

Fig. 3. Architecture of the Generator and Discriminator in our model.

Discriminator Architecture: There are four downsampling modules in the discriminator, and each downsampling module consists of 3×3 convolutions, layer normalization, Leaky ReLu nonlinearlity, and 2×2 max-pooling operations. The discriminator tries to classify whether an input image is real or fake.

4.2   Loss Function

Let x be the input LR image and y be the corresponding HR counterpart. Our ultimate goal is to learn a generator G with parameters θ_G for generating a HR image $\hat{y} = G(x; \theta_G)$ which is as similar to the ground truth HR image y as possible. To learn the parameters (θ_G in the generator and θ_D in the discriminator), we formulate a perceptual loss function as the weighted sum of an adversarial loss and a content loss:

$$L(y, \hat{y}) = L_{adv}(y, \hat{y}) + \alpha L_{con}(y, \hat{y}). \tag{2}$$

Adversarial Loss: The adversarial loss in the GAN encourages the generator to generate images residing on the manifold of the ground truth images by trying to fool the discriminator. From Eq. 1 we can see the adversarial loss is formulated as $\mathbb{E}_{z \sim p_z(z)}[log(1 - D(G(z)))]$. In our case, the generator takes a LR image instead of a noise vector as the input, accordingly the adversarial loss $L_{adv}(y, \hat{y})$ over K training samples can be defined as:

$$L_{adv}(y, \hat{y}) = \frac{1}{K} \sum_{k=1}^{K} [log(1 - D(G(x_k; \theta_G); \theta_D))], \tag{3}$$

Early in training, we can minimize $log(-D(G(x_k; \theta_G); \theta_D))$ instead of $log(1 - D(G(x_k; \theta_G)); \theta_D)$ to mitigate the gradient saturation [6].

Content Loss: In addition to the adversarial loss in the GAN, we also add a content loss $L_{con}(y, \hat{y})$ to our perceptual loss function. Many previous state-of-the-art approaches rely on the widely used pixel-wise mean square error (MSE) loss to learn the parameters of the LR-HR mapping functions [3,15], however, solutions of MSE optimization problems often lack the ability of learning high-frequency contents and result in overly smoothed textures [7,12]. Instead, we propose a new content loss using the DPFs to emphasize the loss on different types of cell regions:

$$L_{con}(y, \hat{y}) = \frac{1}{K} \sum_{k=1}^{K} \sum_{s=1}^{S} \sum_{n=0}^{N-1} \|y_s * DPF_n - \hat{y}_s * DPF_n\|_1, \tag{4}$$

where y_s is the downsampled ground truth image at level s, $\hat{y}_s$ is the generated upscaled LR image at level s (the output layer of the sth module), S is the number of refinement modules in the generator, N is the number of DPFs, and $\| \cdot \|_1$ is the ℓ_1 distance.

4.3   Implementation and Training Details

The number of refinement modules in our generator is decided by the upscaling factor. In our experiments with the upscaling factor of 8×, there are 3 refinement modules, corresponding to a resolution increase from 32×32 to 256×256 in the generator. The Leaky ReLu in the generator and discriminator is with a negative slope of 0.2. Zero-padding is implemented before the convolution to keep the size of all feature maps unchanged in each module. The number of DPFs in our experiment is 12.

To train our networks, we alternate between one gradient descent step on the discriminator, and then one step on the generator. The minibatch stochastic gradient descent (SGD) is used in our experiment and the Adam solver [10] with momentum parameter 0.9 is applied to optimize the SGD. We use the batch size of 1. The learning rate is $1e-4$, and the algorithm is trained for 100 iterations. The weight α in the loss function is 1.

5   Experimental Results

Dataset: 11,500 high-resolution phase contrast microscopy images with different cell densities are captured at the resolution of $256 * 256$ pixels, and the low-resolution images are obtained by downsampling the high-resolution images. After getting the high-resolution and low-resolution image pairs, we randomly select 10,000 pairs of them as the training set, 1,000 as the validation set, and 500 as the testing set.

Evaluation Metrics: We evaluate the proposed super-resolution algorithm with a widely-used image quality metric: Peak Signal-to-Noise Ratio (PSNR).

Evaluation: We compare our algorithm with the baseline bicubic [8] and the current state-of-the-art LapSRN [11] algorithms. Figure 4 presents the visual comparison results on some randomly picked images. The bicubic filtering gives very blurry super-resolution results. LapSRN generates much sharper and clearer high resolution images than bicubic, however, the generated images are over-smoothed. It is mainly because the designed loss function of LapSRN is not suitable for microscopy image super-resolution. By taking the optical property of phase contrast microscopy imaging into consideration and designing a perceptual loss, our proposed algorithm generates HR images with clear cell details.

Given an input phase contrast image with a wide-view (e.g., Fig. 5(a)), we can divide the image into 32×32 patches, super-resolve each patch, and then combine the predicted patches to generate a HR image with megapixel resolutions (Fig. 5(b)).

Ablation Study: First, we investigate the effect of different loss functions. As shown in (Fig. 6(b1, b2)), only using the adversarial loss cannot generate HR images with clear overall contents though some cell details are exhibited. The generated images by only using the content loss (Fig. 6(c1, c2)) are not sharp enough and the cell structures are not presented well.

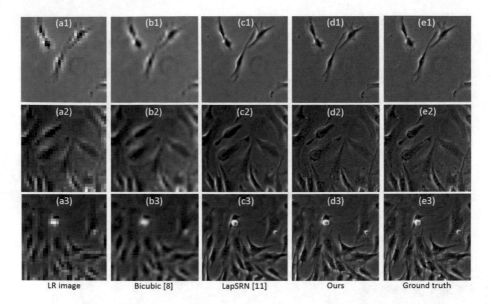

Fig. 4. Upsampling phase contrast images by different algorithms (8× upsampling).

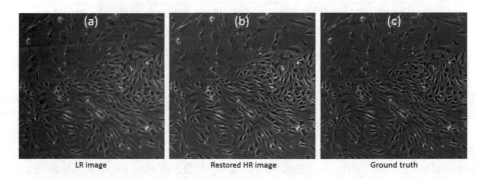

Fig. 5. Upsampling an input phase contrast image with a wide-view. Please zoom-in the online version to observe cell details.

Second, we investigate the effect of the optics-related data enhancement. If using the original image as the input to the generator in Fig. 3 (without enriching the input image by DPFs, the content loss is defined as $\frac{1}{K}\sum_{k=1}^{K}\sum_{s=1}^{S}\|y_s - \hat{y}_s\|$ accordingly), the generated images (Fig. 6(d1, d2)) provide sharp images but with some cell details missed, compared to the images generated using the enriched input (Fig. 6(e1, e2)). The enriched phase contrast images can present more feature information of cells, especially when the original input phase contrast image has low contrast and less textures.

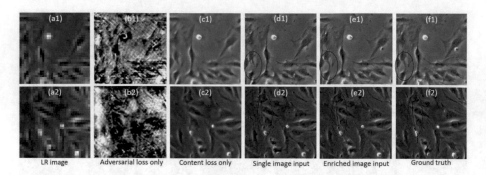

Fig. 6. The effect of different loss functions and the optics-related data enhancement.

The quantitative results of evaluation and ablation study are summarized in Table 1, which shows that our cascaded refinement GAN with optics-related data enhancement and perceptual loss (adversrial loss plus content loss) achieves the best performance.

Table 1. Quantitative evaluation.

	Bicubic [8]	LapSRN [11]	Ours	Content loss only	Adversarial loss only	Single image input
PSNR	20.6039	26.5055	**27.8591**	26.0928	11.6732	26.2914

6   Conclusion

In this paper, we investigate a super resolution algorithm to generate high-resolution phase contrast microscopy images from the low-resolution ones. Instead of upscaling the input image to the desired resolution directly, the proposed algorithm predicts the high resolution image in a coarse-to-fine fashion, i.e., increasing the spatial resolution of the input image progressively. A new loss function is designed for the proposed algorithm which consists of a content loss and an adversarial loss. The content loss forces the prediction of the high-resolution image to be similar to the real image in the feature domain enriched by optics-related data enhancement, while the adversarial loss encourages the prediction to be sharp and with more cell details.

The experiments demonstrate that our algorithm is very effective to recover high resolution phase contrast microscopy images from low resolution ones, and our algorithm outperforms the current state-of-the-art super-resolution algorithm. The research outcome provides a computational solution on achieving a high magnification on individual cells' details and a wide-view on cell populations at the same time, which will benefit the microscopy community.

Acknowledgement. This project was supported by NSF CAREER award IIS-1351049 and NSF EPSCoR grant IIA-1355406.

References

1. Ba, J.L., et al.: Layer normalization. arXiv:1607.06450 (2016)
2. Chen, Q., Koltun, V.: Photographic image synthesis with cascaded refinement networks. In: ICCV (2017)
3. Dong, C., et al.: Image super-resolution using deep convolutional networks. TPAMI (2015)
4. Duchon, C.E.: Lanczos filtering in one and two dimensions. J. Appl. Meteorol. **18**, 1016–1022 (1979)
5. Freedman, G., Fattal, R.: Image and video upscaling from local self-examples. In: ACM TOG (2011)
6. Goodfellow, I., et al.: Generative adversarial nets. In: NIPS (2014)
7. Isola, P., et al.: Image-to-image translation with conditional adversarial networks. In: CVPR (2017)
8. Keys, R.: Cubic convolution interpolation for digital image processing. In: TASSP (1981)
9. Kim, J., Lee, J.K., Lee, K.M.: Accurate image super-resolution using very deep convolutional networks. In: CVPR (2016)
10. Kingma, D., Ba, J.: Adam: a method for stochastic optimization. In: ICLR (2015)
11. Lai, W.S., et al.: Deep laplacian pyramid networks for fast and accurate super-resolution. In: CVPR (2017)
12. Ledig, C., et al.: Photo-realistic single image super-resolution using a generative adversarial network. In: CVPR (2017)
13. Maas, A.L., Hannun, A.Y., Ng, A.Y.: Rectifier nonlinearities improve neural network acoustic models. In: ICML (2013)
14. Odena, A., Dumoulin, V., Olah, C.: Deconvolution and checkerboard artifacts. In: Distill (2016)
15. Shi, W., et al.: Real-time single image and video super-resolution using an efficient sub-pixel convolutional neural network. In: CVPR (2016)
16. Su, H., et al.: Cell segmentation in phase contrast microscopy images via semi-supervised classification over optics-related features. In: Medical Image Analysis (2013)
17. Timofte, R., De Smet, V., Van Gool, L.: Anchored neighborhood regression for fast example-based super-resolution. In: ICCV (2013)
18. Yang, J., Lin, Z., Cohen, S.: Fast image super-resolution based on in-place example regression. In: CVPR (2013)
19. Zernike, F.: How I discovered phase contrast. Science **121**, 345–349 (1955)

Multi-context Deep Network
for Angle-Closure Glaucoma Screening
in Anterior Segment OCT

Huazhu Fu[1], Yanwu Xu[2(✉)], Stephen Lin[3], Damon Wing Kee Wong[1],
Baskaran Mani[4], Meenakshi Mahesh[4], Tin Aung[4], and Jiang Liu[5]

[1] Institute for Infocomm Research, A*STAR, Singapore, Singapore
[2] Guangzhou Shiyuan Electronic Technology Company Limited, Shenzhen, China
ywxu@ieee.org
[3] Microsoft Research, Beijing, China
[4] Singapore Eye Research Institute, Singapore, Singapore
[5] Cixi Institute of Biomedical Engineering, CAS, Ningbo, China

Abstract. A major cause of irreversible visual impairment is angle-closure glaucoma, which can be screened through imagery from Anterior Segment Optical Coherence Tomography (AS-OCT). Previous computational diagnostic techniques address this screening problem by extracting specific clinical measurements or handcrafted visual features from the images for classification. In this paper, we instead propose to learn from training data a discriminative representation that may capture subtle visual cues not modeled by predefined features. Based on clinical priors, we formulate this learning with a presented Multi-Context Deep Network (MCDN) architecture, in which parallel Convolutional Neural Networks are applied to particular image regions and at corresponding scales known to be informative for clinically diagnosing angle-closure glaucoma. The output feature maps of the parallel streams are merged into a classification layer to produce the deep screening result. Moreover, we incorporate estimated clinical parameters to further enhance performance. On a clinical AS-OCT dataset, our system is validated through comparisons to previous screening methods.

1 Introduction

Glaucoma is the foremost cause of irreversible blindness. Since vision loss from glaucoma cannot be reversed, improved screening and detection methods for glaucoma are essential to preserve vision and life quality. A common type of glaucoma is angle-closure, where the anterior chamber angle (ACA) is narrow as shown in Fig. 1, leading to blockage of drainage channels that results in pressure on the optic nerve. Anterior Segment Optical Coherence Tomography (AS-OCT) has been shown to provide an objective method for the evaluation and assessment of ACA structure [12], and thus has been widely used by recent computational techniques for early screening of angle-closure glaucoma.

© Springer Nature Switzerland AG 2018
A. F. Frangi et al. (Eds.): MICCAI 2018, LNCS 11071, pp. 356–363, 2018.
https://doi.org/10.1007/978-3-030-00934-2_40

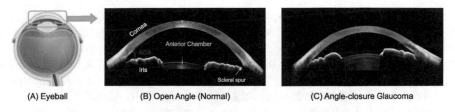

(A) Eyeball   (B) Open Angle (Normal)   (C) Angle-closure Glaucoma

Fig. 1. The example of (B) open angle and (C) angle-closure. The narrow anterior chamber angle (ACA) blocks drainage channels of aqueous fluid.

Recently, several automatic angle-closure glaucoma assessment methods have been studied. Tian *et al.* provided a Schwalbe's line detection method for High-Definition OCT (HD-OCT) to compute ACA measurements [15]. Xu *et al.* localized the ACA region, and then extracted visual features directly to classify the glaucoma subtype [17,18]. Fu *et al.* proposed a data-driven approach to integrate AS-OCT segmentation, measurement, and screening [5,6]. These methods segment the AS-OCT image and then extract the representation based on clinical parameters or visual features which are subsequently used for angle-closure classification. These methods, however, lack sufficiently discriminative representations and are easily affected by noise and low quality of the AS-OCT image. Recently, deep learning has been shown to yield highly discriminative representation that surpass the performance of handcrafted features in many computer vision tasks [8,11]. For example, deep learning has high sensitivity and specificity for detecting referable diabetic retinopathy in retinal fundus photographs [8]. Deep learning has also been shown to be effective in other retinal fundus applications [2–4]. These successes have motivated our examination of deep learning for glaucoma assessment in AS-OCT imagery.

A common limitation of deep learning based approaches is the need to downsample the input image to a low resolution (i.e., 224 × 224) in order for the network size to be computationally manageable [8]. However, this downsampling leads to a loss of image details that are important for discrimination of subtle pathological changes. To address this issue, we propose to supplement the downsampled global image with a local window chosen at a specific ocular region known to be informative for clinical diagnosis of angle-closure glaucoma [13]. The benefit of including this local window is that it is small enough to be processed by a deep network while maintaining the original image details.

Based on this, we propose a Multi-Context Deep Network (MCDN) architecture, which includes two parallel streams that jointly learn predictive representations from the different regions/scales useful for angle-closure estimation. Moreover, an intensity-based data augmentation is utilized to artificially enlarge the AS-OCT training data in order to gain robustness to different AS-OCT imaging devices. The main contributions of this work are as follows: (1) We introduce deep learning to the problem of angle-closure glaucoma screening in AS-OCT imagery, for the purpose of gaining more discriminative representations on different regions for glaucoma screening prediction. (2) A MCDN architecture is developed based on clinical priors about informative image areas. MCDN learns predictive representations for these image regions through processing by separate, parallel network streams. (3) An intensity-based augmentation of training data is presented to deal with intensity variations among AS-OCT images. (4) We also demonstrate that incorporating estimated clinical parameters can be beneficial for final glaucoma screening. (5) A large-scale AS-OCT dataset containing 8270 ACA images is collected for evaluation. Experiments show that our method outperforms the existing screening methods.

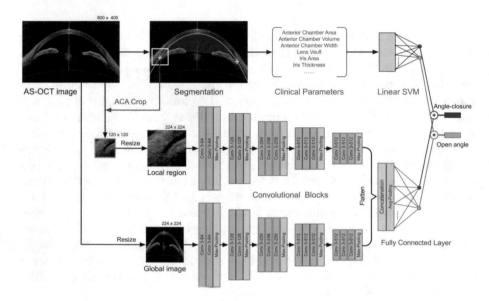

Fig. 2. The framework of our angle-closure glaucoma screening system, which contains AS-OCT structure segmentation and MCDN. The CNN layer parameters are denoted as "Conv (receptive field size)-(number of channels)".

2   Proposed Method

Our angle-closure glaucoma screening system include two stages, AS-OCT structure segmentation and MCDN, as shown in Fig. 2. The AS-OCT structure segmentation is utilized to localize the ACA region and predict the screening result based on clinical parameters, while the MCDN is used to gain the discriminative representation and output the final angle-closure glaucoma screening. Finally, the probability results of clinical parameter and deep learning are averaged to produce the angle-closure glaucoma screening.

2.1 AS-OCT Segmentation and Clinical Parameter

In our system, we implement the data-driven AS-OCT segmentation method in [5], which utilizes marker transfer from labeled exemplars to generate initial markers, and segments the major AS-OCT structure to compute the clinical parameters. A 120×120 patch centered on the detected ACA is cropped and used as the input of the following MCDN. Moreover, we also calculate the clinical parameters (e.g., Anterior Chamber Width, Lens-Vault, Chamber Height, Iris Curvature, and Anterior Chamber Area) and employ a linear Support Vector Machine (SVM) to predict an angle-closure probability. More details of the clinical parameters can be found in [5].

2.2 Multi-context Deep Network Architecture

Our MCDN architecture includes two parallel streams to obtain the representations for different clinical regions in an AS-OCT image, namely the global fundus image and local disc region. As shown as in Fig. 2, each stream consists of a sequence of convolutional units that each contain layers for convolution, batch normalization [9], and Rectified Linear Units (ReLU) activation [10]. The CNN of each stream learns and extracts local feature representations based on patches randomly sampled from its input. The batch normalization aids training the network [9], and the ReLU activation function is defined as $f(x) = \max(0, x)$, where x is the input to the neuron.

The first stream processes the cropped patch centered on the ACA region from the AS-OCT segmentation. This area is the most important for clinical diagnosis, as several major clinical measurements are taken from it [13] (e.g., iris curvature, angle opening distance, and trabecular-iris space area). The second stream of our MCDN architecture learns a global feature map for the complete cornea structure. In the clinical domain, the cornea structure offers various cues associated with risk factors for angle-closure glaucoma [16], such as lens vault and anterior chamber width, area and volume. The input images of the two streams are all resized to 224×224 to enable use of pre-trained parameters from other deep models [10,14] as the initialization for our network. The output maps of these two streams are concatenated into a single feature vector that is fed into a fully connected layer to obtain the final screening result. Here, the angle-closure glaucoma screening is formulated as a binary classification task, and softmax regression is employed as a generalization of the logistic regression classifier. The classifier is trained by minimizing the following binary cross-entropy loss function:

$$Loss = -\frac{1}{N} \sum_{i=1}^{N} \{y_i \log(g(\mathbf{w} \cdot \mathbf{x}_i)) + (1 - y_i) \log(1 - g(\mathbf{w} \cdot \mathbf{x}_i))\}, \qquad (1)$$

where $g(\mathbf{w} \cdot \mathbf{x}_i)$ is the logistic function with weight vector $\mathbf{w}$, $(\mathbf{x}_i, y_i)$ is the training set containing N AS-OCT images, $\mathbf{x}_i$ is the output representation of the i-th image and $y_i \in \{0, 1\}$ is the angle-closure label.

Discussion: A related deep learning model is the Region-based Convolutional Neural Network [7], which classifies object proposals using deep convolutional networks. The object proposal regions are obtained using general object detectors, in contrast to our work where we take advantage of clinical guidance to specifically extract the ACA region for glaucoma diagnosis. Our proposed MCDN architecture is also related to multi-scale or multi-column deep networks [1], which combine features from different scales or receptive field sizes, and generate the final feature map to build a representation. Our network also learns features at different scales, but constructs a more concise representation that focuses on image areas and corresponding scales that are clinically relevant to our problem. Avoiding extraneous information in this way facilitates network training, especially in cases of limited training data. In the following experiment, we also demonstrate that our MCDN architecture outperforms the multi-column network (i.e., [1]) in the AS-OCT screening task.

Moreover, our system utilizes an individual linear SVM for clinical parameter based estimation instead of concatenating them with deep features into the fully connected layer. This is due to two considerations: (1) the dimensionality of clinical parameters (24 D as in [5]) is much lower than that of deep features from the two streams (2×4096 D), which would reduce the impact of the clinical parameters; (2) estimation from clinical parameters with linear SVM has demonstrated satisfactory performance in the previous works [5,13].

2.3   Data Augmentation for AS-OCT

AS-OCT images are captured along the perpendicular direction of the eye, and the structure of the anterior chamber appears at a relatively consistent position among AS-OCT images in practice. Traditional image augmentation, e.g. by rotation and scaling, therefore does not aid in AS-OCT screening. On the other hand, image intensities typically vary among different AS-OCT imaging devices, which may affect screening accuracy. We thus employ an intensity-based augmentation to enlarge the data with varied intensities, by rescaling image intensities by a factor k_I ($k_I \in \{0.5, 1, 1.5\}$ in this paper). To increase the robustness of ACA region localization, we additionally perform data augmentation by shifting the ACA position to extract multiple patches as the input to the ACA stream in our MCDN architecture.

3   Experiments

For experimentation, we collected a total of 4135 Visante AS-OCT images (Model 1000, Carl-Zeiss Meditec) from 2113 subjects to construct a clinical AS-OCT dataset. Since each AS-OCT image contains two ACA regions, each image is split into two ACA images (8270 ACA images in total), with right-side ACA images flipped horizontally to match the orientations of left-side images. For each ACA image, the ground truth label of open-angle or angle-closure is determined from the majority diagnosis of three ophthalmologists. The data contains 7375 open-angle and 895 angle-closure cases. The dataset is divided equally and randomly into training and testing sets based on subject, such that the two ACAs of one patient will not be separated between the training and test sets. We employ several evaluation criteria to measure performance: Sensitivity (Sen), Specificity (Spe), Balanced Accuracy (B-Acc), which are defined as

$$\text{Sen} = \frac{TP}{TP+FN}, \ \text{Spe} = \frac{TN}{TN+FP}, \ \text{B-Acc} = \frac{1}{2}(\text{Sen}+\text{Spe}),$$

where TP and TN denote the number of true positives and true negatives, respectively, and FP and FN denote the number of false positives and false negatives, respectively. Moreover, we additionally report the ROC curves and area under ROC curve (AUC).

We compare our algorithm with several AS-OCT screening and deep learning methods: (1) The clinical-based screening method in [2], which segments the AS-OCT image and calculates several clinical parameters. A linear SVM is added to determine a screening result from the parameters. (2) The visual feature-based screening method in [17], which localizes the ACA based on geometric structure and extracts histograms of oriented gradients (HOG) features to classify the glaucoma subtype. The HOG features are computed on a 150×150 region centered on the ACA, and the classification result is obtained using a linear SVM. (3) The multi-column deep model in [1], which is a state-of-the-art deep learning model with different receptive field sizes for each stream. For our algorithm, we show not only the final screening result (Our MCDN), but also provide results obtained without the clinical parameters (Our MCDN w/o CP), and the individual stream result for the global fundus image (Global Image) and for the local disc region (Local Region). The results are reported in Table 1 and Fig. 3.

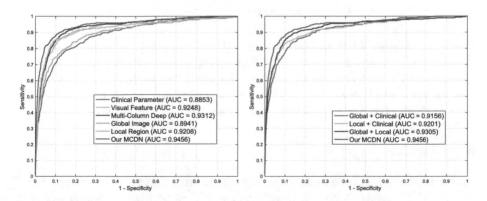

Fig. 3. ROC curves with AUC scores on the Visante AS-OCT dataset.

Clinical parameters are defined by anatomical structure, and most of them have a specific physical significance that clinicians take into consideration in making a diagnosis. By contrast, visual features can represent a wider set of image

Table 1. Performance of different methods on the Visante AS-OCT dataset.

	AUC	B-Accuracy	Sensitivity	Specificity
Clinical Parameter	0.8853	0.8198	0.7914	0.8483
Visual Feature	0.9248	0.8688	0.8503	0.8872
Multi-Column	0.9312	0.8802	0.8821	0.8783
Global Image	0.8941	0.8286	0.7846	0.8726
Local Region	0.9208	0.8790	0.8526	**0.9055**
Global + Clinical	0.9156	0.8508	0.8322	0.8694
Local + Clinical	0.9201	0.8657	0.8322	0.8992
Global + Local	0.9305	0.8786	0.8617	0.8955
Our MCDN	**0.9456**	**0.8926**	**0.8889**	0.8963

properties, beyond what clinicians recognize as relevant. Thus visual features perform better than clinical parameters as expected, and achieve 0.9248 AUC score. The deep learning based Global Image applied to full AS-OCT images does not work well with only 0.8941 AUC. A possible reason for this is that although learned discriminative features are more powerful than handcrafted visual features, they are learned in this case over the entire AS-OCT image. By contrast, the Local Region results in performance similar to handcrafted visual features. For the multi-column deep model [1], the shallow layers can be easier to optimize, giving better results than visual features. Our MCDN outperforms the other baselines, demonstrating that the proposed fusion of significant clinical regions is effective for angle-closure glaucoma screening. Moreover, we also observe that the combination with clinical parameters leads to an obvious improvement, as the AUC score increases from 0.9305 to 0.9456.

Running Time: We implement our MCDN system using the publicly available TensorFlow Library. Each stream is fine-tuned from an initialization with the pre-trained VGG-16 deep model in [14]. The entire fine-tuning phase takes about 5 hours on a single NVIDIA K40 GPU (200 iterations). In testing, it takes 500 ms to output the final screening result for a single AS-OCT image.

4   Conclusion

In this paper, we propose an automatic angle-closure glaucoma screening method for AS-OCT imagery via deep learning. A multi-context deep network architecture is proposed to learn discriminative representations on particular regions of different scales. Experiments on a clinical AS-OCT dataset show that our method outperforms the existing screening methods and other state-of-the-art deep architectures. Our MCDN architecture arises from the use of clinical prior knowledge in designing the deep network, and the intensity-based augmentation can also be used in other OCT-based applications.

References

1. Ciregan, D., Meier, U., Schmidhuber, J.: Multi-column deep neural networks for image classification. In: CVPR, pp. 3642–3649 (2012)
2. Fu, H., Cheng, J., Xu, Y., Wong, D., Liu, J., Cao, X.: Joint optic disc and cup segmentation based on multi-label deep network and polar transformation. IEEE Trans. Med. Imaging **37**(7), 1597–1605 (2018)
3. Fu, H., et al.: Disc-aware ensemble network for glaucoma screening from fundus image. IEEE Trans. Med. Imaging (2018)
4. Fu, H., Xu, Y., Lin, S., Wong, D.W.K., Liu, J.: DeepVessel: Retinal Vessel Segmentation via Deep Learning and Conditional Random Field. In: MICCAI, pp. 132–139 (2016)
5. Fu, H., et al.: Segmentation and quantification for angle-closure glaucoma assessment in anterior segment OCT. IEEE Trans. Med. Imaging **36**(9), 1930–1938 (2017)
6. Fu, H., et al.: Automatic anterior chamber angle structure segmentation in AS-OCT image based on label transfer. In: EMBC, pp. 1288–1291 (2016)
7. Girshick, R., Donahue, J., Darrell, T., Malik, J.: Rich feature hierarchies for accurate object detection and semantic segmentation. In: CVPR (2014)
8. Gulshan, V., Peng, L., Coram, M., et al.: Development and validation of a deep learning algorithm for detection of diabetic retinopathy in retinal fundus photographs. J. Am. Med. Assoc. **304**(6), 649–656 (2016)
9. Ioffe, S., Szegedy, C.: Batch normalization: accelerating deep network training by reducing internal covariate shift. In: ICML, pp. 448–456 (2015)
10. Krizhevsky, A., Sutskever, I., Hinton, G.: Imagenet classification with deep convolutional neural networks. In: NIPS (2012)
11. LeCun, Y., Bengio, Y., Hinton, G.: Deep learning. Nature **521**(7553), 436–444 (2015)
12. Leung, C., Weinreb, R.: Anterior chamber angle imaging with optical coherence tomography. Eye **25**(3), 261–267 (2011)
13. Nongpiur, M., Haaland, B., Friedman, D., et al.: Classification algorithms based on anterior segment optical coherence tomography measurements for detection of angle closure. Ophthalmology **120**(1), 48–54 (2013)
14. Simonyan, K., Zisserman, A.: Very deep convolutional networks for large-scale image recognition. arXiv 1409.1556 (2014)
15. Tian, J., Marziliano, P., Baskaran, M., Wong, H., Aung, T.: Automatic anterior chamber angle assessment for HD-OCT images. IEEE Trans. Biomed. Eng. **58**(11), 3242–3249 (2011)
16. Wu, R., Nongpiur, M., He, M., et al.: Association of narrow angles with anterior chamber area and volume measured with anterior-segment optical coherence tomography. Arch. Ophthalmol. **129**(5), 569–574 (2011)
17. Xu, Y., et al.: Automated anterior chamber angle localization and glaucoma type classification in OCT images. In: EMBC, pp. 7380–7383 (2013)
18. Xu, Y., et al.: Anterior chamber angle classification using multiscale histograms of oriented gradients for glaucoma subtype identification. In: EMBC, pp. 3167–3170 (2012)

Analysis of Morphological Changes of Lamina Cribrosa Under Acute Intraocular Pressure Change

Mathilde Ravier[1]([✉]), Sungmin Hong[1], Charly Girot[2], Hiroshi Ishikawa[3], Jenna Tauber[3], Gadi Wollstein[3], Joel Schuman[3], James Fishbaugh[1], and Guido Gerig[1]

[1] Department of Computer Science, Tandon School of Engineering, Brooklyn, NY, USA
{mor244,gerig}@nyu.edu
[2] Department of Computer Science, CPE Lyon School of Engineering, Lyon, France
[3] Department of Ophthalmology, Langone Medical Center, New York City, NY, USA

Abstract. Glaucoma is the second leading cause of blindness worldwide. Despite active research efforts driven by the importance of diagnosis and treatment of the optic degenerative neuropathy, the relationship between structural and functional changes along the glaucomateous evolution are still not clearly understood. Dynamic changes of the lamina cribrosa (LC) in the presence of intraocular pressure (IOP) were suggested to play a significant role in optic nerve damage, which motivates the proposed research to explore the relationship of changes of the 3D structure of the LC collagen meshwork to clinical diagnosis. We introduce a framework to quantify 3D dynamic morphological changes of the LC under acute IOP changes in a series of swept-source optical coherence tomography (SS-OCT) scans taken under different pressure states. Analysis of SS-OCT images faces challenges due to low signal-to-noise ratio, anisotropic resolution, and observation variability caused by subject and ocular motions. We adapt unbiased diffeomorphic atlas building which serves multiple purposes critical for this analysis. Analysis of deformation fields yields desired global and local information on pressure-induced geometric changes. Deformation variability, estimated with repeated images of a healthy volunteer without IOP elevation, is found to be a magnitude smaller than pressure-induced changes and thus illustrates feasibility of the proposed framework. Results in a clinical study with healthy, glaucoma suspect, and glaucoma subjects demonstrate the potential of the proposed method for non-invasive in vivo analysis of LC dynamics, potentially leading to early prediction and diagnosis of glaucoma.

1 Introduction

Glaucoma is the second leading cause of blindness and visual morbidity worldwide [9]. The optic degenerative neuropathy, characterized by a high eye pressure that damages the optic nerve, is challenging to treat as it has no apparent

© Springer Nature Switzerland AG 2018
A. F. Frangi et al. (Eds.): MICCAI 2018, LNCS 11071, pp. 364–371, 2018.
https://doi.org/10.1007/978-3-030-00934-2_41

symptoms before vision loss. Because damage is irreversible, timely diagnosis of disease and tracking its progression are of paramount importance. Structural deformation of the lamina cribrosa (LC), a connective tissue located in the optic nerve head, is suggested to play an important role in glaucomateous damage [4]. The LC is a collagen meshwork where all retinal axons pass through to the brain. Despite the importance of analyzing structural changes of the LC, there has not been any previous study analyzing full 3D changes of the LC which would give clinicians new insight into the pathology of the disease.

Previous studies of the LC structure generally used *ex vivo* or animals experiments [6,10]. Recently, with the progress of swept-source optical coherence tomography (SS-OCT), a few studies made use of the microscopic resolution imaging of the *in vivo* human LC. Previous studies showed promising results on 3D SS-OCT images for structural analysis of the LC, but results required extensive manual interactions and had aspects of the analysis limited to 2D [7,12], impeded by challenges in SS-OCT imaging such as scan variability due to subject and ocular motions, low signal-to-noise ratio, and an anisotropic voxel size [8]. In [3], a computational framework was proposed to analyze the deformation of the LC but analysis was limited to a single case without a validation study.

In this paper, we propose an unified framework to characterize morphological changes of micro-structures of the human LC *in vivo* by carefully selecting image analysis approaches to tackle the major challenges. This includes image denoising [2], image resampling [11], rigid alignment, and deformation-based analysis. The methodology is tested and validated in intraocular (IOP) experiments for comparative analysis between normal, glaucoma suspect, and glaucoma subjects.

We adopt unbiased diffeomorphic atlas building [5] to construct subject-specific LC atlases, which results in a deformable mapping of the series of pressure-state images to study pressure induced 3D structural changes of the LC, and to quantify delicate interactions of the LC micro-structures as a function of pressure. Variability of imaging and image analysis is assessed with repeated scans of a healthy volunteer without pressure.

2   Methods

2.1   IOP Experiment Setup

To analyze the structural changes induced by IOP elevation, an ophthalmo-dynamometer device was used to apply controlled pressure on the temporal sclera. Anesthetized eyes were imaged twice at baseline, 30g load of ophthalmo-dynamometer, and recovery after five minutes from IOP elevation. All subjects were scanned with a prototype SS-OCT system. Each 3D volume has a field-of-view of $3.5 \times 3.5 \times 1.6mm^3$ with $400 \times 400 \times 861$ voxel resolution. Clinical experts first assessed data quality to exclude severely corrupted images after intra-volume motion artifact correction and also images where the LC area was not fully visible.

2.2   Image Preprocessing

Image Resampling: Images from the prototype SS-OCT imaging system have anisotropic voxel dimensions, $8.75 \times 1.86 \times 8.75 \ \mu m^3$. This anisotropy may lead to incorrect results from 3D image processing methods which assume isotropic voxel grids. We applied B-spline image resampling [11] to up-sample images to an isotropic $2 \times 2 \times 2 \ \mu m^3$ voxel grid.

Noise Reduction: In order to overcome the speckle noise pattern inherent in OCT images, we make use of previously reported results in [3] where six filtering methods for OCT images were tested and compared. We therefore applied the best performing method, the block matching and 3D filtering (BM3D) method [2]. BM3D is based on a collaborative Wiener filtering on 3D groups of 2D image segments. This method preserves detail in local structures in images while reducing speckle noise.

Rigid Intrasubject Image Alignment: One major challenge of the analysis is to cope with patient and intra-ocular motions over the longitudinal series of scans and also scanning variability. Second, the SS-OCT images have a large field of view which covers the entire area of the optic nerve head. To constrain the analysis to the LC, images of a subject were rigidly aligned to correct for motion, and cropped to a region-of-interest of the LC area. Clinical experts define the best quality baseline image as a target reference for rigid alignment of the series.

2.3   Unbiased Atlas Building

To capture dynamic 3D structural changes, we adopt an unbiased diffeomorphic atlas building method [1,5] to create an atlas of each pressure state, baseline, IOP elevation ($30 \ mmHg$), and post pressure recovery, and finally an overall subject-specific atlas. Here, we follow a two-step procedure to overcome low SNR of high-resolution images from the experimental OCT device. For each of the three pressure states, a pressure specific template was estimated from two repeated scans. These pressure specific templates then form the basis for estimating a subject-specific unbiased atlas (Fig. 1). This two-step procedure enables us to improve the image quality of each pressure state under assumption that structural property of same pressure state is homogeneous.

The diffeomorphisms h_1, h_2, and h_3 that map the pressure state averages to the template encode the structural changes as deviations from average. Also, the inverse of $\mathbf{h}$ will be used to map structural information extracted from the atlas to each pressure state, e.g. masking of the LC area. Deformations from baseline to different pressure states are computed directly by composition of diffeomorphisms. For example, deformation from baseline to IOP elevation $\phi_{IOP} = h_2^{-1} \circ h_1$ and from baseline to recovery $\phi_{recovery} = h_3^{-1} \circ h_1$ were finally used for comparative analysis between clinical groups.

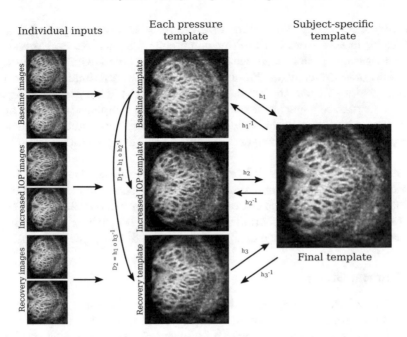

Fig. 1. Overview of subject-specific template construction. Repeated images for each pressure state are used to estimated pressure specific templates, which are used in turn to estimate the final template. Deformations between pressure state averages are calculated by composition of diffeomorphisms.

3   Results

3.1   Validation

We first assessed the stability and repeatability of our method using repeated SS-OCT images. Thirteen repeated scans of a healthy volunteer were acquired.

Scanning Stability: There is inherent scanning variability of the prototype SS-OCT imaging even for the same subject under patient's eyes during scanning and alignment of eyes to an OCT imaging sensor relies on manual adjustment by a technician. To analyze variability of SS-OCT scans, we estimated a template utilizing all 13 images and calculated the magnitude of deformation from template to each image. The deformation can be considered as the square root of Fréchet variance analogous to standard deviation of a scalar data. The Fréchet variance calculated the geometrical variance of all 13 images from a same subject at same baseline state to show the inherent variability of SS-OCT image scans at a same condition.

This study showed low magnitude (mean of 0.006 ± 0.003 mm) of deformation and consistent deformation distribution, indicating that the LC structure in each imaged LC is similar.

Framework Stability: We further assess stability by mimicking the IOP experiment using images from the healthy volunteer under no external pressure, to establish baseline performance without the added complexity of subject variability and pressure changes. From the 13 images, we randomly selected 6 and randomly assigned them to "pressure states" (2 each). This process is repeated 10 times. "Pressure" specific templates and overall templates are estimated as before (Sect. 2.3). Thus, in this validation experiment, the magnitude of deformation represents structural changes due only to scanning variability or ambiguity introduced by our processing.

The average magnitude of deformation of all sets was 0.007 mm with standard deviation 0.003 mm. Mean and standard deviation show that the magnitude of deformation is lower than the one caused by IOP elevation (0.014 ± 0.006 mm). It also shows that the deformation of recovery images (0.009 ± 0.004 mm) from baseline images are in a range of the deformations of the repeated scans.

3.2   Clinical Study

Twenty-two subjects, two healthy, twelve glaucoma, and eight suspect (structural changes in anatomy without vision loss), were scanned using the swept source 3D OCT system. Each subject was imaged as follows: 2 scans at baseline, at increased IOP ($30\ mmHg$) induced by an ophthalmodynameter, at post pressure, after 5 min of recovery. All images underwent an expert quality control where scans corrupted by motion were excluded. When two scans at each pressure state were not available after the quality control, we used a single image in place of a pressure specific template. For both global and local analysis, we used the deformation fields to quantify the deformation that maps the three pressure states into correspondence. Those deformation fields were estimated by composition of the diffeomorphic maps that transform every input image to the average in the template construction.

Global Analysis: Distribution of Deformation Magnitude. To study the global behavior of the LC structure, we calculated the magnitude of deformation from baseline to increased IOP and from baseline to recovery for every subject. We restricted those deformations by masking them to the visible LC only. The results were visualized with histograms.

We plot the distribution of deformation magnitudes integrated over the LC volume to compare changes at different pressure states. Figure 2 illustrates the examples of single subjects from healthy and glaucoma groups. Those subjects show a larger deformation for IOP (in yellow) than for post pressure recovery (in purple). Among the 22 subjects, 21 showed this pattern.

We also compared the distribution of deformation magnitude of all subjects at elevated IOP and studied the distributions of the means of deformation. Figure 3 illustrates those results with respect to the three groups. Due to the limited sample size, the comparison at elevated IOP between the different groups does not lead to any clinical conclusion. However, we can clearly see that elevated IOP has a larger deformation than recovery over the groups (left side figure). This

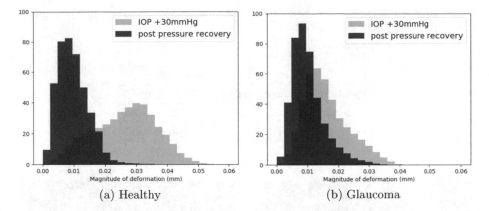

(a) Healthy   (b) Glaucoma

Fig. 2. Single subject examples. Histograms represent distribution of the magnitude of deformation at elevated IOP (yellow) and post pressure recovery (purple) for a healthy and a glaucoma subject. Both subjects show larger deformation at elevated IOP than at recovery.

indicates that the experimental setup and analysis methodology are sensitive to tissue response to pressure and may serve as an *in-vivo* diagnostic or monitoring procedure well suited for routine clinical practice.

Table 1 represents the means of the deformations and their standard deviations for healthy, glaucoma suspect, and glaucoma subjects at elevated IOP and recovery. The healthy group shows a larger difference between elevated IOP and recovery than the other groups. This may indicate that the LC becomes stiffer when glaucoma appears.

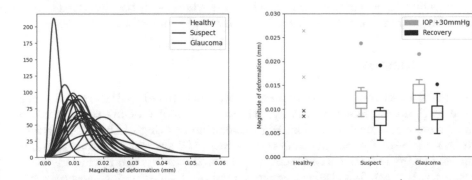

Fig. 3. Group-wise study. Left) Comparison of the distribution of deformation magnitude at elevated IOP for all subjects (green: healthy, blue: suspect, red: glaucoma). Right) The shape of the distribution of the means of deformation magnitude by groups of subjects. Elevated IOP and recovery statistics are represented in yellow and purple, respectively. The healthy group is being composed of two subjects so that the statistics is displayed as dots.

Table 1. Means and standard deviations of deformation magnitude (in mm) per groups of subjects and per pressure states.

Group	Pressure	
	IOP +30 $mmHg$	Recovery
Healthy	0.0216 ± 0.009	0.0091 ± 0.005
Suspect	0.0129 ± 0.006	0.0089 ± 0.004
Glaucoma	0.0128 ± 0.005	0.0095 ± 0.005

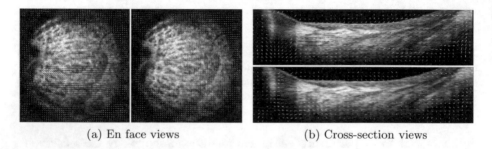

(a) En face views   (b) Cross-section views

Fig. 4. Images of a glaucoma case with local deformations overlaid with the structure of the LC. For each view, the deformations at elevated IOP (left, up) and recovery (right, bottom) are represented.

Local Analysis: Maps of Deformation. Local deformations are seen as maps of deformations overlaid with the structure of the LC (Fig. 4). The arrows show different directions and different lengths which indicate parts of the structure expand while others contract. Interestingly, the whole LC is not deformed homogeneously, rather it is characterized by patterns of local deformations.

4   Conclusions

This paper describes the development of an image-based system to study the cause of glaucoma based on the hypothesis that rigidity of LC contributes to glaucomateous damage to axons. High resolution imaging of the LC structure requires the use of a prototype swept source OCT system. Whereas previous studies mostly reported assessment based on 2D methods on selected cross-sections, this is the first study to make full use of 3D imaging for measurements of pressure-induced deformations. The contribution of this work is a systematic approach to determine best performing methods which were tested and validated to overcome the challenges of image quality and patient and intra-ocular motions over longitudinal scans, moreover as pressure was induced to the eye via an external device. Given the clinical hypothesis and available OCT images from an experimental scanner, unbiased atlas-building was chosen to make best use of the method's inherent capabilities, which include improved quality of the template and use of deformation maps to study global and local rigidity of the LC. Major efforts went into testing and validation, and the demonstration of feasibility in a small clinical study with three groups.

The proposed method captures subtle global and local structural changes in the LC under elevated IOP and recovery. The experimental setup and analysis method allows quantitative study of LC structure dynamics that has the potential to provide clinically useful biomarkers for glaucoma assessment.

Acknowledgements. This research was supported by NIH R01-EY013178 and EY025011.

References

1. Avants, B.B., Tustison, N., Song, G.: Advanced normalization tools (ANTs). Insight J. **2**, 1–35 (2009)
2. Dabov, K., Foi, A., Katkovnik, V., Egiazarian, K.: Image denoising by sparse 3-D transform-domain collaborative filtering. IEEE Trans. Image Process. **16**(8), 2080–2095 (2007)
3. Girot, C., Ishikawa, H., Fishbaugh, J., Wollstein, G., Schuman, J., Gerig, G.: Spatiotemporal analysis of structural changes of the lamina cribrosa. In: Cardoso, M.J., et al. (eds.) FIFI/OMIA-2017. LNCS, vol. 10554, pp. 185–193. Springer, Cham (2017). https://doi.org/10.1007/978-3-319-67561-9_21
4. Inoue, R., et al.: Three-dimensional high-speed optical coherence tomography imaging of lamina cribrosa in glaucoma. Ophthalmology **116**(2), 214–222 (2009)
5. Joshi, S., Davis, B., Jomier, M., Gerig, G.: Unbiased diffeomorphic atlas construction for computational anatomy. NeuroImage **23**, S151–S160 (2004)
6. Lee, E.J., Choi, Y.J., Kim, T.W., Hwang, J.M.: Comparison of the deep optic nerve head structure between normal-tension glaucoma and nonarteritic anterior ischemic optic neuropathy. PloS ONE **11**(4), e0150242 (2016)
7. Nadler, Z., et al.: In vivo three-dimensional characterization of the healthy human lamina cribrosa with adaptive optics spectral-domain optical coherence tomography. Invest. Ophthalmol. Vis. Sci. **55**(10), 6459–6466 (2014)
8. Ortiz, S., et al.: Optical distortion correction in optical coherence tomography for quantitative ocular anterior segment by three-dimensional imaging. Opt. Express **18**(3), 2782–2796 (2010)
9. Quigley, H.A., Broman, A.T.: The number of people with glaucoma worldwide in 2010 and 2020. Br. J. Ophthalmol. **90**(3), 262–267 (2006)
10. Sigal, I.A., Wang, B., Strouthidis, N.G., Akagi, T., Girard, M.J.: Recent advances in OCT imaging of the lamina cribrosa. Br. J. Ophthalmol. **98**(Suppl 2), ii34–ii39 (2014)
11. Unser, M., Aldroubi, A., Eden, M.: Fast B-spline transforms for continuous image representation and interpolation. IEEE Trans. Patt. Anal. Mach. Intell. **13**(3), 277–285 (1991)
12. Wollstein, G., et al.: Optical coherence tomography longitudinal evaluation of retinal nerve fiber layer thickness in glaucoma. Arch. Ophthalmol. **123**(4), 464–470 (2005)

Beyond Retinal Layers: A Large Blob Detection for Subretinal Fluid Segmentation in SD-OCT Images

Zexuan Ji[1]($\boxtimes$), Qiang Chen[1]($\boxtimes$), Menglin Wu[2], Sijie Niu[3], Wen Fan[4], Songtao Yuan[4], and Quansen Sun[1]

[1] School of Computer Science and Engineering, Nanjing University of Science and Technology, Nanjing, China
{jizexuan,chen2qiang}@njust.edu.cn
[2] School of Computer Science and Technology, Nanjing Tech University, Nanjing, China
[3] School of Information Science and Engineering, University of Jinan, Jinan, China
[4] Department of Ophthalmology, The First Affiliated Hospital with Nanjing Medical University, Nanjing, China

Abstract. Purpose: To automatically segment neurosensory retinal detachment (NRD)-associated subretinal fluid in spectral domain optical coherence tomography (SD-OCT) images by constructing a Hessian-based Aggregate generalized Laplacian of Gaussian algorithm without the use of retinal layer segmentation. **Methods:** The B-scan is first filtered into small blob candidate regions based on local convexity by aggregating the log-scale-normalized convolution responses of each individual gLoG filter. Two Hessian-based regional features are extracted based on the aggregate response map. Pooling with regional intensity, the feature vectors are fed into an unsupervised clustering algorithm. By voting the blob candidates into the superpixels, the initial subretinal fluid regions are obtained. Finally, an active contour with narrowband implementation is utilized to obtain integrated segmentations. **Results:** The testing data set with 23 longitudinal SD-OCT cube scans from 12 eyes of 12 patients are used to evaluate the proposed algorithm. Comparing with two independent experts' manual segmentations, our algorithm obtained a mean true positive volume fraction 95.15%, positive predicative value 93.65% and dice similarity coefficient 94.35%, respectively. **Conclusions:** Without retinal layer segmentation, the proposed algorithm can produce higher segmentation accuracy comparing with state-of-the-art methods that relied on retinal layer segmentation results. Our model may provide reliable subretinal fluid segmentations for NRD from SD-OCT images.

Keywords: Spectral domain optical coherence tomography
Subretinal fluid segmentation · Neurosensory retinal detachment
Blob segmentation

This work was supported by the Natural Science Foundation of Jiangsu Province under Grant No. BK20180069, and the National Natural Science Foundation of China under Grants Nos. 61671242, 61701192, 61701222 and 61473310.

© Springer Nature Switzerland AG 2018
A. F. Frangi et al. (Eds.): MICCAI 2018, LNCS 11071, pp. 372–380, 2018.
https://doi.org/10.1007/978-3-030-00934-2_42

1   Introduction

As a chronic disease, central serous chorioretinopathy (CSCR) is one of the leading causes of vision threat among middle-aged male individuals, in which serous retinal detachments such as neurosensory retinal detachment (NRD) are generally presented and treated as a prominent characteristic of CSCR. Spectral-domain optical coherence tomography (SD-OCT) imaging technology can generate 3D cubes and provide more detailed characteristics of disease phenotypes, which has become an important imaging modality for the diagnosis and treatment of CSCR [1]. Because retinal detachment is the separation of the neurosensory retina (NSR) from the underlying retinal pigment epithelium (RPE), state-of-the-art algorithms principally segment NRD regions based on layer segmentation results. For example, Wang et al. [2] utilized fuzzy level-set method to identify the boundaries. Wu et al. [3] presented an OCT Enface fundus-driven subretinal fluid segmentation method. Semi-supervised segmentation methods have also been utilized. Zheng et al. [4] used computerized segmentation combining with minimal expert interaction. Wang et al. [5] proposed a slice-wise label propagation algorithm. Supervised machine learning methods, including random forest [6] and deep learning model [7], have been introduced by treating the fluid segmentation as a binary classification problem. However, most state-of-the-art algorithms rely on the accuracy of retinal layer segmentations.

Because the subretinal fluid in SD-OCT images are typically darker than the surroundings, they can be treated as blob-like structures, which can be efficiently dealt with blob detection algorithms based on scale-space theory. One of the most widely used blob detection algorithm is Laplacian of Gaussian (LoG). The generalized Laplacian of the Gaussian (gLoG) [8] is developed to detect asymmetric structures. To further explore the convexity and elliptic shape of the blobs, Hessian-based LoG (HLoG) [9] and Hessian-based Difference of Gaussians (HDoG) [10] are proposed. Most algorithms mentioned above need to detect the candidate blobs by finding the local optimal within a large range of multi-scale Gaussian scale-space, which is, however, time consuming and sensitive to noise.

In this paper, an unsupervised blob segmentation algorithm is proposed to segment subretinal fluid in SD-OCT images. First, a Hessian-based aggregate generalized Laplacian of Gaussian (HAgLoG) algorithm is proposed by aggregating the log-scale-normalized convolution responses of each individual gLoG filter. Second, two regional features, i.e. blobness and flatness, are extracted based on the aggregate response map. Third, together with the intensity values, the features are fed into the variational Bayesian Gaussian mixture model (VBGMM) [11] to obtain the blob candidates which are voted into the superpixels to get the initial subretinal fluid regions. Finally, an active contours driven by local likelihood image fitting energy (LLIF) [12] with narrowband implementation is utilized to obtain integrated segmentations. Without retinal layer segmentation, the proposed algorithm can obtain higher segmentation accuracy compared to the state-of-the-art methods that rely on the retinal layer segmentation results.

2   Methodology

Figure 1 illustrates the pipeline of our framework. In the preprocessing phase, the B-scan as shown in Fig. 1(a) is firstly smoothed with bilateral filter as shown in Fig. 1(b). Then a mean value based threshold is used to get the region of interest (ROI) as shown in Fig. 1(c). Based on the denoised result, the proposed HAgLoG is carried out with the following three phases: (1) aggregate response construction, (2) Hessian analysis, and (3) post-pruning with VBGMM and LLIF.

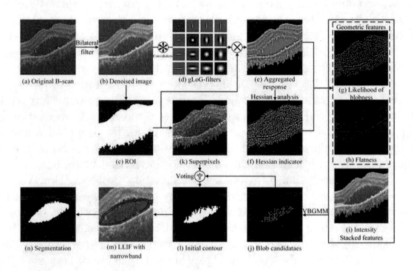

Fig. 1. The pipeline of the proposed automatic subretinal fluid segmentation method.

2.1   Aggregate Response Construction

A blob is a region in an image that is darker (or brighter) than its surroundings with consistent intensity inside. Because the NRD in SD-OCT images are typically darker than the surroundings, in this paper, we only consider the blob with brighter surroundings. We modify the general Gaussian function by setting the kernel angle as 0. Based on the general Gaussian function in Ref. [8], let $G(x, y, \sigma_x, \sigma_y)$ be the 2-D modified general Gaussian function defined as:

$$G(x, y, \sigma_x, \sigma_y) = Ae^{-((\sigma_y^2 x^2 + \sigma_x^2 y^2)/2\sigma_x^2 \sigma_y^2)} \tag{1}$$

where A is a normalization factor, and σ_x and σ_y are the scales on the x-axis and y-axis directions, respectively. The coordinates of the kernel center are set as zeros without losing generality. Based on Ref. [8], for the 2-D image f, the modified gLoG-filter (as shown in Fig. 1(d)) image $\triangledown^2 I(x, y, \sigma_x, \sigma_y)$ can be represented as

$$\triangledown^2 I(x, y, \sigma_x, \sigma_y) = [\triangledown^2 G(x, y, \sigma_x, \sigma_y)] * f(x, y) \tag{2}$$

where $\bigtriangledown^2$ denotes the Laplacian operator, $*$ is the convolution operation. To further improve the estimation accuracy, the convolution response is log-scale normalized [8]:

$$l = (1 + \log(\sigma_x)^\alpha)(1 + \log(\sigma_y)^\alpha) \bigtriangledown^2 I(x, y, \sigma_x, \sigma_y) \tag{3}$$

Finally, as shown in Fig. 1(e), the aggregated response map L is obtained by summing up all intermediate response maps:

$$L(x, y) = \sum_{\sigma_x, \sigma_y} \left[(1 + \log(\sigma_x)^\alpha)(1 + \log(\sigma_y)^\alpha) \bigtriangledown^2 I(x, y, \sigma_x, \sigma_y) \right] \tag{4}$$

2.2 Hessian Analysis

For a pixel (x, y) in the aggregated response L, the Hessian matrix is

$$H\left(L(x, y)\right) = \left[\frac{\partial^2 L(x, y)}{\partial x^2} \quad \frac{\partial^2 L(x, y)}{\partial x \partial y}; \quad \frac{\partial^2 L(x, y)}{\partial x \partial y} \quad \frac{\partial^2 L(x, y)}{\partial y^2} \right] \tag{5}$$

Therefore, we can identify the dark blobs using the following proposition.

Proposition. In an aggregated response 2D image, every pixel of a dark blob has a positive definite Hessian matrix.

Proof. The Ref [13] provided detailed relationships between the eigenvalues of Hessian matrix and geometric shape. Specifically, if a pixel belongs to a dark blob-like structure, all the eigenvalues of the corresponding Hessian matrix are positive, that is, the Hessian matrix of the pixel is positive definite.

However, the above proposition is a necessary but not sufficient property to determine the dark blobs. To further reduce the false detection, similar with Ref. [9], we give the following definition.

Definition. A blob candidate in aggregated response image is a 8-connected component of set $U = \{(x, y) \| (x, y) \in L(x, y), T(x, y) = 1\}$, where $T(x, y)$ is the binary indicator: if the pixel has a positive definite Hessian matrix, then $T(x, y) = 1$; otherwise, $T(x, y) = 0$.

Instead of determining the positive matrix with eigenvalues of H(L(x,y)), we utilize the Sylvester's criterion, which is a necessary and sufficient criterion, to determine whether a Hermitian matrix is positive-definite. In our Hessian matrix, the leading principal minors are $D_1 = \partial^2 L(x, y)/\partial x^2$ and $D_2 = (\partial^2 L(x, y)/\partial x^2)(\partial^2 L(x, y)/\partial y^2) - (\partial^2 L(x, y)/\partial x \partial y)^2$. Therefore, the Hessian matrix is positive definite if and only if $D_1 > 0$ and $D_2 > 0$. As a result, based on Proposition and Definition, we can obtain the dark blob candidates with the two leading principal minors of Hessian matrix as shown in Fig. 1(f).

Based on the eigenvalues λ_1 and λ_2, Refs. [9,13] defined two geometric features for blob detection: the likelihood of blobness R_B and the second-order structureness (flatness) S_B as:

$$R_B = 2\lambda_1\lambda_2/(\lambda_1^2 + \lambda_2^2) = 2det(H(L))/(trace(H(L))^2 - 2det(H(L))) \tag{6}$$

$$S_B = \sqrt{\lambda_1^2 + \lambda_2^2} = \sqrt{trace(H(L))^2 - 2det(H(L))} \tag{7}$$

where $0 < R_B \leq 1$, when $\lambda_1 = \lambda_2$, $R_B = 1$. $0 < S_B \leq 1$. The higher S_B is the more salient the blob is against the local background [10]. Both features are shown in Fig. 1(g) and (h), respectively.

2.3   Post-pruning

The input feature space is constructed by stacking the blob features R_B and S_B with average local intensity A_B, and fed into VBGMM [11] to remove false positive detections and cluster the blob candidates into blob regions and non-blob regions as shown in Fig. 1(j). The detected blob regions are then voted into superpixels (as shown in Fig. 1(k)) obtained by simple linear iterative clustering (SLIC) [14] to get the initial subretinal fluid regions shown in Fig. 1(l). Generally, the subretinal fluid can be observed within several continuous B-scans. Therefore, the segmentation results of three adjacent slices are utilized to make sure the continuity of the subretinal fluid and remove the false detections. Finally, an active contours driven by LLIF [12] with narrowband implementation in Fig. 1(m) is utilized to obtain integrated segmentations in Fig. 1(n).

3   Results

In this paper, 23 longitudinal SD-OCT cube scans with only NRD from 12 eyes of 12 patients acquired with a Cirrus OCT device were used to evaluate the proposed algorithm. All the scans covered a $6 \times 6 \times 2\,\text{mm}^3$ area centered on the fovea with volume dimension $512 \times 128 \times 1024$. This study was approved by the Institutional Review Board (IRB) of the First Affiliated Hospital of Nanjing Medical University with informed consent. Two independent experts manually drew the outlines of NRD regions based on B-scan images, which were used to generate the segmentation ground truths.

Three criteria were utilized to evaluate the performances: true positive volume fraction (TPVF), positive predicative value (PPV) [3] and dice similarity coefficient (DSC). A linear analysis and Bland-Altman approach was applied for statistical correlation and reproducibility analyses.

Six state-of-the-art methods were compared, including a semi-supervised segmentation algorithm using label propagation and higher-order constraint (LPHC) [5], a stratified sampling k-nearest neighbor classifier based algorithm (SS-KNN) [15], a random forest classifier based method (RF) [6], a fuzzy level set with crosssectional voting (FLSCV) [2], a continuous max flow optimization-based method (CMF) [16] and an Enface fundus-driven method (EFD) [3].

In Fig. 2, five example B-scans selected from five patients were used to show the performance of the proposed model. LPHC can hardly obtain satisfactory segmentations without good initializations. SS-KNN may produce obvious false detections, and cannot guarantee the smoothness of the contour. FLSCV suffers from under segmentation, while RF suffers from false positive segmentations.

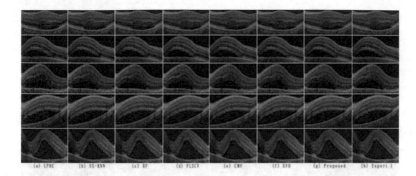

Fig. 2. Comparison of segmentation results overlaid on original B-scan images for five example cases selected from five patients. For each row, the images shown from left to right are the segmenta-tion results obtained by LPHC, SS-KNN, RF, FLSCV, CMF, EFD and the proposed algorithm. The last column shows the manually segmentation results of Expert 1.

Both CMF and EFD are sensitive to low contrast. By contrast, the proposed algorithm effectively avoid the under-segmentation and is more robust to low contrast to produce smooth and accurate segmentation results which are highly consistent with the ground truth.

To further highlight the superior performances of the proposed algorithm, Fig. 3 shows the 3-D segmentation surfaces of three example subjects selected from three different patients. Both RF and FLSCV suffer from insufficient segmentations with smaller segmentation volumes. Moreover, FLSCV may produce more misclassifications. Because of the sensitiveness to the low contrast, the surfaces obtained by CMF and EFD contains obvious protrusions. By contrast, the proposed algorithm apparently outperforms other approaches and generates the segmentation results most similar to the ground truths.

Table 1 summarizes the average quantitative results between the segmentations and manual gold standards. Overall, our model is capable of producing a higher segmentation accuracy than the other comparison methods. It should be noted both CMF and EFD rely on the layer segmentation results. Comparatively, without utilizing any layer information, our algorithm can still obtain better segmentations.

Finally, as shown in Fig. 4, a statistical correlation analysis is carried out by utilizing a linear regression analysis and Bland-Altman approach to compare the segmentation results of the proposed method with the manually segmentations from two experts. From Fig. 4(a) and (c), we can find that the proposed algorithm can produce high correlation with two experts (both $r^2 = 0.99$). The Bland-Altman plots in Fig. 4(b) and (d) also indicate stable agreement between the automated and manual segmentations.

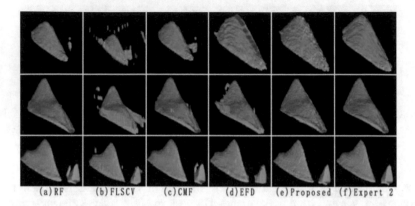

(a)RF   (b)FLSCV   (c)CMF   (d)EFD   (e)Proposed (f)Expert 2

Fig. 3. Comparison of segmentation results overlaid on three 3D example cases selected from three patients. For each row, the images shown from left to right are the segmentation surfaces obtained by RF, FLSCV, CMF, EFD and the proposed algorithm. The last column shows the manually segmentation surfaces of Expert 2.

Table 1. The summarizations of the quantitative results (mean ± standard deviation) between the segmentations and manual gold standards (two individual experts' segmentations).

Methods	Expert 1			Expert 2		
	TPVF	PPV	DSC	TPVF	PPV	DSC
LPHC [5]	81.3 ± 9.4	55.6 ± 13.3	65.3 ± 10.4	81.2 ± 9.3	55.8 ± 12.8	65.7 ± 10.5
SS-KNN [15]	80.9 ± 6.6	91.9 ± 3.8	86.1 ± 4.1	80.3 ± 6.5	91.8 ± 3.8	85.9 ± 4.1
RF [6]	92.6 ± 4.4	92.4 ± 2.0	87.1 ± 4.3	92.5 ± 4.3	91.9 ± 2.2	88.9 ± 4.2
FLSCV [2]	84.4 ± 16.0	86.2 ± 7.3	78.9 ± 21.7	84.4 ± 15.1	86.8 ± 7.3	79.4 ± 2.2
CMF [16]	92.1 ± 4.1	93.0 ± 3.4	93.9 ± 2.5	92.0 ± 3.9	94.0 ± 3.5	94.3 ± 2.6
EFD [3]	94.2 ± 5.2	93.0 ± 4.8	93.7 ± 4.0	94.5 ± 5.1	94.1 ± 5.3	94.6 ± 4.1
Proposed	**95.1 ± 2.3**	**93.1 ± 5.0**	**94.0 ± 3.1**	**95.2 ± 2.2**	**94.2 ± 4.9**	**94.7 ± 3.0**

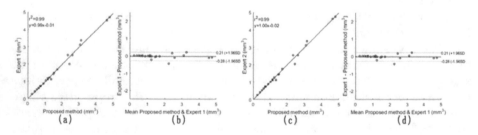

Fig. 4. Statistical correlation analysis. (a) Linear regression analysis between the proposed method and Expert 1. (b) Bland-Altman plot for the proposed method and Expert 1. (c) Linear regression analysis between the proposed method and Expert 2. (d) Bland-Altman plot for the proposed method and Expert 2.

4 Conclusion

In this paper, we propose an automatic and accurate NRD segmentation method in SD-OCT images. Our proposed model moves past the limitations that retinal layer segmentation present, is unsupervised without utilizing any training data, and automatic without using any manual interactions. Consequently, without retinal layer segmentation, the proposed algorithm can produce accurate segmentation results which are highly consistent with the ground truths. Our methods may provide reliable NRD segmentations for SD-OCT images and be useful for clinical diagnosis. Our future work mainly focus on the extension of 3D segmentation.

References

1. Teke, M.Y., et al.: Comparison of autofluorescence and optical coherence tomography findings in acute and chronic central serous chorioretinopathy. Int. J. Ophthalmol. **7**(2), 350 (2014)
2. Wang, J., et al.: Automated volumetric segmentation of retinal fluid on optical coherence tomography. BOE **7**(4), 1577–1589 (2016)
3. Wu, M., et al.: Automatic Subretinal fluid segmentation of retinal SD-OCT images with neurosensory retinal detachment guided by enface fundus imaging. IEEE-TBE **65**(1), 87–95 (2018)
4. Zheng, Y., et al.: Computerized assessment of intraretinal and subretinal fluid regions in spectral-domain optical coherence tomography images of the retina. Am. J. Ophthalmol. **155**(2), 277–286 (2013)
5. Wang, T., et al.: Label propagation and higher-order constraint-based segmentation of fluid-associated regions in retinal SD-OCT images. Info. Sci. **358**, 92–111 (2016)
6. Lang, A., et al.: Automatic segmentation of microcystic macular edema in OCT. BOE **6**(1), 155–169 (2015)
7. Xu, Y., et al.: Dual-stage deep learning framework for pigment epithelium detachment segmentation in polypoidal choroidal vasculopathy. BOE **8**(9), 4061–4076 (2017)
8. Kong, H., et al.: A generalized Laplacian of Gaussian filter for blob detection and its applications. IEEE-TCy **43**(6), 1719–1733 (2013)
9. Zhang, M., et al.: Small blob identification in medical images using regional features from optimum scale. IEEE-TBE **62**(4), 1051–1062 (2015)
10. Zhang, M., et al.: Efficient small blob detection based on local convexity, intensity and shape information. IEEE-TMI **35**(4), 1127–1137 (2016)
11. Bishop, C.M.: Pattern Recognition and Machine Learning. Springer, New York (2006)
12. Ji, Z., et al.: Active contours driven by local likelihood image fitting energy for image segmentation. Info. Sci. **301**, 285–304 (2015)
13. Frangi, A.F., Niessen, W.J., Vincken, K.L., Viergever, M.A.: Multiscale vessel enhancement filtering. In: Wells, W.M., Colchester, A., Delp, S. (eds.) MICCAI 1998. LNCS, vol. 1496, pp. 130–137. Springer, Heidelberg (1998). https://doi.org/10.1007/BFb0056195
14. Achanta, R.: SLIC superpixels compared to state-of-the-art superpixel methods. IEEE-TPAMI **34**(11), 2274–2282 (2012)

15. Xu, X., et al.: Stratified sampling voxel classification for segmentation of intrareti-nal and subretinal fluid in longitudinal clinical OCT data. IEEE-TMI **34**(7), 1616–1623 (2015)
16. Wu, M., et al.: Three-dimensional continuous max flow optimization-based serous retinal detachment segmentation in SD-OCT for central serous chorioretinopathy. BOE **8**(9), 4257–4274 (2017)

Automated Choroidal Neovascularization Detection for Time Series SD-OCT Images

Yuchun Li[1], Sijie Niu[2], Zexuan Ji[1], Wen Fan[3], Songtao Yuan[3], and Qiang Chen[1(✉)]

[1] School of Computer Science and Engineering,
Nanjing University of Science and Technology, Nanjing, China
`chen2qiang@njust.edu.cn`
[2] School of Information Science and Engineering, University of Jinan, Jinan, China
[3] Department of Ophthalmology, The First Affiliated Hospital with Nanjing Medical University, Nanjing, China

Abstract. Choroidal neovascularization (CNV), caused by new blood vessels in the choroid growing through the Bruch's membrane, is an important manifestation of terminal age-related macular degeneration (AMD). Automated CNV detection in three-dimensional (3D) spectral-domain optical coherence tomography (SD-OCT) images is still a huge challenge. This paper presents an automated CNV detection method based on object tracking strategy for time series SD-OCT volumetric images. In our proposed scheme, experts only need to manually calibrate CNV lesion area for the first moment of each patient, and then the CNV of the following moments will be automatically detected. In order to fully represent space consistency of CNV, a 3D-histogram of oriented gradient (3D-HOG) feature is constructed for the generation of random forest model. Finally, the similarity between training and testing samples is measured for model updating. The experiments on 258 SD-OCT cubes from 12 eyes in 12 patients with CNV demonstrate that our results have a high correlation with the manual segmentations. The average of correlation coefficients and overlap ratio for CNV projection area are 0.907 and 83.96%, respectively.

Keywords: Choroidal neovascularization · 3D-HOG features
Image segmentation · Spectral-domain optical coherence tomography

1 Introduction

CNV is characterized by the abnormal growth of blood vessels in the choroid layer in age-related macular degeneration (AMD) [1]. Characterization of CNV

This work was supported by the National Natural Science Foundation of China (61671242, 61701192, 61701222, 61473310), Suzhou Industral Innovation Project (SS201759).

© Springer Nature Switzerland AG 2018
A. F. Frangi et al. (Eds.): MICCAI 2018, LNCS 11071, pp. 381–388, 2018.
https://doi.org/10.1007/978-3-030-00934-2_43

is fundamental in the diagnosis of diabetic retinopathy because it could help clinicians to objectively predict the progression of CNV or make a treatment decision. However, this characterization relies mainly on the accurate detection and their properties, such as area and length. Apart from the challenging and time-consuming, CNV owns more complicated structure characteristics [2]. Thus, effectively automated CNV detection and segmentation are able to assist CNV clinical diagnosis vastly.

Currently, the optical coherence tomography angiography (OCTA) is a novel evolving imaging technology which utilizes motion contrast to visualize retinal and choroidal vessels. It can provide more distinct vascular network that is used to visualize and detect CNV [3]. Additionally, several CNV segmentation methods only target at fluorescein angiography (FA) image sequences [4]. For the quantitative analysis of CNV in OCTA, Jia et al. [5] manually calculated the CNV area and flow index from two-dimensional (2D) maximum projection outer retina CNV angiogram in AMD patients. Recently, for the purpose of calculating the vessel length of CNV network in OCTA, they developed a level set method to segment neovascular vessels within detected CNV membrane, and a skeleton algorithm was applied to determine vessel centerlines [6]. Zhu et al. [7] proposed a CNV prediction algorithm based on reaction diffusion model in longitudinal OCT images. Xi et al. [8] learned local similarity prior embedding active contour model for CNV segmentation in OCT images.

Most of CNV quantitative evaluation methods above are two-dimensional (2D) and only suitable for FA [4] or OCTA [5]. In this paper, we presented an automated CNV detection method based on three-dimensional histogram of oriented gradient (3D-HOG) feature in time series spectral-domain optical coherence tomography (SD-OCT) volumetric images. In summary, our contributions in this paper can be highlighted as: (1) A CNV detection method based on object tracking strategy was proposed for time series SD-OCT images. (2) A 3D-HOG feature was constructed for CNV detection in SD-OCT volumetric images. (3) Aiming at the characteristic changes of CNV along with drug treatment and time variation, a model updating method is proposed.

2   Method

2.1   Method Overview

The whole framework of our method is shown in Fig. 1. In the stage of image pre-processing, noise removal and layer segmentation are performed on each B-scan. Consequently, we divide patches into positive and negative samples and extract 3D-HOG features. Finally, random forest is utilized to train a prediction model. In the testing phase, we first measure the similarity between the testing and training images. If they are similar, we extract 3D-HOG feature and use the trained model to directly predict the location of CNV. Otherwise, the detection results from the previous moments are utilized to update the training samples, and then to obtain the final detection results.

2.2   Preprocessing

To reduce the influence of speckle noise on the layer segmentation, this paper uses bilateral filter to remove noise. Then, we segment internal limiting membrane (ILM) and Bruch membrane (BM) layers based on gradual intensity distance to restrict the region of interest (ROI). Figure 2 shows the preprocessing, where the red and green lines are the ILM and BM layers (Fig. 2(c)), respectively. The blue rectangle in Fig. 2(d) represents the ROI, which is the minimum rectangle containing ILM and BM.

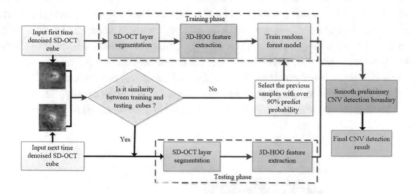

Fig. 1. Framework of the proposed method.

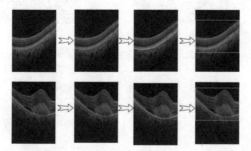

(a) Original image (b) Denoised image (c) Layer segmentation (d) Intercept area

Fig. 2. Preprocessing for one normal and one CNV (second row) SD-OCT images.

2.3   Classification of positive and negative samples

Longitudinal data from 12 eyes in 12 patients with CNV at the First Affiliated Hospital with Nanjing Medical University were included in this paper. Experts manually draw CNV region as the ground truth. The ROIs of each B-scan are extracted to construct training data using sliding window method, and then we can extract 3D HOG features from the ROIs. Experiment has proved 64×128 (width height) is the best image size for extracting HOG feature [9]. Therefore, we resize all the preprocessed images to 512×128. For the z (azimuthal) direction, the slide window size is 1, which means that three continuous B-scans are selected.

As shown in Fig. 3(a), the size of sample is $64 \times 128 \times 3$. For the x direction, the optimum step size is 16. Tiny step size will lead to high similarity between training samples, which will reduce the efficiency and increase time cost. On the contrary, it will affect the accuracy of detection. If the training sample is within the red manual division line we mark it as the positive sample. In contrast, we mark it as the negative sample (Fig. 3(b)). However, when the sliding window contains positive and negative samples (the yellow rectangle in Fig. 3(b)), we mark it as the positive sample if the number of columns containing CNV exceeds the half width of the sliding window, the negative sample or not. Based on the above procedures, we will get 3712 training samples for each SD-OCT volumetric image.

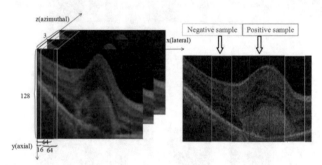

(a) Sample construction (b) Positive and negative samples

Fig. 3. Construct training samples.

2.4   3D-HOG Feature Extraction

HOG descriptors provide a dense overlapping description of image regions [9]. The main idea of HOG feature is that the appearance and shape of local objects can be well described by the directional density distribution of gradients or edges. In this paper, we extend the traditional HOG feature from 2D to 3D by considering adjacent pixel information more effectively. The basic process is as follows:

(1) Gamma space standardization. We firstly normalize the input image with Gamma standardization to adjust image contrast, reduce the influence of

local shadows, and suppress the noise interference.

$$I(x, y, z) = I(x, y, z)^{Gamma} \tag{1}$$

where Gamma is set to 0.5 here.

(2) Image gradient calculation. Then the gradient magnitude is computed by:

$$G(x, y, z) = \sqrt{G_x(x, y, z)^2 + G_y(x, y, z)^2 + G_z(x, y, z)^2} \tag{2}$$

where $G_x(x, y, z)$, $G_y(x, y, z)$ and $G_z(x, y, z)$ represent the image gradients along the x, y and z directions, respectively.

In 2D images, we only need to calculate the gradient direction in x-y plan. However, the gradient direction in x-z plan can also be calculated in 3D images. Considering computational complexity, gradient information in y-z plan is ignored. Then the gradient direction in the x-y and x-z plans are calculated as

$$\alpha(x, y) = tan^{-1}\left(\frac{G_y(x, y, z)}{G_x(x, y, z)}\right) \tag{3}$$

$$\alpha(x, z) = tan^{-1}\left(\frac{G_z(x, y, z)}{G_x(x, y, z)}\right) \tag{4}$$

(3) Construction of gradient orientation histogram. Firstly, the gradient direction of each cell will be divided into 9 directions in x-y and x-z plans. Hence, there are 81 bins of histogram to count the gradient information in each cell. In this way, each pixel in the cell is graded in the histogram with a weighted projection (mapped to a fixed angular range) to obtain a gradient histogram, that is, an 81-dimensional eigenvector corresponding to the cell. The gradient magnitude is used as the weight of the projection. Then, the feature vectors of all cells in a block are concatenated to obtain the 3D-HOG feature. Finally, 3D-HOG features from all overlapping blocks are concatenated to the ultimate features for random forest classification.

2.5   Similarity measurement and model update

For each patient, the CNV characteristic will change along with the medication and time. Therefore, it is necessary to update the trained random forest model. Since OCT volumetric images at different moments will shift, we use en face projection images rather than B-scans to measure the similarity between the training and testing cubes.

Because the brightness, contrast, and structure of the projection image will change along the diversification of CNV, structural similarity index (SSIM) [10] is suitable for similarity measure between projection images. If the similarity between the current and first projection images is larger than the average similarity, we extract 3D-HOG feature and use the trained model to directly predict the location of CNV. Otherwise, the detection results from the previous moment are utilized to construct the training samples in which the corresponding predict probability in the detection result is over 90%. Then the previous trained model is refined with new training data to obtain the final CNV detection results.

2.6   Post-processing

The width of sliding window (Fig. 3(a)) will influence the accuracy of CNV detection. If we reduce the width, the detection accuracy will also be reduced due to high similarity between training samples. To make the detected CNV boundary smoother, the tradeoff between the CNV boundaries of two adjacent cubes is taken as the new CNV boundary of the current cube.

3   Experiments

Our algorithm was implemented in Matlab and ran on a 4.0 GHz Pentium 4 PC with 16.0 GB memory. We obtained 258 SD-OCT volumetric image datasets from 12 eyes in 12 patients with CNV to quantitatively test our algorithm. The SD-OCT cubes are 512 (lateral) × 1024 (axial) × 128 (azimuthal) corresponding to a $6 \times 6 \times 2 \, mm^3$ volume centered at the retinal macular region generated with a Cirrus HD-OCT device.

We quantitatively compared our automated results with the manual segmentations drawn by expert readers. Five metrics were used to assess the CNV area differences: correlation coefficient (cc), p-value of Mann-Whitney U-test (p-value), overlap ratio (Overlap), overestimated ratio (Overest) and underestimated ratio (Underest).

3.1   Quantitative Evaluation

Table 1 shows the agreement of CNV projection area in the axial direction between our automated result and the ground truth. From Table 1, we can observe that the correlation coefficient (0.9070) and overlap ratio (83.96%) are high for CNV projection area. The low p-value (<0.05) indicates that there are significant differences in the segmented CNV projection area between our automated method and the manual rater. The overestimated ratio (8.95%) and underestimated ratio (7.10%) are similar.

Table 1. Correlation coefficients (cc), p-value, Overlap, Overestimated and Underestimated between our detections and the expert detections for CNV projection area.

cc (mean,std)	p-value	Overlap[%] (mean,std)	Overrest[%] (mean,std)	Underrest[%] (mean,std)
0.90 ± 0.082	0.016	83.96 ± 9.05	8.95 ± 6.23	7.10 ± 4.23

3.2   Qualitative Analysis

Figure 4 shows the CNV detection results in B-scan where the green transparent areas represent our automated detection results and the red lines are the manual segmentation. Due to the complex characteristic of CNV, it is difficult for the

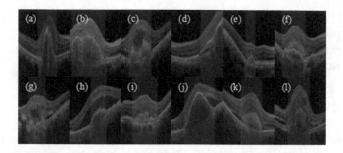

Fig. 4. CNV detection results and each image represents different example of patients.

CNV detection. However, our proposed method is effective to deal with many difficulties, such as (1) non-uniform reflectivity within CNV ((a)(c)(d)(l)), (2) blur
and obscure CNV up boundary ((c)(i)(k)(l)), (3) invisible CNV down boundary
(a)–(e) and (g)–(l), (4) influence of other retinal diseases (cystoid edema (c),
hyper-reflective foci (g), and neurosensory retinal detachment (h) (j)), and (5)
the great difference of CNV sizes ((e)(j)).

Because our detection precision is high and robust in B-scan images, we can
also obtain a relatively high segmentation precision in their projection images.
Figure 5 shows the CNV projection images collected at 25 time points of one

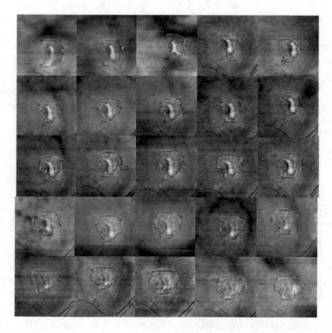

Fig. 5. CNV projection images with result of our method and expert manually for the
right eye of a patient for 25 imaging dates between 2013 and 2015.

patient in two years, corresponding to Fig. 4(a). In Fig. 5, the red lines are the manual segmentation and the green lines are our segmentation in the projection images. It can be seen from Fig. 5 that our automated CNV detection is similar with the manual segmentation.

4   Conclusions

In this paper, we presented an automated CNV detection method based on object tracking strategy for time series SD-OCT volumetric images. In order to fully represent space consistency of CNV in SD-OCT volumetric images, 3D-HOG features are conducted for CNV classification. We update random forest models persistently to make our model more robust, which can improve the accuracy of detection. According to the CNV detection results in B-scans, quantitative evaluation is performed on OCT projection images. The experiments on 258 SD-OCT volumetric images with CNV demonstrate that our method is effective and can achieve a high correlation with the manual segmentations.

References

1. Jager, R.D., Mieler, W.F., Miller, J.W.: Age-related macular degeneration. New Engl. J. Med. **358**(24), 2606–2617 (2008)
2. Donoso, L.A., Kim, D., Frost, A., Callahan, A., Hageman, G.: The role of inflammation in the pathogenesis of age-related macular degeneration. Surv. Ophthalmol. **51**(2), 137–152 (2006)
3. Miyata, M., Ooto, S., Hata, M.: Detection of myopic choroidal neovascularization using optical coherence tomography angiography. Am. J. Ophthalmol. **165**, 108–114 (2016)
4. Abdelmoula, W.M., Shah, S.M., Fahmy, A.S.: Segmentation of choroidal neovascularization in fundus fluorescein angiograms. IEEE Trans. Biomed. Eng. **60**(5), 1439–1445 (2013)
5. Jia, Y., Bailey, S.T., Wilson, D.J.: Quantitative optical coherence tomography angiography of choroidal neovascularization in age-related macular degeneration. Ophthalmology **121**(7), 1435–1444 (2014)
6. Gao, S.S., et al.: Quantificaton of choroidal neovascularization vessel length using optical coherence tomography angiography. J. Biomed. Opt. **21**(7), 76010 (2016)
7. Zhu, S., Shi, F., Xiang, D.: Choroid neovascularization growth prediction with treatment based on reaction-diffusion model in 3-D OCT images. IEEE J. Biomed. Health Inform. **21**(6), 1667 (2017)
8. Xi, X., Meng, X., et al.: Learned local similarity prior embedded active contour model for choroidal neovascularization segmentation in optical coherence tomography images. SCIENCE CHINA Inf. Sci. (2017). https://doi.org/10.1007/s11432-017-9247-8
9. Dalal, N., Triggs, B.: Histograms of oriented gradients for human detection. In: IEEE Computer Society Conference on Computer Vision and Pattern Recognition, pp. 1063–6919 (2005)
10. Wang, Z., Bovik, A.C.: Image quality assessment: from error visibility to structural similarity. IEEE Trans. Image Process. **13**(4), 1057–7149 (2004)

CapsDeMM: Capsule Network for Detection of Munro's Microabscess in Skin Biopsy Images

Anabik Pal[1(✉)], Akshay Chaturvedi[1], Utpal Garain[1], Aditi Chandra[2], Raghunath Chatterjee[2], and Swapan Senapati[3]

[1] CVPR Unit, Indian Statistical Unit, Kolkata 700108, West Bengal, India
anabikpal@gmail.com
[2] Human Genetics Unit, Indian Statistical Unit, Kolkata 700108, West Bengal, India
[3] Consultant Dermatologist, Uttarpara, Hooghly 712258, West Bengal, India

Abstract. This paper presents an approach for automatic detection of Munro's Microabscess in stratum corneum (SC) of human skin biopsy in order to realize a machine assisted diagnosis of Psoriasis. The challenge of detecting neutrophils in presence of nucleated cells is solved using the recent advances of deep learning algorithms. Separation of SC layer, extraction of patches from the layer followed by classification of patches with respect to presence or absence of neutrophils form the basis of the overall approach which is effected through an integration of a U-Net based segmentation network and a capsule network for classification. The novel design of the present capsule net leads to a drastic reduction in the number of parameters without any noticeable compromise in the overall performance. The research further addresses the challenge of dealing with Mega-pixel images (in 10X) vis-à-vis Giga-pixel ones (in 40X). The promising result coming out of an experiment on a dataset consisting of 273 real-life images shows that a practical system is possible based on the present research. The implementation of our system is available at https://github.com/Anabik/CapsDeMM.

Keywords: Psoriasis histopathology · Biopsy image · Neutrophil
Munro's microabscess · Stratum corneum
Convolutional neural network · Capsule network · Super-pixel
Segmentation · Evaluation · Dataset

1 Introduction

Psoriasis is a chronic, immune-mediated, relapsing, inflammatory skin disease with variable morphology, distribution, severity and course [2]. The prevalence of psoriasis varies 1%–12% among different populations worldwide. It is often difficult to differentiate psoriasis from other erythemato-squamous diseases like Seborrheic dermatitis, Leprosy, Lichen planus, Tinea corporis, Pityriasis, Eczema etc. [3,4,6]. Hence, histopathological examination is considered for confirmation.

© Springer Nature Switzerland AG 2018
A. F. Frangi et al. (Eds.): MICCAI 2018, LNCS 11071, pp. 389–397, 2018.
https://doi.org/10.1007/978-3-030-00934-2_44

Psoriasis develops when the immune system mistakes a normal skin cell for a pathogen and sends out faulty signals to yield the over production of new skin cells. Hence, in many cases, neutrophils and nucleated cells infiltrate into stratum corneum (SC). This infiltration occurs either in confluent (throughout the SC layer) or in focal (not confluent) manner. The presence of nucleated cells in SC is termed as parakeratosis and the accumulation of neutrophils in SC along with parakeratosis is termed as Munro's Microabscess (MM). In clinical pathology, Munro's Microabses is considered as the diagnostic hallmark of psoriasis [2].

Challenge in detecting MM lies in the fact that due to staining variation, neutrophils in stratum corneum are often misclassified as nucleated keratinocytes since both of them become dark stained. Several imaging artefacts add further challenges and thus, accurate diagnosis of skin biopsy by eye-inspection is challenging, even for highly experienced pathologists. Figure 1 illustrates the problem.

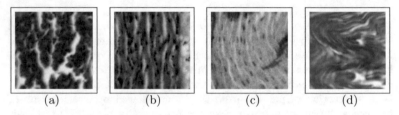

(a)   (b)   (c)   (d)

Fig. 1. Patches cropped from stratum corneum layer of WSIs. Neutrophils are circular shaped and dark blue colored. Nucleus are oval shaped and light blue colored. Here, in (a) and (b) both neutrophils and nucleated cells are present, in (c) only nucleated cells are present and in (d) neither nucleated cells nor neutrophils are present.

In the last two decades, several automatic systems are designed and developed to complement the workload of pathologists from microscopic examination of clinical tissue. But there is a dearth in automatic identification of neutrophils in biopsy images. Some research initiatives are reported for acute inflammation diagnosis [8,9] where Giga-pixel images are used.

The contributions of this paper are many folds. The pathological challenges of detection of MM in skin biopsy have been solved by developing an automated computational framework incorporating the latest advances in deep learning. The capsule network has been designed in such a way that drastically reduces the number of parameters without sacrificing performance. Mega-pixel images are used instead of usual Giga-pixel ones to reduce the computational burden and thereby supporting a low cost imaging system. Preparation of an annotated dataset of 273 whole slide skin biopsy images (WSI) is another important outcome of this research. This dataset[1] not only helps to demonstrate the efficiency of the present approach, but would also facilitate further research.

---

[1] For the dataset contact Prof. Utpal Garain (utpal@isical.ac.in).

2 Proposed Methodology

The goal of this paper is to detect Munro's Microabscess in whole slide skin biopsy images (WSI). We break down the task into three parts (i) Segmentation of SC layer, (ii) Patch extraction from SC layer and (iii) Neutrophil detection in the extracted patches. Note that we are only interested in detecting neutrophils present in the SC layer as opposed to the entire image and the SC layer lies in a small portion of the WSI image (approx. 2–15%). Hence, segmentation of SC layer followed by neutrophil detection is a logical approach. The pictorial representation of the proposed framework is shown in Fig. 2. A brief description about proposed framework is given in the following subsections.

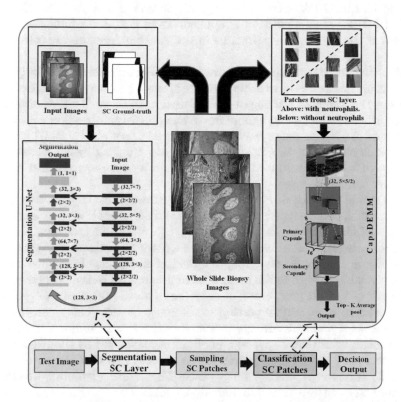

Fig. 2. Proposed system architecture. The green arrows represent convolution layer followed by ReLU activation, red arrows represent max-pooling layer, pink arrows represent up-sampling layer and dark purple arrow represent skip connection.

Stratum Corneum Segmentation. Nowadays, U-Net [5] is the state-of the art for image segmentation. We trained the U-Net given in Fig. 2 for segmenting the SC layer. Given the segmentation output $S_{x,y}$ and the corresponding ground truth $G_{x,y}$, we minimize the dice loss function L_{seg} given by

$$L_{seg} = \frac{2 \times \sum_{x,y} G_{x,y} S_{x,y}}{\sum_{x,y} G_{x,y} + \sum_{x,y} S_{x,y}} \tag{1}$$

where x, y denote the spatial coordinate of the WSI image.

Stratum Corneum Patch Selection. The stratum corneum patches should be selected in such a way that all the pixels of a patch belong to a perceptually similar region as well as their union covers the entire stratum corneum (SC). For dividing the image into perceptual regions, Simple Linear Iterative Clustering (SLIC) [1] super-pixel algorithm is applied. Then a square window around the centroids of the super-pixels which lie in the stratum corneum are selected.

CapsDeMM for Stratum Corneum Patch Classification. Recently, convolutional neural networks have achieved state of the art for several image classification tasks. But the max pooling operation used in traditional convolutional neural network architecture may ignore important spatial information cues which is undesirable. So, in this paper, recently introduced capsule network [7] is adopted for SC patch classification. Capsule network uses "routing by agreement"policy to ensure that significant spatial information in an image is not lost as we go from lower to higher layers.

The capsule network consists of two parts, namely, primary capsule and secondary capsule. We designed the capsule network in such a way that the receptive fields of the capsules in the secondary capsule avoid crowding. Crowding in capsule networks refers to the phenomenon where multiple instances of the same entity is present in the receptive field of a capsule. In such a case, the capsule is unable to encode the instantiation parameters of the concerned entity. The length of the output vector of secondary capsule denotes the probability of neutrophil in a particular portion of the image patch. There can be several neutrophils in a particular image patch. Keeping this in mind, average of the top K probabilities (top-K average pooling) is considered as the probability of neutrophil in the given image patch. Given an image patch I, let p_I denote the probability of neutrophil in the image patch. Then, during training, we minimize the binary cross entropy loss function L_{patch} given by

$$L_{patch} = -y_I * log(p_I) - (1 - y_I) * log(1 - p_I) \tag{2}$$

where y_I is 1 if the image patch contains neutrophil and 0 otherwise. This network is further referred to as CapsDeMM (**Caps**ule network for **De**tection of **M**unro's **M**icroabscess).

3   Dataset

In this research, after clinical confirmation of psoriasis, affected tissues are collected in 10% formalin under the supervision of an expert dermatologist. Formalin fixed tissues are dehydrated and embedded in paraffin blocks. Thin sections (5 μM) are used for slide preparation and then stained with hematoxylin and eosin to prepare the histopathological slides. These slides are kept under a microscope with 10X magnification and the images are collected from the microscope using a digital camera. The images are captured in 10X magnification as this is the highest magnification in which the whole biopsy sample fits adequately in the field of view of the camera. The size of the captured images are 1936 × 2584 pixels. Written informed consents were obtained from all patients before recruiting them for the study. This study is conducted after obtaining ethical approval from the 'Review Committee for Protection of Research Risks to Humans' of Indian Statistical Institute, Kolkata, West Bengal, India.

The skin biopsy samples are collected from 120 patients. Multiple serial sections of skin tissue present in the biopsy slides are imaged. The images where the stratum corneum (SC) layer is lost during tissue processing are discarded. Then the images are labelled by two experts. The images where both experts' agreement match are considered for this research. In our dataset, there are 88 images with Munro's Microabscess and 185 images without Munro's Microabscess. The ground-truth annotation of SC segmentation of the images is done by an expert. In order to construct the SC patch classifier, multiple squared patches (224 × 224 pixel sized) are cropped from SC layer of the biopsy images. Then the existence of neutrophil in these patches are labelled by two experts and the cases where both experts' agreement match are chosen. In total, there are 886 patches with neutrophils and 1700 patches without any neutrophil. In rest of the paper, the SC patches having neutrophils are termed as positive patches and the patches not having neutrophils are termed as negative patches.

4   Experiments

4.1   Experimental Setting

The proposed system is tested with three-fold cross validation. Each fold contains random selection of 91 images from our dataset. Among them, two folds contain 29 images and another fold contains 30 images having Munro's Microabscess. The cropped SC patches are grouped fold-wise (862 patches/fold) to build the fold-wise SC patch classifiers. The validation data is developed by random selection of 10% training images (original WSI) for U-Net and 20% training images (SC patches) for CapsDeMM. The validation data is used for tuning filter number, filter size and other hyper-parameters. The architecture of the used U-Net and capsule network are shown in Fig. 2. In CapsDeMM, each primary capsule contains 8 convolutional units (5 × 5 and stride 2) of 16 channels and the secondary capsule is a convolutional capsule which does routing by agreement between the capsules in the same spatial region of the primary capsule.

For U-Net, keeping the resource constraints in mind, the original images and the corresponding ground-truths are down-sampled to 960×1280. However, the segmentation output is up-scaled to the original dimension and 224×224 pixel sized SC patches are selected for classification. In order to achieve the best performing CapsDeMM network, the value of K for the top-K average pooling layer is tuned (without making any architectural change to the other layers) and the resulting network is named as CapsDeMM-K.

4.2   Results and Discussion

Segmentation Performance: The accurate segmentation of the SC region improves the diagnosis performance of our system. The U-Net produces good segmentation (Dice Coefficient of 0.8493 ± 0.025) but it generates several spurious holes and isolated segmented regions in the SC regions as shown in Fig. 3. To get rid of it, 'hole-filling' algorithm is applied for smoothing such spurious and isolated regions. Figure 3 illustrates that the used smoothing technique is able to remove falsely detected non-SC regions. Final segmentation outcome results in Dice Coefficient of 0.8614 ± 0.014.

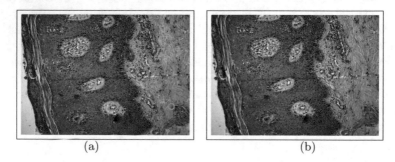

        (a)   (b)

Fig. 3. The yellow line is used to denote the ground-truthed region boundary whereas the green line is used to denote the detected region boundary. (a) Segmentation outcome from the U-Net, (b) Segmentation outcome after post-processing.

Stratum Corneum Patch Classification: The development of stratum corneum patch classification is an important component for the success of the proposed system. The capsule network shown in Fig. 2 is used for this purpose. In $top - K$ average pooling, lower values of K might misclassify an image patch as positive due to some portions of the patches getting high probabilities whereas higher values of K might overcompensate this effect leading to positive samples being classified as negative. To get the optimum value of K, we compare the ROC curves for different values of K. $K = 5$ is chosen for classification since it provides best AUC score (average of three folds). The diagnosis for presence or absence of neutrophils in a patch is made by comparing the cut off value

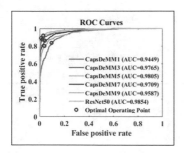

Fig. 4. Comaprison of ROC curves.

Table 1. Performance comparison of patch classifiers. M = Million, s = second.

Metric	ResNet-50	CapsDeMM5
Recall	0.87 ± 0.078	0.84 ± 0.064
Precision	0.95 ± 0.015	0.94 ± 0.027
F1 score	0.91 ± 0.036	0.88 ± 0.027
Accuracy	0.94 ± 0.020	0.92 ± 0.013
Parameters	23.5 M	0.1 M
Load time	2.15 s	0.26 s
Prediction time	0.021 s/img	0.087 s/img

obtained from the ROC analysis. In case the network output for a patch is less than the cut off value, the predicted output is negative, otherwise, the predicted output is positive. The comparison of ROC curves for first fold for five different K values (1, 3, 5, 7 and 9) is shown in Fig. 4.

The classification performance is evaluated with Recall, Precision, F1 Score and classification accuracy (ACC). The average value for all metrics for all three folds are listed in Table 1. Finally, the performance of the proposed capsule network is compared with a trained CNN i.e. ResNet 50, trained on the same dataset. The experimental result shows that Capsule network achieves comparable accuracy to ResNet-50 despite having orders of magnitude less parameters.

Whole Slide Image (WSI) Diagnosis: Ideally, detection of a single positive SC patch should indicate the presence of Munro's microabscess. But there are occasional misclassification in classifying SC patches (see Table 1). So, to develop a robust WSI Classification system, a threshold T is decided from the training set. Only those WSIs which have more than T number of positive patches are diagnosed as having Munro's microabscess. Two different strategies are analysed for selecting the value of T - (I) The system should produce best WSI classification performance: T is selected in such a way that the best WSI classification accuracy is achieved; (II) The system will reduce the workload of pathologists by rejecting the negative cases (slides without having Munro's Microabscess): T is selected in such way that true negative rate is maximized. Strategy I is evaluated with correct classification accuracy (ACC) and strategy II is evaluated with True Negative Rate (TNR) and Precision. Obviously, the value of T varies across the folds depending on the used thresholding strategy.

In order to compare the performance of the proposed diagnostic system on the super-pixel numbers, 3 different number of super-pixels are considered. The performance averaged over all the folds is listed in Table 2. According to Table 2, both capsule network and ResNet-50 produces comparable performances. Note that when Strategy I is considered, CapsDeMM outperforms ResNet-50 but when Strategy II is considered, ResNet-50 outperform CapsDeMM.

Table 2. Performance comparison of WSI classifiers

Number of superpixel	ResNet-50			CapsDeMM5		
	Strategy I	Strategy II		Strategy I	Strategy II	
	ACC (%)	TNR	Precision	ACC (%)	TNR	Precision
300	86.13	1.0000	0.4649	88.71	0.9606	0.4373
500	85.76	0.9837	0.4479	88.70	0.9656	0.4291
700	87.59	0.9651	0.5068	89.06	0.9333	0.4000

5   Conclusion and Future Work

This paper presents the first of its kind system for detection of Munro's Microabscess in skin biopsy images. The drastic reduction of parameters without notable performance degradation justifies the applicability of CapsDeMM for the present problem. The promising performance of the two strategies for WSI classification presented in the paper shows their applicability for reducing the workload of the pathologists by a huge margin. The use of Mega-pixel images not only reduces the overall computational burden but also attests the use of a low cost system consisting of a light microscope (without digital scanner) and a digital camera. The outcome of the present research along with the dataset of WSIs will help in addressing several other important histopathological analysis of psoriasis including classification of parakeratosis (confluent/focal), detection of Kogoj Microabscesses. Efficiency of the present framework can be validated by employing different architectures and the patch classification can also be attempted with patches of different shapes (e.g. rectangular).

Acknowledgments. Authors would like to acknowledge all volunteers who participated in this study.

References

1. Achanta, R., Shaji, A., Smith, K., Lucchi, A., Fua, P., Susstrunk, S.: Slic superpixels compared to state-of-the-art superpixel methods. IEEE Trans. Pattern Anal. Mach. Intell. **34**(11), 2274–2282 (2012)
2. Marks, R.M., Knight, A.G., Laidler, P.: Atlas of Skin Pathology, vol. 11. Springer, Netherlands (2012). https://doi.org/10.1007/978-94-009-4127-4
3. Pal, A., Chaturvedi, A., Garain, U., Chandra, A., Chatterjee, R.: Severity grading of psoriatic plaques using deep CNN based multi-task learning. In: 23rd International Conference on Pattern Recognition (ICPR 2016), pp. 1478–1483, 4–8 December 2016
4. Pal, A., Garain, U., Chandra, A., Chatterjee, R., Senapati, S.: Psoriasis skin biopsy image segmentation using deep convolutional neural network. Comput. Methods Programs Biomed. **159**, 59–69 (2018)
5. Ronneberger, O., Fischer, P., Brox, T.: U-Net: convolutional networks for biomedical image segmentation. In: Navab, N., Hornegger, J., Wells, W.M., Frangi, A.F. (eds.) MICCAI 2015. LNCS, vol. 9351, pp. 234–241. Springer, Cham (2015). https://doi.org/10.1007/978-3-319-24574-4_28

6. Roy, A., Pal, A., Garain, U.: JCLMM: a finite mixture model for clustering of circular-linear data and its application to psoriatic plaque segmentation. Pattern Recognit. **66**, 160–173 (2017)
7. Sabour, S., Frosst, N., Hinton, G.E.: Dynamic routing between capsules. In: Advances in Neural Information Processing Systems, pp. 3859–3869 (2017)
8. Wang, J., MacKenzie, J.D., Ramachandran, R., Chen, D.Z.: Identifying neutrophils in h&e staining histology tissue images. In: MICCAI Proceedings, Boston, USA, pp. 73–80, 14–18 September 2014. https://doi.org/10.1007/978-3-319-10404-1_10
9. Wang, J., MacKenzie, J.D., Ramachandran, R., Chen, D.Z.: Neutrophils identification by deep learning and voronoi diagram of clusters. In: Navab, N., Hornegger, J., Wells, W.M., Frangi, A.F. (eds.) MICCAI 2015. LNCS, vol. 9351, pp. 226–233. Springer, Cham (2015). https://doi.org/10.1007/978-3-319-24574-4_27

Webly Supervised Learning for Skin Lesion Classification

Fernando Navarro[1($\boxtimes$)], Sailesh Conjeti[1,2], Federico Tombari[1],
and Nassir Navab[1,3]

[1] Computer Aided Medical Procedures,
Technische Universität München, Munich, Germany
fernando.navarro@tum.de

[2] German Center for Neurodegenrative Diseases (DZNE), Bonn, Germany

[3] Computer Aided Medical Procedures, Johns Hopkins University, Baltimore, USA

Abstract. Within medical imaging, manual curation of sufficient well-labeled samples is cost, time and scale-prohibitive. To improve the representativeness of the training dataset, for the first time, we present an approach to utilize large amounts of freely available web data through web-crawling. To handle noise and weak nature of web annotations, we propose a two-step transfer learning based training process with a robust loss function, termed as Webly Supervised Learning (WSL) to train deep models for the task. We also leverage *search by image* to improve the search specificity of our web-crawling and reduce cross-domain noise. Within WSL, we explicitly model the noise structure between classes and incorporate it to selectively distill knowledge from the web data during model training. To demonstrate improved performance due to WSL, we benchmarked on a publicly available 10-class fine-grained skin lesion classification dataset and report a significant improvement of top-1 classification accuracy from 71.25% to 80.53% due to the incorporation of web-supervision.

1 Introduction

The success of deep learning in computer vision tasks such as image classification, object detection, segmentation *etc.* is owed to the availability of a large corpus of annotated training data [1–3]. However, translating these developments to medical imaging applications is often challenging as curating a representative dataset is cost-, time- and scale-prohibitive. On the other hand, excessive reliance on a small-sized, well-curated dataset offers limited guarantees on the generalizability to unseen scenarios and could lead to potential overfit on the training data due to excessive over-parameterization of deep networks. In this paper, we propose to leverage freely available data crawled from the web to offset the need for a large dataset and introduce the concept of *Webly Supervised Learning* (WSL) as a potential approach for training neural networks for medical imaging applications. We present a proof of concept for the task of fine-grained classification of skin lesions in dermatological images.

© Springer Nature Switzerland AG 2018
A. F. Frangi et al. (Eds.): MICCAI 2018, LNCS 11071, pp. 398–406, 2018.
https://doi.org/10.1007/978-3-030-00934-2_45

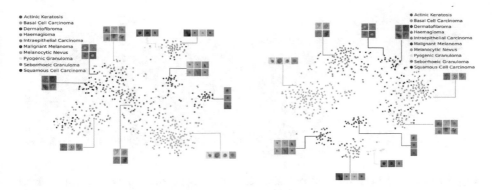

Fig. 1. Comparison of t-SNE embedding space generated from networks trained on limited clean data (Left) against network trained with Webly Supervised Learning (Right) generating compact class clusters with improved separability especially for under-represented classes.

The task of skin lesion classification is a representative example of a medical imaging application in which, annotated training data is limited in availability. However, there is an abundance of freely-available web data. We source our images from multiple publicly-accessible sites such as [4], where pictures of skin lesions are uploaded with the goal of getting feedback on the type of lesion with respect to visual features. Prior work on deep learning for skin lesion classification includes training networks that perform either a two or three-class classification (melanoma, non-cancerous and seborrheic keratosis) [5–7]. Authors in [8] propose a deeply learned network for nine-class categorization using a large dataset of 130000 images extensively curated from hospital archives and from dermatological websites. The data used in this work underwent extensive manual quality control with 23 human experts and filtering prior to fine-tuning InceptionV3 [2]. In contrast to [8], within this paper, we adopt a more unconstrained learning paradigm by focusing on learning in presence of extreme label noise by developing a dedicated robust loss function and employing transfer learning strategies to seamlessly leverage webly sourced data into training without employing any additional heuristics or expert knowledge.

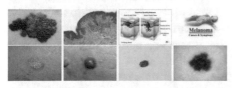

Fig. 2. Type of noise in WSL for Melanoma class as keyword. The images in the first row represent examples of cross-domain noise. The second row represents the cross-category noise.

Harvesting images from the web presents opportunities for abundant availability and the ability to encompass sufficient heterogeneity during training. However, learning from them is challenging due to the presence of different types of noise. These include *cross-domain noise*: retrieved web images may include non-dermatoscopic images such as histology, artistic illustrations, icons *etc.*

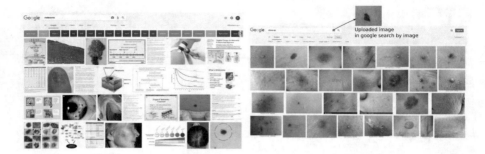

Fig. 3. Comparison of crawled results. The left image shows an example of a search by keyword "melanoma": the resulting images contain high cross-domain noise. The right image shows the results of a search by image, where the cross-domain noise is significantly reduced sharing strong visual similarity to the query image.

and *cross-category noise*: images that are visually similar to the query yet belong to a different class. Cross-domain noise is introduced by bias due to a specific search engine and associated search criterion (such as user tags). Additionally, image-search engines are biased as they often operate in high-precision low-recall regimes and preferentially present objects centered with clean background and a canonical view-point. Figure 2 illustrates different types of noise present in retrieved images upon web-crawling with "melanoma" as the search tag. Learning from web data is one approach for learning under extreme label noise. Methods within the computer vision community that leverage web supervision for training can be broadly categorized as: (1) *Filtering*: approaches that aim to clean or filter the collected web images prior to training [9,10]; (2) *Modeling Relationships*: approaches that model the relationship between web images and noisy labels with a small subset of clean images and utilize the discovered relationships to improve training [11,12] and (3) *Robust Loss Functions*: approaches that learn in the presence of label noise by introducing robustness within their loss-function design [13,14]. Our proposed approach encompasses the best of the aforementioned approaches with the following contributions:

1. **Reduction in Cross-domain Noise:** This is the first work to leverage *search by image* to improve search specificity and reduce cross-domain noise by fetching images that share close visual features to the query image.
2. **Noise Modeling:** We model the noise as a class-transition matrix which is estimated from the bag of retrieved images. This noise modeling approach allows for distillation of knowledge from noisy web-images to train very-deep networks.
3. To the best of our knowledge, this is the first work within the medical image computing that leverages web-supervision to train deep neural networks and specifically targeted at fine-grained ten-class categorization of skin lesions.

2 Methodology

Given a small representative training dataset $\mathcal{C} = \{(\mathbf{x}_c^n, \mathbf{y}_c^n)\}_{n=1}^N$ of dermatological images with expert annotations, we source web-images for WSL by utilizing the *Search by Image* option within standard search engines (here, https://images.google.com/) by submitting each of the *clean* images independently and crawling the top retrieved results. Let the bag of images (of size M) crawled from the web for a query image of $\mathbf{x}_c^n$ be represented as $\mathcal{W}^n = \{\mathbf{x}_w^m \mid \text{Query: } \mathbf{x}_c^n\}_{m=1}^M$. The semantic label associated with the query clean image $\mathbf{y}_c^n$ is given to the corresponding web-crawled bag $\mathcal{W}_n$. Let the complete web-crawled images with their corresponding annotations be denoted as $\mathcal{W} = \{(\mathcal{W}^n, \mathbf{y}_c^n)\}_{n=1}^N$. Contrasting with prior WSL approaches [15,16] that use search by keyword (such as *melanoma*, *keratosis etc.*), we observe that our approach significantly reduces the cross-domain noise by fetching only images that share strong visual features with the query. Figure 3 contrasts the proposed search by image approach against the search by keyword methodology for the construction of a web-dataset for WSL. It must be noted that the labels transferred from $\mathcal{C}$ to $\mathcal{W}$ are extremely noisy as the web-search relies on non-task specific solely visual features for ranking and carries no guarantees on the fetched results sharing the same semantic class as the query. Additionally, in such an uncontrolled setting, multiple queries could fetch the same images thus the web-images could carry potential cross-category noise. With per-image web-crawling, our training dataset is significantly augmented (with at most $M \times N$ unique images) and the resultant dataset is rich in representativeness and heterogeneity but fraught with extreme label noise which needs to be factored out in the subsequent training steps.

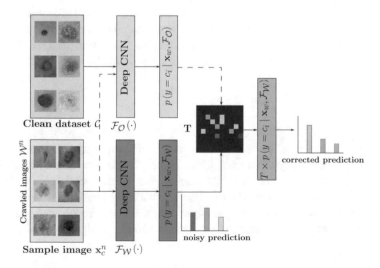

Fig. 4. Overview of the proposed WSL approach consisting of a two-step training. First, training a network on web data, follow by fine-tuning a second network utilizing the latter as strong prior initialization. Noise correction is performed when training on web data.

2.1   Model Learning

Noise Correction: Assuming that we have access to a perfect oracle network $\mathcal{F}_O(\cdot)$, we model the noise within the web images as a class-transition matrix T that can be used to diffuse the predictions on web data across confusing classes. In naïve terms, T models the probability of each class being confused into one another. Considering three classes (c_1, c_2 and c_3), if c_1 and c_2 are visually more similar than c_3, there is a higher probability for cross-category noise across c_1 and c_2 in comparison to c_1 and c_3 (or c_2 and c_3) and this reflects back in the estimated class-transition matrix as $T(c_1, c_2) > T(c_1, c_3)$. From within the web crawled images $\mathcal{W}$, we use the predictions of oracle network $\mathcal{F}_O$ to mine the most representative sample $\hat{\mathbf{x}}_{w,c_i}$ of class c_i from within $\mathcal{W}$ as:

$$\hat{\mathbf{x}}_{w,c_i} = \mathrm{argmax}_{\mathbf{x}_w \in \mathcal{W}} \, p\,(y = c_i \mid \mathbf{x}_w, \mathcal{F}_O),\tag{1}$$

where $p(\cdot)$ is the class posterior probability. This is repeated for all target classes and the class transition matrix for the web-data is estimated as:

$$T_{ij} = p\,(y = c_j \mid \hat{\mathbf{x}}_{w,c_i}, \mathcal{F}_O)\tag{2}$$

The aforementioned approach globally estimates the noise transition matrix across the web-crawled images and allows for selective diffusion across confounding classes associated with that bag. As the availability of a perfect oracle network is highly unlikely in real-world, we use a deep network trained on the limited clean dataset $\mathcal{C}$ as a potential surrogate for $\mathcal{F}_O$.

Webly Supervised Learning: We adopt a transfer-learning like paradigm to train our fine-grained classification network as shown in Fig. 4. From an overall perspective, the web-crawled dataset $\mathcal{W}$ is used to train an initial model $\mathcal{F}_\mathcal{W}(\cdot)$ with weighted-cross entropy loss. Noise correction is modulated by changing the network predictions with the estimated noise transition matrix T from the retrieved web-images $\mathcal{W}$, the modulated cross-entropy loss for training $\mathcal{F}_\mathcal{W}$ is estimated as:

$$\mathcal{L} = -\sum_{\mathbf{x}_c^n \in \mathcal{W}} w(\mathbf{x}_c^n)\, y(\mathbf{x}_c^n)\, log(T \times p(\mathbf{x}_c^n))\tag{3}$$

where $w(\mathbf{x}_c^n)$ is the weight associated with the class, estimated using median-frequency balancing, $y(\mathbf{x}_c^n)$ is the ground truth of sample $\mathbf{x}_c^n$ and $p(\mathbf{x}_c^n)$ provides the estimated probability of sample $\mathbf{x}_c^n$ to belong to class c. The trained network $\mathcal{F}_\mathcal{W}$ is used an initialization for subsequent fine-tuning with clean data $\mathcal{C}$ to obtain the final target model $\mathcal{F}_\mathcal{C}(\cdot)$. Such a training strategy ensures that all available rich information from web-supervision is transferred as a strong prior to $\mathcal{F}_\mathcal{C}$ and that only expert annotated data is used to train the final network.

3   Experiments

Dataset: The limited manually annotated dataset was sourced from the Dermofit Image Library [17], which consists of 1300 high quality skin lesion images annotated by expert dermatologists. The lesions are categorized into ten fine-grained classes including melanomas, seborrhoeic keratosis, basal cell carcinomas, *etc.* The dataset has an extreme class imbalance (*e.g.* the melanocytic nevus (25.4%) *vs.* pyogenic granuloma (1.8%)). The under-representation of these classes further motivates the need for augmentation with web-crawled data. For our experiments, we performed a patient-level split and used 50% of the data for training and the rest for testing. It must be noted that due to the proprietary nature of the Dermofit library, we do not expect any of our test-data to be freely accessible via the web and hence would not be duplicated within the web-data while training the networks.

Networks: To demonstrate the contributions in terms of both the effectiveness of the proposed search by image as well as the introduction of noise correction while model learning, we established three baselines as presented in Table 1. Specifically, BL1 is the *vanilla* version of training exclusively with the clean training dataset, while contrasting with BL2 we can test the hypothesis that creating a web-dataset through *search by image* induces higher search specificity and significantly reduces the cross-domain noise compared to the web data mined with keywords or user tags. We chose to use the Inception V3 deep architecture [2] as the base model for this work. All the aforementioned models were trained with stochastic gradient descent with a decaying learning rate initialized at 0.01, momentum of 0.9 and dropout of 0.8 for regularization and the code was developed in TensorFlow [18].

Table 1. Design parameters and average performance observed for incremental baselines designed to validate WSL for skin lesion classification.

#	Name	Model learning			Performance	
		Training data	Initialization	Noise correction	Average accuracy	Cohen's Kappa
1	BL1	Clean	ImageNet	–	0.713	0.650
2	BL2	Web data	ImageNet	×		
3		Clean	#4		0.799	0.760
4	Proposed	Web data	ImageNet	✓		
5		Clean	#6		**0.805**	**0.768**

4 Results and Discussion

To evaluate the effect of inclusion of WSL and the proposed noise correction, we report the average accuracy across all classes and the Cohens Kappa coefficient in Table 1. The latter metric is particularly motivated due to the presence of significant class imbalance within our dataset. We also report the class-wise area under the curve (ROC) in Table 2. The confusion matrices are visualized in Fig. 5. To contrast the learned intermediate features, we embed them into a two-dimensional subspace using t-Stochastic Neighbor Embedding (t-SNE) illustrated in Fig. 1.

Analyzing the Embedding Space: Comparing the t-SNE embeddings of the test data generated by BL1 and the proposed approach in Fig. 1, we observe that the embeddings in WSL approach cluster examples from the same semantic class more compactly and maintain better class-separability. Within the embedding of BL1, we notice poor separability between the less-frequently occurring classes (represented with ●, ● and ● bullets), which is significantly improved in the embedding of WSL. We also observe that the misclassification of Pyogenic Granuloma(benign) ● class into Basal Cell Carcinoma (malignant) ● in case of BL1 is not observed for WSL. This is quite critical as these classes are mutually exclusive. Meaning that, a vast malignant samples can be classified as benign, leading to a wrong diagnosis.

Effect of Web Supervision: Contrasting BL1 against the proposed method in Table 1 and Fig. 5, we clearly observe a significant improvement in the model performance across all classes, with a more pronounced diagonal in its confusion matrix. This is clearly attributed to a better network initialization derived through transfer learning with web-supervision. This also demonstrates that we are effective in factoring out the cross-domain and cross-category noise within the web-dataset and effectively use it for supervising deep models in the presence of limited manual annotations. In Table 2, contrasting the class-wise performance, we observe that the performance on under-represented classes is significantly improved upon WSL. This is clearly evident in Intraepithelial Carcinoma ● (5.99% Clean data) and Pyogenic Granuloma ● (1.17% Clean data) where the performance improves by 3.6% and 7.3% respectively. Contrasting BL2 with the proposed approach in Table 2, we observe an overall improvement when

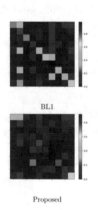

BL1

Proposed

Fig. 5. Confusion matrices showing the effect of the proposed WSL approach compared to BL1.

performing noise correction. The AUC has a slight improvement across the majority of classes. With this observation, it can be concluded that the web-crawled images retrieved in a search by image proposed methodology are so rich in terms of visual features that the effect of noise correction is only marginal when comparing BL2 and the proposed approach.

Table 2. Results showing the AUC for each class and the average overall accuracy for every model.

	C1	C2	C3	C4	C5	C6	C7	C8	C9	C10	Avg AUC
Class % in train	3.42	18.49	4.96	7.53	5.99	5.82	25.51	1.17	19.86	6.67	–
BL1	0.898	0.943	0.976	**0.983**	0.936	0.955	0.979	0.927	0.933	0.872	0.940
BL2	0.873	0.955	0.995	0.966	0.967	0.984	**0.987**	0.991	**0.975**	0.935	0.963
Proposed	**0.920**	**0.966**	**0.995**	0.968	**0.972**	**0.985**	0.983	**0.991**	0.961	**0.957**	**0.970**

5 Conclusions

In this work, we have demonstrated for the first time the effectiveness of webly supervised learning for the task of skin lesion classification. We demonstrate that WSL can be very effective for training in limited data regimens with high-class imbalance as web data can augment under-represented classes and boost the model performance. By crawling the web through search by image to generate the web-dataset, we induce high search specificity and effectively minimize the influence of cross-domain noise. The proposed noise correction approach by modeling cross-category noise helps in learning an effective network initialization from web data.

Acknowledgements. The authors gratefully acknowledge CONACYT for the financial support.

References

1. He, K., Zhang, X., Ren, S., Sun, J.: Deep residual learning for image recognition. In: CVPR (2016)
2. Szegedy, C., Vanhoucke, V., Ioffe, S., Shlens, J., Wojna, Z.: Rethinking the inception architecture for computer vision. In: CVPR (2017)
3. Szegedy, C., Ioffe, S., Vanhoucke, V., Alemi, A.A.: Inception-v4, inception-resnet and the impact of residual connections on learning. In: AAAI (2017)
4. DermQuest. https://www.dermquest.com/
5. Yu, L., Chen, H., Dou, Q., Qin, J., Heng, P.A.: Automated melanoma recognition in dermoscopy images via very deep residual networks. IEEE TMI **36**, 994–1004 (2017)
6. Matsunaga, K., Hamada, A., Minagawa, A., Koga, H.: Image classification of melanoma, nevus and seborrheic keratosis by deep neural network ensemble. arXiv:1703.03108 (2017)
7. Codella, N.C., et al.: Skin lesion analysis toward melanoma detection. arXiv:1710.05006 (2017)
8. Esteva, A., et al.: Dermatologist-level classification of skin cancer with deep neural networks. Nature **542**, 115 (2017)
9. Krause, J., et al.: The unreasonable effectiveness of noisy data for fine-grained recognition. In: Leibe, B., Matas, J., Sebe, N., Welling, M. (eds.) ECCV 2016. LNCS, vol. 9907, pp. 301–320. Springer, Cham (2016). https://doi.org/10.1007/978-3-319-46487-9_19

10. Massouh, N., Babiloni, F., Tommasi, T., Young, J., Hawes, N., Caputo, B.: Learning deep visual object models from noisy web data: how to make it work. arXiv:1702.08513 (2017)
11. Xiao, T., Xia, T., Yang, Y., Huang, C., Wang, X.: Learning from massive noisy labeled data for image classification. In: CVPR (2015)
12. Vahdat, A.: Toward robustness against label noise in training deep discriminative neural networks. In: NIPS (2017)
13. Sukhbaatar, S., Fergus, R.: Learning from noisy labels with deep neural networks. arXiv:1406.2080 (2014). **2**(3), 4
14. Patrini, G., Rozza, A., Menon, A., Nock, R., Qu, L.: Making neural networks robust to label noise: a loss correction approach. arXiv:1609.03683 (2016)
15. Chen, X., Gupta, A.: Webly supervised learning of convolutional networks. In: ICCV (2015)
16. Oquab, M., Bottou, L., Laptev, I., Sivic, J.: Is object localization for free?-weakly-supervised learning with convolutional neural networks. In: CVPR (2015)
17. Ballerini, L., Fisher, R.B., Aldridge, B., Rees, J.: A color and texture based hierarchical K-NN approach to the classification of non-melanoma skin lesions. In: Celebi, M., Schaefer, G. (eds.) Color Medical Image Analysis, pp. 63–86. Springer, Dordrecht (2013). https://doi.org/10.1007/978-94-007-5389-1_4
18. Abadi, M., et al.: TensorFlow: large-scale machine learning on heterogeneous distributed systems. CoRR abs/1603.04467 (2016)

Feature Driven Local Cell Graph (FeDeG): Predicting Overall Survival in Early Stage Lung Cancer

Cheng Lu[1,2(✉)], Xiangxue Wang[2], Prateek Prasanna[2],
German Corredor[2,3], Geoffrey Sedor[4], Kaustav Bera[2],
Vamsidhar Velcheti[5], and Anant Madabhushi[2]

[1] College of Computer Science, Shaanxi Normal University,
Xian, Shaanxi Province, China
cxl884@case.edu
[2] Department of Biomedical Engineering,
Case Western Reserve University, Cleveland, OH, USA
[3] Computer Imaging and Medical Applications Laboratory,
Universidad Nacional de Colombia, Bogota, Colombia
[4] School of Medicine, Case Western Reserve University, Cleveland, USA
[5] Hematology and Medical Oncology Department,
Cleveland Clinic, Cleveland, OH, USA

Abstract. The local spatial arrangement of nuclei in histopathology image has been shown to have prognostic value in the context of different cancers. In order to capture the nuclear architectural information locally, local cell cluster graph based measurements have been proposed. However, conventional ways of cell graph construction only utilize nuclear spatial proximity, and do not differentiate different cell types while constructing a cell graph. In this paper, we present feature driven local cell graph (FeDeG), a new approach to constructing local cell graphs by simultaneously considering spatial proximity and attributes of the individual nuclei (e.g. shape, size, texture). In addition, we designed a new set of quantitative graph derived metrics to be extracted from FeDeGs, in turn capturing the interplay between different local cell clusters. We evaluated the efficacy of FeDeG features in a digitized H&E stained tissue micro-array (TMA) images cohort consists of 434 early stage non-small cell lung cancer for predicting short-term (<5 years) vs long-term (>5 years) survival. Across a 100 runs of 10-fold cross-validation, a linear discriminant classifier in conjunction with the 15 most predictive FeDeG features identified via the Wilcoxon Rank Sum Test (WRST) yielded an average of AUC = 0.68. By comparison, four state-of-the-art pathomic and a deep learning based classifier had a corresponding AUC of 0.56, 0.54, 0.61, 0.62, and 0.55 respectively.

1 Introduction

Changes in distribution, appearance, size, morphology, and arrangement of histologic primitives, e.g., nuclei and glands, can predict tumor aggressiveness. For instance, in the context of lung cancer, it is known that more and less aggressive diseases are characterized

© Springer Nature Switzerland AG 2018
A. F. Frangi et al. (Eds.): MICCAI 2018, LNCS 11071, pp. 407–416, 2018.
https://doi.org/10.1007/978-3-030-00934-2_46

by differences in nuclear shape, morphology and arrangement. For a number of different cancers, the hallmark of presence of disease is the disruption in the cohesion of architecture between nuclei and other primitives belonging to the same family, e.g. nuclei or lymphocytes. Conversely, aggressive tumor tends to exhibit relatively lower degrees of structure and organization between the same class of primitives compared to less aggressive cancers.

There has been recent interest in developing computational graph-based approaches to characterize spatial arrangement of nuclei in histopathology images to be able to predict patient outcome [1–3]. Many of these approaches are based on global graphs such as Voronoi and Delaunay triangulation strategies to connect individual nuclei (representing graph vertices or nodes) and then computing and associating statistics relating to edge length and node density to disease outcome. Lewis et al. proposed cell cluster graphs (CCG) in which the nodes are defined on groups/clusters of nuclei rather than on individual nucleus [3], since there is a growing recognition that tumor aggressiveness might be driven more by the spatial inter-actions of proximally situated nuclei, compared to global interactions of distally located nuclei. While these approaches showed that attributes relating to spatial arrangement of proximal nuclei were prognostic [1–3], the graph connections did not discriminate between different cell populations, e.g. whether the proximal cells were all cancer cells or belonged to other families such as lymphocytes.

In this work we seek to go beyond the traditional way of constructing cell graphs, which focus solely on cell proximity. Instead we seek to incorporate the intrinsic nuclear morphologic features coupled with spatial distance to construct locally and morphologically distinct cell clusters. We introduce a new way of constructing a local cell graph called the Feature Driven Local Cell Graph (FeDeG), along with a corresponding new set of quantitative histomorphometric features. In the context of early stage lung cancer, we demonstrate that FeDeG features extracted from nuclear graphs from digitized pathology images are predictive of overall survival.

2 Brief Overview and Novel Contributions

The novel contributions of this work include: (1) FeDeG is a new way to construct local cell graphs based on the nuclear features. This results in locally packed cell graphs comprising nuclei with similar phenotype. Figure 1 illustrates the global cell graph [1], CCG [3] and FeDeG graph in the same local region contains lymphocytes and cancer cells. One may see that the global graph connects all the nuclei in the image may not allow for capturing of local tumor morphology efficiently. Similarly, the CCG only considers nuclear locations which results in connecting lymphocytes and cancer nuclei into a graph, important information involving local spatial interaction between different cellular clusters may be left unexploited.

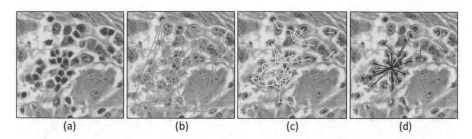

Fig. 1. Illustration of (a) original H&E stained color histology image of non-small cell lung cancer, (b) global cell graph (Delaunay triangulation), (c) CCG, the cell clusters were created based on the proximity of nuclei, (d) FeDeG driven by nuclear intensity and proximity.

The FeDeG incorporates nuclear morphologic feature (nuclear mean intensity in this case) into the graph constructing process, which enable us to interrogate the interaction between different graphs and to reveal more sub-visual information from the underlying tissue image.

(2) In addition to construct local cell graphs using FeDeG, we designed a new set of quantitative histomorphometrics based on the constructed FeDeGs. These features are: Intersection between different FeDeGs, size of FeDeGs, Disorder of nuclear morphology within FeDeG and the spatial arrangement of FeDeG. There features are different compared to standard features extracted from CCG and global graph methods, which only quantify the density of local/global graph, or the local/global distances between cells. The FeDeG features attempt to capture the interactions between and within local cell clusters with similar morphological properties.

(3) We employ the FeDeG and associated quantitative features in conjunction with a linear machine learning classifier to predict risk of recurrence in early stage non-small cell lung cancer (NSCLC). Similar work has been reported by Yu et al. [4] and Wang et al. [5] for predicting recurrence in early stage NSCLC patients, in which the global architecture and shape of nuclei features were found to be predictive. However, the interactions between different local cell clusters have not been explored. In the experiment, we compared the FeDeG with these nuclear features. Figure 2 shows the flowchart of FeDeG construction and associated feature computation, which include nuclei segmentation, FeDeG construction, and FeDeG feature extraction modules.

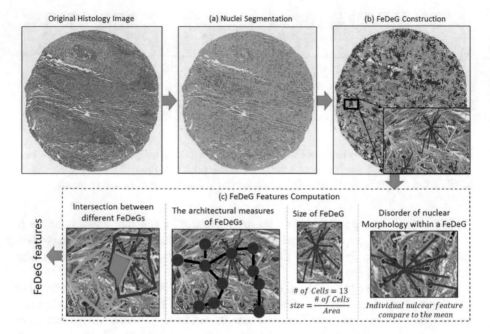

Fig. 2. Flowchart of FeDeG construction and associated feature computation. (a) Green contours indicate the nuclear boundaries (b) FeDeG construction based on the nuclear features (used mean intensity of nuclei in this case). Nuclei that belong to the same FeDeG have connecting edges with the same color. (c) FeDeG feature computation. (Color figure online)

3   Feature Driven Cell Graph

3.1   Nuclei Segmentation and Morphologic Feature Extraction

In order to efficiently segment nuclei a multiple-pass adaptive voting method was employed to detect the cells [6] followed by a local optimal thresholding method that segments nuclei based on analyzing the shape of these cells as well as the area occupied by them. A set of 6 nuclear morphologic features that described the nuclear shape, size and texture were then computed based on these pre-segmented nuclei.

3.2   FeDeG Construction in Nuclear Morphologic Feature Space

In this step, spatial and morphological features of nuclei were used for feature space analysis to construct FeDeG. The mean-shift clustering [7] was applied to perform the feature space analysis for sub-graph construction. It accomplishes this by first estimating the modes (i.e., stationary points of the density of nuclear morphologic feature) of the underlying density function of the nuclear morphologic feature. It then groups nuclei into different sub-graphs based on the corresponding modes.

We denote as N the total number of nuclei in the image, and each nucleus has a corresponding feature vector in d-dimensional Euclidean space $\boldsymbol{R}^d$, so that we have a set of nuclear feature vectors $\boldsymbol{X} = \boldsymbol{x}_1, \boldsymbol{x}_1, \cdots, \boldsymbol{x}_N$, where $\boldsymbol{x}_n \in \boldsymbol{R}^d$. For each feature vector $\boldsymbol{x}_n \in \boldsymbol{X}$, there is a corresponding mode $\boldsymbol{y}_i$. In the beginning, the mode $\boldsymbol{y}_i$ is initialized with the original feature vector $\boldsymbol{x}_n$ i.e., $\boldsymbol{y}_i^o = \boldsymbol{x}_n$. The $\boldsymbol{y}_i^u$ is then recursively updated, based on the neighborhood nuclear characteristics, using the following equation:

$$ \boldsymbol{y}_i^{u+1} = \boldsymbol{y}_i^u + \boldsymbol{m}_G(\boldsymbol{y}_i^u), \ 1 \leq i \leq n \tag{1} $$

where $\boldsymbol{y}_i^{u+1}$ is the updated version of $\boldsymbol{y}_i^u$. The vector $\boldsymbol{m}_G(\boldsymbol{y}_i^u)$ is called the mean-shift vector and calculates the difference between the weighted mean and the center of the kernel. It has been previously shown that the mean-shift vector always points toward the direction of maximum increase in the underlying density function [Comaniciu2002]. At the final step, each nuclear feature vector $\boldsymbol{x}_n$ finds a corresponding mode $\boldsymbol{y}_i$ which will be used for constructing the FeDeG.

In this work, we explored a Q-dimensional feature space which includes 2-D spatial coordinates (i.e., centroid location) of nuclei in the image and Q-2 of the nuclear morphologic features. These features are chosen based on the observation that the same types of nuclei are usually located closely together and have a similar phenotype. The corresponding multivariate kernel is defined as the product of two radially symmetric kernels as follows:

$$ K_{h_s, h_m}(x_i) = \frac{C}{h_s^2 h_m^{Q-2}} k\left(\left\|\frac{x_{i,s}}{h_s}\right\|\right) k\left(\left\|\frac{x_{i,m}}{h_m}\right\|\right) \tag{2} $$

where $k(\cdot)$ is the profile of the kernel, $\boldsymbol{x}_s$ is the spatial component, $\boldsymbol{x}_m$ is the nuclear morphologic component, C is the normalization constant, and h_s and h_m are the kernel bandwidths controlling the size of the kernels. The higher value of the kernel bandwidths h_s and h_m correspond to more neighboring data points that are used to estimate the density in the Q-D feature space. This can be seen in Fig. 2(d), in which the FeDeGs were constructed in a 3-D feature space (2D coordination + nuclear intensity).

3.3   FeDeG Features Computation

Based on the FeDeG created, four groups of features were derived as show in Table 1. These quantitative features were aiming to measure the interaction between FeDeGs, intrinsic nuclear variation within each FeDeG, and spatial arrangement of FeDeGs.

Table 1. FeDeG Feature description (see Fig. 2 bottom panel for illustrations).

Feature groups	# of features	Feature names	Explanation
Intersection between different FeDeGs	44	Portion/number of intersected FeDeGs, mean intersected area	Quantify the interaction between local cell clusters
Size of FeDeG	12	Size of FeDeG, cell number in FeDeG	Quantify the size of local cell clusters
Disorder of nuclear morphology	18	Variations of morphology within a FeDeG	Quantify disorder of nuclear morphology locally
The architectural measures of FeDeGs	102	Global graph measurements	Quantify global architecture of FeDeGs

4   Experimental Design

4.1   Dataset Description

The early stage NSCLC cohort comprises a total of 434 patients in the form of digitized TMA image (scanned at 20X magnification digitally). Long term clinical outcome was available for all patients in this cohort (collected between 2004 and 2014), which ends up with 280 short-term survival patients (<5 years after surgery) and 154 long-term survival patients (>5 years after surgery).

4.2   Comparative Methods

4.2.1   Graph Based and Other Pathomic Strategies

The goal of the experiment is to be able to predict short vs. long term survival in NSCLC patients. By doing that, we built separated predictive models based on pathomic features extracted from the histologic TMA spots. We compared the efficacy of FeDeG features with four states-of-the-art histomorphometric based approaches involving description of cell morphology and architecture which has been reported to have prognostic values [3–5, 8]. For all the feature sets, the nuclear segmentation from Sect. 3.1 was used to calculate the nuclear boundaries and centroids. In total, we investigated the performance of 5 feature sets: (1) 100 features describing nuclear shape [4, 5], (2) 51 features describing global cell architectures [5], (3) 24 features describing cell orientation entropy by COrE [8], (4) 35 CCG features describing local cell cluster arrangement [3], and (5) 176 FeDeG features describing the interaction between local cell clusters comprising nuclei with similar properties. A linear discriminant analysis classier (LDA) was implemented and trained based on the patient labels for samples, under 10-fold cross-validation (CV) with 100 runs. Within each fold, top 10 predictive features for each of the 5 feature groups were selected by using Wilcoxon rank sum test (WRST). The mean area under the receiver operating characteristic curve (AUC), was used to evaluate and compare the different classifiers.

4.2.2   Deep Learning

We also compared the FeDeG features with a deep learning method (DLM). The DLM was implemented using the Alexnet style Convolutional Neural Network (ConvNet). Specifically, a 10-layer ConvNet architecture comprising 1 input layer, 5 convolution layers, 3 fully connected layers and 1 output layer was constructed. The input layer accepts an image patch of 256×256 pixels, and the output layer is a soft-max function which outputs the class probability of being positive or negative. In the DLM, we split each TMA spot image into smaller patches of 200×200 pixels, the class labels for these image patches being assigned the same class label as that of the corresponding TMA spot image it was derived from. The average image size of the TMA spot was 3000×3000 pixels at $20\times$ magnification, which in turn resulted in a total number of about 68,000 patches after filtering out unusable patches. We performed the training and testing using a 10-fold cross-validation approach across each fold, all training and testing being done at the patient and not at the individual image-level. Once each of the individual image patches corresponding to a single patient have been assigned a class label, majority voting was employed to aggregate all the individual predictions to generate a patient-level prediction.

5   Results and Discussion

5.1   Discrimination of Different Graph and Deep Learning Representations

Figure 3(b) show the classification performance comparison based on different types of feature sets. The FeDeG based classifier achieved the highest AUC of 0.68 ± 0.02, outperforming the other feature sets. The Global graph, shape, COrE, CCG, and DL feature classifiers respectively yielded AUCs of $0.56 \pm 0.02, 0.54 \pm 0.03, 0.61 \pm 0.02$,

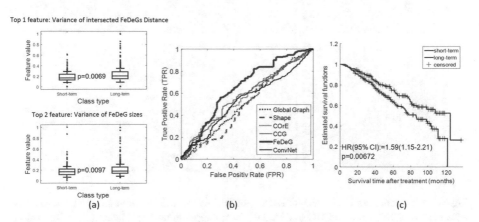

Fig. 3.   (a) The box-plot of top-2 FeDeG features in distinguishing short vs. long-term survival. (b) The ROC curves for all comparative strategies. (c) The KM curves for the FeDeG classifier associated with short and long-term survival under a leave-one-out framework (p = 0.00772, HR (95% CI) = 1.59(1.15–2.21)).

414   C. Lu et al.

0.62 ± 0.03, and 0.55 ± 0.04, respectively. The Receiver operating characteristic (ROC) curves are shown in Fig. 3. The classification results suggested that the locally extracted nuclear features provided better prognostic value than those associated with global architecture. Comparing the performance of CCG and FeDeG based classifiers suggests that the organization of local cell clusters, where cluster membership was defined not solely based off spatial proximity but also on morphologic similarity resulted in more prognostic signatures. Figure 4 shows two representative H&E stained TMA spot images for long-term and short-term survival NSCLC patients along with the corresponding CCG and FeDeG feature representations. The panel inset for FeDeG reveals the grouping of the TIL and cancer nuclei as distinct clusters with associated spatial interaction between these two cell families, unlike the CCG representation which does not distinguish between the nuclei and TILs.

Building a good deep learning model normally requires a large amount of well-annotated training cases. The deep learning approach we employed was constrained by the fact that we had an unbalanced dataset, (280 short-term vs. 154 long-term survivals). It is likely that the relatively few long-term survival patients, coupled with the class imbalance resulted in a sub-optimally trained deep learning network. Also, while DLMs have been reported good at low-level visual object detection and segmentation tasks, it is still unclear now how to use DLMs to summarize the sub-visual information extract from image patches in order to make prognostic predictions.

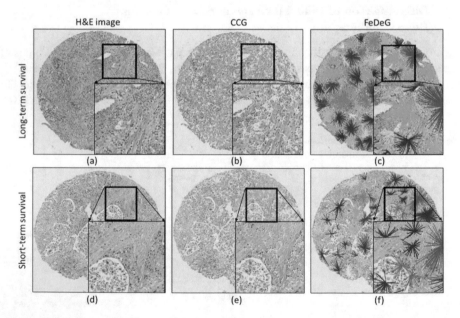

Fig. 4. Representative H&E stained TMA spot images for (a) long-term survival and (d) short-term survival NSCLCs with CCG and FeDeG feature representations. The second column shows the CCG configuration. The third column shows the FeDeG configuration, in which FeDeG graphs were colored. The panel inset for FeDeG reveals the grouping of the TIL and cancer nuclei as distinct clusters with a spatial interaction between these two cell families, unlike the CCG representation which does not distinguish between them.

During feature discovery, we found that measures of the degree of FeDeGs intersection, and the variance of FeDeG graph sizes were the most two frequently selected features by WRST across 100 runs of 10-fold cross-validation (the boxplot of these two FeDeG features are shown in Fig. 3(a)). The top 1 feature reflects the degree of interactions between different local cell families. The boxplot in Fig. 3(a) appears to suggest that tumor outcome is improved with an increase in the total number of local cell cluster interactions. This may in turn reflect increase spatial interplay between tumor infiltrating lymphocytes (TIL) and cancer nuclei clusters. This is also reflected in the FeDeG maps shown in Fig. 4(c) and (f), in which we observe a higher number of intersections between nearby FeDeG graphs in the case of patient with long-term survival (Fig. 4(c)), compared to a short-term survivor (Fig. 4(f)).

5.2   Survival Analysis

In univariate survival analysis, the Log-rank test was performed based on the predicted labels generated by FeDeG classifier. The patients identified as high risk had significantly poorer overall survival, with Hazard Ratio (95% Confident Interval) = 1.59 (1.15–2.21), p = 0.00672. We set the threshold for statistical significance at 0.05, and none of the other comparative were found to be statistically significantly prognostic of survival in NSCLC.

6   Concluding Remarks

We presented a new approach called feature driven local cell graph (FeDeG), which provide a new way to construct local cell graph. A new set of histomorphometric features also derived based on the constructed FeDeGs, the aim of which was to quantify the interaction and arrangement of local cell cluster comprising of nuclei with similar properties. The FeDeG feature based classifier showed a strong correlation with overall survival in non-small cell lung cancer patients and yield superior classification performance compared to the other pathomics. Going forward, we will attempt to validate FeDeG in larger cohorts and other tissue types, such as breast cancer.

References

1. Bilgin, C., et al.: Cell-graph mining for breast tissue modeling and classification. In: International Conference on IEEE Engineering in Medicine and Biology Society, pp. 5311–5314. IEEE (2007)
2. Shin, D., et al.: Quantitative analysis of high-resolution microendoscopic images for diagnosis of esophageal squamous cell carcinoma. Clin. Gastroenterol. Hepatol. 13, 272–279.e2 (2015)
3. Lewis, J.S., et al.: A. A quantitative histomorphometric classifier (QuHbIC) identifies aggressive versus indolent p16-positive oropharyngeal squamous cell carcinoma. Am. J. Surg. Pathol. 38, 128–137 (2014)
4. Yu, K.-H., et al.: Predicting non-small cell lung cancer prognosis by fully automated microscopic pathology image features. Nat. Commun. 7(12474), 1–10 (2016)

5. Wang, X., et al.: Prediction of recurrence in early stage non-small cell lung cancer using computer extracted nuclear features from digital H&E images. Sci. Rep. **7**(1), 13543 (2017)
6. Lu, C., et al.: Multi-pass adaptive voting for nuclei detection. Sci. Rep. **6**(1), 33985 (2016)
7. Comaniciu, D., Meer, P.: Mean shift: a robust approach toward feature space analysis. IEEE Trans. Pattern Anal. Mach. Intell. **24**, 603–619 (2002)
8. Lee, G., et al.: Cell orientation entropy (COrE): predicting biochemical recurrence from prostate cancer tissue microarrays. In: MICCAI, pp. 396–403 (2013)

Cardiac, Chest and Abdominal Applications: Cardiac Imaging Applications

Towards Accurate and Complete Registration of Coronary Arteries in CTA Images

Shaowen Zeng[1,2,3], Jianjiang Feng[1,2,3(✉)], Yunqiang An[4], Bin Lu[4], Jiwen Lu[1,2,3], and Jie Zhou[1,2,3]

[1] Department of Automation, Tsinghua University, Beijing, China
jfeng@tsinghua.edu.cn
[2] State Key Lab of Intelligent Technologies and Systems, Tsinghua University, Beijing, China
[3] Beijing National Research Center for Information Science and Technology, Beijing, China
[4] Fuwai Hospital, Beijing, China

Abstract. Coronary computed tomography angiography (CCTA) has been widely used nowadays. By combining multiple intra-subject CCTA images from different dates or different phases, cardiologists can monitor the disease progress, and researchers can explore the rules of coronary artery motion and changes within a cardiac cycle. For direct comparison and high efficiency, alignment of arteries is necessary. In this paper, we propose an automated method for accurate and complete registration of coronary arteries. Our method includes bifurcation matching, segment registration, and a novel approach to further improve the completeness of registration by combining the previous results and a level set algorithm. Our method is evaluated using 36 CCTA image pairs captured at different dates or different phases. The average distance error is $0.044 \pm 0.008\,\mathrm{mm}$ and the average correct rate of registration is 90.7%.

1 Introduction

Coronary artery disease (CAD) is one of the leading causes for death in the whole world. Coronary computed tomography angiography (CCTA) examinations are growing in use as a non-invasive method for detecting narrowing, calcifications and fatty deposits in coronary arteries, with the ability to display anatomical details. By combining multiple CCTA images of the same patient at different dates (e.g. initial and follow-up visits), cardiologists can monitor CAD progress. Furthermore, based on the combination of CCTA images at different phases within a cardiac cycle (e.g. end-systole and end-diastole), many valuable medical researches can be done, such as exploring the rules of coronary artery motion and lumen changes. Coronary arteries in intra-subject CCTA images, even within the same cardiac cycle, vary in shape and posture due to factors such different

© Springer Nature Switzerland AG 2018
A. F. Frangi et al. (Eds.): MICCAI 2018, LNCS 11071, pp. 419–427, 2018.
https://doi.org/10.1007/978-3-030-00934-2_47

relative positions, cardiac motions and respiratory motions. Therefore, comparative observation and analysis for multiple CCTA images is time-consuming, and an automated registration method of coronary arteries is beneficial.

Medical image registration has been studied a lot in recent years, but most of them are on large organs such as brains and lungs [7]. Existing methods of coronary artery registration take segmented coronary arteries or extracted artery centerlines as objects, rather than whole CCTA images, because the tree-like arteries with small lumen and wide spatial distribution will be severely disturbed by surrounding structures. In [3], point sets sampled on artery centerlines are registered based on the coherent point drift (CPD) algorithm and depending on the temporal consistency of multiple phases covering the whole cardiac cycle. The approach in [6] is limited to register straightened centerlines of left anterior descending artery (LAD), left circumflex artery (LCX) and right coronary artery (RCA) separately. The methods in [3,6] are validated on only 3 and 5 real cases. [4] uses a bigger dataset of 26 cases, whose approach consists of an affine transform and a cubic B-spline transform. In [1], the coronary artery registration is converted to aligning nearby cardiac surface landmarks, so the accuracy highly relies on the performance of heart segmentation and landmark detection. Most studies [1,3,4] focus on cases of multiple phases, only [6] considers images from two dates. The registration accuracy reported in these work is approximately 1–2 mm, measured by average distance of centerlines or manual landmarks. A main challenge for registration is topological difference such as missing branches in segmentation results, which may undermine some methods. Another limitation of these work is that only the common parts of arteries are considered. This is undesirable because missed arteries are usually pathological and important.

In this paper, we propose an automated method to register coronary arterial trees extracted from CCTA images, which can deal with two images from different dates or phases, and can also be extended to register multiple images. The method focuses on both accuracy and completeness of registration. The arterial trees used as input can be obtained from any centerline extraction method. Bifurcation matching is the first and fundamental step, which determines the correspondence of centerline segments. And then correctly matching the sampling points on each segment pair contributes largely to accuracy. When input arteries have different topologies, level set segmentation is used to find missing arteries in one image with the guidance of unmatched arteries in the other image. The registration process is then repeated using the new segmented arteries. The performance is assessed in terms of accuracy and completeness, on a dataset of 36 pairs of CCTA images from 36 patients, among which 9 pairs are acquired with an interval of 3–7 years and 27 pairs are from end-systole and end-diastole.

2   Methods

In this work, the coronary arteries are segmented using a method combining thresholding and region growing. Then the centerlines used as the input of registration are extracted using minimal cost path algorithm. As seen in Fig. 1, the registration is composed of three main steps, including matching coronary bifurcations, matching sampling points on the centerlines, whose results are utilized to compute the parameters of a Thin Plate Spline (TPS) model [2], and further improving the completeness of segmentation and registration.

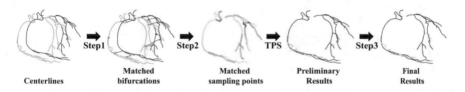

Fig. 1. The flow chart of registration. Step1 is bifurcation matching. Step2 is segment registration. Step3 is further registration. The source and aligned centerlines are shown in blue, the target centerline in green, the matched parts after step2/step3 in red/cyan. The matched/unmatched bifurcations are displayed by black lines/circles.

2.1   Bifurcation Matching

In the first step, the bifurcations on target and source centerlines undergo a point matching process, with properties of location and direction. The direction is defined as the tangent direction of branch before the bifurcation and pointing from the proximal to distal. The matching method takes both similarity and compatibility of pairs into account.

Consider two bifurcation sets: set B_s with n_s bifurcations on source centerline and set B_t with n_t bifurcations on target centerline. Based on the 3D scale-invariant feature transform (SIFT) [8] descriptors, for each point $b_t \in B_t$, we find a point $b_s \in B_s$ with the shortest Euclidean distance from b_t, thus we have n_t point pairs. Then a correspondence graph $G(V, E, M)$ is constructed, in which the node set V represents bifurcation pairs, the edge set E consists of relations between pairs, and M is an attribute matrix. The attribute value $M(i, j)$ assigned to edge $e_{ij} \in E(i \neq j)$ reflects the compatibility of ith and jth pairs, and $M(i, i)$ indicates the similarity of ith pair. Since correct pairs tend to establish links among each other, the matching problem can be formulated as a problem of detecting the main strongly connected cluster in graph G, which can be solved by eigenvector technique [5].

M is related to three geometric parameters. As illustrated in Fig. 2, d is the Euclidean distance between bifurcations, θ is the relative angle of bifurcation directions, and φ is the angle of one bifurcation measured when taking the other as the polar axis. M is defined as:

$$M(i,j) = \begin{cases} Z(i,j), & i \neq j \\ S(i,j), & i = j \end{cases}, \tag{1}$$

$$Z(i,j) = \frac{ratio(i,j) - TH_{\text{dist}}}{1 - TH_{\text{dist}}} \times \left(1 - \frac{|\theta_i - \theta_j|}{TH_\theta}\right) \times \left(1 - \frac{|\varphi_i - \varphi_j|}{TH_\varphi}\right), \tag{2}$$

$$ratio(i,j) = \frac{\min\{d_i, d_j\}}{\max\{d_i, d_j\}}, \tag{3}$$

$$S(i,j) = \begin{cases} 1 - \frac{\|Des_i^{\text{s}} - Des_i^{\text{t}}\|}{\|Des_i^{\text{s}}\| + \|Des_i^{\text{t}}\|}, & i = j \\ 0, & i \neq j \end{cases}, \tag{4}$$

where TH_{dist}, TH_θ and TH_φ are thresholds of the minimum $ratio(i,j)$, the maximum $|\theta_i - \theta_j|$ and the maximum $|\varphi_i - \varphi_j|$, respectively. And $Z(i,j)$ is small when any threshold is approached, representing bad compatibility. Des_i^{s} and Des_i^{t} are SIFT descriptors of ith pair on the source and target centerlines. Here, the SIFT descriptor is composed of $4 \times 4 \times 4$ orientation histograms each with 12 bins, thus having 768 elements.

Here we define a segment as a tree section between two bifurcations or between a bifurcation and an end point (or root point). The input trees may be different in topology due to incomplete segmentation. As illustrated in Fig. 3(a), centerline C_s has bifurcation b_2 while C_t has not. Our algorithm removes b_2 and related segment c_5 as well as merging c_3 and c_4, and then C_s is updated with new topology.

Fig. 2. Illustration of three parameters involved in the attribute matrix M. m_{i1} and m_{i2} are two bifurcations with direction.

Note that which segment to be removed is decided by the continuity and smoothness between c_5, c_4 and c_3. Figure 3(b) shows a real case in which three segments will be removed one by one from the source centerline. All the unmatched bifurcations are processed like this before segment matching, in which segments of two centerlines were considered matched if they share two bifurcation pairs or have one bifurcation pair and similar directions. The unmatched segments will skip the step of segment registration, and undergo the TPS transform directly.

(a) Illustration of C_s and C_t.   (b) A pair of RCA trees.

Fig. 3. Centerlines with different topologies. In (b) the segments to be removed are shown in red.

2.2 Segment Registration

For each segment pair determined as above, refined registration is applied. Segment Seg_s on source centerline and segment Seg_t on target centerline are discretized by evenly sampling points, with intervals of $\triangle_s$ and $\triangle_t$, satisfying $\triangle_t = K\triangle_s$ ($K = 10$ in our work). Suppose that Seg_s and Seg_t have N_s and N_t points respectively, we define a deformation model by a series of status:

$$\mathcal{S} := \{S(i) = j | i \in \{0, 1, \ldots, N_t\}, j \in \{0, 1, \ldots, N_s\}\}, \tag{5}$$

where $S(i)$ is the status of ith point on Seg_t. $S(i) = j$ means that ith point on Seg_t corresponds to jth point on Seg_s. Here $i \in \{0, 1, \ldots, N_t\}$ can be seen as a label assigned to points on Seg_s. Note that some labels may be omitted when Seg_s is shorter than Seg_t.

To determine the parameters (a series of index numbers on Seg_s) of model $\mathcal{S}$, an objective function is defined and maximized. The function consists of image similarity and geometric similarity. We define the image similarity as:

$$Sim1(i) = 1 - \frac{\left\| Des_i^t - Des_{S(i)}^s \right\|}{\left\| Des_i^t \right\| + \left\| Des_{S(i)}^s \right\|}, \tag{6}$$

where Des_i^t and $Des_{S(i)}^s$ are SIFT descriptors (computed as the same way of Sect. 2.1) of ith point on Seg_t and $S(i)$th point on Seg_s respectively. Geometric constraints are imposed to avoid excessive stretching or centerlines folding, and thus geometric similarity for ith point on Seg_t is defined as:

$$Sim2(i) = \begin{cases} 1 - \left| \log\left(\frac{S(i)-S(i-1)}{K} \right) \right|, & S(i) \geq S(i-1) \\ -\infty, & S(i) < S(i-1) \end{cases}, \tag{7}$$

where $K = \triangle_t/\triangle_s$ is 10 as mentioned above. We use logarithm to limit the difference in spacing between corresponding points on two segments, due to its better performance than piecewise linear functions in experiments.

The global objective function is as follows:

$$J(\mathcal{S}) = \sum_{i=1}^{N_t} \omega_1 Sim1(i) + \omega_2 Sim2(i). \tag{8}$$

Since each term of $J(\mathcal{S})$ related to i depends only on status $S(i)$ and status $S(i-1)$, which satisfies Markov property, J can be viewed as a Hidden Markov Model and optimized using Viterbi algorithm [6]. Matching points from all the segment pairs together form the control points of TPS transform, which is used to align the coronary arterial trees.

2.3   Further Segmentation and Registration

After registering common parts of input arterial trees, the third step is to further improve the completeness of segmentation and registration. Assuming that a branch mask BR_s is part of the input segmented arterial tree T_s but has no correspondence on tree T_t, we attempt to segment the missing (potential) branch on tree T_t. Firstly, BR_s is transformed using the TPS model from the previous registration, resulting in a mask BR_a in the other image. We define two volumes of interest (Vs and V_t) surrounding BR_s and BR_a with a 10-pixel margin in each direction parallel to coordinate axes. A B-spline transform model is computed to register Vs and V_t, which is then applied to BR_s, resulting in BR_t^0. Next, a level set algorithm is implemented initialized by BR_t^0, giving the segmentation result BR_t. The level set algorithm implemented is the very efficient sparse field method proposed by Whitaker [9] and the well-known Chan-Vese energy is minimized. Some branches absent in original segmentation can be obtained in this way, because the prior information derived from the other image contributes to overcoming the difficulties such as fuzzy edges and false connection to surrounding structures. Some examples are shown in Fig. 4. However, the method may fail in regions where the image quality is too bad and even experts cannot distinguish the vessels.

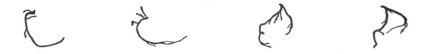

Fig. 4. The original segmentation (blue) and branches segmented by level set (red).

After attempts of further segmentation, new centerlines are extracted from arteries, and the registration process is performed again. The completeness of registration is improved because larger parts of trees can be registered.

3   Experiments and Results

We validated our method using 36 CCTA image pairs from 36 patients, among which 9 pairs (Group 1) are acquired with an interval of 3–7 years and 27 pairs (Group 2) are from end-systole and end-diastole. The method is evaluated from aspects of accuracy and completeness. The accuracy is assessed by the average Euclidian distance between the aligned centerline C_a and target centerline C_t:

$$D\left(C_a, C_t\right) = \frac{1}{2N_a} \sum_{i=1}^{N_a} D\left(c_a^i, C_t\right) + \frac{1}{2N_t} \sum_{i=1}^{N_t} D\left(c_t^i, C_a\right), \qquad (9)$$

$$D\left(c_a^i, C_t\right) = \min\left\{d\left(c_a^i, t\right) : t \in C_t\right\}, \qquad (10)$$

$$D\left(c_t^i, C_a\right) = \min\left\{d\left(c_t^i, a\right) : a \in C_a\right\}, \qquad (11)$$

where $c_a^i \in C_a$, $c_t^i \in C_t$, N_a and N_t are the numbers of dense sampling points on C_a and C_t, and d means Euclidean distance. The completeness is measured by the correct rate of registration, defined as $R^{reg} = \left(N_a^{reg}/N_a + N_t^{reg}/N_t\right)/2$, where N_a^{reg} and N_t^{reg} are the numbers of correctly matched points on C_a and C_t, respectively. Here a point on one centerline is considered correctly matched when the closest point on the other centerline is within 0.5 mm. The preliminary and final results (before and after further registration) of index $D(C_a, C_t)$ and R^{reg} on the dataset are displayed in Table 1. The further registration improves the correct rate of registration. The slight improvement in distance is not surprising as additional registered arteries are usually more noisy.

Table 1. E_{dist} represents the average and standard deviation of $D(C_a, C_t)$. E_{reg} indicates the average of R^{reg}. Superscript 1 and 2 indicate preliminary and final results.

Dataset	E_{dist}^1 (mm)	E_{dist}^2 (mm)	E_{reg}^1	E_{reg}^2
Group 1	0.047 ± 0.009	0.050 ± 0.011	88.0%	90.1%
Group 2	0.040 ± 0.007	0.043 ± 0.007	88.0%	90.8%
All	0.042 ± 0.008	0.044 ± 0.008	88.0%	90.7%

Figure 5(a) and (b) demonstrate the centerlines after preliminary and further registration respectively in two cases. A pair of further registered arteries in case 1 is indicated by arrows in Fig. 5(c), using the presentation method of straighten curved planar reformation (SCPR). The artery segment in the right image acquired in 2012 is missed in initial segmentation due to the serious calcification at the bifurcation, but it is important for reflecting the CAD progress.

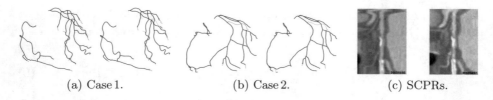

(a) Case 1.   (b) Case 2.   (c) SCPRs.

Fig. 5. (a)(b) The preliminary (left) and further (right) registration results. The preliminary/further matched parts are shown in red/cyan, unmatched parts in blue/green for two trees. (c) A pair of further registered arteries in case 1 is indicated by arrows.

4   Discussion and Conclusion

Our work has two main contributions in registration of coronary arteries. One is the hierarchical strategy for registration, consisting of bifurcation matching and segment registration. Bifurcation matching as the fundamental step properly handles the problem of different topologies, and segment registration contributes to the final accuracy. The other contribution is the improvement in completeness of registration, which is ignored by other related studies. In view of the fact that registration and segmentation are closely coupled problems, a level set method is used to further segment the difficult arteries missed by the initial segmentation algorithm, based on the initial registration results and prior information from the other image where the corresponding arteries are present. Moreover, more complete segmentation results in turn improve the completeness of registration.

Although the control points for TPS are totally on centerlines, the transform can be applied to whole arteries. The registration results can not only assist cardiologists in monitoring CAD progress, but also contribute to exploring the rules of coronary artery motion and changes within a cardiac cycle.

In conclusion, the method proposed for registration of coronary arteries in CCTA images performs well in aspects of accuracy and completeness, which is validated using 36 pairs of intra-subject CCTAs images captured at different dates or different phases. In future work, we will assess the method on larger datasets, and improve the algorithm for registering noisy arteries.

Acknowledgment. This work is supported by the National Natural Science Foundation of China under Grant 61622207.

References

1. Baka, N., et al.: Statistical coronary motion models for 2D+ t/3D registration of X-ray coronary angiography and CTA. Med. Image Anal. **17**(6), 698–709 (2013)
2. Bookstein, F.L.: Principal warps: thin-plate splines and the decomposition of deformations. IEEE Trans. Pattern Anal. Mach. Intell. **11**(6), 567–585 (1989)
3. Habert, S., Khurd, P., Chefd'Hotel, C.: Registration of multiple temporally related point sets using a novel variant of the coherent point drift algorithm: application to coronary tree matching. In: Medical Imaging 2013: Image Processing, vol. 8669, p. 86690M. International Society for Optics and Photonics (2013)

4. Hadjiiski, L., et al.: Coronary CT angiography (cCTA): automated registration of coronary arterial trees from multiple phases. Phys. Med. Biol. **59**(16), 4661 (2014)
5. Leordeanu, M., Hebert, M.: A spectral technique for correspondence problems using pairwise constraints. In: Proceedings of the Tenth IEEE International Conference on Computer Vision (ICCV 2005) Volume 1, vol. 2, pp. 1482–1489, October 2005
6. Luo, Y., Feng, J., Xu, M., Zhou, J., Min, J.K., Xiong, G.: Registration of coronary arteries in computed tomography angiography images using hidden Markov model. In: Proceedings of the 37th Annual International Conference of the IEEE Engineering in Medicine and Biology Society (EMBC), pp. 1993–1996, August 2015
7. Oliveira, F.P., Tavares, J.M.R.: Medical image registration: a review. Comput. Methods Biomech. Biomed. Eng. **17**(2), 73–93 (2014)
8. Scovanner, P., Ali, S., Shah, M.: A 3-dimensional SIFT descriptor and its application to action recognition. In: Proceedings of the 15th ACM International Conference on Multimedia, pp. 357–360. ACM (2007)
9. Whitaker, R.T.: A level-set approach to 3D reconstruction from range data. Int. J. Comput. Vis. **29**(3), 203–231 (1998)

Quantifying Tensor Field Similarity with Global Distributions and Optimal Transport

Arnold D. Gomez[1]([✉]), Maureen L. Stone[2], Philip V. Bayly[3],
and Jerry L. Prince[1]

[1] Electrical and Computer Engineering Department, Jonhs Hopkins University,
Baltimore, USA
adgomez@jhu.edu
[2] Department of Neural and Pain Sciences, University of Maryland, Baltimore, USA
[3] Mechanical Engineering Department, Washington University in St. Louis, St.
Louis, USA

Abstract. Strain tensor fields quantify tissue deformation and are important for functional analysis of moving organs such as the heart and the tongue. Strain data can be readily obtained using medical imaging. However, quantification of similarity between different data sets is difficult. Strain patterns vary in space and time, and are inherently multidimensional. Also, the same type of mechanical deformation can be applied to different shapes; hence, automatic quantification of similarity should be unaffected by the geometry of the objects being deformed. In the pattern recognition literature, shapes and vector fields have been classified via global distributions. This study uses a distribution of mechanical properties (a 3D histogram), and the Wasserstein distance from optimal transport theory is used to measure histogram similarity. To evaluate the method's consistency in matching deformations across different objects, the proposed approach was used to sort strain fields according to their similarity. Performance was compared to sorting via maximum shear distribution (a 1D histogram) and tensor residual magnitude in perfectly registered objects. The technique was also applied to correlate muscle activation to muscular contraction observed via tagged MRI. The results show that the proposed approach accurately matches deformation regardless of the shape of the object being deformed. Sorting accuracy surpassed 1D shear distribution and was on par with residual magnitude, but without the need for registration between objects.

Keywords: Strain · Tensor fields · Tagged MRI · Organ deformation

1 Introduction

Tissue deformation is necessary for vital bodily functions such as cardiac blood pressurization [1], locomotion via the musculoskeletal system [2], and motion in

© Springer Nature Switzerland AG 2018
A. F. Frangi et al. (Eds.): MICCAI 2018, LNCS 11071, pp. 428–436, 2018.
https://doi.org/10.1007/978-3-030-00934-2_48

the tongue (involved in breathing, swallowing, and speech) [3]. The strain tensor quantifies deformation, and can produce biomarkers related to organ function [1,3]. For this reason, many acquisition and processing methods have been developed for using medical imaging to observe motion (as in Fig. 1) and to measure strain. Strain can be reduced to global metrics to simplify clinical or research applications, e.g., radial or circumferential strains in cardiac deformation [1], or fiber strains for analysis of tongue motion [3]. However, the state of deformation across an organ can only be truly captured by a volumetric strain field.

Statistical analysis of mechanical deformation is relevant when studying disease progression and functional mechanisms, particularly with computational models aimed at predicting deformation, such as in traumatic brain injury research [4], speech analysis [5], the study of muscular contraction [2], and for assessing of cardiac contractility [6]. Ideally, these models must agree with experimental data; hence, similarity quantification between tensor fields is useful in: (i) determining the uncertainty of experimental measurements, (ii) measuring the descriptive or predictive power of a simulation, and (iii) assessing the sensitivity of strain results to processing or modeling parameters [7,8]. Strain comparisons are also useful to align data for atlas generation [9].

Similarity measurement between strain fields is challenging [8]. As with scalar fields (e.g., images), the concept of similarity is diverse, encompassing not only correspondence and alignment, but also directionality, magnitude, and orientation [8]. Mechanical deformation also changes in time and across patients, and is defined in many different discretization schemes. For instance, image measurements generally result in pixel wise values [1] while computational models often use finite elements (FE) [10] or (more recently) point clouds [4]. This variety of configurations and formats can make it difficult to compare strain fields by means of evaluating field properties in matching comparison points. (Fields can be defined across different geometric domains, which can have topological or discretization incompatibilities, limiting or even preventing registration.)

This paper describes a novel approach to measure similarity between strain tensor fields. The methodology was developed to overcome the need to register domains, while capturing the spatial distribution of strain within the organ.

2   Background

Assuming that tissue behaves as a continuum for macroscopic deformation, a particle in the reference configuration $\boldsymbol{X} = \boldsymbol{X}(t_o) \in \mathbb{R}^3$ at time t_0 is associated to a single point in the deformed configuration $\boldsymbol{x}(t)$ via a Lagrangian displacement field $\boldsymbol{u}(\boldsymbol{X}, t) = \boldsymbol{X} - \boldsymbol{x}(\boldsymbol{X}, t)$. Displacement information is obtainable via medical imaging e.g., speckle tracking in ultrasound, registration of CINE MRI, or tagged MRI [1,11], and biomechanics simulations [10]. Relative displacement between neighboring particles is related to the deformation gradient tensor

$$\boldsymbol{F} = \boldsymbol{F}(\boldsymbol{X}, \boldsymbol{x}, t) = \frac{\partial \boldsymbol{x}(t)}{\partial \boldsymbol{X}(t_0)} = 1 + \frac{\partial \boldsymbol{u}(t)}{\partial \boldsymbol{X}(t_0)}, \tag{1}$$

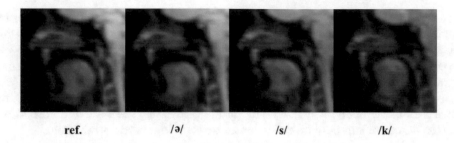

Fig. 1. Sequence from magnetic resonance imaging (MRI) during speech generation (sagittal). Deformation can be seen by comparing the shape of the tongue at the beginning of the sound /ə/ (/ə/ means "a" as in "car"), which is the reference (ref.) versus the shapes during the sounds /ə/, /s/ (as in "sound"), and /k/ (as in "kiosk").

where $\mathbf{1}$ is the identity tensor [12]. $\boldsymbol{F}$ differs from $\mathbf{1}$ in rigid motion and rotation; thus, the direct application of $\boldsymbol{F}$ in quantifying deformation is limited. Instead, we can define strain tensors insensitive to rigid transformations. These include the (left) Cauchy-Green strain tensor

$$C = C(X, x, t) = F^T F, \tag{2}$$

and the Green-Lagrange strain tensor $\boldsymbol{E} = \frac{1}{2}(\boldsymbol{C} - \mathbf{1})$ [12]. Eigenvalue decomposition of these quantities yields principal components along key directions such as the radial and circumferential strains used in cardiac mechanics [1].

Methods for quantification of similarity between strain fields are varied. One common approach is to apply point-wise norms or patch correlations [8]. While this is an effective similarity measure, it requires matching points or regions between two or more geometries. If registration is needed, it can introduce computational expense and (or) registration error. Another common approach is to compare the distributions of scalar metrics [4,8], which does not require registration and is effective in cases where similarity is determined largely by magnitude. However, traditional global distributions are spatially underdetermined resulting in loss of structural information.

In pattern recognition, structural distributions have emerged as a fast and effective means of identifying objects [13,14], and these have also been extended to vector fields [15]. The main idea behind these techniques is the construction of a *structurally sensitive* distribution (a shape or vector field signature), which is populated by sampling properties between points inside each domain. Examples include 1D histograms constructed from the distance between two random points within an object [13], and 2D histograms populated by sampling magnitude and angle differences along streamlines in a vector field [15].

3   Quantifying Tensor Field Similarity

Based on previous work in pattern recognition [13–15], we propose the construction of a structurally sensitive global distribution for each strain field. This distribution acts as a *strain signature* (or a set of features), enabling similarity quantification. In the context of pattern identification, a metric of similarity is derived from a normalized measure of distance between distributions.

The properties f for the construction of features are obtained from points with randomly assigned coordinates $R \in \mathcal{D} \in \mathbb{R}^3$, where $\mathcal{D}$ is the domain in which the strain field is defined. At each point,

$$f(R) = \begin{bmatrix} \gamma_{\max} \\ \theta \\ \bar{\gamma} \end{bmatrix}. \tag{3}$$

The quantity $\gamma_{\max} = \gamma_{\max}(R) = E_1 - E_3$ (where E_1 and E_3 represent the first and third eigenvalues of E) is the maximum shear strain. Since $\gamma_{\max}$ is directly evaluated at R, it provides a *global* component to the distribution. The other two properties are associated with R and $P \in \mathcal{D}$—another point chosen at random. The local state of deformation at these two locations is coupled via $F_{RP} = F(R)^{-1}F(P)$, which is analogous to the distance between random internal points used to construct shape distributions [13]. F_{RP} represents a mechanical deformation; thus, θ is the net rotation from F_{RP} obtained via singular value decomposition. Finally, $\bar{\gamma} = \frac{1}{2}\Sigma(C_{RP})_{ij}$ $(i \neq j)$ is the mean shear strain, which is extracted substituting F_{RP} into (2). Both θ and $\bar{\gamma}$ are relative properties, providing the *structural* component of the distribution. Shear and rotation values are used due to the incompressible nature of tissue, which favors isochoric deformation—this intrinsic feature affects similarity comparison indirectly.

To approximate the distribution of $f(R) \forall R \in \mathcal{D}$, N samples f_i $(i = 1, 2, ..., N)$ are binned into a 3D histogram p_f with d bins. Sample histograms appear in Fig. 2, and show differences based on the deformation pattern, and not necessarily on the orientation and geometry of the object being deformed (Fig. 2(a) is different to Fig. 2(b) given the same object). There are also similarities that can be used to define distance (Fig. 2(a) is closer to Fig. 2(c)).

By edge normalization, any two histograms to be compared, say p_f and p_g, are defined in a common simplex $\Sigma_d = \{x \in \mathbb{R}^d_+ : x^T 1_d = 1\}$ [16]. (1_d denotes an array of ones.) We can thus write the transportation, or coupling, polytope $U(p_f, p_g) = \{Z \in \mathbb{R}^{d \times d}_+ | Z 1_d = p_f, Z^T 1_d = p_g\}$, which allows posing an optimal transport (OT) problem as seen in some registration and shape similarity approaches [16–18]. Letting C be a cost matrix reflecting the l^2 distance between the centers of the histogram bins,

$$W_c(p_f, p_g) = \min_{Z \in U} \langle Z, C \rangle \tag{4}$$

is a discrete transport to measure the distance—or dissimilarity—between p_f and p_g. (Angle brackets denote the Frobenius product.) Specifically, (4) defines the Wasserstein distance after obtaining an optimal transport $Z^\star$.

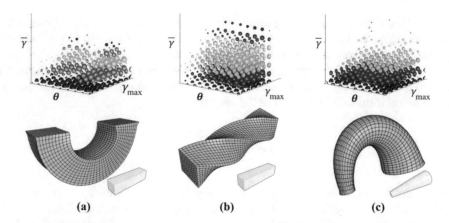

Fig. 2. Field property distributions. The top row shows 3D histograms, where the count scales sphere radii logarithmically, and color indicates height. The corresponding deformed shapes include: (a) a rod with square cross-section being bent upwards, (b) the same rod being twisted, and (c) a cylindrical rod being bent downwards. The undeformed shape appears below.

Computing $Z^\star$ for large multidimensional histograms is computationally prohibitive; thus, we implemented an approximation via the Sinkhorn-Knopp algorithm [16]. This approach uses an entropy constraint enforced by a Lagrangian multiplier λ, i.e., we find $W_c^\lambda(\boldsymbol{p}_f, \boldsymbol{p}_g) = \langle Z^\lambda, C \rangle$, where

$$Z^\lambda = \arg\min_{Z \in U} \langle Z, C \rangle - \frac{1}{\lambda} h(Z), \tag{5}$$

with $h(Z) = -\sum_{ij} Z_{ij}(\log(Z_{ij}) - 1)$. For the experiments in this study, we find that Z^λ is a reasonable approximation of $Z^\star$ for values of λ near 200, while being faster by nearly two orders of magnitude.

4   Experiments and Results

Sorting Test Strain Fields: Similarity-based sorting was used to determine accuracy and consistency against other methods. We created a dictionary of 27 simulated deformation fields containing bending, torsion, and extension (nine cases each). The fields were defined in geometries with different cross-section and discretization primitives using FE software [10]. A reference (or query) deformation pattern was matched to dictionary entries. Ideally, similar deformations will be the closest to the query, not only in top match, but the top $k-1$ matches—as there are $k = 9$ cases with similar deformations. Every field was used as query against all others to quantify the percentage of successes. For comparison, sorting was performed via: (i) 3D distributions using OT distance (3DOT), (ii) 3D distributions using the Euclidean distance (3DEU) [15], and (iii) 1D distributions of γ_{max} using Euclidean distance (1DEU) [4]. Given the random nature of the sampling, the comparisons were performed 10 times using different seeds, and compared using unpaired t-test with significance level at $p = 0.01$.

The 3DOT approach was able to identify strain patterns regardless of geometry and discretization (see Fig. 3). Note that registration between the shapes—e.g., a square and a quarter-circular cross-section—would be difficult to perform. The proposed method was capable of identifying the top five matches with perfect accuracy, which reduced to 55% for the top eight matches. This is in stark contrast compared to 3DEU (accuracy dropped below 80% on the top three, and was 22% for the top eight), which demonstrates the utility of the OT approach. 1DEU was the least accurate likely due to structural information loss. Statistically significant performance differences between 3DOT and the alternatives were observed for $k = 3$ through $k = 8$. Sampling 10^4 points and calculation of W_c^λ took 90 s on a standard 12-core server.

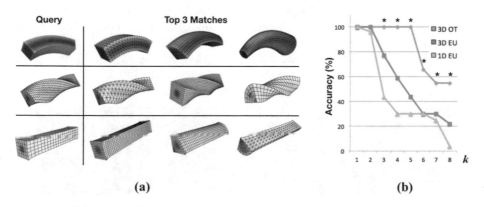

(a)   (b)

Fig. 3. Strain field sorting results. (a) Typical sorting results using the proposed algorithm. (b) Accuracy of the top k results across all simulations. A start denotes statistically significant differences between 3DOT and both of the alternatives.

Relating Image Measurements to Simulations: We used the proposed method to associate strain to muscular activation patterns in the tongue. Activation cannot be reliably measured but can be simulated; thus, it is possible to infer which muscles are active by matching experimental data to simulations. Tongue deformation during the sequence in Fig. 1 was measured via tagged MRI in healthy adult volunteers ($n = 7$, 4 male, 3 female, with informed consent) [5]. Strain fields were sampled and 3DOT was used to compare the experimental results to a dictionary composed of 74 FE simulations. The simulations included muscular activation and deformation as linear combinations of four categories: dorsiflexion (D), which moves the tip of the tongue upwards; protrusion (P), which moves the tip forward; retraction (R), which moves the tip backward; and ventriflexion (V), which lowers it. The experimental data was decomposed into percentages of each category (D, P, R, and V) and overall activation level (AL) based on the top three matches—AL = 0 indicates no activation. Also, the dictionary entries (which are perfectly registered with one another) were sorted within themselves to compare the top matches via 3DOT, 1DEU, and the deformation gradient residual magnitude $||\boldsymbol{F}_i - \boldsymbol{F}_j||$ (sampling was also repeated 10 times).

The decomposition results appear in Fig. 4. Deformation from the reference configuration (early /ə/) to /ə/ was associated largely to retraction ($75 \pm 5\%$) and to a lesser extent to protrusion ($25 \pm 5\%$) with AL = 3.0. This low value of AL indicates a small, retraction-like deformation, as observed in Figs. 1 and 4. Deformation to /s/ was associated largely with protrusion ($64 \pm 10\%$), and less so with retraction and retroflexion ($15 \pm 21\%$ and $17 \pm 11\%$, respectively) with AL = 5.3. This is consistent with that observed forward motion of the tip of the tongue during this sound. During /k/ the observed deformation was associated mostly with retraction ($66 \pm 10\%$), and to a lesser extent with protrusion ($34 \pm 10\%$) with AL = 5. Compared to the reference, the tongue appears to retract during /k/ in the images. Both of the latter sounds result in larger AL values, as more activation is needed to achieve larger deformations. When comparing the top results of dictionary sorting, 3DOT agreed with residual magnitude in $56 \pm 2\%$ of the top results, compared to $22 \pm 3\%$ for 1DEU (statistically significant). Sampling 2×10^4 points and distance measurement took roughly 150 s.

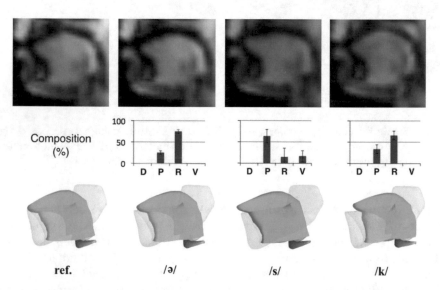

Fig. 4. Decomposition results. The close-up of a typical volunteer (top) is aligned with the decomposition shown as bar charts, and the models with the closest simulation.

5   Discussion

The proposed method is able to discriminate deformation patterns across different geometries and discretizations, its accuracy surpasses the alternatives studied, and it is also fast. Distance measurement via OT also shows clear benefits. The results from motion measurement via tagged MRI are consistent with visual inspection. The tongue shape varies considerably from subject to subject; thus, avoiding registration will simplify analysis of motion as larger datasets are produced. Sorting error was still observed likely indicating that the selection of features has a level of incompleteness via interdependence or data loss [8]. Also the distribution approach has no inverse mapping, which would be useful for machine learning. However, the methodology can be framed in different ways to address these limitations, e.g., via constructing distributions by sampling along hyperstreamlines, or applying OT methodology to tensor entries directly, as done in shape matching [17]. The proposed method remains a viable alternative given the seeding and computational requirements of these potential approaches.

References

1. Ibrahim, E.S.H.: Myocardial tagging by cardiovascular magnetic resonance: evolution of techniques-pulse sequences, analysis algorithms, and applications. J. Cardiovasc. Magn. Reson. **13**(1), 36–42 (2011)
2. Moerman, K.M., Sprengers, A.M.J., Simms, C.K., Lamerichs, R.M., Stoker, J., Nederveen, A.J.: Validation of tagged MRI for the measurement of dynamic 3D skeletal muscle tissue deformation. Med. Phys. **39**(4), 1793–1810 (2012)
3. Parthasarathy, V., Prince, J.L., Stone, M., Murano, E.Z., NessAiver, M.: Measuring tongue motion from tagged cine-MRI using harmonic phase (HARP) processing. J. Acoust. Soc. Am. **121**(1), 491–504 (2007)
4. Ganpule, S., et al.: A 3D computational human head model that captures live human brain dynamics. J. Neurotrauma **34**(13), 2154–2166 (2017)
5. Gomez, A.D., Xing, F., Chan, D., Pham, D.L., Bayly, P., Prince, J.L.: Motion estimation with finite-element biomechanical models and tracking constraints from tagged MRI. In: Wittek, A., Joldes, G., Nielsen, P.M.F., Doyle, B.J., Miller, K. (eds.) Computational Biomechanics for Medicine: From Algorithms to Models and Applications, pp. 81–90. Springer, Cham (2017). https://doi.org/10.1007/978-3-319-54481-6_7
6. Wenk, J.F., et al.: Regional left ventricular myocardial contractility and stress in a finite element model of posterobasal myocardial infarction. J. Biomech. Eng. **133**(4), 1–14 (2011)
7. Henninger, H.B., Reese, S.P., Anderson, A.E., Weiss, J.A.: Validation of computational models in biomechanics. Proc. Inst. Mech. Eng. Part H **224**(7), 801–812 (2010)
8. Tian, Y., Nearing, G.S., Peters-Lidard, C.D., Harrison, K.W., Tang, L.: Performance metrics, error modeling, and uncertainty quantification. Mon. Weather Rev. **144**(2), 607–613 (2016)
9. Woo, J., Xing, F., Lee, J., Stone, M., Prince, J.L.: Construction of an unbiased spatio-temporal atlas of the tongue during speech. In: Ourselin, S., Alexander, D.C., Westin, C.-F., Cardoso, M.J. (eds.) IPMI 2015. LNCS, vol. 9123, pp. 723–732. Springer, Cham (2015). https://doi.org/10.1007/978-3-319-19992-4_57
10. Maas, S.A., Ellis, B.J., Ateshian, G.A., Weiss, J.A.: FEBio: finite elements for biomechanics. J. Biomech. Eng. **134**(1), 011005 (2012)

11. Keszei, A.P., Berkels, B., Deserno, T.M.: Survey of non-rigid registration tools in medicine. J. Digit. Imaging **30**(1), 102–116 (2017)
12. Spencer, A.J.M.: Continuum Mechanics, 1995th edn. Dover Books, Essex (1985)
13. Osada, R., Funkhouser, T., Chazelle, B., Dobkin, D.: Shape distributions. ACM Trans. Graph. **21**(4), 807–832 (2002)
14. Ohbuchi, R., Minamitani, T., Takei, T.: Shape-similarity search of 3D models by using enhanced shape functions. Int. J. Comput. Appl. Technol. **23**(2/3/4), 70–78 (2005)
15. Dinh, H.Q., Xu, L.: Measuring the similarity of vector fields using global distributions. In: da Vitoria, L.N. (ed.) SSPR/SPR 2008. LNCS, vol. 5342, pp. 187–196. Springer, Heidelberg (2008). https://doi.org/10.1007/978-3-540-89689-0_23
16. Cuturi, M.: Sinkhorn distances: lightspeed computation of optimal transportation distances. Adv. Neural Inf. Process. Syst. **26**, 2292–2299 (2013)
17. Su, Z., et al.: Optimal mass transport for shape matching and comparison. IEEE Trans. Pattern Anal. Mach. Intell. **37**(11), 2246–2259 (2015)
18. ur Rehman, T., Haber, E., Pryor, G., Melonakos, J., Tannenbaum, A.: 3D nonrigid registration via optimal mass transport on the GPU. Med. Image Anal. **13**(6), 931–940 (2009)

Cardiac Motion Scoring with Segment- and Subject-Level Non-local Modeling

Wufeng Xue[1,2], Gary Brahm[1], Stephanie Leung[1], Ogla Shmuilovich[1], and Shuo Li[1(✉)]

[1] Department of Medical Imaging, Western University, London, ON, Canada
slishuo@gmail.com
[2] National-Regional Key Technology Engineering Laboratory for Medical Ultrasound, School of Biomedical Engineering, Health Science Center, Shenzhen University, Shenzhen, China

Abstract. Motion scoring of cardiac myocardium is of paramount importance for early detection and diagnosis of various cardiac disease. It aims at identifying regional wall motions into one of the four types including normal, hypokinetic, akinetic, and dyskinetic, and is extremely challenging due to the complex myocardium deformation and subtle inter-class difference of motion patterns. All existing work on automated motion analysis are focused on binary abnormality detection to avoid the much more demanding motion scoring, which is urgently required in real clinical practice yet has never been investigated before. In this work, we propose Cardiac-MOS, the first powerful method for cardiac motion scoring from cardiac MR sequences based on deep convolution neural network. Due to the locality of convolution, the relationship between distant non-local responses of the feature map cannot be explored, which is closely related to motion difference between segments. In Cardiac-MOS, such non-local relationship is modeled with non-local neural network within each segment and across all segments of one subject, i.e., segment- and subject-level non-local modeling, and lead to obvious performance improvement. Besides, Cardiac-MOS can effectively extract motion information from MR sequences of various lengths by interpolating the convolution kernel along the temporal dimension, therefore can be applied to MR sequences of multiple sources. Experiments on 1440 myocardium segments of 90 subjects from short axis MR sequences of multiple lengths prove that Cardiac-MOS achieves reliable performance, with correlation of 0.926 for motion score index estimation and accuracy of 77.4% for motion scoring. Cardiac-MOS also outperforms all existing work for binary abnormality detection. As the first automatic motion scoring solution, Cardiac-MOS demonstrates great potential in future clinical application.

1 Introduction

Cardiac motion scoring is essential for clinical diagnosis of various cardiac disease [4], including coronary artery disease, congestive heart failure, stress-induced cardiomyopathy, myocarditis, stroke, amongst others. However, cardiac

© Springer Nature Switzerland AG 2018
A. F. Frangi et al. (Eds.): MICCAI 2018, LNCS 11071, pp. 437–445, 2018.
https://doi.org/10.1007/978-3-030-00934-2_49

wall motion is a complex deformation procedure with regional wall thickening, circumferential shortening and longitudinal ventricular shortening. It varies a lot in the presence of different types of pathology. In routine clinical practice, motion scoring is often conducted by labor-intensive visual inspection of the dynamic cardiac sequences of MR or Echocardiograms for each segment of left ventricle, following the scoring system of [4]: (1) normal, (2) hypokinetic, (3) akinetic, and (4) dyskinetic. The results obtained in this way are characterized by large inter-rater variability and low reproducibility [8] due to the complex regional motion patterns and the subtle motion difference between segments.

However, automated motion scoring from cardiac MR images has never been investigated despite its clinical significance. Existing work only focused on binary motion abnormality detection [1,2,5–7,9–15], which alleviates a lot the difficulty of differentiating the subtle difference among various motion patterns. In summary, these methods follow a pipeline of: (1) *myocardium segments localization*, by manually or semi-automatically delineating the contours of myocardium [1,2,5,6,9–12,15], (2) handcrafted *motion information extraction*, including spatial-temporal profiles [13,14], inter-frame correlations [1,2,6], or parameter distribution [9–12], and then (3) *motion classification*.

Table 1. Existing methods on *binary* abnormality detection only obtained good performance for small dataset with LOO experiment setting.

Methods	# of subject	Modality	Training/Test	Accuracy (%)	Kappa value
[11]	30	SAX MR	LOO	90.8	0.738
[9]	30	SAX, 2C, 3C, 4C MR	LOO	91.9	0.738
[10]	58	SAX MR	LOO	87.1	0.73
[13,14]	22	SAX Tagged MR	LOO	87.8	-
[6]	17	SAX Basal MR	No split	86.3	0.693
[1]	58	SAX MR	3-fold CV	86	0.73
[15]	89	SAX MR	45/44	65.9	-
[5]	129	2C and 4C Echo	65/64	76.5	-

SAX: short axis view; 2C: two chamber view; 3C: three chamber view; 4C: four chamber view; LOO: leave-one-subject-out; CV: cross validation

While these methods achieved promising accuracy for abnormality detection, they cannot be applied to the task of motion scoring because (1) only heuristic handcrafted feature is not sufficient to capture the complex regional motion information; and (2) absence of dependency modeling between local features of all segments cannot capture the subtle motion difference between segments. Besides, they still suffer from the following limitations: (1) delineation of myocardium border is required, either manually or semi-automatically, introducing inconvenience in clinical practice; (2) multiple classifiers are trained for different segments [1,2,5,6] or slices [9–11,15], complicating their practical application;

(3) only achieves good performance on small dataset (as shown in Table 1), where the diversity of cardiac motion pattern is limited.

In this paper, we take advantage of the deep convolution network and non-local modeling [17], and propose the first reliable solution, Cardiac-MOS for Cardiac MOtion Scoring. While the convolution network extracts discriminative *local* features, non-local modeling allows distant *non-local* responses to contribute to the response at a location, therefore capturing the subtle relative changes of local motion features. In Cardiac-MOS, we (1) design a kernel-interpolation based convolution (conv-KI) layer, which captures motion information by convolution along the temporal dimension, and reuses the kernel by interpolation for sequences of various lengths, and (2) introduce segment- and subject-level non-local modeling to explore the long-range relationships within each segment and across all 16 segments of one subject. With non-local modeling, Cardiac-MOS is capable of extracting the subtle motion difference between segments and thus delivering accurate motion scoring results.

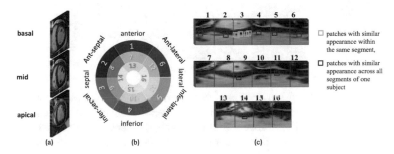

Fig. 1. Myocardium segment re-sampling. The 16 segments obtained from short axis slices (a) according to the AHA 17-segment model [4] of left ventricle (b) are converted into the polar coordinates and re-sampled to rectangular sequences of the same size (c), so that the motion information can be more easily modeled. Appearance similarity between patches within each segment (blue) and patches across all segments (red) underlies our non-local modeling.

2   Cardiac Motion Scoring

The proposed network Cardiac-MOS takes as input the myocardial segment sequences represented in the polar coordinate system. We first describe how to convert the spatial cardiac MR sequences into the polar coordinate system, and then describe how Cardiac-MOS works.

2.1   Myocardium Segment Re-sampling in Polar Coordinate System

To ensure a uniform scoring procedure for all the 16 regions in spite of their position, and to leverage the powerful representation of neural network for motion information extraction, the fan-shaped regions obtained following the AHA 17-segment model of left ventricle [4] (Fig. 1(b)) are converted into the polar coordinate system. For segments of apical slice, we re-sample them along the angular dimension, therefore resulting in segments of the same size with those of basal and mid-slices (Fig. 1(c)). Such conversion and re-sampling make it more convenient to capture the motion information and model the spatial dependencies since most motions fall into the same orientation. Denote the obtained ith ($i = 1, ...16$) segment sequence for patient p as $X_{p,i} \in \mathcal{R}^{r,a,t}$, where r, a are the sampling numbers along the radial and angular dimension, and t is the frame number in the cardiac cycle. In this work, r equals half of the image size, a is 60 for all the segments.

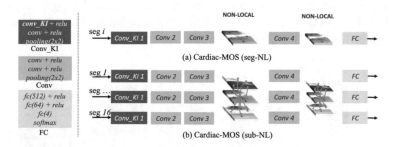

Fig. 2. Our Cardiac-MOS models the distant non-local relationship of convolution features with Non-local neural networks in both segment-level ((a) Cardiac-MOS (seg-NL)) and subject-level ((b) Cardiac-MOS (sub-NL)). Kernel interpolation (conv-KI) is deployed to extract motion information from sequences of various lengths.

2.2   Motion Scoring Neural Network

With the segment sequence $X_{p,i}$, the task of motion scoring aims to rate its motion function following the above mentioned scoring system $\mathbf{s}_{p,i} \in \{0, 1, 2, 3\}$. The proposed Cardiac-MOS (Fig. 2) contains four successive convolution blocks to extract discriminative motion-aware information from each segment sequence. Specifically, to extract the motion information from sequences of various lengths, the first convolution block is equipped with a kernel-interpolation based convolution (conv-KI) layer, which is applied along the temporal dimension. To capture the subtle motion difference between segments, non-local relationship of local convolutional features is modeled with non-local neural network. Finally, a fully connection block with Softmax layer is used for motion scoring.

Motion Extraction with Kernel-Interpolation Based Convolution Layer. For input sequence $X_{p,i}$ with frame number $t = N_0$, we first employ a $1 \times 1 \times t \times n_o$ convolution kernel k_0 with n_o the filter number, to extract its motion information (Fig. 3 left). Each filter in k_0 acts as a template to match the temporal profile in every spatial position. However, such a fixed-shape kernel

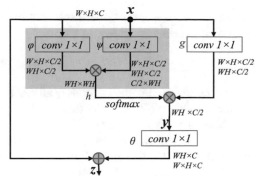

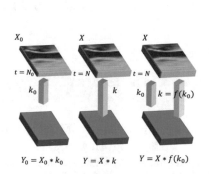

Fig. 3. The proposed conv-KI layer extracts motion information from segment sequences of different lengths by interpolating k_0 to form the new kernel.

Fig. 4. Non-Local block employed in Fig. 2, which explores relationships between distant non-local response in feature maps **x** of the convolution layer.

cannot be applied to the sequence with a different length $t = N$ (Fig. 3 middle). We propose a kernel-interpolation based convolution (conv-KI) layer to reuse k_0 (Fig. 3 right) when the sequence length changes. Denote X and Y the input and output of a convolution layer, then in a conv-KI layer, $Y = X * f(k_0)$, where $k = f(k_0)$ can be any parametric or nonparametric function that makes k match the frame number of the new sequence. With conv-KI layer, the proposed network can be trained with and applied to cardiac sequences of multiple sources. In this work, bilinear interpolation is used for f.

Segment- and Subject-Level Non-local Modeling. Cardiac motion score is determined by the motion patterns within one segment and its relative difference to other segments. As shown in Fig. 1(c), patches with similar appearance exist within one segment (patches in blue) and across all segments (patches in red) of the subject. Only the convolution layer cannot model such relationship due to their local receptive field. To model such long-range relationships, non-local (NL) blocks are deployed in Cardiac-MOS, as shown in Fig. 2(a) and (b) for segment- and subject-level NL properties, respectively. NL operation for neural network [17] was inspired by the non-local means method in computer vision. A general NL operation computes the response **y** at a position i as weighted sum of the features at all positions:

$$\mathbf{y}_i = \frac{1}{\mathcal{C}(\mathbf{x})} \sum_{\forall j} h(\mathbf{x}_i, \mathbf{x}_j) g(\mathbf{x}_j), \tag{1}$$

where the pairwise function h computes the similarity between two positions, g computes a representation of the input feature, and $\mathcal{C}(\mathbf{x}) = \sum_{\forall j} h(\mathbf{x}_i, \mathbf{x}_j)$ is a normalization factor. In this work, we use the embedded Gaussian [17] for h:

$$h(\mathbf{x}_i, \mathbf{x}_j) = \exp^{\phi(\mathbf{x}_i)^T \psi(\mathbf{x}_j)}, \tag{2}$$

which makes $\frac{1}{\mathcal{C}(\mathbf{x})}h(\mathbf{x}_i,\mathbf{x}_j)$ as a softmax function. The computation of a NL block in neural network is shown in Fig. 4:

$$\mathbf{z}_i = \theta(\mathbf{y}_i) + \mathbf{x}_i, \tag{3}$$

where the residual connection $+\mathbf{x}_i$ allows a NL block to be inserted into any pretrained model, while keeping its initial behavior. ϕ, ψ and θ are implemented as convolution with 1×1 kernel.

In this work, NL blocks are innovatively deployed into Cardiac-MOS in two different ways: (1) Cardiac-MOS (seg-NL), as shown in Fig. 2(a), where the position index j traverse all possible positions in one segment, therefore segment-level non-local property is explored; and (2) Cardiac-MOS (sub-NL), as shown in Fig. 2(b), where j traverse all possible positions of all segments in one batch, thus subject-level non-local property is explored. While seg-NL helps capture the motion features robustly for each segment, sub-NL helps capture the relative change of motion patterns between segments. During network training, one batch contains 16 segments, i.e., all segments from one subject.

3   Dataset and Configurations

To validate the proposed Cardiac-MOS, cardiac MR sequences of 90 subjects (5775 images) are collected from scanners of multiple vendors, with spatial resolution of 0.6445–1.9792 mm/pixel, frame number of 20 (65 subjects) or 25 (25 subjects) in one cardiac cycle. Various pathologies are in presence, including dilated cardiomyopathy, ventricular hypertrophy, infarction, ischemia, scar formation, etc. For each subject, three representative short-axis cine sequences are chosen from the basal, mid, and apical left ventricle. Segment-wise ground truth of motion score is obtained from the radiologists' report and expert's visual inspection, resulting in a total of 1440 segments in the dataset. The distribution of motions score is $\{794, 348, 207, 91\}$ for the four motion types $s_{p,i}$.

For each sequence, three landmarks, i.e, the junctions of left and right ventricles, and the center point of cavity, are manually pointed to crop the left ventricle and to align its orientation. Normalization of the myocardium size is conducted by resizing the cropped images to 160×160. Normalization of the intensity is conducted by contrast-limited adaptive histogram equalization.

Our network is implemented in Tensorflow, with cross-entropy loss used during training. Three-fold cross validation (split according to subject, not segment) is used to benchmark the performance. Following [17], we first train a baseline CNN network, where no NL-block is employed, and then finetune the two non-local networks from this pre-trained model.

4   Results and Analysis

The performance of Cardiac-MOS is benchmarked with the task of motion scoring, and motion score index (MSI, calculated as the average of the scores of all segments for each subject [4]) estimation. Classification accuracy (acc_{ms}) and Pearson correlation ρ_{msi} are used for evaluation. To compare with existing work on binary abnormality detection, classification accuracy (acc_{ad}) and Kappa value [16] (κ_{ad}, which is a more convincing index considering the prevalence of positive and negative samples) are also evaluated.

As shown in Table 2, the proposed Cardiac-MOS achieves effective performance, with correlation of 0.926 for MSI estimation, and accuracy of 0.774 for motions scoring. For reference, the only reported inter-observer correlation for MSI is 0.85 [3] for echocardiography. Therefore, the proposed Cardiac-MOS has great potential in clinical practice of cardiac motion analysis. Besides, the non-local modeling effectively improves the performance of Cardiac-MOS upon the baseline CNN model, proving its capability of capturing subtle motion difference between segments. Among the four configurations of NL blocks, Cardiac-MOS (sub-NL-1) performs better than the other configurations, revealing the importance of subject-level non-local modeling for cardiac motion scoring, which explores the mutual dependencies of local features across all 16 segments, therefore is capable of capturing the subtle relative change of motion patterns between segments. This inter-segment dependencies are better modeled with higher level convolution features (with more context information), thus Cardiac-MOS (sub-NL-2) performs slightly inferior to Cardiac-MOS (sub-NL-1). When compared with existing methods for abnormality detection (Table 1), the proposed Cardiac-MOS achieves the best Kappa value among all the competitors despite the unfair settings, proving the effectiveness of Cardiac-MOS.

Table 2. Performance of Cardiac-MOS with various configuration of NL blocks. (seg-NL-1: one segment-level NL block after Conv4; seg-NL-2: two segment-level NL blocks after Conv3 and Conv4.)

	$acc_{ms}(\%)$	ρ_{msi}	$acc_{ad}(\%)$	κ_{ad}
Baseline CNN	74.7	0.913	85.8	0.711
Cardiac-MOS (seg-NL-1)	75.6	0.907	86.3	0.720
Cardiac-MOS (seg-NL-2)	76.1	0.914	87.0	0.735
Cardiac-MOS (sub-NL-1)	**77.4**	**0.926**	**87.8**	**0.749**
Cardiac-MOS (sub-NL-2)	76.4	0.919	87.6	0.746

5 Conclusions

We proposed the first effective solution Cardiac-MOS for automated cardiac motion scoring from MR sequences. Cardiac-MOS is capable of extracting the complex motion information from cardiac sequences of various lengths with a kernel-interpolation based convolution layer, learning discriminative features with hierarchy convolution layers, and capturing subtle differences among motion patterns by modeling long-range spatial dependency with segment- and subject-level non-local networks. Performance of Cardiac-MOS on a MR dataset of 90 subjects demonstrated its great potential in future clinical application.

References

1. Afshin, M., et al.: Regional assessment of cardiac left ventricular myocardial function via MRI statistical features. IEEE TMI **33**, 481–494 (2014)
2. Afshin, M., et al.: Assessment of regional myocardial function via statistical features in MR images. In: Fichtinger, G., Martel, A., Peters, T. (eds.) MICCAI 2011. LNCS, vol. 6893, pp. 107–114. Springer, Heidelberg (2011). https://doi.org/10.1007/978-3-642-23626-6_14
3. Bjørnstad, K., Al Amri, M., Lingamanaicker, J., Oqaili, I., Hatle, L.: Interobserver and intraobserver variation for analysis of left ventricular wall motion at baseline and during low-and high-dose dobutamine stress echocardiography in patients with high prevalence of wall motion abnormalities at rest. J. Am. Soc. Echocardiogr. **9**(3), 320–328 (1996)
4. Lang, R.M., et al.: Recommendations for cardiac chamber quantification by echocardiography in adults: an update from the American society of echocardiography and the european association of cardiovascular imaging. Eur. Hear. J. Cardiovasc. Imaging **16**(3), 233–271 (2015)
5. Leung, K.Y.E., Bosch, J.G.: Localized shape variations for classifying wall motion in echocardiograms. In: Ayache, N., Ourselin, S., Maeder, A. (eds.) MICCAI 2007. LNCS, vol. 4791, pp. 52–59. Springer, Heidelberg (2007). https://doi.org/10.1007/978-3-540-75757-3_7
6. Lu, Y., Radau, P., Connelly, K., Dick, A., Wright, G.: Pattern recognition of abnormal left ventricle wall motion in cardiac MR. In: Yang, G.-Z., Hawkes, D., Rueckert, D., Noble, A., Taylor, C. (eds.) MICCAI 2009. LNCS, vol. 5762, pp. 750–758. Springer, Heidelberg (2009). https://doi.org/10.1007/978-3-642-04271-3_91
7. Mantilla, J., et al.: Classification of LV wall motion in cardiac MRI using kernel dictionary learning with a parametric approach. In: EMBC, pp. 7292–7295 (2015)
8. Paetsch, I., Jahnke, C., Ferrari, V.A., Rademakers, F.E., Pellikka, P.A., Hundley, W.G.: Determination of interobserver variability for identifying inducible left ventricular wall motion abnormalities during dobutamine stress magnetic resonance imaging. Eur. Hear. J. **27**(12), 1459–1464 (2006)
9. Punithakumar, K., Ayed, I.B., Islam, A., Goela, A., Li, S.: Regional heart motion abnormality detection via multiview fusion. In: Ayache, N., Delingette, H., Golland, P., Mori, K. (eds.) MICCAI 2012. LNCS, vol. 7511, pp. 527–534. Springer, Heidelberg (2012). https://doi.org/10.1007/978-3-642-33418-4_65
10. Punithakumar, K., et al.: Regional heart motion abnormality detection: an information theoretic approach. Med. Image Anal. **17**(3), 311–324 (2013)
11. Punithakumar, K., Ben Ayed, I., Islam, A., Ross, I.G., Li, S.: Regional heart motion abnormality detection via information measures and unscented Kalman filtering. In: Jiang, T., Navab, N., Pluim, J.P.W., Viergever, M.A. (eds.) MICCAI 2010. LNCS, vol. 6361, pp. 409–417. Springer, Heidelberg (2010). https://doi.org/10.1007/978-3-642-15705-9_50
12. Punithakumar, K., Ayed, I.B., Ross, I.G., Islam, A., Chong, J., Li, S.: Detection of left ventricular motion abnormality via information measures and bayesian filtering. IEEE Trans. Inf. Technol. Biomed. **14**(4), 1106–1113 (2010)

13. Qian, Z., Liu, Q., Metaxas, D.N., Axel, L.: Identifying Regional cardiac abnormalities from myocardial strains using spatio-temporal tensor analysis. In: Metaxas, D., Axel, L., Fichtinger, G., Székely, G. (eds.) MICCAI 2008. LNCS, vol. 5241, pp. 789–797. Springer, Heidelberg (2008). https://doi.org/10.1007/978-3-540-85988-8_94

14. Qian, Z., Liu, Q., Metaxas, D.N., Axel, L.: Identifying regional cardiac abnormalities from myocardial strains using nontracking-based strain estimation and spatio-temporal tensor analysis. IEEE TMI **30**(12), 2017–2029 (2011)

15. Suinesiaputra, A., et al.: Automated detection of regional wall motion abnormalities based on a statistical model applied to multislice short-axis cardiac MR images. IEEE TMI **28**(4), 595–607 (2009)

16. Viera, A.J., Garrett, J.M.: Understanding interobserver agreement: the kappa statistic. Fam Med **37**(5), 360–363 (2005)

17. Wang, X., Girshick, R., Gupta, A., He, K.: Non-local neural networks. arXiv preprint arXiv:1711.07971 (2017)

Computational Heart Modeling for Evaluating Efficacy of MRI Techniques in Predicting Appropriate ICD Therapy

Eranga Ukwatta[1,2(✉)], Plamen Nikolov[3],
Natalia Trayanova[3], and Graham Wright[4]

[1] Systems and Computer Engineering, Carleton University, Ottawa, ON, Canada
eukwatta@uoguelph.ca
[2] School of Engineering, University of Guelph, Guelph, ON, Canada
[3] Institute of Computational Medicine,
Johns Hopkins University, Baltimore, MD, USA
[4] Department of Medical Biophysics, University of Toronto,
Toronto, ON, Canada

Abstract. The objective of this study is to use individualized heart computer models in evaluating efficacy of myocardial infarct (MI) mass determined by two different MRI techniques in predicting patient risk for post-MI ventricular tachycardia (VT). 27 patients with MI underwent late gadolinium-enhanced MRI using inversion-recovery fast gradient echo (IR-FGRE) and multi-contrast late enhancement (MCLE) prior to implantable cardioverter defibrillators (ICD) implantation and were followed up for 6–46 months. The myocardium, MI core (IC), and border zone (BZ) were segmented from the images using previously validated techniques. The segmented structures were then reconstructed as a high-resolution label map in 3D. Individualized image-based computational models were built separately for each imaging technique; simulations of propensity to VT were conducted with each model. The imaging methods were evaluated for sensitivity and specificity by comparing simulated inducibility of VT to clinical outcome (appropriate ICD therapy) in patients. Twelve patients had at least one appropriate ICD therapy for VT at follow-up. For both MCLE and IR-FGRE, the outcomes of the simulations of VT were significantly different between the groups with and without ICD therapy. Between the IR-FGRE and MCLE, the virtual models built using the latter may have yielded higher sensitivity and specificity in predicting appropriate ICD therapy.

Keywords: T1 mapping · Computational modeling · Myocardial infarct

1 Introduction

Heart attacks often may cause scarring of heart muscle. The resulting myocardial infarct (MI) regions and surrounding tissue may act as substrate for ventricular tachycardia (VT) and fibrillation (VF) [1], which may eventually lead to sudden cardiac death (SCD). In particular, electrical conduction in the heart through the infarcted regions may lead to anatomically defined re-entry circuits causing VT. For individuals at high risk for

© Springer Nature Switzerland AG 2018
A. F. Frangi et al. (Eds.): MICCAI 2018, LNCS 11071, pp. 446–454, 2018.
https://doi.org/10.1007/978-3-030-00934-2_50

SCD, prophylactic insertion of implantable cardioverter defibrillators (ICDs) decreases mortality. Among the non-invasive techniques developed to identify patients with chronic MI at risk for SCD, left ventricular ejection fraction (LVEF), below 35%, remains the primary deciding factor for ICD implantation. However, several studies have shown that LVEF along is not adequate as a criteria for screening patients for ICDs and recent research has focused on developing alternative non-invasive risk stratification strategies based on direct measurement of MI mass or volume.

Previous studies using late gadolinium enhanced cardiac MR (LGE-CMR) imaging using inversion-recovery fast-gradient-echo (IR-FGRE) have demonstrated that both the infarct core (IC) and the surrounding semi-viable tissue, also termed "border zone" (BZ), play an important role in cardiac arrhythmogenesis [4]. However, quantitative assessment of the MIs using IR-FGRE requires precise manual or semi-automated segmentation of the myocardium as a pre-processing step. Due to this dependency on manual myocardial segmentation, the method also has high intra- and inter-observer variability. T1 mapping techniques, as compared to IR-FGRE, have been shown to be more reproducible in determining MI mass. The T1 mapping techniques enable quantitative assessment of myocardial tissue on a voxel-wise basis, reducing the need for manual segmentation of the myocardial boundaries. The multi-contrast late enhancement (MCLE) is a T1 mapping technique, which enables infarct and cardiac wall assessment in a single acquisition with reduced scan times [9]. The MCLE method, as compared to IR-FGRE technique, has been shown to be more sensitive in predicting ICD therapy in patients with MI [4].

Computational modeling of the hearts with MIs has emerged as a promising non-invasive tool to simulate electrical activation of the heart and determine propensity for re-entrant arrhythmias such as VT or VF [7]. The computational models are built based on cardiac MR images, and can be non-invasively interrogated to yield mechanistic insights into the electrical activity of the heart. To accurately represent patient-specific structural changes, these models must incorporate accurate 3D geometric reconstructions of cardiac structure and MI geometry [8]. With the use of computer simulations of VT, there is potential to investigate and compare LGE-MRI using IR-FGRE and MCLE methods in predicting inducibility of VT in post-MI patients. Therefore, the objective of this study was to evaluate individualized computational heart models in determining efficacy of LGE-MRI using IR-FGRE and MCLE techniques in predicting patient risk for post-MI VT.

2 Methods

2.1 Study Subjects and Image Acquisition

Our study consists of twenty-seven patients with prior MI eligible for ICD implantation for primary or secondary prevention. The CMR study protocol was approved by the institutional research ethics board at Anonymous University and all the subjects provided written informed consent. Patients with MR-incompatible implants were excluded from study. After the CMR examination and ICD implantation, the subjects were followed up in an ICD clinic on a quarterly basis. The CMR studies were conducted using a 1.5 T GE Signa HDx system (GE Healthcare, Milwaukee, USA) with ECG gating and using an eight-channel phased-array cardiac coil. The CMR protocol included LV functional parameter assessment using cine steady-state free precession (SSFP), as well as LGE-CMR using an inversion recovery fast gradient echo (IR-FGRE) and MCLE post double-dose Gd injection. For SSFP acquisition, a short-axis oblique 20 phase-resolved images over the whole cardiac cycle were acquired in a breath hold. Ten to twenty minutes after a double-dose intravenous bolus injection of Gd-DTPA, LGE-CMR images using IR-FGRE were acquired followed by MCLE images, using the same short-axis oblique localization as the cine SSFP images. Depending on the null point of normal myocardium, the inversion time (TI) varied from 200 to 300 ms in IR-FGRE. Approximately 20 heartbeats (18-s breath-holds on average) were required to produce a single LGE-CMR image using IR-FGRE. For MCLE, a segmented SSFP readout was used following an inversion recovery pulse, providing 20 cardiac phase-resolved images at different TIs. The MCLE pulse sequence required approximately 13 heartbeats to acquire.

According to clinical guidelines, all the patients received a single or dual ICD implantation. All patients were followed in an ICD clinic at intervals of three months and more frequently (if device shocks were delivered) for 6–46 months with a median follow-up of 30 months. Two experienced electrophysiologists reviewed the ICD data for the relevant ventricular arrhythmic events. The primary outcome measure was appropriate ICD therapy, which was defined as shock for VT, VF, or any ventricular arrhythmic event identified as sustained VT or VF [4]. In this study, appropriate ICD therapy refers to an ICD event which was triggered for a single rhythm episode regardless of the total number of actual shocks that were needed for termination of tachycardia [4].

2.2   Image Processing

In IR-FGRE and MCLE images, the epi- and endo-cardial boundaries of the LV and RV were manually contoured in the image slices by an expert using the ImageJ software program (National Institutes of Health, Bethesda, MD, USA). From the 20 phases of the MCLE images, a diastolic phase after signal recovery was chosen for myocardial segmentation. Due to the inherent differences of IR-FGRE and MCLE, two different approaches were used for MI segmentation.

For the IR-FGRE images, the MI was segmented as IC and BZ using the full-width at half maximum (FWHM) method, for which the pre-segmented LV myocardium was used as the initial region. The expert chooses a region of interest in the remote healthy myocardium and the peak intensity in the MI. The IC was considered as the regions with intensities above the half of the peak intensity of the MI. The BZ was computed as the regions with intensity above peak of the remote region, but below the half of the peak intensity of the MI. The MCLE images were first pre-processed one slice at a time, where curve fitting of signal intensities acquired at multiple inversion times is used to create the T1* and the steady state maps. The MIs were segmented as IC and BZ using a clustering approach based on fuzzy c-means, using both T1* and steady state maps [9]. Unlike the MI segmentation approach for IR-FGRE, the precise segmentation of the myocardial boundaries is not required for MCLE. The algorithm considers four clusters representing the IC, BZ, blood pool, and healthy myocardium. This algorithm determines the probability of each voxel belonging to each of the clusters based on a distance metric in a scatter plot of T1* and steady state values [9]. Figure 1 shows segmentation results of the IC and BZ regions for example IR-FGRE and MCLE images.

2.3 Simulation of Cardiac Electrophysiology

Using the ventricular reconstruction, and the MI reconstructions, two finite element models (FEMs), one incorporating MI geometries reconstructed from IR-FGRE, and the other with MI zone geometries built from the MCLE, were created. Figure 2(c) shows two FEMs created from IR-FGRE and MCLE images of a patient heart, where the geometries of the IC and BZ appears different. The fiber orientations for the models were estimated using a rule-based method [10].

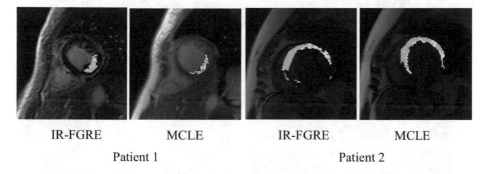

| IR-FGRE | MCLE | IR-FGRE | MCLE |

Patient 1   Patient 2

Fig. 1. Segmentation of the IC and BZ masses in for two example images. The IC is represented as a green region while the BZ is represented as a yellow region.

Electrical propagation was modeled using the monodomain formulation [11]. Intracellular conductivities in the normal myocardium were assigned such that the resulting conduction velocity matched those recorded in human ventricular experiments [12]. To represent connexin 43 remodeling and lateralization in the remodeled BZ, transverse conductivity was decreased by 90%, resulting in increased tissue anisotropy. The IC was modeled as passive tissue with zero conductivity.

The Ten Tusscher human ventricular action potential model was used to represent the membrane kinetics in the healthy myocardium [13]. For the remodeled BZ, the action potential model was modified to represent electrophysiological changes that have been observed experimentally (reduction in peak sodium current to 38% of the normal value, in peak L-type calcium current to 31% of normal, and in peak potassium currents IKr and IKs to 30% and 20% of the maximum, respectively) [5]. These modifications resulted in BZ action potential morphology that had decreased upstroke velocity, decreased amplitude, and increased duration, consistent with experimental recordings.

Simulations of VT induction were also performed in all models by applying at the apex and RV insertion point a programmed electrical stimulation (PES) protocol similar to the one used in the clinic [14]. The PES protocol consisted of six pacing (S1) stimuli with a coupling interval of 350 ms, followed by a premature stimulus (S2) whose cycle length was shortened until sustained VT was initiated or the last stimulus failed to capture. If needed, two additional extra-stimuli were delivered to attempt arrhythmia induction. An arrhythmia was classified as sustained if it persisted for at least two seconds. All simulations were performed using the software package CARP (CardioSolv, LLC) on a parallel computing platform.

A true positive (TP) is considered as simulated sustained VT matching the appropriate ICD therapy (i.e., shocks for VT or VF) at follow-up. A true negative (TN) is considered as non-inducibility of the simulated heart model matching no delivered shocks to the patient. An event is denoted a false positive (FP) when the simulation incorrectly predicts appropriate ICD therapy. An event is considered a false negative (FN) when the simulation fails to predicts an appropriate ICD therapy. For both MI MRI imaging technique, we computed sensitivity (TP/(TP + FN)) and specificity (TN/(TN + FP)) of the simulations of VT.

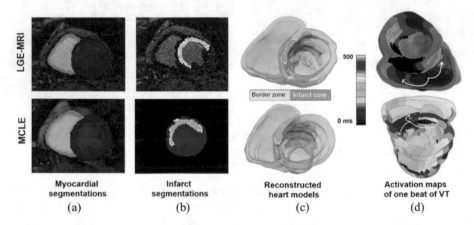

Fig. 2. (a) Manually segmented myocardium of the LV and RV shown in color blue and green respectively. (b) The IC and BZ are shown in green and yellow respectively. (c) Reconstructed heart models. (d) Corresponding activation maps of simulations of VT.

For the patient characteristics and imaging indices, we expressed continuous variables as mean ± SD and categorical data as numbers (percentages). For statistical analysis, we used and the Student's t-test for continuous variables and one-tailed Fisher exact test for categorical data. All statistical analyses were performed using IBM SPSS Statistical version 19 (IBM Corporation 2010), in which results were considered significant when the probability of making a type I error was less than 5% (p < 0.05).

3   Results

Table 1 lists CMR MI heterogeneity measurements for patient groups with and without ICD therapy. The MIs were normalized to LV mass. The BZ mass determined by MCLE was significantly different between the groups with and without ICD therapy. None of the other MI masses determined by both the MRI techniques was significantly different between the patients with and without ICD therapy, although such quantities were typically larger in patients undergoing appropriate ICD therapy.

Figure 2(d) shows activation maps of a single beat of VT for models, corresponding to both MCLE and IR-FGRE images, with re-entry circuit activity shown with white arrows near MI location. The activation maps in simulations were derived by determining, at each node of the finite element meshes, the instant in time at which the upstroke of the action potential at that node reached a threshold of 0 mV.

Table 1. Infarct masses estimated using the MCLE and IR-FGRE techniques, reported separately for the 27 study subjects with and without ICD therapy. The reported masses were normalized by the left-ventricular mass (LVM). From all the reported indices, only the BZ mass determined by MCLE was significantly different between the groups with and without ICE therapy.

	With ICD therapy (n = 12)		Without ICD therapy (n = 15)		P value	
	MCLE	IR-FGRE	MCLE	IR-FGRE	MCLE	IR-FGRE
BZ (%)	17.4 ± 6.5	11.1 ± 6.3	12.0 ± 5.6	9.8 ± 5.3	0.044	0.58
IC (%)	29.8 ± 8.6	22.7 ± 14.9	23.1 ± 12.9	19.5 ± 11.7	0.094	0.60
Total MI (%)	47.2 ± 13.1	33.8 ± 20.7	35.1 ± 18.3	29.7 ± 17.3	0.081	0.54

Table 2. Sensitivity and specificity of predicting appropriate ICD therapy for computer simulations of VT for models built using LGE-MRI using IR-FGRE and MCLE. For both MCLE and IR-FGRE, the simulated VT inducibility was significantly different between the patients with and without ICD therapy.

	MCLE	IR-FGRE
Number of Patients	25	25
TP	10 (40%)	8 (32%)
TN	11 (44%)	10 (40%)
FP	2 (8%)	3 (12%)
FN	2 (8%)	4 (16%)
Sensitivity (%)	83.3	66.7
Specificity (%)	84.6	76.9

Due to errors that occurred in creating the heart models, two patients out of 27 were excluded from further analysis. Sensitivity and specificity for computer simulations of VT for models built with LGE-MRI using IR-FGRE and MCLE are shown in Table 2. For both MCLE and IR-FGRE, the outcomes of simulations of VT were significantly different (p = 0.001 and 0.03) between the patients with and without ICD therapy. The simulations using MCLE images, as compared to the ones using IR-FGRE may have yielded a higher sensitivity and specificity. We also evaluated predictability of appropriate ICD therapy of BZ mass using cut-off thresholds from 10% to 17% as shown in Table 3. Sensitivity and specificity of predicting appropriate ICD therapy from BZ volume at these various thresholds for both MRI techniques were smaller than that of using the simulations of VT.

Table 3. Sensitivity and specificity of predicting appropriate ICD therapy using peri-MI BZ mass cut-off values ranging from 10% to 17% for MCLE and IR-FGRE for 25 study subjects. Due to errors that occurred in creating the heart models, two patients out of 27 were excluded from this analysis.

BZ/LVM (%)	MCLE		IR-FGRE	
	Sensitivity	Specificity	Sensitivity	Specificity
10%	91.7	25	75	50
11%	83.3	33.3	75	58.3
12%	75	33.3	66.7	58.3
13%	75	58.3	58.3	66.7
14%	66.7	75	50	75
15%	50	75	41.7	75
16%	50	75	41.7	75
17%	33.3	83.3	33.3	83.3

4 Discussion and Conclusion

The objective of this study was to evaluate individualized heart computer models in determining efficacy of IR-FGRE and MCLE techniques in predicting patient risk for post-MI VT. In this preliminary study, we demonstrated that computer simulations of VT in patient-specific models could be used in stratifying patient risk for SCD using computer simulations of VT inducibility. Simulations of VT inducibility interrogate the detailed electrical activation of the heart in the MI-remodeled cardiac substrate, which is directly dependent on the reconstruction of the MI and ventricular geometry.

Except for the BZ mass determined by the MCLE technique, none of the other indices was statistically significant between the patients with and without appropriate ICD therapy. However, for both MCLE and IR-FGRE, the outcome of simulations of VT (i.e., simulated VT inducibility) were significantly different between the patients with and without ICD therapy. This indicates that, irrespective of the MI imaging method, the simulations of VT were more sensitive in predicting appropriate ICD therapy in post-MI patients. Furthermore, the simulations of VT inducibility using

MCLE images may have yielded higher sensitivity and specificity in predicting appropriate ICD therapy compared to those using IR-FGRE images. Due to the limited number of data points in our study cohort, the sensitivity and specificity values are sensitive to single data points. Therefore the results should be interpreted as hypothesis generating. Higher sensitivity for MCLE, as compare to the one for IR-FGRE, may be partially due to the larger BZ mass determined by the MCLE technique. Arevalo et al. [15], using computer simulations of VT, have shown that larger BZs in models lead to increased inducibility of VT. Simulations of VT inducibility, as compared to cut-off thresholds defined on peri-MI BZ mass, had a better operating point for sensitivity and specificity irrespective of the MRI technique used to quantify the MI. This is in agreement with the higher predictive capability of mass-based measurement determined by MCLE technique [4].

One of the main errors in MI quantification in IR-FGRE stems from the manual segmentation of the endocardium. The MCLE technique uses SSFP readout immediately after an inversion pulse, which permits visualization of infarction as an area of fast T1 recovery with the simultaneous nulling of blood pool and viable myocardium. A T1 mapping technique, such as MCLE, does not require precise myocardial segmentation and hence may avoid such potential errors in MI quantification.

References

1. Fishman, G.I., et al.: Sudden cardiac death prediction and prevention: Report from a national heart, lung, and blood institute and heart rhythm society workshop. Circulation 122(22), 2335–2348 (2010)
2. Ismail, T.F., Prasad, S.K., Pennell, D.J.: Prognostic importance of late gadolinium enhancement cardiovascular magnetic resonance in cardiomyopathy. Heart 98(6), 438–442 (2012)
3. Schmidt, A., et al.: Infarct tissue heterogeneity by magnetic resonance imaging identifies enhanced cardiac arrhythmia susceptibility in patients with left ventricular dysfunction. Circulation 115(15), 2006–2014 (2007)
4. Yang, Y., et al.: Multi-contrast late enhancement CMR determined gray zone and papillary muscle involvement predict appropriate ICD therapy in patients with ischemic heart disease. J. Cardiovasc. Magn. Reson. 15(1), 57 (2013)
5. Arevalo, H.J., et al.: Arrhythmia risk stratification of patients after myocardial infarction using personalized heart models. Nat. Commun. 7, 11437 (2016)
6. Trayanova, N.A., Pashakhanloo, F., Wu, K.C., Halperin, H.R.: Imaging-based simulations for predicting sudden death and guiding ventricular tachycardia ablation. Circ. Arrhythm. Electrophysiol. 10(7), e004743 (2017)
7. Vadakkumpadan, F., Arevalo, H., Jebb, A., Wu, K.C., Trayanova, N.: Image-based patient-specific simulations of ventricular electrophysiology for sudden arrhythmic death risk stratification. In: Circulation, vol. 128, no. 22 (2013)
8. Ukwatta, E., et al.: Myocardial infarct segmentation from magnetic resonance images for personalized modeling of cardiac electrophysiology. IEEE TMI 35(6), 1408–1419 (2016)
9. Detsky, J.S., Paul, G., Dick, A.J., Wright, G.A.: Reproducible classification of infarct heterogeneity using fuzzy clustering on multicontrast delayed enhancement magnetic resonance images. IEEE TMI 28(10), 1606–1614 (2009)

10. Bayer, J.D.J., Blake, R.C.R., Plank, G., Trayanova, N.A.N.A.: A novel rule-based algorithm for assigning myocardial fiber orientation to computational heart models. Ann. Biomed. Eng. **40**(10), 2243–2254 (2012)
11. Plank, G., et al.: From mitochondrial ion channels to arrhythmias in the heart: computational techniques to bridge the spatio-temporal scales. Philos. Trans. R. Soc. A Math. Phys. Eng. Sci. **366**(1879), 3381–3409 (2008)
12. Moreno, J.D., et al.: A computational model to predict the effects of class I anti-arrhythmic drugs on ventricular rhythms. Sci. Trans. Med. **3**(98), 98ra83 (2011)
13. ten Tusscher, K.H.W.J., Noble, D., Noble, P.J., Panfilov, A.V.: A model for human ventricular tissue. Am. J. Physiol. Circ. Physiol. **286**(4), H1573–H1589 (2004)
14. Wellens, H.J.J., Brugada, P., Stevenson, W.G.: Programmed electrical stimulation of the heart in patients with life-threatening ventricular arrhythmias: what is the significance of induced arrhythmias and what is the correct stimulaton protocol? Circulation **72**(1), 1–7 (1985)
15. Arevalo, H., Plank, G., Helm, P., Halperin, H., Trayanova, N.: Tachycardia in post-infarction hearts: insights from 3D image-based ventricular models. PLoS ONE **8**(7), e68872 (2013)

Multiview Two-Task Recursive Attention Model for Left Atrium and Atrial Scars Segmentation

Jun Chen[1], Guang Yang[2,3], Zhifan Gao[4], Hao Ni[5,6], Elsa Angelini[7],
Raad Mohiaddin[2,3], Tom Wong[2,3], Yanping Zhang[1(✉)], Xiuquan Du[1(✉)],
Heye Zhang[4], Jennifer Keegan[2,3], and David Firmin[2,3]

[1] Anhui University, Hefei, China
zhangyp2@gmail.com,dxqllp@ahu.edu.cn
[2] Cardiovascular Research Centre, Royal Brompton Hospital,
London SW3 6NP, UK
[3] National Heart & Lung Institute, Imperial College London,
London SW7 2AZ, UK
[4] Shenzhen Institutes of Advanced Technology, Chinese Academy of Sciences,
Shenzhen, China
[5] Department of Mathematics, University College London,
London WC1E 6BT, UK
[6] Alan Turing Institute, London NW1 2DB, UK
[7] Faculty of Medicine, Department of Surgery & Cancer, Imperial College London,
London SW7 2AZ, UK

Abstract. Late Gadolinium Enhanced Cardiac MRI (LGE-CMRI) for detecting atrial scars in atrial fibrillation (AF) patients has recently emerged as a promising technique to stratify patients, guide ablation therapy and predict treatment success. Visualisation and quantification of scar tissues require a segmentation of both the left atrium (LA) and the high intensity scar regions from LGE-CMRI images. These two segmentation tasks are challenging due to the cancelling of healthy tissue signal, low signal-to-noise ratio and often limited image quality in these patients. Most approaches require manual supervision and/or a second *bright-blood* MRI acquisition for anatomical segmentation. Segmenting both the LA anatomy and the scar tissues automatically from a single LGE-CMRI acquisition is highly in demand. In this study, we proposed a novel fully automated multiview two-task (MVTT) recursive attention model working directly on LGE-CMRI images that combines a sequential learning and a dilated residual learning to segment the LA (including attached pulmonary veins) and delineate the atrial scars simultaneously via an innovative attention model. Compared to other state-of-the-art methods, the proposed MVTT achieves compelling improvement, enabling to generate a patient-specific anatomical and atrial scar assessment model.

J. Chen, G. Yang—These authors contributed equally to this work.

© Springer Nature Switzerland AG 2018
A. F. Frangi et al. (Eds.): MICCAI 2018, LNCS 11071, pp. 455–463, 2018.
https://doi.org/10.1007/978-3-030-00934-2_51

1   Introduction

Late Gadolinium-Enhanced Cardiac MRI (LGE-CMRI) has been used to acquire data in patients with atrial fibrillation (AF) in order to detect native and post-ablation treatment scarring in the thin-walled left atrium (LA) [1]. This technique is based on the different wash-in and wash-out gadolinium contrast agent kinetics between healthy and scarred tissues [2]. The hyper-enhanced regions in the LGE-CMRI images reflect fibrosis and scar tissue while healthy atrial myocardium is 'nulled' [3]. This has shown promise for stratifying patients, guiding ablation therapy and predicting treatment success. Visualisation and quantification of atrial scar tissue requires a segmentation of the LA anatomy including attached pulmonary veins (PV) and a segmentation of the atrial scars.

Solving these two segmentation tasks is very challenging using LGE-CMRI images, where the nulling of signal from healthy tissue reduces the visibility of the LA boundaries. Moreover, in the AF patient population, prolonged scanning time, irregular breathing pattern and heart rate variability during the scan can result in poor image quality that can further complicate both segmentation tasks. Because of this, previous studies have segmented the LA and PV anatomy from an additional *bright-blood* data acquisition, and have then registered the segmented LA and PV anatomy to the LGE-CMRI acquisition for visualisation and delineation of the atrial scars [4–6]. This approach is complicated by motion (bulk, respiratory or cardiac) between the two acquisitions and subsequent registration errors.

Recent deep learning based methods have been widely used for solving medical image segmentation. A convolutional neural networks (CNN) based approach has been proposed to segment the LA and PV from bright-blood images [7], but not yet applied for LGE-CMRI images. For most previous studies, the LA and PV have been segmented manually although this is time-consuming, subjective and lacks reproducibility [8]. Based on the segmented LA and PV, and the derived LA, the atrial scars is then typically delineated using unsupervised learning based methods, e.g., thresholding and clustering, as described in this benchmarking paper [8].

In this study, a novel fully automated multiview two-task (MVTT) recursive attention model is designed to segment the LA and PV anatomy and the atrial scars directly from the LGE-CMRI images, avoiding the need for an additional data acquisition for anatomical segmentation and subsequent registration. Our MVTT method consists of a sequential learning and a dilated residual learning to segment the LA and proximal PV while the atrial scars can be delineated simultaneously via an innovative attention model.

2   Method

The workflow of our MVTT recursive attention model is summarised as shown in Fig. 1. It performs the segmentations for the LA and PV anatomy and atrial scars simultaneously.

LA and PV Segmentation via a Multiview Learning. Our 3D LGE-MRI data were acquired and reconstructed into a volume with 60–68 2D axial slices with a spatial resolution of $(0.7$–$0.75) \times (0.7$–$0.75) \times 2\,\mathrm{mm}^3$. In this study, we propose a multiview based method to delineate LA and PV that mimics the inspection procedure of radiologists, who view the images by stepping through the 2D axial slices to obtain the correlated information in the axial view (with finer spatial resolution) while also using complementary information from sagittal and coronal views (with lower spatial resolution). We modelled the information extracted from the axial view by a *sequential learning* and for the sagittal and coronal views we designed a *dilated residual learning*.

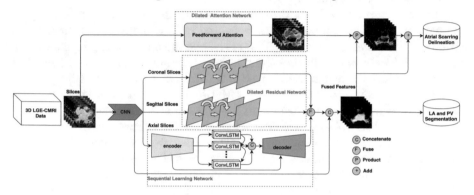

Fig. 1. Workflow of our proposed MVTT recursive attention model (Detailed architecture of each subnetworks can be found in the Supplementary Materials).

Firstly, a 3×3 convolutional layer with 12 kernels is used to extract the high resolution features. We stack the obtained feature maps to 3D maps to slice them into axial, sagittal and coronal slices respectively, which are used to perform multiview learning. Our *sequential learning network* consists of six convolutional layers for the encoder and decoder path, respectively. In the encoder path, each convolutional layer is followed by a rectified linear unit (ReLU) layer and a local response normalisation (LRN) layer to normalise the feature maps. In addition, three max-pooling layers are used to reduce the dimension of the feature maps. In the decoder path, three up-sampling layers are implemented via bilinear interpolation to recover the original image size, and the decoder is also incorporated convolutional and LRN layers. Each convolutional layer contains 12 kernels with size of 3×3 pixels. Furthermore, convolutional long-short term memory (ConvLSTM) [9] layers are embedded into the encoder-decoder network to account for inter-slices correlations. The ConvLSTM is a special recursive neural network architecture that can be defined mathematically as

$$i_t = \sigma(W_{xi} * x_t + W_{hi} * h_{t-1} + W_{ct} \circ c_{t-1} + b_i), \tag{1}$$

$$f_t = \sigma(W_{xf} * x_t + W_{hf} * h_{t-1} + W_{cf} \circ c_{t-1} + b_f), \tag{2}$$

$$c_t = f_t \circ c_{t-1} + i_t \circ \text{ReLU}(W_{xc} * x_t + W_{hc} * h_{t-1} + b_c), \tag{3}$$

$$o_t = \sigma(W_{xo} * x_t + W_{ho} * h_{t-1} + W_{cfo} \circ c_t + b_o), \tag{4}$$

$$h_t = o_t \circ \text{ReLU}(c_t) \tag{5}$$

where '$*$' represents convolutional operator and '$\circ$' denotes the Hadamard product, W terms denote weight matrices, b terms denote bias vectors, σ represents a sigmoid function and ReLU is used in our study instead of tanh. The ConvLSTM uses three gates including the input gate i_t, the forget gate f_t and the output gate o_t, and memory cell c_t represents an accumulator of the state information and h_t denotes the hidden states.

Secondly, in order to learn the complementary information from the sagittal and coronal views, we propose to use a dilated residual network. In the network, we adopt the *dilated convolution* [10] and remove the max-pooling layers to avoid loss of useful information during the pooling operation. The network consists of four 3×3 dilated convolutional layers based on residual architecture [11], and each has 12 kernels and is followed by a ReLU layer and a LRN layer. By using the dilated convolution, the size of the feature maps is remained.

Finally, two 3D volumes are created to store the learned feature maps from the sagittal and coronal view, respectively. Then we slice them into multiple 2D axial slices, and concatenate them with the feature maps derived from the sequential learning at their corresponding channels. Next, a convolutional operation is applied to these concatenated feature maps to get the fused multiview features. Meanwhile, high resolution features from the previous layer are combined with the fused multiview features for localizing LA/PV and atrial scars. At the end, three convolutional layers perform the LA/PV segmentation. Two of them contain 24 kernels with the size of 3×3 and each is followed by a ReLU layer and a LRN layer. At the last layer, a 3×3 convolution is used to map each pixel to the desired segments, and the sigmoid activation function is used.

Atrial Scars Segmentation via an Attention Model. The regions of atrial scars are relatively small and discrete; therefore, in this study we tackle the delineation of atrial scars using the attention mechanism to force the model to focus on the locations of the atrial scars, and enhance the representations of the atrial scars at those locations. Moreover, conventional pooling operations can easily lose the information of these small atrial scars regions. Therefore, a novel dilated attention network is designed to integrate a *feedforward attention structure* [12] with the dilated convolution to preserve the fine information of the atrial scars. In our dilated attention network, the attention is provided by a mask branch, which is changing adaptively according to the fused multiview features. There are four convolutional layers for the mask branch and each of the first three layers is followed by a ReLU layer and a LRN layer. Finally, according to [12], we utilise a sigmoid layer which connects to a 1×1 convolutional layer to normalise the output into a range of [0,1] for each channel and spatial position to get the attention mask. This sigmoid layer can be defined as following

$$AM(x_{i,c}) = \frac{1}{1 + e^{(-x_{i,c})}}, \tag{6}$$

where i ranges over all spatial positions and c ranges over all channels.

Because the soft attention mask can potentially affect the performance of the multiview learning, a residual architecture is also applied to mitigate such influence. The output O of the attention model can be denoted as

$$O(x_{i,c}) = (1 + AM(x_{i,c})) \cdot F(x_{i,c}), \tag{7}$$

in which i ranges over all spatial positions, c ranges over all the channels, $AM(x_{i,c})$ is the attention mask, which ranges from $[0,1]$, $F(x_{i,c})$ represents the fused multiview features, and $\cdot$ denotes the dot product. Finally, based on generated attention maps, three convolutional layers are connected at the end to perform the atrial scars delineation, which are similar to the ones used for the LA and PV segmentation.

Implementation Details. For the implementation, we used the Adam method to perform the optimization with a mean squared error based loss function and decayed learning rate (the initial learning rate was 0.001 and dropped to 0.000445 at the end). Our deep learning model was implemented using Tensorflow 1.2.1 on a Ubuntu 16.04 machine, and was trained and tested on an NVidia Tesla P100 GPU (3584 cores and 16 GB GPU memory).

3   Experimental Results and Discussion

We retrospectively studied 100 3D LGE-CMRI scans acquired in patients with longstanding persistent AF. Both pre- and post-ablation acquisitions were included (detailed LGE-CMRI scanning sequence and patient cohort information can be found in the Supplementary Materials). Manual segmentations of the LA and PV anatomy and atrial scars by an experienced physicist were used as the ground truth for training and evaluation of our MVTT recursive attention model. All patient recruitment and data acquisition were approved by the institutional review board in accordance with local ethics procedures. Ten-fold cross-validation was applied to provide an unbiased estimation of the accuracy, sensitivity, specificity and Dice score of the two segmentations. For comparison studies, we also evaluated the performance of state-of-the-art methods for LA and PV segmentation (using atlas based whole heart segmentation, WHS [13]) and the atrial scars delineation (using unsupervised learning based methods [8] and a re-implementation of the U-Net [14]).

LA and PV Segmentation. The experimental results show that our MVTT framework can accurately segment the LA and PV (Table 1 and Fig. 2). The obtained accuracy, sensitivity, specificity and Dice scores are 98.51%, 90.49%, 99.23% and 90.83%. Figure 2 shows example segmentation results of the LA and PV for a pre-ablation case and a post-ablation case. Both the segmentation result obtained by our MVTT framework (green contours) and the ground truth (red contours) are overlaid on LGE-CMRI images, and our fully automated segmentation has demonstrated high consistency compared to the manual delineated ground truth.

Atrial Scars Segmentation. Our MVTT framework also shows great performance for segmenting the atrial scars (Table 1 and Fig. 3). We achieve an overall segmentation accuracy of 99.90%, with a sensitivity of 76.12%, a specificity of 99.97% and a Dice score of 77.64% (median 83.59% and 79.37% for post- and pre-ablation scans). Segmentation results in Fig. 3(c) and (k) show a great agreement compared to the ground truth. In addition, correlation analysis of the calculated scar percentage between our MVTT and the ground truth as shown in Fig. 4(c). The derived correlation coefficient $r = 0.7401 \in (0.6, 0.8)$ represents a strong correlation between our fully automated segmentation and the manual delineated ground truth. Furthermore, the Bland-Altman plot of the calculated scar percentage (Fig. 4(d)) shows the 94% measurements are in the 95% limits of agreement, which also corroborates the accurate scar percentage measure of our MVTT framework.

Table 1. Quantitative results of the cross-validated LA and PV segmentation and the atrial scars delineation. For the LA and PV segmentation, we compared with the WHS [13], and for the atrial scars delineation we compared with the SD, k-means, Fuzzy c-means [8] and the U-Net [14].

	Accuracy	Sensitivity	Specificity	Dice Score
WHS	0.9978 ± 0.0009	0.8587 ± 0.0415	0.9993 ± 0.0006	0.8905 ± 0.0317
Multi-view	0.9773 ± 0.0127	0.8163 ± 0.1355	0.9924 ± 0.0038	0.8502 ± 0.1033
Axial view+ConvLSTM	0.9778 ± 0.0088	0.8370 ± 0.0802	0.9909 ± 0.0036	0.8609 ± 0.0510
S-LA/PV	0.9845 ± 0.0081	0.8901 ± 0.1012	0.9930 ± 0.0035	0.8999 ± 0.0857
MVTT	0.9851 ± 0.0052	0.9049 ± 0.0487	0.9923 ± 0.0041	0.9083 ± 0.0309
2-SD	0.9984 ± 0.0007	0.5137 ± 0.2497	0.9994 ± 0.0006	0.5277 ± 0.1916
K-means	0.9975 ± 0.0009	0.7777 ± 0.1508	0.9981 ± 0.0010	0.5409 ± 0.1539
Fuzzy c-means	0.9974 ± 0.0010	0.7968 ± 0.1539	0.9979 ± 0.0010	0.5350 ± 0.1601
U-Net	0.9987 ± 0.0008	0.8342 ± 0.1720	0.9992 ± 0.0003	0.7372 ± 0.1326
Multi-view+ConvLSTM	0.9990 ± 0.0008	0.73267 ± 0.1705	0.9997 ± 0.0002	0.7566 ± 0.1396
Multi-view+attention	0.9987 ± 0.0008	0.7928 ± 0.1759	0.9993 ± 0.0002	0.7275 ± 0.1342
Axial view+ConvLSTM+Attention	0.9987 ± 0.0008	0.7861 ± 0.1719	0.9992 ± 0.0003	0.7090 ± 0.1415
S-Scar	0.9989 ± 0.0009	0.7464 ± 0.1675	0.9995 ± 0.0003	0.7441 ± 0.1448
MVTT	0.9990 ± 0.0009	0.7612 ± 0.1708	0.9997 ± 0.0002	0.7764 ± 0.1459

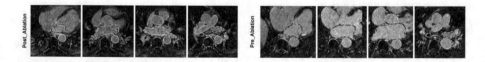

Fig. 2. Qualitative visualisation of the LA and PV segmentation.

Ablation Study I: Multi-View Sequential Learning. To demonstrate the add-on value of our multi-view sequential learning (multi-view+ConvLSTM) for extracting better anatomical features. We replaced the multi-view with axial view only in our MVTT framework (axial view+ConvLSTM). Results in Table 1 show that multi-view sequential learning achieved better performance for the LA and PV segmentation.

Ablation Study II: Attention Mechanism. We introduced an attention mechanism to enforce our model to pay more *attention* to the small atrial scar regions, and enhance their representations. To evaluate the performance of this attention mechanism, we removed the attention architecture from the MVTT framework, and only use the multi-view and ConvLSTM parts to predict the atrial scars. As shown in Table 1, the MVTT trained with attention architecture outperforms the multi-view+ConvLSTM, which proves the effectiveness of our MVTT framework with the attention mechanism.

Comparison Studies. Table 1 tabulates the quantitative comparison results for both the LA and PV segmentation and the atrial scars delineation. Compared to the WHS, our MVTT framework obtained much higher sensitivity (0.905 vs. 0.859) and similar specificity and therefore a higher Dice score. It is of note that the WHS method derived the LA and PV anatomy from additionally acquired *bright-blood* images and that was then registered to the LGE-MRI to derive the scar segmentation. Our MVTT method derived both LA and PV anatomy and scar segmentations from a single 3D LGE-CMRI dataset, which is a more challenging task but one which eliminates the need for an additional acquisition and subsequent registration errors. For the atrial scars delineation, all the unsupervised learning methods, e.g., standard deviation (SD) based thresholding and clustering, obtained high specificities, but very low sensitivities and poor Dice scores. Qualitative visualisation in Fig. 3 shows that the SD method clearly underestimated the atrial scars and both k-means and Fuzzy c-means (FCM) over-estimated the enhanced scar regions. The U-Net based method improved the delineation, but was still struggling to segment the atrial scars accurately. In addition, the experiments with the same architecture but separated two tasks (S-LA/PV, S-scar) illustrated that our simultaneous method showed better results because the two tasks constrain each other.

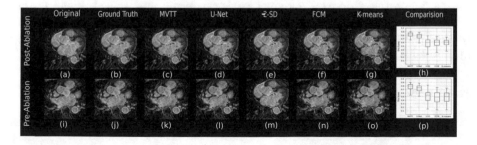

Fig. 3. Qualitative visualisation of the atrial scars delineation.

Limitations. One possible limitation is that our MVTT framework performed less well in some pre-ablation cases that is mainly due to very rare amount of native scar in these AF patients (see the outliers in Fig. 4(c) and (d)). The performance of our proposed MVTT recursive attention model did not rely on a comprehensive network parameters tuning and currently used network parameters defined by test and trials may cause possible overfitting of the trained models (see convergence analysis in Fig. 4(a–b)); however, this could be mitigated via techniques such as early stopping.

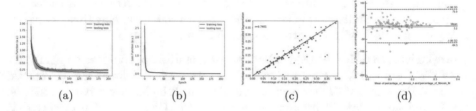

(a)	(b)	(c)	(d)

Fig. 4. (a) Training/testing convergence for the LA and PV segmentation, (b) Training/testing convergence for the atrial scars segmentation, (c) Correlation of the atrial scars percentage, (d) Bland-Altman plot of the measurements of atrial scars percentage.

4   Conclusion

In this work, we propose a fully automatic MVTT to segment both the LA and PV and atrial scars simultaneously from LGE-CMRI images directly. By combining the sequential learning and dilated residual learning for extracting multiview features, our attention model can delineate atrial scars accurately while segmenting the LA and PV anatomy. Validation of our framework has been performed against manually delineated ground truth. Compared to other state-of-the-art methods, our MVTT framework has demonstrated superior performance when using only the LGE-CMRI data. In conclusion, the proposed MVTT framework makes it possible to create a robust patient-specific anatomical model for the LA and PV that is accredited by our efficient and objective segmentation. It has further enabled a fast, reproducible and reliable atrial scarring assessment for individual AF patients.

References

1. Peters, D.C., et al.: Detection of pulmonary vein and left atrial scar after catheter ablation with three-dimensional navigator-gated delayed enhancement MR imaging: initial experience. Radiology **243**(3), 690–695 (2007)
2. Yang, G., et al.: Fully automatic segmentation and objective assessment of atrial scars for longstanding persistent atrial fibrillation patients using late gadolinium-enhanced MRI. Med. Phys. **45**(4), 1562–1576 (2018)

3. Keegan, J., et al.: Dynamic inversion time for improved 3D late gadolinium enhancement imaging in patients with atrial fibrillation. Magn. Reson. Med. **73**(2), 646–654 (2015)
4. Karim, R., et al.: A method to standardize quantification of left atrial scar from delayed-enhancement MR images. IEEE J. Transl. Eng. Health Med. **2**, 1–15 (2014)
5. Tao, Q., et al.: Fully automatic segmentation of left atrium and pulmonary veins in late gadolinium-enhanced MRI: towards objective atrial scar assessment. J. Magn. Reson. Imaging **44**(2), 346–354 (2016)
6. Yang, G., et al.: Multi-atlas propagation based left atrium segmentation coupled with super-voxel based pulmonary veins delineation in late gadolinium-enhanced cardiac MRI. In: SPIE Medical Imaging, vol. 10133, p. 1013313 (2017)
7. Mortazi, A., Karim, R., Rhode, K., Burt, J., Bagci, U.: *CardiacNET*: segmentation of left atrium and proximal pulmonary veins from MRI using multi-view CNN. In: Descoteaux, M., Maier-Hein, L., Franz, A., Jannin, P., Collins, D.L., Duchesne, S. (eds.) MICCAI 2017. LNCS, vol. 10434, pp. 377–385. Springer, Cham (2017). https://doi.org/10.1007/978-3-319-66185-8_43
8. Karim, R., et al.: Evaluation of current algorithms for segmentation of scar tissue from late gadolinium enhancement cardiovascular magnetic resonance of the left atrium: an open-access grand challenge. J. Cardiovasc. Mag. Reson. **15**(1), 105–122 (2013)
9. Xingjian, S., et al.: Convolutional LSTM network: a machine learning approach for precipitation nowcasting. In: NIPS, pp. 802–810 (2015)
10. Yu, F., Koltun, V.: Multi-scale context aggregation by dilated convolutions. In: ICLR (2015)
11. He, K., et al.: Deep residual learning for image recognition. In: CVPR, pp. 770–778 (2016)
12. Wang, F., et al.: Residual attention network for image classification. In: CVPR, pp. 6450–6458 (2017)
13. Zhuang, X., Shen, J.: Multi-scale patch and multi-modality atlases for whole heart segmentation of MRI. Med. Image Anal. **31**, 77–87 (2016)
14. Ronneberger, O., Fischer, P., Brox, T.: U-Net: convolutional networks for biomedical image segmentation. In: Navab, N., Hornegger, J., Wells, W.M., Frangi, A.F. (eds.) MICCAI 2015. LNCS, vol. 9351, pp. 234–241. Springer, Cham (2015). https://doi.org/10.1007/978-3-319-24574-4_28

Learning Interpretable Anatomical Features Through Deep Generative Models: Application to Cardiac Remodeling

Carlo Biffi[1,2]([✉]), Ozan Oktay[1], Giacomo Tarroni[1], Wenjia Bai[1],
Antonio De Marvao[2], Georgia Doumou[2], Martin Rajchl[1], Reem Bedair[2],
Sanjay Prasad[3], Stuart Cook[3,4], Declan O'Regan[2], and Daniel Rueckert[1]

[1] Biomedical Image Analysis Group, Imperial College London, London, UK
c.biffi15@imperial.ac.uk
[2] MRC London Clinical Sciences Centre, Imperial College London, London, UK
[3] National Heart & Lung Institute, Imperial College London, London, UK
[4] Duke-NUS Graduate Medical School, Singapore, Singapore

Abstract. Alterations in the geometry and function of the heart define well-established causes of cardiovascular disease. However, current approaches to the diagnosis of cardiovascular diseases often rely on subjective human assessment as well as manual analysis of medical images. Both factors limit the sensitivity in quantifying complex structural and functional phenotypes. Deep learning approaches have recently achieved success for tasks such as classification or segmentation of medical images, but lack interpretability in the feature extraction and decision processes, limiting their value in clinical diagnosis. In this work, we propose a 3D convolutional generative model for automatic classification of images from patients with cardiac diseases associated with structural remodeling. The model leverages interpretable task-specific anatomic patterns learned from 3D segmentations. It further allows to visualise and quantify the learned pathology-specific remodeling patterns in the original input space of the images. This approach yields high accuracy in the categorization of healthy and hypertrophic cardiomyopathy subjects when tested on unseen MR images from our own multi-centre dataset (100%) as well on the ACDC MICCAI 2017 dataset (90%). We believe that the proposed deep learning approach is a promising step towards the development of interpretable classifiers for the medical imaging domain, which may help clinicians to improve diagnostic accuracy and enhance patient risk-stratification.

1 Introduction

Alterations in the geometry and function of the heart (remodeling) are used as criteria to diagnose and classify cardiovascular diseases as well as risk-stratify

The research was supported by grants from the British Heart Foundation (NH/17/1/32725, RE/13/4/30184).

© Springer Nature Switzerland AG 2018
A. F. Frangi et al. (Eds.): MICCAI 2018, LNCS 11071, pp. 464–471, 2018.
https://doi.org/10.1007/978-3-030-00934-2_52

individual patients [1]. For instance, hypertrophic cardiomyopathy (HCM), a leading cause of sudden death in adults [2], is an inherited disease of the heart muscle which manifests clinically with unexplained left ventricular (LV) hypertrophy and can occur in many different patterns that are not readily quantifiable [3]. Cardiovascular magnetic resonance (CMR) has become the gold-standard imaging technique for quantitative assessment in the diagnosis and risk-stratification of cardiomyopathy [4]. However, image interpretation is often dependent on both clinical expertise and effective diagnostic criteria, making automated data-driven approaches appealing for patient classification - especially as conventional manual analysis is not sensitive to the complex phenotypic manifestations of inherited heart disease. In recent years, large population cohorts have been recruited, such as the UK Biobank study with cardiac imaging in up 100,000 participants [5], requiring new approaches to high-throughput analysis. Learning-based approaches that can capture complex phenotypic variation could offer an objective data-driven means of disease classification without human intervention. Indeed, early work has shown the potential of machine learning algorithms in distinguishing benign from pathological hypertrophy from multiple manually-derived cardiac parameters [6].

Deep learning approaches have recently achieved outstanding results in the field of medical imaging due to their ability to learn complex non-linear functions, but they lack interpretability in the feature extraction and decision processes, limiting their clinical value. In this work, we propose a variational autoencoder (VAE) model [7] based on 3D convolutional layers, which is employed for classification of cardiac diseases associated with structural remodeling. This generative model enables us to visualise and leverage interpretable task-specific anatomical patterns learned from the segmentation data. The performance of the proposed approach is evaluated for the classification of healthy volunteers (HVols) and HCM subjects on our own dataset multi-centre cohort and on the ACDC MICCAI 2017 challenge dataset. This work makes two major contributions. First, we introduce a deep learning architecture which can discriminate between different clinical conditions through task-specific interpretable features, making the classification decision process transparent. Second, we develop a method to visualise and quantify the learned pathology-specific remodeling in the original space of the images, providing a data-driven method to study complex phenotypic manifestations.

1.1   Related Work

Given the high dimensionality of medical images, a popular approach in the literature is to analyze them by constructing statistical shape models of the heart using finite elements models or segmentation and co-registration algorithms to derive subject-specific meshes [8,9]. Similar to brain image analysis, principal component analysis (PCA) is then subsequently performed on these point distribution models to learn their main modes of deformation. These modes are then employed in the discrimination of distinct groups of subjects by their shape differences or to identify the ones mostly associated with diseases [10–12]. However,

PCA shape components do not define the features that differentiate between disease classes. For this purpose, approaches that search for new axes of variation that are clinically-meaningful have been proposed [13,14]. Relevant to this work, in the brain imaging domain, Shakeri et al. [15] employed a VAE model based on two fully connected layers to learn a low-dimensional representation of co-registered hippocampal meshes, which is later employed in a multi-layer perceptron to classify patients with Alzheimer disease. By contrast, the proposed method can exploit a deep convolutional neural network architecture directly on the segmentation maps to learn a discriminative latent space in an end-to-end fashion.

2   Materials and Methods

2.1   Datasets

A multi-centre cohort consisting of 686 HCMs patients (57 $\pm$ 14 years, 27% women, 77% Caucasian, HCM diagnosed using standard clinical criteria) and 679 healthy volunteers (40.6 $\pm$ 12.8 years, 55% women, 69% Caucasian) was considered for this work. Participants underwent CMR at 1.5-T on Siemens (Erlangen, Germany) or Philips (Best, Netherlands) systems. Cine images were acquired with a balanced steady-state free-precession sequence and included a stack of images in the left ventricular short axis plane (voxel size $2.1 \times 1.3 \times 7$ mm^3, repetition time/echo time of 3.2/1.6 ms, and flip angle of 60°). End-diastolic (ED) and end-systolic (ES) phases were segmented using a previously published and extensively validated cardiac multi-atlas segmentation framework [9]. As a first preprocessing step, we improved the quality of the 2D stacks segmentation by a multi-atlas-aided upsampling scheme. For each segmentation, twenty manually-annotated high-resolution atlases at ED and ES were warped to its space using a landmark-based rigid registration. Then a free-form non-rigid registration with a sparse set of control points was applied (nearest-neighbor interpolation) [16] and fused with a majority voting consensus. In a second step, we aligned all the quality-enhanced segmentations onto the same reference space at ED by means of landmark-based and subsequent intensity-based rigid registration to remove pose variations. After extracting the LV myocardium label, we cropped and padded each segmentation to $[x = 80, y = 80, z = 80, t = 1]$ dimension using a bounding box centered at the LV's ED myocardium. The latter operation guarantees shapes to maintain their alignment after cropping. Finally, all the segmentations underwent manual quality control in order to discard scans with strong inter-slice motion or insufficient LV coverage. As an additional testing dataset, 20 HVols and 20 HCMs from the ACDC MICCAI'17 challenge training dataset, consisting of 2D MR image sequences which are annotated at ED and ES phases by a clinical expert, were pre-processed using the same pipeline explained above.

2.2   Deep Generative Model

Architecture. A schematic representation of the proposed architecture is shown in Fig. 1. The network input $\mathbf{X}$ consists of subjects' 3D LV myocardial segmentations at ED and ES phases presented as a two-channel input. A 3D convolutional VAE is employed to learn a d-dimensional probability distribution representing the input segmentations $\mathbf{X}$ in a latent space through an encoder network. In this work, this latent distribution is parametrized as d-dimensional normal distribution $\mathcal{N}(\mu_i, \sigma_i)$ with mean μ_i and standard deviation σ_i, $i = 1, \ldots, d$. During training, a decoder network learns to reconstruct approximations of the input segmentations $\mathbf{X}$, which are denoted as $\hat{\mathbf{X}}$, by sampling vectors $\mathbf{z}$ from the learned latent d-dimensional manifold $\mathcal{Z}$, $\mathbf{z} \in \mathcal{Z} = \mathcal{N}(\boldsymbol{\mu}, \boldsymbol{\sigma})$. Simultaneously, a discriminative network (which is referred to as prediction network in the context of the paper) constructed with a multilayer perceptron (MLP) is connected to the mean vector $\boldsymbol{\mu}$ and trained to discriminate between HVols and HCMs subjects. This architecture is trained end-to-end with a loss function of the form $\mathcal{L} = \mathcal{L}_{rec} + \alpha \mathcal{L}_{KL} + \beta \mathcal{L}_{MLP}$. $\mathcal{L}_{rec}$ is the reconstruction loss and it was implemented as a Sorensen-Dice loss between the input segmentations $\mathbf{X}$ and their reconstruction $\hat{\mathbf{X}}$. $\mathcal{L}_{KL}$ is the Kullback-Leibler divergence loss forcing $\mathcal{N}(\boldsymbol{\mu}, \boldsymbol{\sigma})$ to be as close as possible to its prior distribution $\mathcal{N}(\mathbf{0}, \mathbf{1})$. $\mathcal{L}_{MLP}$ is the cross-entropy loss for the MLP classification task. The latent space dimension was fixed to $d = 64$. At test time, each input segmentation is reconstructed by passing the predicted $\boldsymbol{\mu}$ to $\mathbf{z}$ (without sampling from the latent space), while the classification is performed as in training time.

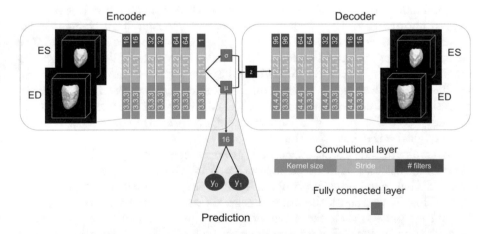

Fig. 1. Generative model architecture. Registered LV segmentations at ED and ES phases are mapped to a low-dimensional latent space. Each latent dimension is forced to be normally distributed with mean $\boldsymbol{\mu}$ and standard deviation $\boldsymbol{\sigma}$. A decoder network is then used to reconstruct the input segmentation from a low-dimensional vector $\mathbf{z}$ sampled from the learned latent distribution (training) or the $\boldsymbol{\mu}$ vector (testing). The $\boldsymbol{\mu}$ latent representation is used as input of a MLP to predict disease status.

Interpreting Learned Features via Navigation in the Latent Space. Our generative model architecture allows for visualization of the features learned by the network in the original segmentation space. For this, the weights learned by the MLP can be exploited to compute the partial derivative of the disease class label C (y_C) w.r.t. to the latent space representation μ of an input X, i.e. $\frac{\partial y_C}{\partial \mu_i}$, by backpropagating the gradient from the class label C to μ_i using chain-rule. Given a randomly selected healthy shape, we can use the derived gradient to move the latent representation of a subject μ along the direction of the latent code variability that maximises the probability of its classification to class C using an iterative algorithm. Starting with the mean latent representation $\mu_0 = \bar{\mu}$ of a healthy shape we can iteratively update μ_i at each step t accordingly to Eq. 1:

$$\mu_{i,t} = \mu_{i,t-1} + \lambda \frac{\partial y_1}{\partial \mu_{i,t-1}}, \quad \forall i = 1, \ldots d \tag{1}$$

Here we use $\lambda = 0.1$. Finally, each latent representation μ_t at each step t can be decoded back to the segmentation space by passing it to $\mathbf{z}$, allowing for the visualization of the corresponding reconstructed segmentations $\hat{\mathbf{X}}$.

3 Results

Our dataset was split into training, evaluation and testing sets consisting of 537 (276 HVols, 261 HCMs), 150 (75 HVols, 75 HCMs) and 200 (100 HVols, 100 HCMs) subjects respectively. The model was developed in Tensorflow, and trained on a Nvidia Tesla K80 GPU using Adam Optimizer, learning rate of 10^{-4} and batch size of 16. After 96k iterations, the total validation loss function stopped improving and the training was stopped. No significant changes in the classification results were found by varying the loss parameters α and β, while α was set to 0.1 as this captured local shape variations without losing the generative model properties. All the 200 subjects in the testing dataset were correctly classified (100% accuracy) by the trained prediction network. The model also correctly classified 36 out of the 40 ACDC MICCAI 2017 segmentations (90% accuracy); of the 4 misclassified cases, 3 did not properly cover the whole LV, which might be the cause for the error.

By employing the proposed method for latent space navigation, we deformed a randomly selected healthy segmentation from the training set towards the direction that maximizes its probability of being classified as HCM. On the right of Fig. 2, we report the original segmentations of the selected subject at ED and ES phases, their reconstruction from the VAE, and the reconstructed segmentations at four different iterations of the latent space navigation method. On the left of Fig. 2, the latent 64-dimensional representation μ of the training set segmentations together with the latent representations μ_t obtained at each iteration t were reduced for visualization purposes to a bi-dimensional space using Laplacian Eigenmaps [17]. This technique allows to build a neighborhood graph of the latent representations that can be used to monitor the transformation (light blue points) of the segmentation under study from the HVol cluster to the HCM cluster. At each reported step, LV mass (LVM) from each segmentation was derived by computing the volume of the myocardial voxels. Moreover, a LV atlas segmentation having also labels for the LV cavity was non-rigidly registered to each segmentation to compute LV cavity volume (LVCV) by computing the volume of the blood pool voxels. Finally, for each iteration we also report the probabilities of being an HVol or HCM as computed by the prediction network. The learned deformations demonstrate a higher LVM and lower LVCV with an asymmetric increase in septal wall thickness in the geometric transition from HVol to HCM - which is the typical pattern of remodeling in this disease [18]. At iteration 8, where the prediction network gives an indeterminate classification probability, LV geometry appears normal at ED but is thickened at ES suggesting that altered contractility may also be a discriminative feature.

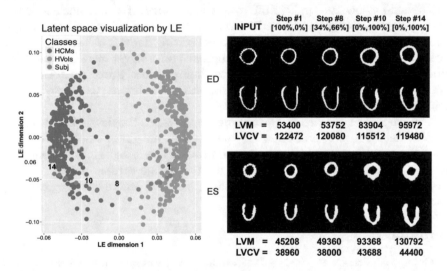

Fig. 2. On the left, Laplacian Eigenmaps (LE) bi-dimensional representation of the latent μ of each subject in the training set (red and green dots) and of the μ_t obtained through latent space navigation (light blue dots) for a random healthy shape. This latter is displayed on the right, together with the decoded segmentations corresponding to the sampled μ_t reported on the left at 4 exemplary iterations. The probabilities of class HVOls and HCM, and the computed LVM and LVCV are also shown.

4   Discussion and Conclusion

We present a deep generative model for automatic classification of heart pathologies associated with cardiac remodeling which leverages explainable task-specific anatomical features learned directly from 3D segmentations. The proposed architecture is specifically designed to enable the visualization and quantification of the learned features in the original segmentation space, making the classification decision process interpretable and potentially enabling quantification of disease severity. In this work we also propose a simple method that allows navigation in the low-dimensional manifold learned by the network, showing the potential clinical utility of the derived latent representation for tracking and scoring patients against a reference population. In the reported exemplar clinical application, the learned features achieved high accuracy in the discrimination of healthy subjects from HCM patients on our unseen testing dataset and on the ACDC MICCAI 17 dataset.

The proposed architecture can be easily extended to other cardiac related clinical tasks by replacing the prediction network with survival, risk score or other clinical models implemented as neural networks. The proposed approach worked successfully on conventional MR acquisitions, showing its potential for using routinely acquired clinical MR imaging. Moreover, the use of segmentation masks could allow its application to a wider range of CMR images such as multi-site images acquired from different machines and using different imaging protocols. We acknowledge that our external testing dataset was small, in future work we plan to evaluate the proposed approach on a bigger unseen dataset from different centres and on various types of cardiomypathies. Further extensions will also include the integration of clinical variables to the latent space as well as the inclusion of other cardiac phases.

The proposed approach is a promising step towards the development of interpretable deep learning classifiers for the medical imaging domain, which may assist clinicians to improve diagnosis and provide new insight into patient stratification. This general approach is not limited to the cardiac domain and can potentially be extended to other image analysis tasks where pathological shape change is prognostically relevant.

References

1. Cohn, J.N., Ferrari, R., Sharpe, N.: Cardiac remodeling concepts and clinical implications: a consensus paper from an international forum on cardiac remodeling. J. Am. Coll. Cardiol. **35**(3), 569–582 (2000)
2. Yancy, C.W., et al.: 2013 ACCF/AHA guideline for the management of heart failure: a report of the American College of Cardiology Foundation/American Heart Association Task Force on Practice Guidelines. J. Am. Coll. Cardiol. **62**(16), e147–239 (2013)
3. Captur, G., et al.: The embryological basis of subclinical hypertrophic cardiomyopathy. Sci. Rep. **6**, 27714 (2016)
4. Authors/Task Force Members, Elliott, P.M., et al.: 2014 ESC Guidelines on diagnosis and management of hypertrophic cardiomyopathy: the Task Force for the Diagnosis and Management of Hypertrophic Cardiomyopathy of the European Society of Cardiology (ESC). Eur. Heart J. **35**(39), 2733–79 (2014)
5. Petersen, S.E., et al.: Imaging in population science: cardiovascular magnetic resonance in 100,000 participants of UK Biobank-rationale, challenges and approaches. J. Cardiovasc. Magn. Reson. **15**(1), 46 (2013)
6. Narula, S., Shameer, K., Omar, A.M., Dudley, J.T., Sengupta, P.P.: Machine-learning algorithms to automate morphological and functional assessments in 2D echocardiography. J. Am. Coll. Cardiol. **68**(21), 2287–2295 (2016)

7. Kingma, D.P., Welling, M.: Auto-encoding variational bayes. arXiv preprint arXiv:1312.6114, 20 December 2013
8. Medrano-Gracia, P., Cowan, B.R., Suinesiaputra, A., Young, A.A.: Atlas-based anatomical modeling and analysis of heart disease. Drug Discov. Today Dis. Models **1**(14), 33–9 (2014)
9. Bai, W., et al.: A bi-ventricular cardiac atlas built from 1000+ high resolution MR images of healthy subjects and an analysis of shape and motion. Med. Image Anal. **26**(1), 133–45 (2015)
10. Remme, E.W., Young, A.A., Augenstein, K.F., Cowan, B., Hunter, P.J.: Extraction and quantification of left ventricular deformation modes. IEEE Trans. Biomed. Eng. **51**(11), 1923–1931 (2004)
11. Ardekani, S., et al.: Computational method for identifying and quantifying shape features of human left ventricular remodeling. Ann. Biomed. Eng. **37**(6), 1043–54 (2009)
12. Zhang, X., et al.: Atlas-based quantification of cardiac remodeling due to myocardial infarction. PLoS One **9**(10), e110243 (2014)
13. Suinesiaputra, A., et al.: Statistical shape modeling of the left ventricle: myocardial infarct classification challenge. IEEE J. Biomed. Health Inform. **22**(2), 503–515 (2017)
14. Zhang, X., et al.: Orthogonal decomposition of left ventricular remodeling in myocardial infarction. GigaScience **6**(3), 1–5 (2017)
15. Shakeri, M., Lombaert, H., Tripathi, S., Kadoury, S.: Deep spectral-based shape features for Alzheimer's disease classification. In: Reuter, M., Wachinger, C., Lombaert, H. (eds.) SeSAMI 2016. LNCS, vol. 10126, pp. 15–24. Springer, Cham (2016). https://doi.org/10.1007/978-3-319-51237-2_2. Alzheimers Disease Neuroimaging
16. Rueckert, D., Sonoda, L.I., Hayes, C., Hill, D.L.G., Leach, M.O., Hawkes, D.J.: Non-rigid registration using free-form deformations: application to breast MR images. IEEE Trans. Med. Imaging **18**(8), 712–721 (1999)
17. Belkin, M., Niyogi, P.: Laplacian eigenmaps for dimensionality reduction and data representation. Neural Comput. **15**(6), 1373–96 (2003)
18. Desai, M.Y., Ommen, S.R., McKenna, W.J., Lever, H.M., Elliott, P.M.: Imaging phenotype versus genotype in hypertrophic cardiomyopathy. Circ. Cardiovasc. Imaging **4**(2), 156–168 (2011)

Joint Learning of Motion Estimation and Segmentation for Cardiac MR Image Sequences

Chen Qin[1]($\boxtimes$), Wenjia Bai[1], Jo Schlemper[1], Steffen E. Petersen[2],
Stefan K. Piechnik[3], Stefan Neubauer[3], and Daniel Rueckert[1]

[1] Department of Computing, Imperial College London, London, UK
c.qin15@imperial.ac.uk
[2] NIHR Biomedical Research Centre at Barts, Queen Mary University of London,
London, UK
[3] Division of Cardiovascular Medicine, Radcliffe Department of Medicine,
University of Oxford, Oxford, UK

Abstract. Cardiac motion estimation and segmentation play important roles in quantitatively assessing cardiac function and diagnosing cardiovascular diseases. In this paper, we propose a novel deep learning method for joint estimation of motion and segmentation from cardiac MR image sequences. The proposed network consists of two branches: a cardiac motion estimation branch which is built on a novel unsupervised Siamese style recurrent spatial transformer network, and a cardiac segmentation branch that is based on a fully convolutional network. In particular, a joint multi-scale feature encoder is learned by optimizing the segmentation branch and the motion estimation branch simultaneously. This enables the weakly-supervised segmentation by taking advantage of features that are unsupervisedly learned in the motion estimation branch from a large amount of unannotated data. Experimental results using cardiac MlRI images from 220 subjects show that the joint learning of both tasks is complementary and the proposed models outperform the competing methods significantly in terms of accuracy and speed.

1   Introduction

Cardiac magnetic resonance imaging (MRI) is one of the reference methods to provide qualitative and quantitative information of the morphology and function of the heart, which can be utilized to assess cardiovascular diseases. Both cardiac MR image segmentation and motion estimation are crucial steps for the dynamic exploration of the cardiac function, which enable the accurate quantification of regional function measures such as changes in ventricular volumes and

Electronic supplementary material The online version of this chapter (https://doi.org/10.1007/978-3-030-00934-2_53) contains supplementary material, which is available to authorized users.

© Springer Nature Switzerland AG 2018
A. F. Frangi et al. (Eds.): MICCAI 2018, LNCS 11071, pp. 472–480, 2018.
https://doi.org/10.1007/978-3-030-00934-2_53

the elasticity and contractility properties of the myocardium [13]. Traditionally, most approaches consider segmentation and motion estimation as two separate problems. However, these two tasks are known to be closely related [6,17], and learning meaningful representations for one problem should be helpful to learn representations for the other one.

In this paper, we propose a joint deep learning network for predicting the segmentation and motion estimation simultaneously for cardiac MR sequences. In particular, the proposed architecture consists of two branches: one is an unsupervised Siamese style spatial transformer network for cardiac motion estimation, which exploits multi-scale features and recurrent units to accurately predict sequences of motion fields while ensuring spatio-temporal smoothness; and the other one is a segmentation branch which takes advantage of the joint feature learning to enable weakly-supervised segmentation for temporally sparse annotated data. We formulate the problem as a composite loss function optimized by training both tasks simultaneously. Using experiments with cardiac MRI from 220 subjects, we show that the proposed models can significantly improve the performance.

1.1   Related Work

In recent years, many works in deep learning domain have been proposed for cardiac MR image segmentation. Most of these approaches employ a fully convolutional network which learns useful features by training on manually annotated images and predicts a pixel-wise label map [2–4,10]. However, in real world applications, normally only end-distolic (ED) and end-systolic (ES) frames are manually annotated in a sequence of cardiac MR images, while information contained in other frames is not exploited in previous works. On the other hand, traditional methods commonly extended classical optical flow or image registration methods for cardiac motion estimation [7,13,14,16]. For instance, De Craene et al. [7] optimized a 4D velocity field parameterized by B-Spline spatio-temporal kernels to introduce temporal consistency, and Shi et al. [14] combined different MR sequences to estimate myocardial motion using a series of free-form deformations (FFD) [12]. In recent years, some deep learning works [15,18] have also been proposed for medical image registration. They either trained networks to learn similarity metrics or simulated transformations as ground truth to learn the regression. In contrast, our proposed method is a unified model for learning both cardiac motion estimation and segmentation, where no motion ground truth is required and only temporally sparse annotated frames in a cardiac cycle are needed. Of particular relevance to our approach are works [6,11] proposed in computer vision domain. Segflow [6] used a joint learning framework for natural video object segmentation and optical flow, and the work [11] propagated labels using the estimated flow to enable weakly-supervised segmentation. In comparison, our method proposes a different way to couple both tasks by learning a joint feature encoder, which exploits the massive information contained in unlabeled data and explores the redundancy of the feature representation for both tasks.

2   Methods

Our goal is to realize the simultaneous motion estimation and segmentation for cardiac MR image sequences. Here we construct a unified model consisting of two branches: an unsupervised motion estimation branch based on a Siamese style recurrent multi-scale spatial transformer network, and a segmentation branch based on a fully convolutional neural network, where the two branches share a joint feature encoder. The overall architecture of the model is shown in Fig. 1.

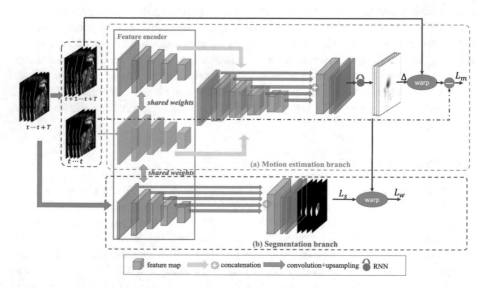

Fig. 1. The overall schematic architecture of proposed network for joint estimation of cardiac motion and segmentation. (a) The proposed Siamese style multi-scale recurrent motion estimation branch. (b) The segmentation branch which shares the joint feature encoder with motion estimation branch. The architecture for feature encoder is adopted from VGG-16 net before FC layer. Both branches have the same head architecture as the one proposed in [4], and the concatenation layers of motion estimation branch are from last layers at different scales of the feature encoder. For detailed architecture, please refer to supplementary material.

2.1   Unsupervised Cardiac Motion Estimation

Deep learning methods normally rely heavily on the ground truth labeled data. However, in problems of cardiac motion estimation, dense transformation maps between frames are rarely available. Inspired by the success of spatial transformer network [5,9,11] which effectively encodes optical flow to describe motion, here we propose a novel Siamese style multi-scale recurrent network for estimating the cardiac motion of MR image sequences without supervision effort. A schematic illustration of the model is shown in Fig. 1(a).

The task is to find a sequence of consecutive optical flow representations between the target frame I_t and the source frames $I_{t+1}, I_{t+2}, ..., I_{t+T}$, where the output is pixel-wise 2D motion fields Δ representing the displacement in x and y directions. In order to realize this, the proposed network mainly consists of four components: a Siamese network for the feature extraction of both target frame and source frame; a multi-scale concatenation of features from pairs of frames; a convolutional recurrent unit (RNN) which propagates information along temporal dimension; and a sampler that warps the source frame to the target one by using the estimated displacement field. In details, inspired by the success of cardiac segmentation network proposed in [4], we determine the Siamese feature encoder as the one in [4] which is adapted from VGG-16 net. For the combination of information from frame pairs, motivated by the traditional multi-level registration method [12], here we propose to concatenate multi-scale features from both streams of Siamese network to exploit information at different scales. This is followed by a convolution and upsampling operation back to the original resolution, and combined using a concatenation layer. In addition, in order to exploit information from consecutive frames and also to ensure the spatio-temporal smoothness of the estimated motion fields, we additionally incorporate a convolutional simple RNN with tanh function at the last layer to propagate motion information along the temporal dimension and to estimate flow with two feature maps $\Delta = (\Delta x, \Delta y; \theta_\Delta)$ corresponding to displacements for the x and y dimensions, where the network is parameterized by θ_Δ. Finally, the source frames I_{t+k} are transformed using bilinear interpolation to the target frame, which can be expressed as $I'_{t+k}(x,y) = \Gamma\{I_{t+k}(x + \Delta_{t+k}x, y + \Delta_{t+k}y)\}$.

To train the spatial transformer, we optimize the network by minimizing the pixel-wise mean squared error between the transformed frames and the target frame. To ensure local smoothness, we penalize the gradients of flow map by using an approximation of Huber loss proposed in [5], namely $\mathcal{H}(\delta_{x,y}\Delta_t) = \sqrt{\epsilon + \sum_{i=x,y}(\delta_x\Delta i^2 + \delta_y\Delta i^2)}$ and similarly, we use a regularization term $\mathcal{H}(\delta_t\Delta) = \sqrt{\epsilon + \sum_{i=x,y,t}\delta_t\Delta i^2}$ to constrain the flow to behave smoothly in temporal dimension, where $\epsilon = 0.01$. Therefore, the loss function can be described as follows:

$$\mathcal{L}_m = \frac{1}{T}\sum_{k=1}^{T}[\|I_t - I'_{t+k}\|^2 + \alpha\mathcal{H}(\delta_{x,y}\Delta_{t+k})] + \beta\mathcal{H}(\delta_t\Delta), \tag{1}$$

where T is the number of sequence, α and β are regularization parameters to trade off between image dissimilarity, local and temporal smoothness.

2.2 Joint Model for Cardiac Motion Estimation and Segmentation

As we know, motion estimation and segmentation tasks are closely related, and previous works in computer vision domain have shown that the learning of one task is able to benefit the other [6,17]. Motivated by the success of self-supervised learning which learns features from intrinsic freely available signals [1,8], here we propose a joint learning model for cardiac motion estimation and segmentation, where features learned from unsupervised (or self-supervised) motion estimation are exploited for segmentation. By coupling the motion estimation and segmentation network, the proposed approach can be viewed as a weakly-supervised method with temporally sparse annotated data while motion estimation facilitates the feature learning by exploring those unlabeled data. The schematic architecture of the unified model is shown in Fig. 1.

In details, the proposed joint model consists of two branches: the motion estimation branch proposed in Sect. 2.1, and the segmentation branch based on the effective network proposed in [4]. Here both branches share the joint feature encoder (Siamese style network) as shown in Fig. 1, so that the features learned can better capture the useful related representations for both tasks. Here a categorical cross-entropy loss $\mathcal{L}_s = -\sum_{l \in L} y_l \log(f(x_l; \Theta))$ on labeled data set L is used for segmentation branch, in which we define x_l as the input data, y_l as the ground truth, and f is the segmentation function parameterized by Θ. In addition, to further exploit the input unlabeled data, we add an additional spatial transformer in segmentation branch, which warps the predicted segmentation to the target frame using the motion fields estimated from motion estimation branch. Similarly, a categorical cross-entropy loss $\mathcal{L}_w = -\sum_{n \in U} y_l \log(f_w(x_n; \Theta))$ is used between the warped segmentations and the target, where U stands for unlabeled data set, and f_w is f plus the warp operation. This component mainly works as a regularization for the motion estimation branch, which is supposed to improve the estimation around boundaries.

As a result, a composite loss function consisting of image similarity error, smoothness penalty of motion fields, and pixel-wise cross entropy segmentation losses with the softmax function can be defined as follows:

$$\mathcal{L} = \mathcal{L}_m + \lambda_1 \mathcal{L}_s + \lambda_2 \mathcal{L}_w, \tag{2}$$

where λ_1 and λ_2 are trade-off parameters for different tasks. To initialize the joint model, we first train the motion estimation branch using all the available data we have. Then we fix the weights of the shared feature encoder, and train the segmentation branch with the available annotated data. Lastly, we jointly train both branches by minimizing the composite loss function on training set.

3   Experiments and Results

Experiments were performed on 220 short-axis cardiac MR sequences from UK Biobank study. Each scan contains a sequence of 50 frames, where manual segmentations of left-ventricular (LV) cavity, the myocardium (Myo) and the right-ventricular (RV) cavity are available on ED and ES frames. A short-axis image stack typically consists of 10 image slices. For pre-processing, all training images were cropped to the same size of 192×192, and intensity was normalized to the range of [0,1]. In our experiments, we split the data into 100/100/20 for training/testing/validation. Parameters used in the loss function were set to be

$\alpha = 0.001$, $\beta = 0.0001$, $\lambda_1 = 0.01$ and $\lambda_2 = 0.001$, which were chosen via validation set. The number of image sequence for RNN during training was $T = 10$, and a learning rate of 0.0001 was used. Data augmentation was performed on-the-fly, with random rotation, translation, and scaling.

Evaluation was performed with respect to both segmentation and motion estimation. We first evaluated the segmentation performance of the joint model by comparing it with the baseline method, i.e., training the segmentation branch only (Seg only). Results reported in Table 1 are Dice scores computed with manual annotations on LV, Myo, and RV. It shows that the proposed joint model significantly outperforms the results of Seg only on all three structures with $p \ll 0.001$ using Wilcoxon signed rank test, especially on Myo where motion normally affects the segmentation accuracy greatly. This indicates the merits of joint feature learning, where features explored by motion estimation are beneficial for segmentation task.

Table 1. Evaluation of segmentation accuracy for the proposed joint model and the baseline (Seg only) method in terms of the Dice Metric (mean and standard deviation).

Method	LV	Myo	RV
Seg only	0.9217 (0.0450)	0.8373 (0.0309)	0.8676 (0.0513)
Joint model	**0.9348 (0.0408)**	**0.8640 (0.0295)**	**0.8861 (0.0453)**

Table 2. Evaluation of motion estimation accuracy for FFD, proposed model in Sect. 2.1 (Motion only) and the proposed joint model in terms of the mean contour distance (MCD) and Hausdorff distance (HD) in mm (mean and standard deviation). Time reported is testing time on 50 frames in a cardiac cycle per slice.

Method	MCD			HD			Time
	LV	Myo	RV	LV	Myo	RV	
FFD	1.83(0.53)	2.47(0.74)	3.53(1.25)	5.10(1.28)	6.47(1.69)	12.04(4.85)	13.22 s
Motion only	1.55(0.49)	1.23(0.30)	3.14(1.12)	4.20(1.04)	3.51(0.88)	11.72(**4.28**)	**1.23 s**
Joint model	**1.30(0.34)**	**1.19(0.26)**	**3.03(1.08)**	**3.52(0.82)**	**3.43(0.87)**	**11.38**(4.34)	2.80 s

We also evaluated the performance of motion estimation by comparing the results obtained using a B-spline free-form deformation (FFD) algorithm[1] [12], network proposed in Sect. 2.1 (Motion only), and the joint model proposed in Sect. 2.2. We warped the segmentations of ES frame to ED frame by using the estimated motion fields, and mean contour distance (MCD) and Hausdorff distance (HD) were computed between the transformed segmentations and the segmentations of ED frame. Table 2 shows the comparison results of these methods.

---

[1] https://github.com/BioMedIA/MIRTK.

It can be observed that both of the proposed methods outperform FFD registration method in terms of MCD and HD on all the three structures ($p \ll 0.001$) and similarly, the joint model shows better performance than the model trained for motion estimation only ($p \ll 0.001$ on LV and RV, and $p < 0.01$ on Myo). Additionally, we compared the test time needed for motion estimation on 50 frames of a single slice in a cardiac cycle, and results indicated a faster speed of proposed methods compared to FFD.

Furthermore, the proposed joint method is capable of predicting a sequence of estimated motion fields and segmentations simultaneously. Here we show a visualization result of the network predictions with segmentations and motions combined on frames in a cardiac cycle in Fig. 2. Myocardial motion indicated by the yellow arrows were established between ED and other time frames. Note that the network predicts dense motion fields, while for better visualization, we only show a sparse representation around myocardium. To further validate the proposed unified model in terms of the motion estimation, Fig. 3(a)(b) shows a labeling results of the LV and RV boundaries along temporal dimension, which is obtained by warping the labeled segmentations available in ED frame to other time points, and Fig. 3(c) calculated the transformed LV volume over the cardiac cycle. These show that the proposed model is able to produce an accurate estimation, which is also smooth and consistent over time.

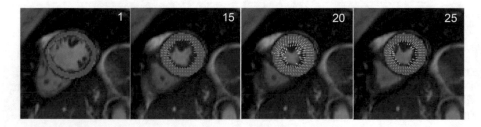

Fig. 2. Visualization results for simultaneous prediction of motion estimation and segmentation. Myocardial motions are from ED to other time points. Please refer to supplementary material for a dynamic video of a cardiac cycle.

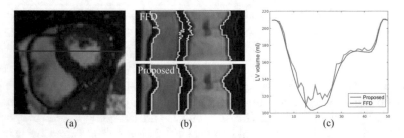

Fig. 3. (a) (b) Labeling results obtained by warping the ED frame segmentation to other time points using FFD and the proposed joint model. Results are shown in temporal views of the red short-axis line. (c) Left ventricular volume (ml) of the subject by warping the ED frame segmentation to other time points in a cardiac cycle. (Color figure online)

4   Conclusion

In this paper, we have presented a novel deep learning model for joint motion estimation and segmentation of cardiac MR image sequence. The proposed architecture is composed of two branches: a proposed unsupervised Siamese style recurrent spatial transformer network for motion estimation and a segmentation branch based on a fully convolutional network. A joint feature encoder is shared between the two branches, which enables the effective feature learning via multi-task training and also the weakly-supervised segmentation in terms of the temporally sparse annotated data. Experimental results showed significant improvements of proposed models against baseline approaches in terms of accuracy and speed. For the future work, we will validate our method on a larger scale dataset, and will also investigate its usefulness on 3D applications.

References

1. Agrawal, P., Carreira, J., Malik, J.: Learning to see by moving. In: ICCV, pp. 37–45 (2015)
2. Avendi, M., Kheradvar, A., Jafarkhani, H.: A combined deep-learning and deformable-model approach to fully automatic segmentation of the left ventricle in cardiac MRI. Med. Image Anal. **30**, 108–119 (2016)
3. Bai, W., et al.: Semi-supervised learning for network-based cardiac MR image segmentation. In: Descoteaux, M., Maier-Hein, L., Franz, A., Jannin, P., Collins, D.L., Duchesne, S. (eds.) MICCAI 2017. LNCS, vol. 10434, pp. 253–260. Springer, Cham (2017). https://doi.org/10.1007/978-3-319-66185-8_29
4. Bai, W., Sinclair, M., Tarroni, G., et al.: Automated cardiovascular magnetic resonance image analysis with fully convolutional networks. J. Cardiovasc. Magn. Reson. (2018)
5. Caballero, J., Ledig, C., Aitken, A., et al.: Real-time video super-resolution with spatio-temporal networks and motion compensation. In: CVPR (2017)
6. Cheng, J., Tsai, Y.H., Wang, S., Yang, M.H.: SegFlow: joint learning for video object segmentation and optical flow. In: ICCV, pp. 686–695 (2017)
7. De Craene, M., Piella, G., Camara, O., et al.: Temporal diffeomorphic free-form deformation: application to motion and strain estimation from 3D echocardiography. Med. Image Anal. **16**(2), 427–450 (2012)
8. Doersch, C., Zisserman, A.: Multi-task self-supervised visual learning. In: ICCV (2017)
9. Jaderberg, M., Simonyan, K., Zisserman, A., et al.: Spatial transformer networks. In: NIPS, pp. 2017–2025 (2015)
10. Ngo, T.A., Lu, Z., Carneiro, G.: Combining deep learning and level set for the automated segmentation of the left ventricle of the heart from cardiac cine magnetic resonance. Med. Image Anal. **35**, 159–171 (2017)
11. Patraucean, V., Handa, A., Cipolla, R.: Spatio-temporal video autoencoder with differentiable memory. In: ICLR Workshop (2016)
12. Rueckert, D., Sonoda, L.I., Hayes, C., et al.: Nonrigid registration using free-form deformations: application to breast MR images. IEEE Trans. Med. Imaging **18**(8), 712–721 (1999)

13. Shen, D., Sundar, H., Xue, Z., Fan, Y., Litt, H.: Consistent estimation of cardiac motions by 4D image registration. In: Duncan, J.S., Gerig, G. (eds.) MICCAI 2005. LNCS, vol. 3750, pp. 902–910. Springer, Heidelberg (2005). https://doi.org/10.1007/11566489_111

14. Shi, W., Zhuang, X., Wang, H., et al.: A comprehensive cardiac motion estimation framework using both untagged and 3-D tagged MR images based on nonrigid registration. IEEE Trans. Med. Imaging **31**(6), 1263–1275 (2012)

15. Simonovsky, M., Gutiérrez-Becker, B., Mateus, D., et al.: A deep metric for multimodal registration. In: MICCAI, pp. 10–18 (2016)

16. Tobon-Gomez, C., De Craene, M., Mcleod, K., et al.: Benchmarking framework for myocardial tracking and deformation algorithms: an open access database. Med. Image Anal. **17**(6), 632–648 (2013)

17. Tsai, Y.H., Yang, M.H., Black, M.J.: Video segmentation via object flow. In: CVPR, pp. 3899–3908 (2016)

18. Uzunova, H., Wilms, M., Handels, H., Ehrhardt, J.: Training CNNs for image registration from few samples with model-based data augmentation. In: Descoteaux, M., Maier-Hein, L., Franz, A., Jannin, P., Collins, D.L., Duchesne, S. (eds.) MICCAI 2017. LNCS, vol. 10433, pp. 223–231. Springer, Cham (2017). https://doi.org/10.1007/978-3-319-66182-7_26

Multi-Input and Dataset-Invariant Adversarial Learning (MDAL) for Left and Right-Ventricular Coverage Estimation in Cardiac MRI

Le Zhang[1]([⊠]), Marco Pereañez[1], Stefan K. Piechnik[2], Stefan Neubauer[2], Steffen E. Petersen[3], and Alejandro F. Frangi[1]

[1] Centre for Computational Imaging and Simulation Technologies in Biomedicine, Department of Electronic and Electrical Engineering, University of Sheffield, Sheffield, UK
le.zhang@sheffield.ac.uk
[2] Oxford Center for Clinical Magnetic Resonance Research (OCMR), Division of Cardiovascular Medicine, University of Oxford, John Radcliffe Hospital, Oxford, UK
[3] Cardiovascular Medicine at the William Harvey Research Institute, Queen Mary University of London and Barts Heart Center, Barts Health NHS Trust, London, UK

Abstract. Cardiac functional parameters, such as, the Ejection Fraction (EF) and Cardiac Output (CO) of both ventricles, are most immediate indicators of normal/abnormal cardiac function. To compute these parameters, accurate measurement of ventricular volumes at end-diastole (ED) and end-systole (ES) are required. Accurate volume measurements depend on the correct identification of basal and apical slices in cardiac magnetic resonance (CMR) sequences that provide full coverage of both left (LV) and right (RV) ventricles. This paper proposes a novel adversarial learning (AL) approach based on convolutional neural networks (CNN) that detects and localizes the basal/apical slices in an image volume independently of image-acquisition parameters, such as, imaging device, magnetic field strength, variations in protocol execution, etc. The proposed model is trained on multiple cohorts of different provenance, and learns image features from different MRI viewing planes to learn the appearance and predict the position of the basal and apical planes. To the best of our knowledge, this is the first work tackling the fully automatic detection and position regression of basal/apical slices in CMR volumes in a dataset-invariant manner. We achieve this by maximizing the ability of a CNN to regress the position of basal/apical slices within a single dataset, while minimizing the ability of a classifier to discriminate image features between different data sources. Our results show superior performance over state-of-the-art methods.

Keywords: Deep learning · Dataset invariance · Adversarial learning Ventricular coverage assessment · MRI

© Springer Nature Switzerland AG 2018
A. F. Frangi et al. (Eds.): MICCAI 2018, LNCS 11071, pp. 481–489, 2018.
https://doi.org/10.1007/978-3-030-00934-2_54

1   Introduction

To obtain accurate and reliable volume and functional parameter measurements in CMR imaging studies, recognizing basal and apical slices for both ventricles is crucial. Unfortunately, current practice to detect basal/or apical slice positions is still carried out by visual inspection of experts on the image. This practice is costly, subjective, error prone, and time consuming [1]. Although significant progress [14] has been made in automatic assessment of full LV coverage in cardiac MRI, to accurately measure volumes and functional parameters for both ventricles where the basal/apical slices are missing, methods to estimate the position of the missing slices are required [10]. Such methods would be critical to prompt the intervention of experts to correct problems in data measurements, or to trigger algorithms that can cope with missing data by, for instance, imputation [5] through image synthesis, or shape based extrapolation. This paves the way to "quality-aware image analysis" [13]. To the best of our knowledge, previous work regarding image quality control has focused solely on coverage detection of the LV, but not on missing slice position estimation.

In medical image analysis, it is sometimes convenient or necessary to infer an image in one modality from another for image quality assessment purposes. One major challenge of basal/apical slice estimation for CMR comes from differences between data sources, which are tissue appearance and/or spatial resolution of images sourced from different physical acquisition principles or parameters. Such differences make it difficult to generalize algorithms trained on specific datasets to other data sources. This is problematic not only when the source and target datasets are different, but more so, when the target dataset contains no labels. In all such scenarios, it is highly desirable to learn a discriminative classifier or other predictor in the presence of a shift between training and test distributions, which is called *dataset invariance*. The general approach of achieving dataset adaptation has been explored under many facets. Among the existing cross-dataset learning works, dataset adaptation has been adopted for re-identification hoping labeled data from a source dataset can provide transferable identity-discriminative information for a target dataset. [7] explored the possibility of generating multimodal images from single-modality imagery. [8,9] employed multi-task metric learning models to benefit the target task. However, these works are focused mainly on linear assumptions.

In this paper, we focus on the non-linear representations and analysis of short-axis (SA) and long-axis (LA) cine MRI for the detection and regression of the basal and apical slices of both ventricles in CMR volumes. To deal with the problem where there is no labeled data for a target dataset, and one hopes to transfer knowledge from a model trained on sufficient labeled data of a source dataset sharing the same feature space, but with a different marginal distribution we present these contributions: (1) We present a unified model (MDAL) for any cross-dataset basal/apical slice estimation problem in CMR volumes; (2) We integrate adversarial feature learning by building an end-to-end architecture of CNNs and transferring non-linear representations from a labeled source dataset to a target dataset where labels are non-existent. Our deep architecture effectively improves the adaptability of learning with data of different databases; (3) A multi-view image extension of the adversarial learning model is proposed and exploited. By making use of multi-view images acquired from short- and long-axis views, one can further improve and constrain the basal/apical slice position. We evaluate our method on three datasets and compare with state-of-the-art methods. Experimental results show the superior performance of our method compared to other approaches.

2   Methodology

2.1   Problem Formulation

The cross-dataset localization of basal or apical slices can be formulated as two tasks: (i) *Dataset Invariance:* given a set of 3D images $\mathcal{X}^s = [\mathbf{X}_1^s, ..., \mathbf{X}_N^s] \in \mathbb{R}^{m \times n \times z^s \times N^s}$ of modality $\mathcal{M}_s$ in the source dataset, and $\mathcal{X}^t = [\mathbf{X}_1^t, ..., \mathbf{X}_N^t] \in \mathbb{R}^{m \times n \times z^t \times N^t}$ of modality $\mathcal{M}_t$ in the target dataset. m, n are the dimensions of axial view of the image, and z^s and z^t denote the size of images along the z-axis, while N^s and N^t are the number of volumes in source and target datasets, respectively. Our goal is to build mappings between the source (training-time) and the target (test-time) datasets, that reduce the difference between the source and target data distributions; (ii) *Multi-view Slice Regression:* In this task, slice localization performance is enhanced by using multiple image stacks, *e.g.* SA and LA stacks, into a single regression task. Let $\mathbf{X}^s = \{\mathbf{x}_i^s, r_i^s\}_{i=1}^{Z^s}$ and $\mathbf{Y}^s = \{\mathbf{y}_i^s, r_i^s\}_{i=1}^{Z^s}$ be a labeled 3D CMR volume from source modality $\mathcal{M}_s$ in short- and long-axis, respectively, and $\mathbf{x}_b^s$, $\mathbf{x}_a^s$, and $\mathbf{y}_b^s$, $\mathbf{y}_a^s$ be the short-axis slices, and long-axis image patches of the basal and apical views; let $\mathbf{X}^t = \{\mathbf{x}_i^t\}_{i=1}^{Z^t}$ and $\mathbf{Y}^t = \{\mathbf{y}_i^t\}_{i=1}^{Z^t}$ represent an unlabeled sample from the target dataset in short- and long-axis, i represents the ith slice and Z is the total number of CMR slices. Our goal is to learn the discriminative features from $\mathbf{x}_b^s$, $\mathbf{x}_a^s$, and $\mathbf{y}_b^s$, $\mathbf{y}_a^s$ to localize the basal and apical slices in two axes for CMR volumes in the target dataset[1]. We use the labeled UK Biobank (UKBB) [11] cardiac MRI data cohort together with the MESA[2] and DETERMINE[3] datasets, and apply our method to cross-dataset basal and apical slice regression tasks.

2.2   Multi-Input and Dataset-Invariant Adversarial Learning

Inspired by Adversarial Learning (AL) [6] and Dataset Adaptation (DA) [12] for cross-dataset transfer, we propose a Dataset-Invariant Adversarial Learning model, which extends the DA formulation into a AL strategy, and performs them jointly in a unified framework. We propose multi-view adversarial learning by

---

[1] **Notation:** Matrices and 3D images are written in bold uppercase (*e.g.*, image $\mathbf{X}$, $\mathbf{Y}$), vectors and vectorized 2D images in bold lowercase (*e.g.*, slice $\mathbf{x}$, $\mathbf{y}$) and scalars in lowercase (*e.g.*, slice position label r).

[2]   http://www.cardiacatlas.org/studies/mesa/.

[3]   http://www.cardiacatlas.org/studies/determine/.

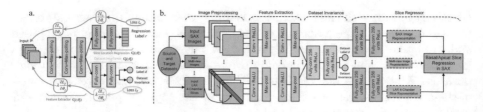

Fig. 1. *a:* Schematic of our dataset-invariant adversarial network; *b:* System overview of our proposed dataset-invariant adversarial model with multi-view input channels for bi-ventricular coverage estimation in cardiac MRI. Each channel contains three conv layers, three max-pooling layers and two fully-connected layers. Additional dataset invariance net (yellow) includes two fully-connected layers. Kernel numbers in each conv layer are 16, 16 and 64 with sizes of 7×7, 13×13 and 10×10, respectively; filter sizes in each max-pooling layer are 2×2, 3×3 and 2×2 with stride 2.

creating multiple input channels (MC) from images which are re-sampled to the same spatial grid and visualize the same anatomy. An overview of our method is depicted in Fig. 1. Given two sets of slices $\{\mathbf{x}_i^s\}_{i=1}^N$, $\{\mathbf{y}_i^s\}_{i=1}^N$ with slice position labels $\{r_i^s\}_{i=1}^N$ for training, to learn a model that can generalize well from one dataset to another, and is used both during training and test time to regress the basal/apical slice position, we optimize this objective in stages: (1) we optimize the label regression loss

$$
\begin{aligned}
\mathcal{L}_r^i &= \mathcal{L}_r(G_{sigm}(G_{conv}(\mathbf{x}_s, \mathbf{y}_s; \theta_f); \theta_r), r_i) \\
&= \sum_i \|r_i - G_{sigm}(G_{conv}(\mathbf{x}_s, \mathbf{y}_s; \theta_f); \theta_r), r_i)\|_2^2 + \frac{1}{2}\left(\|\theta_f\|_2^2 + \|\theta_r\|_2^2\right),
\end{aligned}
\tag{1}
$$

where θ_f is the representation parameter of the neural network feature extractor, which corresponds to the feature extraction layers. θ_r is the regression parameter of the slice regression net, which corresponds to the regression layers. r_i denotes the ith slice position label. θ_f and θ_r are trained for the ith image by using the labeled source data $\{\mathbf{X}_i^s, \mathbf{r}_i^s\}_{i=1}^{N^s}$ and $\{\mathbf{Y}_i^s, \mathbf{r}_i^s\}_{i=1}^{N^s}$. (2) Since dataset adversarial learning satisfies a dataset adaptation mechanism, we minimize source and target representation distances through alternating *minimax* between two loss functions: one is the dataset discriminator loss

$$
\begin{aligned}
\mathcal{L}_d^i &= \mathcal{L}_d(G_{disc}(G_{conv}(\mathbf{x}_s, \mathbf{y}_s, \mathbf{x}_t, \mathbf{y}_t; \theta_f); \theta_d), d_i) \\
&= -\sum_i \mathbb{1}\left[o_d = d_i\right] \log(G_{disc}(G_{conv}(\mathbf{x}_s, \mathbf{y}_s, \mathbf{x}_t, \mathbf{y}_t; \theta_f); \theta_d), d_i),
\end{aligned}
\tag{2}
$$

which classifies whether an image is drawn from the source or the target dataset. o_d indicates the output of the dataset classifier for the ith image, θ_d is the parameter used for the computation of the dataset prediction output of the network, which corresponds to the dataset invariance layers; d_i denotes the dataset that the example slice i is drawn from. The other is the source and target mapping invariant loss

$$
\begin{aligned}
\mathcal{L}_f^i &= \mathcal{L}_f(G_{conf}(G_{conv}(\mathbf{x}_s,\mathbf{y}_s,\mathbf{x}_t,\mathbf{y}_t;\theta_f);\theta_d),d_i) \\
&= -\sum_d \frac{1}{D}\log(G_{conf}(G_{conv}(\mathbf{x}_s,\mathbf{y}_s,\mathbf{x}_t,\mathbf{y}_t;\theta_f);\theta_d),d_i),
\end{aligned}
\tag{3}
$$

which is optimized with a constrained adversarial objective by computing the cross entropy between the output predicted dataset labels, and a uniform distribution over dataset labels. D indicates the number of input channels. Our full method then optimizes the joint loss function

$$
\begin{aligned}
E(\theta_f,\theta_r,\theta_d) &= \mathcal{L}_r(G_{sigm}(G_{conv}(\mathbf{x}_s,\mathbf{y}_s;\theta_f);\theta_r),r) \\
&\quad + \lambda\mathcal{L}_f(G_{conf}(G_{conv}(\mathbf{x}_s,\mathbf{y}_s,\mathbf{x}_t,\mathbf{y}_t;\theta_f);\theta_d),d),
\end{aligned}
\tag{4}
$$

where hyperparameter λ determines how strongly the dataset invariance influences the optimization; $G_{conv}(\cdot)$ is a convolution layer function that maps an example into a new representation; $G_{sigm}(\cdot)$ is a label prediction layer function; $G_{disc}(\cdot)$ and $G_{conf}(\cdot)$ are the dataset prediction and invariance layer functions.

2.3   Optimization

Similar to classical CNN learning methods, we propose to tackle the optimization problem with the stochastic gradient procedure, in which updates are made in the opposite direction of the gradient of Eq. (4) to minimize parameters, and in the direction of the gradient to maximize other parameters [4]. We optimize the objective in the following stages.

Optimizing the Label Regressor: In adversarial adaptive methods, the main goal is to regularize the learning of the source and target mappings, so as to minimize the distance between the empirical source and target mapping distributions. If so then the source regression model can be directly applied to the target representations, eliminating the need to learn a separate target regressor. Training the neural network then leads to this optimization problem on the source dataset:

$$
\arg\min_{\theta_f,\theta_r}\{\frac{1}{N^s}\sum_{i=1}^{N^s}\mathcal{L}_r^i(G_{sigm}(G_{conv}(\mathbf{x}_s,\mathbf{y}_s;\theta_f);\theta_r),r_i)\}.
\tag{5}
$$

Optimizing for Dataset Invariance: This optimization corresponds to the true *minimax* objective ($\mathcal{L}_d$ and $\mathcal{L}_f$) for the dataset classifier parameters and the dataset invariant representation. The two losses stand in direct opposition to one another: learning a fully dataset invariant representation means the dataset classifier must do poorly, and learning an effective dataset classifier means that the representation is not dataset invariant. Rather than globally optimizing θ_d

and θ_f, we instead perform iterative updates for these two objectives given the fixed parameters from the previous iteration:

$$\arg\min_{\theta_d}\{-\frac{1}{\mathcal{N}}\sum_{i=1}^{\mathcal{N}}\mathcal{L}_d^i(G_{disc}(G_{conv}(\mathbf{x}_s,\mathbf{y}_s,\mathbf{x}_t,\mathbf{y}_t;\theta_f);\theta_d),d_i)\}, \qquad (6)$$

$$\arg\max_{\theta_f}\{-\frac{1}{\mathcal{N}}\sum_{i=1}^{\mathcal{N}}\mathcal{L}_f^i(G_{conf}(G_{conv}(\mathbf{x}_s,\mathbf{y}_s,\mathbf{x}_t,\mathbf{y}_t;\theta_f);\theta_d),d_i)\}, \qquad (7)$$

where $\mathcal{N}=N^s+N^t$ being the total number of samples. These losses are readily implemented in standard deep learning frameworks, and after setting learning rates properly so Eq. (6) only updates θ_d and (7) only updates θ_f, the updates can be performed via standard backpropagation. Together, these updates ensure that we learn a representation that is dataset invariant.

2.4 Detection and Regression for Basal/Apical Slice Position

We denote $\hat{\mathcal{H}}_t$, $\hat{\mathcal{G}}_t$ as extracted query features, and $\hat{\mathcal{H}}_s$, $\hat{\mathcal{G}}_s$ as extracted basal/apical slice representations from SAX and LAX, respectively. In order to regress basal and apical slices according to query features, we compute the dissimilarity matrix $\delta_{i,j}$ based on $\hat{\mathcal{H}}_t$, $\hat{\mathcal{G}}_t$ and $\hat{\mathcal{H}}_s$, $\hat{\mathcal{G}}_s$ using the volume's inter-slice distance as: $\delta_{i,j}(\hat{\mathcal{H}}_t,\hat{\mathcal{H}}_s,\hat{\mathcal{G}}_t,\hat{\mathcal{G}}_s)=\sqrt{(\hat{\mathcal{H}}_t^i-\hat{\mathcal{H}}_s^j)^2+(\hat{\mathcal{G}}_t^i-\hat{\mathcal{G}}_s^j)^2}$. Then, ranking can be carried out based on the ascending order of each row of the dissimilarity distance, *i.e.*, the lower the entry value $\delta_{i,j}$ is, the closer the basal/apical slice and the query slice are.

3 Experiments and Analysis

Data Specifications: Quality-scored CMR data is available for circa 5,000 volunteers of the UK Biobank imaging (UKBB) resource. Following visual inspection, manual annotation for SAX images was carried out with a simple 3-grade quality score [2]. 4,280 sequences correspond to quality score 1 for both ventricles, these had full coverage of the heart from base to apex and were the source datasets to construct the ground-truth classes for our experiments. Note that having full coverage should not be confused with having the top/bottom slices corresponding exactly to base/apex. Basal slices including the left ventricular outflow tract, pulmonary valve and right atrium, and apical slices with a visible ventricular cavity were labeled manually. The distance between the actual location of the basal/apical slice to other slices in the volume were used as training labels for the regression. We validated the proposed MDAL on three target datasets: UKBB, DETERMINE and MESA (protocols of the three datasets are shown in Table 1). To prevent over-fitting due to insufficient target data, and to improve the detection rate of our algorithm, we employ data augmentation techniques to artificially enlarge the target datasets. For this purpose we chose a set of realistic rotations, scaling factors, and corresponding mirror images, and applied them to the MRI images. The set of rotations chosen were $-45°$ and $45°$, and the scaling factors 0.75 and 1.25. This increased the number of training samples by a factor of eight. After data augmentation, we had 2400, and 2384 sequences for DETERMINE and MESA datasets, respectively. For evaluating of multi-view models, we defined two input channels, one for SAX images, and another for LAX (4-chamber) from the UKBB, MESA and DETERMINE. The LAX image information was extracted by collecting pixels values along the intersecting line between the 4-chamber view plane and corresponding short-axis plane over the cardiac cycle. We extracted 4 pixels above and below the two plane intersection. We embedded the constructed profile within a square image with zeros everywhere except the profile diagonal (see Fig. 1b bottom channel).

Table 1. Cardiovascular magnetic resonance protocols for UKBB, MESA and DETERMINE Datasets.

Dataset	View	Number of sequences	Cardiac phases	Matrix size	Slice thickness	Slice gap	Slice spacing	Slices per volume
UKB	SAX	4280	50	208×187	8 mm	2 mm	10 mm	ca. 10
	LAX	4280	50	208×187	6 mm	n.a	n.a	1
MESA	SAX	298	20–30	256×160	6 mm	4 mm	10 mm	ca. 10
	LAX	298	20–30	256×160	6 mm	n.a	n.a	1
DETERMINE	SAX	300	25	128×256	$\leqslant 10$ mm	$\leqslant 2$ mm	10 mm	ca. 10
	LAX	300	25	128×256	6 mm	n.a	n.a	1

Experimental Set-Up: The architecture of our proposed method is shown in Fig. 1. To maximize the number of training samples from all datasets, while preventing biased learning of image features from a particular dataset and given that the number of samples from the UKBB is at least an order of magnitude larger than from MESA or DETERMINE, we augmented both the MESA and DETERMINE datasets, to match the resulting number of samples from the UKBB. This way our dataset classification task will not over-fit to anyone sample. Our MDAL method processes images with small blocks (120×120), which are crop-centered on the images to extract specific regions of interest. The experiments here reported were conducted using the ConvNet library [3] on an Intel Xeon E5-1620 v3 @3.50 GHz machine running Windows 10 with 32 GB RAM and Nvidia Quadro K620 GPU. We optimize the network using a learning rate μ of 0.001 and set the hyper-parameter parameter λ to be 0.01, respectively. To evaluate the detection process, we measure classification accuracy, and to evaluate the regression error between the predicted position and the ground truth, we use the Mean Absolute Error (MAE).

Table 2. The comparison of basal/apical slice detection accuracy (Mean ± standard deviation) (%) between adaptation and non-adaptation methods, each with single (SAX)- and multi-view inputs (BS/AS indicate basal/apical slice detection accuracy). Best results are highlighted in bold.

Dataset	No dataset adaptation (BS/AS)		With dataset Adaptation (BS/AS)	
	Single-view [14]	Multi-view [14]	Single-view [4]	Multi-view (Ours)
UKBB	79.0 ± 0.2/76.2 ± 0.3	**89.2 ± 0.1/92.4 ± 0.2**	78.2 ± 0.2/75.4 ± 0.3	88.7 ± 0.1/91.4 ± 0.3
MESA	31.6 ± 0.3/35.1 ± 0.1	61.5 ± 0.2/68.3 ± 0.4	74.2 ± 0.2/72.9 ± 0.4	**87.1 ± 0.3/90.2 ± 0.2**
DETERMINE	48.3 ± 0.2/51.1 ± 0.3	75.6 ± 0.3/78.4 ± 0.3	77.2 ± 0.3/76.5 ± 0.2	**89.0 ± 0.2/91.2 ± 0.2**

Table 3. Regression error comparison between adaptation and non-adaptation methods, each with single (SAX)- and multi-view inputs for cardiac SAX slice position regression in terms of MAE (Mean ± standard deviation)(mm)(BS/AS indicate basal/apical slice regression errors). Best results are highlighted in bold.

Dataset	No dataset adaptation (BS/AS)		With dataset adaptation (BS/AS)	
	Single-view [14]	Multi-view [14]	Single-view [4]	Multi-view (Ours)
UKBB	4.32 ± 1.6/5.73 ± 1.9	**3.42 ± 1.1/3.98±1.7**	5.13 ± 2.1/6.33 ± 2.3	3.64 ± 1.9/4.02 ± 2.0
MESA	7.78 ± 2.0/8.34 ± 2.4	6.47 ± 1.7/6.83 ± 1.4	4.81 ± 1.0/5.73 ± 1.5	**3.98 ± 1.1/4.07 ± 1.3**
DETERMINE	6.43 ± 1.9/6.81 ± 2.0	6.01 ± 1.3/6.17 ± 1.4	4.73 ± 1.6/4.81 ± 1.3	**4.24 ± 1.0/4.45 ± 1.3**

Results: We evaluate the performance of the multi-view basal/apical slice detection and regression tasks with and without dataset invariance (adaptation vs non-adaptation), by transferring object regressors from the UKBB to MESA and DETERMINE. To evaluate performance on MESA and DETERMINE, we manually generated annotations as follows: we checked one slice above and below the detected basal slice to confirm the slice is the basal and record true or false, ditto for apex. We chose the CNN architecture in [14] for single- and multi-view metrics with non-adaptation, and the GTSRB architecture in [4] for single-view adaption method. Table 2 shows the detection accuracy for basal/apical slice of the adaptation and non-adaptation from single and multi-view. For both test datasets, the best improvements are the result of combining both of these features. For MESA the detection accuracy was increased by 64%, and for DETERMINE best improvements are of 44% (right-most column). Table 3 shows the average regression errors of slice locations in millimeter (mm). Even without using the multi-input channels, our dataset invariance framework is able to reduce the slice localization error to less than half the average slice spacing found on our test datasets, $i.e.$, $<5\,mm$. With multi-view we reduced the localization errors to 4.24 and 4.45 mm on average for both basal/apical slices. All the experiences are significantly different at $p < 0.05$.

4   Conclusion

In this paper, we have proposed a Multi-Input and Dataset-Invariant Adversarial Learning (MDAL) framework capable of learning a common image representation, and using it to detect and localize basal and apical CMR slices, we achieve this by: first, using a Dataset-Invariant Adversarial Learning (DIAL) model to fit the joint distribution over the images from different datasets with a minimax game. Second, extending the DIAL model to handle multiple view input scenarios thereby obtaining better results for Left and Right-Ventricular coverage estimation in Cardiac MRI. And third, by introducing a regressor network able to predict the location of basal/apical slices. We evaluated our framework on two large datasets MESA and DETERMINE and found that our approach significantly outperforms state-of-the-art non-dataset-adaptive and single-input methods. Finally, Our MDAL framework can be easily generalized to any anatomical structure or image modality.

References

1. Attili, A.K., Schuster, A., Nagel, E., Reiber, J.H., van der Geest, R.J.: Quantification in cardiac MRI: advances in image acquisition and processing. Int. J. Cardiovasc. Imaging **26**(1), 27–40 (2010)
2. Carapella, V.: Towards the semantic enrichment of free-text annotation of image quality assessment for UK Biobank cardiac cine MRI scans. In: Carneiro, G. (ed.) LABELS/DLMIA 2016. LNCS, vol. 10008, pp. 238–248. Springer, Cham (2016). https://doi.org/10.1007/978-3-319-46976-8_25
3. Demyanov, S.: ConvNet library for Matlab. https://github.com/sdemyanov/ConvNet. Accessed 15 Oct 2017
4. Ganin, Y., Ustinova, E., Ajakan, H., Germain, P., et al.: Domain-adversarial training of neural networks. J. Mach. Learn. Res. **17**(1), 2096–2030 (2016)
5. García-Laencina, P.J., Sancho-Gómez, J.L., Figueiras-Vidal, A.R.: Pattern classification with missing data: a review. Neural Comput. Appl. **19**(2), 263–282 (2010)
6. Goodfellow, I., Pouget-Abadie, J., Mirza, M., Xu, B., Warde-Farley, D., et al.: Generative adversarial nets. In: Advances in Neural Information Processing Systems, pp. 2672–2680 (2014)
7. Huang, Y., Shao, L., Frangi, A.F.: Simultaneous super-resolution and cross-modality synthesis of 3D medical images using weakly-supervised joint convolutional sparse coding. In: IEEE Conference on CVPR, pp. 6070–6079 (2017)
8. Lisanti, G., Masi, I., Bagdanov, A.D., Del Bimbo, A.: Person re-identification by iterative re-weighted sparse ranking. IEEE TPAMI **37**(8), 1629–1642 (2015)
9. Ma, L., Yang, X., Tao, D.: Person re-identification over camera networks using multi-task distance metric learning. IEEE TIP **23**(8), 3656–3670 (2014)
10. Paknezhad, M., Marchesseau, S., Brown, M.S.: Automatic basal slice detection for cardiac analysis. J. Med. Imaging **3**(3), 034004–034004 (2016)
11. Petersen, S.E., Matthews, P.M., Francis, J.M.: UK Biobank's cardiovascular magnetic resonance protocol. J. Cardiovasc. Magn. Reson. **18**(1), 1 (2016)
12. Sharmanska, V., Quadrianto, N.: Learning from the mistakes of others: matching errors in cross-dataset learning. In: IEEE Conference on CVPR, pp. 3967–3975 (2016)
13. Wang, Z., Wu, G., Sheikh, H.R., Simoncelli, E.P., Yang, E.H., Bovik, A.C.: Quality-aware images. IEEE TIP **15**(6), 1680–1689 (2006)
14. Zhang, L., et al.: Automated quality assessment of cardiac MR images using convolutional neural networks. In: Tsaftaris, S.A., Gooya, A., Frangi, A.F., Prince, J.L. (eds.) SASHIMI 2016. LNCS, vol. 9968, pp. 138–145. Springer, Cham (2016). https://doi.org/10.1007/978-3-319-46630-9_14

Factorised Spatial Representation Learning: Application in Semi-supervised Myocardial Segmentation

Agisilaos Chartsias[1(✉)], Thomas Joyce[1], Giorgos Papanastasiou[2],
Scott Semple[2], Michelle Williams[2], David Newby[2], Rohan Dharmakumar[3],
and Sotirios A. Tsaftaris[1]

[1] Institute for Digital Communications, School of Engineering,
University of Edinburgh, West Mains Rd, Edinburgh EH9 3FB, UK
`agis.chartsias@ed.ac.uk`
[2] Edinburgh Imaging Facility QMRI, Centre for Cardiovascular Science,
Edinburgh EH16 4TJ, UK
[3] Cedars Sinai Medical Center, Los Angeles, CA, USA

Abstract. The success and generalisation of deep learning algorithms heavily depend on learning good feature representations. In medical imaging this entails representing anatomical information, as well as properties related to the specific imaging setting. Anatomical information is required to perform further analysis, whereas imaging information is key to disentangle scanner variability and potential artefacts. The ability to factorise these would allow for training algorithms only on the relevant information according to the task. To date, such factorisation has not been attempted. In this paper, we propose a methodology of latent space factorisation relying on the cycle-consistency principle. As an example application, we consider cardiac MR segmentation, where we separate information related to the myocardium from other features related to imaging and surrounding substructures. We demonstrate the proposed method's utility in a semi-supervised setting: we use very few labelled images together with many unlabelled images to train a myocardium segmentation neural network. Specifically, we achieve comparable performance to fully supervised networks using a fraction of labelled images in experiments on ACDC and a dataset from Edinburgh Imaging Facility QMRI. Code will be made available at https://github.com/agis85/spatial_factorisation.

1 Introduction

The effectiveness of any (deep or shallow) learning algorithm lies in learning good feature representations. These must be maximally informative for the task at hand, whilst being invariant to unrelated information (e.g. variations in imaging, noise, etc), so that they can generalise to unseen examples [5]. Invariance to some factors, e.g. translations, can be attributed to the architecture, for instance with the use of convolution and max-pooling, but invariance to more complex factors

© Springer Nature Switzerland AG 2018
A. F. Frangi et al. (Eds.): MICCAI 2018, LNCS 11071, pp. 490–498, 2018.
https://doi.org/10.1007/978-3-030-00934-2_55

is achieved by the learning process, and specifically encouraged by regularisers (explicit regularisation) or data augmentation (implicit regularisation) [1].

At a high level the aim is to keep relevant but discard irrelevant information, however which information is relevant is strongly task dependent. In this paper we are interested in the related task of decomposing the input into meaningful components (or factors), which offers many benefits. Critically it enables preserving factors not directly relevant to the primary task, which may otherwise be discarded when driven by pure supervised learning. It is then possible to reuse parts of a factorised representation for related tasks or for transfer learning to other domains. Further, by capturing specific properties of the data, such representations become easier to interpret, an aspect of currently heated debate in deep learning with dedicated workshops on the topic (e.g. http://interpretable.ml). Finally, finding (and preserving) the factors of variation is *de facto* necessary for generative models, in order to be able to (re)produce realistic results.

Factorised representations are a recent topic in deep learning [6,7,9,11,14,15]. These works focus on decomposing feature representations into discrete or continuous latent vectors. At present, there has not been any work on learning factorised representations that include spatial components, which are of particular interest for spatially equivariant tasks using fully convolutional networks (such as segmentation and registration).[1] Here we propose a spatial decomposition network (SDNet), that decomposes input images into a spatial map containing anatomical information and a latent vector of image intensity information (and residual anatomical information), leveraging the cycle-consistency loss [21], originally proposed for style transfer. Specifically, we train two networks: one that learns a decomposition into spatial and non-spatial latent factors, and one that learns to reconstruct the input image using the decomposed representation. We demonstrate our method in semi-supervised myocardium segmentation, using a small amount of labelled but a large pool of unlabelled cardiac cine MR images. In this application, our method learns to decompose the shape and location of the myocardium from information related to surrounding structures and pixel intensities (related to scanner properties and other imaging characteristics).

In summary, our contributions are the following: (a) We propose a new method for disentangling images into a spatial map and a continuous vector, which is directly applicable to medical images for representing anatomical and non-anatomical information. (b) We show properties of the decomposed latent space by generating examples using latent space arithmetic. (c) We demonstrate the utility of our method in a semi-supervised myocardium segmentation task, where the learned high-level topological knowledge allows the network to retain performance in a low data regime.

---

[1] Concurrent work with ours, introduced auxiliary variables and combined them with a spatial representation for the task of image translation [2,10].

2   Related Work

Learning Factorised Representations: To date interest has centred on representing factors of variation as independent latent variables, using Autoencoders [7] or Variational Autoencoders (VAE) [15] to decompose classification related factors from remaining image reconstruction factors. VAE were used for unsupervised learning of factorised representations, where the factors of variation are discovered throughout the learning process [9,11]. A generative model combining VAE with Generative Adversarial Networks (GAN) was proposed in [14] to decompose the input into image classes and remaining factors. Further, InfoGAN was proposed in [6], in which mutual information between a latent variable and the generated images is maximised. More recently, feature decompositions were proposed for video data to separate foreground from background [19], and motion from content [18]. These methods learn decomposed representations in terms of continuous or discrete variables; however, spatial information could be directly represented in a convolutional map, and this would be useful when the learning task is semantic segmentation. Our proposed method produces a decomposition as a combination of spatial and non-spatial information. This makes our learned representation directly applicable to segmentation tasks.

Semi-supervised Segmentation: Using unlabelled data to guide learning is appealing and has been exploited by the community. In [3] an iterative method was proposed, where a CNN is alternately trained on labelled and post-processed unlabelled sets. GANs were used in [20], for a gland segmentation task, involving supervised and unsupervised adversarial costs. Another approach [4] aims to minimise the distance between embeddings of labelled and unlabelled examples by comparing them in feature space. Semi-supervised learning with GANs was also proposed for semantic segmentation. The discriminator classifies between real and synthetic segmentation masks produced by the generator in [12], while in [17] the generator is used to increase the dataset size and the discriminator performs segmentation. Our method differs from these in that we introduce both adversarial and cycle losses to push mask generation to be spatially aligned with the image and avoid the need for post-processing as in [3]. Also we do not require any pairs of image and masks for discriminator training as in [20], and we retain all information, in contrast to [4] which preserves only task relevant information.

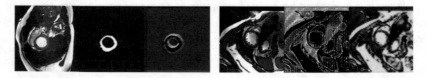

Fig. 1. Input images, segmentation masks and reconstructions produced by a Cycle-GAN. Left: high weight on segmentation, right: high weight on reconstruction.

3 Proposed Approach: The SDNet

Motivation: A useful latent representation is one that describes the data well. Spatial (segmentation) maps can be considered a form of latent variable that allows visual inspection of what a network learns. At the same time, an easy (unsupervised) way to see whether a latent representation captures the data is to use a decoder to reconstruct the input. In fact, even CycleGANs are autoencoders: they encode (and decode) the input via an intermediate output and thus inspire the design of our approach. Yet they have problems particularly when the intermediate output is discretised (a binary mask) and supervised losses are introduced. Their performance heavily depends on the weighting of the losses, as shown in Fig. 1. If the segmentation loss is weighted higher than the reconstruction loss, it is not possible to reconstruct the input since the binary mask does not contain enough information for the transformation. When differently weighted, information is stored in the binary mask ruining semantics. This confirms findings of others, that a CycleGAN resolves the many-to-one/one-to-many problem by storing low-frequency information in the output image [8]. We can see that the two losses are antagonistic, and a standard CycleGAN is not suitable as is. We need to introduce variables that break the many-to-one problem, encouraging a balance between the losses to achieve good segmentation and reconstruction.

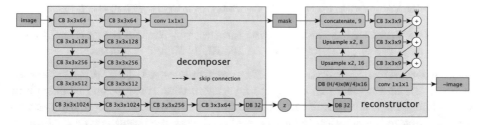

Fig. 2. Schematic of SDNet: an image is decomposed as a spatial representation of anatomy (in our case myocardial mask M) and a latent vector Z that captures other anatomical and imaging characteristics. Both mask and Z are used to reconstruct the input. The model consists of several convolutional (CB) and dense blocks (DB). BatchNormalization and LeakyRelu activations are used throughout.

SDNet: Our model is comprised of two interconnected neural networks, a "decomposer" and a"reconstructor", as illustrated in Fig. 2. The former decomposes an input 2D image (slice in a cine acquisition) into two components: a spatial representation of the myocardium in the form of a binary mask, and a latent representation of the remaining anatomical and imaging features in the form of a vector. Thus, the mask is an image having pixel to pixel correspondences with the input and is inherently spatial, whereas the other representation is a vector representing information in a high level way that is not directly spatial. The reconstructor receives the two representations and aims to synthesise the original input image. Given a successful decomposition, the binary mask acts as a guide defining where the reconstructed myocardium should be. The role of the latent feature variable is then to learn some topology around the myocardium and fill the necessary intensity patterns, and allow for many-to-many mappings.

Costs: More formally, let f and g be the decomposer and reconstructor. Given an image slice X_i, we aim to learn weights of f to decompose into a mask M and a 16 dimensional vector Z, that is $f(X_i) = \{f_M(X_i), f_Z(X_i)\} = \{M, Z\}$, and the weights of g to remap the decomposition back to an image $g(f_M(X_i), f_Z(X_i))$.

In a semi-supervised setup data comes from a labelled set $S_L = \{X_i, M_i\}_{i \in [1,N]}$ and an unlabelled set $S_U = \{X_j\}_{j \in [1,M]}$ where usually $M > N$. We now define the following losses. Firstly, a reconstruction loss from autoencoding an image, $L_{rec}(f, g) = \mathbb{E}_X[\|X - g(f(X))\|_1]$. Secondly, two supervised losses when having images with corresponding masks M_X, $L_M(f) = \mathbb{E}_X[Dice(M_X, f_M(X))]$, and $L_I(f, g) = \mathbb{E}_X[\|X - g(M_X, f_Z(X))\|_1]$. Finally, an adversarial loss using an image discriminator D_X, as $A_I(f, g, D_X) = \mathbb{E}_X[D_X(g(f(X)))^2 + (D_X(X) - 1)^2]$. Networks f and g are trained to maximise this objective against an adversarial discriminator trained to minimise it. Similarly, we define an adversarial loss using a mask discriminator D_M as $A_M(f) = \mathbb{E}_{X,M}[D_M(f_M(X))^2 + (D_M(M) - 1)^2]$. Both adversarial losses are based on [13]. The overall cost function is defined as:

$$\lambda_1 L_M(f) + \lambda_2 A_M(f, D_M) + \lambda_3 L_{rec}(f, g) + \lambda_4 L_I(f, g) + \lambda_5 A_I(f, g, D_X)$$

The loss for images from the unlabelled set does not contain the first and fourth terms. The λ are experimentally set to 10, 10, 1, 10 and 1 respectively.

Implementation Details: The decomposer follows a U-Net [16] architecture (see Fig. 2), and its last layer outputs a segmentation mask of the myocardium via a sigmoid activation function. The model's deep spatial maps contain downsampled image information, which is used to derive the latent vector Z through a series of convolutions and fully connected layers, with the final output being passed through a sigmoid so Z is bounded. Following this, an architecture with three residual blocks is employed as the reconstructor (see Fig. 2).

The spatial and continuous representations are not explicitly made independent, so during training the model could still store all information needed for reconstructing the input as low values in the spatial mask, since finding a mapping from a spatial representation to an image is easier than combining two sources of information, namely the mask and Z. To prevent this, we apply a step function (i.e. a threshold) at the spatial input of the reconstructor to binarise the mask in the forward pass. We store the original values and bypass the step function during back-propagation, and apply the updates to the original non-binary mask. Note that the binarisation of the mask only takes place at the input of the reconstructor network and is not used by the discriminator.

4   Experiments and Discussion

4.1   Data and Baselines

ACDC: We use data from the 2017 ACDC Challenge[2] containing cine-MR images from patients with various disease. Images were acquired in 1.5T or 3T MR scanners, with resolution between 1.22 and $1.68\,\mathrm{mm^2}$/pixel and the number of phases varying between 28 to 40 images per patient. We resample all volumes to $1.37\,\mathrm{mm^2}$/pixel resolution and normalise in the range $[-1, 1]$.

QMRI: We also use cine-MR data acquired at Edinburgh Imaging Facility QMRI with a 3T scanner, of 28 healthy patients, each having a volume of 30 frames. The spatial resolution is $1.406\,\mathrm{mm^2}$/pixels with a slice thickness 6 mm, matrix size 256×216 and field of view 360 mm $\times$ 303.75 mm.

Baselines: We use as a *fully-supervised baseline* a standard U-Net network trained with a Dice loss, similar to most participants of the ACDC challenge. We also consider a *semi-supervised baseline*, shorthanded as GAN below, by adding a GAN loss to the supervised loss to allow adversarial training [12].

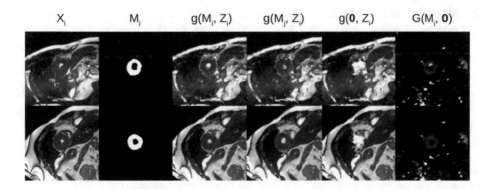

Fig. 3. Reconstructions using different M_i and Z_i combinations (see text for details).

4.2   Latent Space Arithmetic

As a demonstration of our learned representation, in Fig. 3 we show reconstructions of input images from the training set using different combinations of masks and Z components. In the first three columns, we show the original input with the predicted mask and the input's reconstruction. Next, we take the spatial representation M_j from one image and combine it with the Z_i component of the other image, and vice versa. As shown in the figure (4th column) the intensities and the anatomy around the myocardium remains unchanged, but the myocardial shape and position, which are encoded in the mask, change to that of the

---

[2] https://www.creatis.insa-lyon.fr/Challenge/acdc/index.html.

second image. The final two columns show reconstructions using a null mask (i.e. $M_i = \mathbf{0}$) and the correct Z_i in 5th column, or using the original mask with a $Z_i = \mathbf{0}$ in 6th column. In the first case, the produced image does not contain myocardium, whereas in the second case the image contains only myocardium and no other anatomical or MR characteristics.

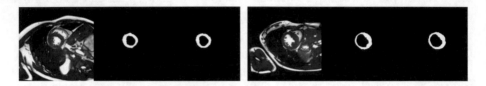

Fig. 4. Two examples of segmentation performance: input, prediction and ground truth.

4.3   Semi-supervised Results

The utility of a factorised representation becomes evident in semi-supervised learning. Qualitatively in Fig. 4 we can see that our method closely follows ground truth segmentation masks (example from ACDC held-out test set).

To assess our performance quantitatively we train a variety of setups varying the number of labelled training images whilst keeping the unlabelled fixed (in both ACDC and QMRI cases). We train SDNet and the baselines (U-Net and GAN), test on held-out test sets, and use 3-fold cross validation (with 70%, 15%, 15% of the volumes used in training, validation and test splits respectively). Results are shown in Table 1. For reference a U-Net trained with supervision on the full ACDC and QMRI datasets achieves a Dice score of 0.817 and 0.686 respectively. We can see that even when the number of labelled images is very low, our method is able to achieve segmentation accuracy considerably higher than the other two methods. As the number of labelled images increases, all models achieve similar accuracy.

Table 1. Myocardium Dice scores on ACDC and QMRI data. For training, 1200 unlabelled and varying numbers of labelled images were used. Masks for adversarial training came from the dataset, but do not correspond to any training images.

	ACDC					QMRI			
Labelled images	284	142	68	34	11	157	78	39	19
U-Net	0.782	0.657	0.581	0.356	0.026	0.686	0.681	0.441	0.368
GAN	**0.787**	0.727	0.648	0.365	0.080	**0.795**	0.756	0.580	0.061
SDNet	0.771	**0.767**	**0.731**	**0.678**	**0.415**	0.794	**0.772**	**0.686**	**0.424**

5   Conclusion

We presented a method that decomposes images into spatial and (non-spatial) latent representations employing the cycle-consistency principle. To the best of our knowledge this is the first work to investigate spatial representation factorisation, in which one factor of the representation is inherently spatial, and thus well suited to spatial tasks. We demonstrated its applicability in semi-supervised myocardial segmentation. In the low-data regime ($\approx 1\%$ of labelled with respect to unlabelled data) it achieves remarkable results, showing the power of the proposed learned representation. We leave as future work generative extensions, where we learn statistical distributions of our embeddings (as in VAEs).

Acknowledgements. This work was supported in part by the US National Institutes of Health (1R01HL136578-01) and UK EPSRC (EP/P022928/1). We also thank NVIDIA Corporation for donating a Titan X GPU.

References

1. Achille, A., Soatto, S.: Emergence of invariance and disentangling in deep representations. In: ICML Workshop Principled Approaches to Deep Learning (2017)
2. Almahairi, A., Rajeswar, S., Sordoni, A., Bachman, P., Courville, A.: Augmented CycleGAN: learning many-to-many mappings from unpaired data. In: Dy, J., Krause, A. (eds.) Proceedings of the 35th International Conference on Machine Learning, Proceedings of Machine Learning Research, vol. 80, pp. 195–204. PMLR, Stockholm (2018). http://proceedings.mlr.press/v80/almahairi18a.html
3. Bai, W., et al.: Semi-supervised learning for network-based cardiac MR image segmentation. In: Descoteaux, M., Maier-Hein, L., Franz, A., Jannin, P., Collins, D.L., Duchesne, S. (eds.) MICCAI 2017. LNCS, vol. 10434, pp. 253–260. Springer, Cham (2017). https://doi.org/10.1007/978-3-319-66185-8_29
4. Baur, C., Albarqouni, S., Navab, N.: Semi-supervised deep learning for fully convolutional networks. In: Descoteaux, M., Maier-Hein, L., Franz, A., Jannin, P., Collins, D.L., Duchesne, S. (eds.) MICCAI 2017. LNCS, vol. 10435, pp. 311–319. Springer, Cham (2017). https://doi.org/10.1007/978-3-319-66179-7_36
5. Bengio, Y., Courville, A., Vincent, P.: Representation learning: a review and new perspectives. IEEE PAMI **35**(8), 1798–1828 (2013)
6. Chen, X., Duan, Y., Houthooft, R., Schulman, J., Sutskever, I., Abbeel, P.: InfoGAN: interpretable representation learning by information maximizing generative adversarial nets. In: NIPS, pp. 2172–2180 (2016)
7. Cheung, B., Livezey, J.A., Bansal, A.K., Olshausen, B.A.: Discovering hidden factors of variation in deep networks. arXiv:1412.6583 (2014)
8. Chu, C., Zhmoginov, A., Sandler, M.: CycleGAN: a Master of Steganography. arXiv:1712.02950 (2017)
9. Higgins, I., et al.: beta-VAE: Learning basic visual concepts with a constrained variational framework. In: ICLR (2017)
10. Huang, X., Liu, M.-Y., Belongie, S., Kautz, J.: Multimodal Unsupervised Image-to-image Translation. In: ECCV (2018)
11. Kim, H., Mnih, A.: Disentangling by factorising. In: ICML (2018)

12. Luc, P., Couprie, C., Chintala, S., Verbeek, J.: Semantic segmentation using adversarial networks. arXiv preprint arXiv:1611.08408 (2016)

13. Mao, X., Li, Q., Xie, H., Lau, R.Y., Wang, Z., Smolley, S.P.: On the Effectiveness of Least Squares Generative Adversarial Networks. arXiv:1712.06391 (2017)

14. Mathieu, M.F., Zhao, J.J., Zhao, J., Ramesh, A., Sprechmann, P., LeCun, Y.: Disentangling factors of variation in deep representation using adversarial training. In: NIPS, pp. 5040–5048 (2016)

15. Narayanaswamy, S., et al.: Learning disentangled representations with semi-supervised deep generative models. In: NIPS, pp. 5927–5937 (2017)

16. Ronneberger, O., Fischer, P., Brox, T.: U-Net: convolutional networks for biomedical image segmentation. In: Navab, N., Hornegger, J., Wells, W.M., Frangi, A.F. (eds.) MICCAI 2015. LNCS, vol. 9351, pp. 234–241. Springer, Cham (2015). https://doi.org/10.1007/978-3-319-24574-4_28

17. Souly, N., Spampinato, C., Shah, M.: Semi and weakly supervised semantic segmentation using generative adversarial network. arXiv:1703.09695 (2017)

18. Tulyakov, S., Liu, M.-Y., Yang, X., Kautz, J.: Mocogan: decomposing motion and content for video generation. arXiv:1707.04993 (2017)

19. Vondrick, C., Pirsiavash, H., Torralba, A.: Generating videos with scene dynamics. In: NIPS, pp. 613–621 (2016)

20. Zhang, Y., et al.: Deep adversarial networks for biomedical image segmentation utilizing unannotated images. In: Descoteaux, M., Maier-Hein, L., Franz, A., Jannin, P., Collins, D.L., Duchesne, S. (eds.) MICCAI 2017. LNCS, vol. 10435, pp. 408–416. Springer, Cham (2017). https://doi.org/10.1007/978-3-319-66179-7_47

21. Zhu, J.-Y., Park, T., Isola, P., Efros, A.A.: Unpaired image-to-image translation using cycle-consistent adversarial networks. In: ICCV, pp. 2242–2251 (2017)

High-Dimensional Bayesian Optimization of Personalized Cardiac Model Parameters via an Embedded Generative Model

Jwala Dhamala[1](✉), Sandesh Ghimire[1], John L. Sapp[2], B. Milan Horáček[2], and Linwei Wang[1]

[1] Rochester Institute of Technology, New York, USA
jd1336@rit.edu
[2] Dalhousie University, Halifax, Canada

Abstract. The estimation of patient-specific tissue properties in the form of model parameters is important for personalized physiological models. However, these tissue properties are spatially varying across the underlying anatomical model, presenting a significance challenge of high-dimensional (HD) optimization at the presence of limited measurement data. A common solution to reduce the dimension of the parameter space is to explicitly partition the anatomical mesh, either into a fixed small number of segments or a multi-scale hierarchy. This anatomy-based reduction of parameter space presents a fundamental bottleneck to parameter estimation, resulting in solutions that are either too low in resolution to reflect tissue heterogeneity, or too high in dimension to be reliably estimated within feasible computation. In this paper, we present a novel concept that embeds a generative variational auto-encoder (VAE) into the objective function of Bayesian optimization, providing an implicit low-dimensional (LD) search space that represents the generative code of the HD spatially-varying tissue properties. In addition, the VAE-encoded knowledge about the generative code is further used to guide the exploration of the search space. The presented method is applied to estimating tissue excitability in a cardiac electrophysiological model. Synthetic and real-data experiments demonstrate its ability to improve the accuracy of parameter estimation with more than 10x gain in efficiency.

Keywords: Parameter estimation · Model personalization
Cardiac electrophysiology · Variational auto-encoder
Bayesian optimization

1 Introduction

Patient-specific cardiac models have shown increasing potential in personalized treatment of heart diseases [9]. A significant challenge in personalizing these

© Springer Nature Switzerland AG 2018
A. F. Frangi et al. (Eds.): MICCAI 2018, LNCS 11071, pp. 499–507, 2018.
https://doi.org/10.1007/978-3-030-00934-2_56

models arises from the estimation of patient-specific tissue properties that vary spatially across the myocardium. To estimate these high-dimensional (HD) tissue properties (in the form of model parameters) is not only algorithmically difficult given indirect and sparse measurements, but also computationally intractable in the presence of computing-intensive simulation models.

Numerous efforts have been made to circumvent the challenge of HD parameter estimation. Many works assume homogeneous tissue property that can be represented by a single global model parameter [7]. To preserve local tissue properties, a common approach is to reduce the parameter space through an explicit partitioning of the cardiac mesh. These efforts can be generally summarized in two categories. In one approach, the cardiac mesh is pre-divided into 3–26 segments, each represented by a uniform parameter value [11]. Naturally, this artificial low-resolution division has a limited ability to represent tissue heterogeneity that is not known *a priori*. It has also been shown that the initialization of model parameters becomes increasingly more critical as the number of segments grows [11]. Alternatively, a multi-scale hierarchy of the cardiac mesh can be defined for a coarse-to-fine optimization, which allows spatially-adaptive resolution that is higher in certain regions than the others [3,4]. However, the representation ability of the final partition is limited by the inflexibility of the multi-scale hierarchy: homogeneous regions distributed across different scales cannot be grouped into the same partition, while the resolution of heterogeneous regions can be limited by the level of scale the optimization can reach [4]. In addition, because these methods involve a cascade of optimizations along the hierarchy of the cardiac mesh, they are computationally expensive. In the presence of models that could require hours or days for a single simulation, these methods could quickly become computationally prohibitive.

In this paper, we present a novel HD parameter optimization approach that replaces the explicit anatomy-based reduction of the parameter space, with an implicit low-dimensional (LD) manifold that represents the generative code for HD spatially-varying tissue properties. This is achieved by embedding within the optimization a generative variational auto-encoder (VAE) model, trained from a large set of spatially-varying tissue properties reflecting regional tissue abnormality with various locations, sizes, and distributions. The VAE decoder is utilized within the objective function of the Bayesian optimization [2] to provide an implicit LD search space for HD parameter estimation. Meanwhile, the VAE-encoded posterior distribution of the generative code is used to guide an efficient exploration of the LD manifold. The presented method is applied to estimating tissue excitability of a cardiac electrophysiological model using non-invasive electrocardiogram (ECG) data. On both synthetic and real data experiments, the presented method is compared against the use of anatomy-based LD [11] or multi-scale representation of the parameter space [4]. Experiments demonstrate that the presented method can achieve a drastic reduction in computational cost while improving the accuracy of the estimated parameters. To the best of our knowledge, this is the first work that utilizes a probabilistic generative model within an optimization framework for estimating HD model parameters. It provides an efficient and general solution to personalizing HD model parameters.

2   Background: Cardiac Electrophysiological System

Cardiac Electrophysiology Model: Among the different types of cardiac electrophysiological models, phenomenological models such as the Aliev-Panfilov (AP) model [1] can explain the macroscopic process of cardiac excitation with a small number of model parameters and reasonable computation. Therefore, the AP model given below is chosen to test the feasibility of the presented method:

$$\partial u/\partial t = \nabla(\mathbf{D}\nabla u) - cu(u - \theta)(u - 1) - uv,$$
$$\partial v/\partial t = \varepsilon(u,v)(-v - cu(u - \theta - 1)). \tag{1}$$

Here, u is the transmembrane action potential and v is the recovery current. The transmural action potential is computed by solving the AP model (1) on a 3D myocardium discretized using the meshfree method [10]. Because u is most sensitive to the value of the parameter θ [4], we focus on its estimation in this study.

Body-Surface ECG Model: The propagation of the spatio-temporal transmural action potential $\mathbf{U}$ to the potentials measured on the body surface $\mathbf{Y}$ can be described by the quasi-static approximation of the electromagnetic theory [8]. Solving the governing equations on a discrete heart-torso mesh, a linear relationship between $\mathbf{U}$ and $\mathbf{Y}$ can be obtained as: $\mathbf{Y} = \mathbf{H}(\mathbf{U}(\boldsymbol{\theta}))$, where $\boldsymbol{\theta}$ is the vector of local parameters θ at the resolution of the cardiac mesh.

3   HD Parameter Estimation

To estimate $\boldsymbol{\theta}$, we maximize the similarity between the measured ECG and those simulated by the combined electrophysiological and ECG model $M(\boldsymbol{\theta})$:

$$\hat{\boldsymbol{\theta}} = \arg \max_{\boldsymbol{\theta}} -||\mathbf{Y} - M(\boldsymbol{\theta})||^2. \tag{2}$$

To enable the estimation of $\boldsymbol{\theta}$ at the resolution of the cardiac mesh, the presented method embeds within the Bayesian optimization framework a stochastic generative model that generates $\boldsymbol{\theta}$ from a LD manifold. It includes two major components as outlined in Fig. 1: (1) the construction of a generative model of HD spatially-varying tissue properties at the resolution of the cardiac mesh, and (2) a novel Bayesian optimization method utilizing the embedded generative model.

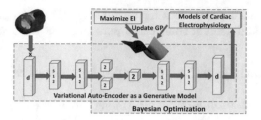

Fig. 1. Outline of the presented method, with the dimension of each VAE layer labeled.

3.1   LD-to-HD Parameter Generation via VAE

Generative VAE Model: We assume that the spatially varying tissue properties at the resolution of a cardiac mesh $\boldsymbol{\theta}$ is generated by a small number of unobserved continuous random variables $\mathbf{z}$ in a LD manifold. To obtain the generative process from $\mathbf{z}$ to $\boldsymbol{\theta}$, the VAE consists of two modules: a probabilistic deep encoder network with parameters $\boldsymbol{\alpha}$ that approximates the intractable true posterior density as $q_{\boldsymbol{\alpha}}(\mathbf{z}|\boldsymbol{\theta})$; and a probabilistic deep decoder network with parameters $\boldsymbol{\beta}$ that can probabilistically reconstruct $\boldsymbol{\theta}$ given $\mathbf{z}$ as $p_{\boldsymbol{\beta}}(\boldsymbol{\theta}|\mathbf{z})$. Both networks consist of three fully-connected layers as shown in Fig. 1.

To train the VAE, we generate $\boldsymbol{\Theta} = \left\{\boldsymbol{\theta}^{(i)}\right\}_{i=1}^{N}$ consisting of N configurations of heterogeneous tissue properties in a patient-specific cardiac mesh. The training involves optimizing the variational lower bound on the marginal likelihood of each training data $\boldsymbol{\theta}^{(i)}$ with respect to network parameters $\boldsymbol{\alpha}$ and $\boldsymbol{\beta}$:

$$\mathcal{L}(\boldsymbol{\alpha}; \boldsymbol{\beta}; \boldsymbol{\theta}^{(i)}) = -D_{\mathrm{KL}}(q_{\boldsymbol{\alpha}}(\mathbf{z}|\boldsymbol{\theta}^{(i)})\|p_{\boldsymbol{\beta}}(\mathbf{z})) + E_{q_{\boldsymbol{\alpha}}(\mathbf{z}|\boldsymbol{\theta}^{(i)})}[\log p_{\boldsymbol{\beta}}(\boldsymbol{\theta}^{(i)}|\mathbf{z})], \qquad (3)$$

where we model $p_{\boldsymbol{\beta}}(\boldsymbol{\theta}|\mathbf{z})$ with a Bernoulli distribution. To optimize Eq. (3), stochastic gradient descent with standard backpropagation can be utilized. Assuming the approximate posterior $q_{\boldsymbol{\alpha}}(\mathbf{z}|\boldsymbol{\theta})$ as a Gaussian density and the prior $p_{\boldsymbol{\beta}}(\mathbf{z}) \sim \mathcal{N}(0,1)$, their KL divergence can be derived analytically as:

$$D_{\mathrm{KL}}(q_{\boldsymbol{\alpha}}(\mathbf{z}|\boldsymbol{\theta}^{(i)})\|p_{\boldsymbol{\beta}}(\mathbf{z})) = -\frac{1}{2}\sum(1 + \log(\sigma_j^2) - \mu_j^2 - \sigma_j^2), \qquad (4)$$

where j is along the dimensions of $\mathbf{z}$, and $\boldsymbol{\mu}$ and $\boldsymbol{\sigma}^2$ are mean and variance from $q_{\boldsymbol{\alpha}}(\mathbf{z}|\boldsymbol{\theta}^{(i)})$. Because stochastic latent variables are utilized, the gradient of the expected negative reconstruction term during backpropagation cannot be directly obtained. The popular re-parameterization trick is utilized to express $\mathbf{z}$ as a deterministic variable as $\mathbf{z}^{(i)} = \boldsymbol{\mu}^{(i)} + \boldsymbol{\sigma}^{(i)}\boldsymbol{\epsilon}$, where $\boldsymbol{\epsilon} \sim \mathcal{N}(0,\mathbf{I})$ is noise [6].

Probabilistic Modeling of the Latent Code: The trained encoder provides an approximated posterior density of the LD latent code $q_{\boldsymbol{\alpha}}(\mathbf{z}|\boldsymbol{\theta})$. This represents valuable knowledge about the probabilistic distribution of $\mathbf{z}$ learned from a large training dataset. To utilize this in the subsequent optimization, we integrate $q_{\boldsymbol{\alpha}}(\mathbf{z}|\boldsymbol{\theta})$ over the training data $\boldsymbol{\Theta}$ to obtain the density $q_{\boldsymbol{\alpha}}(\mathbf{z})$ as a mixture of Gaussians $1/N \sum_i^N \mathcal{N}(\boldsymbol{\mu}^{(i)}, \boldsymbol{\Sigma}^{(i)})$, where $\boldsymbol{\mu}^{(i)}$ and $\boldsymbol{\Sigma}^{(i)}$ are mean and covariance from $q_{\boldsymbol{\alpha}}(\mathbf{z}|\boldsymbol{\theta}^{(i)})$. Because the number of mixture components in $q_{\boldsymbol{\alpha}}(\mathbf{z})$ scales linearly with the number of training data, we approximate $q_{\alpha}(\mathbf{z})$ with a single Gaussian density as $\mathcal{N}\big(1/N \sum_i^N \boldsymbol{\mu}^{(i)}, 1/N \sum_i^N (\boldsymbol{\Sigma}^{(i)} + \boldsymbol{\mu}^{(i)}\boldsymbol{\mu}^{(i)T}) - \boldsymbol{\mu}\boldsymbol{\mu}^T\big)$. Alternatively, we approximate $q_{\alpha}(\mathbf{z})$ with a mixture of Gaussians with $K << N$ components, where k-means clustering with the Bregman divergence [5] as a similarity metric is used to reduce the number of mixture components.

In this way, we obtain a generative model $p_{\beta}(\boldsymbol{\theta}|\mathbf{z})$ of HD tissue properties from an implicit LD manifold, and prior knowledge of the LD manifold $q_{\alpha}(\mathbf{z})$ from the probabilistic encoder. Both will be embedded into Bayesian optimization to enable efficient and accurate HD parameter estimation.

3.2 Bayesian Optimization with Embedded Generative Model

Representing $\boldsymbol{\theta}$ with the expectation of the trained decoder $p_{\beta}(\boldsymbol{\theta}|\mathbf{z})$, we obtain:

$$\hat{\mathbf{z}} = \arg \max_{\mathbf{z}} -||\mathbf{Y} - M\big(\mathrm{E}[p_{\beta}(\boldsymbol{\theta}|\mathbf{z})]\big)||^2, \tag{5}$$

which allow us to optimize the HD parameter $\boldsymbol{\theta}$ in an implicit LD manifold of $\mathbf{z}$. For Bayesian optimization, we assume a zero mean Gaussian process (GP) with an anisotropic Mátern 5/2 kernel as a prior over the objective function (5). The optimization then consists of two iterative steps: (1) select point in the LD manifold that allows the GP to globally approximate Eq. (5) (exploration) while locally refining the area of optimum (exploitation); and (2) update the GP.

VAE-Informed Acquisition Function: To select points on LD manifold, we adopt the expected improvement (EI) function that picks a point with maximum expectation of improvement over the current best objective function value f_m [2]. For a GP posterior $\sim \mathcal{N}(\mu(.), \sigma(.))$, it can be obtained as:

$$\mathrm{EI}(\mathbf{z}) = (\mu(\mathbf{z}) - f_m)\Phi\Big(\frac{\mu(\mathbf{z}) - f_m}{\sigma(\mathbf{z})}\Big) + \sigma(\mathbf{z})\phi\Big(\frac{\mu(\mathbf{z}) - f_m}{\sigma(\mathbf{z})}\Big), \tag{6}$$

where Φ and ϕ are the cumulative distribution function and density function of the standard normal distribution. Here, the first term controls exploitation (through high μ) and the second term controls exploration (through high σ). Because using only f_m can lead to excessive exploitation, it is common to augment f_m with a constant trade-off parameter ε as: $f_m + \varepsilon$ [2]. Here, we utilize the VAE-encoded knowledge about the LD manifold $q_{\alpha}(\mathbf{z})$ to enforce higher exploitation in the areas of high probability density for $\mathbf{z}$, and lower elsewhere. In specific, we define $\varepsilon(\mathbf{z}) = -f_m \sum_i w_i(\mathbf{z} - \boldsymbol{\mu}_i)\boldsymbol{\Sigma}_i^{-1}(\mathbf{z} - \boldsymbol{\mu}_i)$, where w, $\boldsymbol{\mu}$, and $\boldsymbol{\Sigma}$ are the weight, mean, and variance of the K Gaussian mixture components in $q_{\alpha}(\mathbf{z})$.

GP Update: After a new point $\mathbf{z}^{(n)}$ is selected by maximizing the modified EI, the objective function (5) is evaluated at the HD parameter given by the mean of the generative model $p_{\beta}(\boldsymbol{\theta}|\mathbf{z}^{(n)})$. The GP is then updated by adding the new pair of $\mathbf{z}^{(n)}$ and objective function value, and maximizing the log marginal likelihood with respect to kernel parameters: length scales and kernel amplitude.

4   Experiments

Synthetic Experiments: We include 27 synthetic experiments on three CT-derived human heart-torso models. In each case, an infarct sized 2%–40% of the heart was placed at differing locations using various combinations of the AHA segments. The value of the parameter θ in the infarcted and the healthy region is set to 0.5 and 0.15, respectively. 120-lead ECG is simulated and corrupted with 20 dB Gaussian noise as measurement data. We evaluate the accuracy in estimated parameters with two metrics: (1) root mean square error (RMSE) between the true and estimated parameters; and (2) dice coefficient (DC) $=$ $\frac{2(|S_1 \cap S_2|)}{|S_1|+|S_2|}$, where S_1 and S_2 are the sets of nodes in the true and estimated regions of infarct; these regions are determined by *Otsu's thresholding* method.

VAE Architecture and Training: For each heart, we generate a training dataset of tissue properties with various heterogeneous infarcts. Each infarct is generated by random region growing in which, starting with one infarct node, one out of the five closest neighbors of the present infarct is randomly added to the infarct until an infarct of desired size is obtained. It is then added to training data. Because infarcts thus generated tend to be very irregular, we also include infarcts generated by growing the infarct with the node closest to its center. For each heart, we extract 123,896, 155,099, and 116,459 data. The training of VAE with an architecture as shown in Fig. 1 with the *Adam* optimizer on Titan X GPU took 9.77, 13.96, and 9.0 min for each dataset.

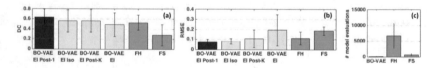

Fig. 2. Comparison of BO-VAE EI Post-1 (blue bar) with: (1) FH and FS (green bars); and (2) BO-VAE using standard EI, EI Isotropic, and EI Post-K (yellow bars) in terms of DC, RMSE, and number of model evaluations (from left to right).

Comparison with Existing Methods: The presented method (termed as BO-VAE) is compared against two common approaches based on explicit LD representation: (1) optimization over fixed 18 segments (fixed-segment (FS) method); and (2) coarse-to-fine optimization along a fixed multi-scale hierarchy (fixed-hierarchy (FH) method). As summarized in Fig. 2(a)(b), BO-VAE (blue bar) is more accurate than the other two methods (green bars) in both DC and RMSE (paired t-tests, $p < 0.012$). This is achieved at a reduction of the computational cost by: 87.57% for the FS method and 98.73% for the FH method (Fig. 2(c)).

The FS method shows the lowest accuracy with some estimated parameters either missing the infarct or including large false positives (Fig. 3) left. The FH method overcomes this issue, although to a limited extent. In the LD representation obtained by the FH method as shown in Fig. 3 right several dimensions

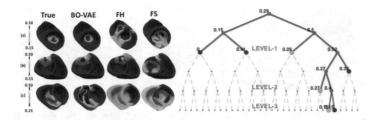

Fig. 3. Left: Examples of estimated parameters with BO-VAE, FH, and FS. Right: Progression of FH on the multi-scale hierarchy for parameter estimation of (a) (green leaf: homogeneous tissues; red leaf: heterogeneous tissues).

are wasted at representing homogeneous healthy regions (green) across different scales, which limits its ability to optimize deeper along the tree. BO-VAE is not limited by such explicitly-imposed anatomy-based structure, allowing it to attain higher accuracy with only 2 latent dimensions and 1–10% of the computation.

The Effect of VAE-Encoded Knowledge About the LD Manifold: To study the effect of incorporating the VAE-encoded $q_\alpha(\mathbf{z})$ in the EI, we compare the standard EI with EI augmented with three types of distributions on $\mathbf{z}$: (1) $p_\beta(\mathbf{z}) \sim \mathcal{N}(0,1)$ (EI Isotropic), (2) approximated $q_\alpha(\mathbf{z})$ with a single Gaussian density (EI Post-1); and (3) approximated $q_\alpha(\mathbf{z})$ with a mixture of 10 Gaussian densities (EI Post-K). As shown in Fig. 2, the accuracy using all three distributions is higher than that without using any, among which EI Post-1 has the highest accuracy. Figure 4(b) illustrates that, when $q_\alpha(\mathbf{z})$ is utilized, the exploration proceeds from the region of high probability density to the region of low probability density. In comparison, with standard EI, the points are spread to reduce overall variance (Fig. 4(a)); this could result in incorrect (Fig. 4(c)) or suboptimal (Fig. 4(d)) solutions.

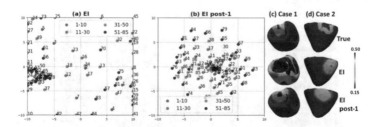

Fig. 4. Comparison of training points selected by EI (a) and EI Post-1 (b), and examples of the estimated parameters by the two acquisition functions (c–d).

We also experimented with HD latent code $\mathbf{z}$. As shown in Fig. 5(a)(b), there was only a marginal improvement in accuracy with a five *vs.* a two dimensional (2d) latent code. It suggests that, given the focus of the training data on local

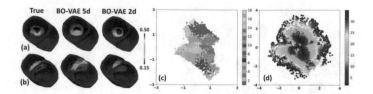

Fig. 5. (a–b): Examples of estimated parameters using five *vs.* two dimensional latent codes. (c–d): Latent code manifold based on (c) infarct location, and (d) infarct size.

infarcts, a 2d latent code may be sufficient to capture the necessary generative factors. The plot of these 2d latent codes in Fig. 5(c)(d) show that they cluster by infarct location and their radial direction accounts for the infarct size.

Real Data Experiments: Real-data studies are conducted on two patients with previous myocardial infraction. Patient-specific heart and torso meshes are constructed from axial CT images. Tissue excitability is estimated from 120-lead ECG data. The results are evaluated by *in-vivo* bipolar voltage data which, although not a direct measure of tissue excitability, provides a reasonable reference about the region of infarcts. The first two columns of Fig. 6 show the original voltage data (red: dense infarct; purple: healthy tissue; green: infarct border) and the same data registered to cardiac meshes.

The voltage map in case 1 (Fig. 6(a)) shows a highly heterogeneous infarct spread over a large region in the lateral LV. The estimated parameters by all methods capture this region of infarct. For this accuracy, the FH and FS methods required 4056 and 1058 model evaluations, whereas BO-VAE required only 105 model evaluations. By contrast, as shown in Fig. 6(b), case 2 has a smaller region of dense scar in the lateral LV. The estimated parameters by BO-VAE and FH correctly reveal this region of scar, whereas the FS method is less accurate. In this case, BO-VAE, FH method, and FS method required 105, 5798, and 1501 model evaluations respectively.

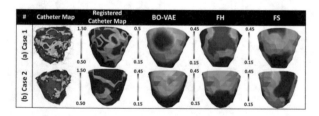

Fig. 6. Model parameter estimated with BO-VAE, FH, and FS on real-data study.

Conclusion: We present a novel approach to estimating HD model parameters, achieved by embedding within the Bayesian optimization a generative model of HD tissue properties from a LD manifold. Experiments show a gain in accuracy with drastically reduced computation. Future works include the incorporation of training data from high resolution 3D imaging and study of alternatives to incorporate the knowledge of latent manifold in Bayesian optimization.

Acknowledgment. This work is supported by the National Science Foundation under CAREER Award ACI-1350374 and the National Institute of Heart, Lung, and Blood of the National Institutes of Health under Award R21Hl125998.

References

1. Aliev, R.R., Panfilov, A.V.: A simple two-variable model of cardiac excitation. Chaos Solitons Fractals **7**(3), 293–301 (1996)
2. Brochu, E., Cora, V.M., De Freitas, N.: A tutorial on Bayesian optimization of expensive cost functions, with application to active user modeling and hierarchical reinforcement learning. arXiv preprint arXiv:1012.2599 (2010)
3. Chinchapatnam, P., Rhode, K.S., Ginks, M.: Model-based imaging of cardiac apparent conductivity and local conduction velocity for diagnosis and planning of therapy. IEEE Trans. Med. Imaging **27**(11), 1631–1642 (2008)
4. Dhamala, J., Sapp, J.L., Horacek, M., Wang, L.: Spatially-adaptive multi-scale optimization for local parameter estimation: application in cardiac electrophysiological models. In: Ourselin, S., Joskowicz, L., Sabuncu, M.R., Unal, G., Wells, W. (eds.) MICCAI 2016. LNCS, vol. 9902, pp. 282–290. Springer, Cham (2016). https://doi.org/10.1007/978-3-319-46726-9_33
5. Garcia, V., Nielsen, F., Nock, R.: Levels of details for Gaussian mixture models. In: Zha, H., Taniguchi, R., Maybank, S. (eds.) ACCV 2009. LNCS, vol. 5995, pp. 514–525. Springer, Heidelberg (2010). https://doi.org/10.1007/978-3-642-12304-7_48
6. Kingma, D.P., Welling, M.: Auto-encoding variational bayes. arXiv preprint arXiv:1312.6114 (2013)
7. Lê, M., Delingette, H., Kalpathy-Cramer, J.: MRI based Bayesian personalization of a tumor growth model. IEEE TMI **35**(10), 2329–2339 (2016)
8. Plonsey, R.: Bioelectric Phenomena. Wiley Online Library, Hoboken (1969)
9. Sermesant, M., Chabiniok, R., Chinchapatnam, P., Mansi, T., et al.: Patient-specific electromechanical models of the heart for the prediction of pacing acute effects in CRT: a preliminary clinical validation. Med. Image Anal. **16**(1), 201–215 (2012)
10. Wang, L., Zhang, H., Wong, K.C., Liu, H., Shi, P.: Physiological-model-constrained noninvasive reconstruction of volumetric myocardial transmembrane potentials. IEEE Trans. Biomed. Eng. **57**(2), 296–315 (2010)
11. Wong, K.C., Sermesant, M., Rhode, K.: Velocity-based cardiac contractility personalization from images using derivative-free optimization. J. Mech. Behav. Biomed. Mater. **43**, 35–52 (2015)

Generative Modeling and Inverse Imaging of Cardiac Transmembrane Potential

Sandesh Ghimire[1(✉)], Jwala Dhamala[1], Prashnna Kumar Gyawali[1],
John L. Sapp[2], Milan Horacek[2], and Linwei Wang[1]

[1] Rochester Institute of Technology, Rochester, NY 14623, USA
sg9872@rit.edu
[2] Dalhouse University, Halifax, NS, Canada
http://www.sandeshgh.com

Abstract. Noninvasive reconstruction of cardiac transmembrane potential (TMP) from surface electrocardiograms (ECG) involves an ill-posed inverse problem. Model-constrained regularization is powerful for incorporating rich physiological knowledge about spatiotemporal TMP dynamics. These models are controlled by high-dimensional physical parameters which, if fixed, can introduce model errors and reduce the accuracy of TMP reconstruction. Simultaneous adaptation of these parameters during TMP reconstruction, however, is difficult due to their high dimensionality. We introduce a novel model-constrained inference framework that replaces conventional physiological models with a deep generative model trained to generate TMP sequences from low-dimensional generative factors. Using a variational auto-encoder (VAE) with long short-term memory (LSTM) networks, we train the VAE decoder to learn the conditional likelihood of TMP, while the encoder learns the prior distribution of generative factors. These two components allow us to develop an efficient algorithm to simultaneously infer the generative factors and TMP signals from ECG data. Synthetic and real-data experiments demonstrate that the presented method significantly improve the accuracy of TMP reconstruction compared with methods constrained by conventional physiological models or without physiological constraints.

Keywords: Inverse problem · ECG imaging
Sequential variational auto-encoder · Bayesian inference

1 Introduction

Noninvasive electrophysiological (EP) imaging involves the reconstruction of cardiac electrical activity from high-density body-surface electrocardiograms (ECGs) [6]. It solves an ill-posed inverse problem that deteriorates as the imaging depth increases from the epicardium to the endocardium [9]. One type of increasingly utilized regularization considers knowledge about the well-defined physiological process of cardiac electrical propagation. This is often realized in

© Springer Nature Switzerland AG 2018
A. F. Frangi et al. (Eds.): MICCAI 2018, LNCS 11071, pp. 508–516, 2018.
https://doi.org/10.1007/978-3-030-00934-2_57

a model-constrained approach, where the optimization or statistical inference of cardiac electrical activity is constrained by a pre-defined model describing local activation/repolarization and its spatial propagation [4,11,12]. Earlier models include step jump functions [10], logistic functions [11], and 3D curve models [4] empirically parameterized to mimic the physiological process. Recently, more expressive cardiac EP simulation models have also been used [7,12].

These model-constrained approaches are afflicted with a common challenge: they are controlled by high-dimensional parameters often associated with local tissue properties and the origin of electrical activation that are unknown *a priori*. The more expressive the model is, the more parameters it has. To fix these model parameters in optimization/inference, as is common in existing approaches [12], model errors may be introduced decreasing the accuracy of the estimated electrical activity [12]. To adapt these model parameters to the observed data, as is desired for accurate inference, is however difficult due to their high-dimensionality and nonlinear relationship with the observed ECG data [3].

In this paper, we introduce a novel model-constrained inference framework that replaces the conventional physiological models with a deep generative model that is trained to generate the spatiotemporal dynamics of transmembrane potential (TMP) from a low-dimensional set of *generative factors*. These generative factors can be viewed as a low-dimensional abstraction of the high-dimensional physical parameters, which allows us to efficiently adapt the prior physiological knowledge to the observed ECG data (through inference of the generative factors) for an improved reconstruction of TMP dynamics.

In specific, the presented method consists of two novel contributions. First, to obtain a generative model that is sufficiently expressive to reproduce the temporal sequence of 3D spatial TMP distributions, we adopt a novel sequence-to-sequence variational auto-encoder (VAE) [2] with cascaded long short-term memory (LSTM) networks. This VAE is trained on a large database of simulated TMP dynamics originating from various myocardial locations and with a wide range of local tissue properties. Second, once trained, the VAE decoder describes the likelihood of the TMP conditioned on a low-dimensional set of generative factors, while the encoder learns the posterior distributions of the generative factors conditioned on the training data. We utilize these two components within the Bayesian inference, and present a variation of the expectation-maximization (EM) algorithm to jointly estimate the generative factors and transmural TMP signals from observed ECG data. In a set of synthetic and real-data experiments, we demonstrate that the presented method is able to improve the accuracy of transmural EP imaging in comparison to statistical inference either constrained by a conventional physiological model [12] or without physiological constraints.

2   Generative Modeling of TMP via Sequential VAE

To learn to generate the spatiotemporal TMP sequences, we use a sequential variation of VAE [8] based on the use of LSTM networks [2].

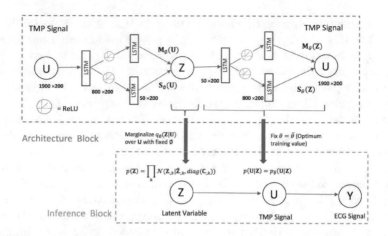

Fig. 1. Red block: VAE architecture. Green block: graphical model in inference.

<u>VAE Architecture:</u> The architecture of the sequential VAE is summarized in the red block in Fig. 1. Both the encoder and the decoder consists of two layers of LSTM, where the second layer includes separate mean and variance networks. The spatial dimension decreases from the original TMP signal $\mathbf{U}$ to the latent representation $\mathbf{Z}$, while the temporal relationship is modeled by the LSTMs. Note that while the random variables in a standard VAE are vectors, a sequential VAE deals with matrices. By defining the conditional distribution of a matrix as the product of distributions over its columns, we obtained the likelihood distribution $p_\theta(\mathbf{U}|\mathbf{Z})$ and the variational posterior distribution $q_\phi(\mathbf{Z}|\mathbf{U})$ as:

$$p_\theta(\mathbf{U}|\mathbf{Z}) = \prod_k \mathcal{N}(\mathbf{U}_{:,k}|\mathbf{M}_\theta(\mathbf{Z})_{:,k}, diag(\mathbf{S}_\theta(\mathbf{Z})_{:,k})) \tag{1}$$

$$q_\phi(\mathbf{Z}|\mathbf{U}) = \prod_k \mathcal{N}(\mathbf{Z}_{:,k}|\mathbf{M}_\phi(\mathbf{U})_{:,k}, diag(\mathbf{S}_\phi(\mathbf{U})_{:,k})) \tag{2}$$

where $\mathbf{M}_\phi(\mathbf{U})$ and $\mathbf{S}_\phi(\mathbf{U})$ are output from the mean and variance networks of the encoder parameterized by ϕ, and $\mathbf{M}_\theta(\mathbf{Z})$ and $\mathbf{S}_\theta(\mathbf{Z})$ are output from mean and variance networks of the decoder parameterized by θ.

<u>VAE Training:</u> Training of the VAE is performed by maximizing the variational lower bound on the likelihood of the training data given as:

$$\mathcal{L}_{ELB}(\theta, \phi; \mathbf{U}^{(i)}) = -KL(q_\phi(\mathbf{Z}|\mathbf{U}^{(i)})||p_\theta(\mathbf{Z})) + E_{q_\phi(\mathbf{Z}|\mathbf{U}^{(i)})}(\log p_\theta(\mathbf{U}^{(i)}|\mathbf{Z})) \tag{3}$$

where $p_\theta(\mathbf{Z})$ is an isotropic Gaussian prior. The calculation of the KL divergence and cross entropy loss for the presented sequential architecture is carried out in a manner similar to that described in [8]. The training data is generated by the Aliev-Panfilov (AP) model [1], simulating spatiotemporal TMP sequences originated from different ventricular locations with different tissue properties.

3   Transmural EP Imaging

The biophysical relationship between cardiac TMP, $\mathbf{U}$ and body-surface ECG, $\mathbf{Y}$ can be described by a linear measurement model: $\mathbf{Y} = \mathbf{HU}$, where $\mathbf{H}$ is specific to the heart-torso model of an individual. To estimate $\mathbf{U}$ from $\mathbf{Y}$ is severely ill-posed and requires the regularization from additional knowledge about $\mathbf{U}$.

Probabilistic Modeling of the Inverse Problem: We formulate the inverse problem in the form of statistical inference. We define the likelihood distribution of $\mathbf{Y}$ given $\mathbf{U}$ by assuming zero-mean measurement errors with variance β^{-1}:

$$p(\mathbf{Y}|\mathbf{U}, \beta) = \prod_k \mathcal{N}(\mathbf{Y}_{:,k}|\mathbf{HU}_{:,k}, \beta^{-1}\mathbf{I}) \tag{4}$$

To incorporate physiological knowledge about $\mathbf{U}$, we model its prior distribution conditioned on $\mathbf{Z}$ using the VAE decoder with trained parameter $\bar{\theta}$:

$$p_{\bar{\theta}}(\mathbf{U}|\mathbf{Z}) = \prod_k \mathcal{N}(\mathbf{U}_{:,k}|\mathbf{M}_{\bar{\theta}}(\mathbf{Z})_{:,k}, diag(\mathbf{S}_{\bar{\theta}}(\mathbf{Z})_{:,k})) \tag{5}$$

To further utilize the knowledge about the generative factor $\mathbf{Z}$ learned by the VAE from a large training dataset, we also utilize the VAE-encoded marginal posterior distribution of $\mathbf{Z}$ as its prior distribution in Bayesian inference. In specific, we approximate samples from this marginalized distribution to be Gaussian:

$$p(\mathbf{Z}) = \prod_k \mathcal{N}(\mathbf{Z}_{:,k}|\bar{\mathbf{Z}}_{:,k}, diag(\mathbf{C}_{:,k})) \tag{6}$$

With this, we complete the statistical formulation of our problem. Our goal is to estimate the joint posterior distributions $p(\mathbf{U}, \mathbf{Z}|\mathbf{Y}) \propto p(\mathbf{Y}|\mathbf{U})p(\mathbf{U}|\mathbf{Z})p(\mathbf{Z})$.

Inference: Due to the presence of a deep neural network, the posterior $p(\mathbf{U}, \mathbf{Z}|\mathbf{Y})$ is analytically intractable. To address this issue, we note that conditioned on $\mathbf{Z}$, the distribution of $\mathbf{U}$ is Gaussian in each column; thus, $p(\mathbf{U}|\mathbf{Y}, \mathbf{Z})$ is analytically available. We leverage this fact and employ a variant of the expectation maximization (EM) algorithm to obtain the *maximum a posteriori* (MAP) estimate of $\mathbf{Z}$ along with the posterior distribution of $\mathbf{U}$ given the MAP estimate of $\mathbf{Z}$.

E-step: Conditioned on an estimated value of $\mathbf{Z}$ (say $\hat{\mathbf{Z}}$), we calculate $\hat{p}(\mathbf{U}|\mathbf{Y}, \hat{\mathbf{Z}}) = \prod_k \mathcal{N}(\mathbf{U}_{:,k}|\hat{\mathbf{U}}_{:,k}, \hat{\boldsymbol{\Sigma}}_{:,:,k})$, with the covariance and mean of the kth column of $\mathbf{U}$ as:

$$\hat{\boldsymbol{\Sigma}}_{:,:,k} = (\beta\mathbf{H}^T\mathbf{H} + \mathbf{D}_k^{-1})^{-1}, \qquad \hat{\mathbf{U}}_{:,k} = \hat{\boldsymbol{\Sigma}}_{:,:,k}(\beta\mathbf{H}^T\mathbf{Y}_{:,k} + \mathbf{D}_k^{-1}\mathbf{m}_k) \tag{7}$$

where $\mathbf{D}_k = diag(\mathbf{S}_\theta(\hat{\mathbf{Z}})_{:,k})$, and $\mathbf{m}_k = \mathbf{M}_{\bar{\theta}}(\hat{\mathbf{Z}})_{:,k}$ and $\mathbf{S}_{\bar{\theta}}(\hat{\mathbf{Z}})_{:,k}$ are the kth column output of the VAE decoder network when $\hat{\mathbf{Z}}$ is input to it.

M-step: Given $\hat{p}(\mathbf{U}|\mathbf{Y}, \hat{\mathbf{Z}})$, we update $\mathbf{Z}$ by maximizing $E_{\hat{p}(\mathbf{U}|\mathbf{Y},\hat{\mathbf{Z}})} \log(p(\mathbf{Y}, \mathbf{U}, \mathbf{Z}))$

$$\mathcal{L} = E_{\prod_k \mathcal{N}(\mathbf{U}_{:,k}|\hat{U}_{:,k}, \hat{\Sigma}_{:,:,k})}[\log(p_{\bar{\theta}}(\mathbf{U}|\mathbf{Z}))] + \log(p(\mathbf{Z})) + constant \qquad (8)$$

Realizing that a complete optimization of $\mathcal{L}$ with respect to $\mathbf{Z}$ would be expensive, we instead take a few gradient descent steps towards the optimum. The gradient of the second term is analytically available. The gradient of the first term is calculated by backpropagation through the decoder network.

The EM steps iterate until convergence, at which we obtain both the MAP value of $\mathbf{Z}$ and the posterior distribution of $\mathbf{U}$ conditioned on $\mathbf{Z}$ and $\mathbf{Y}$.

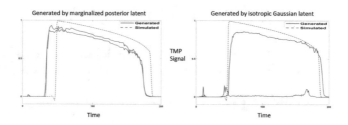

Fig. 2. Examples of TMP signals generated by samples from two different distributions: Left- marginalized posterior density encoded by the VAE; Right- isotropic Gaussian.

4   Results

Synthetic Experiments: Synthetic experiments are carried out on two image-derived human heart-torso models. On each heart, the VAE is trained using around 850 simulated TMP signals considering approximately 50 different origins of ventricular activation in combination with 17 different tissue property configurations. As an initial study, here we focus on tissue properties representing local regions of myocardial scars with varying sizes and locations.

The presented method incorporating the trained VAE model is then tested on simulated 120-lead ECG data from three different settings, each with 20 experiments. The three settings include (1) presence of myocardial scar not included in training data, (2) origin of ventricular activation different from those used in training, and (3) both myocardial scar and activation origin not seen in training. In all experiments, the performance of the presented method is compared to 0-order Tikhonov regularization with temporal constraint (Greensite method) [5] and conventional EP model constrained inference with fixed parameters [12].

The reconstruction accuracy is measured with three metrics: (1) normalized RMSE given by the ratio of Frobenius norm of the error matrix to that of the truth TMP matrix, (2) Euclidean distance between the reconstructed and true origins of ventricular activation, and (3) Dice coefficient of the reconstructed S_1 and true regions of scar S_2 as $= 2|S_1 \cap S_2|/(|S_1|+|S_2|)$. In the two physiologically constrained methods, region of scar is defined based on absence or delay of activation and shortening of action potential duration; in Greensite method, since the reconstructed signal no longer preserves the temporal shape of TMP, the region of scar is defined based on the peak amplitude of the signal.

Computational Cost: Training of the VAE takes approximately 40 h on a 4 GB Nvidia Quadro P1000 GPU. Generation of training data for each heart takes about 7 h and inference around 30 min on Quadcore CPU.

TMP Generation: Fig. 2 shows examples of local TMP signals generated by the trained VAE decoder against TMP signals simulated by the AP model [1]. Note that, when generating from a isotropic Gaussian (Fig. 2 right), noisy rather than meaningful TMP signals may also be generated. In comparison, when sampling from the approximated posterior distribution of $\mathbf{Z}$ as described in Eq. (6), the generated signals closely resemble the simulated TMP signals.

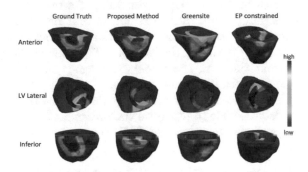

Fig. 3. Snapshots of early TMP pattern reconstructed by the three methods in comparison to the ground truth. The origin of activation is noted on the left in each row.

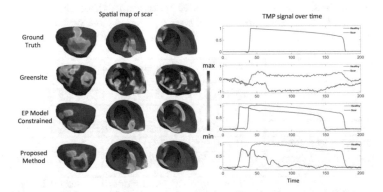

Fig. 4. Spatial distributions of scar tissues and temporal TMP signals obtained by the three methods in comparison to the ground truth.

Imaging TMP from Various Origins: Fig. 3 shows a snapshot from the early stage of ventricular activation reconstructed by the three methods in comparison to the ground truth. Since the EP model constrained approach assumes general sinus-rhythm activation, it introduces model error that incorrectly dominates the results. The simple Greensite method, free from erroneous model assumption, actually does a better job in comparison. By adapting model generative factors to the data, the presented method demonstrates a significantly improved ability to reconstruct TMP sequence resulting from unknown origins.

Imaging TMP at the Presence of Myocardial Scar: Fig. 4 shows the spatial distribution of scar tissue obtained by the three different methods, along with temporal TMP signals reconstructed in healthy and scar regions, in comparison to the ground truth. Without prior physiological knowledge, the Greensite method is not able to preserve the temporal TMP shape, resulting in high RMSE error as shown in Table 1. By thresholding the maximum amplitude of the reconstructed signals, the identified region of scar has high false positives and resembles poorly with the ground truth. The EP model constrained approach does a better job in retaining the temporal TMP shape. However, without prior knowledge about the scar, the model error again affects the accuracy of TMP reconstruction, especially in the early stage of activation when a smaller amount of ECG data is available for correcting the model error. The presented method, in comparison, is able to recognize the presence of scar tissue, adapting the physiological constraint for improved TMP reconstructions and scar identifications.

Summary: Table 1 summarizes the quantitative comparison of the three methods tested in the three settings as described earlier. Although the test cases were not seen by the VAE during training, the proposed method shows a significant improvement in inverse reconstruction (paired t-test, $p < 0.001$) when compared

Table 1. Quantitative accuracy of the three methods in three settings. Test data is simulated with (**1**) **Top**: scar not in VAE training, (**2**) **Middle**: activation origin not in training, (**3**) **Bottom**: both myocardial scar and activation origin not in training.

	Greensite	EP constrained	Proposed Method
Normalized RMSE	1.005 ± 0.006	0.3 ± 0.04	$\mathbf{0.23 \pm 0.05}$
Dice coefficient	0.19 ± 0.04	0.25 ± 0.09	$\mathbf{0.52 \pm 0.2}$

	Greensite	EP constrained	Proposed Method
Normalized RMSE	1.001 ± 0.003	0.28 ± 0.05	$\mathbf{0.11 \pm 0.08}$
Euclidean Distance	18.5 ± 10.96	39.47 ± 6.3	$\mathbf{14.37 \pm 14.0}$

	Greensite	EP constrained	Proposed Method
Normalized RMSE	1.005 ± 0.003	0.39 ± 0.03	$\mathbf{0.29 \pm 0.09}$
Dice coefficient	0.20 ± 0.07	0.21 ± 0.05	$\mathbf{0.48 \pm 0.24}$
Euclidean Distance	18.7 ± 9.3	65.5 ± 11.02	$\mathbf{17.89 \pm 10.6}$

with the other two methods in all settings and metrics except with Euclidean distance using Greensite method, where improvement is only marginal. It shows the importance of physiological knowledge and its adaptation to observed data during model-constrained inference.

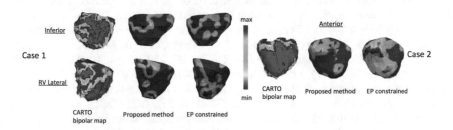

Fig. 5. Real-data experiments: regions of scar tissues identified by the presented method and conventional EP model constrained method, in comparison to bipolar voltage data (red: scar core; green: scar border; purple: healthy tissue).

Real Data Experiments: Two case studies are performed on real-data from patients who underwent catheter ablation due to scar-related ventricular arrhythmia. Spatiotemporal TMP is reconstructed from 120-lead ECG data using the presented method and the EP model constrained method. In Fig. 5, scar regions (red regions with low voltage) identified from the reconstructed TMP are compared with scar regions (red regions) in the *in-vivo* bipolar voltage data. In both cases, while the scar tissue identified by two methods are generally in similar locations, the presented method shows less false positives and higher qualitative consistency with bipolar voltage maps.

5   Discussion and Conclusions:

To our knowledge, this is the first work that integrates a generative network learned from numerous examples into a statistical inference framework to allow the adaptation of prior physiological knowledge via a small number of generative factors. The results show the ability of this concept to improve model-constrained inference. Since the present formulation is in a personalized setting, we intend to extend this architecture to learn a geometry-invariant generative model that can be trained on multiple heart models and applied on a new subject.

Acknowledgement. This work is supported by the National Science Foundation under CAREER Award ACI-1350374.

References

1. Aliev, R.R., Panfilov, A.V.: A simple two-variable model of cardiac excitation. Chaos Solitons Fractals **7**(3), 293–301 (1996)
2. Bowman, S.R., Vilnis, L., Vinyals, O., Dai, A.M., Jozefowicz, R., Bengio, S.: Generating sentences from a continuous space. arXiv preprint arXiv:1511.06349 (2015)
3. Ghimire, Sandesh, Sapp, John L., Horacek, Milan, Wang, Linwei: A variational approach to sparse model error estimation in cardiac electrophysiological imaging. In: Descoteaux, Maxime, Maier-Hein, Lena, Franz, Alfred, Jannin, Pierre, Collins, D.Louis, Duchesne, Simon (eds.) MICCAI 2017. LNCS, vol. 10434, pp. 745–753. Springer, Cham (2017). https://doi.org/10.1007/978-3-319-66185-8_84
4. Ghodrati, A., Brooks, D.H., Tadmor, G., MacLeod, R.S.: Wavefront-based models for inverse electrocardiography. IEEE TBME **53**(9), 1821–1831 (2006)
5. Greensite, F., Huiskamp, G.: An improved method for estimating epicardial potentials from the body surface. IEEE TBME **45**(1), 98–104 (1998)
6. Gulrajani, R.M.: The forward and inverse problems of electrocardiography. IEEE Eng. Med. Biol. Mag. **17**(5), 84–101 (1998)
7. He, B., Li, G., Zhang, X.: Noninvasive imaging of cardiac transmembrane potentials within three-dimensional myocardium by means of a realistic geometry anisotropic heart model. IEEE TBME **50**(10), 1190–1202 (2003)
8. Kingma, D.P., Welling, M.: Auto-encoding variational bayes. arXiv preprint arXiv:1312.6114 (2013)
9. Plonsey, R., Barr, R.C.: Bioelectricity: A Quantitative Approach. Springer, New York (2007). https://doi.org/10.1007/978-0-387-48865-3
10. Pullan, A., Cheng, L., Nash, M., Bradley, C., Paterson, D.: Noninvasive electrical imaging of the heart: theory and model development. Ann. Biomed. Eng. **29**(10), 817–836 (2001)
11. Van Dam, P.M., Oostendorp, T.F., Linnenbank, A.C., Van Oosterom, A.: Noninvasive imaging of cardiac activation and recovery. Ann. Biomed. Eng. **37**(9), 1739–1756 (2009)
12. Wang, L., Zhang, H., Wong, K.C., Liu, H., Shi, P.: Physiological-model-constrained noninvasive reconstruction of volumetric myocardial transmembrane potentials. IEEE Trans. Biomed. Eng. **57**(2), 296–315 (2010)

Pulmonary Vessel Tree Matching for Quantifying Changes in Vascular Morphology

Zhiwei Zhai[1]($\boxtimes$), Marius Staring[1], Hideki Ota[2], and Berend C. Stoel[1]

[1] Division of Image Processing, Department of Radiology,
Leiden University Medical Center, Leiden, The Netherlands
{Z.Zhai,M.Staring,B.C.Stoel}@lumc.nl
[2] Department of Diagnostic Radiology, Tohoku University Hospital, Sendai, Japan
otahide@gmail.com

Abstract. Invasive right-sided heart catheterization (RHC) is currently the gold standard for assessing treatment effects in pulmonary vascular diseases, such as chronic thromboembolic pulmonary hypertension (CTEPH). Quantifying morphological changes by matching vascular trees (pre- and post-treatment) may provide a non-invasive alternative for assessing hemodynamic changes. In this work, we propose a method for quantifying morphological changes, consisting of three steps: constructing vascular trees from the detected pulmonary vessels, matching vascular trees with preserving local tree topology, and quantifying local morphological changes based on Poiseuille's law (changes in $radius^{-4}$, $\triangle r^{-4}$). Subsequently, median and interquartile range (IQR) of all local $\triangle r^{-4}$ were calculated as global measurements for assessing morphological changes. The vascular tree matching method was validated with 10 synthetic trees and the relation between clinical RHC parameters and quantifications of morphological changes was investigated in 14 CTEPH patients, pre- and post-treatment. In the evaluation with synthetic trees, the proposed method achieved an average residual distance of 3.09 ± 1.28 mm, which is a substantial improvement over the coherent point drift method (4.32 ± 1.89 mm) and a method with global-local topology preservation (3.92 ± 1.59 mm). In the clinical evaluation, the morphological changes (IQR of $\triangle r^{-4}$) was significantly correlated with the changes in RHC examinations, $\triangle$sPAP (R $= -0.62$, p-value $= 0.019$) and $\triangle$mPAP (R $= -0.56$, p-value $= 0.038$). Quantifying morphological changes may provide a non-invasive assessment of treatment effects in CTEPH patients, consistent with hemodynamic changes from invasive RHC.

1 Introduction

Computed tomography (CT) pulmonary angiography (CTPA) is an important modality for assessing the severity and treatment effects of pulmonary vascular diseases, such as chronic thromboembolic pulmonary hypertension (CTEPH) [1]. Quantifying density changes in pulmonary vessels, by automatically comparing

© Springer Nature Switzerland AG 2018
A. F. Frangi et al. (Eds.): MICCAI 2018, LNCS 11071, pp. 517–524, 2018.
https://doi.org/10.1007/978-3-030-00934-2_58

CTPA scans of pre- and post-treatment with image registration, can assess treatment effects of CTEPH [2]. CT measurements of pulmonary vascular morphology could reflect the severity of CTEPH disease [3]. However, invasive right-sided heart catheterization (RHC) serves as the gold standard for assessing disease severity and treatment effects of CTEPH [4], since it directly measures blood pressure at the main pulmonary artery. Quantifying morphological changes by matching pulmonary vessel trees of pre- and post-treatment CT scans may provide a non-invasive assessment of treatment effects.

Vascular tree matching can be treated as a point set registration task, in which the point sets represent the vessel trees. Myronenko et al. [5] proposed a coherent point drift (CPD) method for point sets registration based on a Gaussian mixture model (GMM), and with a regularization term for enforcing the motion coherence and preserving the global topology. The regularization is useful to constrain the global topology, however, its capacity to handle local deformation is low. Ge et al. [6] proposed a method with global-local topology preservation (GLTP), where a local topology term was used for regularization, based on a local linear embedding of the K nearest neighbors of each point. The main idea of local topology preservation is that local neighbors in the original point set should be preserved after transformation. The method works well with dense point sets in computer vision, such as data obtained from the Kinect depth sensor, however, the local topology constraint may induce errors in tree-like structures. This is because leaf points, that belong to different sub-trees, may still be located closely to each other. This method would then consider them as genuine neighbors, therefore over-regularizing the deformations of sub-trees.

In this paper, we propose, therefore, a method that preserves the local tree topology during vascular tree matching, and apply this method to quantify morphological changes of pulmonary vessel trees between pre- and post-treatment. The proposed method consists of three steps: (1) pre-processing for converting the detected vessels into tree structures; (2) vascular tree matching with geodesic paths for local tree topology preservation; and (3) quantification of vascular morphological changes on the basis of Poiseuille's law [7]. The vascular tree matching method was validated with a synthetic data set, and a clinical data set consisting of 14 CTEPH patients, with CT scans and invasive RHC examinations before and after treatment.

2   Methods

We aim to align trees T^x and T^y, which can be treated as a point set registration, with reference point set $X = [x_1, ..., x_N]^T$ corresponding to nodes in T^x and template point set $Y = [y_1, ..., y_M]^T$ corresponding to those in T^y, $x_n, y_m \in \mathbb{R}^3$.

2.1   Vascular Tree Construction

For each CT scan, pulmonary vessels were segmented with a graph-cuts method [8]. The skeletons of the pulmonary vessels were extracted with a skeletonization

---

Algorithm 1. Constructing vascular trees

1: **procedure** CONSTRUCTVASCULARTREES(g)   ▷ a graph object g
2:     Initial tree T as empty
3:     **for** node_i in g.allNodes() **do**
4:         Initial node nd as empty
5:         nd.ID = node_i.getID()
6:         [nd.px, nd.py, nd.pz] = node_i.getPosition()
7:         **if** node_i has no InEdges **then**
8:             nd.PreID = -1; nd.Radius = node_i.getRadius()
9:         **else**
10:             e = node_i.getInEdge()
11:             nd.PreID = ID of e.getStartNode(); nd.Radius = average radius of e
12:         Attach nd to T
13:     **return** T

---

method based on a distance transform [9] ('DtfSkeletonization' of MeVisLab), and the radius was recorded at the corresponding voxels on the skeleton. The skeletons were converted into a directed graph g. In the directed graph, an edge e from a start-node a to end-node b, is called an out-edge of node a and an in-edge of node b. The graph g was processed by stripping cyclic edges, so that each node (except for root node) has only one in-edge, and was converted to a tree T. A node, then, represents a bifurcation point or a leaf point, and an edge represents a branch. For each node, the average radius of the in-edge was calculated by iterating along the voxels on that in-edge and was assigned to the corresponding node. The pseudo-code of the algorithm for constructing vascular trees is given in Algorithm 1.

2.2 Vascular Tree Matching

In GMM-based methods, point sets X and Y can be registered by maximizing the likelihood function and an additional regularization term $R(\Theta)$ where Θ represents the deformation parameters. This framework minimizes the energy function:

$$E = -\log\left(p(X)\right) + R(\Theta). \tag{1}$$

X is considered to be distributed from a GMM with centroids Y' and all Gaussians are equally-weighted with the same isotropic variance σ^2, where Y' is deformed from Y, $Y' = Y + GW$, G is a Gaussian kernel matrix with elements $g_{ij} = exp(-\frac{\|y_i - y_j\|^2}{2\beta^2})$ and W is $M \times D$ weight matrix of the Gaussian kernel. W can be calculated by minimizing Eq. (1) when fitting the GMM to X.

The CPD [5] and GLTP [6] use this GMM framework, with different regularization terms. CPD uses a global regularization term $R_{cpd}(W) = \frac{\lambda}{2}\mathrm{Tr}(W^T G W)$ and GLTP [6] adapted the regularization term by adding a term for preserving local topology:

$$R(W) = \frac{\lambda}{2}\mathrm{Tr}(W^T G W) + \frac{\alpha}{2}\mathrm{Tr}\{(Y + GW)^T M(Y + GW)\}, \tag{2}$$

where M is an $M \times M$ kernel matrix for preserving local deformation obtained by minimizing local linear cost function embedded with K nearest neighbors [10]. Instead of using K nearest neighbors, we compute a geodesic path with K connected nodes N^g for local topology preservation, which is more suitable for the vascular trees' deformation. $M = (I - H)^T(I - H)$, where H_{ij} is calculated by minimizing: $\Phi(Y) = \sum_i |y_i - \sum_{j \in N_i^g} H_{ij}y_j|^2$ [10]. For each node, a geodesic path is generated by iteratively searching the parent node and child node with a depth-first strategy, the pseudo-code is described in Algorithm 2. E is optimized with the EM algorithm, by minimizing its upper bound is:

$$Q = \sum_{n=1}^{N}\sum_{m=1}^{M} p^{prev}(y'_m|x_n)\frac{\| x_n - y_m - G(m,.)W \|^2}{2\sigma^2} + R(W), \tag{3}$$

where $p^{prev}(y'_m|x_n) = p(y'_m)p(x_n|y'_m)/p(x_n)$ is the posterior probability computed with the parameters from the previous step. For optimizing Eq. (3), the derivative of Q with respect to W is:

$$\frac{\partial Q}{\partial W} = \frac{1}{\sigma^2}G(diag(P \cdot 1)(Y + GW) - PX) + \lambda GW + \alpha GM(Y + GW), \tag{4}$$

in which P is an $M \times N$ matrix with elements $p^{prev}(y'_m|x_n)$. By setting the function 4 to zero and right multiplying it by $\sigma^2 G^{-1}$, we have:

$$\{diag(P \cdot 1) + \sigma^2\lambda I + \sigma^2\alpha MG\}W = PX - diag(P \cdot 1)Y + \sigma^2\alpha MY. \tag{5}$$

In the M-step of the EM algorithm, W is calculated by solving Eq. (5). In the E-step, P is updated with the weight W. After optimizing the energy function, the matching pair C between X and Y can be built by searching point x_n that maximizes the posterior probability, $C(m) = \operatorname*{argmax}_n\{p(y'_m|x_n)\}$.

2.3   Quantitative Analysis

The nodes of the vascular trees in pre-treatment CT scans can be compared with those in post-treatment CT scans based on C. As the average radius of a branch is assigned to its end-node, morphological changes in each branch can be quantified based on C between vascular trees. Poiseuille's law [7] describes the relation between the resistance (ratio between pressure difference and flow rate, $\triangle P/F$) and the radius r in a tube:

$$\triangle P/F = \frac{8\eta L}{\pi r^4}, \tag{6}$$

Algorithm 2. Searching geodesic paths with a deep first strategy

---
1: **procedure** GEODESICPATHSEARCHING(T, K)
2:     Initial N with the number of nodes in T; $Neighbors$ as an $N \times K$ zeros matrix
3:     **for** $i = 1$ to N **do**
4:         $kfind = 0$
5:         ID $= T(i)$.ID; PreID $= T(i)$.PreID
6:         **while** $kfind < K$ & not (PreID==-1& ID==0) **do**
7:             **if** PreID $\neq$ -1 **then**
8:                 [preind, PreID]=findPreID(T,PreID)   ▷ find the ID of pre-Node
9:                 $kfind = kfind + 1$; $Neighbors(i, kfind)$=preind
10:            [postind, ID]=findPostID(T, ID)   ▷ randomly pick a post-Node
11:            **if** ID $\neq 0$ **then**
12:                $kfind = kfind + 1$; $Neighbors(i, kfind)$=postind
13:    **return** $Neighbors$ as N^g

---

where L is the length of the tube and η is the fluid viscosity. Assuming that L and η of a local branch do not change after treatment, its resistance changes can be estimated by the changes in r^{-4} ($\triangle r^{-4}$). Thus, the morphological changes of vascular trees are quantified based on $\triangle r^{-4}$ of matched branches. The median and interquartile range (IQR) of the $\triangle r^{-4}$ are calculated over all branches and are used as global assessments of morphological changes.

3   Experiment

The method for constructing pulmonary vascular trees was implemented as a module in MeVisLab 2.7.1, the methods for matching vascular trees and quantifying morphological changes were implemented in Matlab, which is benefiting from the open source tools of CPD [5]. The experiments were performed on a local PC, with a 2.67 GHz CPU, 24 GB memory and a 64-bit Windows 7 system.

To evaluate the performance of vascular tree matching, synthetic vascular trees were obtained with a tree editing method [11]. In short, an initial tree T^0 with 3176 nodes was obtained from the left lung of a clinical CT scan and 10 synthetic trees $T^i, i = 1, ..., 10$ were generated by randomly removing $30 * i$ leaf nodes and deformed with Elastix using different non-rigid transformation parameters [12]. To simulate both deletions and additions, the synthetic tree T^5 and T^i were matched with the proposed method (settings: MaxIteration $= 100$, $\beta = 1, \lambda = 3$, outlier $= 0.05, \alpha = 100, K = 5$), furthermore, CPD [5] (MaxIteration $= 100$, $\beta = 1, \lambda = 3$, outlier $= 0.05$) and GLTP [6] (MaxIteration $= 100$, $\beta = 1, \lambda = 3$, outlier $= 0.05, \alpha = 100, K = 5$) were adopted for comparison. The Euclidean distance between nodes in T^5 and T^i were calculated, based on the corresponding point pairs. The average and standard deviation (STD) of the residual distances were used for evaluation.

The quantification of morphological changes was validated with 14 CTEPH patients [2], who were treated with balloon pulmonary angioplasty (BPA), referred to the Tohoku University Hospital. All patients underwent both CTPA

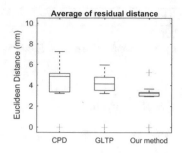
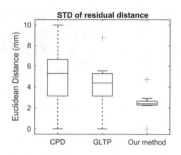

Fig. 1. Evaluation for vascular tree matching, average and STD of distance.

Table 1. Pearson's correlation R (p-value) between morphological changes and hemo-dynamic changes.

	$\triangle$sPAP	$\triangle$dPAP	$\triangle$mPAP	$\triangle$PVR
median of $\triangle r^{-4}$	0.19 (0.506)	0.04 (0.901)	0.16 (0.576)	0.07 (0.815)
IQR of $\triangle r^{-4}$	−0.62 (0.019)	−0.46 (0.097)	−0.56 (0.038)	−0.47 (0.088)

scans and RHC examinations, pre- and post-BPA treatment. The invasive RHC examinations, including pulmonary artery pressure (PAP, systolic, diastolic and mean; sPAP, dPAP and mPAP) and pulmonary vascular resistance (PVR), are examined at the main pulmonary artery. The RHC parameters changes ($\triangle$PAP and $\triangle$PVR) were used as reference measurements for assessing treatment effects. The morphological changes in vascular trees were quantified with the proposed method. The relation between the quantifications of morphological changes and hemodynamic changes ($\triangle$sPAP, $\triangle$dPAP, $\triangle$mPAP, $\triangle$PVR) were validated with Pearson's correlation.

4   Results

The proposed method obtained an average residual distance of 3.09 ± 1.28 mm, while CPD and GLTP obtained an average distance of 4.32 ± 1.89 mm and 3.92 ± 1.59 mm, respectively. In comparison with CPD and GLTP, the proposed method achieved a substantial improvement, as shown in Fig. 1. The 3D visualization of vascular tree matching can be found in the supplement.

The relation between morphological changes in pulmonary vascular trees and changes in RHC measurements were investigated with 14 CTEPH patients. The IQR of $\triangle r^{-4}$ significantly correlated with $\triangle$sPAP (R = −0.62, p-value = 0.019) and $\triangle$mPAP(R = −0.56, p-value = 0.038), but the median of $\triangle r^{-4}$ did not have a significant correlation with hemodynamic changes. Quantitative analysis of vascular morphological changes in two selected patients are shown in Fig. 2. Pearson's correlation results are given in Table 1, and scatter plots are shown in Fig. 3.

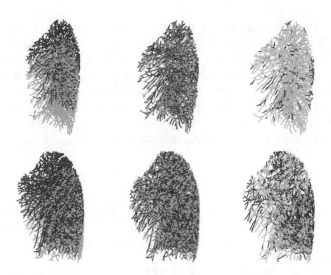

Fig. 2. Morphological changes of pulmonary vessels for two patients, patient A in the first row and B in the second row. Left column, initial position of vascular trees; middle column, matched vascular trees; right column, color-coded vascular trees, based on morphological changes (red: a large increase in r^{-4}; blue: a large decrease; green small changes).

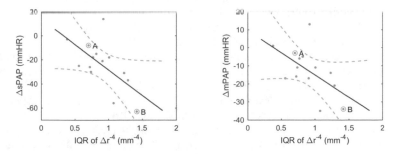

Fig. 3. Scatter plot for IQR of $\triangle r^{-4}$ against $\triangle$sPAP and $\triangle$mPAP (A and B are corresponding to patient A and B in Fig. 2).

5   Discussion and Conclusion

We present a method for quantifying morphological changes in pulmonary vascular trees, pre- and post-treatment, using vascular tree matching. The vascular tree matching method with geodesic paths for local topology preservation showed a better performance, in comparison with methods of CPD and GLTP. The IQR of $\triangle r^{-4}$, calculated based on Poiseuille's law, had a significant negative correlation with the $\triangle$sPAP and $\triangle$mPAP, which implies that a higher variation in $\triangle r^{-4}$ corresponds to a bigger treatment effect of decreasing pulmonary arterial pressure. This finding is consistent with a previous observation that a higher variation in density changes was related to bigger drop in pressure. In future work, we will focus on a more detailed validation of the vascular tree matching with manually annotated corresponding point pairs. By applying methods of artery-vein separation, the quantification of morphological changes may become more specific for CTEPH, since that is an arterial disease.

In conclusion, morphological changes can reflect hemodynamic changes, and quantifying morphological changes by matching vascular trees can provide a non-invasive assessment of treatment effects in CTEPH patients.

References

1. Liu, M., Ma, Z., Guo, X., Zhang, H., Yang, Y., Wang, C.: Computed tomographic pulmonary angiography in the assessment of severity of chronic thromboembolic pulmonary hypertension and right ventricular dysfunction. Eur. J. Radiol. **80**(3), e462–e469 (2011)
2. Zhai, Z., et al.: Treatment effect of balloon pulmonary angioplasty in chronic thromboembolic pulmonary hypertension quantified by automatic comparative imaging in computed tomography pulmonary angiography. Investig. Radiol. **53**(5), 286–292 (2018)
3. Rahaghi, F., et al.: Pulmonary vascular morphology as an imaging biomarker in chronic thromboembolic pulmonary hypertension. Pulm. Circ. **6**(1), 70–81 (2016)
4. Kim, N.H., et al.: Chronic thromboembolic pulmonary hypertension. J. Am. Coll. Cardiol. **62**(25 Supplement), D92–D99 (2013)
5. Myronenko, A., Song, X.: Point set registration: coherent point drift. IEEE Trans. Pattern Anal. Mach. Intell. **32**(12), 2262–2275 (2010)
6. Ge, S., Fan, G., Ding, M.: Non-rigid point set registration with global-local topology preservation. In: 2014 IEEE Conference on Computer Vision and Pattern Recognition Workshops (CVPRW), pp. 245–251. IEEE (2014)
7. Kirby, B.J.: Micro-and Nanoscale Fluid Mechanics: Transport in Microfluidic Devices. Cambridge University Press, New York (2010)
8. Zhai, Z., Staring, M., Stoel, B.C.: Lung vessel segmentation in CT images using graph-cuts. In: Medical Imaging 2016: Image Processing, vol. 9784. International Society for Optics and Photonics (2016). 97842K
9. Selle, D., Preim, B., Schenk, A., Peitgen, H.O.: Analysis of vasculature for liver surgical planning. IEEE Trans. Med. Imaging **21**(11), 1344–1357 (2002)
10. Saul, L.K., Roweis, S.T.: An Introduction to Locally Linear Embedding (2000, unpublished). http://www.cs.toronto.edu/~roweis/lle/publications.html
11. Pinzón, A.M., Hoyos, M.H., Richard, J.C., Flórez-Valencia, L., Orkisz, M.: A tree-matching algorithm: application to airways in CT images of subjects with the acute respiratory distress syndrome. Med. Image Anal. **35**, 101–115 (2017)
12. Klein, S., Staring, M., Murphy, K., Viergever, M.A., Pluim, J.P.: Elastix: a toolbox for intensity-based medical image registration. IEEE Trans. Med. Imaging **29**(1), 196–205 (2010)

MuTGAN: Simultaneous Segmentation and Quantification of Myocardial Infarction Without Contrast Agents via Joint Adversarial Learning

Chenchu Xu[1], Lei Xu[2], Gary Brahm[1], Heye Zhang[3(✉)], and Shuo Li[1(✉)]

[1] Western university, London, ON, Canada
slishuo@gmail.com
[2] Beijing AnZhen Hospital, Beijing, China
[3] Shenzhen Institutes of Advanced Technology, Chinese Academy of Sciences, Shenzhen, China
hy.zhang@siat.ac.cn

Abstract. Simultaneous segmentation and full quantification (estimation of all diagnostic indices) of the myocardial infarction (MI) area are crucial for early diagnosis and surgical planning. Current clinical methods still suffer from high-risk, non-reproducibility and time-consumption issues. In this study, the multitask generative adversarial networks (MuTGAN) is proposed as a contrast-free, stable and automatic clinical tool to segment and quantify MIs simultaneously. MuTGAN consists of generator and discriminator modules and is implemented by three seamless connected networks: spatio-temporal feature extraction network comprehensively learns the morphology and kinematic abnormalities of the left ventricle through a novel three-dimensional successive convolution; joint feature learning network learns the complementarity between segmentation and quantification through innovative inter- and intra-skip connection; task relatedness network learns the intrinsic pattern between tasks to increase the accuracy of estimations through creatively utilized adversarial learning. MuTGAN minimizes a generalized divergence to directly optimize the distribution of estimations by using the competition process, which achieves pixel segmentation and full quantification of MIs. Our proposed method yielded a pixel classification accuracy of 96.46%, and the mean absolute error of the MI centroid was 0.977 mm, from 140 clinical subjects. These results indicate the potential of our proposed method in aiding standardized MI assessments.

Electronic supplementary material The online version of this chapter (https://doi.org/10.1007/978-3-030-00934-2_59) contains supplementary material, which is available to authorized users.

© Springer Nature Switzerland AG 2018
A. F. Frangi et al. (Eds.): MICCAI 2018, LNCS 11071, pp. 525–534, 2018.
https://doi.org/10.1007/978-3-030-00934-2_59

1   Introduction

Simultaneous segmentation and quantification (*including pixel segmentation and full quantification of all indices such as the infarct size, segment percentage, perimeter, centroid, major axis length, minor axis length and orientation*) of a myocardial infarction (MI) are crucial to clinical treatment of the MI [1]. It segments MI to predict the recovery of dysfunctional segments in chronic ischemic heart diseases or to select therapeutic options; it estimates all indices that indicate the presence, location, and transmurality of acute and chronic MI. The combination can obtain all information required for a thorough understanding of the extent of the MI to prevent further heart failure [2].

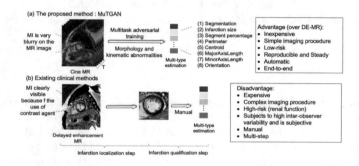

Fig. 1. (a) MuTGAN can accurately segment and quantify an infarction in one step without contrast agents compared to (b) the high-risk, non-reproducible and time-consuming current clinical methods.

Current clinical methods still suffer from high-risk, non-reproducibility and time-consumption issues [3]. The clinical standards include two steps: (1) delayed enhancement (DE) imaging by using magnetic resonance (MR) with gadolinium contrast agents and (2) manual segmentation and quantification of all indices of the MI from DE -MR image [2]. The high risk comes from the use of contrast agents, which are fatal with regard to the kidney disease that accompanies more than 20% of MI patients [3]. The non-reproducibility comes from the manual process that is subject to high inter-observer variability and is subjective. The time-consumption factor comes from the imaging process itself that requires multiple imaging techniques and a two-step process. Therefore, there is an urgent clinical desire to obtain a non-contrast agent, stable and automated clinical tool. However, while it is widely believed that an MI can be identified and localized vaguely without a contrast agent through the detection of morphological and kinematic abnormalities of the left ventricle (LV) directly from blurry cine MR [4], it is still challenging to build a unified model for segmenting and quantifying the MI simultaneously: (1) Effective learning of the relationship between segmentation and quantification. Segmentation and quantification as two related tasks sharing the same factors can share the information during the learning process to produce a beneficial interaction [5]. However, it is difficult to uniformly learn this beneficial interaction because of huge differences in the dimensions and distribution between the two. (2) Comprehensive learning of the spatio-temporal information inside of and between images. Extracting spatio-temporal information from the myocardium and surrounding tissues in sequential images is highly effective for building the intrinsic representation of the MI [6]. However, it is still difficult to systematically learn the asymmetry of the spatial and temporal motion over different time steps from 2D+T image sequences [7]. (3) Efficient leveraging of the relationship between quantification indices. Accurate full quantification is highly dependent on the ability to leverage the important relationship that exists between the different indices to directly optimize the estimations [8]. However, it is difficult to train this relationship properly to reduce the distribution error of the estimation due to the different locally optimal and probability distributions of the different indices [9].

In this study, the multitask generative adversarial networks (MuTGAN) is proposed for joint segmentation and quantification of MI directly from cine MR without contrast agents. MuTGAN formulates the segmentation and seven quantification indices into eight tasks that can be estimated simultaneously under combined multitask and adversarial learning. To accomplish this, a novel three dimensional (3D) successive convolutional framework that takes spatial correlation over different time steps into consideration is proposed for extracting the comprehensive spatio-temporal feature of MI from 2D+T images. An innovative joint learning architecture as multitask learning that fuses the feature maps of different level layers is proposed for achieving a reciprocal representation that has a beneficial interaction between segmentation and quantification. A creative task relatedness adversarial learning that models the substantial pattern between tasks is proposed for exploiting the inductive bias of the task's relevance to approximate the estimation distribution to the real data. In the end, our MuTGAN not only simultaneously segments and quantifies MI for the first time but also effectively exploits the trait of multitask to improve itself.

2   Methodology

MuTGAN was implemented by two competing modules: the generator (Sect. 2.2) and discriminator (Sect. 2.3), as shown in Fig. 2. The two modules interact with each other and consist of three seamlessly connected networks. The generator first builds the spatio-temporal feature extraction network based on novelty stacks of 3D convolution (Conv) and ConvLSTMs [10] to learn a comprehensive representation of the 2D+T data through successive convolution over different time steps in replacing the pooling layer; it then builds joint feature learning network based on new skip architecture [11] to share the representation of the segmentation and quantification by multiple skip connections between inter- and intra-networks. The discriminator builds task relatedness network based on bidirectional (Bi) -LSTMs [12] to creatively use adversarial training that takes the complete contextual pattern between tasks as a criterion for measuring the accuracy of estimations.

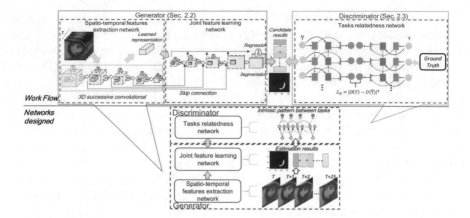

Fig. 2. The architecture of MuTGAN: the generator combines spatio-temporal feature extraction network and joint feature learning network for multitask learning; the discriminator uses task relatedness network for adversarial learning.

2.1 MuTGAN Formulation

The output of MuTGAN is multitask result $Y \in (y_1, y_2, ..., y_n, n = 8)$ including one segmentation task y_1 and seven quantification tasks $y_2, ..., y_n$. The objective of MuTGAN is to simultaneously estimate Y from cine MR, which consists of $2D + T$ image sequences $X \in (x_1, x_2, ..., x_T, \mathbb{R}^{H \times W \times T})$, where H and W are the height and width of each temporal frames respectively ($H = W = 64$), and T is the temporal step, $T = 25$. X can be considered as special 3D data ($H \times W \times T$). Given the discriminator and generator parameters θ_D and θ_G, each updated by minimizing the losses $\mathcal{L}_G$ and $\mathcal{L}_D$, MuTGAN can be express as:

$$\begin{cases} \mathcal{L}_D = \mathcal{L}(d(Y)) - \lambda \mathcal{L}(d(g(X))) & \text{for } \theta_D \\ \mathcal{L}_G = \mathcal{L}(g(X)) & \text{for } \theta_G \end{cases} \tag{1}$$

Where $g(.)$ and $d(.)$ are the generator and discriminator function, and $\lambda \in [0, 1]$.

2.2 Generator

The generator module uses spatio-temporal feature extraction network and joint feature learning network to generate candidate multitask estimations directly from cine MR.

Spatio-Temporal Features Extraction Network (SFEN). The network innovatively stacks ConvLSTMs and 3DConvs for accurate extraction of the left ventricular morphology and kinematic abnormalities. ConvLSTMs and 3DConvs are both effective tools for learning spatial and temporal information from 2D+T data and are usually used separately. In our work, for a better handle on the asymmetry distortion that is a unique myocardial motion pattern caused by MI, special integration of ConvLSTMs and 3DConvs is used to consider spatial correlation over different time steps. The benefit of this integration is two-fold:

first, by using successive Convs instead of the pooling layers, temporal and spatial information can be extracted simultaneously and equally. Second, multiple temporal ranges with different spatial scales can be extracted by adjusting the size of the Conv kernel over different layers. ConvLSTMs uses its internal memory to process 2D+T images, which creates an internal state that can discover the dynamic temporal behavior between frames and allows for persistence [10]. Given that i_t, f_t, $\tilde{c}_t$, and o_t represent the input, forget, cell, and output gates, respectively, the ConvLSTMs are:

$$\begin{cases} i_t = \sigma(x_t * w_{xi} + h_{t-1} * w_{hi} + w_{i\text{bias}}) \\ f_t = \sigma(x_t * w_{xf} + h_{t-1} * w_{hf} + w_{f\text{bias}}) \\ \tilde{c}_t = \tanh(x_t * w_{x\tilde{c}} + h_{t-1} * w_{h\tilde{c}} + w_{\tilde{c}\text{bias}}) \\ c_t = \tilde{c}_t \odot i_t + c_{t-1} \odot f_t \\ o_t = \sigma(x_t * w_{xo} + h_{t-1} * w_{ho} + w_{o\text{bias}}) \\ h_t = o_t \odot \tanh(c_t) \end{cases} \tag{2}$$

Where c and h are the memory and output activations; σ and tanh are the sigmoid and hyperbolic tangent non-linearities; $*$ represents the convolution operation, and $\odot$ the Hadamard product. 3DConvs are inserted between each ConvLSTMs, which stride $2\times2\times3$ downsampling to reduce the resolution both spatially and temporally. In the last of this networks (Conv13), each X maps into a fixed-length vector $\mathcal{F}_{Conv13} = f_{encoding}(X) \approx \arg\min_{H} p((H - X) \mid$

$x_1, \dots, x_t), H \in (h_1, \dots, h_t), \mathcal{F}_{Conv13} \in \mathbb{R}^{4\times4\times512}$.

Joint Feature Learning Network. A new multiple skip connection is used to forcibly connect the segmentation and quantification, and joint learning beneficial interactions to promote the learning mutually. This network combines upsampling and the same successive Convs as SFEN uses the skip architecture to integrate SFEN and learn a shared representation of the segmentation and quantification. The skip architecture that fused feature maps of different layers to avoid spatial information loss and gradient dispersion has gained great success in U-Net and ResNet. In our work, for segmentation, the skip architecture symmetrically connects the SFEN and joint feature learning network $(Conv12 \rightarrow Conv18, Conv8 \rightarrow Conv22, Conv4 \rightarrow Conv26)$ to contain the full context available in time series data and learn a more precise segmentation. For regression, the skip architecture combines the $\mathcal{F}_{Conv13}$ and each feature map before the filters change in the joint learning network to integrate coarse, high layer information with fine, low layer information to produce accurate and detailed quantification. Two parallel, fully connected layers generate candidate results $\widetilde{Y} \approx g_{predicting}(\mathcal{F}_{Conv13}) = g_{predicting}(\widetilde{y}_1, \dots, \widetilde{y}_n \mid f_{encoding}(x_1, \dots, x_t))$, including $\widetilde{y}_1$, a binary 64×64 image and seven indices $\widetilde{y}_n$.

Loss for Generator Training. Dice loss takes tackle class imbalance into consideration is employed for the segmentation and mean absolute error (MAE) for the quantification:

$$\mathcal{L}_G = \mathcal{L}_{dice}(g(X), y_1) + \sum_{i=2}^{n} \mathcal{L}_{mae}(g(X), y_i) = \frac{2|y_1 \cap g(X)|}{|y_1| + |g(X)|} + \sum_{i=2}^{n} |y_i - g(X)|^\eta \tag{3}$$

Where η is the target norm, $\eta \in \{1, 2\}$.

2.3   Discriminator

The discriminator creatively uses a task relatedness network to determine whether the candidate multitask estimations fit the ground truth and directly optimizes the candidate to improve MuTGAN performance based on the inherent pattern between tasks.

Task Relatedness Network. The network utilize Bi-LSTMs to learn the inherent pattern between tasks. LSTMs provides a general framework for learning this pattern. However, Bi-LSTMs consider more complete contextual relationships than LSTMs because of replacing each hidden sequence h^l with the forward and backward sequences $\overrightarrow{h^l}$ and $\overleftarrow{h^l}$, ensuring that every hidden layer receives input from both the forward and backward layers at the level below. In our work, Bi-LSTMs regulates task relatedness by gates structures, which remove or add information to the cell state by processing different tasks [12].

$$h_n^l = f_{LSTM}(W_{h^{l-1}h^l}h_n^{l-1} + W_{h^lh^l}h_{n-1}^l + b_h^l) \tag{4}$$

where the hidden vector sequences h_n^l are iteratively computed from $\tilde{Y} = \tilde{y}_1, \ldots, \tilde{y}_n$ and all L ($l = 1$ to L) are layers in the stack. The network output is $\hat{Y}_l = W_{h^L\hat{y}}h_l^N + b_{\hat{y}}$

Loss for Discriminator Training. For efficiently converging GANs, the discriminator module is equivalent to minimizing the following MAE loss:

$$\mathcal{L}_D = \sum_{n=1}^{N} \mathcal{L}_{mae}(d(\tilde{y}_n), y_n) = \sum_{n=1}^{N} |y_n - d(\tilde{y}_n)|^\eta \tag{5}$$

3   Materials and Implementation Details

A total of 140 patients were retrospectively selected between May 2015 and May 2017 and completed cine and DE-MR imaging scans. MR imaging was performed using a 3T MR system (MAGNETOM Verio, Siemens). SSFP cine images were acquired during repeated breath holds: TR 3.1 ms, TE 1.3 ms, FA 45°, FOV (276×340) mm^2, matrix 156×192, slice thickness 6 mm, and 25 cardiac phases. DE-MR imaging was performed in the same orientations and with the same slice thickness as cine imaging ten minutes after the intravenous injection of gadolinium (Magnevist, 0.2 m mol/kg): TR $= 10.5$ ms, TE $= 5.4$ ms, and FA $= 30°$. Two radiologists with more than 10 years of experience manually segmented and quantified the MI (syngo MR B17) in the DE-CMR images. If there was disagreement, a consensus between the two experts must be reached. In our experiments, a network with heart localization layers, described in [6], was used to automatically crop cine MR to 64 × 64 region-of-interest sequences including the LV. All experiments were assessed with a 10-fold cross-validation test.

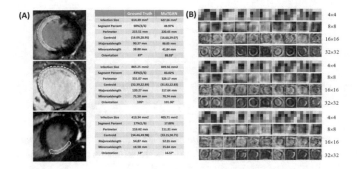

Fig. 3. (A) The infarction areas segmented and quantified by our method (green zone) are consistent with the ground truth (yellow dotted line). (B) The different resolution feature maps indicate that MuTGAN effectively extracts spatio-temporal motion information of different myocardial regions at different time steps.

4   Experiments and Results

MutGAN produces high performance with a pixel classification accuracy of 96.46%, the MAE of the centroid point is 0.97 mm with the ground truth obtained manually by human experts, which demonstrates this method's effectiveness for segmentation and quantification of MI.

Accurate MI Segmentation. The experiment's result shows that MuTGAN can accurately locate the MI, as shown in Fig. 3. We achieve an overall pixel classification accuracy of 96.46%, with a sensitivity of 91.82% and a specificity of 98.21%; the Dice coefficient is $90.27 \pm 0.05\%$; the ROCs and PRs curves are shown in Fig. 4. The ground truth and result are binary images; each pixel is assessed for infarction or normality (0 or 1).

Precise MI Quantification. MuTGAN can also obtain good quantification of the MI, as shown in Fig. 3 and Table 1. The MAE computed between the ground truth and our estimation of the infarction size is $22.311 \pm 18.39 \, \text{mm}^2$, the segment percentage is $1.04 \pm 0.62\%$, the perimeter is $5.392 \pm 4.66 \, \text{mm}$, the centroid is $0.977 \pm 0.78 \, \text{mm}$, the major axis length is $2.303 \pm 1.88 \, \text{mm}$, the minor axis length is $1.030 \pm 0.76 \, \text{mm}$, and the orientation is $7.242 \pm 3.63°$.

Advantage of GANs Architecture. Figure 4 and Table 1 show that MuTGAN has better segmentation and quantification performance in comparison to those frameworks because of its combined ability for joint learning (Joi) and adversarial learning (Adv). To evaluate this ability, MuTGAN (Joi+Adv), Generator (Joi) and separately estimated tasks by SFEN are implemented individually.

Advantages of the Spatio-temporal Feature Extraction Network. Table 2 indicates that SFEN (3DConvs + ConvLSTMs) achieved better performance than all other the frameworks because of its learned spatial correlation over different time steps. To evaluate the performance of extraction, we replaced

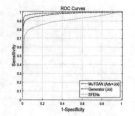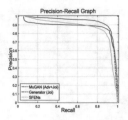

Fig. 4. ROCs and PRs demonstrate that MuTGAN can accurately segment infarct areas by combining joint learning (Joi) and adversarial learning (Adv).

Table 1. MuTGAN works best in comparison with frameworks that do not utilize the joint learning and adversarial learning.

	MuTGAN	Generator	SFEN
Accuracy	**96.46%**	95.83%	94.13%
Sensitivity	**91.82%**	90.74%	81.86%
Specificity	**98.21%**	98.17%	96.64%
Dice (%)	**90.27%**	89.76%	83.13%
Infarct Size (mm^2)	**22.31**	30.91	54.91
segments percentage	**1.04%**	2.05%	1.05%
Perimeter (mm)	**5.39**	10.26	7.53
Centroid (mm)	**0.97**	3.87	1.42
Majoraxislength (mm)	**2.30**	4.83	7.65
Minoraxislength (mm)	**1.03**	3.26	5.34
Orientation (°)	**7.24**	8.51	8.47

the 3DConvs + ConvLSTMs with 3DConvs, ConvLSTMs, 3DConvs + LSTMs, CNNs and LSTMs in our framework.

Comparison with Some Existing Methods. Table 3 demonstrates that MuTGAN achieved higher segmentation and quantification accuracy compared with existing classical methods in segmentation/quantification (Seq/Qua).

Table 2. MuTGAN works best in comparison with other frameworks.

	MuTGAN	ConvLSTMs	3DConvs	3DConvs+LSTM	CNNs	LSTMs
Accuracy	**96.46%**	96.31%	93.32%	94.48%	90.64%	90.63%
Dice	**0.90**	0.89	0.81	0.82	0.73	0.77
Infarct size	**22.31**	47.35	92.54	79.94	224.28	176.46

Table 3. MuTGAN realized segmentation and quantification of MI simultaneously without a contrast agent and yielded higher performance than some existing methods.

	Seg/Qua	Accuracy	Dice	Infarct size	Centroid
MuTGAN	**Seg and Qua**	**96.46%**	**90.27%**	**22.31**	**0.97**
Xu et al. [6]	Seg only	94.35%	89.87%	92.02*	7.98*
Popescu et al. [7]	Seg only	85.68%	74.45%	176.28*	10.46*
Bleton et al. [13]	Seg only	84.78	71.62	224.28*	12.93*

* The quantification result estimate from segmentation result.

5 Conclusions

Multitask generative adversarial networks have been proposed and, for the first time, used for simultaneous segmentation and quantification of MI without contrast agents. MuTGAN was conducted on 140 subjects and yielded a pixel classification accuracy of 96.46%; the MAE of the infarction size was $22.31\,\mathrm{mm^2}$. All of these results demonstrate that MuTGAN can aid in the clinical diagnosis of MI assessments.

References

1. Bijnens, B., Claus, P., Weidemann, F.: Investigating cardiac function using motion and deformation analysis in the setting of coronary artery disease. Circulation **116**(21), 2453–2464 (2007)
2. Ordovas, K.G., Higgins, C.B.: Delayed contrast enhancement on MR images of myocardium: past, present, future. Radiology **261**(2), 358–374 (2011)
3. Fox, C.S., Muntner, P.: Use of evidence-based therapies in short-term outcomes of ST-Segment elevation myocardial infarction and Non-ST-Segment elevation myocardial infarction in patients with chronic kidney disease. Circulation **121**(3), 357–365 (2010)
4. Lipton, M.J., Bogaert, J., Boxt, L.M., Reba, R.C.: Imaging of ischemic heart disease. Eur. Radiol. **12**(5), 1061 (2001)
5. Wollmann, T., Ivanova, J., Gunkel, M.: Multi-channel deep transfer learning for nuclei segmentation in glioblastoma cell tissue images. Bildverarbeitung für die Medizin **2018**, 316–321 (2018)
6. Xu, C., et al.: Direct detection of pixel-level myocardial infarction areas via a deep-learning algorithm. In: Descoteaux, M., Maier-Hein, L., Franz, A., Jannin, P., Collins, D.L., Duchesne, S. (eds.) MICCAI 2017. LNCS, vol. 10435, pp. 240–249. Springer, Cham (2017). https://doi.org/10.1007/978-3-319-66179-7_28
7. Popescu, I.A., Irving, B., Borlotti, A., Dall'Armellina, E., Grau, V.: Myocardial scar quantification using SLIC supervoxels - parcellation based on tissue characteristic strains. In: Mansi, T., McLeod, K., Pop, M., Rhode, K., Sermesant, M., Young, A. (eds.) STACOM 2016. LNCS, vol. 10124, pp. 182–190. Springer, Cham (2017). https://doi.org/10.1007/978-3-319-52718-5_20

8. Xue, W., Lum, A., Mercado, A., Landis, M., Warrington, J., Li, S.: Full quantification of left ventricle via deep multitask learning network respecting intra- and inter-task relatedness. In: Descoteaux, M., Maier-Hein, L., Franz, A., Jannin, P., Collins, D.L., Duchesne, S. (eds.) MICCAI 2017. LNCS, vol. 10435, pp. 276–284. Springer, Cham (2017). https://doi.org/10.1007/978-3-319-66179-7_32

9. Ogawa, R., Kido, T.: Diagnostic capability of feature-tracking cardiovascular magnetic resonance to detect infarcted segments: a comparison with tagged magnetic resonance and wall thickening analysis. Eur. Radiol. **72**(10), 828–834 (2017)

10. Xingjian, S.H.I., Chen, Z.: Convolutional LSTM network: a machine learning approach for precipitation nowcasting. In: NIPS, pp. 802–810 (2015)

11. Long, J., Shelhamer, E., Darrell, T.: Fully convolutional networks for semantic segmentation. In: CVPR, pp. 3431–3440 (2015)

12. Graves, A., Schmidhuber, J.: Framewise phoneme classification with bidirectional LSTM and other neural network architectures. Neural Netw. **18**(5–6), 602–610 (2005)

13. Bleton, H., Margeta, J., Lombaert, H., Delingette, H., Ayache, N.: Myocardial infarct localization using neighbourhood approximation forests. In: Camara, O., Mansi, T., Pop, M., Rhode, K., Sermesant, M., Young, A. (eds.) STACOM 2015. LNCS, vol. 9534, pp. 108–116. Springer, Cham (2016). https://doi.org/10.1007/978-3-319-28712-6_12

14. Karim, R., Housden, R.J., Balasubramaniam, M.: Evaluation of current algorithms for segmentation of scar tissue from late gadolinium enhancement cardiovascular magnetic resonance of the left atrium: an open-access grand challenge. JCMR **15**(1), 105 (2013)

More Knowledge Is Better: Cross-Modality Volume Completion and 3D+2D Segmentation for Intracardiac Echocardiography Contouring

Haofu Liao[1]([✉]), Yucheng Tang[3], Gareth Funka-Lea[2], Jiebo Luo[1], and Shaohua Kevin Zhou[4]

[1] Department of Computer Science, University of Rochester, Rochester, USA
hliao6@cs.rochester.edu
[2] Medical Imaging Technologies, Siemens Healthineers, Princeton, USA
[3] Department of Electrical and Computer Engineering, New York University, New York, USA
[4] Institute of Computing Technology, Chinese Academy of Sciences, Beijing, China

Abstract. Using catheter ablation to treat atrial fibrillation increasingly relies on intracardiac echocardiography (ICE) for an anatomical delineation of the left atrium and the pulmonary veins that enter the atrium. However, it is a challenge to build an automatic contouring algorithm because ICE is noisy and provides only a limited 2D view of the 3D anatomy. This work provides *the first automatic solution* to segment the left atrium and the pulmonary veins from ICE. In this solution, we demonstrate the benefit of building a *cross-modality framework* that can leverage a database of diagnostic images to supplement the less available interventional images. To this end, we develop a novel deep neural network approach that uses the (i) *3D geometrical information* provided by a position sensor embedded in the ICE catheter and the (ii) *3D image appearance information* from a set of computed tomography cardiac volumes. We evaluate the proposed approach over 11,000 ICE images collected from 150 clinical patients. Experimental results show that our model is significantly better than a direct 2D image-to-image deep neural network segmentation, especially for less-observed structures.

1 Introduction

Atrial fibrillation (AF) affects about 2% to 3% of the population in Europe and North America as of 2014 [13]. One of its treatments is to perform catheter ablation to destroy the cardiac tissues causing the abnormal electrical signal. During catheter ablation, intracardiac echocardiography (ICE) is often used to guide the intervention. Compared with other imaging modalities such as transoesophageal echocardiography, ICE provides better patient tolerance, requiring no general

---

S. K. Zhou—The work was done when Liao, Tang, and Zhou were with Siemens.

© Springer Nature Switzerland AG 2018
A. F. Frangi et al. (Eds.): MICCAI 2018, LNCS 11071, pp. 535–543, 2018.
https://doi.org/10.1007/978-3-030-00934-2_60

anesthesia [2]. The junction (ostia) of the pulmonary veins with the left atrium (LA) (see Fig. 1(a)) is usually where the catheter ablation is performed [8]. However, due to the limitations of 2D ICE, these 3D anatomical structures may only be partially viewed. This can introduce difficulties for the electrophysiologists as well as for automated analysis algorithms. Fortunately, modern ICE devices are equipped with an embedded position sensor that measures the 3D location of the ICE transducer. The spatial geometry information associated with the ICE image is key to this study.

Existing approaches to 2D echocardiogram segmentation only focus on single cardiac chamber such as left ventricle (LV) [5,9,11] or LA [1]. They are designed to distinguish between the blood tissues and the endocardial structures which is relatively easy due to the significant difference in appearance. When it comes to multiple cardiac components (chambers and their surrounding structures), where the boundaries cannot be clearly recognized, these methods may fail. To the best of our knowledge, this paper is the first to handle the multi-component echocardiogram segmentation from 2D ICE images.

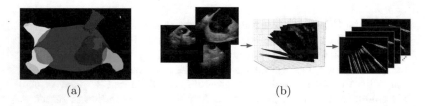

(a)   (b)

Fig. 1. (a) Graphical illustration of LA and its surrounding structures: blue-LA, green-left atrial appendage (LAA), red-left inferior pulmonary vein (LIPV), purple-left superior pulmonary vein (LSPV), white-right inferior pulmonary vein (RIPV), yellow-right superior pulmonary vein (RSPV). (b) 3D sparse ICE volume generation using the location information associated with each ICE image.

Recently, deep convolutional neural networks (CNNs) have achieved unprecedented success in medical image analysis, including segmentation [12]. However, our baseline method of training a CNN to directly generate segmentation masks from 2D ICE images does not demonstrate satisfactory performance, especially for the less-observed pulmonary veins. Such a baseline solely relies on the brute force of big data to cover all possible variations, which is difficult to achieve. To go beyond brute force, we further integrate knowledge to boost contouring performance. Such knowledge stems from two sources: (i) *3D geometry information* provided by a position sensor embedded inside an ICE catheter, and (ii) *3D image appearance information* exemplified by cross-modality computed tomography (CT) volumes that contain the same anatomical structures.

2 Method

The proposed method consists of three parts. Using the 3D geometry knowledge, we first form a 3D sparse volume based on the 2D ICE images. Then, to tap into the 3D image appearance knowledge, we design a multi-task 3D network with an adversarial formulation. The network performs cross-modality volume completion and sparse volume segmentation simultaneously for collaborative structural understanding and consistency. Finally, taking as inputs both the original 2D ICE image and the 2D mask projected from the generated 3D mask, we design a network to refine the 2D segmentation results.

We form a 3D sparse ICE volume from a set of 2D ICE images with each including part of the heart in its field of view and its 3D position from a magnetic localization system. As shown in Fig. 1, we use the location information to map all ICE images (left) to 3D space (middle), thus forming a sparse ICE volume (right). The generated sparse ICE volume keeps the spatial relationships among individual ICE views. A segmentation method based on the sparse volume can take this advantage for better anatomical understanding and consistency.

2.1 3D Sparse Volume Segmentation and Completion

The architecture of the proposed 3D segmentation and completion network (3D-SCNet) is illustrated in Fig. 2(a). The network consists of a generator G_{3d} and two discriminators D_{3d}^s and D_{3d}^c. Taking the sparse ICE volume $\mathbf{x}$ as input, G_{3d} performs 3D segmentation and completion simultaneously, and outputs a segmentation map $G_{3d}^s(\mathbf{x})$ as well as a dense volume $G_{3d}^c(\mathbf{x})$. During training, the ground truth of $G_{3d}^c(\mathbf{x})$ is a CT volume instead of a dense ICE volume as we lack the training data of the latter. The ICE images and the CT volumes are from *completely different* patients. This inherently creates a challenging *cross-modality volume completion* problem with unpaired data. We target this problem through adversarial learning and mesh pairing (See Sect. 3). The two discriminators judge the *realness* of the outputs from the generator. When trained adversarially together with a generator, they make sure the generator's outputs are more perceptually realistic. Following conditional GAN [4], we also allow the discriminators to take $\mathbf{x}$ as the input to further improve adversarial training.

Adversarial Loss. The segmentation task s and completion task c are trained jointly in a multi-task learning (MTL) fashion [3]. The adversarial loss for a task $t \in \{s, c\}$ can be written as

$$\mathcal{L}_{adv}^t = \mathbb{E}_{\mathbf{x}, y_t \sim p(\mathbf{x}, y_t)}[\log D_{3d}^t(\mathbf{x}, y_t)] + \mathbb{E}_{\mathbf{x} \sim p(\mathbf{x})}[1 - \log D_{3d}^t(\mathbf{x}, G_{3d}^t(\mathbf{x}))], \quad (1)$$

where p denote the data distributions. For a real data y_t, i.e., the ground truth segmentation map or CT volume, D_{3d}^t is trained to predict a "real" label. For the generated data $G_{3d}^t(\mathbf{x})$, D_{3d}^t learns to give a "fake" label. On the other hand, the generator G_{3d} is trained to deceive D_{3d}^t by making $G_{3d}^t(\mathbf{x})$ as "real" as possible.

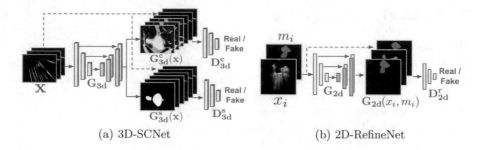

(a) 3D-SCNet   (b) 2D-RefineNet

Fig. 2. The network architectures of the proposed method.

Reconstruction Loss. Adversarial loss alone, however, does not give a strong structural regularization to the training [6]. Hence, we use reconstruction loss to measure the pixel-level error between the generator outputs and the ground truths. For the segmentation task, we first convert the score map to a multichannel map with each channel denoting the binary segmentation map of a target anatomy and then apply an L2 loss $\mathcal{L}_{rec}^s$ between $G_{3d}^s(\mathbf{x})$ and y_s. For the completion task, the L1 loss $\mathcal{L}_{rec}^c$ between $G_{3d}^c(\mathbf{x})$ and y_c is measured. We use L1 loss instead of L2 loss for this task due to the observation that outputs from L2 losses are usually overly smoothed. The total loss of the sparse volume segmentation and completion network is given by

$$\mathcal{L}_{3d} = \sum_{t \in \{c,s\}} \lambda_{rec}^t \mathcal{L}_{rec}^t + \lambda_{adv}^t \mathcal{L}_{adv}^t, \tag{2}$$

where λ_{rec}^t and λ_{adv}^t balance the importance of the reconstruction loss and reconstruction loss, respectively.

Architecture Details. We use a 3D UNet-like network [7] as the generator. There are 8 consecutive downsampling blocks followed by 8 consecutive upsampling blocks in the network. We use skip connections to shuttle feature maps between two symmetric blocks. Each downsampling block contains a 3D convolutional layer, a batch normalization layer and a leaky ReLU layer. Similarly, each upsampling layer contains a 3D deconvolutional layer, a batch normalization layer and a ReLU layer. The convolutional and deconvolutional layers have the same parameter settings: $4 \times 4 \times 4$ kernel size, $2 \times 2 \times 2$ stride size and $1 \times 1 \times 1$ padding size. Finally, a tanh function is attached at the end of the generator to bound the network outputs. The two discriminators D_{3d}^s and D_{3d}^c have identical network architecture with each of them having 3 downsampling blocks followed by a 3D convolutional layer and a sigmoid layer. The downsampling blocks for the discriminators are the same as the ones used in the generator. The final 3D convolutional layer ($3 \times 3 \times 3$ kernel size, $1 \times 1 \times 1$ stride size and $1 \times 1 \times 1$ padding size) and sigmoid layer are used for realness classification.

2.2   2D Contour Refinement

As shown in Fig. 2(b), the 2D refinement network (2D-RefineNet) has a similar structure to the 3D-SCNet. Actually, G_{2d} and D_{2d}^r have almost the same structure as their 3D counterparts except that the convolutional and deconvolutional layers are now in 2D. The inputs to the 2D-RefineNet is a 2D ICE image x_i together with its corresponding 2D segmentation map m_i, where m_i is obtained by projecting $G_{3d}^s(\mathbf{x})$ onto x_i. The training of the 2D-RefineNet is also performed in an adversarial fashion and conditional GAN is used to allow D_{2d}^r observing the generator inputs. We compute the adversarial loss L_{adv}^r the same way as Eq. (1) and use the L2 distance between the refinement network output $G_{2d}(x_i, m_i)$ and the ground truth 2D segmentation map y_r as the reconstruction loss L_{rec}^r. The total loss is

$$\mathcal{L}_{2d} = \lambda_{rec}^r \mathcal{L}_{rec}^r + \lambda_{adv}^r \mathcal{L}_{adv}^r, \tag{3}$$

where λ_{rec}^r and λ_{adv}^r are the corresponding balancing coefficients.

3   Experiments

Dataset and Preprocessing. The left atrial ICE images used in this study are collected using a clinical system with each image associated with a homogeneous matrix that projects the ICE image to a common coordinate system. We perform both 2D and 3D annotations on the ICE images for the cardiac components of interest, i.e., LA, LAA, LIPV, LSPV, RIPV and RSPV. For the 2D annotations, contours of all the plausible components in the current view are annotated. For the 3D annotations, ICE images, from the same patient and at the same cardiac phase [1], are first projected to 3D, and 3D mesh models of the target components are then manually annotated. 3D segmentation masks are generated using these mesh models. In total, the whole database has 150 patients. For each patient, there are 20–80 gated frames for use. We have 3D annotations for all 150 patients. For 2D annotations, we annotated 100 patients, resulting in a total of 11,782 annotated ICE images. By anatomical components, we have in 2D 4669 LA, 1104 LAA, 1799 LIPV, 1603 LSPV, 1309 RIPV, and 1298 RSPV annotations. So, the LA is mostly observed and the LAA and PVs are less observed. For a subset of 1568 2D ICE images, we have 2–3 expert annotations per image to compute the inter-rater reliability (IRR).

As we do not have dense ICE volumes available for training, we use CT volumes instead as the ground truth for the completion task. Each CT volume has an annotated LA mesh model. To pair with a sparse ICE volume, we pick the CT volume whose LA mesh model is closest to that of the targeting sparse ICE volume using Procrustes analysis [10]. In total, 414 CT volumes are available, which gives enough anatomical variability for the mesh pairing. All the data used

---

[1] While in clinical practice multiple 2D ICE clips are acquired to dynamically image a patient's LA anatomy, here we focus on a stack of 2D ICE images, with often one gated frame per clip, and leave dynamic modeling for future study.

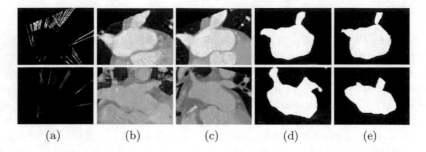

(a)   (b)   (c)   (d)   (e)

Fig. 3. Sparse volume segmentation and completion results for 2 cases. (a) Sparse ICE volume; (b) Completed CT volume; (c) the paired "ground truth" CT volume; (d) Predicted and (e) Ground truth 3D segmentation map.

for 3D training are augmented with random perturbations in scale, rotation and translation to increase the generalizability of the model.

Training and Evaluation. We train the 3D-SCNet and 2D-RefineNet using Adam optimization with $lr = 0.005$, $\beta_1 = 0.5$, $\beta_2 = 0.999$. The 3D-SCNet is trained for about 25 epochs with $\lambda^s_{adv} = 0.2$, $\lambda^c_{adv} = 1$, $\lambda^s_{rec} = 1000$, $\lambda^c_{rec} = 100$. The 2D-RefineNet is also trained for about 25 epochs with $\lambda^r_{adv} = 1$, $\lambda^r_{rec} = 1000$. All λs are chosen empirically and we train the models using 5-fold cross-validation. The segmentation results are evaluated using the Dice metric and average symmetric surface distance (ASSD).

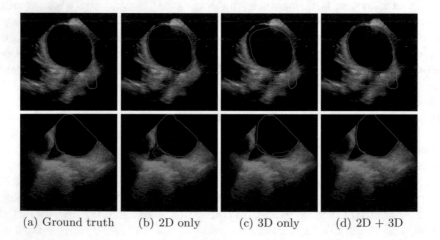

(a) Ground truth   (b) 2D only   (c) 3D only   (d) 2D + 3D

Fig. 4. Samples of 2D ICE contouring results from different models.

Results. The outputs from the 3D network model are shown in Fig. 3. We can observe that the model not only gives satisfying segmentation outputs, Fig. 3(d), but also gives a good estimation about the CT volume, Fig. 3(b). Especially, we note that the estimated completion outputs do not give structurally exact results as the "ground truth" but instead try to match the content from the sparse volume. Since the "ground truth" CT volume is paired based on mesh models, this difference is expected. It demonstrates that the completion outputs are based on the sparse volume and the system only tries to complete the missing region such that it looks like a "real" CT volume. We also quantitatively evaluate the performance of the 3D sparse volume segmentation (before projecting on 2D) and obtain the following Dice scores: LA (89.5%), LAA (50.0%), LIPV (52.9%), LSPV (43.4%), RIPV (62.43%), RSPV (57.6%) and overall (86.1%). This shows that using the limited information from sparse volumes our model still can achieve a satisfactory 3D segmentation performance. As we will show in later experiments, the segmentation accuracy, actually, is even higher in the region where 2D ICE images are presented. We also notice that *it is vital to use the 3D appearance information* – the training fails to converge in our experiment of learning the 3D network without using the 3D appearance information from CT.

Figure 4 shows the 2D ICE contouring results using different models: the "2D only" model that is trained directly with the 2D ICE images, the "3D only" model by projecting the predicted 3D segmentation results onto the corresponding ICE image, and the "2D + 3D" model by refining the outputs from 3D-SCNet using 2D-RefineNet. We observe from the first row that the "3D only" outputs give better estimation about the PVs (red and orange) than the "2D only" outputs. This is because the PVs in the current 2D ICE view are not clearly visible which is challenging for the "2D only" model. While for the "3D only" model, it makes use of the information from other views and hence predicts better the PV locations. Finally, we see that the outputs from the "2D + 3D" model combines the knowledge from both the 2D and 3D models and generally gives superior outputs than these two models. Similar results can also be found in the second row where we see the "2D + 3D" model not only predicts the location of the PVs (purple and brown) better by making use of the 3D information but also refines the output according to the 2D view.

Table 1. 2D segmentation accuracy of different models. The results are evaluated in terms of Dice metric (%) and ASSD (mm).

	Dice	ASSD	Dice	ASSD	Dice	ASSD	Dice	ASSD
LA	94.3	0.623	93.5	0.693	**95.4**	**0.537**	89.6	1.340
LAA	68.2	1.172	66.5	1.206	**71.2**	**1.106**	68.8	1.786
LIPV	70.1	0.918	71.7	0.904	**72.4**	**0.856**	69.9	1.459
LSPV	65.9	1.275	67.8	**0.916**	**71.1**	1.197	62.9	1.582
RIPV	69.6	0.927	71.7	0.889	**73.8**	**0.786**	71.4	1.378
RSPV	63.3	0.872	70.4	**0.824**	**70.5**	0.862	57.8	1.633
Total	91.0	0.839	89.8	0.834	**92.1**	**0.791**	88.6	1.432

The quantitative results of these models are given in Table 1. The "3D only" model in general has better performance in PVs and worse performance in LA and LAA than the "2D only" model. This is because LA and LAA usually have a clear view in 2D ICE images, unlike the PVs. The "2D + 3D" model combines the advantages of the "2D only" and "3D only" model and in general yields the best performance. The IRR scores from human experts are relatively lower, especially for the LSPV and RSPV. This is expected as these two structures are difficult to view with ICE and there is variability in how far distally experts do their annotation. The IRR scores are generally lower than those from our models, which demonstrates the benefit of using an automatic segmentation model – better consistency.

4   Conclusions and Future Work

We present a knowledge fusion + deep learning approach to ICE contouring of multiple LA components. It uses 3D geometry and cross-modality appearance knowledge for better anatomical understanding and structural consistency. Then, it refines the contours in 2D by exploiting the detailed 2D appearance information. We show that the proposed model indeed benefits from the integrated knowledge and gives superior performance to the models trained individually. In the future, we will investigate the use of temporal information for better modeling and the clinical utility of the generated dense 3D cross-modality views.

References

1. Allan, G., et al.: Simultaneous analysis of 2D echo views for left atrial segmentation and disease detection. IEEE TMI **36**(1), 40–50 (2017)
2. Bartel, T., Müller, S., Biviano, A., Hahn, R.T.: Why is intracardiac echocardiography helpful? Benefits, costs, and how to learn. Eur. Hear. J. **35**(2), 69–76 (2013)
3. Caruana, R.: Multitask learning. In: Thrun, S., Pratt, L. (eds.) Learning to Learn, pp. 95–133. Springer, Boston (1998). https://doi.org/10.1007/978-1-4615-5529-2_5
4. Isola, P., Zhu, J.Y., Zhou, T., Efros, A.A.: Image-to-image translation with conditional adversarial networks. In: Proceedings of the CVPR, pp. 1125–1134 (2017)
5. Lin, N., Yu, W., Duncan, J.S.: Combinative multi-scale level set framework for echo image segmentation. Med. Image Anal. **7**(4), 529–537 (2003)
6. Pathak, D., Krahenbuhl, P., Donahue, J., Darrell, T., Efros, A.A.: Context encoders: feature learning by inpainting. In: Proceedings of tne CVPR, pp. 2536–2544 (2016)
7. Ronneberger, O., Fischer, P., Brox, T.: U-Net: convolutional networks for biomedical image segmentation. In: Navab, N., Hornegger, J., Wells, W.M., Frangi, A.F. (eds.) MICCAI 2015. LNCS, vol. 9351, pp. 234–241. Springer, Cham (2015). https://doi.org/10.1007/978-3-319-24574-4_28
8. Sánchez-Quintana, D., López-Mínguez, J.R., Macías, Y., Cabrera, J.A., Saremi, F.: Left atrial anatomy relevant to catheter ablation. Cardiology Research and Practice (2014)

9. Sarti, A., Corsi, C., Mazzini, E., Lamberti, C.: Maximum likelihood segmentation of ultrasound images with rayleigh distribution. IEEE Trans. Ultrason. Ferroelectr. Freq. Control. **52**(6), 947–960 (2005)
10. Schönemann, P.H.: A generalized solution of the orthogonal procrustes problem. Psychometrika **31**(1), 1–10 (1966)
11. Zhou, S.K.: Shape regression machine and efficient segmentation of left ventricle endocardium from 2D B-mode echocardiogram. Med. Image Anal. **14**(4), 563–581 (2010)
12. Zhou, S., Shen, D., Greenspan, H. (eds.): Deep Learning for Medical Image Analysis. Academic Press, Cambridge (2017)
13. Zoni-Berisso, M., Lercari, F., Carazza, T., Domenicucci, S.: Epidemiology of atrial fibrillation: european perspective. Clinical Epidemiol. **6**, 213–20 (2014)

Unsupervised Domain Adaptation for Automatic Estimation of Cardiothoracic Ratio

Nanqing Dong[1,2]([✉]), Michael Kampffmeyer[3], Xiaodan Liang[4], Zeya Wang[1], Wei Dai[1], and Eric Xing[1]

[1] Petuum, Inc., Pittsburgh, USA
[2] Cornell University, Ithaca, USA
nd367@cornell.edu
[3] UiT The Arctic University of Norway, Tromsø, Norway
[4] Carnegie Mellon University, Pittsburgh, USA

Abstract. The cardiothoracic ratio (CTR), a clinical metric of heart size in chest X-rays (CXRs), is a key indicator of cardiomegaly. Manual measurement of CTR is time-consuming and can be affected by human subjectivity, making it desirable to design computer-aided systems that assist clinicians in the diagnosis process. Automatic CTR estimation through chest organ segmentation, however, requires large amounts of pixel-level annotated data, which is often unavailable. To alleviate this problem, we propose an unsupervised domain adaptation framework based on adversarial networks. The framework learns domain invariant feature representations from openly available data sources to produce accurate chest organ segmentation for unlabeled datasets. Specifically, we propose a model that enforces our intuition that prediction masks should be domain independent. Hence, we introduce a discriminator that distinguishes segmentation predictions from ground truth masks. We evaluate our system's prediction based on the assessment of radiologists and demonstrate the clinical practicability for the diagnosis of cardiomegaly. We finally illustrate on the JSRT dataset that the semi-supervised performance of our model is also very promising.

1 Introduction

Cardiomegaly, also referred to as heart enlargement, is ranked as the most frequent disease code among a public collection of radiology reports from the National Library of Medicine (NLM) according to a National Institutes of Health (NIH) study on medical information retrieval [4]. Cardiomegaly can result from other diseases or medical conditions, such as coronary artery disease and hypertension. It is suggested that cardiomegaly is associated with a high risk of sudden cardiac death [13]. The prevention of cardiomegaly starts from early detection and CTR measured from posterior-anterior (PA) CXR is an important indicator for cardiomegaly [5]. CTR is calculated as the ratio of maximal horizontal cardiac diameter to maximal horizontal thoracic diameter, and CTR greater than

© Springer Nature Switzerland AG 2018
A. F. Frangi et al. (Eds.): MICCAI 2018, LNCS 11071, pp. 544–552, 2018.
https://doi.org/10.1007/978-3-030-00934-2_61

0.5 is commonly considered as cardiomegaly [3,5]. Manual measurement of CTR requires domain knowledge in radiology and extensive human labor in annotating CXRs, with results being error-prone due to observational error. This motivates the automation of CTR calculation and cardiomegaly detection. One common approach to estimating CTR is lung field segmentation [2].

Recent advances in Convolutional Neural Networks (CNNs) have brought breakthroughs in the field of semantic segmentation, achieving state-of-the-art performance [1,9]. Compared to traditional semantic segmentation, the annotated data for medical image segmentation is more difficult to be acquired, because of the limited available data and the tremendous cost of collecting and labeling it. Transfer learning is a common approach to solve tasks with data scarcity, utilizing the fact that CNNs generally learn feature representations that are robust across a variety of tasks [14]. However, as segmentation predictions based on these representations do not generalize very well to different datasets because of the dataset shift phenomena [7], it is commonly required to fine-tune the network based on a set of labels for the target domain. In particular, CXRs from different hospitals are often taken with different imaging protocols and commonly exhibit differences in noise levels, contrast and resolution. So it is impractical to directly use transfer learning techniques. See Figs. 1 and 3 for the differences between CXRs obtained at different hospitals.

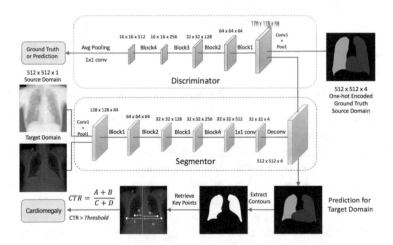

Fig. 1. Illustration of the architecture. In our proposed adversarial training procedure, the segmentor produces segmentations for the input images and the discriminator attempts to distinguish these predictions from ground truth annotations. A post-processing step (bottom part of figure) is used to predict cardiomegaly based on the predicted lung segmentation masks.

In this paper, we propose an unsupervised domain adaptation (UDA) framework based on adversarial networks, which allows us to learn domain invariant feature representations from openly available data sources in order to produce accurate chest organ segmentation for unlabeled datasets. Domain adaptation methods aim to reduce the problems of dataset shift, commonly, by aligning the learned source and target representation in a joint embedding space [12,14]. Adversarial networks have become a popular choice to achieve this alignment, by introducing a discriminator that is trained to distinguish between the source and the target domain and by forcing the model to learn representations that can fool the discriminator. We propose an alternative training scheme where we utilize a discriminator that enforces our intuition that prediction masks should be domain independent by discriminating segmentation predictions from ground truth masks. We evaluate our system's performance based on the assessment of radiologists on a CTR estimation dataset. Our approach outperforms the state-of-the-art UDA and shows the clinical practicability for the diagnosis of cardiomegaly. We finally illustrate that our approach can also be used for semi-supervised chest organ segmentation of the JSRT benchmark dataset.

2   Methodology

The complete pipeline is shown in Fig. 1. The adversarial neural network consists of a discriminator and a segmentor. To demonstrate the generalization and simplicity of the methodology, we use ResNet18 as a backbone architecture [8]. The discriminator is a standard ResNet classifier and the segmentor is inspired by the Fully Convolutional Network (FCN) [9], but uses an output stride of 16, following the example of [1]. Provided the predicted labels for the two lungs, the CTR is calculated in a post-processing step.

2.1   Adversarial Training for Supervised Semantic Segmentation

Adversarial learning was first introduced in the Generative Adversarial Network (GAN) [6] as a two-model zero-sum game, in which one model generates candidates for the other network to evaluate. Inspired by [10], who used adversarial learning to improve semantic segmentation results, we let S be the segmentor and D be the discriminator. S is trained to produce realistic prediction masks in order to fool D, which in turn is attempting to discriminate these predictions from ground truth images in a binary classification. D is encouraged to learn a complex loss between the higher-order label statistics, which in practice cannot be explicitly formulated. Medical domain knowledge is being implicitly incorporated into this formulation as part of the annotated ground truth data.

An alternative training scheme is applied to train the segmentor and discriminator. Given D, the loss to be minimized for S is a multi-class cross-entropy loss for semantic segmentation, in addition to the binary cross-entropy loss for segmentation prediction $S(\boldsymbol{x})$ being classified as ground truth by D [10].

$$J_{seg}(S(\boldsymbol{x}), \boldsymbol{y}) = -\frac{1}{B_S} \sum_s \frac{1}{HW} \sum_i \sum_c y_{s,i,c} \log S(x_{s,i,c}) \tag{1}$$

$$J_S(S(\boldsymbol{x}), \boldsymbol{y}) = J_{seg}(S(\boldsymbol{x}), \boldsymbol{y}) - \lambda_{adv} \frac{1}{B_S} \sum_s \log D(S(x_s)) \qquad (2)$$

We use x_s and y_s to denote the input image and the ground truth, respectively, where x_s is of shape $[H, W, 1]$ and y_s is of shape $[H, W, C]$ for C-class one-hot encoded labels. B_S denotes the batch size for the segmentor training and i ranges over all the spatial positions. Given S, D is optimized to maximize the probability of correctly distinguishing $S(\boldsymbol{x})$ from $\boldsymbol{y}$ as

$$J_D(S(\boldsymbol{x}), \boldsymbol{y}) = -\frac{1}{B_D} \sum_s \left[\log(D(y_s)) + \log(1 - D(S(x_s))) \right], \qquad (3)$$

where B_D is the batch size for the discriminator training.

2.2   Unsupervised Domain Adaption

Our approach to unsupervised domain adaptation is illustrated in Fig. 1 and is based on the idea that prediction masks, unlike input images and intermediate feature representations, can be considered domain independent. Unlike in [10], we do not only make use of a discriminator to judge the quality of the segmentation mask, but also use it to align both source and target segmentation results with the domain-independent prediction mask. We propose an alternative training scheme, where we present the discriminator with real ground truth images from our source domain, y_s, and with segmentation mask predictions from both the source and the target domain, x_s and x_t, respectively. In order to learn domain invariant feature representations, we exploit the fact that we can train the segmentor using both the segmentation and the discriminator loss in the source domain to produce accurate segmentation prediction masks. However, simultaneously we enforce the fact that the segmentation masks for the target domain need to be of high quality. The updated losses are

$$J_{S-DA}(S(\boldsymbol{x}), \boldsymbol{y}) = J_S(S(\boldsymbol{x}), \boldsymbol{y}) - \lambda_{adv} \frac{1}{B_S} \sum_t \log D(S(x_t)), \qquad (4)$$

$$J_{D-DA}(S(\boldsymbol{x}), \boldsymbol{y}) = J_D(S(\boldsymbol{x}), \boldsymbol{y}) - \frac{1}{B_D} \sum_t \log(1 - D(S(x_t))). \qquad (5)$$

2.3   Estimation of CTR

CTR is the ratio of maximal horizontal cardiac diameter to maximal horizontal thoracic diameter, as formulated in the Danzer Method [3]. The diameters are the horizontal distance between horizontal coordinates of corresponding key points on the lung contours. As shown in Fig. 2, the maximal horizontal cardiac diameter and maximal horizontal thoracic diameter can only be achieved by points above cardiodiaphragmatic angles and costophrenic angles, which can be retrieved by the use of a convex hull algorithm. With a hypothetical central line, the Danzer Method could be reinterpreted as $\frac{A+B}{C+D}$, while line segments A, B, C, D are all maximized independently. The constraints of maximizing $A+B$ are that the points of intersection between lung contours and A and B must be above cardiodiaphragmatic angles. The points of intersection between the lung contours and the maximized A, B, C, and D are the key points. Provided the estimated CTR, cardiomegaly can be predicted under different thresholds for different age groups. Following [2], the threshold, T, is chosen to be 0.5.

2.4   Semi-Supervised Semantic Segmentation

We further illustrate our model's ability for the task of semi-supervised learning. As the annotated data are limited, it is common in medical image segmentation to have only a subset of training data labeled. Provided with a set of labeled and unlabeled datapoints $\{\{(x_1,\ y_1),...,(x_l, y_l)\}, \{\tilde{x}_1,...,\tilde{x}_u\}\}$, the task of semi-supervised learning aims to exploit the underlying data properties of the unlabeled data in addition to the labeled data. l and u correspond to the number of labeled and unlabeled examples, respectively. Similar to our unsupervised domain adaptation, we adopt an alternating training strategy, where the model is presented with both labeled and unlabeled data. We optimize S and D using Eqs. 4 and 5 and treat the labeled data as the source domain and the unlabeled data as the target domain. This lets us leverage the unlabeled data to align the distribution of segmentation predictions with the distribution of ground truth labels, effectively regularizing the model and improving overall performance.

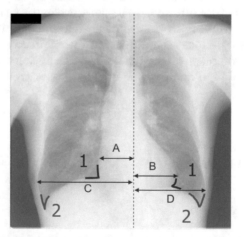

Fig. 2. Contour landmarks for lower lungs: cardiodiaphragmatic angles (1) and costophrenic angles (2).

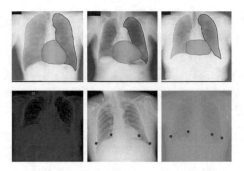

Fig. 3. Example images of the two datasets. The three images in the top row correspond to examples of the JSRT dataset, overlaid with the segmentation annotation. The three images in the second row originate from the Wingspan dataset overlaid with the key points for the CTR calculation.

3   Experimental Results

The **JSRT** dataset is released by the Japanese Society of Radiological Technology (JSRT) [11] and is a benchmark dataset for lung and heart segmentation. JSRT contains 247 grayscale CXRs with annotated lung and heart pixel-wise labels, where 154 have lung nodules and 93 don't have lung nodules. Each CXR has a size of 2048 × 2048 and the pixel spacing is 0.175 mm. In this paper, JSRT is used as the source domain for the unsupervised domain adaption. See Fig. 3 for examples from the dataset overlaid with the ground truth annotation.

The **Wingspan** dataset is provided by a private research institute, Wingspan Technology. The dataset contains 221 grayscale CXRs for adult patients with annotated key points for calculation of CTR. Each image was annotated by two licensed radiologists independently, and the annotations were accepted by both annotators and an independent reviewer. The de-identified data were collected from 6 hospitals, which have different imaging protocols. The image sizes, pixel spacing and clinical setup vary for each CXR. See Fig. 3 for examples from the dataset with key point annotations and the differences to the JSRT dataset and Fig. 4 for the large variety in the data modalities, which is not present in the available public benchmark datasets.

In our work, we use the Wingspan dataset as the target domain. We investigate the potential of our proposed approach for unsupervised domain adaptation for the task of CTR estimation. For this, we utilize the segmentation masks of the source domain (JSRT) to perform segmentation on our target domain (Wingspan) and use the predicted segmentation result to compute the CTR. We then show how our method can be easily adapted to semi-supervised semantic segmentation. We evaluate our approach on JSRT and illustrate that we can use the information encoded in our unlabeled data. The adversarial networks are trained using the Adam optimizer with a learning rate of 10^{-3}. The discriminator is updated twice before the segmentor is updated, and λ_{adv} is 10^{-4}. We use $B_S = B_D = 8$. JSRT is randomly split into 80% for training and 20% for testing. For all the experiments in this paper, no data augmentation is used, which further shows the robustness of our approach.

Table 1. Results for the unsupervised domain adaptation of CTR estimation experiments. APE denotes average percentage error, MAE denotes mean absolute error, and RMSE denotes root mean square error.

Method	APE	MAE	RMSE
TL-SEG	$16.0\% \pm 16.1\%$	$8.9\% \pm 9.3\%$	0.13
TL-ADV	$11.4\% \pm 11.2\%$	$5.9\% \pm 5.9\%$	0.08
ADDA	$9.2\% \pm 9.9\%$	$5.1\% \pm 5.8$	0.08
DA-ADV	$5.8\% \pm 8.5\%$	$3.3\% \pm 5.1\%$	0.06

Unsupervised Domain Adaptation: To assess our performance for unsupervised domain adaptation, we compare our approach (DA-ADV) to three alternative approaches and present the quantitative results for the CTR estimation in Table 1. The baseline uses the segmentor trained on the source domain directly on the target domain. This corresponds to transfer learning without fine-tuning on the target domain (TL-SEG). The baseline segmentor can be improved by adding a discriminator with an adversarial training scheme (TL-ADV). Finally, we compare with one of the state-of-the-art approaches for domain adaptation, ADDA [14], which trains a segmentation network and then utilizes an adversarial loss to align the source and the target domain feature representations in order to minimize data shift. However, ADDA's performance is highly dependent on the quality of the segmentation network, which is not robust. We observe that our method outperforms the alternative approaches, providing considerable improvements for CTR estimation. Qualitative results for the predicted segmentation masks and the key points for images from the Wingspan dataset can be seen in Fig. 4. Based on the threshold of 0.5, we predict cardiomegaly with our pipeline and achieve 87.78% in accuracy, 97.72% in precision, 84.21% in sensitivity and 95.57% in specificity.

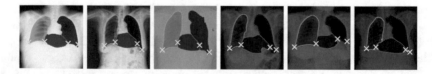

Fig. 4. Visualization of the segmentation and key point results for the Wingspan dataset for our proposed domain adaptation method.

Semi-Supervised Semantic Segmentation: As a baseline we train the model respectively on 10%, 25% and 50% of annotated data in a supervised manner.

Table 2. Results for the semi-supervised segmentation experiments. IoU denotes the Intersection over Union.

Method	IoU (Lungs)	IoU (Heart)
Human Observer [15]	94.6% ± 1.8%	87.8% ± 5.4%
Supervised	95.5% ± 0.3%	90.2% ± 0.5%
Supervised (50%)	82.9% ± 3.5%	71.2% ± 7.6%
Supervised (25%)	75.4% ± 5.7%	62.4% ± 11.9%
Supervised (10%)	60.1% ± 9.6%	39.4% ± 14.7%
Semi-Supervised (50%)	90.4% ± 3.1%	81.2% ± 2.5%
Semi-Supervised (25%)	89.9% ± 3.3%	75.5% ± 5.4%
Semi-Supervised (10%)	81.7% ± 4.6%	69.4% ± 7.2%

As a comparison, we train the model on the whole dataset in a semi-supervised manner, while only portions of the data used in the supervised setting are provided with the labels. Table 2 provides the results of our semi-supervised experiments. Our approach clearly makes use of the unlabeled data, achieving large performance gains. To put our results into perspective and to illustrate the performance that can be achieved when all training labels are available, we also train the model on the fully labeled training dataset.

4   Conclusions

In this paper, we present an approach to unsupervised domain adaptation for the task of CTR estimation that is based on the intuition that prediction masks should be domain independent. Using an adversarial training approach, we show that we can predict cardiomegaly from a dataset without segmentation annotations. We further illustrate how our approach can be adapted for semi-supervised learning.

Acknowledgements. We thank Wingspan Technology for collecting and annotating the data for this study.

References

1. Chen, L., Papandreou, G., Kokkinos, I., Murphy, K., Yuille, A.: DeepLab: semantic image segmentation with deep convolutional nets, atrous convolution, and fully connected crfs. In: IEEE TPAMI (2017)
2. Dallal, A.H., Agarwal, C., Arbabshirani, M.R., Patel, A., Moore, G.: Automatic estimation of heart boundaries and cardiothoracic ratio from chest x-ray images. In: Proceedings of the SPIE, vol. 10134, id. 101340K 10, p. 134 (2017)
3. Danzer, C.S.: The cardiothoracic ratio. Am. J. Med. Sci. **157**, 513–554 (1919)
4. Demner-Fushman, D., et al.: Preparing a collection of radiology examinations for distribution and retrieval. JAMIA **23**(2), 304–10 (2016)

5. Dimopoulos, K., et al.: Cardiothoracic ratio from postero-anterior chest radiographs: a simple, reproducible and independent marker of disease severity and outcome in adults with congenital heart disease. Int. J. Cardiol. **166** (2011)
6. Goodfellow, I., et al.: Generative adversarial nets. In: NIPS, pp. 2672–2680 (2014)
7. Gretton, A., Smola, A., Huang, J., Schmittfull, M., Borgwardt, K., Schölkopf, B.: Covariate shift and local learning by distribution matching, pp. 131–160. MIT Press, Cambridge (2009)
8. He, K., Zhang, X., Ren, S., Sun, J.: Deep residual learning for image recognition. In: CVPR, pp. 770–778 (2016)
9. Long, J., Shelhamer, E., Darrell, T.: Fully convolutional networks for semantic segmentation. In: CVPR, pp. 3431–3440 (2015)
10. Luc, P., Couprie, C., Chintala, S., Verbeek, J.: Semantic segmentation using adversarial networks. In: NIPS Workshop on Adversarial Training (2016)
11. Shiraishi, J., et al.: Development of a digital image database for chest radiographs with and without a lung nodule: receiver operating characteristic analysis of radiologists' detection of pulmonary nodules. Am. J. Roentgenol. **174**(1), 71–74 (2000)
12. Shu, R., Bui, H., Narui, H., Ermon, S.: A DIRT-T approach to unsupervised domain adaptation. In: ICLR (2018)
13. Tavora, F., et al.: Cardiomegaly is a common arrhythmogenic substrate in adult sudden cardiac deaths, and is associated with obesity. Pathology **44**, 187–91 (2012)
14. Tzeng, E., Hoffman, J., Saenko, K., Darrell, T.: Adversarial discriminative domain adaptation. In: CVPR, pp. 2962–2971. IEEE (2017)
15. Van Ginneken, B., Stegmann, M.B., Loog, M.: Segmentation of anatomical structures in chest radiographs using supervised methods: a comparative study on a public database. Med. Image Anal. **10**(1), 19–40 (2006)

TextRay: Mining Clinical Reports to Gain a Broad Understanding of Chest X-Rays

Jonathan Laserson[1(✉)], Christine Dan Lantsman[2], Michal Cohen-Sfady[1],
Itamar Tamir[3], Eli Goz[1], Chen Brestel[1], Shir Bar[4], Maya Atar[5],
and Eldad Elnekave[1]

[1] Zebra Medical Vision LTD, Shefayim, Israel
`jonil@zebra-med.com`
[2] Sheba Medical Center and Tel Aviv University, Ramat Gan, Israel
[3] Rabin Medical Center, Petah Tikva, Israel
[4] Technion, Israel Institute of Technology, Haifa, Israel
[5] Ben Gurion University, Beersheba, Israel

Abstract. The chest X-ray (CXR) is by far the most commonly performed radiological examination for screening and diagnosis of many cardiac and pulmonary diseases. There is an immense world-wide shortage of physicians capable of providing rapid and accurate interpretation of this study. A radiologist-driven analysis of over two million CXR reports generated an ontology including the 40 most prevalent pathologies on CXR. By manually tagging a relatively small set of sentences, we were able to construct a training set of 959k studies. A deep learning model was trained to predict the findings given the patient frontal and lateral scans. For 12 of the findings we compare the model performance against a team of radiologists and show that in most cases the radiologists agree on average more with the algorithm than with each other.

Keywords: Radiology · Chest x-ray · Deep learning

1 Introduction

Chext X-rays (CXR's) are the most commonly performed radiology examination world-wide, with over 150 million obtained annually in the United States alone. CXR's are a cornerstone of acute triage as well as longitudinal surveillance. Despite the ubiquity of the exam and its apparent technical simplicity, the chest x ray is widely regarded among radiologists as among the most difficult to master [1].

Due to a shortage in supply of radiologists, radiographic technicians are increasingly called upon to provide preliminary interpretations, particularly in Europe and Africa. In the US, non-radiology physicians often provide preliminary

Electronic supplementary material The online version of this chapter (https:// doi.org/10.1007/978-3-030-00934-2_62) contains supplementary material, which is available to authorized users.

ⓒ Springer Nature Switzerland AG 2018
A. F. Frangi et al. (Eds.): MICCAI 2018, LNCS 11071, pp. 553–561, 2018.
https://doi.org/10.1007/978-3-030-00934-2_62

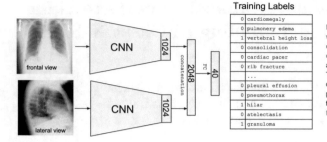

Fig. 1. TextRay Model Illustration. Frontal (PA) and lateral view images each go through a separate CNN. A fully-connected layer is applied on their concatenated feature vectors and emits the confidence for each finding. Training labels were extracted by analyzing the report sentences. Negative (green) and positive (red) sentences identified. Findings in positive sentences receive a positive training label. Negative or unmentioned findings receive a negative label.

or definitive readings of CXRs, decreasing the waiting interval at the nontrivial expense of diagnostic accuracy.

Even among expert radiologists, clinically substantial errors are made in 3–6% of studies [1,2], with minor errors seen in 30% [3]. Accurate diagnosis of some entities is particularly challenging: early lung cancer for example is missed in 19–54% of cases, with similar sensitivity figures described for pneumothorax and rib fracture detection. The likelihood for major diagnostic errors is directly correlated with both shift length and volume of examinations being read [4], a reminder that diagnostic accuracy varies substantially even at different times of the day for a given radiologist.

Hence there exists an immense unmet need and opportunity to provide immediate, consistent and expert-level insight into every CXR. In the present work we describe a novel methodology employed in this endeavor and we present the results achieved using a robust method of clinical validation.

2 Materials and Methods

Data. All Patient Health Information (PHI) was removed from the data prior to acquisition in compliance with HIPAA standards. We utilized a dataset of 2.1 million CXRs with their respective diagnostic reports. All postero-anterior (PA) CXR films of individuals aged 18 and above were procured. Corresponding lateral views were present in 85% of the CXR examinations and were included in the study data.

Textual Analysis. A standardization process was employed whereby all CXR reports were reduced to a set of distinct canonical labels. First, a sentence boundary detection algorithm was applied to the 2.1M reports, yielding a pool of 827k unique sentences. Three expert radiologists and two medical students categorized the most occurring sentences with respect to their pertinence to CXR images.

Three categories emerged: sentences that report the presence or absence of a finding, for example *"the heart is enlarged"*, or *"normal cardiac shadow"*, and could be used as labels; neutral sentences, which referenced information not derived from or inherently related to the image itself, for example: *"84 year old man with cough"*, *"lung nodule follow up"*, or *"comparison made to CT chest"*.

A third category of sentences could render the study unreliable for training due to ambiguity regarding the relationship of the text to the image, for example *"no change in the appearance of the chest since yesterday"*.

After filtering out neutral and negative sentences using a few hand-crafted regular expressions, it was possible to fully cover 826k reports using just the 20k most prevalent positive sentences. The same expert radiologists reviewed each of these sentences and mapped them to an initial ontology of 60 findings which covered 99.99% of all positive sentence volume.

In making the final ontology, we focused on visual findings rather than clinical interpretations or diagnoses. We chose to merge some categories: osteoporosis was merged into *osteopenia*, twisted and uncoiled aorta into *abnormal aorta*, and bronchial markings into *interstitial markings*, since it is often impossible to differentiate these based on the image alone. Although visually distinct, all tubes and venous lines were consolidated into two respective categories. The resulting 40 categories are presented in Table 1.

Table 1. Number of studies with each finding in our data. 596k (62%) of the total 959k studies had no reported findings.

#	Finding	Total	%	#	Finding	Total	%
1	Abnormal aorta	15,932	1.66	21	Mass	633	0.07
2	Aortic calcification	11,508	1.20	22	Mediastinal widening	1,639	0.17
3	Artificial valve	5,847	0.61	23	Much bowel gas	441	0.05
4	Atelectasis	5,492	0.57	24	Nodule	553	0.06
5	Bronchial wall thickening	2,773	0.29	25	Orthopedic surgery	717	0.07
6	Cardiac pacer	17,378	1.81	26	Osteopenia	5,585	0.58
7	Cardiomegaly	95,137	9.92	27	Pleural effusion	16,688	1.74
8	Central line	3,802	0.40	28	Pleural thickening	8,164	0.85
9	Consolidation	34,260	3.57	29	Pneumothorax	741	0.08
10	Costophrenic angle blunting	13,673	1.43	30	Pulmonary edema	8,637	0.90
11	Degenerative changes	18,545	1.93	31	Rib fracture	4,607	0.48
12	Elevated diaphragm	21,913	2.28	32	Scoliosis	4,907	0.51
13	Fibrotic changes	11,027	1.15	33	Soft tissue calcifications	1,086	0.11
14	Fracture	526	0.05	34	Sternotomy wires	45,002	4.69
15	Granuloma	1,475	0.15	35	Surgical clips noted	8,147	0.85
16	Hernia diaphragm	8,892	0.93	36	Thickening of fissure	1,714	0.18
17	Hilar prominence	10,407	1.08	37	Trachea deviation	601	0.06
18	Hyperinflation	37,319	3.89	38	Transplant	5,180	0.54
19	Interstitial markings	97,703	10.18	39	Tube	2,025	0.21
20	Kyphosis	5,531	0.58	40	Vertebral height loss	1,212	0.13

Training Set Generation. On completion of sentence labeling, we set out to design the appropriate training set. A conservative approach would only include studies whose report sentences were *fully-covered*, i.e. every potentially positive sentence in them was manually reviewed and mapped to a finding. A more permissive *any-hit* approach would include any study with a recognized positive sentence in its report, ignoring other unrecognized sentences, with the risk that some of them also mention abnormalities that would be mislabeled as negatives.

The *fully-covered* approach yielded 596k normal studies (no positive findings), and 230k abnormal studies. The *any-hit* approach, while noisier, added 58% more abnormal studies, for a total of 363k. Hence our final training set had 826k studies in the *fully-covered* approach, and 959k studies in the *any-hit* approach.

Additionally, many radiologists will omit mention of normal structures in favor of brevity, thereby implying a negative label. This bias extends to many studies in which even mildly abnormal or senescent changes are omitted. For example, the same CXR may produce a single-line report of *"No acute disease"* by one radiologist and descriptions of cardiomegaly, and degenerative changes by another radiologist. Inherently, this omission bias introduces noise into the labeling process, particularly for findings which are not deemed critical, even in the more conservative *fully-covered* training set.

We decided to compare both approaches, and took the larger *any-hit* training set as our baseline. To the best of our knowledge, this is the largest training set ever assembled for chest X-ray, both in terms of the number of studies and the number of labels (see Table 1 for its composition). We partitioned the training set into *training*, *validation*, and *testing* (80%/10%/10% respectively), based on the (anonymized) patient identity. From the 10% of studies designated as *validation* we compiled a validation set of size 994 with at least 25 positives from each finding. We picked the model with lowest validation loss.

2.1   Model

Our model, called TextRay, is illustrated in Fig. 1. We start by applying a CNN (DenseNet121 [5]) on the Lateral and PA views (separately). We removed the last fully connected layer from each CNN and concatenated their outputs (just after the average pooling layer). We then applied our own fully-connected layer resulting in $K = 40$ outputs, one for each finding, followed by a sigmoid activation. Hence, our model treats each study as a "bag of findings", reporting the confidence for each one. We used the mean of the binary cross-entropy losses as our main loss function:

$$loss = \frac{1}{K} \sum_{k=1}^{K} y_k \log(p_k) + (1 - y_k) \log(1 - p_k)$$

where p_k is the value of the k-th output unit and y_k is the binary label for the k-th finding.

Our model receives two inputs of size 299×299. When lateral view was unavailable, we fed the network with random noise instead. Each X-Ray image (up to 3000×3000 pixels in raw format) was zero-mean-normalized, rescaled to a size of $330(1 + a)$ x $330(1 + b)$, and rotated c degrees. A random patch of 299×299 was taken as input. For training augmentation, we sampled a, b uniformly from ± 0.09 and c from ± 9, randomly flipping each image horizontally. For balance, we replaced the PA view with random noise in 5% of the samples. For test we used $a = b = c = 0$ and took the central patch as input, without flipping.

We trained on two 1080Ti GPUs, putting each CNN on a different GPU. We used the built-in Keras 2.1.3 implementation of DenseNet121 over Tensorflow 1.4. We used the Adam optimizer with Keras' default parameters, and a batch size of 32. We sorted the studies in two queues, normals and abnormals, and filled each batch with 95% abnormal studies on average. An epoch was defined as 150 batches. We started with a learning rate of 0.001 and multiplied it by 0.75 if validation loss hadn't improved for 30 epochs. We trained for 2000 epochs.

2.2   Evaluation Sets

We chose 12 of the 40 findings and prepared evaluation sets for them, using studies from the *test* partition. Most sets focused on a single finding except *cardiomegaly, hilar prominence*, and *pulmonary edema*, which were lumped together as they are commonly seen in the setting of congestive heart failure. In each set, the studies were derived from two pools: *pos-pool* are studies that the reports indicated as positive for that finding. These studies were obtained by a manual textual search for terms indicative for each finding, independently of our sentence-tagging operation; *neg-pool* are randomly sampled studies, which are mostly negative for any finding (see Table 2 for the sets composition).

Each set was evaluated by three expert radiologists. In each set, the radiologist reviewed the shuffled studies and indicated the presence or absence of the relevant finding, using a web-based software operated on a desktop. The radiologists were shown both PA and Lateral view in their original resolutions.

We considered the report as a fourth expert opinion. To measure the accuracy of the label-extraction process, we cross referenced the report opinion with the training set labels. The positive labels in the training set were accurately mentioned the report; frequently, positive findings mentioned in the reports were mislabeled as negatives as would be expected in the *any-hit* training set, but this was also observed to lesser degree even in the *fully-covered* set.

3   Results

We performed pairwise analysis of the radiologist agreement following the procedure in [6], except we used the agreement rate between two taggers (e.g. accuracy) instead of the F1 score, because (a) it also measures agreement on the negatives; and (b) it is easier to interpret. The *average agreement rate* (AAR) for a radiologist (or a model) is the average of the agreement rates achieved against the other two (three for a model) radiologists. The *avg. radiologist rate* is the mean of the three radiologists' AARs. We used the bootstrap method ($n = 10000$) to obtain 95% confidence intervals over the difference between TextRay and the average radiologist agreement rates. As TextRay's threshold for each finding, we used the one that maximized the AAR on the validation set.

Table 2. Evaluation Sets. The number of studies taken from the *pos-pool* (finding is positive in report) and *neg-pool* (random sample) are indicated, along with the average agreement rate (AAR) of the 3 radiologists (rads) assigned to each set vs. the report. The AAR between our model and the rads (column *textray*) is compared against the AAR between any radiologist and the other rads (*avg. rad.*). Confidence intervals are computed over the difference (Δ = textray − avg. rad.).

Finding	Pool		Avg. agreement w/ rads			Δ (CI)
	pos	neg	Report	Avg. rad	Textray	Textray vs. rads
Pulmonary edema	128	482	0.613	0.639	0.730	+0.09 (0.07, 0.11)
Elevated diaphragm	202	77	0.731	0.675	0.754	+0.08 (0.05, 0.10)
Abnormal aorta	198	80	0.736	0.693	0.771	+0.08 (0.05, 0.11)
Hyperinflation	95	80	0.678	0.619	0.657	+0.04 (−0.02, 0.10)
Vertebral height loss	126	55	0.781	0.742	0.757	+0.02 (−0.02, 0.06)
Atelectasis	201	78	0.778	0.756	0.767	+0.01 (−0.03, 0.04)
Cardiomegaly	238	372	0.755	0.861	0.866	+0.01 (−0.02, 0.03)
Pleural effusion	207	73	0.905	0.893	0.896	+0.00 (−0.02, 0.03)
Consolidation	194	78	0.690	0.730	0.707	−0.02 (−0.07, 0.02)
Pneumothorax	111	124	0.830	0.855	0.823	−0.03 (−0.08, 0.01)
Rib fracture	183	76	0.683	0.799	0.745	−0.05 (−0.10, −0.01)
Hilar prominence	184	426	0.552	0.797	0.736	−0.06 (−0.09, −0.03)

Table 2 shows that TextRay is on par with human radiologists (within the 95% CI) on 10 out of 12 findings, with the exception of *rib fracture* and *hilar prominence*. On some findings (*elevated diaphragm*, *abnormal aorta*, and *pulmonary edema*), radiologists agree significantly more with our algorithm than with each other (e.g. the CI does not include 0). Table 2 also shows the average agreement of the radiologists with the report. Here as well, this agreement is often higher than the average agreement among the radiologists themselves. This provides evidence that the noise added by using the reports as labels is no larger than the noise added by training a radiologist to do the tagging.

Using our text-based labels as ground-truth, TextRay's performance was then tested over all 40 findings. To create the test set, a random sample of 5,000 studies was chosen from the *test* partition. Then, more studies were added from the partition until each finding had at least 100 positive cases, for a total of

7,030 studies. The ROCs (in the Supp. material) have AUCs ranging between 0.7 and 1.0 (average 0.892). At the top of the chart, artificial objects (i.e. pacers, lines, tubes, wires, and implants) are detected with AUCs approaching 1.0, much better than all diseases.

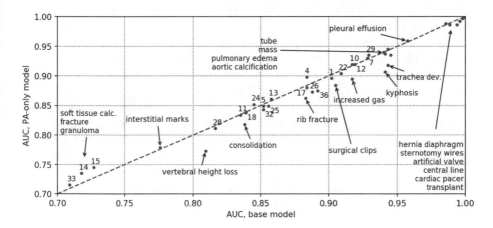

Fig. 2. Area under the ROC curve (AUC) of our base model vs. the PA-only variant over 40 chest X-ray findings. The numbers refer to the index of Table 1. A cluster of labels should be mapped left-to-right.

Figure 2 shows the area under the ROC curve (AUC) achieved by our model compared to a variant that was trained only with the PA view of each study (the approach used in [6,7]). We see that in most findings, the performance is similar, but *vertebral height loss, consolidation, rib fracture*, and *kyphosis* stand out as findings in which the lateral view improved detection. These findings are expected from a clinical radiographic perspective.

For comparison, we also trained a variant of TextRay with the *fully-covered* training set, but it achieved significantly lower results in almost all findings (see Supp. material), suggesting that the additional abnormal studies in the *any-hit* set more than compensated for the higher label noise. Finally, we draw heat maps based on the procedure presented in [7] (presented in Supp. material).

4   Discussion

The extraction of labels from full CXR reports has been recognized as essential for efficient and robust CNN training on large datasets. Shin et al. [8] extracted labels from the 3,955 CXR reports in the OpenI dataset, using the MeSH system [9]. The ChestX-ray14 dataset released by Wang et al. [7] contains 112k PA images loosely labeled using a combination of NLP and hand-crafted rules. Rajpurkar et al. [6] team of four radiologists reported a high degree of disagreement with the provided ChestX-ray14 labels in general, although they demonstrate the ability to achieve expert-level prediction for the presence of pneumonia after training upon a DenseNet121 CNN.

Utilizing several public datasets with image labels and reports provided, Jing et al. [10] built a system that can generate a natural appearing radiology report using a hierarchical RNN. The high-level RNN generates sentence embeddings that seed low-level RNNs that produce the words of each sentence. As part of their report generation, they also produce tags representing the clinical finding present in the image. Interestingly, the model trained using these tags and the text of the reports did not predict the tags better than the model that was trained just using the tags. The ultimate accuracy of the system however remains poorly defined due to lack of clinical radiologic validation.

To the best of our knowledge, the present study is the first to utilize extensive radiology expertise for both multi-label generation and visual validation of algorithmic results. Study labels were generated bottom-up via ontology-based methodology which was rooted in the text rather than pre-existing categories or tags (i.e. MeSH). We trained upon the largest dataset of CXRs described to date, achieving results on twelve distinct visual findings which are on par with inter-radiologist agreement and in some cases, better.

5   Conclusion

In this work we attempt to broadly cover all findings radiologists usually report when reviewing a PA and Lateral chest X-ray. Since a relatively small set of sentences is heavily re-used in CXR reports, we were able to generate organic labels for millions of reports by examining and indexing twenty thousand individual sentences. This massive amount of data allowed us to obtain radiology-level detection performance on various of findings using a single model, in essence distilling the insight of millions of radiographic interpretations into software code. Application of a similar technique upon AP chest X-ray scans, musculoskeletal and abdominal radiographies is currently ongoing.

References

1. Robinson, P.J., Wilson, D., Coral, A., Murphy, A., Verow, P.: Variation between experienced observers in the interpretation of accident and emergency radiographs. Br. J. Radiol. **72**(856), 323–30 (1999)
2. Brady, A., Laoide, R., McCarthy, P., McDermott, R.: Discrepancy and error in radiology: concepts, causes and consequences. Ulster Med. J. **81**(1), 3–9 (2012)
3. Bruno, M.A., Walker, E.A., Abujudeh, H.H.: Understanding and confronting our mistakes: the epidemiology of error in radiology and strategies for error reduction. RadioGraphics **35**(6), 1668–1676 (2015)
4. Hanna, T.N., Lamoureux, C., Krupinski, E.A., Weber, S., Johnson, J.O.: Effect of shift, schedule, and volume on interpretive accuracy: a retrospective analysis of 2.9 million radiologic examinations. Radiology (2017) 170555
5. Huang, G., Liu, Z., van der Maaten, L., Weinberger, K.Q.: Densely connected convolutional networks. In: Proceedings of the IEEE Conference on Computer Vision and Pattern Recognition (2017)

6. Rajpurkar, P., et al.: CheXNet: radiologist-level pneumonia detection on chest X-rays with deep learning (2017)
7. Wang, X., et al.: Chestx-ray8: hospital-scale chest x-ray database and benchmarks on weakly-supervised classification and localization of common thorax diseases (2017). openaccess.thecvf.com
8. Shin, H.C., Roberts, K., Lu, L., Demner-Fushman, D., Yao, J., Summers, R.M.: Learning to read chest x-rays: recurrent neural cascade model for automated image annotation. In: Computer Vision and Pattern Recognition (CVPR), June 2016
9. Demner-Fushman, D., Shooshan, S.E., Rodriguez, L., Antani, S., Thoma, G.R.: Annotation of chest radiology reports forindexing and retrieval, pp. 99–111 (2015)
10. Jing, B., Xie, P., Xing, E.: On the automatic generation of medical imaging reports, November 2017

Localization and Labeling of Posterior Ribs in Chest Radiographs Using a CRF-regularized FCN with Local Refinement

Alexander Oliver Mader[1,2,3(✉)], Jens von Berg[3], Alexander Fabritz[2], Cristian Lorenz[3], and Carsten Meyer[1,2,3]

[1] Institute of Computer Science, Kiel University of Applied Sciences, Kiel, Germany
`alexander.o.mader@fh-kiel.de`
[2] Department of Computer Science, Faculty of Engineering, Kiel University, Kiel, Germany
[3] Department of Digital Imaging, Philips Research Hamburg, Hamburg, Germany

Abstract. Localization and labeling of posterior ribs in radiographs is an important task and a prerequisite for, e.g., quality assessment, image registration, and automated diagnosis. In this paper, we propose an automatic, general approach for localizing spatially correlated landmarks using a fully convolutional network (FCN) regularized by a conditional random field (CRF) and apply it to rib localization. A reduced CRF state space in form of localization hypotheses (generated by the FCN) is used to make CRF inference feasible, potentially missing correct locations. Thus, we propose a second CRF inference step searching for additional locations. To this end, we introduce a novel "refine" label in the first inference step. For "refine"-labeled nodes, small subgraphs are extracted and a second inference is performed on all image pixels. The approach is thoroughly evaluated on 642 images of the public Indiana chest X-ray collection, achieving a landmark localization rate of 94.6%.

Keywords: Posterior ribs · Localization and labeling
Chest radiography · Fullyconvolutional network
Conditional random field

1 Introduction

Segmenting ribs in chest radiographs is used for the analysis of the lung parenchyma, as the overlaid ribs may obscure important findings. Rib shadows may be either excluded from the automatic analysis [1] or suppressed from the image [2] to minimize their impact. Ribs may also be used as an anatomical reference

Electronic supplementary material The online version of this chapter (https://doi.org/10.1007/978-3-030-00934-2_63) contains supplementary material, which is available to authorized users.

© Springer Nature Switzerland AG 2018
A. F. Frangi et al. (Eds.): MICCAI 2018, LNCS 11071, pp. 562–570, 2018.
https://doi.org/10.1007/978-3-030-00934-2_63

to automatically locate findings like lung lesions or to establish correspondence between different images (e.g., in follow-up acquisition). Further on, counting the ribs in the lung field is a standard radiological procedure used to assure proper inhalation state in chest X-ray quality assessment. Unlike the previous two, these applications require the ribs not only to be segmented, but also to be anatomically labeled correctly.

There is a number of methods described in literature to segment ribs in chest radiographs using either pixel classification [3], atlas registration [1], or a mixture of methods [4]. But there is no method described yet that does a robust anatomical labeling of posterior ribs. Even the atlas-based method did not use rib labels. Unlike CT where this task could be solved easier [5,6], the upper ribs are often overlaid in a chest radiograph (by, e.g., clavicles and other ribs) in a way that may prevent an algorithm from identifying and counting all the upper ribs properly. Also using the lung field as reference space appears not to be sufficient to unambiguously assign an anatomic label to a detected rib.

In this paper, we propose an automatic and general approach for localizing and labeling spatially correlated point landmarks. We apply our approach specifically to rib localization and labeling in posterior-anterior chest radiographs, by formulating the problem as finding a key point on each rib near the rib center. Unlike previous methods, it is a general approach and does not make or need any assumption about the task. Instead, all model parameters are automatically learned from annotated training data. First, the fully convolutional network (FCN) U-Net [7] is used to generate localization hypotheses. Then, a conditional random field (CRF) is applied to assess spatial information between landmarks. For feasibility, the CRF state space is combinatorically defined by the U-Net-generated localization hypotheses. Since the CRF has no means to select other than these localization hypotheses, we introduce a novel "refine" label. This allows the CRF to select this label instead of any of the localization hypotheses in case, e.g., none of them presents a viable option w.r.t. the CRF model. A second inference is performed for all "refine"-labeled nodes on a local subgraph over all image pixels rather than the set of localization hypotheses. Applying our approach to 642 images of the publicly available Indiana chest X-ray collection [8], we are able to localize and label 94.6% of the 16 individual landmarks correctly, corresponding to 83.0% fully correct cases. A median distance to the rib centerline of 0.7 mm is achieved.

2   Method

We formulate the problem as predicting $N = 16$ labeled key points for each posterior rib (2nd to 9th) close to its centerline (see Fig. 3a) in posterior-anterior chest radiographs. Our approach to solve this problem is split into three steps (compare Fig. 1): First, a FCN is used to regress heat maps to derive $n = 15$ localization hypotheses $\hat{\mathcal{X}}_i = \{\hat{\mathbf{x}}_{i,1}, \ldots, \hat{\mathbf{x}}_{i,n}\}$ for each key point $i \in [1 .. N]$ (Fig. 1a). Second, the unary information of the localizer is combined with binary information assessing spatial features between key point localization hypotheses. Both are jointly modeled in a CRF with key points being the nodes and the corresponding localization hypotheses the respective states. An additional "refine" label is introduced for each node to be selected if no localization hypotheses is plausible (given the CRF model). CRF A* inference [9] is applied to find the best selection $\hat{\mathbf{S}} = (\hat{s}_1, \ldots, \hat{s}_N) \in [0..n]^N$ out of all possible selections $|\mathcal{S}| = (n+1)^N$. For each key point i, the inference either selects a localization hypothesis $\hat{\mathbf{x}}_{i,\hat{s}_i}$ if $\hat{s}_i \in [1..n]$, or the "refine" label if $\hat{s}_i = 0$ (Fig. 1b). In the third step, we derive positions for the "refine"-labeled nodes. We fix all nodes with predicted positions and optimize each "refine" node in a small subgraph over all image pixels rather than over the n localization hypotheses only (Fig. 1c). The following three subsections describe each step in detail.

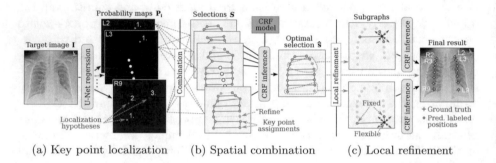

(a) Key point localization   (b) Spatial combination   (c) Local refinement

Fig. 1. Schematic illustration of our three-step approach: (a) Generation of localization hypotheses using a U-Net, (b) followed by a CRF modelling spatial relations between key points and (c) a final local refinement based on a subgraph considering the whole image domain.

2.1   Generating Localization Hypotheses Using a U-Net

The goal of the first step is to predict candidate positions for each key point. The basic idea is to transform an image $\mathbf{I} : \mathbb{R}^2 \rightarrow \mathbb{R}$ into pseudo (not normalized) probability maps $\widetilde{\mathbf{P}}_i : \mathbb{R}^2 \rightarrow \mathbb{R}^+$ (for each target key point i) in which the location of the highest value $\hat{\mathbf{x}}_{i,1} = \arg\max_{\mathbf{x}} \widetilde{\mathbf{P}}_i(\mathbf{x})$ corresponds to the most likely predicted position of key point i.

To do so, we use U-Net [7], which has proven to deliver good results in the medical domain. However, its architecture is designed for pixel-wise segmentation, while we aim at localizing points to combine it with a CRF. Therefore, we directly formulate the problem as a pixel-wise heat map regression. This is achieved by dropping the soft-max classification and extending the final layer to N feature maps. Each feature map corresponds to a key point specific heat map that we want to regress. Assuming that high values in these heat maps correspond to likely positions of the searched key point, we can simply apply non-maximum suppression to each heat map to generate n localization hypotheses $\hat{\mathcal{X}}_i = \{\hat{\mathbf{x}}_{i,1}, \ldots, \hat{\mathbf{x}}_{i,n}\}$ (we use $n = 15$) for each key point i. This setup allows to generate localization hypotheses jointly for all key points in a single network.

Training. The modified U-Net is trained using stochastic gradient descent in the form of the Adam [10] algorithm using standard parameters with a mini-batch size of 8 and a sum-squared-error loss function. The target regression values are defined by a multivariate Gaussian distribution $\mathcal{N}(\mathbf{x}_i^*, 1/91r^2)$ with its mean located at the key point's true position $\mathbf{x}_i^*$. This provides high values close to the true position and very low values outside a small neighborhood ($r = 6$). As advocated in [7], we also perform data augmentation in form of elastic transformations of the training images, effectively increasing the training set size by the factor 11. We stop the training after 1000 epochs.

2.2   Selecting Reasonable Localization Hypotheses Using a CRF

To compensate for potentially incorrect first best localization hypotheses $\hat{\mathbf{x}}_{i,1}$ for arbitrary key points i, we use a CRF to model geometric relationships between key points. Each key point $i \in [1..N]$ is represented by a node in the graph with the corresponding localization hypotheses $\hat{\mathcal{X}}_i$ being the respective labels. We introduce an additional "refine" label for the CRF to choose during inference to compensate for cases where none of the localization hypotheses is plausible (and might negatively influence the selection of neighboring nodes). This "refine" label is used in our third step (Sect. 2.3) to still derive an accurate prediction in case CRF inference assigned the "refine" label to any node.

An energy-based formulation is applied where a low energy $E(\mathbf{S})$ of a selection $\mathbf{S} = (s_1, \ldots, s_N)$ implies a large posterior probability. For each node, either a localization hypothesis $\hat{\mathbf{x}}_{i,s_i}$ is assumed if $s_i > 0$, or the "refine" label if $s_i = 0$. The energy $E(\mathbf{S})$ of the CRF is parameterized by a set of J unary and binary potential functions $\Phi = \{\phi_1(\cdot), \ldots, \phi_J(\cdot)\}$ with corresponding weights $\mathbf{\Lambda} = (\lambda_1, \ldots, \lambda_J)$ and missing potential values $\boldsymbol{\beta} = (\beta_1, \ldots, \beta_J)$ for the "refine" label $s_i = 0$:

$$E(\mathbf{S}) = \sum_{j=1}^{J} \lambda_j \cdot \begin{cases} \beta_j & \text{if } s_i = 0 \text{ for any } i \in \text{Scope}(\phi_j) \\ \phi_j(\mathbf{S}) & \text{else} \end{cases} . \tag{1}$$

The inclusion of the missing energy values $\boldsymbol{\beta}$ is necessary, because it is not possible to compute potential values for the "refine" label $s_i = 0$. We use the same four potential types as introduced in [11]: For each key point i, an unary potential $\phi_i^{\text{loc}}(\mathbf{S})$ corresponding to the localizer's respective heat map value is introduced (see Fig. 2a). For each key point pair i and j, a distance 0potential $\phi_{i,j}^{\text{dist}}(\mathbf{S})$, an angle potential $\phi_{i,j}^{\text{ang}}(\mathbf{S})$ and a vector potential $\phi_{i,j}^{\text{vec}}(\mathbf{S})$ are used to model the geometric relations. The probability densities of estimated Gaussian, von Mises and multivariate Gaussian distributions, respectively, are used as potential values (see Fig. 2b). Finally, to efficiently find the best selection $\hat{\mathbf{S}} = \arg\min_{\mathbf{S} \in \mathcal{S}} E(\mathbf{S})$, exact inference in form of the A* algorithm [9] is applied.

Training. The weights $\boldsymbol{\Lambda}$ and the missing energies $\boldsymbol{\beta}$ are automatically learned in a training phase using a gradient descent scheme minimizing a max-margin hinge loss L over data $\mathcal{D} = \{\mathbf{d}_1, \ldots, \mathbf{d}_K\}$. The idea is to increase the energy gap between the "correct" selection $\mathbf{S}^+$ and the best (lowest energy) "incorrect" selection $\mathbf{S}^-$ until a certain margin m is satisfied. Let our loss function be defined as

$$L(\boldsymbol{\Lambda}, \boldsymbol{\beta}) = \frac{1}{K} \sum_{k=1}^{K} \delta(\mathbf{S}_k^+, \mathbf{S}_k^-) \cdot \max\left(0, m + E(\mathbf{S}_k^+) - E(\mathbf{S}_k^-)\right) + \theta \cdot \|\boldsymbol{\Lambda}\|_1 \quad (2)$$

subject to $\lambda_j \geq 0$ for $j = 1, \ldots, J$, with

$$\delta(\mathbf{S}_k^+, \mathbf{S}_k^-) = \frac{1}{NR}\left(e(\mathbf{S}_k^-) - e(\mathbf{S}_k^+)\right) \in [0, 1] \quad (3)$$

weighting each training sample k w.r.t. the reduction in error (capped at $R = 100$)

$$e(\mathbf{S}) = \sum_{i=1}^{N} \begin{cases} 0 & \text{if "refine"}(s_i = 0) \text{ predicted and true,} \\ \min\left(R, \|\hat{\mathbf{x}}_{i,s_i} - \mathbf{x}_i^*\|_2\right) & \text{if "non-refine"}(s_i > 0) \text{ pred. and true,} \\ R & \text{else,} \end{cases} \quad (4)$$

going from the incorrect selection $\mathbf{S}_k^-$ to the correct selection $\mathbf{S}_k^+$. The "refine" label ($s_i = 0$) is assumed true, if none of the localization hypotheses ($s_i > 0$) is correct (the localization criterion is defined in Sect. 3). An additional θ-weighted L1 regularization term w.r.t. $\boldsymbol{\Lambda}$ was added to further accelerate the sparsification of terms. To optimize the loss function from Eq. (2), we apply again the Adam algorithm [10] starting from a grid-structured (Fig. 1b) graph. Once all CRF parameters are estimated, we remove unnecessary potentials where $\lambda_j = 0$, effectively optimizing the graph topology and improving the inference time while simultaneously improving the localization performance.

2.3 Going Beyond Potentially Incorrect Localization Hypotheses

After finding the optimal selection $\hat{\mathbf{S}}$ using CRF inference, we look at all key points $\{i \mid s_i = 0\}$ that have the "refine" label $s_i = 0$ instead of a localization hypothesis assigned. In order to assign those nodes a position, we start by fixing all nodes $\{i \mid s_i > 0\}$ with a properly selected localization hypothesis $\hat{\mathbf{x}}_{i,s_i}$. Then, we individually optimize each "refine"-labeled node by considering all connected binary potentials $\Phi_i = \{\phi_j \mid i \in \text{Scope}(\phi_j) \wedge \exists i' : (i' \in \text{Scope}(\phi_j) \wedge s_{i'} > 0)\}$ that are fully specified (except for the current node). Given that this second inference

$$\widetilde{\mathbf{x}}_i = \arg\min_{\mathbf{x} \in \mathbf{I}} \sum_{\phi_j' \in \Phi_i} \lambda_j \cdot \phi_j'(\mathbf{x}) \quad (5)$$

is performed on a very small subgraph, we can increase the search space to all possible pixel positions $\mathbf{x} \in \mathbf{I}$ for that node, rather than the set of localization hypotheses, which would be intractable on the full problem. Note that we used some handwavy notation ϕ'_j to indicate that the (binary) potentials are computed by solely altering the position of key point i, since all others are known and fixed. By optimizing all "refine" nodes in decreasing order of the number of connected potentials $|\Phi_i|$, we can use previously refined positions in the next optimization in terms of more usable potentials. This also prevents the case that a node may not have any usable potential. How this approach can overcome the limitation of the fixed state space is illustrated on a test case in Fig. 2. Note that this final step does not require any training.

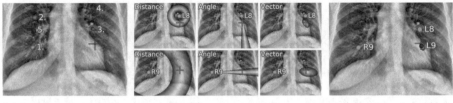

(a) Localizer hypotheses   (b) Binary potentials   (c) Combined result

Fig. 2. Illustration of the refinement process for L9 (true key point indicated as red cross). The "refine" label was chosen by the CRF inference for L9 because all n localizer hypotheses – shown enumerated in (a), heat map overlaid on cropped original image – yield large total energies $E(\mathbf{S})$. Utilizing the connected (b) binary potentials from L8 and R9, we are still able to (c) predict a correct position (red point) for L9 by evaluating over all image pixels instead of just the (here incorrect) localization hypotheses.

3   Experiments and Results

We evaluated our approach on 1000 consecutive images of various quality of the publicly available anonymized Indiana chest X-ray collection from the U.S. National Library of Medicine [8], downsampled to an isotropic resolution of $1 \times 1\text{mm/px}$. To derive key points for the unlabeled images for training and evaluation, we started by generating unlabeled posterior rib centerlines using an automatic approach based on [4]. The generated centerlines were then manually checked for quality, i.e., the line should be properly located within the rib, and correctly labeled, potentially discarding images. Following this approach, we generated labeled centerlines for the posterior ribs $L2, \ldots, L9, R2, \ldots, R9$ for 642 images. The middle points on the centerlines (w.r.t. the x-axis) have been selected as point annotations for each key point (except for the second and third rib where a factor of ±0.3 and ±0.4, respectively, instead of 0.5 was chosen). A corresponding predicted point is treated correct (localization and labeling criterion) if it is close to the annotated point (distance $\leq 15\,mm$) and very close to the centerline (distance $\leq 7.5\,mm$). This resembles the test whether the point lays on the rib while allowing for some translation along the rib. An example annotation as well as this localization criterion are depicted in Fig. 3a.

Note that correct point localizations also mean correct labels for the previously generated unlabeled centerlines, which effectively means the automatic generation of labeled centerlines as well.

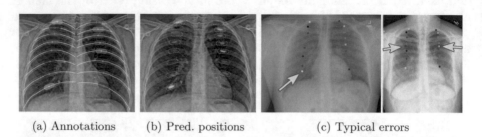

(a) Annotations   (b) Pred. positions   (c) Typical errors

Fig. 3. (a) Illustration of the centerline and key point annotations and the resulting localization criterion, i.e., the area where a localization hypothesis is considered correct. Images in (a) and (b) are cropped and have been enhanced using adaptive histogram equalization. (b) Predicted positions in 642 test images visualized in a single image by registering the images using the true positions (affine and b-spline) and warping the predicted positions. Labels are shown color coded. (c) Typical errors involve an incorrect localization in the abdomen (first image) and chain errors caused by intermediate mistakes (second image).

We used a 3-fold cross-validation setup in our experiments, which provided us with 428 training images in each fold. Each training corpus was divided into three non-overlapping subsets $\mathcal{D}_{\text{pot}}$, $\mathcal{D}_{\text{weights}}$ and $\mathcal{D}_{\text{val}}$, containing 50%, 40%, 10% randomly selected training images, respectively. $\mathcal{D}_{\text{pot}}$ was used to train the localizer (Scct. 2.1) and to estimate the statistics of the CRF potential functions (means, variances). $\mathcal{D}_{\text{weights}}$ was used to optimize the CRF potential weights $\mathbf{\Lambda}$ and to estimate the missing energies $\boldsymbol{\beta}$. The last subset $\mathcal{D}_{\text{val}}$ was used as validation corpus to select unknown meta parameters like learning rate and regularization parameter θ.

Applying our method, 94.6% of the key points were labeled correctly, corresponding to 83.0% of the images where all 16 key points were correct. The rates for individual key points and for the different steps in our chain are depicted in Fig. 4. First, we see that the CRF improves upon the plain U-Net results, especially in terms of the number of correct cases. Second, we see that the U-Net provides few good alternative localization hypotheses, which is apparent in a bad upper bound of the CRF of just 59.7% and justifies our third step. Third, we see that the additional CRF refinement step improves upon the CRF, where the percentage of correct cases increases dramatically from 57.3% to 83.0%. Fourth, the performance slightly decreases towards the lower ribs, which is probably caused by low contrast, higher variability and fewer meaningful surrounding structures (Fig. 3c). Errors in terms of Euclidean distance to the true position as well as distance to the centerline are listed in Table 1. The resulting median values of 2.8 mm and 0.7 mm, respectively, are in line with the visualization of the prediction results depicted in Fig. 3b. The overall average runtime of our approach per case comes down to 36 ms U-Net + 61 ms CRF + 73 ms refinement = 170 ms running our unoptimized Python implementation on an Intel Xeon CPU E5-2650 in combination with an NVIDIA Titan X.

See supplement 1 for supporting content.

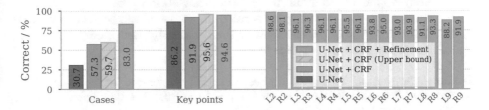

Fig. 4. Rates for correct cases (i.e., all 16 key points localized correctly) and correctly localized key points for our three steps in percent. Upper bound indicates the theoretical maximal performance of the CRF, caused by the limitation of the state space to the set of localization hypotheses. 100% corresponds to 642 cases and individual key points (L2-R9), and 642 · 16 = 10272 total key points.

Table 1. Median and mean Euclidean distance between true and predicted position (error) as well as median and mean distance between centerline and predicted position (line distance) for individual and all key points in mm.

Metric	L2	R2	L3	R3	L4	R4	L5	R5	L6	R6	L7	R7	L8	R8	L9	R9	All
Error / mm																	
Median	3.3	3.4	3.0	3.0	2.1	2.6	2.0	2.1	2.3	2.3	2.5	2.6	3.4	2.8	4.6	3.8	**2.8**
Mean	4.1	4.3	3.9	4.0	3.4	3.6	3.3	3.5	4.0	3.9	4.6	4.8	6.4	5.6	8.4	6.8	**4.7**
Line distance / mm																	
Median	0.8	0.9	0.8	0.9	0.6	0.6	0.5	0.5	0.5	0.5	0.6	0.6	0.9	0.8	1.2	1.1	**0.7**
Mean	1.2	1.2	1.6	1.6	1.7	1.4	1.6	1.5	2.1	1.9	2.6	2.7	3.9	3.3	4.8	4.0	**2.3**

4   Discussion and Conclusions

We presented a general approach for localization and labeling of spatially corre-lated key points and applied it to the task of rib localization. The state-of-the-art FCN U-Net has been used as localizer, which was regularized by a CRF incorpo-rating spatial information between key points. The limitation of a reduced CRF state space in form of localization hypotheses imposed by the exact CRF infer-ence in large graphs has been overcome with a novel "refine" node label. After a first CRF inference, a second inference is performed on small subgraphs formed by the marked "refine" nodes to refine the respective key points over all image pixels (rather than the set of localization hypotheses). Applying our approach to 624 images of the publicly available Indiana chest X-ray collection [8], we were able to correctly localize and label 94.6% of the 16 key points, corresponding to 83.0% fully correct cases. The introduced refinement allowed for an increase of 25.7 percent points in fully correct cases over the global CRF alone. Note that this was achieved without domain-specific assumptions; all CRF model parameters were automatically learned from annotated training data. Our approach is thus directly applicable to other anatomical localization tasks.

In future work, we are going to increase the rotation and scaling invariance by incorporating ternary potentials over the commonly used binary ones, with tractability being the main challenge.

Acknowledgements. This work has been financially supported by the Federal Ministry of Education and Research under the grant 03FH013IX5. The liability for the content of this work lies with the authors.

References

1. Candemir, S., et al.: Atlas-based rib-bone detection in chest X-rays. CMIG **51**, 32–39 (2016)
2. von Berg, J., et al.: A novel bone suppression method that improves lung nodule detection. IJCARS **11**(4), 641–655 (2016)
3. Loog, M., Ginneken, B.: Segmentation of the posterior ribs in chest radiographs using iterated contextual pixel classification. T-MI **25**(5), 602–611 (2006)
4. von Berg, J., et al.: Decomposing the bony thorax in X-ray images. In: ISBI, pp. 1068–1071 (2016)
5. Staal, J., Ginneken, B., Viergever, M.: Automatic rib segmentation and labeling in computed tomography scans using a general framework for detection, recognition and segmentation of objects in volumetric data. MIA **11**(1), 35–46 (2007)
6. Wu, D., et al.: A learning based deformable template matching method for automatic rib centerline extraction and labeling in CT images. In: CVPR, pp. 980–987. IEEE (2012)
7. Ronneberger, O., Fischer, P., Brox, T.: U-Net: convolutional networks for biomedical image segmentation. In: Navab, N., Hornegger, J., Wells, W.M., Frangi, A.F. (eds.) MICCAI 2015. LNCS, vol. 9351, pp. 234–241. Springer, Cham (2015). https://doi.org/10.1007/978-3-319-24574-4_28
8. U.S. National Library of Medicine (NLM): Open-i Open Access Biomedical Image Search Engine (2017). https://openi.nlm.nih.gov. Accessed 14 Feb 2018
9. Bergtholdt, M., Kappes, J.H., Schnörr, C.: Learning of graphical models and efficient inference for object class recognition. In: Franke, K., Müller, K.-R., Nickolay, B., Schäfer, R. (eds.) DAGM 2006. LNCS, vol. 4174, pp. 273–283. Springer, Heidelberg (2006). https://doi.org/10.1007/11861898_28
10. Kingma, D.P., Ba, J.: Adam: a method for stochastic optimization. In: ICLR (2014)
11. Mader, A.O., et al.: Detection and localization of landmarks in the lower extremities using an automatically learned conditional random field. In: GRAIL (2017)

Evaluation of Collimation Prediction Based on Depth Images and Automated Landmark Detection for Routine Clinical Chest X-Ray Exams

Julien Sénégas[1]([✉]), Axel Saalbach[1], Martin Bergtholdt[1],
Sascha Jockel[2], Detlef Mentrup[2], and Roman Fischbach[3]

[1] Philips Research, Roentgenstrasse 24, 22335 Hamburg, Germany
julien.senegas@philips.com
[2] Philips Medical Systems, Roentgenstrasse 24, 22335 Hamburg, Germany
[3] Asklepios Klinik Altona, Paul-Ehrlich-Str. 1, 22763 Hamburg, Germany

Abstract. The aim of this study was to evaluate the performance of a machine learning algorithm applied to depth images for the automated computation of X-ray beam collimation parameters in radiographic chest examinations including posterior-anterior (PA) and left-lateral (LAT) views. Our approach used as intermediate step a trained classifier for the detection of internal lung landmarks that were defined on X-ray images acquired simultaneously with the depth image. The landmark detection algorithm was evaluated retrospectively in a 5-fold cross validation experiment on the basis of 89 patient data sets acquired in clinical settings. Two auto-collimation algorithms were devised and their results were compared to the reference lung bounding boxes defined on the X-ray images and to the manual collimation parameters set by the radiologic technologists.

Keywords: Boosted tree classifiers · Gentle AdaBoost
Anatomical landmarks · Detection · Constellation model
Multivariate regression · X-ray beam collimation

1 Introduction

Conventional X-ray radiography is still the most frequently performed X-ray examination. According to the ALARA[1] principle [1], the radiographic technologist is requested to collimate the X-ray beam to the area of interest to avoid overexposure and to reduce scattered radiation. However, as a consequence of time pressure and training level of the technologists, a significant number of X-ray acquisitions need to be retaken, with numbers varying from 3%–10% [2–4] to 24,5% [5]. In the study published in [5], it was found that errors in patient positioning and/or collimation were the main reason for retake in 67,5% of the cases, while retakes in chest X-ray exams accounted for 37,7% of the total number of retakes. Optical-based methods haven been proposed in a

---

[1] ALARA: As Low As Reasonably Achievable

© Springer Nature Switzerland AG 2018
A. F. Frangi et al. (Eds.): MICCAI 2018, LNCS 11071, pp. 571–579, 2018.
https://doi.org/10.1007/978-3-030-00934-2_64

number of medical imaging applications as a way to automatically assess patient position and morphology and to derive optimal acquisition parameters [6, 7]. More recently, Singh et al. [8] demonstrated significant advances in the detection of anatomical landmarks in depth images acquired by a 3D camera by means of deep convolutional networks. While they used an extensive patient dataset consisting of CT volumetric scans for validation, their results were restricted to the evaluation of landmark detection and body mesh fitting and did not cover automating the CT acquisition itself. In the context of X-ray radiography, MacDougall et al. [9] used a 3D camera to automatically derive patient thickness measurements and detect motion of the examined body part in order to provide guidance to the technologist. Their work did not address the automated computation of system acquisition parameters.

In this paper, we present a method to automatically compute the X-ray beam collimation parameters for posterior-anterior (PA) and lateral (LAT) chest X-ray acquisitions on the basis of 3D camera data. The proposed algorithm detects lung landmarks in the depth image and applies a statistical model to derive patient-specific collimation parameters. Landmarks and regression models were learned from reference data generated on the basis of X-ray and depth image pairs acquired simultaneously during routine clinical exams. The algorithm results are evaluated in a 5-fold cross-validation experiment and compared to the parameters manually set by the radiographic technologists.

2 Methods

A 3D camera (Asus Xtion Pro) was mounted on the side of a clinical X-ray system and connected to a PC for data acquisition. For each patient undergoing an upright chest X-ray exam and having given written consent to participate to the study, a video sequence of depth images covering the duration of the examination was acquired. A total of 89 chest X-ray examinations (PA and LAT views) were acquired over a period of 15 days. The camera was used solely as by-stander, i.e. the depth images were not used in the routine workflow. X-ray retakes were present in 6 out of 89 PA cases and in 1 out of 80 LAT cases leading to 96 PA and 81 LAT acquisitions in total.

2.1 Data Pre-processing

For the retrospective analysis, the following datasets were used: raw X-ray images, depth image series, logfiles from the X-ray system comprising system geometry parameters and collimation parameters selected by the radiographic technologists during the examinations. Based on the timestamps of X-ray release, pairs of X-ray and depth images acquired almost simultaneously were created for each X-ray acquisition and used as basis for the subsequent data analysis. An example is shown in Fig. 1.

Calibration of Camera Extrinsic Parameters. For each examination, the extrinsic camera parameters describing camera position and orientation with respect to the reference coordinate system of the X-ray system were computed. A template matching approach based on the known 3D template of the detector front-cover and an iterative closest point algorithm [10] was applied for this calibration procedure. An example of calibration result is given in Fig. 1.

Reformatting of Depth Images. Based on the extrinsic camera parameters, reformatted depth images were computed from the original depth images by applying a geometry transformation in which the coordinate system of the X-ray tube was taken as reference. For this purpose, a virtual camera was placed at the position of the X-ray focal point, with the main axes of the camera aligned with the axes of the tube coordinate system, and each depth pixel on the original depth image was re-projected onto this geometry. An example of original and corresponding reformatted depth image is shown in Fig. 1.

This approach offered the advantages to eliminate the variability due to the position of the 3D camera, and to facilitate the projection of landmarks defined in the X-ray image onto the depth image (see below for further details).

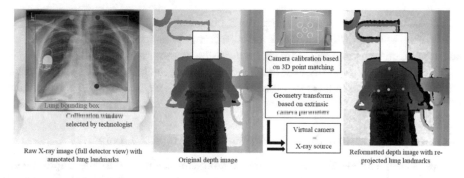

Fig. 1. Overview of the pre-processing steps: the raw X-ray image with manually annotated lung landmarks (colored dots), lung bounding box (blue rectangle) and collimation window selected by the technologist (purple rectangle) and the corresponding original depth image are shown on the left. The calibrated extrinsic camera parameters, computed on the basis of a 3D point matching approach (middle, top), are applied to compute a reformatted depth image corresponding to a virtual camera located at the X-ray source (right). The annotated lung landmarks are mapped onto this reformatted depth image. (Color figure online)

2.2   Annotation of Reference Lung Landmarks and Lung Bounding Box

The anatomical extents of the lung were manually annotated in all PA and LAT X-ray images to provide a reference with which to compare the collimation parameters selected by the technologist on the one side and those computed by the auto-collimation algorithm on the other side. For this purpose, 6 anatomical landmarks were defined on PA X-ray views and 5 landmarks were defined on LAT X-ray views (Table 1). Landmark annotation was done by a technical expert, not by a clinical expert. The variability due to inaccurate landmark localization was not quantified within this study.

Table 1. Overview of lung landmarks defined on X-ray PA and LAT views

Landmark label	View	Localization on X-ray image
LeftLungApexPA	PA	Upper extremity of the left lung apex
LeftLungBaseLatPA	PA	Lower left lateral extremity of the left lung apex
LeftLungBaseMedPA	PA	Lower medial extremity of the left lung apex
RightLungApexPA	PA	Upper extremity of the right lung apex
RightLungBaseLatPA	PA	Lower right lateral extremity of the right lung apex
RightLungBaseMedPA	PA	Lower medial extremity of the right lung apex
LungApexLL	LAT	Upper extremity of the lung apex
LungBaseAntLL	LAT	Lower anterior extremity of the lungs
LungBasePostLL	LAT	Lower posterior extremity of the lungs
LungSpineLL	LAT	Most posterior extremity of the lungs, ca. T6/T7
LungSternumLL	LAT	Anterior lung position, ca. sternum

In each case, parameters of the lung bounding box ($LungBB_{Left}$, $LungBB_{Right}$, $LungBB_{Top}$, and $LungBB_{Bottom}$) were derived from the annotated landmarks using min and max operations on the landmark coordinates, without additional margins.

In order to train a classifier for the detection of lung landmarks on the depth images, the lung landmarks annotated in the X-ray images were mapped onto the corresponding reformatted depth images using the calibrated extrinsic camera parameters.

2.3   Trained Classifier for the Detection of Anatomical Landmarks

In this study, the identification of the anatomical landmarks in the depth images employed a classification-based detection approach similar to the technique proposed by Shotton et al. [11], in combination with a constellation model for the estimation of the most plausible landmark configuration and the prediction of missing landmarks [12]. The detection framework was implemented in C++ using OpenCV 3.3.

Using a fixed sampling pattern generated from a uniform sampling distribution, depth values at single positions as well as pair-wise depth differences within a sliding window were used as classification features to characterize the landmarks. To increase robustness against changes in patient position, the size of the pattern was adjusted dynamically based on the depth value of the current pixel.

During the training phase, features were extracted in the vicinity of the annotated landmarks (positive samples), as well as randomly from the remainder of the depth image (negative samples). These data were then used to train landmark-specific classifiers (i.e. boosted tree classifiers based on Gentle AdaBoost [13]). Here, for all landmarks, a single feature descriptor with 2500 elements was employed, while the classifiers were trained with 25 decision trees with a maximum depth of 5. During the detection phase, a mean-shift clustering algorithm [14] was applied as post-processing to reduce the number of candidates classified as possible landmarks.

Finally, the most plausible landmark combination was identified by evaluating all landmark configurations on the basis of a multivariate Gaussian distribution model and retaining only the configuration with the highest probability. If a particular landmark was not detected during the classification step, its most likely position was predicted based on the conditional distribution of the constellation model, as described in [12]. The parameters of the constellation model, which consisted of the Gaussian distribution of the relative landmark coordinates, were estimated from the training data.

For the evaluation of the classifier trained with the patient data, a 5-fold cross-validation approach was chosen to make sure that the detection results were not generated with the same data as used for training.

2.4   Statistical Models for the Computation of Collimation Parameters

Anatomical landmarks detected in the depth images using the classifiers described in Sect. 2.3 were projected onto the coordinate system of the X-ray detector, using the X-ray source as center of projection. In this way, lung landmarks detected by the classifiers, collimation parameters selected by the technologist, and reference lung landmarks and bounding boxes were all available in the same coordinate system.

Multivariable linear regression analysis was then performed to compute prediction models based on the coordinates of the detected landmarks using the function lm of the statistical software R. The left and right X-coordinates of the reference lung bounding box ($LungBB_{Left}$ and $LungBB_{Right}$), respectively upper and lower Y-coordinates ($LungBB_{Top}$ and $LungBB_{Bottom}$), were fitted using the X-coordinates, respectively the Y-coordinates, of the detected landmarks. The regression models were of the form:

$$y = a + \sum_{1 \leq i \leq n} b_i \cdot x_i$$

where y is the bounding box parameter to be predicted, $(x_i)_{1 \leq i \leq n}$ are the landmark coordinates in the X-ray detector coordinate system, a is the intercept parameter of the regression analysis, and $(b_i)_{1 \leq i \leq n}$ are the regression coefficients.

To compute a collimation window that will contain the lung with high certainty, safety margins were added to the bounding box coordinates. Denoting ROX_{Left}, ROX_{Right}, ROX_{Top}, and ROX_{Bottom} the collimation parameters corresponding to the X- and Y-coordinates of the collimation window, the following formula were applied:

$$ROX_{\{Left,Right,Top,Bottom\}} = LungBB_{\{Left,Right,Top,Bottom\}} + Offset_{\{Left,Right,Top,Bottom\}}$$

Two approaches were applied to compute the offset parameters:

1. QuantileBasedPrediction: Each offset parameter was computed as the 99% quantile of the regression residuals.
2. SDBasedPrediction: Each offset parameter was computed as the standard deviation of the regression residuals multiplied by a given factor (1.65 in this study).

Cases with detection outliers, identified as landmarks with coordinates outside the field-of-view of the X-ray detector, were removed from the regression analysis.

3 Results

Examples of lung landmark detection results obtained with the trained classifier in four randomly selected cases with both PA and LAT views are shown on Fig. 2. Landmark detection outliers were found in one PA case (for which the distance between patient and 3D camera was significantly larger than for all other cases) and eight LAT cases (which were predominantly due to artefacts induced by clothes hanging loose). These cases were excluded from the subsequent statistical analysis.

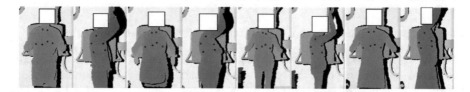

Fig. 2. Example of lung landmark detection results (circles) in 4 cases for PA and LAT views

Figure 3 summarizes the statistics of the landmark detection errors, computed in the coordinate system of the X-ray images. The largest detection variability was found for the Y-coordinates of lung basal landmarks in both PA and LAT views, which are known to have the largest inter-subject variability because of the influence of the internal organs such as the liver and because of possible different breathing status.

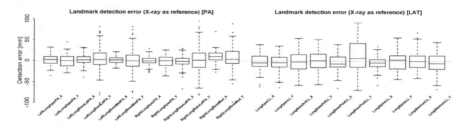

Fig. 3. Boxplot of the landmark detection errors (X- and Y-coordinates separately) for all landmarks associated with PA (left) and LAT (right) views

The results of the multivariable regression analysis to predict the parameters of the lung bounding box are summarized in Table 2. Here again, the largest variability is found for the prediction of the lower edge of the lung bounding box in both PA and LAT cases, as well as for the anterior edge in LAT cases. Interestingly, the regression models based on the detected landmarks resulted in a noticeable larger correlation with the lung bounding box parameters than the collimation parameters selected by the technologists. This is an indication that the models were able to infer to some extent the internal lung anatomy from the depth data while the technologists used external morphological landmarks, such as the shoulders, to adjust the collimation parameters.

Table 2. Root-mean-squared error (RMSE) and correlation between reference lung bounding box and regression prediction from the detected landmarks. The correlation between reference parameters and collimation parameters selected by the technologist is indicated for comparison.

Bounding box parameter	RMSE [mm] PA/LAT	Correlation PA/LAT	Correlation of technologist settings PA/LAT
$LungBB_{Left}$	11.3/13.9	0.77/0.74	0.55/0.60
$LungBB_{Right}$	11.6/20.6	0.78/0.56	0.54/0.25
$LungBB_{Top}$	11.4/12.8	0.56/0.41	0.10/− 0.05
$LungBB_{Bottom}$	24.3/27.2	0.77/0.67	0.44/0.44

The difference between the area of the collimation window predicted by the two statistical models, respectively selected by the technologists, and the area of the lung bounding box was computed for each case as an indication of the area unnecessary exposed to direct X-rays. The corresponding statistics are represented as boxplot on Fig. 4. The distribution of cases in which the collimation settings led/would lead to the lung being cropped on at least one edge of the bounding box (i.e. negative margin) is represented as bar-plot on Fig. 4.

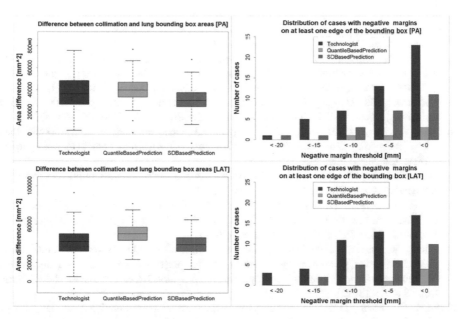

Fig. 4. Boxplots of the area unnecessary exposed to X-ray (left) and bar-plots of distribution of cases with cropped lung (right) for PA (top) and LAT (bottom) views.

4   Discussion/Conclusions

The results summarized in this paper showed the feasibility of training a fully automated algorithm for the detection of internal lung landmarks in depth images acquired during upright chest X-ray examinations and for the subsequent computation of X-ray beam collimation parameters. By using the depth information provided by the 3D camera and the extrinsic camera parameters, the projection of the landmarks onto the X-ray detector could be computed and further processed to estimate the X-ray collimation parameters. As shown by the comparison between the two statistical models computed via regression analysis, decreasing the average area unnecessary exposed to X-rays over the patient population could only be achieved at the risk of increasing the probability of cropping the lungs. Hence, in practice, a trade-off needs to be made between these two conflicting requirements. Interestingly, both statistical models achieved an overall comparable collimation accuracy to the technologists, but led to less variability in over-exposure to X-rays and to noticeably less cases with cropped lungs on the same patient data. In practice, the proposed approach could help reducing the number of X-ray retakes and standardizing the image acquisition process.

References

1. Recommendation of the International Commission on Radiological Protection. IRCP Publication 26, Pergamon Press, Oxford (1977)
2. Foos, D.H., Sehnert, W.J., Reiner, B., Siegel, E.L., Segal, A., Waldman, D.L.: Digital radiography reject analysis: data collection methodology, results, and recommendations from an in-depth investigation at two hospitals. J. Digit. Imaging **22**(1), 89–98 (2009)
3. Hofmann, B., Rosanowsky, T.B., Jensen, C., Wah, K.H.: Image rejects in general direct digital radiography. Acta. Radiol. Open **4** (2015). https://doi.org/10.1177/2058460115604339
4. Jones, A.K., Polman, R., Willis, C.E., Shepard, S.J.: One year's results from a server-based system for performing reject analysis and exposure analysis in computed radiography. J. Digit. Imaging **24**(2), 243–255 (2011)
5. Little, K.J., et al.: Unified database for rejected image analysis across multiple vendors in radiography. J Am Coll Radiol **14**(2), 208–216 (2016)
6. Brahme, A., Nyman, P., Skatt, B.: 4D laser camera for accurate patient positioning, collision avoidance, image fusion and adaptive approaches during diagnostic and therapeutic procedures. Med. Phys. **35**(5), 1670–1681 (2008)
7. Grimm, R., Bauer, S., Sukkau, J., Hornegger, J., Greiner, G.: Markerless estimation of patient orientation, posture and pose using range and pressure imaging for automatic patient setup and scanner initialization in tomographic imaging. Int. J. Comput. Assist. Radiol. Surg. **7**(6), 921–929 (2012)
8. Singh, V., et al.: DARWIN: deformable patient avatar representation with deep image network. In: Descoteaux, M., Maier-Hein, L., Franz, A., Jannin, P., Collins, D.L., Duchesne, S. (eds.) MICCAI 2017. LNCS, vol. 10434, pp. 497–504. Springer, Cham (2017). https://doi.org/10.1007/978-3-319-66185-8_56
9. MacDougall, R., Scherrer, B., Don, S.: Development of a tool to aid the radiologic technologist using augmented reality and computer vision. Pediatr. Radiol. **48**(1), 141–145 (2018)

10. Chen, Y., Medioni, G.: Object modeling by registration of multiple range images. In: IEEE International Conference on Robotics and Automation, vol. 3, pp. 2724–2729 (1991)
11. Shotton, J., et al.: Efficient human pose estimation from single depth images. IEEE Trans. Pattern Anal. Mach. Intell. **35**(12), 2821–2840 (2013)
12. Pham, T., Smeulders, A.: Object recognition with uncertain geometry and uncertain part detection. Comput. Vis. Image Underst. **99**(2), 241–258 (2005)
13. Friedman, J., Hastie, T., Tibshirani, R.: The Elements of Statistical Learning. Springer Series in Statistics. Springer, New York (2001)
14. Cheng, Y.: Mean shift, mode seeking, and clustering. IEEE Trans. Pattern Anal. Mach. Intell. **17**(8), 790–799 (1995)

Efficient Active Learning for Image Classification and Segmentation Using a Sample Selection and Conditional Generative Adversarial Network

Dwarikanath Mahapatra[1]([⊠]), Behzad Bozorgtabar[2], Jean-Philippe Thiran[2], and Mauricio Reyes[3]

[1] IBM Research Australia, Melbourne, Australia
dwarim@au1.ibm.com
[2] Ecole Polytechnique Federale de Lausanne, Lausanne, Switzerland
{behzad.bozorgtabar,jean-philippe.thiran}@epfl.ch
[3] University of Bern, Bern, Switzerland
mauricio.reyes@istb.unibe.ch

Abstract. Training robust deep learning (DL) systems for medical image classification or segmentation is challenging due to limited images covering different disease types and severity. We propose an active learning (AL) framework to select most informative samples and add to the training data. We use conditional generative adversarial networks (cGANs) to generate realistic chest xray images with different disease characteristics by conditioning its generation on a real image sample. Informative samples to add to the training set are identified using a Bayesian neural network. Experiments show our proposed AL framework is able to achieve state of the art performance by using about 35% of the full dataset, thus saving significant time and effort over conventional methods.

1 Introduction

Medical image classification and segmentation are essential building blocks of computer aided diagnosis systems where deep learning (DL) approaches have led to state of the art performance [13]. Robust DL approaches need large labeled datasets which is difficult for medical images because of: (1) limited expert availability; and (2) intensive manual effort required for curation. Active learning (AL) approaches overcome data scarcity with existing models by incrementally selecting the most informative unlabeled samples, querying their labels and adding them to the labeled set [7]. AL in a DL framework poses the following challenges: (1) labeled samples generated by current AL approaches are too few to train or finetune convolution neural networks (CNNs); (2) AL methods select informative samples using hand crafted features [9], while feature learning and model training are jointly optimized in CNNs.

© Springer Nature Switzerland AG 2018
A. F. Frangi et al. (Eds.): MICCAI 2018, LNCS 11071, pp. 580–588, 2018.
https://doi.org/10.1007/978-3-030-00934-2_65

Recent approaches to using AL in a DL setting include Bayesian deep neural networks [1], leveraging separate unlabeled data with high classification uncertainty and high confidence for computer vision applications [14], and fully convolution networks (FCN) for segmenting histopathology images [16]. We propose to generate synthetic data by training a conditional generative adversarial network (cGAN) that learns to generate realistic images by taking input masks of a specific anatomy. Our model is used with chest xray images to generate realistic images from input lung masks. This approach has the advantage of overcoming limitations of small training datasets by generating truly informative samples. We test the proposed AL approach for the key tasks of image classification and segmentation, demonstrating its ability to yield models with high accuracy while reducing the number of training samples.

2 Methods

Our proposed AL approach identifies informative unlabeled samples to improve model performance. Most conventional AL approaches identify informative samples using uncertainty which could lead to bias as uncertainty values depend on the model. We propose a novel approach to generate diverse samples that can contribute meaningful information in training the model. Our framework has three components for: (1) sample generation; (2) classification/segmentation model; and (3) sample informativeness calculation. An initial small labeled set is used to finetune a pre-trained $VGG16$ [12] (or any other classification/segmentation model) using standard data augmentation (DA) through rotation and translation. The sample generator takes a test image and a manually segmented mask (and its variations) as input and generates realistic looking images (details in Sect. 2.1). A Bayesian neural network (BNN) [6] calculates generated images' informativeness and highly informative samples are added to the labeled image set. The new training images are used to fine-tune the previously trained classifier. The above steps are repeated till there is no change in classifier performance.

2.1 Conditional Generative Adversarial Networks

GANs [3] learn a mapping from random noise vector z to output image y: $G : z \rightarrow y$. In contrast, conditional GANs (cGANs) [5] learn a mapping from observed image x and random noise vector z, to y: $G : \{x, z\} \rightarrow y$. The generator G is trained to produce outputs that cannot be distinguished from "real" images by an adversarially trained discriminator, D. The cGAN objective function is:

$$L_{cGAN} = E_{x,y\ p_{data}(x,y)} \left[\log D(x,y)\right] + E_{x\ p_{data}(x),z\ p_z(z)} \left[\log \left(1 - D(x, G(x,z))\right)\right], \quad (1)$$

where G tries to minimize this objective against D, that tries to maximize it, i.e. $G^* = \arg\min_G \max_D L_{cGAN}(G, D)$. Previous approaches have used an additional $L2$ loss [10] to encourage the generator output to be close to ground truth in an $L2$ sense. We use $L1$ loss as it encourages less blurring [8], and defined as:

$$L_{L1}(G) = E_{(x,y)\ p_{data}(x,y),z\ p_z(z)} \left[\|y - G(x,z)\|_1\right]. \quad (2)$$

Thus the final objective function is :

$$G^* = \arg \min_G \max_D L_{cGAN}(G, D) + \lambda L_{L1}(G), \tag{3}$$

where $\lambda = 10$, set empirically, balances the two components' contributions.

Synthetic Image Generation: The parameters of G, θ_G, are given by,

$$\widehat{\theta} = \arg \min_{\theta_G} \frac{1}{N} \sum_{n=1}^{N} l\left(G_{\theta_G}(x, z), x, z\right), \tag{4}$$

N is the number of images. Loss function l combines content loss and adversarial loss (Eqn. 1), and $G(x, z) = y$. Content loss ($l_{content}$) encourages output image y to have different appearance to x. z is the latent vector encoding (obtained from a pre-trained autoencoder) of the segmentation mask. $l_{content}$ is,

$$l_{content} = NMI(x, y) - VGG(x, y) - MSE(x, y). \tag{5}$$

NMI denotes the normalized mutual information (NMI) between x and y, and is used to determine similarity of multimodal images. VGG is the $L2$ distance between two images using all 512 feature maps of Relu $4 - 1$ layer of a pretrained $VGG16$ network [12]. The VGG loss improves robustness by capturing information at different scales from multiple feature maps. MSE is the intensity mean square error. For similar images, NMI gives higher value while VGG and MSE give lower values. In practice $l_{content}$ is measuring the similarity (instead of dissimilarity in traditional loss functions) between two images, and takes higher values for similar images. Since we are minimizing the total loss function, $l_{content}$ encourages the generated image y to be different from input x.

The generator G (Fig. 1(a)) employs residual blocks having two convolution layers with 3×3 filters and 64 feature maps, followed by batch normalization and ReLU activation. It takes as input the test Xray image and the latent vector encoding of a mask (either original or altered) and outputs a realistic Xray image whose label class is the same as the original image. The discriminator D (Fig. 1(b)) has eight convolution layers with the kernels increasing by a factor of 2 from 64 to 512. Leaky ReLU is used and strided convolutions reduce the image dimension when the number of features is doubled. The resulting 512 feature maps are followed by two dense layers and a final sigmoid activation to obtain a probability map. D evaluates similarity between x and y. To generate images with a wide variety of information we modify the segmentation masks of the test images by adopting one or more of the following steps:

1. **Boundary Displacement**: The boundary contours of the mask are displaced to change its shape. We select 25 continuous points at multiple boundary locations, randomly displace each one of them by $\pm[1, 15]$ pixels and fit a b-spline to change the boundary shape. The intensity of pixels outside the original mask are assigned by linear interpolation, or by generating intensity values from a distribution identical to that of the original mask.

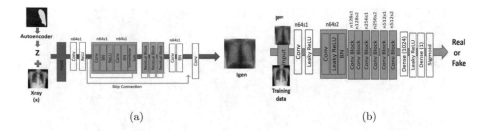

(a)   (b)

Fig. 1. (a) Generator Network; (b) Discriminator network. $n64s1$ denotes 64 feature maps (n) and stride (s) 1 for each convolutional layer.

2. The intensity values of the lung region are changed by generating values from a uniform distribution modeled as $\alpha\mu + \beta\sigma$, where μ is the original distribution's mean, σ is its standard deviation, and $\alpha = [1,5], \beta = [2,10]$ (varied in steps of 0.2).
3. Other conventional augmentation techniques like flipping, rotation and translation are also used.

For every test image we obtain up to 200 synthetic images with their modified masks. Figure 2 (a) shows an original normal image (bottom row) and its mask (top row), and Figs. 2 (b, c) show generated 'normal' images. Figure 2 (d) shows the corresponding image mask for an image with nodules, and Figs. 2 (e, f) show generated 'nodule' images. Although the nodules are very difficult to observe with the naked eye, we highlight its position using yellow boxes. It is quite obvious that the generated images are realistic and suitable for training.

2.2 Sample Informativeness Using Uncertainty Form Bayesian Neural Networks

Each generated image's uncertainty is calculated using the method described in [6]. Two types of uncertainty measures can be calculated from a Bayesian neural network (BNN). Aleotaric uncertainty models the noise in the observation while epistemic uncertainty models the uncertainty of model parameters. We adopt [6] to calculate uncertainty by combining the above two types. A brief description is given below and refer the reader to [6] for details. For a BNN model f mapping an input image x, to a unary output $\widehat{y} \in R$, the predictive uncertainty for pixel y is approximated using:

$$Var(y) \approx \frac{1}{T}\sum_{t=1}^{T}\widehat{y}_t^2 - \left(\frac{1}{T}\sum_{t=1}^{T}\widehat{y}_t\right)^2 + \frac{1}{T}\sum_{t=1}^{T}\widehat{\sigma}_t^2 \qquad (6)$$

$\widehat{\sigma}_t^2$ is the BNN output for the predicted variance for pixel y_t, and $\widehat{y}_t, \widehat{\sigma}_t^2{}_{t=1}^{T}$ being a set of T sampled outputs.

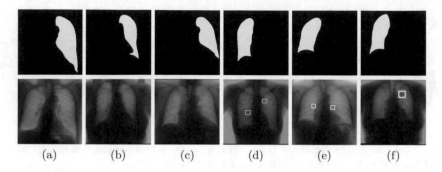

Fig. 2. Mask (Top Row 1) and corresponding informative xray image (Bottom Row); (a)–(c) non-diseased cases; (d)–(f) images with nodules of different severity at the center of yellow box. (a), (d) are the original images while others are synthetic images generated by altering the mask characteristics.

2.3 Implementation Details

Our initial network is a $VGG16$ network [12] or $ResNet18$ [4] pre-trained on the Imagenet dataset. Our entire dataset had 93 normal images and 154 nodule images. We chose an initially labeled dataset of 16 (chosen empirically) images from each class, augment it 200 times using standard data augmentation like rotation and translation, and use them to fine tune the last classification layer of the $VGG16$. The remaining test images and their masks were used to generate multiple images using our proposed cGAN approach (200 synthetic images for every test image as described earlier), and each generated image's uncertainty was calculated as described in Sect. 2.2. We ranked the images with highest uncertainty score and the top 16 images from each class were augmented 200 times (rotation and translation) and used to further fine-tune the classifier. This ensures equal representation of normal and diseased samples in the samples to add to the training data. This sequence of steps is repeated till there is no further improvement of classifier accuracy when tested on a separate test set of 400 images (200 images each of nodule and normal class). Our knowledge of image label allows quantitative analysis of model performance.

3 Experiments

Dataset Description: Our algorithm is trained on the SCR chest XRay database [2] which has Xrays of 247 (93 normal and 154 nodule images, resized to 512 × 512 pixels) patients along with manual segmentations of the clavicles, lungs and heart. The dataset is augmented 500 times using rotation, translation, scaling and flipping. We take a separate test set of 400 images from the NIH dataset [15] with 200 normal images and 200 images with nodules.

3.1   Classification Results

Here we show results for classifying different images using different amounts of labeled data and demonstrate our method's ability to optimize the amount of labeled data necessary to attain a given performance, as compared to conventional approaches where no sample selection is performed. In one set of experiments we used the entire training set of 247 images and augmentation to fine tune the $VGG16$ classifier, and test it on the separate set of 400 images. We call this the fully supervised learning (FSL) setting. Subsequently, in other experiments for AL we used different number of initial training samples in each update of the training data. The batch size is the same as the initial number of samples.

The results are summarized in Table 1 where the classification performance in terms of sensitivity ($Sens$), specificity ($Spec$) and area under the curve (AUC) are reported for different settings using $VGG16$ and $ResNet18$ [4] classifiers. Under FSL, 5–fold indicates normal 5 fold cross validation; and 35% indicates the scenario when 35% of training data was randomly chosen to train the classifier and measure performance on test data (the average of 10 such runs). We ensure that all samples were part of the training and test set atleast once. In all cases AL classification performance reaches almost the same level as FSL when the number of training samples is approximately 35% of the dataset. Subsequently increasing the number of samples does not lead to significant performance gain. This trend is observed for both classifiers, indicating it is not dependent upon classifier choice.

Table 1. Classification and Segmentation results for active learning framework of Xray images. DM-Dice metric and HD- Hausdorff distance

| | Active learning (% labeled + Classifier) | | | | | | | | | | FSL | | | |
| | 10% | | 15% | | 25% | | 30% | | 35% | | 5-fold | | 35% | |
	VGG16 [12]	ResNet18 [4]	[12]	[4]	[12]	[4]	[12]	[4]	[12]	[4]	[12]	[4]	[12]	[4]
Sens	70.8	71.3	75.3	76.2	89.2	89.7	91.5	91.8	91.7	91.9	92.1	92.4	78.1	78.5
Spec	71.1	71.9	76.0	76.8	89.9	90.5	92.1	92.4	92.4	92.5	92.9	93.1	78.4	78.7
AUC	74.3	75.0	78.7	79.4	92.5	93.0	94.9	95.1	95.2	95.3	95.7	95.9	80.6	81.0
DM	68.2		74.1		86.4		90.4		91.0		91.3		79.3	
HD	18.7		14.3		9.3		8.1		7.9		7.5		15.1	

3.2   Segmentation Performance

Using the labeled datasets at different stages we train a UNet [11] for segmenting both lungs. The trained model is then evaluated on the separate set of 400 images from the NIH database on which we manually segment both lungs. The segmentation performance for FSL and different AL settings is summarized in Table 1 in terms of Dice Metric (DM) and Hausdorff Distance (HD). We observe that the segmentation performance reaches the same level as FSL at a fraction of the full dataset - in this case between $30-35\%$, which is similar for classification.

Figure 3 shows the segmentation results for different training models. When the number of training samples are less than 10% the segmentation performance is quite bad in the most challenging cases. However the performance improves steadily till it stabilizes at the 35% threshold.

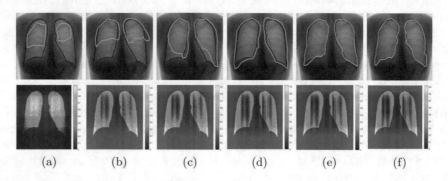

(a)   (b)   (c)   (d)   (e)   (f)

Fig. 3. Segmentation (top row) and uncertainty map (bottom row) results for different numbers of labeled examples in the training data (a) 5%; (b) 10%; (c) 20%; (d) 30%; (e) 35%; (f) 40%. Red contour is manual segmentation and green contour is the UNet generated segmentation.

3.3   Savings in Annotation Effort

Segmentation and classification results demonstrate that with the most informative samples, optimum performance can be achieved using a fraction of the dataset. This translates into significant savings in annotation cost as it reduces the number of images and pixels that need to be annotated by an expert. We calculate the number of pixels in the images that were part of the AL based training set at different stages for both classification and segmentation. At the point of optimum performance the number of annotated pixels in the training images is 33%. These numbers clearly suggest that using our AL framework can lead to savings of nearly 67% in terms of time and effort put in by the experts.

4   Conclusion

We have proposed a method to generate chest Xray images for active learning based model training by modifying the original masks of associated images. A generated image's informativeness is calculated using a bayesian neural network, and the most informative samples are added to the training set. These sequence of steps are continued till there is no additional information provided by the labeled samples. Our experiments demonstrate that, with about $33-35\%$ labeled samples we can achieve almost equal classification and segmentation performance as obtained when using the full dataset. This is made possible by selecting the most informative samples for training. Thus the model sees all the informative samples first, and achieves optimal performance in fewer iterations. The performance of the proposed AL based model translates into significant savings in annotation effort and clinicians' time. In future work we aim to further investigate the realism of the generated images.

Acknowledgement. The authors acknowledge the support from SNSF project grant number 169607.

References

1. Gal, Y., Islam, R., Ghahramani, Z.: Deep Bayesian active learning with image data. In: Proceedings of the International Conference on Machine Learning (2017)
2. van Ginneken, B., Stegmann, M., Loog, M.: Segmentation of anatomical structures in chest radiographs using supervised methods: a comparative study on a public database. Med. Image Anal. **10**(1), 19–40 (2006)
3. Goodfellow, I., et al.: Generative adversarial nets. In: Proceedings of the NIPS, pp. 2672–2680 (2014)
4. He, K., Zhang, X., Ren, S., Sun, J.: Deep residual learning for image recognition. In: Proceedings of the CVPR (2016)
5. Isola, P., Zhu, J., Zhou, T., Efros, A.: Image-to-image translation with conditional adversarial networks. In: CVPR (2017)
6. Kendall, A., Gal, Y.: What uncertainties do we need in bayesian deep learning for computer vision? In: Advances in Neural Information Processing Systems (2017)
7. Li, X., Guo, Y.: Adaptive active learning for image classification. In: Proceedings of the CVPR (2013)
8. Mahapatra, D., Bozorgtabar, B., Hewavitharanage, S., Garnavi, R.: Image super resolution using generative adversarial networks and local saliency maps for retinal image analysis. In: Descoteaux, M., Maier-Hein, L., Franz, A., Jannin, P., Collins, D.L., Duchesne, S. (eds.) MICCAI 2017. LNCS, vol. 10435, pp. 382–390. Springer, Cham (2017). https://doi.org/10.1007/978-3-319-66179-7_44
9. Mahapatra, D., Schüffler, P.J., Tielbeek, J.A.W., Vos, F.M., Buhmann, J.M.: Semi-supervised and active learning for automatic segmentation of Crohn's disease. In: Mori, K., Sakuma, I., Sato, Y., Barillot, C., Navab, N. (eds.) MICCAI 2013. LNCS, vol. 8150, pp. 214–221. Springer, Heidelberg (2013). https://doi.org/10.1007/978-3-642-40763-5_27
10. Pathak, D., Krähenbühl, P., Donahue, J., Darrell, T., Efros, A.: Context encoders: feature learning by inpainting. In: Proceedings of the CVPR, pp. 2536–2544 (2016)
11. Ronneberger, O., Fischer, P., Brox, T.: U-Net: convolutional networks for biomedical image segmentation. In: Navab, N., Hornegger, J., Wells, W.M., Frangi, A.F. (eds.) MICCAI 2015. LNCS, vol. 9351, pp. 234–241. Springer, Cham (2015). https://doi.org/10.1007/978-3-319-24574-4_28
12. Simonyan, K., Zisserman, A.: Very deep convolutional networks for large-scale image recognition. CoRR abs/1409.1556 (2014)
13. Tajbakhsh, N., et al.: Convolutional neural networks for medical image analysis: full training or fine tuning? IEEE Trans. Med. Imaging **35**(5), 1299–1312 (2016)
14. Wang, K., Zhang, D., Li, Y., Zhang, R., Lin, L.: Cost-effective active learning for deep image classification. IEEE Trans. CSVT **27**(12), 2591–2600 (2017)

15. Wang, X., Peng, Y., Lu, L., Lu, Z., Bagheri, M., Summers, R.: Chestx-ray8: hospital-scale chest x-ray database and benchmarks on weakly-supervised classification and localization of common thorax diseases. In: Proceedings of the CVPR (2017)
16. Yang, L., Zhang, Y., Chen, J., Zhang, S., Chen, D.Z.: Suggestive annotation: a deep active learning framework for biomedical image segmentation. In: Descoteaux, M., Maier-Hein, L., Franz, A., Jannin, P., Collins, D.L., Duchesne, S. (eds.) MICCAI 2017. LNCS, vol. 10435, pp. 399–407. Springer, Cham (2017). https://doi.org/10. 1007/978-3-319-66179-7_46

Iterative Attention Mining for Weakly Supervised Thoracic Disease Pattern Localization in Chest X-Rays

Jinzheng Cai[1](✉), Le Lu[2], Adam P. Harrison[2], Xiaoshuang Shi[1],
Pingjun Chen[1], and Lin Yang[1]

[1] University of Florida, Gainesville, FL 32611, USA
jimmycai@ufl.edu
[2] AI-Infra, NVIDIA Corp, Bethesda, MD 20814, USA

Abstract. Given image labels as the only supervisory signal, we focus on harvesting/mining, thoracic disease localizations from chest X-ray images. Harvesting such localizations from existing datasets allows for the creation of improved data sources for computer-aided diagnosis and retrospective analyses. We train a convolutional neural network (CNN) for image classification and propose an attention mining (AM) strategy to improve the model's sensitivity or saliency to disease patterns. The intuition of AM is that once the most salient disease area is blocked or hidden from the CNN model, it will pay attention to alternative image regions, while still attempting to make correct predictions. However, the model requires to be properly constrained during AM, otherwise, it may overfit to uncorrelated image parts and forget the valuable knowledge that it has learned from the original image classification task. To alleviate such side effects, we then design a knowledge preservation (KP) loss, which minimizes the discrepancy between responses for X-ray images from the original and the updated networks. Furthermore, we modify the CNN model to include multi-scale aggregation (MSA), improving its localization ability on small-scale disease findings, *e.g.*, lung nodules. We validate our method on the publicly-available ChestX-ray14 dataset, outperforming a class activation map (CAM)-based approach, and demonstrating the value of our novel framework for mining disease locations.

1 Introduction

Automatic analysis of chest X-rays is critical for diagnosis and treatment planning of thoracic diseases. Recently, several methods applying deep learning for automatic chest X-ray analysis [5,7,8,11,14] have been proposed. In particular, much work has focused on the ChestX-ray14 dataset [11], which is an unprecedentedly large-scale and rich dataset but only provides image-level labels for the

---

Electronic supplementary material The online version of this chapter (https:// doi.org/10.1007/978-3-030-00934-2_66) contains supplementary material, which is available to authorized users.

© Springer Nature Switzerland AG 2018
A. F. Frangi et al. (Eds.): MICCAI 2018, LNCS 11071, pp. 589–598, 2018.
https://doi.org/10.1007/978-3-030-00934-2_66

far majority of the samples. On the other hand, harvesting abnormality locations in this dataset is an important goal, as that provides an even richer source of data for training computer-aided diagnosis system and/or performing retrospective data analyses. Harvesting disease locations can be conducted through a weakly supervised image classification approach [11]; or, in our case we reformulate it as a label supervised *pattern-mining problem*, to gain higher localization accuracy. Toward this end, we propose an integrated and novel framework that combines attention mining, knowledge preservation, and multi-scale aggregation that improves upon current efforts to accurately localize disease patterns.

Recent work on chest X-rays have focused on both classification and localization. Along with the ChestX-ray14 dataset, Wang *et al.* [11] also propose a class activation map (CAM)-based [16] approach using convolutional neural network (CNNs) to perform weakly supervised disease localization. To improve image classification accuracy, Rajpurkar *et al.* [8] introduce an ultra-deep CNN architecture while Yao *et al.* [14] design a new learning objective that exploits dependencies among image labels. Other work investigate methods to automatically generate X-ray reports [4,10]. The proposed framework is a complementary or orthogonal development from the above advances [8,14] since we mine "free" disease locations in the form of bounding boxes given image-level labels. It also can further benefit downstream applications like [4,10].

In terms of related work, our attention mining (AM) approach is closely related to an adversarial erasing scheme proposed in [12] that forces the network to discover other salient image regions by erasing the most representative area of the object class in question. In a similar spirit, we propose AM to locate multiple suspicious disease regions inside a chest X-ray. However, different from [12], AM drops out corresponding pixels in the activation maps so as to leave the original X-ray images unchanged. More importantly, AM is designed to seamlessly couple with multi-label classification, where activation maps are required to be blocked in a class-wise manner. Next, to alleviate the side effects caused by dropping out activation maps, we exploit methods to prevent the network from forgetting its originally learned knowledge on recognizing and localizing disease patterns. Distilling a network's knowledge is proposed in [2] to transfer the learned parameters from multiple models to a new, typically smaller sized, model. A similar technique is used in [9] to regularize the CNN model for incremental learning with new image categories, keeping the network's output of old image categories mostly unchanged. In our method, we minimize the ℓ_2-distance of output logits between the original and updated networks to achieve knowledge preservation (KP). Distinct from [2,9], we use the logits not only from the last output layer but also the intermediate network layers, in order to introduce stronger regularizations. Finally, we propose a multi-scale aggregation (MSA) because we notice that the localization accuracy of lung nodules in [11] is not as good as the other disease findings, which we believe results from the coarse resolution of the attention maps, *i.e.*, CAMs. Inspired by recent work [6,15] we modify the CNN to generate attention maps with doubled resolution, improving the detection performance of small-scale targets.

2   Methods

Our framework is visually depicted in Fig. 1.

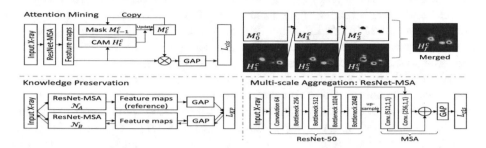

Fig. 1. Architectures of the proposed attention mining (AM), knowledge preservation (KP), and multi-scale aggregation (MSA). Red arrows in the KP module indicate the path of back-propagation. The convolution parameters for MSA are shown as (number of filters, kernel size, stride). See Sect. 2 for details.

2.1   Disease Pattern Localization with Attention Mining

Starting from the output of CNN's last convolutional layer, we denote the feature map as $X \in R^{N \times W \times H \times D}$, where N, W, H, and D are the mini-batch size, width, height, and feature map channel, respectively. We then split the classification layer of the CNN into C branches because feature map erasure is required to be class specific. For now, we assume a binary erasure mask is available, which is defined as $M^c \in R^{N \times W \times H \times 1}$, where $c \in C = \{1, \ldots, C\}$ is the index of a specific disease type (see Sect. 3.2 for details to generate M^c). Zeroed regions in M^c mark spatial regions to drop out of X. For the cth disease, M^c first replicated across its 4th dimension D times as $\hat{M}^c$, and then the erased feature map is,

$$\hat{X}^c = X \odot \hat{M}^c, \tag{1}$$

where $\odot$ is element-wise multiplication. The new feature map $\hat{X}^c$ is then fed into the cth network branch for binary classification, with the loss defined as,

$$L^c = \frac{1}{N} \left[h \left(\sigma \left((w^c)^T g(\hat{X}^c) \right), y^c \right) \right], \tag{2}$$

where $g(\cdot)$ is global average pooling (GAP) [16] over the W and H dimensions, $w^c \in R^{D \times 1}$ is the network parameter of the cth branch, $\sigma(\cdot)$ is the sigmoid activation function, $y^c \in \{0, 1\}^N$ are the labels of class c in a mini-batch, and $h(\cdot)$ is the cross entropy loss function. Thus, the total classification loss is defined as,

$$L_{cls} = \frac{1}{C} \sum_{c \in C} L^c. \tag{3}$$

While AM can help localize pathologies, the CNN model may overfit to spurious regions after erasure, causing the model to classify an X-ray by remembering its specific image part rather than actual disease patterns. We address this with a knowledge preservation (KP) method described below.

2.2 Incremental Learning with Knowledge Preservation

We explore two methods of KP. Given a mini-batch of N images, a straightforward way to preserve the learned knowledge is to use only the first n images for AM and leave the later $N - n$ untouched. If the ratio n/N is set to be small enough (*e.g.*, 0.125 in our implementation), the CNN's updates can possibly be alleviated from overfitting to uncorrelated image parts. We refer to this vanilla implementation of knowledge preservation as KP-Vanilla.

We investigate a stronger regularizer for KP by constraining the outputs of intermediate network layers. Our main idea is to make the CNN's activation to the later $N - n$ images be mostly unchanged. Formally, we denote the original network before AM updates as $\mathcal{N}_A$ and the updated model as $\mathcal{N}_B$. Initially, $\mathcal{N}_A$ and $\mathcal{N}_B$ are identical to each other, but $\mathcal{N}_B$ is gradually altered as it learns to classify the blocked feature maps during AM. Considering outputs from the kth layer of $\mathcal{N}_A$ and $\mathcal{N}_B$ as $X_{A(k)}, X_{B(k)} \in R^{(N-n) \times W \times H \times C}$ for the later $N - n$ images, we define the distance between $X_{A(k)}$ and $X_{B(k)}$ as the ℓ_2-distance between their GAP features as,

$$L^k = \frac{1}{N - n} \|g(X_{A(k)}) - g(X_{B(k)})\|_2. \tag{4}$$

When multiple network layers are chosen, the total loss from KP is,

$$L_{KP} = \frac{1}{|\mathcal{K}|} \sum_{k \in \mathcal{K}} L^k, \tag{5}$$

where $\mathcal{K}$ is the indices set of the selected layers, and $|\mathcal{K}|$ is its cardinality. Finally, the objective for $\mathcal{N}_B$ training is a weighted combination of L_{cls} and L_{KP},

$$L = L_{cls} + \lambda L_{KP}, \tag{6}$$

where λ balances the classification and KP loss. Empirically we find the model updates properly when the value of λL_{KP} is roughly a half of L_{cls}, *i.e.*, $\lambda = 0.5$.

2.3 Multi-scale Aggregation

Our final contribution uses multi-scale aggregation (MSA) to improve the performance of locating small-scale objects, *e.g.*, lung nodules. Taking ResNet-50 [3] as the backbone network, we implement MSA using the outputs of the last two bottlenecks, and refer to the modified network as ResNet-MSA. Given the output of the last bottleneck, denoted as $X_k \in R^{N \times W/2 \times H/2 \times 2048}$, we feed it into a 1×1 convolutional layer to reduce its channel dimension to 512 and also upsample its width and height by 2 using bilinear interpolation. The resulting feature map is denoted as $\bar{X}_k \in R^{N \times W \times H \times 512}$. Similarly, the output of the penultimate bottleneck, $X_{k-1} \in R^{N \times W \times H \times 1024}$, is fed into another 1×1 convolutional layer to lower its channel dimension to 256, producing $\bar{X}_{k-1} \in R^{N \times W \times H \times 256}$. Finally, we concatenate them to produce an aggregated feature map $X = [\bar{X}_k, \bar{X}_{k-1}]$ for AM.

However, MSA is not restricted to bilinear upsampling, as deconvolution [6] can also be used for upsampling, where we use 3×3 convolutions. However, as our experiments will demonstrate, the improvements are marginal, leaving bilinear as an efficient option. On the other hand, the channel dimensions of X_k and X_{k-1} are largely reduced in order to fit the models into limited GPU memory.

3   Experimental Results and Analysis

The proposed method is evaluated on the ChestX-ray14 dataset [11], which contains $51,709$ and $60,412$ X-ray images of subjects with thoracic and no diseases, respectively. 880 images are marked with bounding boxes (bboxs) corresponding to 984 disease patterns of 8 types, i.e., atelectasis (AT), cardiomegaly (CM), pleural effusion (PE), infiltration (Infiltrat.), mass, nodule, pneumonia (PNA), and pneumothorax (PTx). We first use the same data split as [11] to train base models, i.e., ResNet-50, and ResNet-MSA. Later during AM, the 880 bbox images are then incorporated into the training set to further fine-tune models. We notice that the AM strategy is originally designed to mine disease locations in training images. However, for the purpose of conducting quantitative analysis, we use the bbox images during AM, but only using image labels for training, while leaving the bboxs aside to evaluate localization results.

For ease of comparison, we use the same evaluation metrics as [11]. Given the ground truth and the localized bboxs of a disease, its localization accuracy (Acc.) and average false positive (AFP) is calculated by comparing the intersection over union (IoU) ratios with a predefined threshold, i.e., T(IoU). Finally, all of our deep learning implementations are built upon Tensorflow [1] and Tensorpack [13].

3.1   Multiple Scale Aggregation

We first test the impact of MSA prior to the application of AM and KP, implementing the bilinear interpolation and deconvolution variants. We also test two different input image resolutions: 1024×1024 and 512×512, where the latter is downsampled from the original images using bilinear interpolation. Before applying MSA, we fine-tune the base network ResNet-50 with a learning rate of 0.1 for 50 epochs. Mini-batch sizes for 1024 and 512 inputs are 32 and 64, respectively. Then, to initialize MSA, we fix the network parameters below MSA and tune the other layers for 10 epochs. Finally, we have the whole ResNet-MSA updated end-to-end until the validation loss plot plateaus. Since we mainly focus on investigating AM and KP, no further modification has been taken for the network architecture, and thus the ResNet-MSA achieves similar classification performance as reported in [11] (see supplementary materials for details).

The results of different MSA setups are reported in Table 1, where the "baseline" refers to the original ResNet-50, the "bilinear" and "deconv." refer to ResNet-MSA with bilinear upsampling, and deconvolution operation, respectively. Prefixes denote the input resolution. As can be seen, the 512 variants perform better than their 1024 counterparts. This is likely because the receptive field size of the MSA layers with "1024-" input is too small to capture sufficient contextual information. Note that for the "512-" input, the two MSA configurations outperform the baseline by a large margin for the infiltration, mass, and nodule categories. This is supporting our design intuition that MSA can help locate small-scale disease patterns more accurately. Because of the efficiency of bilinear upsampling, we select it to be MSA variant of choice, which will be further fine-tuned with AM and KP using Eq. (6).

Table 1. To compare different MSA setups, each table cell show localization *Acc.* given T(IoU)=0.3 using all bboxs in $\mathcal{B}$. (See Sects. 3.1 and 3.2 for details.)

Method	AT	CM	PE	Infiltrat.	Mass	Nodule	PNA	PTx
512-baseline	0.21	**0.81**	**0.37**	0.37	0.21	<u>0.04</u>	**0.38**	**0.35**
512-bilinear	0.21	0.62	0.34	**0.54**	**0.35**	<u>0.24</u>	0.37	0.29
512-deconv	**0.28**	0.55	0.35	0.50	0.32	0.20	0.35	0.27
1024-baseline	0.21	0.19	0.33	0.37	0.35	0.09	0.23	0.09
1024-bilinear	0.11	0.10	0.30	0.30	0.15	0.22	0.05	0.08
1024-deconv	0.07	0.10	0.23	0.40	0.13	0.01	0.05	0.03

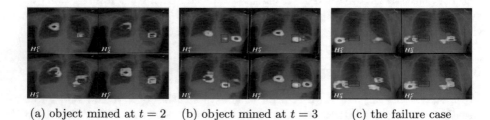

(a) object mined at $t=2$ (b) object mined at $t=3$ (c) the failure case

Fig. 2. Visualization of heatmaps generated during attention mining. The ground truth and the automatic bboxs are colored in red and green, respcetively.

3.2   Disease Pattern Localization with AM and KP

In our implementation, we develop the attention mining (AM) basing on the class activation map (CAM) approach [16] that obtains class-specific heat maps. Specifically, the binary erasure mask, M^c is initialized to be all 1, denoted as M_0^c. The AM procedure is then iteratively performed T times, and at time step t, the intermediate CAMs are generated as,

$$H_t^c = (X \odot \hat{M}_{t-1}^c)w^c, \tag{7}$$

Table 2. Comparsion of localization results, which are reported in the form of "Acc.-AFP". The "ref." and "base." are presenting the referred method proposed by Wang *et al.* [11] and the baseline method presented in Sect. 3.2 in the manuscript, respectively. The proposed method is presented as "ours". The best performance, which has the highest Acc. and lowest AFP is presented in bold.

T(IoU)	Method	AT	CM	Effusion	Infiltra.	Mass	Nodule	PNA	PTx
0.1	ref.	0.69–0.89	0.94–0.59	0.66–0.83	0.71–0.62	0.40–0.67	0.14–0.61	0.63–1.02	0.38–0.49
	base.	0.55–0.88	**0.99–0.08**	0.57–0.82	0.47–0.61	0.36–0.65	0.25–0.59	**0.73–1.01**	0.42–0.48
	ours	0.68–0.88	0.97–0.18	0.65–0.82	0.52–0.61	**0.56–0.65**	**0.46–0.59**	0.65–1.01	**0.43–0.48**
0.2	ref.	0.47–0.98	0.68–0.72	0.45–0.91	0.48–0.68	0.26–0.69	0.05–0.62	0.35–1.08	0.23–0.52
	base.	0.36–0.97	**0.99–0.08**	0.33–0.90	0.22–0.67	0.26–0.68	0.09–0.61	0.48–1.07	**0.36–0.50**
	ours	**0.51–0.97**	0.90–0.28	**0.52–0.90**	0.44–0.67	**0.47–0.68**	**0.27–0.61**	**0.54–1.07**	0.24–0.50
0.3	ref.	0.24–1.40	0.46–0.78	0.30–0.95	0.28–0.72	0.15–0.71	0.04–0.62	0.17–1.11	0.13–0.53
	base.	0.22–1.38	**0.96–0.12**	0.18–0.93	0.13–0.71	0.19–0.69	0.04–0.61	0.31–1.09	**0.21–0.52**
	ours	**0.33–1.38**	0.85–0.35	**0.34–0.93**	**0.28–0.71**	**0.33–0.69**	**0.11–0.61**	0.39–1.09	0.16–0.52
0.4	ref.	0.09–1.08	0.28–0.81	0.20–0.97	0.12–0.75	0.07–0.72	0.01–0.62	0.07–1.12	0.07–0.54
	base.	0.12–1.06	**0.92–0.15**	0.05–0.95	0.02–0.73	0.12–0.71	**0.03–0.61**	0.17–1.11	**0.12–0.53**
	ours	**0.23–1.06**	0.73–0.47	0.18–0.95	**0.20–0.73**	**0.18–0.71**	0.03–0.61	**0.23–1.11**	0.11–0.53
0.5	ref.	0.05–1.09	0.18–0.84	0.11–0.99	0.07–0.76	0.01–0.72	0.01–0.62	0.03–1.13	0.03–0.55
	base.	0.06–1.07	**0.68–0.39**	0.02–0.97	0.02–0.74	0.06–0.71	0.01–0.61	0.06–1.12	**0.08–0.53**
	ours	**0.11–1.07**	0.60–0.60	0.10–0.97	**0.12–0.74**	**0.07–0.71**	0.03–0.61	**0.17–1.12**	0.08–0.53
0.6	ref.	0.02–1.09	0.08–0.85	0.05–1.00	0.02–0.76	0.00–0.72	0.01–0.62	0.02–1.13	0.03–0.55
	base.	0.01–1.08	**0.48–0.60**	0.00–0.99	0.02–0.75	0.04–0.71	**0.01–0.61**	0.03–1.12	0.06–0.53
	ours	**0.03–1.08**	0.44–0.76	**0.05–0.99**	**0.06–0.75**	**0.05–0.71**	0.01–0.61	**0.05–1.12**	**0.07–0.53**
0.7	ref.	0.01–1.10	0.03–0.06	0.02–1.01	0.00–0.77	0.00–0.72	0.00–0.62	0.01–1.13	0.02–0.55
	base.	0.00–1.08	**0.18–0.84**	0.00–0.99	0.01–0.75	**0.01–0.71**	0.00–0.61	0.01–1.12	0.01–0.53
	ours	**0.01–1.08**	0.17–0.84	0.01–0.99	**0.02–0.75**	**0.01–0.71**	**0.00–0.61**	0.02–1.12	0.02–0.53

Table 3. Ablation study of attention mining (AM) and knowledge preservation (KP). Each table cell shows the *Acc.* by using all of the bboxs in $\mathcal{B}$ (in Sect. 3.2).

	T(IoU)	Method	AT	CM	PE	Infiltrat.	Mass	Nodule	PNA	PTx
AM	0.1	t = 1	0.57	0.96	**0.84**	0.78	0.58	**0.65**	0.66	0.68
		t = 2	0.65	**0.97**	0.82	0.77	0.60	0.61	0.72	**0.72**
		t = 3	**0.68**	**0.97**	0.83	**0.79**	**0.62**	0.57	**0.73**	**0.72**
	0.3	t = 1	**0.34**	0.73	0.47	0.40	**0.36**	**0.33**	0.33	0.30
		t = 2	0.32	0.82	0.47	0.40	0.34	0.25	0.42	0.36
		t = 3	0.33	**0.85**	**0.48**	**0.42**	0.34	0.20	**0.44**	**0.38**
KP	0.1	w/o KP	0.67	**1.00**	0.48	0.58	0.54	0.47	0.70	0.71
		KP-Vanilla	0.65	0.97	0.78	**0.87**	0.61	0.48	**0.73**	**0.72**
		KP	**0.68**	0.97	**0.83**	0.79	**0.62**	**0.57**	0.73	0.72
	0.3	w/o KP	0.22	**0.99**	0.11	0.20	0.20	0.06	0.29	0.34
		KP-Vanilla	0.26	0.73	0.41	**0.46**	0.32	0.10	0.42	0.36
		KP	**0.33**	0.85	**0.48**	0.42	**0.34**	**0.20**	0.44	**0.38**

where the inner product is executed across the channel dimension. These CAMs are then normalized to [0,1] and binarized with a threshold of 0.5. M_t^c is then updated from $M_{(t-1)}^c$, except that pixel locations of the connected component that contains the global maximum of the binarized CAM are now set to 0.

There are different options to generate a final heatmap aggregated from all T CAMs. We choose to have them averaged. However, when $t > 1$ regions have been erased, as per Eq. (7). Thus, we fill in these regions from the corresponding un-erased regions from prior heatmaps. If we define the complement of the masks as $\bar{M}_t^c = (1 - \hat{M}_t^c)$, then the final heatmap H_f^c is calculated using

$$H_f^c = \frac{1}{T} \sum_{t=1}^{T} \left[H_t^c + \sum_{t'=1}^{t-1} (H_{t'}^c \odot \bar{M}_{t'}^c) \right]. \tag{8}$$

Empirically, we find $T = 3$ works best in our implementation.

Bbox Generation: To convert CAMs into bboxs, we have 3 bboxs generated from each H_f^c by adjusting the intensity threshold. For image i, the bboxs are then ranked as $\{bbox_i^c(1), bbox_i^c(2), bbox_i^c(3)\}$ in descending order based on the mean H_f^c intensity values inside the bbox areas. These are then arranged into an aggregated list across all test images from the cth category:

$$\mathcal{B} = \{bbox_1^c(1), \ldots, bbox_N^c(1), bbox_1^c(2), \ldots, bbox_N^c(2), bbox_1^c(3), \ldots, bbox_N^c(3)\}.$$

Thereafter, these bboxs are sequentially selected from $\mathcal{B}$ to calculate $Acc.$ until the AFP reaches its upper bound, which is the corresponding AFP value reported in [11]. Here, we choose to generate 3 bboxs from each image as it is large enough to cover the corrected locations, while an even larger alternate will greatly increase the AFP value. However, in some cases, H_f^c would just allow to generate fewer than 3 bboxs, for instance, see Fig. 2(a).

Since Wang et al. [11] were not tackling the disease localization in the way as data-mining, direct comparison to their results is not appropriate as they incorporated the bbox images in their test set. Instead, we use our method prior to the application of AM steps as the baseline, which is, for all intents and purposes, Wang et al.'s approach [11] applied to the data-mining problem. It is presented as the "baseline" method in Table 2. More specifically, it is set up as the 1st time step of AM with KP-Vanilla and then fine-tuned until it is converged on the bbox images. As shown in Table 2, our method reports systematic and consistent quantitative performance improvements over the "baseline" method, except slightly degrades on the category of CM, demonstrating the impact of our AM and KP enhancements. Meanwhile, comparing with the results in [11], our method achieves significant improvements by using no extra manual annotations. More Importantly, the results in Table 2 indicate our method would also be effective when implemented to mine disease locations in the training images.

Figure 2 depicts three atelectasis cases visualizing the AM process. As can be seen, AM improves upon the baseline results, H_1^c, by discovering new regions after erasing that correlate with the disease patterns. More qualitative results can be found in the supplementary materials.

Ablation Study: We further investigate the impact of AM and KP. First, we compare the three steps in AM. Since the erasure map M_0^c is initialized with all 1s, then the time step $t = 1$ is treated as the baseline. Table 3 shows the localization results at two IoU thresholds, 0.1 and 0.3. As can be seen, significant improvements of AM are observed in the AT, CM, mass, PNA, and PTx disease patterns. Next, we compare the KP, KP-Vanilla and an implementation without KP, where the ResNet-MSA is tuned in AM using only the bbox images. In particular, we set $\mathcal{K}$ by using the outputs of the 3rd and 4th bottleneck, the MSA, and the classification layers. As Table 3 presents, KP performs better than KP-Vanilla in the AT, PE, mass, nodule, PNA and PTx categories.

4 Conclusion

We present a novel localization data-mining framework, combining AM, KP, and MSA. We introduce a powerful means to harvest disease locations from chest X-ray datasets. By showing improvements over a standard CAM-based approach, our method can mine localization knowledge in existing large-scale datasets, potentially allowing for the training of improved computer-aided diagnosis tools or more powerful retrospective analyses. Future work includes improving the MSA, possibly by using the atrous convolution [15]. Additionally, we find that when the activation map fails to localize disease in none of the AM steps, our method will not locate the correct image region as demonstrated in Fig. 2(c). To address this issue, we may consider semi-supervised learning, like the use of bboxs in [5], as a complementary means to discover those difficult cases.

References

1. Abadi, M., Agarwal, A., Barham, P., et al.: TensorFlow: large-scale machine learning on heterogeneous systems (2015). https://www.tensorflow.org/
2. Geoffrey, H., et al.: Distilling the knowledge in a neural network. In: NIPS (2014)
3. He, K., et al.: Deep residual learning for image recognition. In: IEEE CVPR (2016)
4. Jing, B., Xie, P., Xing, E.: On the automatic generation of medical imaging reports. arXiv:1711.08195 (2017)
5. Li, Z., Wang, C., Han, M., Xue, Y., et al.: Thoracic disease identification and localization with limited supervision. In: IEEE CVPR (2018)
6. Noh, H., Hong, S., Han, B.: Learning deconvolution network for semantic segmentation. In: IEEE ICCV, pp. 1520–1528 (2015)
7. Pesce, E., Ypsilantis, P.P., et al.: Learning to detect chest radiographs containing lung nodules using visual attention networks. arXiv:1712.00996 (2017)
8. Rajpurkar, P., Irvin, J., Zhu, K., et al.: Chexnet: radiologist-level pneumonia detection on chest x-rays with deep learning. arXiv:1711.05225 (2017)
9. Shmelkov, K., Schmid, C., Alahari, K.: Incremental learning of object detectors without catastrophic forgetting. In: IEEE ICCV, pp. 3420–3429 (2017)
10. Wang, X., Peng, Y., et al.: Tienet: text-image embedding network for common thorax disease classification and reporting in chest x-rays. In: IEEE CVPR (2018)

11. Wang, X., Peng, Y., Lu, L., Lu, Z., Bagheri, M., Summers, R.M.: Chestx-ray8: hospital-scale chest x-ray database and benchmarks on weakly-supervised classification and localization of common thorax diseases. In: IEEE CVPR (2017)
12. Wei, Y., et al.: Object region mining with adversarial erasing: a simple classification to semantic segmentation approach. In: IEEE CVPR, pp. 6488–6496 (2017)
13. Wu, Y., et al.: Tensorpack (2016). https://github.com/tensorpack/
14. Yao, L., Poblenz, E., Dagunts, D., et al.: Learning to diagnose from scratch by exploiting dependencies among labels. arXiv:1710.10501 (2017)
15. Yu, F., Koltun, V.: Multi-scale context aggregation by dilated convolutions. In: ICLR (2016)
16. Zhou, B., Khosla, A., Lapedriza, A., Oliva, A., Torralba, A.: Learning deep features for discriminative localization. In: IEEE CVPR, pp. 2921–2929 (2016)

Task Driven Generative Modeling for Unsupervised Domain Adaptation: Application to X-ray Image Segmentation

Yue Zhang[1,2](✉), Shun Miao[1], Tommaso Mansi[1], and Rui Liao[1]

[1] Medical Imaging Technologies, Siemens Healthineers Technology Center, Princeton, NJ 08540, USA
yxz772@case.edu
[2] Department of Mathematics, Applied Mathematics and Statistics, Case Western Reserve University, Cleveland, OH 44106, USA

Abstract. Automatic parsing of anatomical objects in X-ray images is critical to many clinical applications in particular towards image-guided invention and workflow automation. Existing deep network models require a large amount of labeled data. However, obtaining accurate pixel-wise labeling in X-ray images relies heavily on skilled clinicians due to the large overlaps of anatomy and the complex texture patterns. On the other hand, organs in 3D CT scans preserve clearer structures as well as sharper boundaries and thus can be easily delineated. In this paper, we propose a novel model framework for learning automatic X-ray image parsing from labeled CT scans. Specifically, a Dense Image-to-Image network (DI2I) for multi-organ segmentation is first trained on X-ray like Digitally Reconstructed Radiographs (DRRs) rendered from 3D CT volumes. Then we introduce a Task Driven Generative Adversarial Network (TD-GAN) architecture to achieve simultaneous style transfer and parsing for unseen real X-ray images. TD-GAN consists of a modified cycle-GAN substructure for pixel-to-pixel translation between DRRs and X-ray images and an added module leveraging the pre-trained DI2I to enforce segmentation consistency. The TD-GAN framework is general and can be easily adapted to other learning tasks. In the numerical experiments, we validate the proposed model on 815 DRRs and 153 topograms. While the vanilla DI2I without any adaptation fails completely on segmenting the topograms, the proposed model does not require any topogram labels and is able to provide a promising average dice of 85% which achieves the same level accuracy of supervised training (88%).

Keywords: Unsupervised domain adaptation · Deep learning
Image parsing · Generative adversarial networks · Task driven

---

Disclaimer: This feature is based on research, and is not commercially available. Due to regulatory reasons its future availability cannot be guaranteed.

© Springer Nature Switzerland AG 2018
A. F. Frangi et al. (Eds.): MICCAI 2018, LNCS 11071, pp. 599–607, 2018.
https://doi.org/10.1007/978-3-030-00934-2_67

1   Introduction

Semantic understanding of anatomical objects in X-ray images is critical to many clinical applications, such as pathological diagnosis, treatment evaluation and surgical planning. It serves as a fundamental step for computer-aided diagnosis and can enable intelligent workflows including organ-based autocollimation, infinite-capture range registration, motion compensation and automatic reporting. In this paper, we study one of the most important problems in semantic understanding of X-ray image, i.e., multi-organ segmentation.

While X-ray understanding is of great clinical importance, it remains a very challenging task, mainly due to the projective nature of X-ray imaging, which causes large overlapping of anatomies, fuzzy object boundaries and complex texture patterns. Conventional methods rely on prior knowledge of the procedure (e.g., anatomical motion pattern from a sequence of images [1]) to delineate anatomical objects from X-ray images. Modern approaches utilize deep convolutional networks and have shown superior performance [2]. However, they typically require a large amount of pixel-level annotated training data. Due to the heterogeneous nature of X-ray images, accurate annotating becomes extremely difficult and time-consuming even for skilled clinicians. On the other hand, large pixel-level labeled CT data are more accessible. Thousands of X-ray like images, the so-called Digitally Reconstructed Radiographs (DRRs), are generated from labeled CTs and used in [3] to train an X-ray depth decomposition model. While using automatically generated DRRs/labels for training has merits, the trained model cannot be directly applied on X-ray images due to their appearance

Generalization of image segmentation models trained on DRRs to X-ray images requires *unsupervised domain adaptation*. While many effective models [4,5] have been studied, most of them focus on feature adaptation which naturally suits for recognition and detection. However, segmentation task desires pixel-wise classification which requires delicate model design and is substantially different. Recently, pixel-level adaptation models [6,7] have been proposed which utilize generative adversarial networks and achieve promising results on image synthesis and recognition. Still, continuing study on image segmentation especially for medical applications remains blank.

In this paper, we present a novel model framework to address this challenge. Specifically, we first create DRRs and their pixel-level labeling from the segmented pre-operative CT scans. A Dense Image-to-Image network (DI2I) [8,9] is then trained for multi-organ (lung, heart, liver, bone) segmentation over these synthetic data. Next, inspired by the recent success of image style transfer by cycle generative adversarial network (cycle-GAN) [7], we introduce a task driven generative adversarial network (TD-GAN) to achieve simultaneous image synthesis and automatic segmentation on X-ray images, see Fig. 1 for an overview. We emphasize that the training X-ray images are **unpaired** with previous DRRs and are totally **unlabeled**. TD-GAN consists of a modified cycle-GAN substructure for pixel-to-pixel translation between DRRs and X-ray images. Meanwhile, TD-GAN incorporates the pre-trained DI2I to obtain deep supervision and enforce consistent performance on segmentation. The intuition behind TD-

GAN is indeed simple: we transfer X-ray images in the same appearance as DRRs and hence leverage the pre-trained DI2I model to segment them. Furthermore, the entire transfer is guided by the segmentation supervision network.

The contributions of our work are: (1) We propose a novel model pipeline for X-ray image segmentation from unpaired synthetic data (DRRs). (2) We introduce an effective deep architecture TD-GAN for simultaneously image synthesis and segmentation without any labeling effort necessary from X-ray images. To our best knowledge, this is the first end-to-end framework for unsupervised medical image segmentation. (3) The entire model framework can be easily adjusted for unsupervised domain adaptation problem where labels from one domain is completely missing. (4) We conduct numerical experiments and demonstrated the effectiveness of the proposed model with over 800 DRRs and 150 X-ray images.

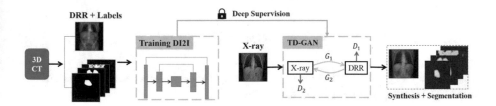

Fig. 1. Overview of the proposed task driven generative model framework.

2 Methodology

2.1 Problem Overview

In this paper, our goal is to learn a multi-organ segmentation model on unlabeled X-ray images using pixel-wise annotated DRRs data. Furthermore, these images are not paired, which means they are not taken from the same group of patients. We collected X-ray images that contain targeted organs such lung, heart, liver and bone (or a subset of them). The DRRs of the same region of interest (ROI) are generated by placing 3D labeled CT volumes in a virtual imaging system that simulates the actual X-ray geometry. Meanwhile, the pixel-level labeling of DRRs are generated by projecting 3D CT labels along the same trajectories. While most public datasets for multi-organ segmentation only consists of tens of cases, our dataset covers a richer variety of scanning ranges, contrast phases as well as morphological differences. In the next subsections, we first train a DI2I on the DRRs and then adapt it to the X-ray images with TD-GAN to provide deep segmentation supervision during the image synthesis.

2.2　Dense Image to Image Network for Segmentation on DRRs

We train a Dense Image-to-Image network (DI2I) on the labeled DRRs data. As is depicted in Fig. 2, the network employs an encoder-decoder UNet structure with dense blocks [2,8,9]. The network consists of dense blocks which are generalizations from ResNets [10] by iteratively concatenating all feature outputs in a feed-forward fashion. This helps alleviating the vanishing gradient problem and thus can obtain a deeper model with higher level feature extraction. Despite these appealing properties, empirically we found that it achieved superior performance than classical UNet. The final output feature map has five channels which consists of a background channel x_0 and four channels $x_1, ..., x_4$ corresponding to the four organs. By doing so, we alleviate the challenge of segmenting overlapped organs and simplify the problem into binary classifications. We further use a customized loss term which is a weighted combination of binary cross entropies between each organ channel and background channel,

$$\mathcal{L}_{seg} = -\sum_{i=1}^{4} w_i(y_i \log(p_i) + (1 - y_i) \log(1 - p_i)) \tag{1}$$

where y_i is the ground truth binary label map for each organ and p_i is calculated as $\exp(x_i)/(\exp(x_0) + \exp(x_i))$ for $i = 1, 2, 3, 4$.

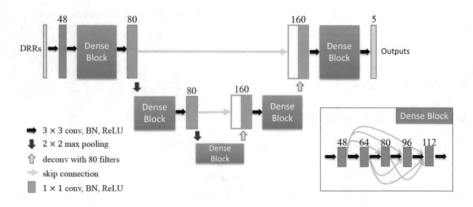

Fig. 2. Illustration of the DI2I for segmentation on DRRs.

2.3　Task Driven Generative Adversarial Networks (TD-GAN)

We now describe the main deep architecture of TD-GAN. The network has a modified cycle-GAN [7] sub-structure with add-on segmentation supervisions. As is depicted in Fig. 3, the base structure consists of two generators G_1, G_2 and two discriminators D_1, D_2 to achieve pixel-to-pixel image synthesis. The generators try to synthesize images in the appearance of the other protocol while

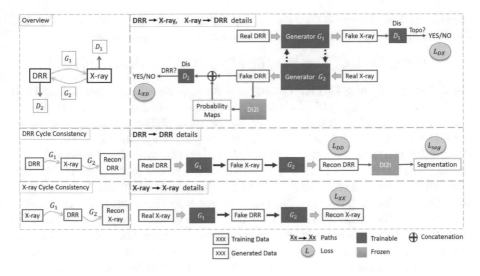

Fig. 3. Proposed TD-GAN architecture. Real X-ray images and DRRs are passed through 4 different paths for simultaneously synthesis and segmentation.

the discriminators need to distinguish the generated images (**fake**) against the reals. When the cyclic training converges to optimal, the network will be able to transfer X-ray images to DRRs through G_2 and transfer back through G_1. This also holds for DRRs. However, image synthesis only serves for a general purpose of appearance transfer and is not segmentation focused. Important prior knowledge such as organ boundaries, shapes and local variations are not carefully treated and could possibly lose during the synthesis process. We therefore add supervision modules to enforce the segmentation consistency, that is, during the transfer process we require the X-ray images that *not only* have the appearance of DRRs *but also* can be segmented by the pre-trained DI2I network. This is done by introducing conditional adversarial training on the translation of X-ray images and cycle segmentation consistency on DRRs. We detail this later on.

The proposed TD-GAN involves 4 different paths that transfer and reconstruct images between the two protocols: real DRR → fake X-ray, real X-ray → fake DRR, real X-ray → reconstructed X-ray and real DRR → reconstructed DRR. Different losses are proposed for each path. We discuss the meaning of these paths in a top-down topological order that is shown in Fig. 3. We denote the data distribution $d \sim p_d$ and $x \sim p_x$ for DRRs and X-ray images. Our main contribution comes in the segmentation driven losses in path real X-ray → fake DRR and real DRR → reconstructed DRR.

Real DRR → Fake X-ray. Given a real DRR image, the generator G_1 tries to produce the corresponding image in the appearance of X-ray images. The discriminator D_1 will need to distinguish the generated fake X-ray image and the real. Since we do not have any paired X-ray images with the DRRs, this real X-ray image is randomly selected from the training dataset. A successful generation from G_1 will confuse D_1 to make the wrong prediction. The loss function involved is a standard GAN loss for image style transfer,

$$\mathcal{L}_{DX} := \mathbb{E}_{t \sim p_x} \left\{ \log \left[D_1(x) \right] \right\} + \mathbb{E}_{d \sim p_d} \left\{ \log \left[1 - D_1(G_1(d)) \right] \right\}.$$

Real X-ray $\rightarrow$ Fake DRR. The other generator G_2 will produce a fake DRR to challenge D_2. We could also randomly select a real DRR in the training of D_2. However, this is suboptimal since the labels of DRRs will be unused which contain important organ information such as size, shape and location and are crucial to our final segmentation task. Inspired by the conditional GANs [11], we leverage the pre-trained DI2I to predict the organ labels on the fake DRRs. The fake DRRs combined with their predicted labels are then fed into D_2 to compare with the real pairs. Therefore D_2 needs to not only distinguish the fake DRRs and the reals but also determine whether the image-label pairs are realistic. To confuse D_2, the generator G_2 will particularly focus on the organs of interest during the image transfer. We hence will obtain a more powerful generator in the task of segmentation. Finally, to make the involved loss function differentiable, we only obtain the predicted probability map from the DI2I and do not binarize them. Denote $U(\cdot)$ as the pre-trained DI2I, we have the following loss function for this path,

$$\begin{aligned} \mathcal{L}_{XD} := & \mathbb{E}_{d \sim p_d} \left\{ \log \left[D_2(d|U(d)) \right] \right\} \\ & + \mathbb{E}_{x \sim p_x} \left\{ \log \left[1 - D_2(G_2(x)|U(G_2(x))) \right] \right\}. \end{aligned} \tag{2}$$

We remark that the pre-trained DI2I is frozen during the training of TD-GAN, otherwise the supervision will be disturbed by the fake DRRs. Furthermore, TD-GAN can be easily adapted to other tasks by replacing $U(\cdot)$.

Real X-ray $\rightarrow$ Reconstructed X-ray. The idea behind this path is that once we transferred a X-ray image to a fake DRR through G_2, we should be able to transfer this DRR back to X-ray image through G_1. The final (reconstructed) X-ray image should be the same as the original one. This is called cycle-consistency. The corresponding loss function is calculated by l_1 distance,

$$\mathcal{L}_{XX} := \mathbb{E}_{x \sim p_x} \left\{ \|G_1(G_2(x)) - x\|_1 \right\}$$

Real DRR $\rightarrow$ Reconstructed DRR. Same argument also applies to the DRR reconstruction. Moreover, we enforce the reconstructed DRR to maintain cycle segmentation consistency by adding a segmentation loss as a regularization term. The implies that we would like that the reconstructed DRR is not only close to the original but maintain the same segmentation performance under DI2I. The two losses involved in this path are as follows,

$$\begin{aligned} \mathcal{L}_{DD} &:= \mathbb{E}_{d \sim p_d} \left\{ \|G_2(G_1(d)) - d\|_1 \right\}, \\ \mathcal{L}_{seg} &:= \mathcal{L}_{seg}, \end{aligned} \tag{3}$$

where the segmentation loss $\mathcal{L}_{seg}$ is the same as in Eq. (1).

The total loss for TD-GAN is then a weighted summation of all the losses in the above paths. We demonstrate the effectiveness of these two losses in the experiments. We employ the same parameter setting as is suggested in [7]. The generator G_1 and G_2 utilize a same Resnet20 structure. The discriminator D_1 and D_2 contains four consecutive convolutional layers with increasing number of filters from 64 to 512 and a final output layer with sigmoid activation.

3   Experiments and Results

In this section we validate our methodology on a dataset of 815 labeled DRRs and 153 topograms. The topograms are acquired before the CT scan for isocentering and therefore co-registered with the CT. The CT scans are labeled pixelwisely and the labels of topograms are generated in a same way as the aforementioned DRRs masks. The co-registered CT is not used in training and the labels on topograms are used only for evaluation purpose. Our model is among the first approaches to address unsupervised domain adaptation for segmentation with unpaired data. We compare with the state-of-the-art image synthesis model cycle-GAN [7] since both can be used in our problem except ours are task driven. To further show the effectiveness of the deep architecture and the proposed losses, we also compare our models with TD-GAN adversarial (TD-GAN-A) and TD-GAN reconstruction segmentation (TD-GAN-S) by enabling either one of the conditional adversarial loss (2) and the cycle segmentation consistency loss (3).

We first train a DI2I for multi organ segmentation on the labeled DRRs. A standard 5 fold cross-validation scheme is used to find the best learned weights. We evaluate the dice score on the testing dataset, summarized as follows (mean ± std): lung 0.9417 ± 0.017, heart 0.923 ± 0.056, liver 0.894 ± 0.061 and bone 0.910 ± 0.020. All the experiments are run on an 12GB NVIDIA TITAN X GPU.

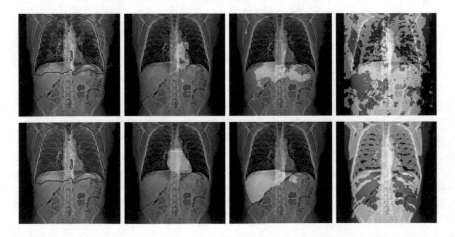

Fig. 4. Visualization of segmentation results on topograms (bottom) against direct application of DI2I (top). The red curves stands for the boundary of the ground truth. The colored fill-in parts are the predictions by TD-GAN and DI2I.

Next we load the pretrained DI2I into TD-GAN with weights all frozen and train the model to segment the topograms. We use all the DRRs as well as 73 topograms for training, 20 topograms for validation and 60 for testing. We visualize one example and compare the proposed method against vanilla setting (where the DI2I is tested directly on topograms) in Fig. 4. For better visualization purpose, we only show the ground the truth labeling for lung, heart and liver. The numerical results are summarized in Table 1. To better understand the performance of our model, we also train the DI2I on the topograms using their labels under the same data splitting setting, listed as Supervised in Table 1.

While the direct application of the learned DI2I on topograms fails completely, it can be seen that our model significantly improved the segmentation accuracy and even provided the same level of accuracy compared with the supervised training with labeled topograms. Compared with the cycle-GAN which only performs image style transfer, both the partially task driven nets TD-GAN-A and TD-GAN-S can improve the performance. Furthermore, the final TD-GAN combines the advantages of all the three models and achieves the best.

Table 1. Average Dice results of segmentation on topograms.

Objects	Vanilla	CGAN	TD-GAN-A	TD-GAN-S	TD-GAN	Supervised
Bone	0.401	0.808	0.800	0.831	**0.835**	0.871
Heart	0.233	0.816	0.846	0.860	**0.870**	0.880
Liver	0.285	0.781	0.797	0.804	**0.817**	0.841
Lung	0.312	0.825	0.853	0.879	**0.894**	0.939
mean	0.308	0.808	0.824	0.844	**0.854**	0.883

4   Discussions and Conclusions

In this paper, we studied the problem on multi-organ segmentation over totally unlabeled X-ray images with labeled DRRs. Our model leverages a cycle-GAN substructure to achieve image style transfer and carefully designed add-on modules to simultaneously segment organs of interest. The proposed model framework is general. By replacing the DI2I with other types of supervision networks, it can be easily adapted to many scenarios in computer-aided diagnosis such as prostate lesion classification, anatomical landmark localization and abnormal motion detection. We leave this for the future direction.

References

1. Zhu, Y., Prummer, S., Wang, P., Chen, T., Comaniciu, D., Ostermeier, M.: Dynamic layer separation for coronary DSA and enhancement in fluoroscopic sequences. In: Yang, G.-Z., Hawkes, D., Rueckert, D., Noble, A., Taylor, C. (eds.) MICCAI 2009. LNCS, vol. 5762, pp. 877–884. Springer, Heidelberg (2009). https://doi.org/10.1007/978-3-642-04271-3_106

2. Ronneberger, O., Fischer, P., Brox, T.: U-Net: convolutional networks for biomedical image segmentation. In: Navab, N., Hornegger, J., Wells, W.M., Frangi, A.F. (eds.) MICCAI 2015. LNCS, vol. 9351, pp. 234–241. Springer, Cham (2015). https://doi.org/10.1007/978-3-319-24574-4_28

3. Albarqouni, S., Fotouhi, J., Navab, N.: X-Ray in-depth decomposition: revealing the latent structures. In: Descoteaux, M., Maier-Hein, L., Franz, A., Jannin, P., Collins, D.L., Duchesne, S. (eds.) MICCAI 2017. LNCS, vol. 10435, pp. 444–452. Springer, Cham (2017). https://doi.org/10.1007/978-3-319-66179-7_51

4. Bousmalis, K., et al.: Domain separation networks. In: NIPs (2016)

5. Tzeng, E., et al.: Adversarial discriminative domain adaptation. In: CVPR (2017)

6. Bousmalis, K., et al.: Unsupervised pixel-level domain adaptation with generative adversarial networks. In: CVPR (2017)

7. Zhu, J.Y., et al.: Unpaired image-to-image translation using cycle-consistent adversarial networks. arXiv preprint arXiv:1703.10593 (2017)

8. Huang, G., et al.: Densely connected convolutional networks. In: CVPR (2017)

9. Jégou, S., et al.: The one hundred layers tiramisu: fully convolutional densenets for semantic segmentation. In: CVPRW (2017)

10. He, K., et al.: Deep residual learning for image recognition. In: CVPR (2016)

11. Mirza, M., et al.: Conditional generative adversarial nets. arXiv preprint arXiv:1411.1784 (2014)

Cardiac, Chest and Abdominal Applications: Colorectal, Kidney and Liver Imaging Applications

Towards Automated Colonoscopy Diagnosis: Binary Polyp Size Estimation via Unsupervised Depth Learning

Hayato Itoh[1(✉)], Holger R. Roth[1,2], Le Lu[2], Masahiro Oda[1], Masashi Misawa[3], Yuichi Mori[3], Shin-ei Kudo[3], and Kensaku Mori[1,4,5]

[1] Graduate School of Informatics, Nagoya University, Nagoya, Japan
hitoh@mori.m.is.nagoya-u.ac.jp
[2] AI-Infra, NVIDIA Corporation, Santa Clara, USA
[3] Digestive Disease Center, Showa University Northern Yokohama Hospital, Yokohama, Japan
[4] Information Technology Center, Nagoya University, Nagoya, Japan
[5] Research Center for Medical Bigdata, National Institute of Informatics, Tokyo, Japan

Abstract. In colon cancer screening, polyp size estimation using only colonoscopy images or videos is difficult even for expert physicians although the size information of polyps is important for diagnosis. Towards the fully automated computer-aided diagnosis (CAD) pipeline, a robust and precise polyp size estimation method is highly desired. However, the size estimation problem of a three-dimensional object from a two-dimensional image is ill-posed due to the lack of three-dimensional spatial information. To circumvent this challenge, we formulate a relaxed form of size estimation as a binary classification problem and solve it by a new deep neural network architecture: BseNet. This relaxed form of size estimation is defined as a two-category classification: under and over a certain polyp dimension criterion that would provoke different clinical treatments (resecting the polyp or not). BseNet estimates the depth map image from an input colonoscopic RGB image using unsupervised deep learning, and integrates RGB with the computed depth information to produce a four-channel RGB-D imagery data, that is subsequently encoded by BseNet to extract deep RGB-D image features and facilitate the size classification into two categories: under and over 10 mm polyps. For the evaluation of BseNet, a large dataset of colonoscopic videos of totally over 16 h is constructed. We evaluate the accuracies of both binary polyp size estimation and polyp detection performance since detection is a prerequisite step of a fully automated CAD system. The experimental results show that our proposed BseNet achieves 79.2 % accuracy for binary polyp-size classification. We also combine the image feature extraction by BseNet and classification of short video clips using a long short-term memory (LSTM) network. Polyp detection (if the video clip contains a polyp or not) shows 88.8 % sensitivity when employing the spatio-temporal image feature extraction and classification.

© Springer Nature Switzerland AG 2018
A. F. Frangi et al. (Eds.): MICCAI 2018, LNCS 11071, pp. 611–619, 2018.
https://doi.org/10.1007/978-3-030-00934-2_68

Keywords: Size estimation · Depth estimation · Deep neural networks · Long short-term memory (LSTM) · Polyp detection

1 Introduction

Size information of detected polyps is an essential factor for diagnosis in colon cancer screening. For example, the U.S. guideline for colonoscopy surveillance defines what treatments should be acted after a physicians find polyps with respect to their size estimations [1]. Whether the size of a polyp is over or under 10 mm is important. The guideline [1] defines that patients with only 1 or 2 small (≤10 mm) tubular adenomas with only low-grade dysplasia should have their next follow-up in 5–10 years; and patients with 3 to 10 adenomas, or any adenoma >10 mm, or any adenoma with villous features or high-grade dysplasia will have follow-ups in 3 years. However, polyp size estimation using only colonoscopy is quite difficult even for expert physicians so that automated size estimation techniques would be desirable.

In general, size estimation of a 3D object from a 2D image is an ill-posed problem due to the lack of three-dimensional spatial information. Figure 1 demonstrates the challenge of the polyp-size estimation from a colonoscopic image. Polyps with different diameters from 2 mm to 16 mm may have the similar image sizes or ranges. The image size of a polyp depends on both the true 3D polyp size and the physical distance from colonoscope to the polyp. Our key question is that will the recovered image depth information augmented with original colonoscopic RGB images be helpful for polyp size estimation and detection. Depth maps from monocular colonoscopic RGB images can be computed through unsupervised deep neural network [2,3].

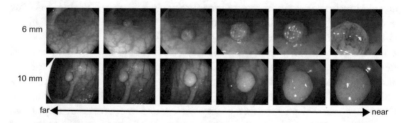

Fig. 1. Examples of polyps on colonoscopic images. Top and bottom rows show images that capture polyps with diameters of 6 mm and 10 mm, respectively. From left to right, columns show images with different (long to short) distances from colonoscope to polyps.

Previous techniques have been proposed for 3D scene reconstruction and camera pose recovery out of 2D images [4,5]. Reference [4] extracts invariant geometry features of rigid objects and complies them to the geometrical constraints of cameras to reconstruct 3D information. In colonoscopy, there is only one light source where shading based 3D object shape reconstruction [5] is possible. However these 3D reconstruction methods may not work well in colonoscopy due to the non-rigidness and complex textures the colon wall.

We propose a new method for binary polyp size estimation or classification from a single colonoscopic image. The problem of size estimation is relaxed into a binary size classification task according to guidelines [1]. We propose the binary-size estimation network (BseNet) to solve two-category polyp classification. First, BseNet estimates depth maps from three-channel (RGB) colonoscopic images via unsupervised depth recovery convolutional neural networks [2,3], and integrates all channels into RGB-D imagery. Second, RGB-D image features from the newly integrated imagery are extracted. Third, the two-category classification for binary size estimation is performed by classifying these RGB-D image features. Finally, For a complete and automated computer-aided polyp diagnosis system, we exploit the polyp detection performance based on spatio-temporal deep features by leveraging a large dataset of colonoscopic videos.

2   Methods

2.1   Spatio-temporal Video Based Polyp Detection

Before estimating binary polyp sizes, polyp detection is a prerequisite processing step with no de facto standard methods [6,7]. In this paper, we adopt scene classification representation to classify the existence status of polyps in any colonoscopic video sub-clips: as *positive* when at least one polyp exists, or *negative* when there is no polyp. Polyp detection in colonoscope imagery requires the extraction of spatio-temporal image feature from videos. Successive colonoscopic image frames usually include similar objects of the same scene category. In particular, for the positive category, a polyp should appear in successive frames. Therefore, polyp detection as scene classification needs to handle the temporal context in addition to the spatial structure of 2D images.

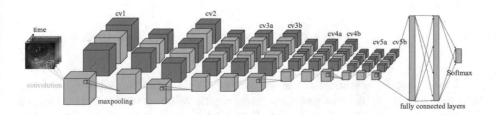

Fig. 2. Architecture of spatio-temporal classification for polyp detection. C3dNet extracts deep image spatial-temporal features via 3D convolutional and pooling procedures.

To extract and classify spatio-temporal image features for polyp detection, we use the 3D convolutional neural network (C3dNet) [8]. Figure 2 illustrates the C3dNet network architecture. The input for C3dNet is a set of successive 16 frames extracted from colonoscopic videos. We set all 3D convolutional filters as $3\times3\times3$ with $1\times1\times1$ stride. All 3D pooling layers are $2\times2\times2$ with $2\times2\times2$ stride, except for the first pooling layer which has kernel size of $1\times2\times2$. The output of C3dNet are the probability scores of two categories. If the output probability for positive category is larger than the criterion, polyp detection CAD system concludes that the input frames represent the scene where polyp exists. Note that before classification, we empirically search the best hyper-parameters of C3dNet to be optimized for polyp detection using the training dataset.

2.2   Two-Category Polyp Size Estimation

Our main purpose is to achieve the binary polyp size estimation (over 10 mm in diameter or not) from a 2D colonoscopic image $\mathcal{X} \in \mathbb{R}^{H \times W \times 3}$ of three channels with height H and width W. The straightforward estimation of polyp size s is defined as

$$\min \|s - s^*\|_2 \text{ w.r.t. } s = f(\mathcal{X}), \tag{1}$$

where $\|\cdot\|_2$ is the Euclidean norm, and s^* is the ground truth. This minimization problem is solved as regression that minimizes the square root error. However, this is an ill-posed problem since a 2D colonoscopic frame represents the appearance of a polyp on an image plane without available depth information. Therefore, we consider the function $f(\mathcal{X}, \boldsymbol{D}^*)$ with the depth image $\boldsymbol{D}^* \in \mathbb{R}^{H \times W}$ that minimizes

$$\|s - s^*\|_2 \text{ w.r.t. } s = f(\mathcal{X}, \boldsymbol{D}^*). \tag{2}$$

We need annotated data with high precision to solve this minimization problem accurately. Note that polyp size annotation on images usually include small errors.

To make the polyp size estimation problem more practical and robust, we define the following relaxed minimization function with ground truth $s_B \in \{0, 1\}$ and $\mathcal{L}_0$-norm $\|\cdot\|_0$ as

$$\|f(\mathcal{X}, D^*) - s_B\|_0 \tag{3}$$

with respect to

$$f(\mathcal{X}, \boldsymbol{D}^*) = \begin{cases} 1, & \text{a polyp on an image is larger than 10 mm,} \\ 0, & \text{otherwise.} \end{cases} \tag{4}$$

Depth map information $\boldsymbol{D}^*$ is necessary in this definition although colonoscope device is not able to measure image depth values directly. In this relaxed form, we compute the depth image $D \in \mathbb{R}^{H \times W}$ that represents only relative depth information in an image, such like far and near. This type of depth cue $\boldsymbol{D}$ is not the physical distance from colonoscope to an object. Our depth images are obtained by adopting the unsupervised deep learning method of depth estimation from [2,3]. Using Depth or Disparity CNNs [2,3], we define a depth estimation function $g(\mathcal{X})$ that satisfies

$$\min \|g(\mathcal{X}) - \boldsymbol{D}^*/\|\boldsymbol{D}^*\|_{\mathrm{F}}\|_{\mathrm{F}}, \tag{5}$$

where $\| \cdot \|_F$ is Frobenius norm, through unsupervised learning. This neural network need only colonoscopic videos for training, without ground truth of depth information (which is infeasible to acquire annotations for colonoscopic videos, if not entirely impossible).

Our proposed BsdNet shown in Fig. 3 intends to satisfy

$$\min \| f(\mathcal{X}, g(\mathcal{X})) - s_B \|_0 \text{ and } \min \| g(\mathcal{X}) - \boldsymbol{D}^* / \| \boldsymbol{D}^* \|_F \|_F. \tag{6}$$

The BseNet output the estimated size label $s \in \{0, 1\}$ for an input colonoscopic image. The right term of Eq. (6) is minimized by Depth CNN. The left term of Eq. (6) is minimized by RGB-D CNN shown in Fig. 4. The RGB-D CNN extracts RGB-D image features that minimizes the softmax loss function of two-category classification, that is, classification of polyps whether over or under 10 mm in diameter.

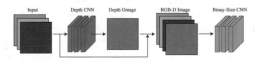

Fig. 3. Architecture of the binary polyp size estimation network (BseNet). BseNet first estimates the depth map from an RGB colonoscopic image by employing depth CNN. The estimated depth image is then combined with the input RGB channels to form an RGB-D image. BsdNet then classifies the newly composite RGB-D image into two categories: polyp over and under 10 mm in diameter.

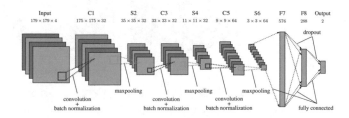

Fig. 4. Architecture of RGB-D CNN. Input is an RGB-D image of four channels.

3   Experimental Results

Dataset: We construct a new dataset to validate our proposed polyp detection and binary size estimation method. We collect 73 colonoscopic videos, captured by CF-HQ290ZI (Olympus, Tokyo, Japan), with IRB approval. All frames of these videos are annotated by expert endoscopists. The total time of these videos is about 16 h 37 min. The total video run time is 4 h 55 min (where 152 polyps are present or exist). These videos are captured under the different observation conditions of white light, narrow band imaging, and staining. Each frame is annotated and checked by two expert colonoscopists with experience over 5000 cases. Labels of pathological types, shape types, size (2, 3, . . . , 16 mm) and observation types are given.

3.1   Polyp Detection

We extract only the polyp frames that are captured under the white light condition. For non-polyp frames, we obtain images where polyps do not exist under several observation conditions. We divide these extracted frames into the training and testing datasets. The training dataset consist of polyp frames of 30 min 30 s and non-polyp frames of 24 min 12 s. The testing dataset represents of polyp frames of 18 min 1 s and non-polyp frames of 18 min 23 s. The training and testing datasets include different 102 and 50 polyps, respectively. Only training dataset is used for searching of optimal hyper-parameters of C3dNet with Adam optimizer. The testing dataset is used for validation of the classification accuracy of polyp and non-polyp frames. In both training and test datasets, colonoscopic images are rescaled into the resolution of 112×112 pixels. Therefore, the size of input data for c3dNet [8] is $112 \times 112 \times 16$. Figure 5 summarizes the validation results on the testing dataset.

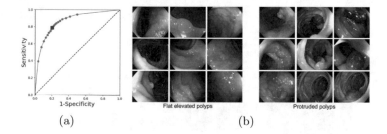

(a)   (b)

Fig. 5. Results for polyp detection. (a) Receiver Operating Characteristic (ROC) curve. (b) and (c) illustrate difficult and easy types, respectively, for detection.

Table 1. Results for each frame

	Accuracy for each frame
BseNet	79.2 %
CNN	77.5 %

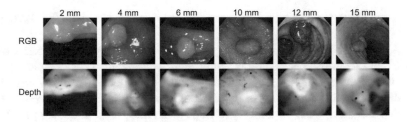

Fig. 6. The results of colonoscopic depth image estimation by unsupervised depth CNNs. White and black pixels represent near and far distances, respectively, from colonoscope.

Table 2. Results for each video clip

	RGB feature	RGB-D feature
Mean	55.3 %	73.7 %
LSTM	73.7 %	79.0

3.2 Polyp Size Estimation

Single Image Based Polyp Size Classification: We evaluated accuracy of the polyp size estimation as a frame classification problem for colonoscopic videos. We extracted 34,396 and 13,093 images of protrude polyps from 73 colonoscopic videos for training and test dataset for size estimation. The training and test datasets include different protrude polyps without duplication.

The training of BseNet is divided to two procedures. At the first training, we trained Depth CNN by using the polyp frames of 30 min 30 s in the previous subsection. For the second training, we estimated depth images of the training and test dataset and generated RGB-D images for training and test respectively. Figure 6 shows the depth images and original RGB images. At the second training, we trained RGB-D CNN with Adam for the generated RGB-D images. We evaluate the ratio of correct estimation as accuracy by using test dataset. For the comparison, we also trained RGB CNN and estimate polyp sizes by using the same training and test dataset of RGB-images. Table 1 summalizes the results of RGB-CNN and BseNet.

Video Clip Based Polyp Size Classification: We evaluated the polyp size estimation as a sequence classification problem with long-short term memory (LSTM) recurrent neural networks [9]. Given the per-frame predictions $P(\mathcal{X}_t) \in [0, 1]$ for over 10 mm size and per-frame penultimate feature response $\boldsymbol{F}(\mathcal{X}_t) \in \mathbb{R}^{288}$ of our size estimation of BseNet (F8 layer in Fig. 4) for a time sequence $t = 1, 2, \ldots,$, we build a sequence of feature vectors $\boldsymbol{f}_s = [P(\mathcal{X}_1), \boldsymbol{F}(\mathcal{X}_1)^\top, \ldots P(\mathcal{X}_n), \boldsymbol{F}(\mathcal{X}_n)^\top]^\top$ for LSTM classification. In our case, this results in a 289 length real valued vector for each frame of the sequence. We standardize all sequences to have zero-mean and std. dev. of one based on our training set. We furthermore limit the total length of a sequence to 1,000 by either truncating the longer or padding the shorter polyp video clip feature vectors.

LSTM Model: We firstly use a stack of two LSTM layers consisting of 128 and 64 memory units each. The outputs from the second LSTM layer are then fed to two fully connected layers with 64 and 32 units, each employing batch normalization followed ReLU activations. A final fully connected layer predicts the polyp size from each sequence vector f_s with a *sigmoid* activation for binary classification.

Results are summarized in Table 2 and compared to using the average prediction value $|P(\mathcal{X}_t)|$ of all frames in the polyp sequence. As we can observe, both RGB and RGB-D cases experience an improved prediction accuracy using the LSTM model with the RGB-D model outperforming the model only based on color channels.

4   Discussion

When using the threshold criterion of 0.5 for polyp detection (see red square on Fig. 5), accuracy, sensitivity and specificity scores are 74.7%, 88.1% and 61.7%, respectively. The area under ROC curve (AUC) value is 0.83. In the current results, specificity is smaller than sensitivity, which implies the wider or broader varieties of patterns in the negative class of non-polyp frames for polyp detections. In these experiments, the detection rate of flat elevated polyp as shown in Fig. 5(b) is smaller than the detection rate of protruded polyps, demonstrated in Fig. 5(c).

The experimental results for size estimations show that our proposed BseNet (using RGB+D) achieves 79.2% accuracy for binary polyp-size classification that is about 2% larger than the accuracy of CNN (only using RGB). This results imply the validity of relaxed form of size estimation. We also combine the image feature extraction by BseNet and classification of short video clips using a long short-term memory (LSTM) network. The results of LSTM classifications also show that RGB+D features that extracted by BseNet achieves 5.3% higher accuracy than RGB features alone. These results show the validity of RGB-D features extracted by BseNet.

5   Conclusions

We formulated the relaxed form of polyp size estimation from colonoscopic video as the binary classification problem and solve it by proposing the new deep learning-based architecture: BseNet towards automated colonoscopy diagnosis. BseNet estimates the depth map image from an input colonoscopic RGB image using upsupervised deep learning, and integrates RGB with the computed depth information to produce four-channel RGB-D imagery data. This RGB-D data is subsequently encoded by BseNet to extract deep RGB-D image features and facilitate the size classification into two categories: under and over 10 mm polyps.

Our experimental results show the validity of the relaxed form of the size estimation and the promising performance of the proposed BseNet.

This research was partially supported by AMED Research Grant (18hs0110006 h0002, 18hk0102034h0103), and JSPS KAKENHI (26108006, 17H00867, 17K20 099).

References

1. Winawer, S.: Guidelines for colonoscopy surveillance after polypectomy: a consensus update by the us multi-society task force on colorectal cancer and the american cancer society. Gastroenterology **130**, 1872–1885 (2006)
2. Mayer, N., et al.: A large dataset to train convolutional networks for disparity, optical flow, and scene flow estimation. In: Proceedings of the CVPR (2016)
3. Zhou, T., Brown, M., Snavely, N., Lowe, D.: Unsupervised learning of depth and ego-motion from video. In: Proceedings of the CVPR (2017)
4. Hartley, R., Zisserman, A.: Multiple View Geometry in Computer Vision, 2nd edn. Cambridge University Press, Cambridge (2011)
5. Visentini-Scarzanella, M., Stoyanov, D., Yang, G.Z.: Metric depth recovery from monocular images using shape-from-shading and specularities. In: Proceedings of the IEEE ICIP (2012)
6. Bernal, J., Sánchez, J., Vilariño, F.: Towards automatic polyp detection with a polyp appearance model. Pattern Recognit. **45**(9), 3166–3182 (2012)
7. Bernal, J.: Comparative validation of polyp detection methods in video colonoscopy: results from the MICCAI 2015 endoscopic vision challenge. IEEE Trans. Med. Imaging **36**(6), 1231–1249 (2017)
8. Tran, D., Bourdev, L., Fergus, R., Torresani, L., Paluri, M.: Learning spatiotemporal features with 3d convolutional networks. In: Proceedings of the ICCV (2015)
9. Hochreiter, S., Schmidhuber, J.: Long short-term memory. Neural Comput. **9**(8), 1735–1780 (1997)

RIIS-DenseNet: Rotation-Invariant and Image Similarity Constrained Densely Connected Convolutional Network for Polyp Detection

Yixuan Yuan[1,2(✉)] ⓘ, Wenjian Qin[3], Bulat Ibragimov[2], Bin Han[2], and Lei Xing[2]

[1] Department of Electronic Engineering, City Univeristy of Hong Kong, Hong Kong, China
yxyuan.ee@cityu.edu.hk
[2] Department of Radiation Oncology, Stanford University, Stanford, USA
[3] Shenzhen Institutes of Advanced Technology, Chinese Academy of Sciences, Shenzhen, China

Abstract. Colorectal cancer is the leading cause of cancer-related deaths. Most colorectal cancers are believed to arise from benign adenomatous polyps. Automatic methods for polyp detection with Wireless Capsule Endoscopy (WCE) images are desirable, but the results of current approaches are limited due to the problems of object rotation and high intra-class variability. To address these problems, we propose a rotation invariant and image similarity constrained Densely Connected Convolutional Network (RIIS-DenseNet) model. We first introduce Densely Connected Convolutional Network (DenseNet), which enables the maximum information flow among layers by a densely connected mechanism, to provide end-to-end polyp detection workflow. The rotation-invariant regularization constraint is then introduced to explicitly enforce learned features of the training samples and the corresponding rotation versions to be mapped close to each other. The image similarity constraint is further proposed by imposing the image category information on the features to maintain small intra-class scatter. Our method achieves an inspiring accuracy 95.62% for polyp detection. Extensive experiments on the WCE dataset show that our method has superior performance compared with state-of-the-art methods.

1 Introduction

Polyps are important precursors to the colorectal cancer, which is the third most common cancer diagnosed in both men and women [8]. It is reported that there will be 140,250 new colorectal cancer cases in United States in 2018. Wireless capsule endoscope (WCE) [4] has revolutionized the diagnostic inspection of the Gastrointestinal (GI) polyps and remains the first-line tool for screening of abnormalities. It provides a noninvasive, direct visualization of the whole GI

© Springer Nature Switzerland AG 2018
A. F. Frangi et al. (Eds.): MICCAI 2018, LNCS 11071, pp. 620–628, 2018.
https://doi.org/10.1007/978-3-030-00934-2_69

tract. Despite sustained technical advancements, WCE videos are still manually reviewed, which is extremely laborious and time-consuming.

Many computational methods have been developed to automatically detect polyps from WCE images [1,7,9–12]. Gueye et al. [1] introduced scale-invariant feature transform descriptor algorithm with bag of word approach for feature extraction. With the support vector machine (SVM) classification method, they discriminated polyp tissues from the normal images. Zhang et al. [12] proposed a novel transfer learning application for automatic polyp image detection using Convolutional Neural Network (CNN) features learned from non-medical domain. Segui et al. [6] fused the original RGB images and corresponding Laplacians and Hessians transformations together as an input of the network, and utilized basic CNN architecture with three convolution-max pooling layers followed by a fully connected layer to conduct polyp detection task. The existing methods [1,7,9,10,12] utilized low level hand-craft features or traditional CNN models to represent information of WCE images. It is reported that traditional features, designed for natural images, could not achieve good performance for medical images due to their poor generalization capability. Although deep CNN networks usually extract better features than shallow network and lead to better performance, the gradient vanish problem may occur and impede the convergence of the network as the layer of CNN goes deeper. The recent Densely Connected Convolutional Network (DenseNet) [3] demonstrated inspiring performance in image classification. It connects each layer to every other layer in a feed forward fashion to learn features. In this regard, it ensures maximum information flow between layers in the network, and alleviates the vanishing-gradient problem, strengthens feature propagation and encourages feature reuse. While the DenseNet has shown impressive success, they still could not effectively deal with the specific challenges in polyp detection, such as object rotation and intra-class variability. The WCE has no active motor and it is propelled by peristalsis along the GI tract. Therefore, the same polyp may exist in different positions of the collected images. Moreover, the polyps may be located at any location of the GI tract with different mucosa surfaces and they are usually small, thus the collected polyps demonstrate large intra-class variance.

In this paper, we propose a novel rotation-invariant and image similarity constrained Densely Connected Convolutional Network (RIIS-DenseNet) to differentiate the polyps from normal WCE images. We first introduce the DenseNet to build the deep learning model. Then we elaborate the DenseNet by introducing rotation invariant constraint, which enforces the training samples and their corresponding rotation ones to share the similar feature representations and hence achieving rotation-invariance. Moreover, a novel image similarity constraint is proposed to enable images to be coincident with corresponding category directions in the learned feature space. With the joint loss function, our model could learn discriminative features of WCE images and further promote the performance of polyp detection.

2   Method: RIIS-DenseNet Model

In this paper, we propose a novel RIIS-DenseNet model to differentiate the polyp images from normal ones. The workflow of our method is shown in Fig. 1. Our method consists of following four steps. First, we rotate the collected training WCE image to augment the datasets. Then we introduce DenseNet, which connects each layer to every other layer in a feed-forward fashion, to learn features from WCE images. The joint loss function including softmax loss, the rotation-invariant constraint and the image similarity constraint is proposed to evaluate loss values in the training procedure. The fourth part of our RIIS-DenseNet model fuses these three loss function together in the DenseNet model to obtain the final discriminative WCE image features and further detect polyps.

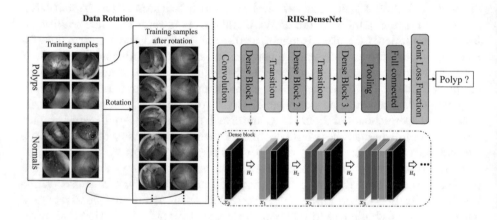

Fig. 1. Workflow of our proposed RIIS-DenseNet. It consists of two parts: data rotation augmentation and RIIS-DenseNet. The RIIS-DenseNet includes three denseblocks, two transitions, one convolution layer, one pooling layer and a novel joint loss function layer.

2.1   Data Rotation Augmentation

Given a set of initial polyps and normal WCE training samples $X = \{X_1, X_2\}$, we generate a new set of training samples $X_{new} = \{X, T_\phi X\}$. T_ϕ represents a group of K rotation transformations and we consider $\phi = \{45°, 90°, 135°, 180°, 225°, 270°, 315°\}$. N defines the original number of training images, then the size of new training images is $N \times (K+1)$. In this way, we enlarge the training data to deal with limited WCE images. The corresponding labels of X_{new} are defined as $L_{new} = \{l_{x_i} | x_i \in X_{new}\}$ where l_{x_i} with only one element being 1 at the mth position ($m = 1 \; or \; 2$).

2.2   DenseNet

A deep network usually extracts better features than shallow network and leads to better performance [2]. However, as the network goes deeper, the gradient vanish problem may occur and impede the convergence of the network. In this work, we utilize the DenseNet [3] to alleviate the vanishing-gradient problem and strengthen feature propagation.

The principal characteristic of DenseNet is the dense connectivity. That is, each layer of the structure is directly connected to every other layer in a feed-forward way. This strategy encourages the direct supervision signal for all layers, enables the reuse of features among layers and strengthens feature propagation. Given x_{l-1} represents the output of the $l - 1^{th}$ layer, $H_l(x)$ denotes a series of transformations, the output of the lth layer x_l is calculated as follows,

$$x_l = H_l([x_0, x_1, ..., x_{l-1}]), \tag{1}$$

where [.] refers to the concatenation operation. Suppose that each function H_l produce k features, then the number of features maps for the lth layer is $k_0 + k \times (l - 1)$, where k_0 represents the number of channels in the input layer. The parameter k defines the growth rate and controls the number of parameters in the model. The DenseNet has fewer parameters than traditional networks because it avoids learning redundant features.

Specific, our proposed workflow includes three denseblocks as shown in Fig. 1. Each denseblock is comprised of 6 densely connections transformation layers and the transformation consists of a batch normalization, a rectified linear unit, and a convolution layer with a 3×3 kernel. The transition layer connects two denseblocks, and it includes of a 1×1 convolution followed by a 2×2 max pooling transformation. Following the last dense block, we set a global max pooling layer and a fully connected layer. Then a joint loss function classifier is attached to conduct the polyp detection problem.

2.3   Joint Loss Function

To achieve better characterization of WCE images and improve the polyp detection performance, our proposed RIIS-DenseNet model introduces a novel joint loss function to evaluate loss values between the predict labels and true ones, further learn discriminative features.

Traditional Softmax Function. The most widely used classification loss function is softmax loss, which tends to minimize the misclassification errors for the given training samples. This loss function $D(X_{new}, L_{new})$ is presented by

$$D(X_{new}, L_{new}) = \frac{1}{N \times (K + 1)} \sum_{x_i \in X_{new}} l_{x_i} \log(\hat{l_{x_i}}), \tag{2}$$

where $\hat{l_{x_i}}$ indicates the probability of image x_i being correctly classified as class l_{x_i}. The Eq. (2) represents the dissimilarity of the approximated output distribution from the true distribution of labels.

Rotation-Invariance Regularization Constraint. The traditional DenseNet model only uses softmax loss function to minimize classification errors in the training process, this strategy ignores the specific rotation variance in the polyp images, which will inevitably result in misclassification of images that belong to the same category. In order to obtain discriminative deeply learned features, we introduce rotation-invariance regularization $D(X, T_\phi X)$, which enforces the training samples X and the ones after rotating $T_\phi X$, to share similar features. This regularization term is defined as follows,

$$D(X, T_\phi X) = \frac{1}{N} \sum_{i=1}^{N} \|f(x_i) - Mean(f(T_\phi x_i))\|^2 \tag{3}$$

where $f(x_i)$ represents the learned feature of the training sample x_i. $Mean(f(T_\phi x_i))$ denotes the average feature of rotated versions of the training sample x_i and it is calculated as

$$Mean(f(T_\phi x_i)) = \frac{1}{K} \sum_{\phi=1}^{K} f(T_\phi x_i) \tag{4}$$

We can find that the rotation-invariance regularization constraint effectively minimizes the distances between the learned features and the average feature representation of its rotated versions. In this regard, it highly enhances the rotation-invariance power of the deeply learned features.

Image Similarity Regularization Constraint. It is intuitive that if two images are in some category, the learned features should be close to each other in the learned feature space. Therefore, the image similarity constraint is introduced to help discover more accurate features. The cosine similarity measurement defines the angle of the feature and its intra-class center. To this end, we propose the image similarity loss constraint $D(X)$ with cosine measurement to emphasize the image similarity.

$$D(X) = \frac{1}{N} \sum_{i=1}^{N} (1 - \frac{f^T(x_i)c_m}{\|f(x_i)\|\|c_m\|}), \tag{5}$$

where $c_m = \frac{1}{N_{x_i \in T_m}} \sum_{x_i \in T_m} f(x_i)$ defines the center of features for the mth category. The introduced loss function tends to minimize the angle of the feature and its intra-class center and keep the intra-class features close to each other.

Final Joint Loss Function. Based on the above three observations, we adopt the joint supervision of softmax loss, rotation-invariance loss and image similarity loss to train the RIIS-DenseNet for discriminative features. The formulation of the joint loss function is given as follows,

$$D_{final} = \frac{1}{N(K+1)} \sum_{x_i \in X_{new}} l_{x_i} \log(\hat{l_{x_i}}) + \frac{1}{N} \sum_{i=1}^{N} \|f(x_i) - Mean(f(T_\phi x_i))\|^2$$

$$+ \frac{1}{N} \sum_{i=1}^{N} (1 - \frac{f^T(x_i)c_m}{\|f(x_i)\|\|c_m\|}),$$

(6)

The softmax loss globally forces the learned feature vectors of different categories to stay away while the introduced image similarity loss effectively pulls the deep features of the same category to be coincident. Equation (6) also imposes a regularization constraint to achieve rotation invariance. With this joint supervision, the discriminative power of the deeply learned features can be highly enhanced.

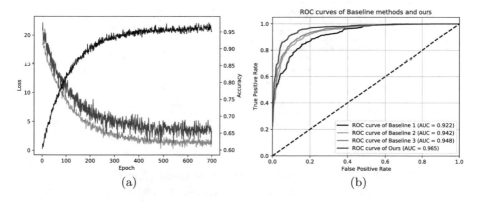

(a)   (b)

Fig. 2. (a) Loss and accuracy values for different iterations. The blue color represents the test loss while the orange color shows the training loss. The black line represents the test accuracy. (b) ROC curves for different baseline methods and ours.

3   Experiment Setup and Results

Our WCE dataset consists of 3000 WCE images, including 1500 polyp frames and 1500 normal ones. These images were extracted from 62 different WCE videos and manually annotated by expert physicians. The original size of each WCE image was $578 \times 578 \times 3$. The input image size of RIIS-DenseNet model was set as $256 \times 256 \times 3$ to reduce the computational complexity. The data set was randomly divided into three subsets: a training (80%), a validation (10%), and a test (10%) set to conduct experiment. Data augmentation, including randomly cropping and scaling [5], was implemented to enlarge the training images for the proposed RIIS-DenseNet model.

We implemented our model using Tensorflow on a desktop with Intel Core i7-7700@3.6 GHz processors and a NVIDIA GeForce Titan X with 128 GB of RAM. All training steps used mini-batches of 80 samples. The learning rate, weight decay and momentums of the RIID-DenseNet model were set as 0.01, 0.005 and 0.9, respectively. The performance of polyp detection was evaluated by accuracy (Acc), recall (Rec), precision (Pre) and F1-score (F1). In addition, the receiver operating characteristic (ROC) curve was plotted for evaluation.

We first analyzed the learning process of the proposed RIIS-DenseNet model. The training loss, test loss and test accuracy are shown in Fig. 2(a). The training loss and test loss converge after iterations indicating that the network is successfully optimized to learn the discriminative features for the polyp detection task. Moreover, the test loss consistently decreases as the training loss goes down, demonstrating that no serious over-fitting is observed with our WCE datasets.

Table 1. Comparison with different polyp detection methods.

	Methods	Acc (%)	Rec (%)	Pre (%)	F1 (%)
Beseline	Comparison 1	89.67	88.17	91.69	89.91
Methods	Comparison 2	94.06	93.18	95.07	94.12
Comparison	Comparison 3	93.75	92.81	94.76	93.77
	Our Method	**95.62**	**94.97**	**96.26**	**95.59**
Existing	Gueye et al. [1]	85.84	83.91	86.25	85.06
polyp recognition	Shin et al. [7]	87.43	86.25	87.79	87.01
Methods	Segui et al. [6]	88.43	86.68	90.94	88.76
	Zhang et al. [12]	89.92	90.64	89.53	90.08

We then analyzed the influence of introduced constraints for the polyp detection. The first baseline experiment was original DenseNet model, which learned image features without utilizing two proposed loss items: rotation invariant and image similarity constraints. The second and third baseline experiments directly applied the DenseNet method with the single rotation invariant loss or image similarity loss to conduct the polyp detection in WCE images. The corresponding criteria of polyp detection are recorded in Table 1. The ROC curves of our method and three comparison methods are shown in Fig. 2(b). Our RIIS-DenseNet achieves an accuracy of 95.62%, recall of 94.97% and precision of 96.26%, showing significant improvements compared with comparison experiments. This result validates the introduced regularized items: RI and IS constraints have critical roles in learning discriminative features for improving detection performance.

We further assessed the performance of the proposed method by comparing it with the state-of-the-art polyp diagnosis methods: the hand-craft feature based methods [1,7] and deep learning based methods [6,12]. We implemented these methods on our datasets and the average accuracy, recall and precision achieved by the existing methods and ours are shown in Table 1, respectively. We found that the deep learning based methods achieve better performance than the methods based on hand-crafted features, suggesting that the high-level features learned from networks are more discriminative than the hand-crafted features. The proposed method shows superior performance with an improvement of 7.19%, 5.70% in accuracy, 8.29%, 4.33% in recall compared with the existing deep learning based methods [6,12], respectively. This result validates the proposed RIIS-DenseNet model possesses superior ability to characterize WCE images as compared with existing methods.

4   Conclusion

We proposed a novel RIIS-DenseNet model for automatic computer-aided polyp detection with WCE videos. Our method is fundamentally different from the previous works since it does not rely on hand-designed features or traditional CNN model. Instead, it utilizes Dense Convolutional Neural Network to learn more discriminative features from the raw images directly and automatically. The image similarity constraint was introduced in the feature learning procedure to enable the intra-class features similar to each other by minimizing the angle of the feature and its intra-class center in the learned feature space. In addition, a rotation invariant constraint was also proposed in our network to deal with the rotation variance of the WCE images. The accuracy of our methods for polyp detection achieves 95.62%. Our intensive evaluations based on the annotated polyp database demonstrate our method has a superior performance over existing state-of-the-art methods.

References

1. Gueye, L., Yildirim-Yayilgan, S., Cheikh, F.A., Balasingham, I.: Automatic detection of colonoscopic anomalies using capsule endoscopy. In: IEEE ICIP, pp. 1061–1064 (2015)
2. He, K., Zhang, X., Ren, S., Sun, J.: Deep residual learning for image recognition. In: IEEE: CVPR, pp. 770–778 (2016)
3. Huang, G., Liu, Z., Weinberger, K.Q., van der Maaten, L.: Densely connected convolutional networks. In: CVPR, pp. 4700–4708. IEEE (2017)
4. Iddan, G., Meron, G., Glukhovsky, A., Swain, P.: Wireless capsule endoscopy. Nature **405**, 417 (2000)
5. Krizhevsky, A., Sutskever, I., Hinton, G.E.: Imagenet classification with deep convolutional neural networks. In: NIPS, pp. 1097–1105 (2012)
6. Seguí, S., et al.: Generic feature learning for wireless capsule endoscopy analysis. Comput. Biol. Med. **79**, 163–172 (2016)
7. Shin, Y., Balasingham, I.: Comparison of hand-craft feature based SVM and CNN based deep learning framework for automatic polyp classification. In: IEEE EMBC, pp. 3277–3280 (2017)
8. American Cancer Society: Key statistics for colorectal cancer. http://www.cancer.org/cancer/colonandrectumcancer/detailedguide/colorectal-cancer-key-statistics/. Accessed 15 Jan 2018

9. Tajbakhsh, N., Gurudu, S.R., Liang, J.: Automatic polyp detection in colonoscopy videos using an ensemble of convolutional neural networks. In: IEEE ISBI, pp. 79–83 (2015)

10. Yu, L., Chen, H., Dou, Q., Qin, J., Heng, P.A.: Integrating online and offline three-dimensaional deep learning for automated polyp detection in colonoscopy videos. IEEE J. Biomed. Health Inform. **21**(1), 65–75 (2017)

11. Yuan, Y., Meng, M.Q.H.: Deep learning for polyp recognition in wireless capsule endoscopy images. Med. Phys. **44**(4), 1379–1389 (2017)

12. Zhang, R., et al.: Automatic detection and classification of colorectal polyps by transferring low-level cnn features from nonmedical domain. IEEE J. Biomed. Health Inform. **21**(1), 41–47 (2017)

Interaction Techniques for Immersive CT Colonography: A Professional Assessment

Daniel Simões Lopes[1,2]([✉]), Daniel Medeiros[1,2], Soraia Figueiredo Paulo[1],
Pedro Brasil Borges[2], Vitor Nunes[3], Vasco Mascarenhas[4], Marcos Veiga[5],
and Joaquim Armando Jorge[1,2]

[1] INESC-ID Lisboa, Lisboa, Portugal
daniel.lopes@inesc-id.pt
[2] Instituto Superior Técnico, Universidade de Lisboa, Lisboa, Portugal
[3] Surgery Department, Hospital Prof. Dr. Fernando Fonseca, E.P.E.,
Amadora, Portugal
[4] Department of Radiology, Hospital da Luz, Lisboa, Portugal
[5] Neuroradiology Department, Centro Hospitalar de Lisboa Central, Lisboa, Portugal

Abstract. CT Colonography (CTC) is considered the leading imaging technique for colorectal cancer (CRC) screening. However, conventional CTC systems rely on clumsy 2D input devices and stationary flat displays that make it hard to perceive the colon structure in 3D. To visualize such anatomically complex data, the immersion and freedom of movement afforded by Virtual Reality (VR) systems bear the promise to assist clinicians to improve 3D reading, hence, enabling more expedite diagnoses. To this end, we propose iCOLONIC, a set of interaction techniques using VR to perform CTC reading. iCOLONIC combines immersive Fly-Through navigation with positional tracking, multi-scale representations and mini-maps to guide radiologists and surgeons while navigating throughout the colon. Contrary to stationary VR solutions, iCOLONIC allows users to freely walk within a work space to analyze both local and global 3D features. To assess whether our non-stationary VR approach can assist clinicians in improving 3D colon reading and 3D perception, we conducted a user study with three senior radiologists, three senior general surgeons and one neuroradiology intern. Results from formal evaluation sessions demonstrate iCOLONIC's usability and feasibility as the proposed interaction techniques were seen to improve spatial awareness and promote a more fluent navigation. Moreover, participants remarked that our approach shows great potential to speed up the screening process.

1 Introduction

CRC is the second leading cause of cancer-related death in the western world, with an estimated 1.4 million new cases every year worldwide, half of which end in death [1]. Screening procedures are the most important preventive methods. Although optical colonoscopy is the preferred screening examination [2], CTC

© Springer Nature Switzerland AG 2018
A. F. Frangi et al. (Eds.): MICCAI 2018, LNCS 11071, pp. 629–637, 2018.
https://doi.org/10.1007/978-3-030-00934-2_70

offers a significantly reduced number of side effects [2, 7] as well as a less invasive alternative (e.g., does not require bowel cleansing nor general anesthesia). The CTC also has the advantage of generating subject-specific 3D colon models. Within these models, standard CTC navigation is performed via Fly-Through visualization [3], which simulates conventional optical colonoscopy as the camera follows antegrade (rectum→cecum) or retrograde (cecum→rectum) paths.

From a geometric point of view, a 3D colon model is a complex structure with several inflections and numerous haustral folds. This makes 3D colon navigation a difficult task *per se* and an even more exacerbated task when performed using conventional workstations: the radiologist is seated at a desk in front of a stationary flat display and interacting with complex radiological data using mouse and keyboard interfaces. However, using a 2D display to analyze 3D structures can lead to missing critical 3D information and time consuming screening procedures, hence, resulting in incomplete or lower number of CTC reports [6]. Moreover, conventional systems negatively affect productivity by providing insufficient space and reduced number of monitors [10].

VR appears as an interesting paradigm for CTC navigation since it has been reported that immersion benefits scientific data set analysis [5]. Moreover, previous studies explore the potential of VR in radiologic settings [4,6,8,12] demonstrating that VR solves several ambient lighting issues, forces users to adopt an ergonomically correct posture, and promotes a far more superior camera control when compared to conventional mouse and keyboard based interfaces. Immersion also promotes a greater visual bandwidth and improves 3D perception. Consequently, immersion can improve the colon anatomy reading and spatial understanding of lesions, such as occult polyps that typically hide behind haustra or folds, leading to faster screening practices and improved lesion counting.

Previous studies considered the application of VR technologies to CTC. Mirhosseini et al. [6] used a *Cave Automatic Virtual Environment* to project the gastrointestinal walls onto the display's physical walls. Although its use lead to improvements in medical diagnostics (examination time and accuracy), such displays are unpractical in real clinical settings when compared to head mounted displays (HMDs). On the other hand, Randall et al. [8] resorted on a HMD (i.e., Oculus Rift) to examine the immersiveness of VR to analyze and interpret CTC content. However, the work lacked positional tracking, did not allow users to signalize lesions, was devoid of navigational signs apart from not exploring different navigation techniques. Even with a HMD, the interaction did not allow more interesting movements such as walking inside the colon or adopting postures to control users' point of view towards the anatomical content.

In this work, we present iCOLONIC, a set of interaction techniques for navigating inside and outside the colon. The main objective of this work is to explore how non-stationary VR can help navigation and readability of 3D colon models in CTC. We contribute with novel interaction techniques for immersive CTC navigation, which provide freedom of movement while standing and moving in the work space, but also greater camera control in comparison to conventional systems. Furthermore, we performed a user study to better understand how specialists respond to these interaction techniques.

2 Immersive CT Colonography System

A VR system called iCOLONIC (Immersive CT Colonography Navigation Interaction Techniques) was developed to navigate both exo- and endoluminal spaces of a virtual 3D colon. Several tools were developed to assist 3D immersive navigation and to perform radiologic measurements. All the code was developed in C# using the SteamVR Plugin and Unity game engine (version 5.5.1f1).

2.1 Apparatus

Our setup relies on the off-the-shelf solution embodied by HTC Vive (Fig. 1). It consists of a binocular Head-Mounted Display, two game controllers and a Lighthouse Tracking System composed by two cameras with emitting pulsed IR lasers that track all 6 degrees-of-freedom of head and handheld gear. The tracking system generates an acquisition volume that enables users to move freely within a $4.5 \times 4.5 \times 2.5$ m^3 space. User tests were performed on an Asus ROG G752VS Laptop with an Intel® Core™ i7-6820 HK Processor, 64 GB RAM and NVIDIA GeForce GTX1070. iCOLONIC runs at 60 frames per second.

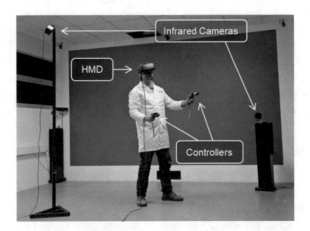

Fig. 1. Virtual Reality setup of the iCOLONIC interactive system.

2.2 3D Data

A single CTC data set from *The Cancer Imaging Archive* [11] was considered (subject ID *CTC-3105759107*), which had almost no liquid, acquired in a supine position, presented large (>10 mm) and quite visible polyps along with several

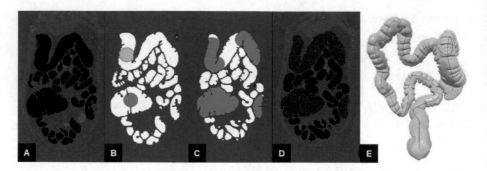

Fig. 2. 3D colon reconstruction: (A) original CTC image; (B) global threshold image with two active contours (red); (C) active contour model progression; (D) segmented colon overlapped with CTC image; (E) reconstructed 3D model with centerline [14]. (Color figure online)

diverticula. The 3D model was reconstructed using the image-based geometric modelling pipeline that is composed by freeware tools [9] (Fig. 2).

The high contrast between luminal space (air: black) and colon luminal surface (colon wall: light grey) facilitates 3D reconstruction (Fig. 2(A)). Firstly, the 3D colon structure is segmented using the active contours method based on region competition (Fig. 2(B-D)), which depends on the intensity values estimated via a simple global threshold filter (ITK-SNAP 3.6). Secondly, a 3-D surface mesh of the segmented data is generated using marching cubes. Thirdly, undesired mesh artifacts were attenuated through a cycle of smoothing and decimating operations (ParaView 5.3.0) and exported into a *.ply (ASCII) file. Finally, the mesh file was converted to *.obj (Blender 2.78) and imported into Unity (version 5.5.1f1). To compute the 3D centerline of the colon mesh, we used the algorithm proposed by Tagliasacchi et al. [14] which solves the 3D mesh skeletonization problem by resorting on mean curvature flow (Fig. 2(E)).

2.3   Interaction Design

From an anatomical point of view, the colon is a complex structure where lesions, anatomical deviations and/or conditions can occur on either sides of the luminal surface. Therefore, iCOLONIC's interaction techniques allow users to navigate on both spaces and to switch between Exo-Luminal View (*ExoV*) and Endo-Luminal View (*EndoV*) for outer and inner colon navigation, respectively. In *ExoV*, the 3D colon is up scaled to the size of an average adult and is placed floating above the ground (Fig. 3(A-B)). As for *EndoV*, the user is down scaled to fit inside the luminal space and experiences the colon confined from within (Fig. 3(C)).

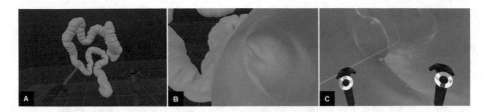

Fig. 3. Representing the colon in different scales and views: **(a)** up scaled colon in *ExoV*; **(b)** clipped view of up scaled colon in *ExoV*; **(c)** down scaled colon in *EndoV*.

The motivation behind *ExoV* came from colonic conditions, such as diverticulosis, that can be better diagnosed when viewed from the outside. To take advantage of the virtual space made available in VR, we consider an up scaled representation so that the user can instantly withdraw the overall geometry and also local landmarks that are now magnified. In *ExoV*, users can freely move around the 3D colon or rotate the model using the non-dominant hand (NDH) controller. Alternatively, users can also stick their heads beyond the colon wall to get a glimpse of the endo-luminal space (Fig. 3(B)). In a less meddlesome fashion, a user can also opt for a target-based travel by selecting a point from outside the colon with the NDH controller to be transported to the closest point on the centerline (Fig. 4), hence, the user is down scaled into the endo-luminal space where the view immediately switches to *EndoV* similarly to the *World In Miniature* metaphor [13].

Following conventional CTC practices, endo-luminal navigation can also be performed in a more orderly fashion, where the user begins navigating from the rectum towards the cecum and *vice versa*. In *EndoV*, the user is placed inside the colon and travels via Fly-Through navigation techniques [8] at a self-controlled smooth pace. Inside the colon lumen, navigation follows the path defined by the colon's centerline. By default, the user is anchored to the centerline to avoid unwanted intersections against the colon walls or, *in extremis*, to avoid exiting the luminal surface. Users can freely move their heads and/or body to look around and behind the virtual colonic scenery. However, users can opt to abandon the centerline by physically walking towards the colon wall and reach the lumen limits to better examine local features. After exploring the colon wall, users can reposition themselves by moving back towards the centerline. To assist navigation, two arrows pointing in opposite directions are placed in front of (green: antegrade) and behind (red: retrograde) the user accompanying the centerline.

iCOLONIC provides navigational and diagnostic tools (only in *EndoV*) that are managed through two HTC Vive controllers (Fig. 4(A)). A menu appears every time the touchpad is touched and tools are activated by pressing the corresponding widget button. The dominant hand (DH) controller handles up- and down-stream navigation as well as tagging and measurement tasks, while the

NDH controller showcases either CTC slices (axial, sagittal, coronal) (Fig. 4(B)), a list of tagged lesions with dimension and C-Rad type information (Fig. 4(C)) or a colon mini-map with current location and lesions tags (Fig. 4(D)).

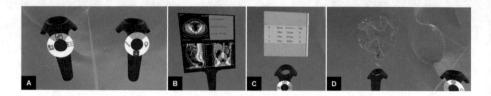

Fig. 4. iCOLONIC tools: **(A)** circular touchpad menus; **(B)** CTC slices of the user's location inside the colon; **(C)** polyp list of tagged lesions with size and C-Rad type; **(D)** colon mini-map with location and tagged lesions.

3   Evaluation with Professionals

We conducted an evaluation with seven medical professionals, two of which were female, ages ranged between 29 and 55 years old. The group included two radiologists with specific training in CTC (each with 3 years of experience), one senior radiologist (10 years of experience), one neuroradiology intern and three general surgeons (1, 8, and 26 years of surgical experience). Four of these professionals regularly examine CTC images, and only one reported previous VR experience. With the exception of the intern, all reported that they read CTC images on a daily basis.

Evaluation sessions comprised four stages: (1) Introduction, (2) Free Experimentation, (3) Questionnaire and (4) Guided Interview. After a thorough demonstration of all available functions and their application, all professionals were asked to test iCOLONIC alone. Participants tested the interaction techniques for 35 min, with 10 min to familiarize themselves with the interface and interaction techniques. The only restriction being they had to experiment each available function at least once. After Free Experimentation participants filled a small profile form along with a questionaire regarding the quality of their experience with the interface and interaction techniques (6-point Likert Scale: 1 - totally disagree; 6 - totally agree). Afterwards, we conducted a semi-structured interview where participants gave insights about the experience, their preferences and suggested improvements. None of the participants reported discomfort, dizziness or fatigue.

(Table 1) reports the participants opinions regarding usefulness and performance of the proposed interaction techniques and tools. In general, users considered the navigation interaction techniques easy to execute and to remember. Navigation tools were considered highly useful with adequate feedback although the CTC slices tool was given a slightly lower score compared to mini-map (Table 1). The participants were able to identify several polyps and diverticula, even though none was prompted to do so. Most participants referred that the color contrast could be slightly improved, specially in *EndoV* mode. With the exception of the intern, all participants mentioned that the non-stationary VR environment clearly improved on the tedious and complex movements performed with mouse and keyboard based CTC interfaces. Even though participants had access to the 3D colon surface and images, two radiologists trained in CTC referred that data was missing as they performed screening with both prone and supine models. The senior radiologist and one senior surgeon referred that larger CT slices with arbitrary orientation could help understand the relation between colon conditions (e.g., polyps, diverticula) and the adjacent tissues. Furthermore, participants were unanimous with the need to paint suspicious areas with different colors, a feature yet to be implemented.

Table 1. Questionnaire results regarding user experience and preferences. NV - up- and down-stream navigation; DM - distance measurement; TG - Tagging; MM - colon mini-map; CS - CTC slices; PL - polyp list; TT - target-based travel from *ExoV* to *EndoV*. Median (Interquartile Range).

Was it	NV	DM	TG	MM	CS	PL	TT
Useful	6(1.5)	6(1)	6(1.5)	6(1.5)	5(1.5)	6(1.5)	5(1.5)
Easy to execute	6(1.5)	5(1.5)	6(1.5)	5(1.5)	4(2)	6(1.5)	5(1.5)
Easy to remember	6(1)	6(1.5)	6(1.5)	6(1)	5(1.5)	6(1.5)	6(1.5)

In general, professionals felt immersed and believed that this kind of interactive visualization will become a future standard. In their opinion, the main advantage of our approach is the speed at which radiologists will be able to examine CTC data. In their words, *"conventional CTC is cumbersome and slow"*, besides the fact that the software and hardware used are expensive. Despite the novelty and early enthusiasm, their opinions are encouraging as they uncover the possibility of radiologists and surgeons to adopt non-stationary VR-based approaches as novel diagnostic and surgical planning tools. Finally, participants mentioned that once the missing features were implemented they would be prone to use iCOLONIC in their day-to-day work.

4   Conclusions

In this work, we explore the potential of VR immersion and freedom of movement to assist CTC navigation. Our approach addresses issues intrinsically associated to conventional CTC screening interfaces that are known to limit camera control, 3D perception and visual bandwidth. Results strongly indicate that the combination of immersion, freedom of movement and World In Miniature metaphors is a feasible way to overcome limited camera control and assists the professional to more rapidly detect lesions and other conditions. Furthermore, participants in our evaluation were positively impressed and suggested that the interaction techniques were adequate. However, several features need to be implemented to provide a more complete diagnostic tool, namely inclusion of both prone/supine 3D data, computer-assisted detection and fecal tagging. To clinically validate the interaction techniques, future research will focus on quantifying user fatigue, polyp count effectiveness and screening efficiency using several CTC data sets.

Acknowledgements. Authors thank the financial support from the Portuguese Foundation for Science and Technology through grants UID/CEC/50021/2013, IT-MEDEX PTDC/EEI-SII/6038/2014, SFRH/BPD/97449/2013 and also the CAPES Foundation, Ministry of Education of Brazil, through grant 9040/13-7.

References

1. Ferlay, J., et al.: Cancer incidence and mortality worldwide: sources, methods and major patterns in GLOBOCAN 2012. Int. J. Cancer **136**(5), E359–E386 (2015). https://doi.org/10.1002/ijc.29210
2. de Haan, M.C., van Gelder, R.E., Graser, A., Bipat, S., Stoker, J.: Diagnostic value of CT-colonography as compared to colonoscopy in an asymptomatic screening population: a meta-analysis. Eur. Radiol. **21**(8), 1747–1763 (2011). https://doi.org/10.1007/s00330-011-2104-8
3. Hong, L., Kaufman, A., Wei, Y.C., Viswambharan, A., Wax, M., Liang, Z.: 3D virtual colonoscopy. In: Biomedical Visualization, Proceedings, pp. 26–32. IEEE (1995). https://doi.org/10.1109/BIOVIS.1995.528702
4. King, F., et al.: An immersive virtual reality environment for diagnostic imaging. J. Med. Rob. Res. **1**(01), 1640003 (2016). https://doi.org/10.1142/S2424905X16400031
5. Kuhlen, T.W., Hentschel, B.: Quo vadis CAVE: does immersive visualization still matter? IEEE Comput. Graph. Appl. **34**(5), 14–21 (2014). https://doi.org/10.1109/MCG.2014.97
6. Mirhosseini, K., Sun, Q., Gurijala, K.C., Laha, B., Kaufman, A.E.: Benefits of 3D immersion for virtual colonoscopy. In: 2014 IEEE VIS International Workshop on 3DVis (3DVis), pp. 75–79, November 2014. https://doi.org/10.1109/3DVis.2014.7160105
7. Pickhardt, P.J., Hassan, C., Halligan, S., Marmo, R.: Colorectal Cancer: CT colonography and colonoscopy for detection—systematic review and meta-analysis. Radiology **259**(2), 393–405 (2011). https://doi.org/10.1148/radiol.11101887
8. Randall, D., et al.: The oculus rift virtual colonoscopy: introducing a new technology and initial impressions. J. Biomed. Graph. Comput. **6**(1) (2015). https://doi.org/10.5430/jbgc.v6n1p34
9. Ribeiro, N., Fernandes, P., Lopes, D., Folgado, J., Fernandes, P.: 3-D solid and finite element modeling of biomechanical structures-a software pipeline. In: 7th EUROMECH Solid Mechanics Conference, September 2009
10. Rumreich, L.L., Johnson, A.J.: From traditional reading rooms to a soft copy environment: radiologist satisfaction survey. J. Digit. Imaging **16**(3), 262–269 (2003). https://doi.org/10.1007/s10278-003-1734-z
11. Smith, K., et al.: Data from CT_COLONOGRAPHY (2015). https://doi.org/10.7937/K9/TCIA.2015.NWTESAY1. Accessed 23 April 2017

12. Sousa, M., Mendes, D., Paulo, S., Matela, N., Jorge, J., Lopes, D.S.: VRRRRoom: virtual reality for radiologists in the reading room. In: Proceedings of the 2017 CHI Conference on Human Factors in Computing Systems, pp. 4057–4062. ACM (2017). https://doi.org/10.1145/3025453.3025566
13. Stoakley, R., Conway, M.J., Pausch, R.: Virtual reality on a WIM: interactive worlds in miniature. In: Proceedings of the SIGCHI Conference on Human Factors in Computing Systems, pp. 265–272. ACM Press/Addison-Wesley Publishing Co. (1995). https://doi.org/10.1145/223904.223938
14. Tagliasacchi, A., Alhashim, I., Olson, M., Zhang, H.: Mean curvature skeletons. Comput. Graph. Forum **31**, 1735–1744 (2012). https://doi.org/10.1111/j.1467-8659.2012.03178.x

Quasi-automatic Colon Segmentation on T2-MRI Images with Low User Effort

B. Orellana[1]([✉]), E. Monclús[1], P. Brunet[1], I. Navazo[1], Á. Bendezú[2], and F. Azpiroz[3]

[1] ViRVIG Group, UPC-BarcelonaTech, Barcelona, Spain
{orellana,Emonclus,pere,isabel}@cs.upc.edu
[2] Digestive Department, Hospital General de Catalunya, Barcelona, Spain
roger.bendezu@clinicavalles.com
[3] Digestive System Research Unit, University Hospital Vall d'Hebron, Barcelona, Spain
fazpiroz@vhebron.net

Abstract. About 50% of the patients consulting a gastroenterology clinic report symptoms without detectable cause. Clinical researchers are interested in analyzing the volumetric evolution of colon segments under the effect of different diets and diseases. These studies require non-invasive abdominal MRI scans without using any contrast agent. In this work, we propose a colon segmentation framework designed to support T2-weighted abdominal MRI scans obtained from an unprepared colon. The segmentation process is based on an efficient and accurate quasi-automatic approach that drastically reduces the specialist interaction and effort with respect other state-of-the-art solutions, while decreasing the overall segmentation cost. The algorithm relies on a novel probabilistic tubularity filter, the detection of the colon medial line, probabilistic information extracted from a training set and a final unsupervised clustering. Experimental results presented show the benefits of our approach for clinical use.

1 Introduction

About 50% of the patients consulting a gastroenterology clinic report symptoms without detectable cause. Colonic content is a potential mechanism involved in their symptoms. The research of colonic metabolic activity and its variations provoked by digestive dysfunctions or diets requires non-invasive measurement of colonic volumes and contents based on medical imaging.

Although diseases under study can be particularly disturbing, they are not life-threatening, and therefore irradiation —if used at all— is to be kept to a minimum. Hence, non-ionizing imaging techniques play an important role as they allow acquiring data from patients with low-severity diseases or healthy

This work has been supported by the Spanish *MINECO* Ministry and by FEDER funds under Grant No. TIN2017-88512-C2 1 R.

© Springer Nature Switzerland AG 2018

A. F. Frangi et al. (Eds.): MICCAI 2018, LNCS 11071, pp. 638–647, 2018.
https://doi.org/10.1007/978-3-030-00934-2_71

volunteers. Furthermore, some clinical studies expressly reject preparation (fasting and/or edema) neither contrast administration. For all these reasons, CT imaging, which has been traditionally used for colon analysis, is not a choice.

The clinical analysis of colon is typically performed on MRI T2-weighted modality, and its goal is to distinguish the specific volumes of the colon segments (ascending S_{asc}, transverse S_{trv}, descending S_{dsc} and sigma-rectum S_σ).

Experts make use of specific tools for engaging colon segmentation on MRI, but it is a complex task due to the high level of variability of its anatomy (specially S_σ segment) and the adjacency of regions with similar intensity levels, such as small bowel, liver or muscular tissues. Techniques used for CT colon segmentation are not applicable for MRI since there is not a fixed correspondence between tissues types and intensities. Furthermore, MRI suffers from higher levels of noise and artifacts that have an impact on segmentation algorithms.

There are few references in the bibliography for T2-MRI colon segmentation on unprepared subjects, here we will review the most relevant. In [1] the authors opted for the simplest segmentation strategy: slice-per-slice manual selection. In order to ease the selection within slices, [2] improved the usability by providing a seed region growing mechanism combined with the ability to add stop markers for prevent leaking. A different proposal is presented in [3], which requires the user to define a Region Of Interest (ROI) by outlining the colon manually with a polygonal in all coronal slices. Their approach is based on k-means clustering on the intensity space within the ROI to separate *colon* from *background*. The authors do not provide comparison metrics against ground truth, only overlapping measures of segmentations obtained from different users on the same image.

In another category of applications, Mahapatra et al. [4] describe a full automatic segmentation of colon areas affected by Crohn's disease on T1-FS under fasting condition and contrast administration. The authors build a Random Forest classificator that permits discriminating healthy and diseased colon regions. Finally, authors in [5] segment only one 2D colon section along a temporal sequence of T2-HS (cine-MRI). Their strategy is based on a set of user marks placed inside and outside the colon image of the first frame. Segmentation is driven by 2D graph-cuts.

As far as we know, there is a lack of algorithms for T2 colon segmentation on MRI images acquired without contrast neither colon preparation. Summarizing, the contributions of this paper are outlined below:

- A new approach for colon segmentation based on the detection of the colon medial line and the usage of a colon probability model that is used on a 3D graph cuts algorithm to produce the final result. Our dual probabilistic model uses training information for a preliminary segmentation and unsupervised clustering for the final segmentation.
- A set of novel probabilistic tubularity filters that allow detecting generalized tubular structures with large radius and non-circular sections. Moreover, a set of fast algorithms to segment a coarse voxel model for adjacent colon areas

and to reduce the search space (liver, psoas, spine and fat inner abdominal layer) have been developed.

- Our segmentation algorithm is suitable for clinical use since it provides a low-effort, accurate colon segmentation in MRI T2-weighted images without neither colon preparation nor contrast administration.
- Our approach achieves a remarkable improvement in the experts interaction. The full colon segmentation requires 5 min of user interaction (UI), and 5 min of CPU processing. In contrast, current manual-based solutions require times that range from 20 up to 40 min of intensive work.

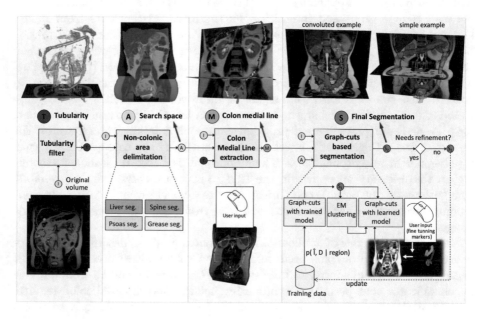

Fig. 1. Overview of the segmentation pipeline. Four stages are shown: (T) Tubularity filter aimed to detect colon candidate areas. (A) Search space delimitation discards adjacent regions. (M) Medial line extraction is based on a set of points provided by the user and information on (T) + (A). (S) is the segmentation stage, which combines (M) + (A) with training data to obtain the final segmentation in a two-phase graph-cuts.

2   Method Overview

Our segmentation strategy consists in modeling the colon as a generalized tube with a characteristic probabilistic distribution of intensities and radius differentiated for each colon segment. Complementary, it is convenient to exclude some adjacent organs from the search space, since their similar intensities cause low contrast boundaries. Our algorithm combines both approaches with a simple user input to obtain the precise colon segmentation. It is remarkable that the algorithm is fully 3D, working on a 3D voxel model built from the acquired images. Figure 1 shows the segmentation pipeline, which relies on four stages:

1. **Tubularity filter**: We propose a tubularity filter evolved from ideas in [6,7] aimed to detect generalized non-uniform tubes. Since the filter has a high tolerance to be able to detect large deviations from perfect tubularity, the output is noisier than regular tubularity filters, and its result alone is not sufficient for colon segmentation. The tubularity feature of each voxel includes its direction, a tubularity measure and an estimated radius, which are used in subsequent stages for the selection of colon candidate areas and for spinal cord detection.

2. **Non-colonic area delimitation**: In this stage, fast tailored algorithms coarsely segment voxel models for four anatomic structures which are closer to the colon: liver, psoas+pelvic muscles, spinal cord + spine and the inner abdominal fat capsule. Therefore, its location is valuable for preventing leaks that may be caused by low contrast boundaries. The output of this stage is a set of binary masking volumes delimiting the segmented structures.

3. **Colon medial line extraction**: The estimation of the colon medial line is the starting point of our segmentation strategy. The user has to provide a minimal set of 5 anatomical reference points along the colon path that are easily located by specialists on MRI: cecum, hepatic angle, splenic angle, descending-sigma interface and anus. Depending on the anatomical complexity of the case under study, further points can be added to guide the location of the medial path.

   On this basis, we build a graph where nodes represent connected sets of voxels with similar intensities. Graph edge cost penalizes paths of low tubularity, tube direction changes and high intensities. The medial path is obtained as the union of the lowest cost paths between pairs of consecutive points provided by the user.

4. **Colon graph-cuts based segmentation**: Last stage performs the colon segmentation. It requires information from the previous stages (medial line (M), search space (A) and intensity (I)) and information from a training database, which is computed in a pre-process and updated after each new performed segmentation.

   In the training phase, we use the golden truth segmentations (see Sect. 3) to estimate $p(D, \hat{I})$, which is the joint probability function of the normalized intensity $\hat{I}$, and the distance to the colon medial, D.

   The intervals of $\hat{I}$ and D are quantized, and the probability function is stored into our training database as a 2D histogram. The probability is analyzed within a ROI defined by those voxels having D below $1.5 \cdot CMR$, where CMR denotes the Colon Maximum Radius (30 mm).

The intensity is normalized using the range of values along the medial path, $\hat{I} = (I - \mu_{medial})/\sigma_{medial}$, redressing this way the effects of MRI intensity variability. $p(D, \hat{I})$ is analyzed independently within each colon segment and outside the colon ($\overline{C}$). Hence, we obtain 5 probability distributions denoted by $p(D, \hat{I}|region)$ where $region \in \{\overline{C}, C_{S_{asc}}, C_{S_{trv}}, C_{S_{dsc}}, C_{S_\sigma}\}$. Figure 2 shows the distribution of $p(D, \hat{I}|C_{S_{trv}})$ in the transverse colon. The training also pro-

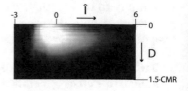

Fig. 2. Probability distribution $p(D, \hat{I}|C_{S_{trv}})$ of transverse colon.

vides statistics of D for the voxels on the colon boundaries per segment $\{DB_\mu^{sg}, DB_\sigma^{sg}\}$.

Now we describe the three steps of the last segmentation stage:

(a) From $p(D, \hat{I}|region)$ obtained in the training and the colon medial (M), we derive the probability of a voxel to be colon $p(C|D, \hat{I}, sg)$ and to be not-colon $p(\overline{C}|D, \hat{I}, sg)$ depending on its normalized intensity, medial distance and nearest segment $sg \in \{C_{S_{asc}}, C_{S_{trv}}, C_{S_{dsc}}, C_{S_\sigma}\}$. At this point we engage the preliminary segmentation. A graph $\mathcal{G}_1$ is created where nodes represent ROI voxels and graph edges represent voxel neighborhoods. In order to segment via graph-cuts we add two extra nodes, sink (colon) and source (not-colon), and use $p(C|D, \hat{I}, sg)$ and $p(\overline{C}|D, \hat{I}, sg)$ to build sink and source costs in the regional term R of graph cuts algorithm. The result is the preliminary colon segmentation, S_1.

(b) S_1 happens to be a conservative colon segmentation, but is not accurate enough. In the second step we cluster intensities in the area outside S_1 within the ROI, using an Expectation Maximization (EM) algorithm. We look for two modalities, one corresponding to fat tissues (high intensity) and the other corresponding to other organs or misclassified colon (medium intensity). At the end of the process we obtain the probabilies of a voxel to be C or $\overline{C}$ as functions of the intensity: $p(C|I)$ and $p(\overline{C}|I)$. The model is based on the mixture of three gaussians, the two obtained from EM and the gaussian model from S_1 intensities.

(c) Using boundary distance statistics $\{DB_\mu^{sg}, DB_\sigma^{sg}\}$ from training, we derive $p(C|D, sg)$ and $p(\overline{C}|D, sg)$, which describe the probability of a voxel to be colon/not-colon depending on its medial distance (Eq. 1) and the corresponding colon segment.

$$p(C|D, sg) = \frac{1}{2}(1 - erf(\frac{D - DB_\mu^{sg}}{\sqrt{2}DB_\sigma^{sg}})) \quad ; \quad p(\overline{C}|D, sg) = 1 - p(C|D, sg)$$
(1)

In the last stage we merge the colon/not-colon probabilities (Eq. 2) based on intensity (from clustering) with the probabilities based on the medial distance (from training) in order to build the probabilities of a voxel to be colon/not colon as functions of intensity, medial distance and segment:

$p(C|D, I, sg)$ and $p(\overline{C}|D, I, sg)$ (Eq. 3). In a similar way that in step (a), we build a graph $\mathcal{G}_2$ using these new probabilities in the regional terms of graph cuts.

The new result, S_2, is more accurate than S_1. If the segmentation S_2 is not satisfactory, the user can add markers (positive or negative) on misclassified areas. Marker information is used to update the regional term costs of the affected nodes of the graph. Graph-cuts is run again to obtain a new corrected version of the segmentation. The refinement is accomplished in near real-time, which allows the user to add markers interactively.

$$\mathcal{M}(p_D, p_I) = p_D(1 + 2(1 - p_D)(p_I - 0.5)) \tag{2}$$

$$p(c|D, I, sg) = \mathcal{M}(p(c|D, sg), p(c|I)) \quad \text{where} \quad c \in \{C, \overline{C}\} \tag{3}$$

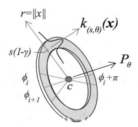

Fig. 3. Ring filter

2.1 Tubularity Detection Filter

We propose a new Tubularity Detection Filter (TDF) that is built as a combination of two filters: the ring filter (RF) that computes for each voxel a tubularity measure RF and its associated radius s, and the directional filter (DF), which estimates the tube direction P_θ. By applying TDF to a certain voxel $\boldsymbol{v}$, it gets characterized by $(\mathrm{RF}(\boldsymbol{v})$, $s(\boldsymbol{v})$ and $P_\theta(\boldsymbol{v}))$.

The Ring Filter (RF) works on a set of planar ring-shaped vectorial kernels $k_{(s,\theta)}(\boldsymbol{x})$ that lie in a plane orthogonal to P_θ and have a scale s, Fig. 3. Multiple kernels are necessary to cover different tube sizes and 3D orientations. On this purpose 13 scales s ($s \in [7\,\mathrm{mm}, 31\,\mathrm{mm}]$ in steps of $2\,\mathrm{mm}$) and 13 directions θ (pointing to the 26 neighbour voxels) are used. Kernel values are 0 outside the P_θ plane and show a radial Gaussian distribution on the P_θ plane as $k_{(s,\theta)}(\boldsymbol{x}) = \mathcal{N}_{(\mu=0,\sigma=\frac{\gamma 2s}{3})}(\|\boldsymbol{x}\| - s(1 - \gamma))$, where $\gamma = 0.25$.

The tubularity measure $RF(\boldsymbol{v})$ of a certain voxel $\boldsymbol{v}$ is computed as $RF(\boldsymbol{v}) = max_{s,\theta}(M_{ring}^{s,\theta}(\boldsymbol{v}) \cdot M_{sym}^{s,\theta}(\boldsymbol{v}))$, where this maximum is computed for all 13 scales and 13 directions, and its associated radius is computed as $s(\boldsymbol{v}) = \arg\max_{s,\theta}(M_{ring}^{s,\theta}(\boldsymbol{v}) \cdot M_{sym}^{s,\theta}(\boldsymbol{v}))$.

$M_{ring}^{s,\theta}$ is the result of computing the well-known convolution of the filter kernel $k_{(s,\theta)}(x)$ with the magnitude of the projection of the intensity gradient at v on the P_θ plane. The symmetry measure M_{sym} weights M_{ring} with the objective to punish partly open areas. We compute the symmetry measure M_{sym} by analysing partial convolutions $M_{ringsectors}$ on angular sections ϕ on the P_θ plane, see Fig. 3. We group sections by pairs P, each pair including one section and its opposite symmetric. For each P, we calculate the symmetry pair value (SPV) as the square of geometric mean divided by the arithmetic mean of P. M_{sym} is the mean of all SPV.

Finally, the DF filter is used to improve the estimation of the tube direction. To this end, we trace 92 uniformly spaced directions from v plus 45 even spaced sample directions in the coronal plane. The tube direction $D(v)$ is estimated by the ray direction that has minimum average squared difference to the central voxel v.

3   Evaluation and Results

The evaluation experiments tested our segmentation approach from three different perspectives, its accuracy with respect manual golden truth segmentations, its computational and user interaction cost, and its usability.

The data set used for the accuracy evaluation includes 30 T2-weighted HASTE volumes ($256 \times 256 \times 50$). Images were obtained from 15 healthy volunteers after and before defecation as part of a clinical experiment to determine the effect of diet on colonic content volume. These data set were segmented accurately by experienced specialists using BowelMetryRM (BMRM) software (its description is explained in [2]). This manual segmentation is considered the golden standard, and is used both for training and validation, using one-left-out methodology.

Dice Similarity Coefficient (DSC) and Sensitivity ($SENS$) measures were selected for comparing our segmentation results against the golden standard. Both measures are studied with respect the number of points introduced by the specialist in the stage M (see Fig. 1) of our approach. Figure 5 shows the evolution of DSC and $SENS$ from 5 up to 16 path points. Segmentation with 5 points reaches a mean DSC above 0.73, but the variability of the results ($\sigma_{DSC} = 0.17$) advises using a larger number of points. The segmentation accuracy saturates near 12 points, reaching medians around 0.85 for DSC and 0.86 for $SENS$, with standard deviation (SD) values $\sigma_{DSC} = 0.05$ and $\sigma_{SENS} = 0.07$ respectively.

In the last stage of the approach (S), the addition of user markers for segmentation correction can improve the accuracy of the results as show in Fig. 6. After the addition of 5 markers, the overall median DSC reaches 0.913, with $\sigma_{DSC} = 0.016$ (Fig. 6).

From a clinical point of view, we have compared the effort of manual segmentation using BMRM software with our proposal. First, a BMRM expert segmented three new cases not included in the validation experiments using our algorithm, after ten minutes briefing on how operating the software. Next,

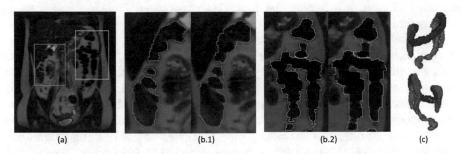

(a)   (b.1)   (b.2)   (c)

Fig. 4. Details on segmentation results for a case of sigma colon highly convoluted. (a) original image and two ROI. (b.1) and (b.2) depict ROIs, with golden truth segmentation (left) and our segmentation (right). (c) shows volume rendering (front view, back view) of our segmentation.

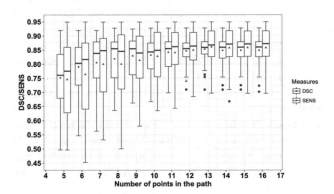

Fig. 5. Tukey boxplot for *DSC* and *SENS* measures for our segmentation against golden standard and its relationship with the number of used path points.

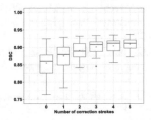

Fig. 6. *DSC* improvement with the addition of manual correction markers.

the specialist segmented the volumes again using BMRM. Note that for fair the learning effect can only benefit the manual segmentation. Time and mouse usage were tracked along the execution.

The results show that manual segmentation takes on average 25' of full user interaction, with 1230 mouse wheel turns, and 122 cm of mouse drag. In contrast, our proposal averages 5' for user interaction, of which 2' correspond to point placement in stage (M) and 3' to review and correct, if needed, the proposed segmentation; CPU computational cost was 5' with an i7 5820 K processor. Mouse usage drops to 500 wheel turns and 36 cm of mouse drag. These results show that our proposal clearly performs much better in terms of time and effort than BMRM. Qualitatively, the users declared to feel highly relieved with the simplicity of the new approach when compared with manual segmentation, emphasizing that the visual fatigue is drastically reduced.

4   Conclusions

We have presented a quasi-automatic pipeline for colon segmentation on T2-weighted MRI images obtained from unprepared colon. Our proposal achieves an important reduction of the segmentation time with respect state-of-the-art solutions, also reducing the user interaction up to a 80% and the usage effort. The segmentation accuracy is comparable to manual experts one. Medical experts found that this new algorithm improves efficiency and it is suitable for its use in clinical practice due to its easy-to-use, low interaction and improves the objectivity of the segmentations.

Segmentation pipeline relies on a new Tubularity filter that allows the detection of irregular tubular structures, such as the colon. The combination of tubularity, a reduced search space and a probabilistic model based on intensity and radius per segment have demonstrated its suitability for accurate colon segmentation.

References

1. Pritchard, S.E., et al.: Fasting and postprandial volumes of the undisturbed colon: normal values and changes in diarrhea-predominant irritable bowel syndrome measured using serial mri. Neurogastroenterol. Motil. **26**(1), 124–130 (2014)
2. Bendezú, R., et al.: Colonic content: effect of diet, meals, and defecation. Neurogastroenterol. Motil. **29**(2) (2017)
3. Sandberg, T.H., et al.: A novel semi-automatic segmentation method for volumetric assessment of the colon based on magnetic resonance imaging. Abdom. Imaging **40**(7), 2232–2241 (2015)
4. Mahapatra, D., et al.: Automatic detection and segmentation of crohn's disease tissues from abdominal MRI. IEEE Trans. Med. Imaging **32**(12), 2332–2347 (2013)
5. Yigitsoy, M., Reiser, M.F., Navab, N., Kirchhoff, S.: Dynamic graph cuts for colon segmentation in functional cine-MRI. In: 2012 9th IEEE International Symposium on Biomedical Imaging (ISBI), pp. 1268–1271. IEEE (2012)

6. Krissian, K., Malandain, G., Ayache, N., Vaillant, R., Trousset, Y.: Model-based detection of tubular structures in 3D images. Comput. Vis. Image Underst. **80**(2), 130–171 (2000)
7. Smistad, E., Brekken, R., Lindseth, F.: A new tube detection filter for abdominal aortic aneurysms. In: Yoshida, H., Näppi, J., Saini, S. (eds.) International MICCAI Workshop on Computational and Clinical Challenges in Abdominal Imaging, pp. 229–238. Springer, Cham (2014). https://doi.org/10.1007/978-3-319-13692-9_22

Ordinal Multi-modal Feature Selection for Survival Analysis of Early-Stage Renal Cancer

Wei Shao[1], Jun Cheng[2], Liang Sun[1], Zhi Han[4], Qianjin Feng[3],
Daoqiang Zhang[1(✉)], and Kun Huang[4(✉)]

[1] College of Computer Science and Technology, Nanjing University of Aeronautics
and Astronautics, Nanjing 211106, China
dqzhang@nuaa.edu.cn
[2] School of Biomedical Engineering, Shenzhen University, Shenzhen 518073, China
[3] School of Biomedical Engineering, Southern Medical University, Guangzhou
510515, China
[4] School of Medicine, Indiana University, Indianapolis, IN 46202, USA
kunhuang@iu.edu

Abstract. Existing studies have demonstrated that combining genomic
data and histopathological images can better stratify cancer patients
with distinct prognosis than using single biomarker, for different
biomarkers may provide complementary information. However, these
multi-modal data, most high-dimensional, may contain redundant features that will deteriorate the performance of the prognosis model, and
therefore it has become a challenging problem to select the informative
features for survival analysis from the redundant and heterogeneous feature groups. Existing feature selection methods assume that the survival
information of one patient is independent to another, and thus miss the
ordinal relationship among the survival time of different patients. To
solve this issue, we make use of the important ordinal survival information among different patients and propose an ordinal sparse canonical
correlation analysis (i.e., OSCCA) framework to simultaneously identify
important image features and eigengenes for survival analysis. Specifically, we formulate our framework basing on sparse canonical correlation
analysis model, which aims at finding the best linear projections so that
the highest correlation between the selected image features and eigengenes can be achieved. In addition, we also add constrains to ensure that
the ordinal survival information of different patients is preserved after
projection. We evaluate the effectiveness of our method on an early-
stage renal cell carcinoma dataset. Experimental results demonstrate
that the selected features correlated strongly with survival, by which we
can achieve better patient stratification than the comparing methods.

This work was supported in part by the National Natural Science Foundation of
China (61473149,61732006), the NCI ITCR (U01CA188547) and Shenzhen Peacock
Plan (KQTD2016053112051497).

© Springer Nature Switzerland AG 2018
A. F. Frangi et al. (Eds.): MICCAI 2018, LNCS 11071, pp. 648–656, 2018.
https://doi.org/10.1007/978-3-030-00934-2_72

1   Introduction

Cancer is the most common form of diseases worldwide. It is reported that the number of affected people in developing country will reach 20 million annually as early as 2025 [1]. Effective and accurate prognosis prediction of human cancer, especially at its early stage has attracted much attention recently. So far, many biomarkers have been shown to be associated with the prognosis of cancers, including the histopathological images, genomic signatures, proteomics makers and demographical information.

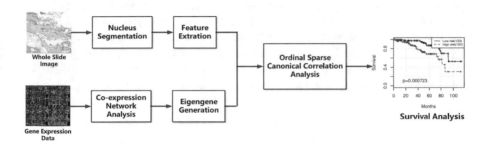

Fig. 1. The flowchart of the proposed method.

Early studies on the prognosis of cancer often focus on using single-modality biomarker (*e.g.,* imaging or genomic data). However, in these studies, some useful complementary information across different modalities of data is ignored. Recently, some studies explored to combine both imaging and genomic biomarkers for survival analysis [2–4]. For instance, Cheng *et al.* [2] constructed a novel framework that can predict the survival outcomes of patients with renal cell carcinoma by using a combination of quantitative image features and gene expression feature. Yuan [3] *et al.* integrated both image data and genomic data to improve the survival prognosis for breast cancer patients. These existing studies have suggested that different modalities of data complement with each other and provide better patient stratification when used together.

Although integrating imaging and genomic features can better predict the clinical outcome for cancer patients, simply combing these features may bring redundant features that will deteriorate the prediction performance, and thus feature selection is a key step for multi-modal feature fusion. In the existing studies [2,3], the authors usually simply concatenate multi-modal data together at first, and then apply traditional feature selection methods (*e.g.,* LASSO) to select components that are related to cancer prognosis. However, these feature selection methods assume that the survival time of one patient is independent to another, and thus missing the strong ordinal relationship among the survival time of different patients, *e.g.,* the survival time of patient A is longer than that of patient B. In addition, most of the studies [2,3] directly combine morphological and genomic data together for survival analysis, which neglects correlation among the multi-modal data. As a matter of fact, the exploitation of multi-modal association has been widely accepted as a key component of the state-of-the-art multi-modality based machine learning approaches [5].

Based on the above consideration, in this paper, we take advantage of the ordinal survival information among different cancer patients, and propose an ordinal sparse canonical correlation analysis (OSCCA) framework that can select features from multi-modal data for survival analysis. Specifically, we formulate our framework based on sparse canonical correlation analysis (*i.e.*, SCCA), which is a powerful association method that can identify linear projections to achieve the highest correlation between the selected imaging and genomic components. In addition, we add constrains to ensure that the ordinal information of different groups of patients is preserved, *i.e.*, the average projection of the patients from the long-term survival groups should be larger than that of short-term survival groups. The experimental results on a public available early-stage clear cell renal cell carcinoma (ccRCC) dataset demonstrate that the proposed method outperforms comparing methods in terms of patient stratification.

Table 1. Demographics and clinical characteristics

Characteristics	Summary	Characteristics	Summary
Patients		Stage	
Censored	188	Stage I	201
Non-censored	55	Stage II	42
Age (Y):	59.1 ± 12.2	Follow-up (M):	43.2 ± 25.2

2   Method

Figure 1 shows the flowchart of our framework, which includes three major steps, *i.e.*, feature extraction, ordinal sparse canonical correlation analysis based feature selection (OSCCA), and prognostic prediction. Before giving the detailed descriptions of these steps, we will firstly introduce the dataset used in this study.

Dataset: The Cancer Genome Atlas (TCGA) project has generated multimodal genomic and imaging data for different types of cancer. Renal cell carcinoma is the most common type of cancer arising from kidney. In this study, we test our method on an early-stage (*i.e.*, stage I and stage II) ccRCC dataset [2] derived from TCGA. Specifically, this dataset contains pathological imaging, genomic, and clinical data for 243 early-stage renal cell carcinoma patients. Of the 243 samples, 188 patients are censored, which means that the death events of them were not observed during the follow-up period, and their exact survival times are longer than the recorded data. The remaining 55 samples are non-censored patients, and their recorded survival times are the exact time from initial diagnosis to death. Table 1 summarizes the demographics of all the samples.

Feature Extraction: For each image, we firstly apply the method in [6] to segment the nucleus in the whole-slide image, and then for each segmented nucleus, we extract ten different features [2], *i.e.*, nuclear area (denoted as area), lengths of the major and minor axes of cell nucleus, and the ratio of major axis length to minor axis length (major, minor, and ratio), mean pixel values of nucleus in RGB channels respectively (rMean, gMean, and bMean), and mean, maximum, and minimum distances (distMean, distMax, and distMin) to its neighboring nuclei. Next, for each type of feature, a 10-bin histogram and five statistic measurements (*i.e.*, mean, SD, skewness, kurtosis, and entropy) are used to aggregate the cell-level features into patient-level features, and thus a 150-dimensional imaging feature for each patient can be obtained. Here, we use area_bin1 to represent the percentage of very small nuclei while area_bin10 indicates the percentage of very large nuclei in the patient sample. As to gene expression data, we firstly use co-expression network analysis algorithms to cluster genes into co-expressed modules, and then summarize each module as an eigengene (gene modules are shown in Supplementary Materials). This algorithm yields 15 coexpressed gene modules. More details about the genomic feature extraction can be found in [2].

Sparse Canonical Correlation Analysis: For the derived imaging and eigengene features, we implement our feature selection model under SCCA framework. Specifically, let $\boldsymbol{X}_H \in R^{N \times p}$ be the histopathological imaging data, and $\boldsymbol{X}_G \in R^{N \times q}$ be the extracted eigengenes data, where N is the number of the patients, and p and q are the feature number of imaging data and eigengene data, respectively. The objective function of SCCA is:

$$\min_{\boldsymbol{\omega}_H, \boldsymbol{\omega}_G} - (\boldsymbol{\omega}_H)^T (\boldsymbol{X}_H)^T \boldsymbol{X}_G \boldsymbol{\omega}_G + r_1 \|\boldsymbol{\omega}_H\|_1 + r_2 \|\boldsymbol{\omega}_G\|_1$$
$$s.t. \|\boldsymbol{X}_G \boldsymbol{\omega}_G\|_2^2 \leq 1; \|\boldsymbol{X}_H \boldsymbol{\omega}_H\|_2^2 \leq 1 \tag{1}$$

where the first term in Eq. (1) seeks linear transformations (*i.e.*, $\boldsymbol{\omega}_H, \boldsymbol{\omega}_G$) to achieve the maximal correlation between imaging and eigengene data, the second and third L1-norm regularized terms are used to select a small number of feature that can maximize the association between the multi-modal data.

Ordinal Sparse Canonical Correlation Analysis: In the SCCA model, we only consider the mutual dependency between imaging and genomic data, and thus ignore the survival information of patients. Although the study in [2] used the survival information for feature selection, they assume that the survival information of one patient is independent to another, and thus miss the strong ordinal relationship among the survival time of different patients. To address this problem, we propose an ordinal sparse canonical correlation analysis (OSCCA) method to simultaneously identify important features from the multi-modal data. Specifically, we divide $\boldsymbol{X} = [\boldsymbol{X}_H, \boldsymbol{X}_G] \in R^{N \times (p+q)}$ into $\boldsymbol{X}^C$ and $\boldsymbol{X}^{NC}$, where $\boldsymbol{X}^C \in R^{k \times (p+q)}$ and $\boldsymbol{X}^{NC} \in R^{(N-k) \times (p+q)}$ correspond to the multi-modal features for censored and non-censored patients,respectively, and k denotes the number of censored patients. We also define $\boldsymbol{Y} = [\boldsymbol{Y}^C, \boldsymbol{Y}^{NC}]$, where $\boldsymbol{Y}^C \in R^k$ and $\boldsymbol{Y}^{NC} \in R^{(N-k)}$ indicate the recorded survival time for censored and non-censored patients, respectively. In order to reduce the chance that all patients in one group are censored, we divide all the patients (include both censored and non-censored patients) into four groups with equal size based on the quartiles of their recorded survival time, where each patient in group $i(i = 1, 2, 3, 4)$ has longer survival time than that in group j if $i > j$. We denote the mean imaging and eigengene feature for censored patients in group i as $\boldsymbol{u}_H^i$ and $\boldsymbol{u}_G^i$, and those for non-censored patients in group i as $\boldsymbol{v}_H^i$ and $\boldsymbol{v}_G^i$, respectively. We show the objective function of the OSCCA model as:

$$\min_{\boldsymbol{\omega}_H, \boldsymbol{\omega}_G} - (\boldsymbol{\omega}_H)^T (\boldsymbol{X}_H)^T \boldsymbol{X}_G \boldsymbol{\omega}_G + r_1 \|\boldsymbol{\omega}_H\|_1 + r_2 \|\boldsymbol{\omega}_G\|_1 + r_3 \left\| \boldsymbol{X}^{NC} \boldsymbol{\omega} - \boldsymbol{Y}^{NC} \right\|_2^2 \quad (2)$$

$$s.t. \quad (\boldsymbol{v}_G^{i+1} - \boldsymbol{v}_G^i)\boldsymbol{\omega}_G > 0, \qquad (\boldsymbol{v}_H^{i+1} - \boldsymbol{v}_H^i)\boldsymbol{\omega}_H > 0 \quad (3)$$

$$(\boldsymbol{u}_G^{i+1} - \boldsymbol{v}_G^i)\boldsymbol{\omega}_G > 0, \qquad (\boldsymbol{u}_H^{i+1} - \boldsymbol{v}_H^i)\boldsymbol{\omega}_H > 0 \quad (4)$$

where the first three terms in Eq. (2) are as same as they are stated in the SCCA model, the forth part is a regression term, where $\boldsymbol{\omega} = [\boldsymbol{\omega}_H, \boldsymbol{\omega}_G] \in R^{p+q}$. We use this term to estimate the relationship between the multi-modal data and the survival time for non-censored patients, since their survival information are accurate. We add two linear inequalities in (3) to ensure that the ordinal survival information of different groups of non-censored patients is preserved after the projections are adopted on both imaging and eigengenes data. In addition, since the genuine survival time for censored patients are longer than the recorded data, it is easy to infer that the average projection for the censored patients in groups $i+1$ should be larger than that for non-censored patients in group i, and we also add this ordinal relationship for both eigengene and imaging data by adding two inequality constrains shown in (4).

Optimization: We adopt an alternating strategy to optimize $\boldsymbol{\omega}_H$ and $\boldsymbol{\omega}_G$ in the proposed OSCCA model. Specifically, given the fixed $\boldsymbol{\omega}_H$, the optimization problem for $\boldsymbol{\omega}_G$ can be reformulated as:

$$\min_{\boldsymbol{\omega}_G} \frac{1}{2}(\boldsymbol{\omega}_G)^T \boldsymbol{A} \boldsymbol{\omega}_G + (\boldsymbol{\omega}_G)^T \boldsymbol{B} + r_2 \|\boldsymbol{\omega}_G\|_1$$

$$s.t. \quad \boldsymbol{C}\boldsymbol{\omega}_G > 0 \quad (5)$$

where $\boldsymbol{B} = -(\boldsymbol{X}_G)^T \boldsymbol{X}_H \boldsymbol{\omega}_H + 2r_3 (\boldsymbol{X}_G^{NC})^T (\boldsymbol{X}_H^{NC} \boldsymbol{\omega}_H - \boldsymbol{Y}^{NC})$, in which $\boldsymbol{X}_G^{NC} \in R^{(N-k) \times p}$ and $\boldsymbol{X}_H^{NC} \in R^{(N-k) \times q}$ correspond to the imaging and eigengene data for non-censored patients, respectively. Also, $\boldsymbol{A} = 2r_3 (\boldsymbol{X}_G^{NC})^T \boldsymbol{X}_G^{NC}$, and $\boldsymbol{C} = [\boldsymbol{v}_G^4 - \boldsymbol{v}_G^3; \boldsymbol{v}_G^3 - \boldsymbol{v}_G^2; \boldsymbol{v}_G^2 - \boldsymbol{v}_G^1; \boldsymbol{u}_G^4 - \boldsymbol{v}_G^3; \boldsymbol{u}_G^3 - \boldsymbol{v}_G^2; \boldsymbol{u}_G^2 - \boldsymbol{v}_G^1] \in R^{6 \times q}$. For the optimization problem in (5), we adopt the alternating direction method of multipliers (i.e., ADMM) algorithm to solve it. To change the problem in (5) into ADMM form, we introduce variables $\boldsymbol{J} \in R^q$ and non-negative vector $\boldsymbol{\theta} \in R^6$, which is used to transform the inequality constraints $\boldsymbol{C}\boldsymbol{\omega}_G > 0$ into equality constrains $C\omega_G - \theta = 0$, Eq. (5) can be reformulated as:

$$\min_{\omega_G} \frac{1}{2}(\omega_G)^T A\omega_G + (\omega_G)^T B + r_2\|J\|_1$$
$$s.t. \quad J = \omega_G, \quad C\omega_G - \theta = 0 \tag{6}$$

Then, the augmented Lagrangian form of Eq. (6) can be written as:

$$L(\omega_G, J, \theta, Q, R) = \frac{1}{2}(\omega_G)^T A\omega_G + (\omega_G)^T B + r_2\|J\|_1 + <Q, \omega_G - J>$$
$$+ \frac{\rho_1}{2}\|\omega_G - J\|_2^2 + <R, C\omega_G - \theta> + \frac{\rho_2}{2}\|C\omega_G - \theta\|_2^2 \tag{7}$$

where Q and R are Lagrange multipliers. A general ADMM scheme for Eq. (7) repeats the following 5 steps until convergence: (1) $\omega_G \leftarrow \arg\min_{\omega_G} L(\omega_G, J, \theta, Q, R)$: It is a convex problem with respect to ω_G and we can solve it via gradient descent method. (2) $J \leftarrow \arg\min_J L(\omega_G, J, \theta, Q, R)$: This optimization problem can be formulated as: $\min_J \frac{\rho_1}{2}\|\omega_G - J\|_2^2 + r_2\|J\|_1 - (Q)^T J$. Since the L1-norm is non-differentiable at zero, a smooth approximation has been estimated for L1 term by including an extremely small value. Then, by taking the derivative regarding to J and let it to be zero, we can obtain $J = (r_2 D + \rho_1 I)^{-1}(Q + \rho_1\omega_G)$, where D is a diagonal matrix with the k-th element as $1/\|J_k\|_1$. Here, J_k denotes the k-th element in J. (3) $\theta \leftarrow \arg\min_\theta L(\omega_G, J, \theta, Q, R)$: It has a close form solution with the k-th element $\theta_k = \max(0, T_k)$, where T_k corresponds to the k-th element in $T = C\omega_G + \frac{1}{\rho_2}R$. (4) $Q = Q + \rho_1(\omega_G - J)$. (5) $R = R + \rho_2(C\omega_G - \theta)$. After ω_G is determined, we use similar method to optimize ω_H.

Prognostic Prediction: We build Cox proportional hazards model [2] for survival analysis. Specifically, we firstly divide all patients into 10 folds, with 9 folds used for training the proposed OSCCA model and the remaining for testing, then the Cox proportional hazards model is built on the selected features in the training set. After that, the median risk score predicted by the cox proportional hazards model is used as a threshold to split patients into low-risk and high-risk groups. Finally, we test if these two groups has distinct survival outcome using Kaplan-Meier estimator and log-rank test [2].

3   Experimental Results

Experimental Settings: The parameters r_1, r_2, r_3 in the OSCCA model are tuned from $\{2^{-4}, 2^{-5}\}$, $\{2^{-5}, 2^{-6}\}$ and $\{2^{-5}, 2^{-6}\}$, respectively, ρ_1 and ρ_2 in Eq. (7) are fixed as 2^{-3}. All the algorithms are implemented using MATLAB 2017.

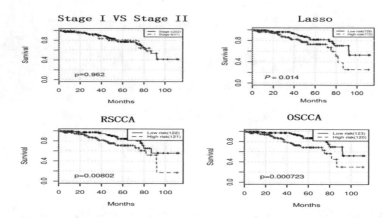

Fig. 2. Comparisons of the survival curves by applying different feature methods.

Results and Discussion: We compare the prognostic power of our proposed OSCCA method with several other methods, including LASSO [2] and RSCCA, as well as tumor staging. Compared to the proposed OSCCA model, RSCCA method has the same objective function (shown in Eq. (2)), but neglect to take the ordinal survival information (shown in the inequalities in (3) and (4)) into consideration We show the survival curves of these four methods in Fig. 2. It is observed that on one hand, the Kaplan-Meier curves for tumor Stage I and Stage II are intertwined (log-rank test $P = 0.962$), which demonstrates that the stratification of the early-stage renal cell carcinoma patients is a challenging task, on the other hand, OSCCA could achieve significantly better patient stratification (log-rank test $P = 7.2e - 3$) than the comparing methods, which shows the advantage of using ordinal survival information for feature selection. In addition, it is worth noting that the proposed RSCCA could provide better prognostic prediction than the LASSO method, this is because RSCCA considers the correlation among different modalities for feature selection, which is better than the direct combination strategy.

Next, in order to investigate the association between the selected imaging feature and eigengenes, the spearman coefficients between $X_H\omega_H$ and $X_G\omega_G$ on 10-fold testing data are shown in Fig. 3. Obviously, OSCCA generally outperforms the comparing methods in term of identifying high correlation between imaging data and genomic data, and the better exploration of the inherent correlation within multi-modal data may be the reason for the better patient stratification performance of the proposed OSCCA method.

Lastly, we compare the features selected by OSCCA with those selected by [2] in Table 2. We find that our method can identify new types of image features (*i.e.*, area_bin10) that are related to large nuclei. It has been demonstrated that the ccRCC patients with large values of nuclei size have worse prognosis [7] than other patients. As to genomic features, two novel eigengenes (*i.e.*, eigengene 9, eigengene 14) are identified. The enrichment analysis on eigengene 9 shows that it is related to mitotic cell cycle process and genome stability, and genes in this

Table 2. Comparisons of the selected features by the method in [2] and OSCCA.

	Image feature	Eigengenes
LASSO [2]	rMean_bin8, rMean_mean, distMean_bin10, rMean_mean	Eigengene3, Eigengene13
OSCCA	rMean_bin9, major_kurtosis, *area_bin10*, distMin_bin1, bMean_bin8	Eigengene3, *Eigengene9*, *Eigengene14*

module are frequently observed to co-express in multiple types of cancers [8]. In addition, eigengene 14 is enriched with genes that are associated with immune response, and it is reported that the deregulation of the immune response genes are associated with the initiation and progression of cancers [9], and our discovery can potentially shed light on the emerging immunotherapics. These results further shows the promise of OSCCA to identify biologically meaningful biomarkers for the prognosis of early-stage renal cancer patients.

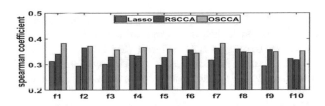

Fig. 3. The spearman coefficients between $X_H \omega_H$ and $X_G \omega_G$ on 10-fold testing data.

4   Conclusion

In this paper, we develop OSCCA which is an effective multimodal feature selection method for patient stratification aiming at identifying subgroups of cancer patients with distinct prognosis. The strength of our approach is its capability of utilizing the ordinal survival information among different patients to identify features that are associated with patient survival time. Experimental results on an early-stage multi-modal renal cell carcinoma dataset have demonstrated that the proposed OSCCA can identify new types of image features and gene modules that are associated with patient survival, by which we can achieve significantly better patients stratification than the comparing methods. Such prediction is particularly important for early stage patients when the prediction is important yet staging information from pathologists is not sufficient to meet the needs. OSCCA is a general framework and can be used to find multi-modal biomarkers for other cancers or predict response of specific treatment, which allow for better patients management and cancer care in precision medicine.

References

1. Torre, L., Bray, F., Siegel, R.: Global cancer statistics. Cancer J. Clin. **65**(2), 87–108 (2012)
2. Cheng, J., Zhang, J., Han, Y., Huang, K.: Integrative analysis of histopathological images and genomic data predicts clear cell renal cell carcinoma prognosis. Cancer Res. **77**(21), 91–100 (2017)
3. Yuan, Y., Failmezger, H., Rueda, O.: Quantitative image analysis of cellular heterogeneity in breast tumors complements genomic profiling. Sci. Transl. Med. **4**(157), 143–157 (2012)
4. Yao, J., Zhu, X., Zhu, F., Huang, J.: Deep correlational learning for survival prediction from multi-modality data. In: Descoteaux, M., Maier-Hein, L., Franz, A., Jannin, P., Collins, D.L., Duchesne, S. (eds.) MICCAI 2017. LNCS, vol. 10434, pp. 406–414. Springer, Cham (2017). https://doi.org/10.1007/978-3-319-66185-8_46
5. Liu, F., Chen, H., Shen, D.: Inter-modality relationship constrained multi-modality multi-task feature selection for alzheimer's disease and mild cognitive impairment identification. Neuroimage **84**(1), 466–475 (2014)
6. Phoulady, H., Goldgof, D., Mouton, P.: Nucleus segmentation in histology images with hierarchical multilevel thresholding. In: Proceedings of SPIE 2016, pp. 1–8 (2016)
7. Kanamaru, H., Akino, H., Suzuki, Y.: Prognostic value of nuclear area index in combination with the world health organization grading system for patients with renal cell carcinoma. Urology **57**(2), 257–261 (2001)
8. Zhang, J., Lu, K., Xiang, Y., Huang, K.: Weighted frequent gene co-expression network mining to identify genes involved in genome stability. Plos Comput. Biol. **8**(8), 1–14 (2012)
9. Kim, S., Park, C., Kim, H., Kang, M.: Deregulation of immune response genes in patients with epstein-barr virus-associated gastric cancer and outcomes. Gastroenterology **148**(1), 137–147 (2015)

Noninvasive Determination of Gene Mutations in Clear Cell Renal Cell Carcinoma Using Multiple Instance Decisions Aggregated CNN

Mohammad Arafat Hussain[1]($\boxtimes$), Ghassan Hamarneh[2], and Rafeef Garbi[1]

[1] BiSICL, University of British Columbia, Vancouver, BC, Canada
{arafat,rafeef}@ece.ubc.ca
[2] Medical Image Analysis Lab, Simon Fraser University, Burnaby, BC, Canada
hamarneh@sfu.ca

Abstract. Kidney clear cell renal cell carcinoma (ccRCC) is the major sub-type of RCC, constituting one the most common cancers world-wide accounting for a steadily increasing mortality rate with 350,000 new cases recorded in 2012. Understanding the underlying genetic mutations in ccRCC provides crucial information enabling malignancy staging and patient survival estimation thus plays a vital role in accurate ccRCC diagnosis, prognosis, treatment planning, and response assessment. Although the underlying gene mutations can be identified by whole genome sequencing of the ccRCC following invasive nephrectomy or kidney biopsy procedures, recent studies have suggested that such mutations may be noninvasively identified by studying image features of the ccRCC from Computed Tomography (CT) data. Such image feature identification currently relies on laborious manual processes based on visual inspection of 2D image slices that are time-consuming and subjective. In this paper, we propose a convolutional neural network approach for automatic detection of underlying ccRCC gene mutations from 3D CT volumes. We aggregate the mutation-presence/absence decisions for all the ccRCC slices in a kidney into a robust singular decision that determines whether the interrogated kidney bears a specific mutation or not. When validated on clinical CT datasets of 267 patients from the TCIA database, our method detected gene mutations with 94% accuracy.

1 Introduction

Kidney cancer, or renal cell carcinomas (RCC) are a common group of chemotherapy resistant diseases that accounted for an estimated 62,000 new patients and 14,000 deaths in the United States in 2015 alone [1]. North America and Europe have recently reported the highest numbers of new cases of RCC in the world [2]. The most common histologic sub-type of RCC is clear cell RCC (ccRCC) [3], which is known to be a genetically heterogeneous disease [4]. Recent studies [5,6] have identified several mutations in genes associated with

© Springer Nature Switzerland AG 2018
A. F. Frangi et al. (Eds.): MICCAI 2018, LNCS 11071, pp. 657–665, 2018.
https://doi.org/10.1007/978-3-030-00934-2_73

ccRCC. For example, the von Hippel-Lindau (VHL) tumor suppressor gene, BRCA1-associated protein 1 (BAP1) gene, polybromo 1 (PBRM1) gene, and SET domain containing 2 (SETD2) gene have been identified as the most commonly mutated genes in ccRCC [5].

Traditionally, ccRCC underlying gene mutations are identified by genome sequencing of the ccRCC of the kidney samples after invasive nephrectomy or kidney biopsy [5]. This identification of genetic mutations is clinically important because advanced stages of ccRCC and poor patient survival have been found to be associated with the VHL, PBRM1, BAP1, SETD2, and lysine (K)-specific demethylase 5C (KDM5C) gene mutations [5,7]. Therefore, knowledge of the genetic make-up of a patient's kidney ccRCC has great prognostic value that is helpful for treatment planning [5,7]. Correlations between mutations in genes and different ccRCC features seen in patient CT images has been shown in recent work [4,8]. For example, an association between well-defined tumor margin, nodular enhancement and intratumoral vascularity with the VHL mutation has been reported [8]. Ill-defined tumor margin and renal vein invasion were also reported to be associated with the BAP1 mutation [4] whereas PBRM1 and SETD2 mutations are mostly seen in solid (non-cystic) ccRCC cases [8]. Such use of radiological imaging data as a noninvasive determinant of the mutational status and a complement to genomic analysis in characterizing disease biology is refereed to as 'Radiogenomics' [4,8]. Radiogenomics requires robust image feature identification, which is typically performed by expert radiologists. However, relying on human visual inspection is laborious, time consuming, and suffers from high intra/inter-observer variability.

A number of machine learning (ML) tools have been used to facilitate the processes of high-throughput quantitative feature extraction from volumetric medical images, with some subsequently used in treatment decision support [9]. This practice is generally known as 'Radiomics'. Radiomics uses higher order statistics (on the medical images) combined with clinical and radiogenomic data to develop models that may potentially improve cancer diagnostic, prognostic, and predictive accuracy [9,10]. The typical tumor radiomic analysis workflow has 4 distinct steps: (1) 3D imaging, (2) manual or automatic tumor detection and segmentation, (3) tumor phenotype quantification, and (4) data integration (i.e. phenotype+genotype+clinical+proteomic) and analysis [10]. Discriminant features needed for proper mutation detection are often not seen in the marginal ccRCC cross-sections (e.g. axial slices in the top and bottom regions of a ccRCC). This scenario makes 'single-instance' ML approaches, especially convolutional neural network (CNN) very difficult to train, as some of the input slices do not contain discriminating features, thus do not correspond to the assigned mutation label. Another solution is to use the full 3D volume as a single instance. However, 3D CNNs are considerably more difficult to train as they contain significantly more parameters and consequently require many more training samples, while the use of the 3D volume itself severely reduces the available number of training samples than its 2D counterpart. An alternative approach is multiple-instance learning (MIL) [11], where the learner receives a set of labeled bags (e.g. mutation present/absent), each containing multiple instances (e.g. all the ccRCC slices in a kidney). A MIL model labels a bag with a class even if some or most of the instances within it are not members of that class.

We propose a deep CNN approach that addresses the challenge of automatic mutation detection in kidney ccRCC. Our method is a variant of the conventional MIL approach, where we use multiple instances for robust binary classification, while using single instances for training the CNN to facilitate higher number and variation of training data. The CNN automatically learns the ccRCC image features and the binary decisions (i.e. presence/absence of a mutation) for all the ccRCC slices in a particular kidney sample are aggregated into a robust singular decision that ultimately determines whether an interrogated kidney sample has undergone a certain mutation or not. Our method can be incorporated in the Radiomics step-3 given that the tumor boundary is already known in step-2. The estimated mutation data can subsequently be integrated in the step-4. The frequency of occurrence of various mutations in ccRCC varies significantly, e.g. VHL, PBRM1, BAP1, SETD2 and KDM5C were found in 76%, 43%, 14%, 14% and 8% of kidney samples of our dataset, respectively. In this study we consider the four most prevalent gene mutations (i.e. VHL, PBRM1, BAP1 and SETD2). We achieve this via four multiple instance decisions aggregation CNNs, however, our approach is directly extendable to more mutation types depending on the availability of sufficient training data.

2   Materials and Methods

2.1   Data

We obtained access to 267 patients' CT scans from The Cancer Imaging Archive (TCIA) database [12]. In this dataset, 138 scans contained at least one mutated gene because of ccRCC. For example, 105 patients had VHL, 60 patients had PBRM1, 60 patients had SETD2, and 20 patients had BAP1 mutations. In addition, some of the patients had multiple types of mutations. However, 9 patients had CT scans acquired after nephrectomy and, therefore, those patients' data were not usable for this study. The images in our database included variations in CT scanner models, contrast administration, field of view, and spatial resolution. The in-plane pixel size ranged from 0.29 to 1.87 mm and the slice thickness ranged from 1.5 to 7.5 mm. Ground truth mutation labels were collected from the *cBioPortal for Cancer Genomics* [7].

We show the number of kidney samples used in the training, validation and testing stages in Table 1. During training, validation and testing, we use only those slices of the kidney that contain ccRCC as our CNNs aim to learn ccRCC features. We form a 3-channel image from each scalar-valued CT slice by generating channel intensities [I, I-50, I-100] HU, where I represents the original intensities in a CT image slice tightly encompassing a kidney+ccRCC cross-section (Fig. 1), whereas I-50 and I-100 represent two variants of I with different

Table 1. Number of kidney samples used in training, validation and testing per mutation case. Acronym used: M: mutation.

Genes	# Training Samples		# Validation Samples		# Test Samples	
	M-Present	M-Absent	M-Present	M-Absent	M-Present	M-Absent
VHL	74	74	10	10	15	15
PBRM1	35	35	6	6	10	10
SETD2	11	11	3	3	5	5
BAP1	10	10	3	3	4	4

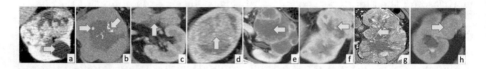

Fig. 1. Illustration of CT features of ccRCC seen in the data of this study. (a) Cystic tumor architecture, (b) calcification, (c) exophytic tumor, (d) endophytic tumor, (e) necrosis, (f) ill-defined tumor margin, (g) nodular enhancement, and (h) renal vein invasion. Arrow indicates feature of interest in each image.

HU values. We add these variations in channel intensity values as similar ccRCC features may have different X-ray attenuation properties across patients [4]. We resized all the image data by resampling into a size of $227 \times 227 \times 3$ pixels. We augmented the number of training samples by a factor of 24 by flipping and rotating the 3-ch image slices as well as by re-ordering the 3 channels in each image. We normalized the training and validation data before training by subtracting the image mean and dividing by the image standard deviation.

2.2   Multiple Instance Decision Aggregation for Mutation Detection

Typically, ccRCC grows in different regions of the kidney and is clinically scored on the basis of their CT slice-based image features, such as size, margin (well- or ill-defined), composition (solid or cystic), necrosis, growth pattern (endophytic or exophytic), calcification etc. [4]. Some of these features seen in our dataset are shown in Fig. 1. We propose to learn corresponding features from the CT images using four different CNNs: VHL-CNN, PBRM1-CNN, SETD2-CNN and BAP1-CNN, each for one of the four mutations (VHL, PBRM1, SETD2 and BAP1). Using a separate CNN per mutation alleviates the problem of data imbalance among mutation types, given that the mutations are not mutually exclusive.

CNN Architecture: All the CNNs in this study (i.e. VHL-CNN, PBRM1-CNN, SETD2-CNN and BAP1-CNN) have similar configuration but are trained separately (Fig. 2). Each CNN has twelve layers excluding the input: five convolutional (Conv) layers; three fully connected (FC) layers; one softmax layer; one average pooling layer; and two thresholding layers. All but the last three layers contain trainable weights. The input is the $227 \times 227 \times 3$ pixel image slice containing the kidney+ccRCC. We train these CNNs (layers 1–9) using a balanced dataset for each mutation case separately (i.e. a particular mutation-present and absent). During training, images are fed to the CNNs in a randomly shuffled single instance fashion. Typically, Conv layers are known for sequentially learning the high-level non-linear spatial image features (e.g. ccRCC size, orientation, edge variation, etc.). We used five Conv layers as the 5th Conv layer typically grabs an entire object (e.g. ccRCC shape) in an image even if there is a significant pose variation [13]. Subsequent FC layers prepare those features for optimal classification of an interrogated image. In our case, three FC layers are deployed to make the decision on the learned features from the 3-ch images to decide if a particular gene mutation is probable or not. The number of FC layers plays a vital role as the overall depth of the model is important for obtaining good performance [13], and we achieve optimal performance with three FC layers. Layers 10, 11 and 12 (i.e. two thresholding and one average pooling layers) of the CNNs are used during the testing phase and do not contain any trainable weights.

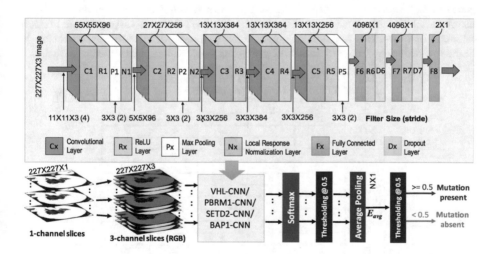

Fig. 2. Multiple instance decisions aggregated CNN for gene mutation detection.

Solver: These networks were trained by minimizing the softmax loss between the expected and detected labels (1: mutation present and 0: mutation absent). We used the *Adam* optimization method [14]. All the parameters for this solver were set to the suggested (by [14]) default values, i.e. $\beta_1 = 0.9$, $\beta_2 = 0.999$ and $\epsilon = 10^{-8}$. We also employed a Dropout unit (Dx) that drops 50% of units in both F6 and F7 layers (Fig. 2) and used a weight decay of 0.005. The base learning rate was set to 0.01 and was decreased by a factor of 0.1 to 0.0001 over 250,000 iterations with a batch of 256 images processed at each iteration. Training was performed on a workstation with Intel 4.0 GHz Core-i7 processor, an Nvidia GeForce Titan Xp GPU with 12 GB of VRAM, and 32 GB of RAM.

Mutation Detection: After all the CNNs are trained (from layer 1 to 9), we use the full configuration (from layer 1 to 12) in the testing phase. Although we use only ccRCC containing kidney slices during training and validation, often not all the ccRCC cross-sections contains the discriminating features for proper mutation detection. Therefore, our trained CNN (from layer 1 to 9) often miss-classifies the interrogated image slice based on the probability estimated at the layer 9 (i.e. softmax layer). In order to address this misclassification by our CNNs, we adopt a multiple instance decision aggregation procedure. In this procedure, we feed all the candidate image slices of a particular kidney to the trained CNN and accumulate the slice-wise binary classification labels (0 or 1) at layer 10 (the thresholding layer). These labels are then fed into a $N \times 1$ average pooling layer, where N is the total number of 3-channel axial slices of an interrogated kidney. Finally, the estimated average (E_{avg}) from layer 11 is fed to the second thresholding layer (layer 12), where $E_{avg} \geq 0.5$ indicates the presence of the mutation in that kidney, and no-mutation otherwise (see Fig. 2).

Table 2. Automatic gene mutation detection performance of different methods. We use acronyms as: M: mutation, x: one of VHL/PBRM1/SETD2/BAP1, Aug: augmentation, SI: single instance, MI: multiple instance, 3ch: 3-channel data with augmentation by channel re-ordering, F: augmentation by flipping, and R: augmentation by rotation.

Methods	Genes x	# Test Samples		# Correct Detection		Overall Error (%)	Mean Error (%)
		M-present	M-absent	M-present	M-absent		
Random Forest (SI+1ch) No Aug	VHL	15	15	5	7	60	53.75
	PBRM1	10	10	4	5	55	
	SETD2	5	5	2	3	50	
	BAP1	4	4	2	2	50	
x-CNN (SI+1ch) No Aug	VHL	15	15	7	8	50	41.88
	PBRM1	10	10	6	6	40	
	SETD2	5	5	3	3	40	
	BAP1	4	4	2	3	37.50	
x-CNN (SI+3ch)	VHL	15	15	12	9	30	29.38
	PBRM1	10	10	4	7	45	
	SETD2	5	3	4	4	30	
	BAP1	4	4	3	4	12.5	
x-CNN (SI+1ch +F+R)	VHL	15	15	11	13	20	21.88
	PBRM1	10	10	8	7	25	
	SETD2	5	5	3	4	30	
	BAP1	4	4	4	3	12.50	
x-CNN (SI+3ch +F+R)	VHL	15	15	15	11	13.33	13.96
	PBRM1	10	10	9	9	10	
	SETD2	5	5	5	3	20	
	BAP1	4	4	3	3	12.50	
Proposed (MI+3ch +F+R +Average)	VHL	15	15	14	13	**10**	**6.25**
	PBRM1	10	10	9	10	**5**	
	SETD2	5	5	5	4	**10**	
	BAP1	4	4	4	4	**0**	

3   Results

We compare the mutation detection performance by a wide range of methods. At first, we tested the performance using a single instance (SI)-based random forest (RF) approach, where hand-engineered image features were used. In a typical SI-based classification approach, the class-label is decided from the maximum among the predicted class-probabilities [15]. Similarly in our SI-based approaches, presence or absence of a certain mutation is decided from the maximum among the estimated probabilities associated with all the ccRCC image slices in a particular kidney. Then we demonstrate the effectiveness of automatic feature learning compared to the hand-engineered features generation using the CNN approach. Afterwards, we show the effect of incorporating augmented data in the training dataset and compared the mutation detection performance for three different types of augmentation (i.e. image flipping+rotation, 3-ch re-ordering and those combined). Finally, we demonstrated the effectiveness of using multiple instance decisions aggregation in our proposed method.

In row 1 of the comparison Table 2, we show results of a traditional RF approach with hand-engineered image features shown to be effective in anatomy classification task [15]: histogram of oriented gradient, Haar features, and local binary patterns. Here, we did not augment any manually transformed data to the training samples. We trained four RFs for the four different mutation cases and as we see in Table 2, the resulting mean detection error was the highest (∼54%) among all contrasted methods. Row 2 shows the results of a deep CNN (namely, x-CNN, where x: VHL/PBRM1/SETD2/BAP1 (see Fig. 2)) approach with no data augmentation. Since the CNN learns the image features automatically, it may have helped this CNN method perform better (mean error ∼42%) than that of the hand-engineered features-based RF approach. Row 3 shows results for x-CNN, where we used data augmentation by deploying 3-ch data and re-ordering of channels (see Sect. 2.1). These data were fed to x-CNN and it can be seen how the SI-based mutation detection performance by this approach (mean error ∼29%) outperformed that with no data augmentation. Thus, including channels with different intensity ranges, mimicking the tumor intensity variation across patients, have shown positive impact on the mutation detection task. Row 4 shows results for x-CNN with a different augmentation process, which deploys the flipping and rotating of the 1-ch training samples. This approach (mean error ∼22%) outperformed that with 3-ch augmentation. So it is clear that the flipping+rotation-based augmentation introduced more variation in the training data than that by the 3-ch augmentation, resulting in better generalization of the model. In the method shown in row 5, we combined the flipping+rotation augmentation with the 3-ch re-ordering augmentation. The performance of the x-CNN with these data was better in mutation detection (mean error ∼14%) than that of flipping+rotation or 3-ch augmentation alone (see Table 2). Finally, row 6 demonstrates results of our proposed method, where flipping, rotation and 3-ch re-ordering augmentations were used. In addition, binary classification was performed based on the multiple instance decisions aggregation. We see in the Table 2 that the mean mutation detection error by our method is ∼6%, which is the lowest tested. In addition, detection errors for individual mutation cases were also low and in the range of 10%. Thus, our multiple instance decisions aggregation procedure made our CNN models more robust on SI-based miss-classification.

4   Conclusions

In this paper, we proposed a multiple instance decision aggregation-based deep CNN approach for automatic mutation detection in kidney ccRCC. We have shown how our approach automatically learned discriminating ccRCC features from CT images and aggregated the binary decisions on the mutation-presence/absence for all the ccRCC slices in a particular kidney sample. This aggregation produced a robust decision on the presence of a certain mutation in an interrogated kidney sample. In addition, our multiple instance decision aggregation approach achieved better accuracy in mutation detection than that of a typical single instance-based approach. On the other hand, better performance by conventional MIL approaches is subject to the availability of sufficient number of data, while in applications such as ours, there are usually very few data samples for some of the mutation cases. Therefore, an end-to-end MIL approach will most likely fail for those mutation cases with few data samples. However, this paper included a number of meaningful comparisons to highlight the effects of different augmentation, pooling schemes etc. within the context of insufficient data, which we believe provide more interesting findings and appears to be suitable for ccRCC Radiomics, where the learned mutations would aid in better ccRCC diagnosis, prognosis and treatment response assessment. Our experimental results demonstrated an approximately 94% accuracy in kidney-wise mutation detection.

References

1. Siegel, R.L., Miller, K.D., Jemal, A.: Cancer statistics, 2015. CA Cancer J. Clin. **65**(1), 5–29 (2015)
2. Ridge, C.A., Pua, B.B., Madoff, D.C.: Epidemiology and staging of renal cell carcinoma. Semin. Interv. Radiol. **31**, 3–8 (2014)
3. Lam, J.S., Shvarts, O., Leppert, J.T., Figlin, R.A., Belldegrun, A.S.: Renal cell carcinoma 2005: new frontiers in staging, prognostication and targeted molecular therapy. J. Urol. **173**(6), 1853–1862 (2005)
4. Shinagare, A.B., Vikram, R., Jaffe, C., Akin, O., Kirby, J.: Radiogenomics of clear cell renal cell carcinoma: preliminary findings of the cancer genome atlas-renal cell carcinoma (TCGA-RCC) imaging research group. Abdom. Imaging **40**(6), 1684–1692 (2015)
5. The Cancer Genome Atlas Research Network: Comprehensive molecular characterization of clear cell renal cell carcinoma. Nature **499**(7456), 43 (2013)
6. Guo, G., et al.: Frequent mutations of genes encoding ubiquitin-mediated proteolysis pathway components in clear cell renal cell carcinoma. Nat. Genet. **44**(1), 17 (2012)

 7. Gao, J., et al.: Integrative analysis of complex cancer genomics and clinical profiles using the cBioPortal. Sci. Signal. **6**(269) pl1 (2013)
 8. Karlo, C.A., Di Paolo, P.L., Chaim, J., Hakimi, A.A.: Radiogenomics of clear cell renal cell carcinoma: associations between CT imaging features and mutations. Radiology **270**(2), 464–471 (2014)
 9. Gillies, R.J., Kinahan, P.E., Hricak, H.: Radiomics: images are more than pictures, they are data. Radiology **278**(2), 563–577 (2015)
10. Aerts, H.J.: The potential of radiomic-based phenotyping in precision medicine: a review. JAMA Oncol. **2**(12), 1636–1642 (2016)
11. Dietterich, T.G., Lathrop, R.H., Lozano-Pérez, T.: Solving the multiple instance problem with axis-parallel rectangles. Artif. Intell. **89**(1–2), 31–71 (1997)
12. Clark, K.: The cancer imaging archive (TCIA): maintaining and operating a public information repository. J. Digit. Imaging **26**(6), 1045–1057 (2013)
13. Zeiler, M.D., Fergus, R.: Visualizing and understanding convolutional networks. In: Fleet, D., Pajdla, T., Schiele, B., Tuytelaars, T. (eds.) ECCV 2014. LNCS, vol. 8689, pp. 818–833. Springer, Cham (2014). https://doi.org/10.1007/978-3-319-10590-1_53
14. Kingma, D.P., Ba, J.: Adam: a method for stochastic optimization. arXiv preprint arXiv:1412.6980 (2014)
15. Wang, H., Moradi, M., Gur, Y., Prasanna, P., Syeda-Mahmood, T.: A multi-atlas approach to region of interest detection for medical image classification. In: Descoteaux, M., Maier-Hein, L., Franz, A., Jannin, P., Collins, D.L., Duchesne, S. (eds.) MICCAI 2017. LNCS, vol. 10435, pp. 168–176. Springer, Cham (2017). https://doi.org/10.1007/978-3-319-66179-7_20

Combining Convolutional and Recurrent Neural Networks for Classification of Focal Liver Lesions in Multi-phase CT Images

Dong Liang[1], Lanfen Lin[1(✉)], Hongjie Hu[2],
Qiaowei Zhang[2], Qingqing Chen[2], Yutaro Iwamoto[3],
Xianhua Han[3], and Yen-Wei Chen[1,3]

[1] Department of Computer Science and Technology,
Zhejiang University, Hangzhou, China
llf@zju.edu.cn
[2] Department of Radiology, Sir Run Run Shaw Hospital, Hangzhou, China
[3] College of Information Science and Engineering,
Ritsumeikan University, Kusatsu, Shiga, Japan

Abstract. Computer-aided diagnosis (CAD) systems are useful for assisting radiologists with clinical diagnoses by classifying focal liver lesions (FLLs) based on multi-phase computed tomography (CT) images. Although many studies have conducted in the field, there still remain two challenges. First, the temporal enhancement pattern is hard to represent effectively. Second, the local and global information of lesions both are necessary for this task. In this paper, we proposed a framework based on deep learning, called ResGL-BDLSTM, which combines a residual deep neural network (ResNet) with global and local pathways (ResGL Net) with a bi-directional long short-term memory (BD-LSTM) model for the task of focal liver lesions classification in multi-phase CT images. In addition, we proposed a novel loss function to train the proposed framework. The loss function is composed of an inter-loss and intra-loss, which can improve the robustness of the framework. The proposed framework outperforms state-of-the-art approaches by achieving a 90.93% mean accuracy.

Keywords: Deep learning · ResGLNet · BD-LSTM
Liver lesions classification · Computer-aid diagnosis (CAD) system

1 Introduction

Liver cancer is the second most common cause of cancer-related deaths worldwide among men, and the sixth among women [1]. Radiological examinations, such as computed tomography (CT) images and magnetic resonance images (MRI) are the primary methods of detecting liver tumors. Computer-aided diagnosis (CAD) systems play an important role in the early and accurate detection and classification of FLLs.

Currently, multi-phase CT images, which are also known as dynamic CT images, are widely used to detect, locate and diagnose focal liver lesions. Multi-phase CT scans are generally divided into four phases (i.e. non-contrast phase, arterial phase, portal phase, delay phase). Between the non-contrast phase and the delay phase, the vascularity and

© Springer Nature Switzerland AG 2018
A. F. Frangi et al. (Eds.): MICCAI 2018, LNCS 11071, pp. 666–675, 2018.
https://doi.org/10.1007/978-3-030-00934-2_74

the contrast agent enhancement patterns of the liver masses can be assessed. We observe that, when human experts diagnose the type of FLLs, they tend to zoom out the CT images to figure out the detail of lesions [2], and they also need to look back or forward in different phases. The observation interprets the importance of the combination of local with global information and the temporal enhancement pattern.

Some published studies have reported on the characterization of FLLs using multiphase images to capture the temporal information among phases. Roy et al. [3] proposed a framework to extract spatiotemporal features from multiphase CT volumes for the characterization of FLLs. In addition to conventional density features (the normalized average intensity of a lesion) and texture features (the gray-level co-occurrence matrix [GLCM]), temporal density and texture features (the intensity and texture enhancement over the three enhancement phases compared with the non-contrast phase), were employed. Compared with low-level features, the mid-level features such as bag-of-visual-words (BoVW) and its variants have proven to be considerably more effective for classifying FLLs [4–9]. In most of the BoVW-based methods, the histograms in each phase are separately extracted and then they are concatenated as a spatiotemporal feature [5, 8, 9] or the averaged histogram over multiple phases is used to represent the multi-phase images [4]. They ignore the temporal enhancement information and relationship among phases.

In recent years, the high-level feature representation of deep convolutional neural networks (DCNN) has proven to be superior to hand-crafted low-level features and mid-level features [10]. Deep learning techniques have also been applied to medical image analysis and computer-aided detection and diagnosis. However, there have been very few studies on the classification of focal liver lesions. Frid-Arar et al. [11] proposed a multi-scale patch-based classification framework to detect focal liver lesions. Yasaka et al. [12] proposed a convolutional neural network with three channels corresponding to three phases (NC, ART and DL) for the classification of liver tumors in dynamic contrast-enhanced CT images. The method can extract high-level temporal and spatial features, resulting in a higher classification accuracy compared with the state-of-the-art methods. The limitation is that it lacks information on image pattern enhancements.

In this paper, we propose a framework based on deep learning, called ResGL-BD-LSTM, which combines a residual network (ResNet) with global and local pathways (ResGLNet) [13] and a bi-directional long short-term memory (BD-LSTM) model for the classification of focal liver lesion. The main contributions are summarized as follows:

(1) We extract features from each single phase CT image via the ResGLNet. The input of the ResGLNet is a pair (patch and ROI) that represent the local and global information, respectively, to handle inter-class similarities.

(2) We extract an enhancement pattern, hidden in multi-phase CT images, via the BD-LSTM block, to represent each patch. To the best of our knowledge, expressing temporal features (enhancement patterns) among multiphase images using deep learning has not been investigated previously.

(3) We propose a new loss function to train our model, and provide a more robust and accurate deep model. The loss function is composed of an inter-loss and intra-loss. The inter-loss minimizes the inter-class variations and the intra-loss minimizes the intra-class variations, updating the center value using a back-propagation process.

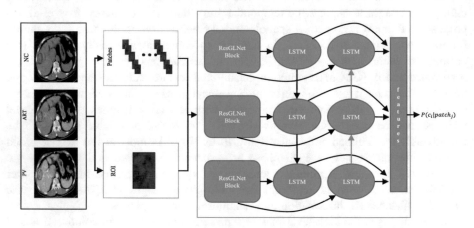

Fig. 1. The flowchart of our framework

2   Methodology

A flowchart of the proposed framework is shown in Fig. 1. The ResGLNet block, which extracts local and global information from each single phase, will be described in detail in Sect. 2.1. The BD-LSTM block, which extracts the enhancement pattern, will be described in detail in Sect. 2.2. The method combining the ResGLNet block and BD-LSTM block will be described in Sect. 2.3. We will introduce the loss function and training strategy of the framework in Sect. 2.4. In Sect. 2.5, we describe the features extracted from the label map, and how we accomplish the lesion-based classification.

2.1   ResGLNet

In this sub-section, we describe ResGLNet block, which was proposed in our previous work [13]. The ResGLNet involves a local pathway and global pathway. Intuitively, these extract local and global information, respectively. The employed ResGLNet is an extension of the ResNet proposed by [10]. We utilize three ResGLNet blocks, which each have the same architecture but do not share weights with each other, to extract the information of the three respective phases. In each ResNet block, we used 19 convolutional layers, one pooling layer (avg-pooling), and one fully connected layer. Each convolution layer was followed by a rectified linear unit (ReLU) activation function and a batch normalization layer.

Global Pathway. First, we apply a random walk-based interactive segmentation algorithm [14] to segment healthy tissue and focal liver lesions. The segmented results were checked by two experienced radiologists. The segmentation was performed for each phase image separately. During a clinical CT study, the spatial placement of tissues formed in multiple phases exhibits some aberration, owing to differences in a patient's body position, respiratory movements, and the heartbeat. Therefore, to obtain a factual variation of the density over phases, a non-rigid registration technique in order to localize a reference lesion in other phases [15]. Each segmented lesion image (i.e., 2D slice image) was resized to 128×128. The resized images were then used as input for global pathway training and testing.

Local Pathway. Patches were extracted from ROIs. Each patch has a label, $c \in \{c_0, c_1, c_2, c_3\}$ where c_0 represents a cyst, c_1 represents an focal nodular hyperplasia (FNH), c_2 represents an hepatocellular carcinoma (HCC) and c_3 represents an hemangioma (HEM). Owing to the different lesions varying significantly in size, extreme imbalances occur among the patch categories. To solve this problem, the pace value is derived in Eq. (1):

$$
pace_i = \begin{cases} floor\left(\sqrt{\frac{w_i * h_i}{\epsilon}}\right), & w_i * h_i > \epsilon \\ 1, & w_i * h_i \leq \epsilon \end{cases} \tag{1}
$$

where i represents the i-th ROI; $pace_i$ is the pace of i-th ROI for extracting the patches, w_i and h_i respectively represent the width and height of the i-th ROI, ϵ represents a threshold that can limit the number of patches, and the floor function represents rounding-down. For the testing dataset, we still set the pace to 1. As in the global pathway approach, we resized the patches to 64×64.

2.2 BD-LSTM

A recurrent neural network (RNN) can maintain self-connected status acting as a memory to remember previous information when it processes sequential data. Long-short term memory (LSTM) is a class of RNN that can avoid the vanishing gradient problem.

Bi-directional LSTM (BD-LSTM), which stacks two layers of LSTM, is an extension of LSTM. The two layers of LSTM, which are illustrated in Fig. 1, work in two opposite directions to extract useful information from sequential data. The enhancement information carried in the two layers of LSTM is concatenated as the output. One layer is in the z^--direction, and extracts the enhancement pattern from the NC phase through the PV phase and the other is in the z^+-direction and extracts the anti-enhancement pattern from the PV phase through the NC phase.

2.3   Combining ResGLNet and BD-LSTM

The motivation of performing focal liver lesions classification based on multi-phases CT images by combining ResGLNet and BD-LSTM is to employ multi-phases CT images as sequential data. The ResGLNet extracts the information (i.e., intra-phase information) based on a single phase. The BD-LSTM distills enhancement information (i.e., inter-phase information) among three phases, and the length of sequential data is a constant number (i.e., 3). The two blocks work in coordination, as follows.

The output of the three ResGLNet blocks, as a sequential data, constitutes the input of the BD-LSTM. Furthermore, the output of the two layers LSTM (i.e., BD-LSTM), representing patches, constitutes the input of the fully connected layer. The softmax layer following the last fully connected layer produces output that gives the result of the patch-based classification.

2.4   Training Strategy

Loss Function. Let N be the batch size and ω^t be the weights in the t-th ($t = 1, 2, \ldots T$) layer. We use W to denote the weights of the mainstream network (involving three ResGLNet blocks and a BD-LSTM block). We used $\widehat{W}_{local}$ and $\widehat{W}_{global}$ to represent the weights of the local and global pathways (involving three ResGLNet blocks, the same below), respectively. Furthermore, $p(j \mid x_i; W)$ represents the probability of the i-th patch belonging to the j-th class. We define $p\left(j \mid x_i; \widehat{W}_{global}\right)$ and $p\left(j \mid x_i; \widehat{W}_{local}\right)$ similarly. The definitions of cross-entropy are as follows:

$$\mathcal{L}_{last} = \frac{1}{N} \sum_{i=1}^{N} \sum_{c=1}^{K} -p(j \mid x_i; W) * \log(p(j \mid x_i; W)) \tag{2}$$

Thus, we can obtain the definition of $\mathcal{L}_{local}$ and $\mathcal{L}_{global}$ for the same reason. And the definition of the inter-loss that as follows:

$$\mathcal{L}_{inter} = \frac{1}{2} * \mathcal{L}_{last} + \frac{1}{4} * \mathcal{L}_{local} + \frac{1}{4} * \mathcal{L}_{global} \tag{3}$$

The definition of the intra-loss (i.e. center loss [16]) is as follows:

$$\mathcal{L}_{intra} = \frac{1}{2} \sum_{i=1}^{N} \|f_i - c_{y_i}\|^2 \tag{4}$$

Here f_i is the representation feature of the i-th patch and c_{y_i} denotes the y_i-th class center of features. In the course of training c_{y_i} should be updated using the process of back-propagation. To accelerate our training, we conduct the update operation based on each batch, instead of basing it on the entire training set. Note that, in this case, some of the centers may not change. The method employed to update the centers is described as follows:

$$
\begin{aligned}
c_j = c_j - \Delta c_j &= c_j - \frac{\partial \mathcal{L}}{\partial c_j} \\
&= c_j - \alpha * \frac{\sum_{i=1}^{N} \delta(y_i == j)(f_i - c_j)}{1 + \sum_{i=1}^{N} \delta(y_i == j)}
\end{aligned}
\tag{5}
$$

Here $\delta(y_i == j) = 1$ if the $y_i == j$ holds, and $\delta(y_i == j) = 0$ otherwise. Furthermore, α can restrict the learning rate of the centers, where the range of α is $(0, 1)$.

Finally, we adopt a joint loss that combines the intra-loss and inter-loss to train the frameworks. The formulation of the optimized loss is given in Eq. 6.

$$
\mathcal{L} = \mathcal{L}_{inter} + \lambda \mathcal{L}_{intra}
\tag{6}
$$

Training Process. Our framework is split into two phases. The first is the training phase, and the second is the testing phase. During training, we first trained the part of our framework that involves the deep learning components and then aggregated the label maps. The effectiveness of the patches from the validation dataset determines when the training stop. We aggregated the label maps belonging to the training and validation datasets after the model was trained. Next, we used the training and validation label maps as input to the support vector machine (SVM) classifier. Then, we also determined the parameters of the SVM (classifier of lesions) using the effectiveness of label map of the validation dataset.

2.5   Post-processing of Label Map and Classification of Lesions

After training, we aggregated the label map of each lesion. Then, we extracted features from the label map. The features are as follows:

$$
feature_i = \{\beta_{i0}, \beta_{i1}, \beta_{i2}, \beta_{i3}\}
\tag{7}
$$

Here $feature_i$ represents the feature vector of i-th label map, and β_{ij}, is derived in Eq. (8), denotes the proportion of pixels belonging to the j-th category of in the i-th label map. Then we use the SVM to achieve lesion-based classification.

$$
\beta_{ij} = \frac{the \; number \; of \; pixels \; belong \; to \; jth \; category}{the \; total \; pixels \; in \; ith \; label \; map}
\tag{8}
$$

3 Experiments

3.1 Data and Implementation

A total of 480 CT liver slice images were used, containing four types of lesions confirmed by pathologists, (i.e., Cyst, HEM, FNH, and HCC). The distribution of our dataset is shown in Table 1. The CT images in our dataset are abdominal CT scans taken from 2015 through 2017. The CT scans were acquired with a slice collimation of 5–7 mm, a matrix of 512×512 pixels, and an in-plane resolution of $0.57 - 0.89$. In our experiment, we randomly split our dataset into a training dataset, a validation dataset, and a testing dataset. In order to eliminate the effect of randomness, we conduct the partition operation twice, and form two groups of dataset.

Table 1. The distribution of database.

Type	Cyst		FNH		HCC		HEM	
	Set1	Set2	Set1	Set2	Set1	Set2	Set1	Set2
Training	61	69	71	60	75	69	62	79
Validation	23	17	25	23	31	36	36	17
Testing	26	24	18	31	26	27	26	28
Total	110		114		132		124	

Our framework was implemented using the Tensorflow library. We initialized the parameters via the Gaussian distribution. We used a momentum optimizer to update our parameters by setting the learning rate initialized as 0.01 and the momentum coefficient to 0.9. We set the batch size as 100. The parameters for our algorithm were $\lambda = 0.1$, $\alpha = 0.2$, $\epsilon = 128$, and *patch size* = 7.

3.2 Results

In order to validate the effectiveness of or proposed methods. We compared our results with the state-of-art methods with low-level features [2], mid-level features [4–8] and CNN with local information [10] and global information [11]. We also compared our proposed methods with different architectures: ResNet with local patch (w/o intra-loss), ResGLNet [13], ResGL-BDLSTM (w/o intra-loss), and ResGL-BDLSTM (with intra-loss). The comparison results (classification accuracy) are summarized in Table 2. It can be seen that our proposed methods outperformed the state-of-the-art methods [3, 5–9, 11, 12]. The ResNet with local and global pathways outperformed the ResNet with local patch only. The classification accuracy was significantly improved by adding the BD-LSTM model, as well as the intra-loss.

Table 2. Comparison results (classification accuracy (%) is represented as mean and standard deviation)

Method	Cyst	FNH	HCC	HEM	Total Accuracy
Roy et al. [3]	97.81 ± 3.1	77.27 ± 6.43	58.83 ± 2.39	56.41 ± 14.5	71.84 ± 0.04
Yang et al. [5]	88.30 ± 10.6	74.64 ± 28.1	75.50 ± 2.0	81.32 ± 6.2	78.81 ± 3.4
Wang et al. [8]	85.90 ± 3.6	65.14 ± 32.8	83.12 ± 7.5	67.99 ± 20.0	74.06 ± 5.7
Xu et al. [9]	68.75 ± 2.9	73.53 ± 4.1	87.25 ± 1.3	76.92 ± 10.8	77.04 ± 3.1
Diamant et al. [6]	82.21 ± 7.4	70.00 ± 18.8	85.04 ± 10.2	76.90 ± 20.3	77.82 ± 1.2
Xu et al. [7]	92.15 ± 5.21	69.08 ± 20.1	85.04 ± 10.2	84.31 ± 0.4	82.11 ± 7.4
Frid-Adar et al. [11] (CNN with local)	100.0 ± 0.0	78.20 ± 0.5	84.37 ± 16.6	40.67 ± 16.2	76.16 ± 0.6
Yasaka et al. [12] (CNN with global)	97.92 ± 2.9	82.26 ± 25.1	86.82 ± 2.32	85.16 ± 0.7	87.26 ± 7.7
ResNet_Local	100.0 ± 0.0	71.27 ± 6.5	80.89 ± 11.18	85.41 ± 8.8	84.12 ± 6.1
ResGLNet [13]	97.92 ± 2.9	81.99 ± 5.9	85.11 ± 15.6	85.42 ± 2.9	88.05 ± 4.8
ResGL-BDLSTM (without intra-loss)	98.08 ± 2.2	90.19 ± 8.9	88.74 ± 5.0	81.25 ± 8.8	89.77 ± 3.59
ResGL-BDLSTM	100.0 ± 0.0	86.74 ± 4.1	88.82 ± 10.3	87.75 ± 5.5	90.93 ± 0.7

4 Conclusions

In this paper, we proposed a method using combined residual local and global path-ways and bi-directional long short-term memory (ResGL-BDLSTM), to tackle the classification of focal liver lesions. The ResGLNet extracts the most representative features from each single phase CT image, and the BD-LSTM helps to extract the enhancement patterns in multi-phases CT images. The experimental results demonstrated that our framework outperforms other state-of-the-art methods. In the future work, we are going to build a large scale liver lesions dataset and to construct an end-to-end framework that achieves lesion-based classification via one model. We believe that our proposed framework can be applied to other contrast-enhanced multi-phases CT images.

Acknowledgements. This work was supported in part by the National Key R&D Program of China under the Grant No. 2017YFB0309800, in part by the Key Science and Technology Innovation Support Program of Hangzhou under the Grant No. 20172011A038, and in part by the Grant-in Aid for Scientific Research from the Japanese Ministry for Education, Science, Culture and Sports (MEXT) under the Grant No. 18H03267 and No. 17H00754.

References

1. Ryerson, A.B., et al.: Annual report to the nation on the status of cancer, 1975–2012, featuring the increasing incidence of liver cancer. Cancer **122**(9), 1312–1337 (2016)
2. Chen, J., et al.: Combining fully convolutional and recurrent neural networks for 3D biomedical image segmentation. In: Advances in Neural Information Processing Systems (2016)
3. Roy, S., et al.: Three-dimensional spatiotemporal features for fast content-based retrieval of focal liver lesions. IEEE Trans. Biomed. Eng. **61**(11), 2768–2778 (2014)
4. Yu, M., et al.: Extraction of lesion-partitioned features and retrieval of contrast-enhanced liver images. Comput. Math. Meth. Med. **2012**, 12 (2012)
5. Yang, W., et al.: Content-based retrieval of focal liver lesions using bag-of-visual-words representations of single-and multiphase contrast-enhanced CT images. J. Digital Imaging **25**(6), 708–719 (2012)
6. Diamant, I., et al.: Improved patch-based automated liver lesion classification by separate analysis of the interior and boundary regions. IEEE J. Biomed. Health Inform. **20**(6), 1585–1594 (2016)
7. Xu, Y., et al.: Bag of temporal co-occurrence words for retrieval of focal liver lesions using 3D multiphase contrast-enhanced CT images. In: Proceedings of 23rd International Conference on Pattern Recognition (ICPR 2016), pp. 2283–2288 (2016)
8. Wang J., et al.: Sparse codebook model of local structures for retrieval of focal liver lesions using multiphase medical images. Int. J. Biomed. Imaging **2017**, 13 p. (2017)
9. Xu, Y., et al.: Texture-specific bag of visual words model and spatial cone matching-based method for the retrieval of focal liver lesions using multiphase contrast-enhanced CT images. Int. J. Comput. Assist. Radiol. Surg. **13**(1), 151–164 (2018)
10. He, K., et al.: Deep residual learning for image recognition. In: Proceedings of the IEEE Conference on Computer Vision and Pattern Recognition (2016)
11. Frid-Adar, M., Diamant, I., Klang, E., Amitai, M., Goldberger, J., Greenspan, H.: Modeling the intra-class variability for liver lesion detection using a multi-class patch-based CNN. In: Wu, G., Munsell, Brent C., Zhan, Y., Bai, W., Sanroma, G., Coupé, P. (eds.) Patch-MI 2017. LNCS, vol. 10530, pp. 129–137. Springer, Cham (2017). https://doi.org/10.1007/978-3-319-67434-6_15
12. Yasaka, K., et al.: Deep learning with convolutional neural network for differentiation of liver masses at dynamic contrast-enhanced CT: a preliminary study. Radiology **286**(3), 887–896 (2017)
13. Liang, D., et al.: Residual convolutional neural networks with global and local pathways for classification of focal liver lesions. In: Geng, X., Kang, B.H. (eds.) PRICAI 2018: Trends in Artificial Intelligence. PRICAI 2018. LNCS, vol. 11012, pp. 617–628. Springer, Cham (2018). https://doi.org/10.1007/978-3-319-97304-3_47

14. Dong, C., et al.: Simultaneous segmentation of multiple organs using random walks. J. Inf. Process. **24**(2), 320–329 (2016)
15. Dong, C., et al.: Non-rigid image registration with anatomical structure constraint for assessing locoregional therapy of hepatocellular carcinoma. Comput. Med. Imaging Graph. **45**, 75–83 (2015)
16. Wen, Y., Zhang, K., Li, Z., Qiao, Yu.: A discriminative feature learning approach for deep face recognition. In: Leibe, B., Matas, J., Sebe, N., Welling, M. (eds.) ECCV 2016. LNCS, vol. 9911, pp. 499–515. Springer, Cham (2016). https://doi.org/10.1007/978-3-319-46478-7_31

Construction of a Spatiotemporal Statistical Shape Model of Pediatric Liver from Cross-Sectional Data

Atsushi Saito[1]([✉]) [iD], Koyo Nakayama[1] [iD], Antonio R. Porras[2] [iD],
Awais Mansoor[2] [iD], Elijah Biggs[2], Marius George Linguraru[2,3] [iD],
and Akinobu Shimizu[1] [iD]

[1] Tokyo University of Agriculture and Technology, Tokyo, Japan
a-saito@go.tuat.ac.jp
[2] Sheikh Zayed Institute for Pediatric Surgical Innovation,
Children's National Health System, Washington, D.C., USA
[3] School of Medicine and Health Sciences, George Washington University,
Washington, D.C., USA

Abstract. This paper proposes a spatiotemporal statistical shape model of a pediatric liver, which has potential applications in computer-aided diagnosis of the abdomen. Shapes are analyzed in the space of a level set function, which has computational advantages over the diffeomorphic framework commonly employed in conventional studies. We first calculate the time-varying average of the mean shape development using a kernel regression technique with adaptive bandwidth. Then, eigenshape modes for every timepoint are calculated using principal component analysis with an additional regularization term that ensures the smoothness of the temporal change of the eigenshape modes. To further improve the performance, we applied data augmentation using a level set-based nonlinear morphing technique. The proposed algorithm was evaluated in the context of a spatiotemporal statistical shape modeling of a liver using 42 manually segmented livers from children whose age ranged from approximately 2 weeks to 95 months. Our method achieved a higher generalization and specificity ability compared with conventional methods.

Keywords: Spatiotemporal analysis · Statistical shape model
Pediatric · Liver

1 Introduction

Statistical shape models (SSMs) [1] of abdominal organs have played important roles in computer-aided diagnosis applications, including image segmentation and assessment of the degree of abnormality. Despite considerable research on SSMs for adult organs, infant abdominal organs have not been extensively investigated. The limitation of conventional SSMs is that intersubject variability is not separated from the age-related shape variation that is not negligible in pediatric datasets. Therefore, we propose a method to construct a spatiotemporal

© Springer Nature Switzerland AG 2018
A. F. Frangi et al. (Eds.): MICCAI 2018, LNCS 11071, pp. 676–683, 2018.
https://doi.org/10.1007/978-3-030-00934-2_75

SSM, or temporally varying SSM, which we refer to as stSSM, that reflects both the intersubject and temporal sources of variation.

Over the last decade, there has been considerable research on spatiotemporal shape and image analysis [2–8]. Its main objective is longitudinal atlas construction that represents the trend of anatomical changes of the population. One of the most successful approaches is the kernel regression-based technique. Davis et al. [2] performed kernel regression on the Riemannian manifold of diffeomorphisms. Serag et al. [3] improved the kernel regression method using adaptive bandwidth selection to deal with non-uniformly distributed ages. Another approach is to utilize subject-specific longitudinal information (i.e., same subject taken at different timepoints) using the spatiotemporal atlas construction process as described by Durrlemann et al. [4], which would be the better choice if longitudinal data is available.

Analysis of intersubject shape variability is also required for stSSM, which can be even more challenging as intersubject change is also a function of time that has not been addressed in [2–4]. An early study dealing with stSSM is found in [5], where principal component analysis (PCA) was first applied to all samples, and then correlation analysis was performed to find the mode best describing the temporal change. Qiu et al. [6] performed a subject-wise analysis by registering all images to a common reference frame under the assumption that the individual change of a specific point of time can be propagated by a parallel transportation method [9]. Kishimoto et al. [7] developed a spatiotemporal statistical model of the anatomical landmarks of human embryos, where group-wise PCA was first applied to build the statistical models of each developmental stage. These statistical models were then smoothly interpolated between neighboring stages to define a continuous subspace. Similarly, Alam et al. [8] employed subject-weighted PCA instead of group-wise PCA to construct a neonatal brain shape model. The main weakness of these methods [7,8] is that independent PCA does not ensure the consistency of the principal modes of shape variation among different timepoints.

In this paper, we propose a novel stSSM construction method for the pediatric liver based on level set shape representation. The key contributions of this paper are summarized below:

1. While most related studies depend on diffeomorphic registration technique [2–6], we employ a level set-based shape representation that can be analyzed without registration and can intrinsically deal with topological changes.
2. We use kernel regression with adaptive bandwidth to compute the average and covariance matrices at given timepoints, which can be seen as a generalization of the method by [8]. We employ an adaptive bandwidth method to overcome inhomogeneous distributions due to patient age.
3. The principal modes of shape variation are calculated by PCA with an additional regularization term to ensure the temporal consistency of the principal modes that is not considered in conventional studies [7,8].
4. We use nonlinear shape interpolation based on level set morphing for data augmentation [10,11].

5. The effectiveness of the proposed method is quantitatively verified based on generalization, specificity [12], and the smoothness of the shape evolution.

We note that level set is just one example of shape representation method we employed to demonstrate the concept of our spatiotemporal SSM. In principle, our statistical analysis method is applicable to other shape representations such as point distribution model and diffeomorphism-based model [2–6].

2   Methods

Let us denote a set of n training data as $\{(S_i, t_i)\}_{i \in \{1,...,n\}}$ where $S_i \subset \Omega$ ($i \in \{1,...,n\}$) is the i-th training shape in the m-dimensional image domain $\Omega \subset \mathbb{R}^m$ and $t_i \in [t_{min}, t_{max}]$ is the associated patient age ranging between t_{min} and t_{max}. In order to provide a linear operation between shapes, they are represented as the zero sublevel set of the function: $\phi_i : \boldsymbol{r} \in \Omega \mapsto \mathbb{R}$ that satisfies:

$$S_i = \{\boldsymbol{r} \in \Omega | \phi_i(\boldsymbol{r}) < 0\}. \tag{1}$$

Specifically, ϕ_i is the signed distance function of S_i in this study. Sampling ϕ_i on every grid point in an image domain $\{\boldsymbol{r}_1, \boldsymbol{r}_2, \ldots, \boldsymbol{r}_p\} \in \Omega$ yields the p-dimensional shape representation vector $\boldsymbol{\phi}_i$:

$$\boldsymbol{\phi}_i = [\phi_i(\boldsymbol{r}_1), \phi_i(\boldsymbol{r}_2), \ldots, \phi_i(\boldsymbol{r}_p)]^\mathsf{T}. \tag{2}$$

For the sake of computational efficiency, instead of $\boldsymbol{\phi}_i$, we use a compact representation of the level set function: $\boldsymbol{x}_i \approx P^\mathsf{T}(\boldsymbol{\phi}_i - \overline{\boldsymbol{\phi}}) \in \mathbb{R}^q$ in the following process, where: $\overline{\boldsymbol{\phi}} = \sum_{i=1}^n \boldsymbol{\phi}_i$ is the mean and $P \in \mathbb{R}^{p \times q}$ is the matrix with q ($\leq n-1$) eigenmodes of the shape variation derived from spatially-weighted PCA [13].

The goal of stSSM is to decompose the shape variation into temporal and individual modes. To this end, inspired by [4], we assume that each shape $\boldsymbol{x}_i$ is an instance of a random process:

$$\boldsymbol{x}_i = \boldsymbol{X}(\boldsymbol{\alpha}_i; t_i) + \boldsymbol{\epsilon}_i, \tag{3}$$

where $\boldsymbol{X}(\boldsymbol{\alpha}; t)$ is a time-dependent shape model with the subject-specific shape parameter: $\boldsymbol{\alpha} = [\alpha_1, \ldots, \alpha_d]^\mathsf{T}$, and $\boldsymbol{\epsilon}_i$ is a Gaussian random noise i.i.d. over $\boldsymbol{\alpha}$ and t. In this study, we consider a linear model:

$$\boldsymbol{X}(\boldsymbol{\alpha}; t) = \boldsymbol{\mu}(t) + \sum_{j=1}^d \boldsymbol{v}_j(t)\sigma_j(t)\alpha_j, \tag{4}$$

where $\boldsymbol{\mu}(t) \in \mathbb{R}^q$, $\boldsymbol{v}_j(t) \in \mathbb{R}^q$ and $\sigma_j(t) \in \mathbb{R}$ are the mean, eigenmode and standard deviation of the j-th ($j \in \{1, \ldots, d\}$) principal mode of the shape variation at time point t, respectively.

We estimate the spatiotemporal trajectory $\boldsymbol{\mu}(t)$ via the Nadaraya-Watson kernel regression method [14], where we employ an adaptive-kernel width strategy in order to achieve stability against an inhomogeneous distribution of the patient age. Instead of the time-varying kernel width used in [3], we employ a subject-wise kernel width inspired by [15] in order to make it differentiable with respect to time (which is required to calculate the tangent of $\boldsymbol{\mu}(t)$, cf. Eq.(6)):

$$\boldsymbol{\mu}(t) = \sum_{i=1}^{n} w_i(t)\boldsymbol{x}_i, \text{ where } w_i(t) = \frac{\frac{1}{\lambda_i}k\left(\frac{t_i-t}{\lambda_i h}\right)}{\sum_{i=1}^{n}\frac{1}{\lambda_i}k\left(\frac{t_i-t}{\lambda_i h}\right)}, \tag{5}$$

where $k(y) = \frac{1}{\sqrt{2\pi}}\exp\left(-\frac{y^2}{2}\right)$ is the Gaussian kernel function and $h > 0$ is a global bandwidth parameter. The bandwidth is adaptively changed by a subject-specific factor $\lambda_i > 0$, which is calculated as: $\lambda_i = \left\{\tilde{f}(t_i)/\sum_{i=1}^{n}\tilde{f}(t_i)\right\}^{-\beta}$, where $\tilde{f}(t) = \frac{1}{nh}\sum_{i=1}^{n}k\left(\frac{t_i-t}{h}\right)$ is a prior kernel estimator with a fixed bandwidth h. The coefficient $\beta \in [0,1]$ is the sensitivity parameter and we used $\beta = 0.5$, which has been reported to achieve good results [15]. The derivative of $\boldsymbol{\mu}(t)$ with respect to time is given as: $\dot{\boldsymbol{\mu}}(t) = \dot{w}_i(t)\boldsymbol{x}_j$ where

$$\dot{w}_i(t) = \frac{\frac{1}{\lambda_i}k'\left(\frac{t_i-t}{\lambda_i h}\right)\left\{\sum_{i=1}^{n}\frac{1}{\lambda_i}k\left(\frac{t_i-t}{\lambda_i h}\right)\right\} - k\left(\frac{t_i-t}{\lambda_i h}\right)\left\{\sum_{i=1}^{n}\frac{1}{\lambda_i^2}k'\left(\frac{t_i-t}{\lambda_i h}\right)\right\}}{\lambda_i h\left\{\sum_{i=1}^{n}\frac{1}{\lambda_i}k\left(\frac{t_i-t}{\lambda_i h}\right)\right\}^2}, \tag{6}$$

which will be used as the 0-th principal component (see Sect. 2.1).

Owing to the fact that kernel regression demonstrates some estimation difficulty for timepoints around the boundary of range $[t_{min}, t_{max}]$, this is generally referred to as a boundary problem. Hence, we assume that our model supports the range of $T = [t_{min} + h, t_{max} - h]$.

2.1 PCA with Temporal Regularization

After the average trajectory is obtained, the kernel weighted covariance matrix at time point t is computed as:

$$C(t) = \frac{\sum_{i=1}^{n} w_i(t)(\boldsymbol{x}_i - \boldsymbol{\mu}(t))(\boldsymbol{x}_i - \boldsymbol{\mu}(t))^\mathsf{T}}{1 - \sum_{i=1}^{n} w_i(t)^2}. \tag{7}$$

We then propose an objective function of PCA with temporal regularization. The j-th time-dependent principal mode $\boldsymbol{v}_j$ for $j \geq 1$ is calculated as:

$$\boldsymbol{v}_j = \arg\max_{\boldsymbol{u}} \int_T \left\{\boldsymbol{u}(t)^\mathsf{T} C(t)\boldsymbol{u}(t) - \gamma \|\dot{\boldsymbol{u}}(t)\|_2^2\right\} dt$$

$$\text{s.t.} \quad \boldsymbol{u}(t)^\mathsf{T}\boldsymbol{u}(t) = 1, \ \boldsymbol{u}(t)^\mathsf{T}\boldsymbol{v}_l(t) = 0 \quad \forall l \in \{0, \ldots, j-1\}, \forall t \in T, \tag{8}$$

where we assume that the direction of the 0-th principal mode is the tangent of the average trajectory, i.e., $\boldsymbol{v}_0(t) = \dot{\boldsymbol{\mu}}(t)/\|\dot{\boldsymbol{\mu}}(t)\|$. When $\gamma = 0$, this is equivalent to applying sample weighted PCA for each point of time independently. The calculation of the unit vector $\boldsymbol{u}(t)$ that maximizes $\boldsymbol{u}(t)^\mathsf{T} C(t)\boldsymbol{u}(t)$ is equivalent to the objective of PCA. The second term evaluates the squared magnitude of the first derivative of the coordinate change, which imposes the temporal smoothness of the coordinate change.

Given that $u(t)$ is a unit vector, the second term is approximated as $\|\dot{u}(t)\|_2^2 \approx \frac{2}{\Delta t^2}(1 - u(t)^{\mathsf{T}}u(t + \Delta t))$ with a sufficiently small interval Δt. Therefore, given regularly-sampled time points $\mathcal{T} = \{\tau_k\}_{k=1}^m \subset T$ with interval $\Delta t = \frac{t_{max} - t_{min}}{m-1}$, Eq. (8) can be reformulated as:

$$(v_j(\tau_1), \ldots, v_j(\tau_m)) = \arg\max_u \left\{ \sum_{k=1}^m u(\tau_k)^{\mathsf{T}}C(\tau_k)u(\tau_k) + \gamma' \sum_{k=1}^{m-1} u(\tau_k)^{\mathsf{T}}u(\tau_{k+1}) \right\}$$

$$\text{s.t.}\quad u(t)^{\mathsf{T}}u(t) = 1,\ u(t)^{\mathsf{T}}v_l(t) = 0\ \forall l \in \{0, \ldots, j-1\},\ \forall t \in \mathcal{T}. \tag{9}$$

where $\gamma' = \frac{2}{\Delta t^2}\gamma$. This type of problem is known to be a non-convex quadratically-constrained quadratic program (QCQP). To minimize the risk of getting trapped in local minima, we initialize $\{v_1, \ldots, v_d\}$ with the optimal solution for $\gamma' = 0$, which can be calculated by pure PCA. Then, the optimal solution is obtained via an internal point algorithm [16] implemented in MATLAB Optimization Toolbox. Finally, the standard deviation along the j-th axis at the k-th time point is calculated in analogy with standard PCA:

$$\sigma_j(\tau_k) = \sqrt{v_j(\tau_k)^{\mathsf{T}}C(\tau_k)v_j(\tau_k)}. \tag{10}$$

2.2 Data Augmentation

To overcome the shortage of training data, data augmentation was performed based on level set morphing [10], which is a nonlinear morphing technique and was successfully applied to improve the performance of SSM for abdominal organs [11]. Level set morphing is applied to the pairs of cases (S_i, S_j) whose age difference $|t_i - t_j|$ is 1–2 years. A sequence of three intermediate shapes with equal surface distance is generated for each pair of shapes. Patient ages for the intermediate shapes are given by linear interpolation.

3 Experiments

We collected 42 healthy CT volumes from children aged 2 weeks to 95 months with manual annotations of the liver. The image size was: $512 \times 512 \times (109 - 747)$ voxels and the resolution was: $(0.291 - 0.625) \times (0.291 - 0.625) \times (0.625 - 3.000)$ mm^3. The patient age in days ranged from $t_{min} = 16$ to $t_{max} = 2912$. The global kernel width and the regularization parameter were empirically determined and set as $h = 300$ [days] and $\gamma = 2 \times 10^5$, respectively. In order to validate the study, 42 cases were separated into two groups: G_{in} and G_{out}, which are 34 and 8 cases inside and outside the age range supported by the kernel regression $T = [t_{min} + h, t_{max} - h]$, respectively. The group G_{out} was used for training purposes only during the two-fold cross validation study on G_{in}. Prior to statistical shape analysis, spatial standardization with rigid transformation was performed based on four manual landmarks on the bone, i.e., the spinous processes of the 8th and 10th vertebrae, and the left and right 8th rib tips. The image size after

Table 1. Comparison of the generalization and the specificity measures between three SSMs. Brackets indicate the statistical significance ($**: p < 0.01$, $*: p < 0.05$).

Method	Generalization	Specificity
stSSM	**0.7741**	**0.7755**
stSSM ($\gamma = 0$)	0.7647	0.7759
SSM	0.7579	0.7495

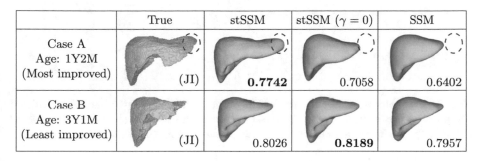

	True	stSSM	stSSM ($\gamma = 0$)	SSM
Case A Age: 1Y2M (Most improved)	(JI)	**0.7742**	0.7058	0.6402
Case B Age: 3Y1M (Least improved)	(JI)	0.8026	**0.8189**	0.7957

Fig. 1. Comparison of the shape reconstruction ability between different SSMs. The cases A and B are the most-improved and least-improved cases in terms of the reconstruction ability by use of the regularization term, respectively.

standardization was $256 \times 256 \times 256$ voxels with 1.0 mm isotropic voxel size. The number of modes q was set to achieve at least 90% of the cumulative contribution ratio (CCR), and the number of modes for the time-dependent principal modes was fixed to $d = 2$ for which CCR was around 80%. The performance of the model was evaluated using generalization and specificity, which assess the ability of the model to reconstruct unknown shapes and to generate acceptable instances, respectively, where Jaccard index (JI) was used for the similarity measure.

Table 1 summarizes the performance indices obtained by the three models in the cross validation study. The proposed stSSM achieved the best generalization with a statistically significant difference when compared to the other models. In summary, our stSSM performed the best out of the three models.

Figure 1 displays the comparison of the reconstructed liver surface between different models focusing on two cases, the most improved and the least improved cases in JI by use of the proposed stSSM compared with the case without a regularization term ($\gamma = 0$), respectively. Case A showed a large improvement ($+6.8$ pt; $0.7058 \rightarrow 0.7742$) with a large difference around the left lobe of the liver (see the red circle in Fig. 1). Even for the worst case B, the drop in JI was relatively small (-1.6 pt; $0.8189 \rightarrow 0.8026$) and had a less visual difference between the constructed surfaces. We also found that the reconstruction ability of the conventional SSM was consistently lower. These findings are consistent with the generalization value in Table 1.

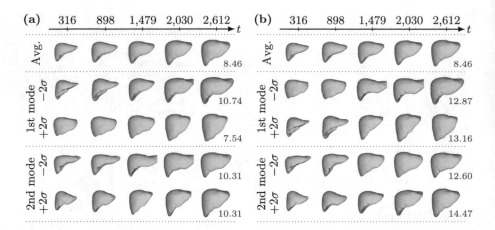

Fig. 2. Liver shapes generated form (a) the proposed stSSM and (b) the stSSM without temporal regularization ($\gamma = 0$). The red numerals on each row show the accumulated value of the surface distance in [mm] between the neighboring time points.

Shapes generated by stSSM with and without temporal regularization are shown in Fig. 2(a) and (b), respectively. Since we expect that changes along time t for the fixed shape parameter α represent the shape development for the specific patient, the shape deformation displayed in each row should be smooth. We measured and displayed in Fig. 2 the smoothness of temporal change by accumulating the surface distance between neighboring time points for each row (shape parameters). We found that our stSSM showed a consistently lower value in accumulated surface distance, which suggests the applicability of our SSM to predict shape development for unknown subjects.

4   Conclusion

In this paper, we proposed a method to construct an stSSM of a pediatric liver. The temporal change of the average shape is calculated using kernel regression with an adaptive bandwidth, and the time-dependent shape variation is learned using PCA with a regularization term to improve the temporal consistency of the temporal variation. The proposed model achieved a generalization of 0.7741 and specificity of 0.7755, which are superior to the stSSM without temporal regularization and the non-spatiotemporal SSM.

In the future, we will collect more samples including longitudinal data for further improvement and evaluation of the performance of stSSM. We also plan to develop computer-aided diagnosis applications including automated organ segmentation and assessment of the degree of abnormality for pediatrics.

Acknowledgments. This work is partly supported by KAKENHI (No. 26108002, 16H06785 and 18H03255) and the Sheikh Zayed Institute at Children's National Health System.

References

1. Heimann, T., Meinzer, H.P.: Statistical shape models for 3D medical image segmentation: a review. Med. Image Anal. **13**(4), 543–563 (2009)
2. Davis, B.C., Fletcher, P.T., Bullitt, E., Joshi, S.: Population shape regression from random design data. Int. J. Comput. Vis. **90**(2), 255–266 (2010)
3. Serag, A., et al.: Construction of a consistent highdefinition spatio-temporal atlas of the developing brain using adaptive kernel regression. Neuroimage **59**(3), 2255–2265 (2012)
4. Durrleman, S., Pennec, X., Trouvé, A., Braga, J., Gerig, G., Ayache, N.: Toward a comprehensive framework for the spatiotemporal statistical analysis of longitudinal shape data. Int. J. Comput. Vis. **103**(1), 22–59 (2013)
5. Mansi, T., et al.: A statistical model of right ventricle in tetralogy of fallot for prediction of remodelling and therapy planning. In: Yang, G.-Z., Hawkes, D., Rueckert, D., Noble, A., Taylor, C. (eds.) MICCAI 2009. LNCS, vol. 5761, pp. 214–221. Springer, Heidelberg (2009). https://doi.org/10.1007/978-3-642-04268-3_27
6. Qiu, A., Albert, M., Younes, L., Miller, M.I.: Time sequence diffeomorphic metric mapping and parallel transport track time-dependent shape changes. Neuroimage **45**(1), S51–S60 (2009)
7. Kishimoto, M., et al.: A spatiotemporal statistical model for eyeballs of human embryos. IEICE Trans. Inf. Syst. **100**(7), 1505–1515 (2017)
8. Alam, S., Kobashi, S., Nakano, R., Morimoto, M., Aikawa1, S., Shimizu, A.: Spatiotemporal statistical shape model construction for longitudinal brain deformation analysis using weighted PCA. In: Computer Assisted Radiology and Surgery (CARS) 2016, vol. 11, p. S204 (2016)
9. Younes, L.: Jacobi fields in groups of diffeomorphisms and applications. Q. Appl. Math. **65**(1), 113–134 (2007)
10. Breen, D.E., Whitaker, R.T.: A level-set approach for the metamorphosis of solid models. IEEE Trans. Vis. Comput. Graph. **7**(2), 173–192 (2001)
11. Saito, A., Nakada, M., Oost, E., Shimizu, A., Watanabe, H., Nawano, S.: A statistical shape model for multiple organs based on synthesized-based learning. In: Yoshida, H., Warfield, S., Vannier, M.W. (eds.) ABD-MICCAI 2013. LNCS, vol. 8198, pp. 280–289. Springer, Heidelberg (2013). https://doi.org/10.1007/978-3-642-41083-3_31
12. Styner, M.A.: Evaluation of 3D correspondence methods for model building. In: Taylor, C., Noble, J.A. (eds.) IPMI 2003. LNCS, vol. 2732, pp. 63–75. Springer, Heidelberg (2003). https://doi.org/10.1007/978-3-540-45087-0_6
13. Uchida, Y., Shimizu, A., Kobatake, H., Nawano, S., Shinozaki, K.: A comparative study of statistical shape models of the pancreas. In: Computer Assisted Radiology and Surgery (CARS) 2010, vol. 5, pp. S385–S387 (2010)
14. Nadaraya, E.A.: On estimating regression. Theory Probab. Appl. **9**(1), 141–142 (1964)
15. Demir, S., Toktamiş, Ö.: On the adaptive Nadaraya-Watson kernel regression estimators. Hacet. J. Math. Stat. **39**(3), 429–437 (2010)
16. Byrd, R.H., Gilbert, J.C., Nocedal, J.: A trust region method based on interior point techniques for nonlinear programming. Math. Program. **89**(1), 149–185 (2000)

Deep 3D Dose Analysis for Prediction of Outcomes After Liver Stereotactic Body Radiation Therapy

Bulat Ibragimov[1]([✉]), Diego A. S. Toesca[1], Yixuan Yuan[1,2], Albert C. Koong[3], Daniel T. Chang[1], and Lei Xing[1]

[1] Department of Radiation Oncology, Stanford University, Stanford, USA
bulat@stanford.edu
[2] Department of Electronic Engineering, City Univeristy of Hong Kong, Hong Kong, China
[3] Department of Radiation Oncology, MD Anderson Cancer Center, Houston, USA

Abstract. Accurate and precise dose delivery is the key factor for radiation therapy (RT) success. Currently, RT planning is based on optimization of oversimplified dose-volume metrics that consider all human organs to be homogeneous. The limitations of such an approach result in suboptimal treatments with poor outcomes: short survival, early cancer recurrence and radiation-induced toxicities of healthy organs. This paper pioneers the concept of deep 3D dose analysis for outcome prediction after liver stereotactic body RT (SBRT). The presented work develops tools for unification of dose plans into the same anatomy space, classifies dose plan using convolutional neural networks with transfer learning form anatomy images, and assembles the first volumetric liver atlas of the critical-to-spare liver regions. The concept is validated on prediction of post-SBRT survival and local cancer progression using a clinical database of primary and metastatic liver SBRTs. The risks of negative SBRT outcomes are quantitatively estimated for individual liver segments.

1 Introduction

With estimated 40,710 new cases and 28,920 deaths in 2017, liver cancer remains one of the deadliest cancers in the US [1]. The modern treatment approach called - stereotactic body radiation therapy (RT) (SBRT) - has been growing into one of the main treatment option for liver cancer patients, especially for patients suffering from unresectable and multifocal tumors. Treatment fractionation allows higher doses to be delivered to the tumor during SBRT in comparison to other RT types. Higher doses to the tumor are however accompanied by irradiation of the healthy organs-at-risks (OARs) located in the close proximity to the tumor [2]. Designing a dose delivery plan, where the tumor control probabilities are maximized while the risks of radiation-induced side effects are kept on the clinically acceptable level, is the main goal of SBRT planning.

In practice, dose delivery optimization is based on computing dose/volume histograms (DVHs), which estimate the volumes of organs receiving certain dose

© Springer Nature Switzerland AG 2018
A. F. Frangi et al. (Eds.): MICCAI 2018, LNCS 11071, pp. 684–692, 2018.
https://doi.org/10.1007/978-3-030-00934-2_76

levels. A clinically acceptable liver SBRT plan must spare ≥ 700 cm^3 of liver from receiving ≥ 15 Gy and ≥ 500 cm^3 of liver from receiving ≥ 7 Gy. These two and other similar constraints can be encoded through the DVH models. Despite it universality and applicability, the DVH concept suffers from several shortcomings. First, DVHs are averaged over the patient population and therefore do not take into account the anatomic and morphological properties of a patient. Second, DVHs tacitly assume that all organs are homogenous tissues and two dose plans with same DVHs are expected to impose the same risks. Limitations of DVHs compromise the quality of RT treatments with up to 27% of liver RT and more than 50% of head-and-neck RT resulting in radiation-induced toxicities of healthy OARs [2]. Toxicities eventually reduce the quality of patients' post-RT life and increase morbidity and mortality rates. Recently, the existence of critical-to-spare regions of OARs has been demonstrated on the example of head-and-neck RT, where sparing of the specific regions of parotid glands with stem cells reduces the risks of post-RT xerostomia toxicity [3]. Similar biochemical analysis is very time consuming and therefore unlikely to be repeated for abdominal OARs in the recent future. At the same time, identification of critical-to-spare regions is urgently needed for the next generation RTs.

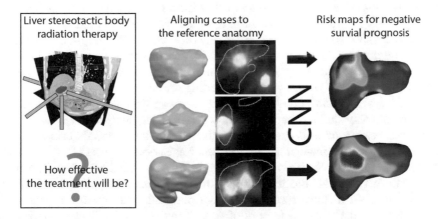

Fig. 1. A schematic illustration of the proposed framework for the analysis of radiation therapy dose patterns associated with negative post-treatment outcomes.

This paper pioneers the concept of deep 3D dose analysis for survival and local cancer progression prediction after liver SBRTs (Fig. 1). Our first innovation is adaptation of convolutional neural networks (CNNs) for detection of consistent patterns in three-dimensional (3D) dose plans computed over patients' livers, and associating such patterns with post-SBRT outcomes. Our second innovation is identification of critical liver regions irradiation of which is associated with the poorest prognosis. Finally, the critical regions are assembled into the first radiation-sensitivity liver atlases for both primary and metastatic cancer.

2   Methodology

During SBRT treatment planning, clinical specialists annotate tumors and surrounding OARs that may be affected by radiation during the treatment, prescribe the optimal doses and SBRT fractionation and finally develop the optimal dose delivery plan. As a results, a 3D dose plan superimposed with patient's
anatomy image, and the anatomy segmentation are generated. To account for
dose SBRT fractionation, the absolute delivered doses are converted into biologically effective doses, and the dose values are normalized according to the
biological properties of individual OARs. The intensity of a voxel with x coordinate in the 3D dose plan indicates how much dose a tissue at the same x
coordinate in the anatomy image is expected to receive during the treatment.

2.1   Registration of 3D Dose Plans into Anatomy-Unified Space

The 3D CNNs that can potentially be used for classification of 3D anatomy
images cannot straightforwardly be applied for classification of 3D dose plan.
First, a 3D dose plan by itself is not sufficient for treatment outcome prediction,
as the dose plan must be paired with the patient's anatomy, and the same dose
plan cannot be delivered to a patient other than the patient for which the plan
was generated. Second, the location of dose hot spots in the plan is critical, and
shifting a hot spot to few centimeters in any directions will completely invalidate
the treatment plan. At the same time, CNNs are generally translation-invariant
and would predict the same outcome from a dose plan even if a hot spot is
repositioned from the tumor to a surrounding structure.

   To address the above mentioned obstacles, we first registered all cases to
the same anatomy defined by a randomly selected segmentation I_{REF}. All liver
masks were registered and the corresponding dose plans were deformed according to the obtained transformation matrices. Registration consisted of two linear,
namely affine and similarity, transformations and one nonlinear B-spline transformation with mutual information used as the registration similarly measure.
Registration used a multi-resolution image pyramid with smoothing sigmas of
4, 2, 1 and 0 and shrinking factors of 4, 2, 2 and 1. To facilitate repetition of
the framework, the publicly available ANTs toolbox [4] was utilized with the
parameters similar to the parameters that won EMPIRE10 challenge [5]. The
dose plan for a case M was then deformed according to the registration results:

$$D'_M \leftarrow T_M(D_M) : T_M = \arg\min_T \left(S(I_{REF}, T(I_M)) \right), \tag{1}$$

where function S estimates similarity between two images, function T transforms
images, T_M is the optimal transformation of liver mask I_M to the reference liver
mask I_{REF}, D_M is the 3D dose plan delivered to I_M and D'_M is the deformed dose
plan aligned towards the anatomy of I_{REF}. After registering all segmentations
and deforming the corresponding dose plans, we obtained the set of anatomically-
aligned dose plans D' where the dose at voxel x on different dose plans is always
delivered to the similar anatomical location of the liver.

All registered dose plan are cropped to the same size that corresponds to the smallest bounding box encompassing all registered liver volumes. A non-zero padding was artificially added around each dose plan. The purpose of the padding is to compensate for translation invariance of CNNs and allow CNNs to learn the consistent dose patterns of dose plans with respect to the plan borders. As all plans are registered, the plan borders approximately correspond to the same anatomical locations near the liver, and therefore knowing the location of a dose pattern with respect to the padding is equivalent to knowing the location of the pattern against the liver anatomy. Registration and padding serve to address the obstacles towards CNN-based analysis of 3D dose plans.

2.2   CNN Transfer Learning for Outcome Prediction After Liver SBRTs

We designed a CNN to discover the consistent dose patterns in registered dose plans and associate these patterns with SBRT outcomes. To account for a potentially limited number of SBRTs, we utilized the CNN transfer learning mechanism. The CNN was first trained on a large collection of general 3D medical images and then tuned on dose plans. The CNN architecture consisted of three sets of convolution, rectified linear unit and dropout layers, separated by two max-pooling layers. All convolution layers have filters of 2^3 size with 15 filters for the first and third layers and 10 filters for the second bottle-neck convolution layer. All max-pooling layers have the size of 3^3. The last network layers were fully-connected layers with softmax activation. The parameters of the CNN were set as follows: learning rate = 0.001, momentum = 0.9 and dropout rate = 0.33. To facilitate repetition of the proposed research, the Computational Network Toolkit (CNTK) developed by Microsoft was used for CNN implementation [6].

The database for transfer learning consisted of 3D CT images of 2644 human organs of 28 types, collected at our institution for RT planning, and additionally using three public databases [7,8]. The database included the following organs (number of samples): aorta (50), adrenal gland (100), bladder (50), chest wall (25), duodenum (53), esophagus (105), eye globe (93), gall bladder (50), inferior vena cava (50), kidney (394), large bowel (51), larynx (45), liver (173), mandible (50), optic chiasm (46), optic nerve (94), pancreas (132), parotid gland (91), pharynx (39), portal and splenic veins (175), rectum (50), small bowel (72), spinal cord (205), spleen (78), stomach (126), submandibular gland (62), uterus (50) and vertebra (135). From these organ images, we generated 26440 samples of 19^3 size of $5\,mm^3$ resolution depicting different parts of each organ. The CNN was trained to recognize which organ is depicted in each sample.

After training the CNN to recognize organs in abdominal, spine and head-and-neck regions, the network was tuned on the registered dose plans. Each dose plan selected for training was duplicated 10 times with added up Gaussian noise from the interval $0.02 \cdot \max(D)$ where $\max(D)$ is the maximum delivered dose, up to $5\,mm$ random shift, and were isotropically rescaled into $2\,cm^3$ resolution. The survival and local progression from the SBRT database were converted into binary values using predefined cut-off thresholds. The generated CNNs then made predictions from the dose plans from unfamiliar-to-it liver SBRTs.

2.3   Treatment Outcome Atlases

Apart from making predictions about SBRT outcomes, we estimated which regions of the liver are most critical to be spared during SBRT. To understand how irradiation of different liver regions and different tumor positioning affects treatment outcome, we created a set of artificial treatment plans with artificial liver tumors. Let's D_0 be an empty dose map and I_{REF} is the reference liver anatomy. An artificial tumor is defined as a spherical region of a size s located at an arbitrary position $\boldsymbol{x}$ in I_{REF}. The artificial doses delivered to the artificial tumor volume were generated according to the following equation:

$$D_{s,x}(\boldsymbol{y}) = p\left(\left(1 - \frac{\|\boldsymbol{y} - \boldsymbol{x}\|}{s}\right)(p_{max} - p_{min}) + p_{min}\right) d_{max}, \qquad (2)$$

where $\forall \boldsymbol{y} \in Sphere(s, \boldsymbol{x})$, $D_{s,x}(\boldsymbol{y})$ is an artificial dose at point $\boldsymbol{y}$, $p(t)$ is a binary variable of Bernoulli distribution, and p_{min} and p_{max} are predefined constants representing probabilities that maximal prescribed dose d_{max} is applied to point $\boldsymbol{y}$. As a result, artificial doses $D_{s,x}$ delivered to the tumor $(s, \boldsymbol{x})$ are represented by a homogeneous sphere of d_{max} intensity with impulse noise occurring more often closer to the borders of the tumor. To finalize the artificial doses to the tumor, $D_{s,x}$ was smoothed with a Gaussian kernel $\mathbf{G}$:

$$D'_{s,x} = \mathbf{G}(D_{s,x}, 1), \qquad (3)$$

Apart from the tumor doses $(s, \boldsymbol{x})$, we needed to add doses to the surrounding structures to create a realistic treatment plan. Such surrounding doses were defined by the Gaussian distribution with sigma $= 1.5s$. The doses to the tumor $D'_{s,x}$ and its surroundings formed the complete artificial dose plan $D''_{s,x}$.

The artificial dose volumes were generated for all possible positionings of the tumor inside the reference liver mask I_{REF}. The CNN-based predictions were then calculated from the corresponding artificial treatments:

$$V_{s,x} = f\left(D''_{s,x}\right), \qquad (4)$$

into the volumetric outcome atlas V. The risk of a negative outcome from treating a tumor centered at point $\boldsymbol{x}$ is stored at the corresponding point of the atlas V. The reference CT image corresponding to liver mask I_{REF} was manually segmented into eight liver segments and the CNN-predicted risks for tumors located at different liver segments were summarized.

3   Experiments and Results

We assembled a database of patients treated with liver SBRT from 2004 to 2015 at our institution. The database consisted of 125 (63 males and 62 females) patients with complete follow-ups, where 58 were treated for liver metastases, 36 for hepatocellular carcinoma, 27 for cholangiocarcinoma and 4 for other primary liver cancers. Each patient was treated in 1–5 SBRT fractions with the total prescribed dose ranging from 25 to 54 Gy. During treatment planning, all doses were converted into biologically effective doses (BED_{10}) using the linear quadratic model with an α/β ratio of 10. Patients were followed for 1 to 98 months after the treatment with the median time of 13 months. Framework validation followed 20-fold cross-validation schema, ensuring that traning and testing was always perfromed on different non-intersection subsets of patients.

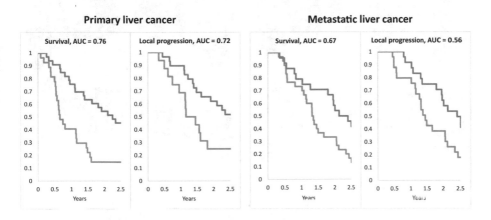

Fig. 2. Kaplan-Meier plots showing separation of patients into classes with positive and negative post-treatment outcome prediction on the $[0, 2.5]$ year time frame.

3.1   Post-SBRT Survival and Local Progression Prediction

The SBRT outcomes of interest were survival time and local progression start after the treatment. The CNNs were designed as binary classifiers with the 2 year cut-off time separating positive and negative survival outcomes, and the 1 year cut-off time separating positive and negative local progression outcomes. A couple of patients who were alive at the time of the last follow-up and whose last follow-ups took place less than 2 years after the treatment were removed from the survival prediction analysis. Similarly, a couple of patients who died less than 1 year from the SBRT and did not develop local cancer progression were removed from the local progression prediction analysis.

The accuracy of CNN-based outcome prediction for primary cancer cases was of 0.76 and 0.67 for survival and local progression prediction, respectively, estimated by the area under the ROC curve (AUC). For metastatic cancer, CNN resulted in AUC of 0.68 and 0.56 for survival and local progression prediction, respectively. Figure 2 presents the Kaplan-Meier estimators.

3.2   Survival and Local Progression Atlases

Prior to evaluating the developed dose atlases, we computed the average distribution of doses and tumor locations for primary and metastatic liver cancers. The doses delivered to eight liver segments significantly correlated ($\rho = 0.02$) for primary and metastatic cancer cases. The occurrence of tumors at individual liver segments also significantly correlated ($\rho = 0.02$) for both cancers.

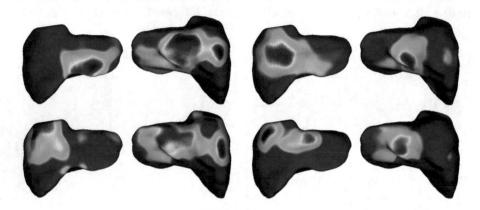

Fig. 3. The CNN-generated risk maps superimposed over liver mesh, where the red colors correspond to the critical-to-spare regions for survival (1st row) and local progression (2nd row) for primary (1st column) and metastatic (2nd column) liver cancer.

The risk scores associated with negative outcomes were computed for individual liver segments for both primary and metastatic cancers. Risk scores are defined on the interval $[0, 1]$ where 0 corresponds to the lowest risks of negative treatment outcome. The risk scores are summarized in Table 1. To additionally visualize the liver regions associated with high risks of negative treatment outcome, we superimposed the liver mesh generated from liver segmentation I_{REF} with the atlas V. The color of a mesh face with the coordinate $\boldsymbol{x}$ shows the predicted risk score from the dose delivered to the coordinate $\boldsymbol{x}$. Figure 3 shows such colored meshes computed for primary and metastatic cancer cases.

4   Discussion and Conclusion

In this paper, we investigated the possibilities to adapt CNNs for prediction of RT outcomes from 3D volumetric dose plans. We developed a framework consisting of the dose plans registration and CNN-based plans classification steps and validated it on a clinical database of SBRTs with follow-ups. We additionally assembled a large collection of 3D CT images for CNN transfer learning.

Our first conclusion is that the outcome prediction accuracy is higher for primary liver cancer than for metastatic liver cancer. We attribute this to the fact that survival of patients with liver metastases considerably depends on the primary cancer site, which is not indicated on the liver SBRT dose plans. The risks score for survival and local progression (Table 1) correlated with each other for both primary (coefficient = 0.56) and metastatic (coefficient = 0.85) cases. This observation is in agreement with clinical studies showing correlation between survival and progression-free survival [9]. As expected, the survival risks scores for primary and metastatic cancers do not correlate with each other (coefficient = 0.19). The tumors and doses are distributed in a statistically similar ways for both primary and metastatic cancer, so we cannot attribute the observed lack of correlation to the database being biased towards some cancer type.

In summary, we pioneered the concept of 3D dose analysis for prediction of RT outcomes. The only previous attempt of studying dose patterns with deep learning was developed for 2D dose plans and was therefore limited to the OARs with the simple cylindrical shape [10]. Highly promising results were observed on the example of liver SBRTs. The deep dose analysis concept is a fundamentally new approach in RT planning, which has potential to move the field from population-averaged to anatomy-driven personalized treatments.

Table 1. The predicted post-SBRT outcome computed for each liver segment. Lower values correspond to lower risks of negative SBRT outcomes.

		Liver segments							
		I	II	III	IV	V	VI	VII	VIII
Primary cancer	Survival	0.34	0.88	0.49	0.51	0.92	0.57	0.44	0.85
	Local progression	0.65	0.95	0.79	0.63	0.76	0.65	0.76	0.73
Metastatic cancer	Survival	0.16	0.54	0.76	0.76	0.80	0.77	0.73	0.39
	Local progression	0.42	0.83	0.89	0.81	0.99	0.91	0.97	0.81

References

1. Siegel, R.L., et al.: Cancer statistics, 2017. Cancer J. Clin. **67**, 7–30 (2017)
2. Toesca, D.A.S., Osmundson, E.C., von Eyben, R., Shaffer, J.L., Lu, P., Koong, A.C., Chang, D.T.: Central liver toxicity after SBRT: an expanded analysis and predictive nomogram. Radiother. Oncol. **122**(1), 130–136 (2016)
3. van Luijk, P., et al.: Sparing the region of the salivary gland containing stem cells preserves saliva production after radiotherapy for head and neck cancer. Sci. Transl. Med. **7**(305), 147 (2015)
4. Avants, B.B., Tustison, N.J., Song, G., Cook, P.A., Klein, A., Gee, J.C.: A reproducible evaluation of ANTs similarity metric performance in brain image registration. Neuroimage **54**(3), 2033–2044 (2011)
5. Murphy, K., et al.: Evaluation of registration methods on Thoracic CT: the EMPIRE10 challenge. IEEE Trans. Med. Imaging **30**(11), 1901–1920 (2011)

6. Agarwal, A., et al.: An introduction to computational networks and the computational network toolkit. Microsoft Technical report MSR-TR-2014-112 (2014)
7. Ibragimov, B., Likar, B., Pernus, F., Vrtovec, T.: Shape representation for efficient landmark-based segmentation in 3D. IEEE Trans. Med. Imaging **33**, 861–874 (2014)
8. Multi-atlas labeling beyond the cranial vault - workshop and challenge - syn3193805. https://www.synapse.org/#!Synapse:syn3193805/wiki/. Accessed 14 Sep 2017
9. Andratschke, N.H., Nieder, C., Heppt, F., Molls, M., Zimmermann, F.: Stereotactic radiation therapy for liver metastases: factors affecting local control and survival. Radiother. Oncol. **10**, 69 (2015)
10. Zhen, X., et al.: Deep convolutional neural network with transfer learning for rectum toxicity prediction in cervical cancer radiotherapy: a feasibility study. Phys. Med. Biolog. **62**(21), 8246–8263 (2017)

Liver Lesion Detection from Weakly-Labeled Multi-phase CT Volumes with a Grouped Single Shot MultiBox Detector

Sang-gil Lee[1], Jae Seok Bae[2,3], Hyunjae Kim[1], Jung Hoon Kim[2,3,4], and Sungroh Yoon[1(✉)]

[1] Electrical and Computer Engineering, Seoul National University, Seoul, Korea
sryoon@snu.ac.kr
[2] Radiology, Seoul National University Hospital, Seoul, Korea
[3] Radiology, Seoul National University College of Medicine, Seoul, Korea
[4] Institute of Radiation Medicine, Seoul National University Medical Research Center, Seoul, Korea

Abstract. We present a focal liver lesion detection model leveraged by custom-designed multi-phase computed tomography (CT) volumes, which reflects real-world clinical lesion detection practice using a Single Shot MultiBox Detector (SSD). We show that grouped convolutions effectively harness richer information of the multi-phase data for the object detection model, while a naive application of SSD suffers from a generalization gap. We trained and evaluated the modified SSD model and recently proposed variants with our CT dataset of 64 subjects by five-fold cross validation. Our model achieved a 53.3% average precision score and ran in under three seconds per volume, outperforming the original model and state-of-the-art variants. Results show that the one-stage object detection model is a practical solution, which runs in near real-time and can learn an unbiased feature representation from a large-volume real-world detection dataset, which requires less tedious and time consuming construction of the weak phase-level bounding box labels.

Keywords: Deep learning · Liver lesions · Detection · Multi-phase CT

1 Introduction

Liver cancer is the sixth most common cancer in the world and the second most common cause of cancer-related mortality with an estimated 746,000 deaths worldwide per year [1]. Of all primary liver cancers, hepatocellular carcinoma (HCC) represents approximately 80% and most HCCs develop in patients with chronic liver disease [2]. Furthermore, early diagnosis and treatment of HCC is known to yield better prognosis [3]. Therefore, it is of critical importance to be able to detect focal liver lesions in patients with chronic liver disease.

© Springer Nature Switzerland AG 2018
A. F. Frangi et al. (Eds.): MICCAI 2018, LNCS 11071, pp. 693–701, 2018.
https://doi.org/10.1007/978-3-030-00934-2_77

Among the various imaging modalities, computed tomography (CT) is the most widely utilized tool for HCC surveillance owing to its high diagnostic performance and excellent availability. A dynamic CT protocol of the liver consists of multiple phases [21], including precontrast, arterial, portal, and delayed phases to aid in the detection of the HCCs that have different hemodynamics from surrounding normal liver parenchyma. However, as a result, dynamic CT of the liver produces a large number of images, which require much time and effort for radiologists to interpret. In addition, early stage HCCs tend to be indistinct or small and sometimes it is difficult to distinguish them from adjacent hepatic vasculatures or benign lesions, such as arterioportal shunts, hemangioma, etc. Hence, diagnostic performance for early stage HCCs using CT is low compared to large, overt HCCs [4]. If focal liver lesions could be automatically pre-detected from CT images, radiologists would be able to avoid the laborious work of reading all images and focus only on the characterization of the focal liver lesions. Consequently, interpretation of liver CT images would be more efficient and expectedly also more accurate owing to focused reading.

Most publicly available CT datasets contain only the portal phase with per-pixel segmentation labeling [19,20]. On the contrary, images of multiple phases are required to detect and diagnose the liver lesions. Representatively, HCC warrants diagnostic imaging characteristics of arterial enhancement and portal or delayed washout as stated by major guidelines [5]. Thus, the representational power of deep learning-based models [6–8] is bounded by the data distribution itself. For example, specific variants of the lesion are difficult to see from the portal phase (Fig. 1). Therefore, a variety of hand-engineered data pre-processing techniques are required for deep learning with medical images.

Furthermore, from a clinical perspective, it is of practical value to detect lesion candidates by flagging them in real-time with a bounding box region of interest, which supports focused reading rather than pixel-wise segmentation, [6,8] which consumes a considerable amount of compute time. Considering the current drawbacks of the public datasets, we constructed a multi-phase detection CT dataset, which better reflects a real-world scenario of liver lesion diagnosis. While the segmentation dataset is more information-dense than the detection dataset, per-pixel labeling is less practical in terms of the scalability of the data, especially for medical images, which require skilled experts for clinically valid labelling. We show that the performance of our liver lesions detection model improves further when using multi-phase CT data.

We design an optimized version of the Single Shot MultiBox Detector (SSD) [10], a state-of-the-art deep learning-based object detection model. Our model incorporates grouped convolutions [12] for the multi-phase feature map. Our model successfully leverages richer information of the multi-phase CT data, while a naive application of the original model suffers from overfitting, which is where the model overly fits the training data and performs poorly on unobserved data.

2   Multi-phase Data

We constructed a 64 subject axial CT dataset, which contains four phases, for liver lesion detection. The dataset is approved by the international review board of Seoul National University Hospital. For image slices that contained lesions, we labeled such lesions in all phases with a rectangular bounding box. All the labels were determined by two expert radiologists. To enable the model to recognize information from the z-axis, we stacked three consecutive slices for each phase to create an input for the model. This resulted in a total of 619 data points, each of them having four phases aligned with the z-axis, and each of the phases having $3 \times 512 \times 512$ image slices of the axial CT scan.

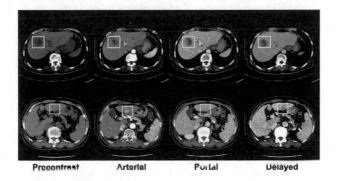

Procontrast   Artorial   Portal   Delayed

Fig. 1. Examples of the multi-phase CT dataset. Top: Lesions are visible from all phases. Bottom: Specific variants of lesions are visible only from specific phases. Note that the lesions are barely visible from the portal phase.

Since the volume of our dataset is much lower than the natural image datasets, the model unavoidably suffers more from overfitting, which is largely due to weakly-labeled ground truth bounding boxes. We labeled the lesions *phase-wise*, rather than *slice-wise*; for all slices that contain lesions in each phase, the coordinates of the bounding box are the same. While this method renders less burden on large-volume dataset construction, we get a skewed distribution of the ground truth, which hinders generalization of the trained model. To compensate for this limitation, we introduced a data augmentation for the ground truth, where we injected a uniform random noise to the bounding boxes to combat overfitting of the model while preserving the clinical validity of the labels. Formally, for each bounding box $\mathbf{y} = \{x_{min}, y_{min}, x_{max}, y_{max}\}$, we apply the following augmentation:

$$\mathbf{y}_{noise} = \mathbf{y} \odot \mathbf{z}, \; z_i \sim U(1 - \alpha, 1 + \alpha), \tag{1}$$

where $\odot$ is an element-wise multiplication, and $\alpha > 0$ is set to a small value in order to preserve label information. We sample the noise on-the-fly while training the model.

We followed a contrast-enhancement pre-processing pipeline for the CT data in [6]. We excluded the pixels outside the Hounsfield Unit (HU) range [−100, 400] and normalized them to [0, 1] for the model to concentrate on the liver and exclude other organs. Since our dataset contains CT scans from several different vendors, we manually matched the HU bias of the vendors before pre-processing.

3   Grouped Single Shot MultiBox Detector

Here, we describe the SSD model and our modifications for the liver lesions detection task. In contrast to two-stage models [13], one-stage models [14], such as SSD, detect the object category and bounding box directly from the feature maps. One-stage models focus on the speed-accuracy trade-off [9], where they aim to achieve a similar performance to two-stage models but with faster training and inference.

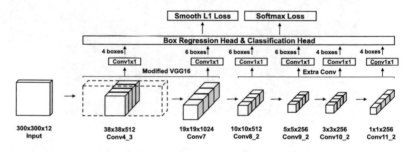

Fig. 2. Schematic diagram of grouped Single Shot MultiBox Detector. Solid lines of the convolutional feature map at the bottom indicate grouped convolutions. Digits next to upper arrows from the feature maps indicate the number of default boxes for each grid of the feature map. Intermediate layers and batch normalization are omitted for visual clarity.

SSD is a one-stage model, which enables object detection at any scale by utilizing multi-scale convolutional feature maps (Fig. 2). SSD can use any arbitrary convolutional neural networks (CNNs) as base networks. The model attaches bounding box regression and object classification heads to several feature maps of the base networks. We use the modified VGG16 [11] architecture as in the original model implementation to ensure a practical computational cost for training and inference. The loss term is a sum of the confidence loss from the classification head and the localization loss from the box regression head:

$$L(x, c, l, g) = \frac{1}{N}(L_{conf}(x, c) + L_{loc}(x, l, g)), \qquad (2)$$

where N is the number of matched (pre-defined) default boxes, $x_{ij}^{p} = \{1, 0\}$ is an indicator for matching the i-th default box to the j-th ground truth box of category p, L_{conf} is the softmax loss over class confidences c and L_{loc} is the smooth L1 loss between the predicted box l and the ground truth box g.

Grouped Convolutions. Our custom liver lesions detection dataset consists of four phases, each of them having three continuous slices of image per data point, which corresponds to 12 "channels" for each input. We could apply the model naively by increasing the input channel of the first convolutional layer to 12. However, this renders the optimization of the model ill-posed, since the convolution filters need to learn a generalized feature representation from separate data distributions. This also runs the risk of exploiting a specific phase of the input, and not fully utilizing the rich information from the multi-phase input. Naive application of the model causes severe overfitting, which means the model fails to generalize to the unobserved validation dataset.

To this end, we designed the model to incorporate grouped convolutions. For each convolutional layer of the base networks, we applied convolution with separate filters for each phase by splitting the original filters, and concatenated the outputs to construct the feature map. Before sending the feature map to the heads, we applied additional 1×1 convolutions. This induces parts of the model to have separate roles, where the base networks learn to produce the best feature representation for each phase of the input, while the 1×1 convolutions act as a channel selector by fusing the grouped feature map [22,23] for robust detection.

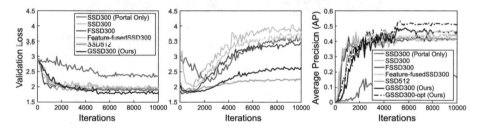

Fig. 3. Performance comparison from the five-fold cross validation set. Left: Localization loss curves. Middle: Confidence loss curves. Right: Average precision scores. All models except GSSD300-opt used 1:1 OHNM (Table 1).

4   Experiments

We trained the modified SSD models with our custom liver lesion detection dataset. For unbiased results, we employed five-fold cross validation. We applied all on-the-fly data augmentation techniques that were used in the original SSD implementation, but excluding hue and saturation randomization of the photometric distortion technique. We randomly cropped, mirrored, and scaled each input image (from 0.5 to 1.5). We trained the model over 10,000 iterations with a batch size of 16. We used a stochastic gradient descent optimizer with a learning rate of 0.0005, a momentum of 0.9, and a weight decay of 0.0005. We scheduled the learning rate adjustment with 1/10 scaling after 5,000 and 8,000 iterations for fine-tuning. We trained the models from scratch without pre-training, and initialized them using the Xavier method. We applied a batch normalization technique to the base networks for the grouped feature maps to have a normalized distribution of activations. We set the uniform random noise α for the ground truth in Eq. (1) to 0.01 for all experiments.

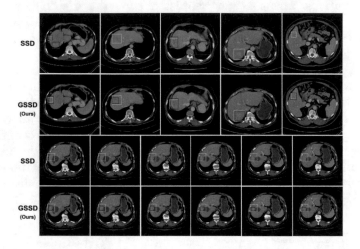

Fig. 4. Qualitative results from the validation set with a confidence threshold of 0.3. Yellow: Ground truth box. Red: Model predictions. Portal images shown. Top: GSSD accurately detects lesions, whereas the original model contains false positives or fails to detect. Bottom: A case of continuous slices. GSSD successfully tracks the exact location of lesions even with the given weak ground truth, whereas SSD completely fails.

The performance definitively improved when using the multi-phase data. For comparison, the single-phase model received portal phase images copied four times as inputs. The model trained with only the portal phase data obviously underfitted (Fig. 3), since several variants of the ground truth lesions are barely visible from the portal CT images.

By significantly suppressing overfitting of the class confidence layers (Fig. 3), our grouped SSD (GSSD) outperformed the original model as well as recently proposed state-of-the-art variants (Table 1) [17, 18]. Figure 4 demonstrates qualitative detection results. The best configuration achieved a 53.3% average precision (AP) score (Table 1). The model runs approximately 40 slices per second and can go through an entire volume of 100 slices in under three seconds on an NVIDIA Tesla P100 GPU. Note that the 1×1 convolutions play a key role as channel selectors. GSSD failed to perform well without the module. Stacking the 1×1 convolutions on top of the original model did not improve its performance, which proved that the combination of grouped convolutions and the channel selector module best harnesses the multi-phase data distribution.

Table 1. Performance comparison of various configurations of SSD models. OHNM: The positive:negative ratio of Online Hard Negative Mining (OHNM) [10]. 2xBase: Whether the model uses 2x feature maps in the base networks. # 1×1 Conv: The number of layers for each feature map before sending to the heads. Best AP scores after 5,000 iterations reported.

Model	OHNM	2xBase	# 1×1 Conv	AP
SSD300 [10] (Portal Only)	1:1			0.208
SSD300 (in Fig. 3)	1:1			0.444
SSD300	1:3			**0.448**
SSD300	1:1		1	0.408
SSD512 (in Fig. 3)	1:1			0.428
SSD512	1:3			0.433
FSSD300 [18]	1:1			0.432
Feature-fusedSSD300 [17]	1:1			0.437
GSSD300	1:1			0.445
GSSD300	1:1		2	0.459
GSSD300	1:1	✓	2	0.468
GSSD300	1:1	✓	1	**0.529**
GSSD300	1:3	✓	1	0.499
GSSD300 (in Fig. 3)	1:1		1	0.487
GSSD300-opt (in Fig. 3)	1:3		1	**0.533**

5   Discussion and Conclusions

This study has shown that our optimized version of the SSD can successfully learn an unbiased feature representation from a weakly-labeled multi-phase CT dataset, which only requires phase-level ground truth bounding boxes. The system can detect liver lesions in a volumetric CT scan in near real-time, which provides practical merit for real-world clinical applications. The framework is also flexible, which gives it strong potential for pushing the accuracy of the model further by using more sophisticated CNNs as the base networks, such as ResNet [15] and DenseNet [16].

We believe that the construction of large-scale detection datasets is a promising direction for fully leveraging the representational power of deep learning models from both machine learning and clinical perspectives. In future work, we plan to increase the size of the dataset to thousands of subjects, combined with a malignancy score label for the ground truth box for an end-to-end malignancy regression task.

Acknowledgements. This work was supported by the National Research Foundation of Korea (NRF) grant funded by the Korea government (Ministry of Science and ICT) [2018R1A2B3001628], the Interdisciplinary Research Initiatives Program from College of Engineering and College of Medicine, Seoul National University (800-20170166), Samsung Research Funding Center of Samsung Electronics under Project Number SRFC-IT1601-05, the Creative Industrial Technology Development Program [No. 10053249] funded by the Ministry of Trade, Industry & Energy (MOTIE, Korea), and the Brain Korea 21 Plus Project in 2018.

References

1. Stewart, B.W., Wild, C.P.: World cancer report 2014. Health (2017)
2. McGlynn, K.A., London, W.T.: Epidemiology and natural history of hepatocellular carcinoma. Best Pract. Res. Clin. Gastroenterol. **19**(1), 3–23 (2005)
3. Bruix, J., Reig, M., Sherman, M.: Evidence-based diagnosis, staging, and treatment of patients with hepatocellular carcinoma. Gastroenterology **150**(4), 835–853 (2016)
4. Kim, B.R., et al.: Diagnostic performance of gadoxetic acid-enhanced liver MR imaging versus multidetector CT in the detection of dysplastic nodules and early hepatocellular carcinoma. Radiology **285**(1), 134–146 (2017)
5. Heimbach, J.K., et al.: AASLD guidelines for the treatment of hepatocellular carcinoma. Hepatology **67**(1), 358–380 (2018)
6. Christ, P.F.: Automatic liver and lesion segmentation in CT using cascaded fully convolutional neural networks and 3D conditional random fields. In: Ourselin, S., Joskowicz, L., Sabuncu, M.R., Unal, G., Wells, W. (eds.) MICCAI 2016. LNCS, vol. 9901, pp. 415–423. Springer, Cham (2016). https://doi.org/10.1007/978-3-319-46723-8_48
7. Vorontsov, E., Chartrand, G., Tang, A., Pal, C., Kadoury, S.: Liver lesion segmentation informed by joint liver segmentation. arXiv preprint arXiv:1707.07734
8. Bi, L., Kim, J., Kumar, A., Feng, D.: Automatic liver lesion detection using cascaded deep residual networks. arXiv preprint arXiv:1704.02703
9. Huang, J., et al.: Speed/accuracy trade-offs for modern convolutional object detectors. In: CVPR (2017)
10. Liu, W., et al.: SSD: single shot multibox detector. In: Leibe, B., Matas, J., Sebe, N., Welling, M. (eds.) ECCV 2016. LNCS, vol. 9905, pp. 21–37. Springer, Cham (2016). https://doi.org/10.1007/978-3-319-46448-0_2
11. Simonyan, K., Andrew, Z.: Very deep convolutional networks for large-scale image recognition. In: ICLR (2015)
12. Alex, K., et al.: ImageNet classification with deep convolutional neural networks. In: NIPS (2012)
13. Ren, S., He, K., Girshick, R., Sun, J.: Faster R-CNN: towards real-time object detection with region proposal networks. In: NIPS (2015)
14. Redmon, J., Divvala, S., Girshick, R., Farhadi, A.: You only look once: unified, real-time object detection. In: CVPR (2016)
15. He, K., Zhang, X., Ren, S., Sun, J.: Deep residual learning for image recognition. In: CVPR (2016)
16. Huang, G., Liu, Z., Weinberger, K. Q., van der Maaten, L.: Densely connected convolutional networks. In: CVPR (2017)
17. Cao, G., et al.: Feature-fused SSD: fast detection for small objects. arXiv preprint arXiv:1709.05054

18. Li, Z., Zhou, F.: FSSD: feature fusion single shot multibox detector. arXiv preprint arXiv:1712.00960
19. Soler, L., et al.: 3D image reconstruction for comparison of algorithm database: a patient-specific anatomical and medical image database (2012)
20. Christ, P.F.: LiTS: liver tumor segmentation challenge. In: ISBI and MICCAI (2017)
21. Diamant, I., Goldberger, J., Klang, E., Amitai, M., Greenspan, H.: Multi-phase liver lesions classification using relevant visual words based on mutual information. In: ISBI (2015)
22. Szegedy, C., et al.: Going deeper with convolutions. In: CVPR (2015)
23. Lin, M., Chen, Q., Yan, S.: Network in network. arXiv preprint arXiv:1312.4400

A Diagnostic Report Generator from CT Volumes on Liver Tumor with Semi-supervised Attention Mechanism

Jiang Tian, Cong Li, Zhongchao Shi, and Feiyu Xu[✉]

AI Lab, Lenovo Research, Beijing, China
{tianjiang1,licong17,shizc2,fxu}@lenovo.com

Abstract. Automatically generating diagnostic reports with interpretability for computed tomography (CT) volumes is a new challenge for the computer-aided diagnosis (CAD). In this paper, we propose a novel multimodal data and knowledge linking framework between CT volumes and textual reports with a semi-supervised attention mechanism. This multimodal framework includes a CT slices segmentation model and a language model. Semi-supervised attention mechanism paves the way for visually interpreting the underlying reasons that support the diagnosis results. This multi-task deep neural network is trained end-to-end. We not only quantitatively evaluate our system performance (76.6% in terms of BLEU@4), but also qualitatively visualize the attention heat map for this framework on a liver tumor dataset.

1 Introduction

Every working day, a Chinese radiologist in Beijing in a regular hospital has to review more than 100 CT volumes[1] and to write many corresponding diagnostic reports, which is time-consuming and prone to inter- and intra-rater variations. There have been continuous efforts and progresses in the automatic recognition and localization of specific diseases and organs, mostly on radiology images. Nonetheless, generating a description about the content of a medical image automatically like a report written by a human radiologist might have a big impact for countries like China where doctors have a very big work load. The full power of this field has vast potentials to renovate medical CAD, but very little related work has been done [1–3]. Recent joint visual content and language modeling by deep learning enables the generation of semantic descriptions, which provide more intelligent predictions [4, 11].

The principles of deep neural networks during training and testing are difficult to interpret and justify. In some scenarios, predictions and metrics calculated on these predictions do not suffice to characterize the model. On the other hand, interpretability of a CAD system is highly needed, due to medical diagnosis mission critical application nature. In comparison, human decision-makers are

---

[1] Typically tens to hundreds of slices per volume.

© Springer Nature Switzerland AG 2018
A. F. Frangi et al. (Eds.): MICCAI 2018, LNCS 11071, pp. 702–710, 2018.
https://doi.org/10.1007/978-3-030-00934-2_78

themselves interpretable because they can explain their actions. Consequently, doctors must feel confident in the reasoning behind the program, and it is difficult to trust systems that do not explain or justify the conclusions.

Inspired by this fact, in this paper, we propose a framework which can train a fully convolutional neural network (FCN) to segment CT slices, and a separate Long-Short Term Memory (LSTM) language model, to generate captions, which might be regarded as interpretations that accompany segmentation. Meanwhile, ability to visualize what the model "sees" may determine qualitatively what a model has learned. Attention is such a main component supporting the visual interpretability of deep neural networks. We integrate two attention mechanisms into this framework. Segmentation may be regarded as a supervised approach to let the network capture visual information on "targeted" regions of interest. Another attention mechanism dynamically computes a weight vector along the axial direction to extract partial visual features supporting word prediction. While these interpretations may not elucidate precisely how a model works, they may nonetheless confer useful information for doctors.

More specifically, we apply this interpretable diagnostic report generator to CT volumes of liver. The liver is a common site of primary or secondary tumor development [12]. Until now, only interactive methods achieved acceptable results on segmenting liver tumors. In comparison, in this work, our framework provides explanations and justifications for its diagnosis prediction and makes the process interpretable to radiologists.

2 Model

In this section, as shown in Fig. 1(c), we describe a general approach, based on the encoder-decoder framework [7], to generate diagnostic report. Throughout the paper, we will denote by $LSTM(\mathbf{h}_{t-1}, \mathbf{y}_t)$ the LSTM operation on vectors $\mathbf{h}_{t-1}$ and $\mathbf{y}_t$ to achieve $\mathbf{h}_t$, wherein, $\mathbf{h}_t$ denotes hidden states from LSTM, $\mathbf{y}_t$ denotes word embedding at time t.

Encoder-Decoder Framework. The encoder network encodes the CT slices into a set of vectors as $a = \{\mathbf{a}_0, \cdots, \mathbf{a}_{\Pi-1}\}$, where Π is the total number of slices in a CT volume. Automatic liver and tumor segmentation from the contrast-enhanced CT volumes is a very challenging task due to the low intensity contrast between the liver and other neighboring organs. To tackle these difficulties, strong ability for extracting visual features is required. Recently, FCNs have achieved remarkable success on segmentation tasks [9]. We build the encoder upon this elegant architecture. The architecture of FCN is illustrated in Fig. 1(a). The final layer consists of two branches for predicting segmentation masks for liver and tumor separately. A 1×1 convolution is used to map each 128-component feature vector to the desired number of classes in each branch.

As shown in Fig. 1(b), the feature maps corresponding to liver and tumor, which represent categorical probability distributions, will be forwarded to a convolutional neural network (CNN) to embed the segmentation results. With prior knowledge that a liver tumor is inside the liver, an element-wise multiplication

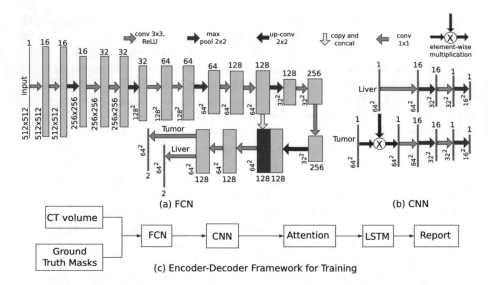

Fig. 1. FCN (a), CNN (b), and overall illustration (c) of the proposed encoder-decoder framework for training (best viewed in color). Each blue box corresponds to a multi-channel feature map. The number of channels is denoted either on top of or below the box. The x-y size is provided at the lower left edge of the box. Red box represents copied feature maps. The arrows denote different operations. Based on input CT slices and resized ground truth masks, the FCN model generates a segmentation mask to pass to CNN to embed the visual features, attention mechanism combines these features with LSTM's hidden state, the resulting vectors are then fed into LSTM in the form of task tuple. LSTM executes prediction tasks according to a specified start token.

of liver mask and tumor one is conducted to eliminate the tumor pixels outside the liver. The resulting two 16×16 feature maps will be the visual features for each input slice. Note that $\mathbf{a}_i$ is defined as reshaping only one 16×16 feature map, either for liver or for tumor depending on a specific task, into a vector.

Visual features are used as the input into $LSTM$ through attention mechanism for subsequently predicting words sequentially within a sentence. The prediction stops when #*end*, which designates the end of a sentence, is emitted. The decoding process is summarized as follows.

$$\mathbf{h}_t = LSTM(\mathbf{h}_{t-1}, \mathbf{y}_t, \mathbf{z}_t), \qquad p(word|\mathbf{h}_t) \propto exp(\mathbf{h}_t, \mathbf{y}_t, \mathbf{z}_t), \qquad (1)$$

where $\mathbf{z}_t = \sum_{i=0}^{\Pi-1} \alpha_{ti}\mathbf{a}_i$, it is a dynamic vector that represents the relevant part of image feature at time step t, α_{ti} is a scalar weighting of visual vector $\mathbf{a}_i$ at time step t, defined as follows.

$$\alpha_{ti} = exp(e_{ti})/\sum_{k=0}^{\Pi-1} exp(e_{tk}), \qquad (2)$$

$$e_{ti} = f_{attention}(\mathbf{a}_i, \mathbf{h}_{t-1}). \qquad (3)$$

$f_{attention}$ is a function that determines the amount of attention allocated to image feature $\mathbf{a}_i$, conditioned on the LSTM hidden state $\mathbf{h}_{t-1}$. This function is implemented as a multilayer perceptron as follows.

$$f_{attention} = \mathbf{w}^T tanh(U_a \mathbf{h}_{t-1} + W_a \mathbf{a}_i + \mathbf{b}_a). \tag{4}$$

Note that by construction $\sum_{i=0}^{\Pi-1} \alpha_{ti} = 1$.

Rather than compress an entire CT volume into a static representation, attention allows for salient features to dynamically come to the forefront as needed. It can be viewed as a type of alignment between image space and language one. Improving such alignment can be achieved by adding supervision on attention maps [2,8]. In our approach, we propose to tackle this problem by utilizing segmentation networks to support image-language alignment. Specifically, we perform two FCN based segmentation tasks (one for liver, the other for tumor). The purpose of the segmentation task here is two-fold. First, it is a supervised attention mechanism. Second, it helps the gradients back-propagation during training.

Report Generation. A radiologist narrates findings in a report from observations of a liver CT imaging study, wherein, an observation is a distinctive area compared to background liver at imaging.[2] The task of report generation is traditionally solved for X-ray or pathology images by learning to map a set of diverse image measurements to a set of semantic descriptor values (or class labels). In comparison, our model is an end-to-end one which avoids managing a complex sequential pipeline.

In this work, a report is structured as *shape, contour,* and *intensity* sections to communicate information (e.g., volumetric, morphometric) with regard to region of interests. Take the descriptions of tumor symptoms on the right lobe of liver as an example, we have English translations as follows. *There are multiple low density regions with large area on the right lobe of liver. There are multiple low density regions on the right lobe of liver. There is one low density region on the right lobe of liver. There is one low density region with large area on the right lobe of liver. There is no abnormal region on the right lobe of liver.* Note that our method localizes the right lobe of liver and produces free-text descriptions.

A report describes multiple symptoms of observing CT volumes. It has more regular linguistic structure than natural image captions [2]. We let one LSTM focus on mining discriminative information for a specific description. All description modelings share LSTM weights. In this way, complete report generation becomes a function of modeling of each specific feature description.

In the training stage, given a mini-batch of CT slices and report, after forwarding the CT slices to the image model, we duplicate each sample inside, resulting in a size of five mini-batch as the input of LSTM. Each duplication takes one of the image features either for liver or for tumor, and one particular symptom description extracted from the report. Note that we denote by #*start* a special start word and #*end* a special stop one which designate the start and

---

[2] https://www.acr.org/Clinical-Resources/Reporting-and-Data-Systems/LI-RADS.

end of a sentence. Each particular feature description has unique start and end tokens. In this way, we use particular signal to inform LSTM the start and end of a targeting task.

In testing, the first element of every input sequence is always a special start token #start, the network therefore makes a prediction corresponding to a special aspect of the visual features based on the LSTM state and the previous word. If #end token is emitted, the prediction will stop.

3   Experiments

To the best of our knowledge, there is no benchmark for generating diagnostic report from CT volumes on liver tumor. In this section, we describe our experimental methodology, run a number of ablations to analyze the framework, and show the corresponding results.

Dataset. We use a publicly available dataset of MICCAI 2017 LiTS Challenge [12], which contains 131 and 70 contrast-enhanced abdominal CT scans for training and testing, respectively. The diagnostic reports (with segmentation masks as reference) for the training dataset were collected in collaboration between two experts on medical imaging and a doctor focused on abdominal surgery in a top hospital in Beijing. A paragraph in Chinese[3] is provided to describe observations to address three types of appearance features, namely the shape, contour, and intensity. We clip all CT scans with a window $[-75, 175]$ HU (Hounsfield scale) according to radiologist's advice to ignore irrelevant abdominal organs for both training and testing. We perform a 3-fold cross validation on the training dataset.

Implementation. All models are trained and tested with Tensorflow on NVIDIA Tesla P100 (with $16276M$ memory) GPUs. Due to the GPU memory constraint, each CT volume has been pooled along the axial direction into 96 slices, if the number of its slices is smaller than 96, they will be zero padded. We implement this average pooling in a sliding window manner as $win = \lceil \Pi/96 \rceil$ and $str = \lfloor \Pi/96 \rfloor$, where win is the window size, str is the stride. $\lceil \cdot \rceil$ and $\lfloor \cdot \rfloor$ denote ceiling and floor operations, respectively. In comparison, we take the union rather than average of the ground truth segmentation masks in the win scope for not missing information. We train the full model end-to-end by stochastic gradient descent (SGD) with momentum. We use a mini-batch size of 1 CT volume and 5 sentences, and a fixed learning rate of 10^{-2}. We use a momentum of 0.9. The model is trained with random initialized weights.

Ablation Study. We are more interested in whether supervised attention model has better captioning performance. In this section we give experimental support. Figure 2 denotes a baseline structure incorporating neither liver nor tumor segmentation structures for visual embedding. In order to make fair comparison, we only make minor modifications of the visual embedding structure shown in

---

[3] It has the same processing pipeline as English report once embedded.

Fig. 1(a). The implicit attention refers to the alignment between the visual feature space and the textual one, it is still in effect for the baseline architecture shown in Fig. 2. Semi-supervised attention refers to segmentation supervision on the visual feature for the aforementioned implicit attention.

Table 1. BLEU@n and ROUGE(R) scores of our methods on liver tumor dataset. All values are reported as percentage (%).

Method	B1	B2	B3	B4	R
S1024	88.3	83.7	79.8	75.6	89.2
I1024	88.1	83.0	78.7	74.0	88.6
S512	88.9	84.5	80.7	76.6	89.8
I512	88.8	83.9	79.7	75.2	89.4
S256	88.8	84.1	80.1	75.9	89.2
S128	86.9	81.5	76.9	71.0	87.9

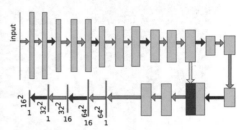

Fig. 2. Baseline architecture for visual embedding. The arrows denote same operations as shown in Fig. 1. The number of channels and x-y size are omitted if they are the same with Fig. 1(a).

We quantitatively evaluate the report generation performance on BLEU(B) [5] and ROUGE(R) [6] scores. The results are given in Table 1. The first column in the table lists the LSTM hidden units number, wherein, S stands for semi-supervised attention, and I depicts implicit attention, the number after S or I lists the corresponding LSTM hidden state size.

The unigram BLEU scores are to account for how much information is retained. The longer n-gram BLEU scores account for to what extent it reads like "diagnostic report". The comparison between S# and I# indicates not only that model using semi-supervised attention improves over the baseline model with only implicit attention mechanism, but also that the longer the n-gram, the bigger the performance difference between S# and I#. It suggests that our framework provides better alignment from natural language words to provided visual features, and semi-supervised mechanism becomes particular necessary.

At the same time, increasing the hidden layer size can generally lead to performance improvements except hidden state size of 1024, which means overfitting occurs here. Meanwhile, the number of parameters increase exponentially. Therefore, in our experiments, the hidden layer size is empirically set to 512 as it has a better tradeoff between performance and model complexity.

Generating Visual Interpretations. One common approach to generate interpretations is to render visualizations in the hope of determining qualitatively what a model has learned. As shown in Fig. 3, by visualizing the attention component learned by the model, we are able to add an extra layer of interpretability to the output of the model. In the computer vision community, these approaches have been explored to investigate what information is retained at various layers of a neural network [10].

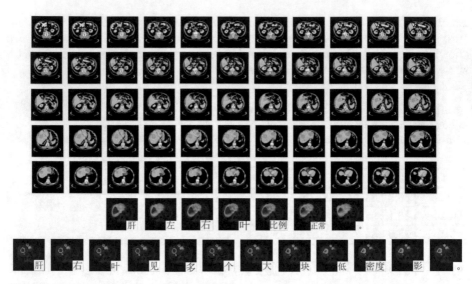

Fig. 3. An example of generating interpretations. The first five rows list a sequence of CT slices, the patient has symptoms of liver cancer as indicated by low density regions on a series of slices. The sixth row shows the attention heat maps for liver superposed onto the averaged CT image. English translation for the description is "The ratio between left lobe of liver and right lobe of liver is normal". The seventh row shows the attention heat maps for tumor superposed onto the averaged CT image. English translation is "There are multiple low density regions with large area on the right lobe of liver", whereas that for visual embedding defined in Fig. 2 is "There are multiple low density regions on the right lobe of liver". The semi-supervised attention captures information about the size (*large area*) compared with the implicit one.

In order to visualize the attention weights for the model, we record down each α_{ti}, a scalar weighting of visual vector $\mathbf{a}_i$ at time step t, in Eq. (2). Heat map for attention at 64×64 scale is calculated as $hm = \sum_{i=0}^{H-1} \alpha_{ti} S_c(i)$, where $S_c(i)$ corresponds to the c-th class (either liver or tumor) of the segmentation output for the i-th input. We up-sample the hm by a factor of 8, which is then superposed onto the averaged image through all CT slices in a volume. As shown in Fig. 3, the model learns alignments that correspond very strongly to the "targeted" regions. We see that it is possible to exploit such visualizations to get an intuition as to why the text explanations were made.

Evaluation on Test Set. Based on BLEU@4, we select the best model from cross validation for the test set. We let the state-of-the-art results from the challenge[4] be ground truth for the segmentation task in our framework. We pre-process the ground truth masks using the aforementioned pooling along the axial direction, and resize them to the dimension of 64×64. Finally, for test set, the Dice per case (an average Dice per volume score) for liver is 0.942, and for tumor is 0.549.

---

[4] We are the MICCAI 2017 LiTS Challenge first place team.

In addition to the automated evaluation metrics, we present human evaluations on the test results. We randomly select 30 report predictions from the test set, and conduct a paid doctor evaluation. A rating scale (1: definite accept, 5: definite reject) is adopted here for each report. Average score is 2.33.

4 Conclusion

This paper investigates multimodal knowledge sharing between CT volumes and diagnostic reports with semi-supervised attention mechanisms. It focuses on introducing a system to assist doctors in medical imaging interpretation. Textual descriptions communicate facts in CT images to doctors. These descriptions are regarded as interpretations. The second objective is to visually interpret the underlying reasons that support the diagnosis results. Showing image attention to interpret how the network uses visual information will support its diagnostic prediction. Furthermore, through experiments, we show that using segmentation supervision on the visual feature for the implicit attention improves the captioning performance.

References

1. Xu, T., Zhang, H., Huang, X., Zhang, S., Metaxas, D.N.: Multimodal deep learning for cervical dysplasia diagnosis. In: Ourselin, S., Joskowicz, L., Sabuncu, M.R., Unal, G., Wells, W. (eds.) MICCAI 2016. LNCS, vol. 9901, pp. 115–123. Springer, Cham (2016). https://doi.org/10.1007/978-3-319-46723-8_14
2. Zhang, Z., Xie, Y., Xing, F., Mcgough, M., Yang, L.: Mdnet: a semantically and visually interpretable medical image diagnosis network. In: CVPR, pp. 6428–6436 (2017)
3. Zhang, Z., Chen, P., Sapkota, M., Yang, L.: TandemNet: distilling knowledge from medical images using diagnostic reports as optional semantic references. In: Descoteaux, M., Maier-Hein, L., Franz, A., Jannin, P., Collins, D.L., Duchesne, S. (eds.) MICCAI 2017. LNCS, vol. 10435, pp. 320–328. Springer, Cham (2017). https://doi.org/10.1007/978-3-319-66179-7_37
4. Vinyals, O., Toshev, A., Bengio, S., Erhan, D.: Show and tell: a neural image caption generator. In: CVPR, pp. 3156–3164 (2015)
5. Papineni, K., Roukos, S., Ward, T., Zhu, W.J.: BLEU: a method for automatic evaluation of machine translation. In: ACL, pp. 311–318 (2002)
6. Lin, C.-Y.: Rouge: a package for automatic evaluation of summaries, pp. 74–81. In: ACL Workshop (2004)
7. Yao, L., et al.: Describing videos by exploiting temporal structure. In: ICCV, pp. 4507–4515 (2015)
8. Liu, C., Mao, J., Sha, F., Yuille, A.: Attention correctness in neural image captioning. In: AAAI, pp. 4176–4182 (2017)
9. Ronneberger, O., Fischer, P., Brox, T.: U-Net: convolutional networks for biomedical image segmentation. In: Navab, N., Hornegger, J., Wells, W.M., Frangi, A.F. (eds.) MICCAI 2015. LNCS, vol. 9351, pp. 234–241. Springer, Cham (2015). https://doi.org/10.1007/978-3-319-24574-4_28

10. Zintgraf, L.M., Cohen, T.S., Welling, M.: A new method to visualize deep neural networks. arXiv preprint arXiv:1603.02518 (2016)
11. Xu, K., et al.: Show, attend and tell: Neural image caption generation with visual attention. In: ICML, pp. 2048–2057 (2015)
12. MICCAI 2017 LiTS Challenge. https://competitions.codalab.org/competitions/ 17094

Less is More: Simultaneous View Classification and Landmark Detection for Abdominal Ultrasound Images

Zhoubing Xu[1(✉)], Yuankai Huo[2], JinHyeong Park[1], Bennett Landman[2], Andy Milkowski[3], Sasa Grbic[1], and Shaohua Zhou[1]

[1] Medical Imaging Technologies, Siemens Healthineers, Princeton, NJ, USA
zhoubing.xu@siemens-healthineers.com
[2] Electrical Engineering, Vanderbilt University, Nashville, TN, USA
[3] Ultrasound, Siemens Healthineers, Issaquah, WA, USA

Abstract. An abdominal ultrasound examination, which is the most common ultrasound examination, requires substantial manual efforts to acquire standard abdominal organ views, annotate the views in texts, and record clinically relevant organ measurements. Hence, automatic view classification and landmark detection of the organs can be instrumental to streamline the examination workflow. However, this is a challenging problem given not only the inherent difficulties from the ultrasound modality, e.g., low contrast and large variations, but also the heterogeneity across tasks, i.e., one classification task for all views, and then one landmark detection task for each relevant view. While convolutional neural networks (CNN) have demonstrated more promising outcomes on ultrasound image analytics than traditional machine learning approaches, it becomes impractical to deploy multiple networks (one for each task) due to the limited computational and memory resources on most existing ultrasound scanners. To overcome such limits, we propose a multi-task learning framework to handle all the tasks by a single network. This network is integrated to perform view classification and landmark detection simultaneously; it is also equipped with global convolutional kernels, coordinate constraints, and a conditional adversarial module to leverage the performances. In an experimental study based on 187,219 ultrasound images, with the proposed simplified approach we achieve (1) view classification accuracy better than the agreement between two clinical experts and (2) landmark-based measurement errors on par with inter-user variability. The multi-task approach also benefits from sharing the feature extraction during the training process across all tasks and, as a result, outperforms the approaches that address each task individually.

1 Introduction

Ultrasound scanning is widely used for safe and non-invasive clinical diagnostics. Given a large population with gastrointestinal diseases (60–70 million in USA

Z. Xu and Y. Huo—Equal Contribution.

© Springer Nature Switzerland AG 2018
A. F. Frangi et al. (Eds.): MICCAI 2018, LNCS 11071, pp. 711–719, 2018.
https://doi.org/10.1007/978-3-030-00934-2_79

[1]), the abdomen is one of the most commonly screened body parts under ultrasound examinations. During an abdominal examination session, a sonographer needs to navigate and acquire a series of standard views of abdominal organs, annotate the view information in texts, adjust the caliper to desirable locations through a track ball, and record measurements for each clinically relevant organ. The substantial manual interactions not only become burdensome for the user, but also decrease the workflow efficiency.

Automatic view classification and landmark detection of the abdominal organs on ultrasound images can be instrumental to streamline the examination workflow. However, it is very challenging to accomplish the full automation from two perspectives. First, analytics of the ultrasound modality are inherently difficult due to the low contrast and large variations throughout ultrasound images, which are sometimes confusing even to experienced ultrasound readers. Second, the associated tasks are typically handled individually, i.e., one classification task for all views, and then one landmark detection task for each relevant view, due to their heterogeneities between each other; this is very hard to fulfill on most existing ultrasound scanners, restricted by limited computational and memory resources. Convolutional neural networks (CNN) have demonstrated superior performance to traditional machine learning methods given large-scale datasets in many medical imaging applications [2]. They provide a favorable option to address ultrasound problems. Based on CNN, multi-task learning (MTL) has been investigated to improve outcomes for each single task with the assumption that common hidden representations are shared among multiple tasks. In MTL, a single neural network is used instead of one network per task so that the requirement for computational and memory resources is substantially reduced. Therefore, we pursue a highly integrated MTL framework to perform simultaneous view classification and landmark detection automatically to increase the efficiency of abdominal ultrasound examination workflow.

Current researches on MTL are quite diversified given the task varieties. Kokkinos et al. [3] presented a unified framework to accomplish seven vision tasks on a single image. The tasks are highly correlated, but differ from each other by focusing on different levels of image details. Given these tasks, it turns out helpful to extract comprehensive image features by sharing every level of convolutional layers, and then branching out for task-specific losses at each level and each resolution. Ranjan et al. [4] introduced another unified framework for detection of face attributes. With empirical knowledge of what level of features can best represent each face attribute, the branching location for each task is customized in this all-in-one network to maximize the synergy across all the tasks. Xue et al. [5] demonstrated full quantification of all size-related measurements of left ventricle in cardiac MR sequences. They also incorporated the phase information as an additional task, through which they regularized the intra- and inter-task relatedness along sequences. While these studies achieved successes in their applications, they cannot be easily adapted to our problem. They are mostly designed for estimating variable attributes of a single object or on a single image, while our scenario is to predict multiple attributes (view and landmarks) on different objects (e.g., liver, spleen, kidney) that are not in the same image for most cases. Moeskops et al. [6] used a single network architecture to perform diverse segmentation tasks (brain MR, breast MR, and cardiac CTA) without task-specific training; this is similar to our problem for handling different organs, but simpler with only segmentation tasks.

In this study, we propose an end-to-end MTL network architecture tailored for abdominal ultrasound analytics to synergize the extraordinary heterogeneous tasks. To the best of our knowledge, we are the first to present an integrated system with fully automated functionalities for the abdominal ultrasound examination.

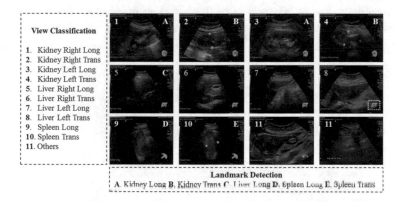

Fig. 1. An overview of the tasks for abdominal ultrasound analytics. In each image, the upper left corner indicates its view type. If present, the upper right corner indicates the associated landmark detection task, and the pairs of long- and short-axis landmarks are colored in red and green, respectively. An icon is circled on one image; such icons are masked out when training the view classification.

2   Methods and Results

2.1   Data and Task Definitions

During a typical abdominal ultrasound session, ten standard views are of major interests, including five structures from two orientations, i.e., liver right lobe, liver left lobe, right kidney, left kidney, and spleen, from longitudinal and transverse directions. On certain views, two longitudinal ("Long") or four transverse ("Trans") landmarks are placed for measurements, where each measurement is derived from a pair of landmarks along the long- or short- axis. These processes are summarized as an 11-view classification task (with an addition of the "others" view) and 5 landmark detection tasks with a total of 14 landmarks (Fig. 1). Note that we combine the left and right views of kidneys for landmark detection. A total of 187,219 ultrasound images from 706 patients were collected. Some images are acquired in sequence, while others are as single frames. The view information was manually assigned to each image as a routine during acquisition, where a representative icon was placed at the corner of the image. Landmark annotations were performed by experienced ultrasound readers on 7,012 images (1921, 1309, 1873, 1711, and 198 for the five landmark detection tasks listed in Fig. 1), and further verified by the ultrasound specialist. Duplicated annotations were performed by a second ultrasound expert for inter-user variabilities on 1999 images for views and 30 50 images for each pair of landmarks. The datasets were separated on the patient level into training and testing sets by an 80%/20% split for all tasks. Any patients with data included in the training set were excluded from the testing set. During preprocessing, the images were resampled into 0.5 mm isotropic resolution, and zero-padded to 512×512. For each image used for training the view classification, a mask was applied to block view-informative icons and texts. The landmark annotations were converted into distance-based Gaussian heat maps centered to the landmark locations.

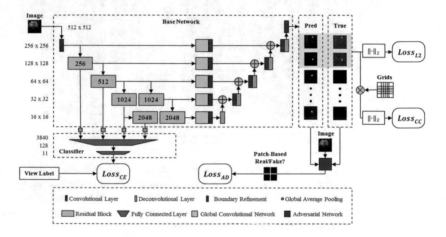

Fig. 2. An illustration of the proposed MTL Framework.

2.2   MTL Framework

In the proposed MTL network architecture (Fig. 2), we construct an encoder that follows ResNet50 [7]. The first convolutional layer is modified to take a single channel input. While the first two residual blocks are shared across all tasks for low level feature extraction, two copies of the 3rd and 4th residual blocks are used, one for view classification, and the other for landmark detection.

Cross Entropy Loss for View Classification: For view classification, each residual block of its encoder is connected with a global average pooling (GAP) layer, and a feature vector is composed by concatenating the pooled features from multiple levels; two fully connected layers are used as the classifier based on the pooled features. A traditional cross entropy loss is defined as

$$Loss_{CE} = -\sum_{c} y_c \log p_c \tag{1}$$

where y_c represents the binary true value, and p_c indicates the probability of an image being view class c, respectively.

Regression Loss for Landmark Detection: For landmark detection, we form a single decoder shared across the landmarks from all views instead of one branch per view, and the decoder follows the skip-connection style in Fully Convolutional Network (FCN) [8], where the output channel of each level is kept the same as the total number of landmarks, i.e., N_L. On each level of skip connection between encoder and decoder, we append Global Convolutional Network (GCN) [9] and boundary refinement modules to capture larger receptive fields. Consider $L = \{0, 1, \ldots, N_L - 1\}$ as the complete set of landmarks, let $\hat{H} \in \mathbb{R}^{N_L \times N_I}$ and $H \in \mathbb{R}^{N_L \times N_I}$ be the Gaussian heat maps for the prediction and truth, respectively, including all N_L channels of images (indexed with l), each with N_I pixels (indexed with i), an L2-norm is computed only on a selective subset $L' \subset L$ with $N_{L'}$ landmarks associated to each image so that only relevant information gets back-propagated

$$Loss_{L2} = \frac{1}{N_I N_{L'}} \sum_i \sum_{l \in L'} \left(\hat{H}_{li} - H_{li}\right)^2 \tag{2}$$

Landmark Location Error: A coordinate-based constraint is applied to regularize the heat map activation. Consider the image grid coordinates as $S \in \mathbb{R}^{N_I \times 1}$ and $T \in \mathbb{R}^{N_I \times 1}$ for the two dimensions, the predicted landmark location $(\hat{s}_l, \hat{t}_l)$ can be derived as a weighted average, i.e., $\hat{s} = \frac{\sum_{i \in \Omega_l} H_{li} S_i}{\sum_{i \in \Omega_l} H_{li}}, \hat{t} = \frac{\sum_{i \in \Omega_l} H_{li} T_i}{\sum_{i \in \Omega_l} H_{li}}$, where Ω_l indicates the area above a threshold k, i.e., $H_l > k$. Unlike identifying the point with maximum value, this weighted averaging is a differentiable process to maintain the end-to-end training workflow. Then Euclidean distance error is computed against the true landmark location (s_l, t_l),

$$Loss_{CC} = \frac{1}{N_{L'}} \sum_{l \in L'} \sqrt{(s_l - \hat{s}_l)^2 + \left(t_l - \hat{t}_l\right)^2} \tag{3}$$

Adversarial Loss: Following PatchGAN [10], an adversarial network $\mathbf{D}$: $\mathbb{R}^{N_I \times (N_L+1)} \mapsto \mathbb{R}^{N_M \times 1}$ is defined; it takes both the input image and the output prediction from the base network to identity the real and fake outputs on the basis of N_M patches. From the perspective of the base network, it regularizes the output with binary cross entropy

$$Loss_{AD} = \frac{1}{N_M} \sum_m [- \sum_{i \in m} (y_i \log p_i + (1 - y_i) \log 1 - p_i)] \tag{4}$$

where m indicates a single patch, y is the real true/false, and p is the probability of true/false prediction. This effectively enforces the output heat maps to follow a reasonable landmark distribution.

Implementation: The landmark detection tasks are trained first with a batch size of 4 for 30 epochs, where each batch can include a mixture of different

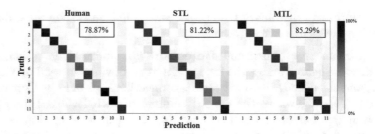

Fig. 3. Confusion matrices for the view classification task of STL, MTL, and between humans. The numbers on x and y axes follow the view definitions in Fig. 1. The overall classification accuracy is overlaid for each approach. The diagonal entries indicate correct classifications.

organs. The base network is optimized by stochastic gradient decent (SGD) with a learning rate (LR) of 1E-6. The adversarial network uses the Adam optimizer with a LR of 2E-4. We take $k = 0.75$ as the threshold for the coordinate derivation. The regression, location, and adversarial losses are equally weighted as an empirical configuration. The view classification task is trained afterwards with a batch size of 8 for 5 epochs, and optimized by Adam with a LR of 5E-4, while the shared parameters pre-trained with landmark detection tasks are kept locked. During testing, the image can be forwarded though the network for all tasks by one shot. The experiments are performed on a Linux workstation equipped with an Intel 3.50 GHz CPU and a 12 GB NVidia Titan X GPU using the PyTorch framework. Single-task learning (STL) approaches and ablation studies are performed for comparison using the same configuration as the proposed method as much as possible. The STL view classification takes the default ResNet50 pre-trained from ImageNet [11] with the data pre-processed accordingly. For evaluation based on clinical standards, we use the classification accuracy for view classification, and the absolute differences of the long- and short-axis measurements for landmark detection.

2.3   Results

For view classification, we achieve a 4.07% improvement compared to STL, and we also outperform the second human expert, especially for distinguishing the non-others classes (Fig. 3). Please note that we use the annotations from one expert with more ultrasound experience as the ground truth for training, and those from the other less experienced expert for reference. For landmark detection, we reduce each landmark-based measurement error by a large margin compared to every other benchmark approaches (Table 1). For most measurements, we also achieve errors below 1.5 times of the inter-user variability. The two measurements for Spleen Trans are slightly worse due to lack of samples ($< 3\%$ of total). Going directly from STL to MTL (SFCN→MFCN) provides implicit data augmentation for tasks with limited data, while the accuracies on other tasks seem to be compromised. Using GCN, the variabilities from multiple tasks are better captured, which leads to improved results (MFCN→MGCN). With the coordinate-based constraint and patch-based adversarial regularization on the outputs, the outliers of landmark detection can be substantially reduced (MGCN→MGCN_R), and thus boosts the performance (Fig. 4). With the GPU implementation, the average time consumption is 90 ms to load and pre-process the data, classify the view, detect landmarks, and derive measurements. The model parameters to handle all the tasks are reduced from 539 MB to 100 MB.

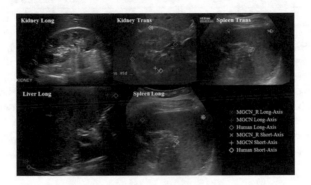

Fig. 4. Qualitative comparison of landmark detection results with and without regularization for the proposed approach. Images are zoomed into region of interest for better visualization

3   Discussion

In this paper, we propose an end-to-end MTL framework that enables efficient and accurate view classification and landmark detection for abdominal ultrasound examination. The main novelty lies in (1) the integration of the heterogeneous tasks into a single network, (2) the design of two regularization criteria to improve MTL performance, and (3) the first systematic design of a streamlined end-to-end workflow for abdominal ultrasound examination.

It is critical to determine where to share and diversify the heterogeneous tasks integrated in a single network. The landmark detection of different views can be considered a MTL problem by itself. Formulating the network with multiple decoders seems straightforward, but not favorable in this study, we observe overwhelming outliers with such network design in our preliminary tests. Our experiment demonstrates that sharing all landmark tasks with one decoder together with a selective scheme for back-propagation provides an effective training platform for the heterogeneous tasks of landmark detection. As the landmarks are defined similarly on the long- and short- axis endpoints of organs even though distributed on different views, it makes sense to share how the output heat maps are reconstructed from the extracted features with a single decoder. The share-it-all design also enables mixed organ types in one mini-batch to get back-propagated together, and thus augments the data implicitly; this is not simple

Table 1. Quantitative comparison for landmark-based measurements in mm.

	KL_LA	KT_LA	KT_SA	LL_LA	SL_LA	ST_LA	ST_SA
Human	4.500	5.431	4.283	5.687	6.104	4.578	4.543
PBT [12]	11.036	9.147	8.393	11.083	7.289	9.359	12.308
SFCN	7.044	7.332	5.189	10.731	8.693	91.309	43.773
MFCN	10.582	16.508	15.942	17.561	8.856	49.887	29.167
MGCN	10.628	5.535	5.348	9.46	7.718	12.284	19.79
MGCN_R	**4.278**	**4.426**	**3.437**	**6.989**	**3.610**	**7.923**	**7.224**

Note that LA and SA represent for long- and short-axis measurements. KL, KT, LL, SL, and ST stand for Kidney Long, Kidney Trans, Liver Long, Spleen Long, and Spleen Trans, respectively. For the methods, the prefix S and M represent single-task and multi-task, respectively, while FCN and GCN are both based on ResNet50 except that the later embeds large kernels and boundary refinement in skip connection. MGCN_R is the proposed method that includes two additional regularization modules. PBT is a traditional machine learning approach. The human statistics are computed on a subset of images for reference.

with the multi-decoder design. View classification, on the other hand, is less compatible with the landmark detection tasks; there are also additional views involved. However, it still benefits from sharing the low level features. The classification accuracy gets improved by combining these shared low level features with the high level features learned by the view classification individually.

Disclaimer: This feature is based on research, and is not commercially available. Due to regulatory reasons its future availability cannot be guaranteed.

References

1. Peery, A.F., et al.: Burden of gastrointestinal disease in the united states: 2012 update. Gastroenterology **143**(5), 1179–1187 (2012)
2. Ronneberger, O., Fischer, P., Brox, T.: U-Net: convolutional networks for biomedical image segmentation. In: Navab, N., Hornegger, J., Wells, W.M., Frangi, A.F. (eds.) MICCAI 2015. LNCS, vol. 9351, pp. 234–241. Springer, Cham (2015). https://doi.org/10.1007/978-3-319-24574-4_28
3. Kokkinos, I.: Ubernet: training a universal convolutional neural network for low-, mid-, and high-level vision using diverse datasets and limited memory. In: CVPR, pp. 6129–6138 (2017)
4. Ranjan, R., et al.: An all-in-one convolutional neural network for face analysis. In: 2017 12th IEEE International Conference on Automatic Face & Gesture Recognition (FG 2017), pp. 17–24. IEEE (2017)
5. Xue, W., Lum, A., Mercado, A., Landis, M., Warrington, J., Li, S.: Full quantification of left ventricle via deep multitask learning network respecting intra- and inter-task relatedness. In: Descoteaux, M., Maier-Hein, L., Franz, A., Jannin, P., Collins, D.L., Duchesne, S. (eds.) MICCAI 2017. LNCS, vol. 10435, pp. 276–284. Springer, Cham (2017). https://doi.org/10.1007/978-3-319-66179-7_32

6. Moeskops, P., et al.: Deep learning for multi-task medical image segmentation in multiple modalities. In: Ourselin, S., Joskowicz, L., Sabuncu, M.R., Unal, G., Wells, W. (eds.) MICCAI 2016. LNCS, vol. 9901, pp. 478–486. Springer, Cham (2016). https://doi.org/10.1007/978-3-319-46723-8_55

7. He, K., et al.: Deep residual learning for image recognition. In: CPVR, pp. 770–778 (2016)

8. Long, J., et al.: Fully convolutional networks for semantic segmentation. In: CVPR, pp. 3431–3440 (2015)

9. Peng, C., et al.: Large kernel matters-improve semantic segmentation by global convolutional network. In: CVPR, pp. 4353–4361 (2017)

10. Isola, P., et al.: Image-to-image translation with conditional adversarial networks. In: CVPR, pp. 1125–1134 (2017)

11. Russakovsky, O.: Imagenet large scale visual recognition challenge. Int. J. Comput. Vis. **115**(3), 211–252 (2015)

12. Tu, Z.: Probabilistic boosting-tree: Learning discriminative models for classification, recognition, and clustering. In: ICCV, vol. 2, pp. 1589–1596. IEEE (2005)

Cardiac, Chest and Abdominal Applications: Lung Imaging Applications

Deep Active Self-paced Learning for Accurate Pulmonary Nodule Segmentation

Wenzhe Wang[1], Yifei Lu[1], Bian Wu[2], Tingting Chen[1], Danny Z. Chen[3], and Jian Wu[1(✉)]

[1] College of Computer Science and Technology, Zhejiang University,
Hangzhou 310027, China
`wujian2000@zju.edu.cn`
[2] Data Science and AI Lab, WeDoctor Group Limited, Hangzhou 311200, China
[3] Department of Computer Science and Engineering, University of Notre Dame,
Notre Dame, IN 46556, USA

Abstract. Automatic and accurate pulmonary nodule segmentation in lung Computed Tomography (CT) volumes plays an important role in computer-aided diagnosis of lung cancer. However, this task is challenging due to target/background voxel imbalance and the lack of voxel-level annotation. In this paper, we propose a novel deep region-based network, called Nodule R-CNN, for efficiently detecting pulmonary nodules in 3D CT images while simultaneously generating a segmentation mask for each instance. Also, we propose a novel Deep Active Self-paced Learning (DASL) strategy to reduce annotation effort and also make use of unannotated samples, based on a combination of Active Learning and Self-Paced Learning (SPL) schemes. Experimental results on the public LIDC-IDRI dataset show our Nodule R-CNN achieves state-of-the-art results on pulmonary nodule segmentation, and Nodule R-CNN trained with the DASL strategy performs much better than Nodule R-CNN trained without DASL using the same amount of annotated samples.

1 Introduction

Lung cancer is one of the most life-threatening malignancies. A pulmonary nodule is a small growth in the lung which has the risk of being a site of cancerous tissue. The boundaries of pulmonary nodules have been regarded as a vital criterion for lung cancer analysis [1], and lung Computed Tomography (CT) is one of the most common methods for examining the presence and boundary features of pulmonary nodules. Automated segmentation of pulmonary nodules in CT volumes will promote early diagnosis of lung cancer by reducing the need for expensive human expertise.

Deep learning has become a powerful tool for a variety of medical imaging applications. However, to achieve good performance on 3D image segmentation, sufficient voxel-level annotations are commonly needed to train a deep

© Springer Nature Switzerland AG 2018
A. F. Frangi et al. (Eds.): MICCAI 2018, LNCS 11071, pp. 723–731, 2018.
https://doi.org/10.1007/978-3-030-00934-2_80

network, which is both time-consuming and costly to obtain. As an effort to tackle this predicament, recent studies [2,3] conducted pulmonary nodule segmentation using weakly labeled data. However, restricted by rough annotations in lung CT volumes, these methods did not perform very well, usually producing rough boundary segmentation of pulmonary nodules and incurring considerable false positives. On the other hand, a deep active learning framework [4] was proposed to annotate samples during network training. Although being able to make good use of fully-annotated samples, this approach did not utilize abundant unannotated samples in model training.

In this paper, we propose a novel deep region-based network, called Nodule R-CNN, for volumetric instance-level segmentation in lung CT volumes, and a novel Deep Active Self-paced Learning (DASL) strategy to reduce annotation effort based on bootstrapping [4,5]. Due to the sparse distribution of pulmonary nodules in CT volumes [6], employing 3D fully convolutional networks (e.g., [7,8]) to semantically segment them may suffer the class imbalance issue. Built on 3D image segmentation work [8,9] and Mask R-CNN [10], our 3D region-based network provides an effective way for pulmonary nodule segmentation. Further, to alleviate the lack of fully-annotated samples and make use of unannotated samples, we propose a novel DASL strategy to improve our Nodule R-CNN by combining Active Learning (AL) [11] and Self-Paced Learning (SPL) [12] schemes. To our best knowledge, this is the first work on pulmonary nodule instance segmentation in 3D images, and the first work to train 3D CNNs using both AL and SPL.

Figure 1 outlines the main steps of our framework. Starting with annotated samples, we train our Nodule R-CNN, and use it to predict on unannotated samples. After ranking the confidence and uncertainty of each test sample, we utilize high-confidence and high-uncertainty samples in self-paced and active annotation learning [13], respectively, and add them to the training set to fine-tune Nodule R-CNN. The testing and fine-tuning of Nodule R-CNN repeat until Active Learning process is terminated.

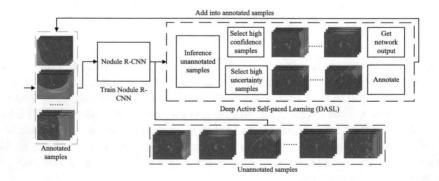

Fig. 1. Our weakly-supervised pulmonary nodule segmentation model.

Experimental results on the LIDC-IDRI dataset [6] show (1) our Nodule R-CNN can achieve state-of-the-art pulmonary nodule segmentation performance, and (2) our weakly-supervised segmentation approach is more effective than common fully supervised methods [3] and other weakly labeled methods [2,3].

2   Method

Our framework consists of two major components: (1) a novel region-based network (Nodule R-CNN) for pulmonary nodule instance segmentation; (2) a Deep Active Self-paced Learning (DASL) strategy for 3D CNN training.

2.1   Nodule R-CNN

Building on recent advances of convolutional neural networks such as Region Proposal Networks (RPN) [14], Feature Pyramid Networks (FPN) [15], Mask R-CNN [10], and DenseNet [16], we develop a novel deep region-based network for pulmonary nodule instance segmentation in 3D CT images.

Figure 2 illustrates the detailed architecture of our proposed Nodule R-CNN. Like Mask R-CNN [10], our network has a convolutional backbone architecture for feature extraction, a detection branch that outputs class labels and bounding-box offsets, and a mask branch that outputs object masks. In our backbone network, we extract diverse features in different levels by exploring an FPN-like architecture, which is a top-down architecture with lateral connections to build an in-network feature pyramid from a single-scale input. Three 3D DenseBlocks [9] with a growth rate 12 are used to ease network training by preserving maximum information flow between layers and to avoid learning redundant feature maps by encouraging feature reuse. Deconvolution is adopted to ensure that the size of the feature map is consistent with the size of the input volume. Our model employs an RPN-like architecture to output classification results and bounding-box regression results. The architecture provides three anchors for each detected location. We use a patch-based training and testing strategy instead of using RoIAlign to extract feature maps from RoIs due to limited GPU memory. In the mask branch, we utilize RoIPool to extract a small feature map from each RoI, and a Fully Convolutional Network (FCN) to generate the final label map of pulmonary nodule segmentation. In the final label map, the value of each voxel a represents the probability of a being a voxel of a pulmonary nodule.

We define a multi-task loss on each sampled RoI as $L = L_{cls} + L_{box} + L_{mask}$, where the classification loss L_{cls} and the bounding-box loss L_{box} are defined as in [17]. We define our segmentation loss L_{mask} as Dice loss (since the output of the models trained with Dice loss is almost binary, it appears visually cleaner [8,18]). Specifically, the Dice loss is defined as:

$$L_{Dice} = -\frac{2\sum_i p_i y_i}{\sum_i p_i + \sum_i y_i},\tag{1}$$

where $p_i \in [0,1]$ is the i-th output of the last layer in the mask branch passed through a sigmoid non-linearity and $y_i \in \{0,1\}$ is the corresponding label.

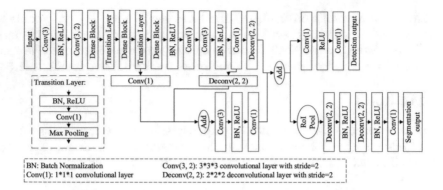

Fig. 2. The detailed architecture of our Nodule R-CNN.

2.2   The Deep Active Self-paced Learning Strategy

Active Learning Scheme. Active Learning attempts to overcome the annotation bottleneck by querying the most confusing unannotated instances for
further annotation [11]. Different from [4] which applied a set of FCNs for confusing sample selection, we utilize a straightforward strategy to select confusing
samples during model training. To do so, a common approach is to calculate the
uncertainty of each unannotated sample, and filtrate the most uncertain ones.
The calculation of uncertainty is defined as:

$$U_d = \frac{1}{n} \sum_{i=1}^{n} (1 - \max(p_i, 1 - p_i)), \tag{2}$$

where U_d denotes the uncertainty of the d-th sample and n denotes the voxel
number of the d-th sample.

Note that the initial training set is often too small to cover the entire population distribution. Thus, there are usually a lot of samples which a deep learning
model is not (yet) trained with. It is not advisable to extensively annotate those
samples of similar patterns in one iteration. As in [4], we use cosine similarity to
estimate the similarity between volumes. Therefore, the uncertainty of the d-th
volume is defined as:

$$U_d = \frac{1}{n} \sum_{i=1}^{n} (1 - \max(p_i, 1 - p_i)) \times \left(\frac{\sum_{j=1}^{D} \text{sim}(P_d, P_j) - 1}{D - 1} \right)^{\beta}, \tag{3}$$

where D denotes the number of unannotated volumes, sim() denotes cosine similarity, P_d and P_j denote the output of the d-th and j-th volumes, respectively,
and β is a hyper-parameter that controls the relative importance of the similarity term. Note that when $\beta = 0$, this definition degenerates to the *least confident*
uncertainty as defined in Eq. (2). We set $\beta = 1$ in our experiments.

In each iteration, after acquiring the uncertainty of each unannotated sample,
we select the top N samples for annotation and add them to the training set for
further fine-tuning.

Self-paced Learning Scheme. Self-Paced Learning (SPL) was inspired by the learning process of humans/animals that gradually incorporates easy-to-hard samples into training [12]. It utilizes unannotated samples by considering both prior knowledge known before training and the learning progress made during training [13].

Formally, let $L(\mathbf{w}; \mathbf{x}_i, p_i)$ denote the loss function of Nodule R-CNN, where $\mathbf{w}$ denotes the model parameters inside the model, $\mathbf{x}_i$ and p_i denote the input and output of the model, respectively. SPL aims to optimize the following function:

$$\min_{\mathbf{w}, \mathbf{v} \in [0,1]^n} \mathbb{E}(\mathbf{w}, \mathbf{v}; \lambda, \Psi) = C \sum_{i=1}^{n} v_i L(\mathbf{w}; \mathbf{x}_i, p_i) + f(\mathbf{v}; \lambda), \quad s.t. \quad \mathbf{v} \in \Psi \qquad (4)$$

where $\mathbf{v} = [v_1, v_2, \ldots, v_n]^T$ denotes the weight variables reflecting the samples' confidence, $f(\mathbf{v}; \lambda)$ is a self-paced regularization term that controls the learning scheme, λ is a parameter for controlling the learning pace, Ψ is a feasible region that encodes the information of predetermined curriculum, and C is a standard regularization parameter for the trade-off of the loss function and the margin. We set $C = 1$ in our experiments.

Note that a self-paced function should satisfy three conditions [19]. (1) $f(\mathbf{v}; \lambda)$ is convex with respect to $\mathbf{v} \in [0,1]^n$. (2) The optimal weight of each sample v_i^* should be monotonically decreasing with respect to its corresponding loss l_i. (3) $\|\mathbf{v}\|_1 = \sum_{i=1}^{n} v_i$ should be monotonically increasing with respect to λ.

To linearly discriminate the samples with their losses, the regularization function of our learning scheme is defined as follows [19]:

$$f(\mathbf{v}; \lambda) = \lambda \left(\frac{1}{2} \|\mathbf{v}\|_2^2 - \sum_{i=1}^{n} v_i \right), \qquad (5)$$

With $\Psi = [0,1]^n$, the partial gradient of Eq. (4) using our learning scheme is equal to

$$\frac{\partial \mathbb{E}}{\partial v_i} = Cl_i + v_i \lambda - \lambda = 0, \qquad (6)$$

where $\mathbb{E}$ denotes the objective in Eq. (4) with a fixed $\mathbf{w}$, and l_i denotes the loss of the i-th sample. The optimal solution for $\mathbb{E}$ is given by Eq. (8) below. Note that since the labels of unannotated samples are unknown, it is challenging to calculate their losses. We allocate each "pseudo-label" by Eq. (7).

$$y_i^* = \operatorname*{argmin}_{y_i = \{0,1\}} l_i, \qquad (7)$$

$$v_i^* = \begin{cases} 1 - \dfrac{Cl_i}{\lambda}, & Cl_i < \lambda \\ 0, & \text{otherwise,} \end{cases} \qquad (8)$$

For pace parameter updating, we set the initial pace as λ^0. For the t-th iteration, we compute the pace parameter λ^t as follows:

$$\lambda^t = \begin{cases} \lambda^0, & t = 0 \\ \lambda^{(t-1)} + \alpha \times \eta^t, & 1 \le t < \tau \\ \lambda^{(t-1)}, & t \ge \tau, \end{cases} \tag{9}$$

where α is a hyper-parameter that controls the pace increasing rate, η^t is the average accuracy in the current iteration, and τ is a hyper-parameter for controlling the pace update. Note that based on the third condition defined above, $\|\mathbf{v}\|_1 = \sum_{i=1}^n v_i$ should be monotonically increasing with respect to λ. Since $\mathbf{v} \in [0,1]^n$, the updating of the parameter λ should be stopped after a few iterations. Thus, we introduce the hyper-parameter τ to control the pace updating.

3   Experiments and Results

We evaluate our proposed approach using the LIDC-IDRI dataset [6]. Our experimental results are given in Table 1.

The LIDC-IDRI dataset contains 1010 CT scans (see [6] for more details of this dataset). In our experiments, all nodules are used except those with a diameter < 3mm, and each scan is resized to $512 \times 512 \times 512$ voxels by linear interpolation. The inputs of our model are 3D patches in the size of $128 \times 128 \times 128$ voxels, which are cropped from CT volumes. 70% of the input patches contain at least one nodule. For this part of the inputs, segmentation masks are cropped to $32 \times 32 \times 32$ voxels with nodules centering in them. We obtain the rest of the inputs by randomly cropping scans that very likely contain no nodule. The output size of the detection branch is $32 \times 32 \times 32 \times 3 \times 5$, where the second last dimension represents 3 anchors and the last dimension corresponds to the classification results and bounding-box regression results. In our experiments, 10% of the whole dataset are randomly selected as the validation set. We use a small subset of the remaining scans to train the initial Nodule R-CNN and the rest samples are gradually added to the training set during the DASL process.

First, we evaluate our Nodule R-CNN for pulmonary nodule instance segmentation. As shown in Table 1, its Dice achieves 0.64 and TP Dice (Dice over truly detected nodules) achieves 0.95, both of which are best results among state-of-the-art methods.

We then evaluate the combination of Nodule R-CNN and the DASL strategy. In our experiments, α is set to 0.002 and λ^0 is set to 0.005, due to the high confidence of positive prediction. To verify the relationship between AL and SPL in DASL, we use a sequence of "SPL-AL-SPL" to fine-tune Nodule R-CNN. To verify the impact of different amounts of initial annotated samples, we conduct three experiments with 50, 100, and 150 initial annotated samples, respectively. Figure 3 summarizes the results. We find that, in DASL, when using less initial annotated samples to train Nodule R-CNN, SPL tends to incorporate more unannotated samples. This makes sense since the model trained with less samples does not learn enough patterns and is likely to allocate high confidence to more unseen samples. One can see from Fig. 3 that although the amount of samples selected by AL is quite small ($N = 20$ in our experiments), AL does help achieve higher Dice. Experimental results are shown in Table 1. We find that more initial annotated samples bring better results, and the experiment with 150 initial annotated samples gives the best results among our experiments on DASL, which is comparable to the performance of Nodule R-CNN trained with all samples.

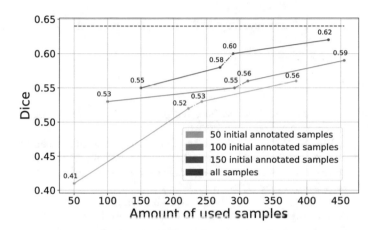

Fig. 3. Comparison using different amounts of initial annotated inputs for DASL: The solid lines are for the SPL process, the dotted lines are for the AL process, and the dashed line is for the current state-of-the-art result using full training samples.

Table 1. Results on the LIDC-IDRI dataset for pulmonary nodule segmentation.

Method	Dice mean ± SD	TP Dice mean ± SD
Method in [3]	0.55(±0.33)	0.74(±0.14)
Nodule R-CNN (full training samples)	**0.64(±0.44)**	**0.95(±0.12)**
Nodule R-CNN with DASL (50 initial annotated samples)	0.56(±0.45)	0.87(±0.09)
Nodule R-CNN with DASL (100 initial annotated samples)	0.59(±0.45)	0.90(±0.05)
Nodule R-CNN with DASL (150 initial annotated samples)	0.62(±0.43)	0.92(±0.03)

4   Conclusions

We have developed a novel Deep Active Self-paced Learning framework for pulmonary nodule instance segmentation in 3D CT images by combining our proposed Nodule R-CNN and Deep Active Self-paced Learning. Our new approach makes two main contributions: (1) A Nodule R-CNN model that attains state-of-the-art pulmonary nodule segmentation performance; (2) a weakly-supervised method that can make good use of annotation effort as well as information of unannotated samples.

Acknowledgement. The research of D.Z. Chen was supported in part by NSF Grant CCF-1617735.

References

1. Gonçalves, L., Novo, J.: Hessian based approaches for 3D lung nodule segmentation. Expert Syst. Appl. **61**, 1–15 (2016)
2. Messay, T., Hardie, R.C.: Segmentation of pulmonary nodules in computed tomography using a regression neural network approach and its application to the lung image database consortium and image database resource initiative dataset. Med. Image Anal. **22**(1), 48–62 (2015)
3. Feng, X., Yang, J., et al.: Discriminative localization in CNNs for weakly-supervised segmentation of pulmonary nodules. In: MICCAI, pp. 568–576 (2017)
4. Yang, L., Zhang, Y., et al.: Suggestive annotation: a deep active learning framework for biomedical image segmentation. In: MICCAI, pp. 399–407 (2017)
5. Li, X., Zhong, A., et al.: Self-paced convolutional neural network for computer aided detection in medical imaging analysis. In: International Workshop on Machine Learning in Medical Imaging, pp. 212–219 (2017)
6. Armato, S.G., McLennan, G.: The lung image database consortium (LIDC) and image database resource initiative (IDRI): a completed reference database of lung nodules on CT scans. Med. Phy. **38**(2), 915–931 (2011)
7. Çiçek, Ö., Abdulkadir, A., Lienkamp, S.S., Brox, T., Ronneberger, O.: 3D U-Net: learning dense volumetric segmentation from sparse annotation. In: Ourselin, S., Joskowicz, L., Sabuncu, M.R., Unal, G., Wells, W. (eds.) MICCAI 2016. LNCS, vol. 9901, pp. 424–432. Springer, Cham (2016). https://doi.org/10.1007/978-3-319-46723-8_49
8. Milletari, F., Navab, N., et al.: V-Net: fully convolutional neural networks for volumetric medical image segmentation. In: 4th IEEE International Conference on 3D Vision, pp. 565–571 (2016)
9. Yu, L., et al.: Automatic 3D cardiovascular MR segmentation with densely-connected volumetric convnets. In: Descoteaux, M., Maier-Hein, L., Franz, A., Jannin, P., Collins, D.L., Duchesne, S. (eds.) MICCAI 2017. LNCS, vol. 10434, pp. 287–295. Springer, Cham (2017). https://doi.org/10.1007/978-3-319-66185-8_33
10. He, K., Gkioxari, G., et al.: Mask R-CNN. In: ICCV, pp. 2980–2988 (2017)
11. Settles, B.: Active learning literature survey. Computer Sciences Technical Report 1648, University of Wisconsin - Madison (2009)
12. Kumar, M.P., Packer, B., et al.: Self-paced learning for latent variable models. In: NIPS, pp. 1189–1197 (2010)

13. Lin, L., Wang, K., et al.: Active self-paced learning for cost-effective and progressive face identification. IEEE TPAMI **40**(1), 7–19 (2018)
14. Ren, S., He, K., et al.: Faster R-CNN: towards real-time object detection with region proposal networks. In: NIPS, pp. 91–99 (2015)
15. Lin, T.Y., Dollár, P., et al.: Feature pyramid networks for object detection. In: CVPR, vol. 1, p. 4 (2017)
16. Huang, G., Liu, Z., et al.: Densely connected convolutional networks. In: CVPR, vol. 1, p. 3 (2017)
17. Girshick, R.: Fast R-CNN. In: ICCV, pp. 1440–1448 (2015)
18. Drozdzal, M., Vorontsov, E., et al.: The importance of skip connections in biomedical image segmentation. In: Deep Learning and Data Labeling for Medical Applications, pp. 179–187 (2016)
19. Jiang, L., Meng, D.: Self-paced curriculum learning. In: AAAI, vol. 2, p. 6 (2015)

CT-Realistic Lung Nodule Simulation from 3D Conditional Generative Adversarial Networks for Robust Lung Segmentation

Dakai Jin, Ziyue Xu[(✉)], Youbao Tang, Adam P. Harrison,
and Daniel J. Mollura

National Institutes of Health, Bethesda, MD, USA
ziyue.xu@nih.gov

Abstract. Data availability plays a critical role for the performance of deep learning systems. This challenge is especially acute within the medical image domain, particularly when pathologies are involved, due to two factors: (1) limited number of cases, and (2) large variations in location, scale, and appearance. In this work, we investigate whether augmenting a dataset with artificially generated lung nodules can improve the robustness of the progressive holistically nested network (P-HNN) model for pathological lung segmentation of CT scans. To achieve this goal, we develop a 3D generative adversarial network (GAN) that effectively learns lung nodule property distributions in 3D space. In order to embed the nodules within their background context, we condition the GAN based on a volume of interest whose central part containing the nodule has been erased. To further improve realism and blending with the background, we propose a novel multi-mask reconstruction loss. We train our method on over 1000 nodules from the LIDC dataset. Qualitative results demonstrate the effectiveness of our method compared to the state-of-art. We then use our GAN to generate simulated training images where nodules lie on the lung border, which are cases where the published P-HNN model struggles. Qualitative and quantitative results demonstrate that armed with these simulated images, the P-HNN model learns to better segment lung regions under these challenging situations. As a result, our system provides a promising means to help overcome the data paucity that commonly afflicts medical imaging.

Keywords: Lung nodule · CT · GAN · Dataset bottleneck
Lung segmentation

Z. Xu—This work is supported by NIH Intramural Research. We also thank NVidia for the donation of a Tesla K40 GPU.

© Springer Nature Switzerland AG 2018
A. F. Frangi et al. (Eds.): MICCAI 2018, LNCS 11071, pp. 732–740, 2018.
https://doi.org/10.1007/978-3-030-00934-2_81

1   Introduction

Deep learning has achieved significant recent successes. However, large amounts of training samples, which sufficiently cover the population diversity, are often necessary to produce high quality results. Unfortunately, data availability in the medical image domain, especially when pathologies are involved, is quite limited due to several reasons: significant image acquisition costs, protections on sensitive patient information, limited numbers of disease cases, difficulties in data labeling, and large variations in locations, scales, and appearances. Although efforts have been made towards constructing large medical image datasets, options are limited beyond using simple automatic methods [8], huge amounts of radiologist labor [1], or mining from radiologist reports [14]. Thus, it is still an open question on how to generate effective and sufficient medical data samples with limited or no expert-intervention.

One enticing alternative is to generate synthetic training data. However, historically synthetic data is less desirable due to shortcomings in realistically simulating true cases. Yet, the advent of generative adversarial networks (GANs) [4] has made game-changing strides in simulating real images and data. This ability has been further expanded with developments on fully convolutional [13] and conditional [10] GANs. In particular, Isola *et al.* extend the conditional GAN (CGAN) concept to predict pixels from known pixels [6]. Within medical imaging, Nie *et al.* use a GAN to simulate CT slices from MRI data [11], whereas Wolterink *et al.* introduce a bi-directional CT/MRI generator [15]. For lung nodules, Chuquicusma *et al.* train a simple GAN to generate simulated images from random noise vectors, but do not condition based on surrounding context [2].

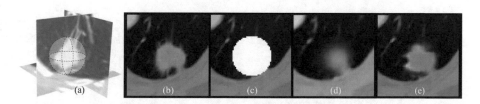

Fig. 1. Lung nodule simulation using the 3D CGAN. (a) A VOI centered at a lung nodule; (b) 2D axial view of (a); (c) same as (b), but with central sphere region erased; (d-e) simulated lung nodule using a plain $L1$ reconstruction loss and the 3D CGAN with multi-mask $L1$ loss coupled with adversarial loss, respectively.

In this work, we explore using CGAN to augment training data for specific tasks. For this work, we focus on pathological lung segmentation, where the recent progressive holistically nested network (P-HNN) has demonstrated state of the art results [5]. However, P-HNN can struggle when there are relatively large (*e.g.*, >5 mm) peripheral nodules touching the lung boundary. This is mainly because these types of nodule are not common in Harrison *et al.*'s [5] training set. To improve P-HNN's robustness, we generate synthetic 3D lung nodules of different sizes and appearances, at multiple locations, that naturally blend with surrounding tissues (see Fig. 1 for an illustration). We develop a 3D CGAN model that learns nodule shape and appearance distributions directly in 3D space. For the generator, we use a U-Net-like [3] structure, where the input to our CGAN is a volume of interest (VOI) cropped from the original CT image with the central part, containing the nodule, erased (Fig. 1(c)). We note that filling in this region with a realistic nodule faces challenges different than generating a random 2D nodule image from scratch [2]. Our CGAN must generate realistic and natural 3D nodules conditioned upon and consistent with the surrounding tissue information. To produce high quality nodule images and ensure their natural blending with surrounding lung tissues, we propose a specific multi-mask reconstruction loss that complements the adversarial loss.

The main contributions of this work are: (1) we formulate lung nodule generation using a 3D GAN conditioned on surrounding lung tissues; (2) we design a new multi-mask reconstruction loss to generate high quality realistic nodules alleviating boundary discontinuity artifacts; (3) we provide a feasible way to help overcome difficulties in obtaining data for "edge cases" in medical images; and (4) we demonstrate that GAN-synthetized data can improve training of a discriminative model, in this case for segmenting pathological lungs using P-HNN [5].

2   Methods

Figure 2 depicts an overview of our method. Below, we outline the CGAN formulation, architecture, and training strategy used to generate realistic lung nodules.

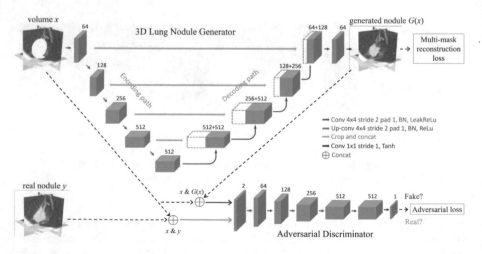

Fig. 2. 3D CGAN architecture for lung nodule generation. The input is the original CT VOI, y, containing a real nodule and the same VOI, x, with the central region erased. Channel numbers are placed next to each feature map.

2.1   CGAN Formulation

In their original formulation, GANs [4] are generative models that learn a mapping from a random noise vector z to an output image y. The generator, G, tries to produce outputs that fool a binary classifier discriminator D, which aims to distinguish real data from generated "fake" outputs. In our work, the goal is to generate synthetic 3D lung nodules of different sizes, with various appearances, at multiple locations, and have them naturally blend with surrounding lung tissues. For this purpose, we use a CGAN conditioned on the image x, which is a 3D CT VOI cropped from a specific lung location. Importantly, as shown in Fig. 1(c), we erase the central region containing the nodule. The advantage of this conditional setting is that the generator not only learns the distribution of nodule properties from its surrounding context, but it also forces the generated nodules to naturally fuse with the background context. While it is possible to also condition on the random vector z, we found it hampered performance. Instead, like Isola *et al.* [6], we use dropout to inject randomness into the generator.

The adversarial loss for CGANs can then be expressed as

$$L_{CGAN}(G, D) = \mathrm{E}_{x,y}[\log D(x, y)] + \mathrm{E}_x[\log (1 - D(x, G(x)))], \qquad (1)$$

where y is the original VOI and G tries to minimize this objective against an adversarial discriminator, D, that tries to maximize it. Like others [6,12], we also observe that an additional reconstruction loss is beneficial, as it provides a means to learn the latent representation from surrounding context to recover the missing region. However, reconstruction losses tend to produce blurred results because it tends to average together multiple modes in the data distribution [6]. Therefore, we combine the reconstruction and adversarial loss together, making the former responsible for capturing the overall structure of the missing region while the latter learns to pick specific data modes based on the context. We use the $L1$ loss, since the $L2$ loss performed poorly in our experiments.

Since the generator is meant to learn the distribution of nodule appearances in the erased region, it is intuitive to apply $L1$ loss only to this region. However, completely ignoring surrounding regions during generator's training can produce discontinuities between generated nodules and the background. Thus, to increase coherence we use a new multi-mask $L1$ loss. Formally, let M be the binary mask where the erased region is filled with 1's. Let N be a dilated version of M. Then, we assign a higher $L1$ loss weight to voxels where $N - M$ is equal to one:

$$L_{L1}(G) = \mathrm{E}_{x,y}[M \odot \|y - G(x)\|_1] + \alpha \mathrm{E}_{x,y}[(N - M) \odot \|y - G(x)\|_1], \qquad (2)$$

where $\odot$ is the element-wise multiplication operation and $\alpha >= 1$ is a weight factor. We find that a dilation of 3 to 6 voxels generally works well. By adding the specific multi-mask $L1$ loss, our final CGAN objective is

$$G^* = \arg \min_G \max_D L_{CGAN}(G, D) + \lambda L_{L1}(G), \qquad (3)$$

where α and λ are determined experimentally. We empirically find $\alpha = 5$ and $\lambda = 100$ works well in our experiments.

2.2   3D CGAN Architecture

Figure 2 depicts our architecture, which builds off of Isola *et al.*'s 2D work [6], but extends it to 3D images. More specifically, the generator consists of an encoding path with 5 convolutional layers and a decoding path with another 5 deconvolutional layers where short-cut connections are added in a similar fashion to U-net [3]. The encoding path takes an input VOI x with missing regions and produces a latent feature representation, and the decoding path takes this feature representation and produces the erased nodule content. We find that without shortcut connections, our CGAN models do not converge, suggesting that they are important for information flow across the network and for handling fine-scale 3D structures, confirmed by others [7]. To inject randomness, we apply dropout on the first two convolutional layers in the decoding path.

The discriminator also contains an encoding path with 5 convolutional layers. We also follow the design principles of Radford *et al.* [13] to increase training stability, which includes strided convolutions instead of pooling operations, LeakyReLu's in the encoding path of G and D, and a Tanh activation for the last output layer of G.

2.3   CGAN Optimization

We train the CGAN model end-to-end. To optimize our networks, we use the standard GAN training approach [4], which alternates between optimizing G and D, as we found this to be the most stable training regimen. As suggested by Goodfellow *et al.* [4], we train G to maximize $\log D(x, G(x))$ rather than minimize $\log(1 - D(x, G(x)))$. Training employs the Adam optimizer [9] with a learning rate 0.0001 and momentum parameters $\beta_1 = 0.5$ and $\beta_2 = 0.999$ for both the generator and discriminator.

3   Experiments and Results

We first validate our CGAN using the LIDC dataset [1]. Then, using artificially generated nodules, we test if they can help fine-tune the state-of-the-art P-HNN pathological lung segmentation method [5].

3.1   3D CGAN Performance

The LIDC dataset contains 1018 chest CT scans of patients with observed lung nodules, totaling roughly 2000 nodules. Out of these, we set aside 22 patients and their 34 accompanying nodules as a test set. For each nodule, there can be multiple radiologist readers, and we use the union of the masks for such cases. True nodule images, y, are generated by cropping cubic VOIs centered at each nodule with 3 random scales between 2 and 2.5 times larger than the maximum dimension of the nodule mask. All VOIs are then resampled to a fixed size of $64 \times 64 \times 64$. Conditional images, x, are derived by erasing the pixels within a sphere of diameter 32 centered at the VOI. We exclude nodules whose diameter is less than 5 mm, since small nodules provide very limited contextual information after resampling and our goal is to generate relatively large nodules. This results in roughly 4300 training sample pairs. We train the cGAN for 12 epochs.

We tested against three variants of our method: (1) only using an all-image $L1$ loss; (2) using both the adversarial and all-image $L1$ loss. This is identical to Isola *et al.*'s approach [6], except extended to 3D; (3) using the same combined objective in (3), but not using the multi-mask version, *i.e.*, only using the first term of equation (2). As reconstruction quality hinges on subjective assessment [6], we visually examine nodule generation on our test set. Selected examples are shown in Fig. 3. As can be seen, our proposed CGAN produces realistic nodules of high quality with various shapes and appearances that naturally blend with surrounding tissues, such as vessels, soft tissue, and parenchyma. In contrast, when only using the reconstruction $L1$ loss, results are considerably blurred with very limited variations in shape and appearance. Results from Isola *et al.*'s method [6] improve upon the $L1$ only loss; however, it has obvious inconsistencies/misalignments with the surrounding tissues and undesired sampling artifacts that appear inside the nodules. It is possible that by forcing the generator to reconstruct the entire image, it distracts the generator from learning the nodule appearance distribution. Finally, when only performing the $L1$ loss on the erased region, the artifacts seen in Isola *et al.*'s are not exhibited; however, there are stronger border artifacts between the M region and the rest of the VOI. In contrast, by incorporating a multi-mask loss, our method can produce nodules with realistic interiors and without such border artifacts.

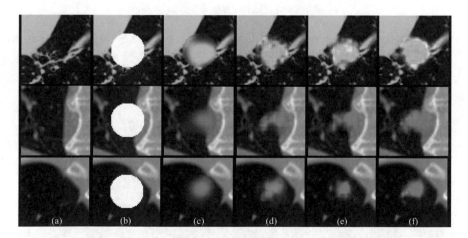

Fig. 3. Examples results: (a) original images; (b) input after central region erased; (c) only $L1$ loss, applied to the entire image; (d) Isola *et al.*'s method [6]; (e) CGAN with $L1$ loss, applied only to the erased region; (f) our CGAN with multi-mask $L1$ loss.

3.2   Improving Pathological Lung Segmentation

With the CGAN trained, we test whether our CGAN benefits pathological lung segmentation. In particular, the P-HNN model shared by Harrison *et al.* [5] can struggle when peripheral nodules touch the lung boundary, as these were not well represented in their training set. Prior to any performed experiments, we selected 34 images from the LIDC dataset exhibiting such peripheral nodules. Then, we randomly chose 42 LIDC subjects from relatively healthy subjects with no large nodules. For each of these, we pick 30 random VOI locations, centering within (8,20)mm to the lung boundary with random size ranging (32, 80)mm. VOIs are resampled to $64 \times 64 \times 64$ voxels and simulated lung nodules are generated in each VOI, using the same process as in Sect. 3.1, except the trained CGAN is only used for inference. The resulting VOIs are resampled back to their original resolution and pasted back to the original LIDC images, and then the axial slices containing the simulated nodules are used as training data ($\sim$10000 slices) to fine-tune the P-HNN model for 4–5 epochs. For comparison, we also fine-tune P-HNN using images generated by the $L1$-only loss and also Isola *et al.*'s CGAN.

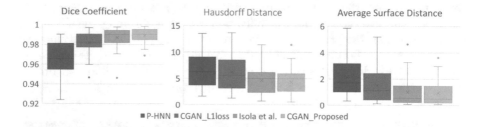

Fig. 4. Lung segmentation results on LIDC patients with peripheral lung nodules. All metrics are measured on a size 64 pixel VOI centered on the nodule.

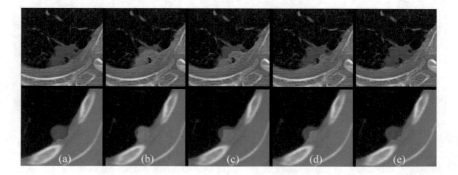

Fig. 5. Examples P-HNN lung segmentations. (a) ground truth; (b) original model; (c-e) fine-tuned with $L1$ loss only, Isola *et al.* [6], and proposed CGAN, respectively.

Figure 4 depicts quantitative results. First, as the chart demonstrates, fine-tuning using *all* CGAN variants improves P-HNN's performance on peripheral lung nodules. This confirms the value in using simulated data to augment training datasets. Moreover, the quality of nodules is also important, since the results using nodules generated by only an all-image $L1$ loss have the least improvement. Importantly, out of all alternatives, our proposed CGAN produces the greatest improvements in Dice scores, Hausdorff distances and average surface distances. For instance, our proposed CGAN allows P-HNN's mean Dice scores to improve from 0.964 to 0.989, and reduces the Hausdorff and average surface distance by 2.4 mm and 1.2 mm, respectively. In particular, worse case performance is also much better for our proposed system, showing it can help P-HNN deal with edge cases. In terms of visual quality, Fig. 5 depicts two examples. As these examples demonstrate, our proposed CGAN allows P-HNN to produce considerable improvements in segmentation mask quality at peripheral nodules, allowing it to overcome an important limitation.

4   Conclusion

We use a 3D CGAN, coupled with a novel multi-mask loss, to effectively generate CT-realistic high-quality lung nodules conditioned on a VOI with an erased central region. Our new multi-mask $L1$ loss ensures a natural blending of the generated nodules with the surrounding lung tissues. Tests demonstrate the superiority of our approach over three competitor CGANs on the LIDC dataset, including Isola *et al.*'s state-of-the-art method [6]. We further use our proposed CGAN to generate a fine-tuning dataset for the published P-HNN model [5], which can struggle when encountering lung nodules adjoining the lung boundary. Armed with our CGAN images, P-HNN is much better able to capture the true lung boundaries compared to both its original state and when it is fine-tuned using the other CGAN variants. As such, our CGAN approach can provide an effective and generic means to help overcome the dataset bottleneck commonly encountered within medical imaging.

References

1. Armato, S.G., McLennan, G., Bidaut, L.: The lung image database consortium (LIDC) and image database resource initiative (IDRI): a completed reference database of lung nodules on ct scans. Med. Phy. **38**(2), 915–931 (2011)
2. Chuquicusma, M.J., Hussein, S., Burt, J., Bagci, U.: How to fool radiologists with generative adversarial networks? a visual turing test for lung cancer diagnosis. In: Proceedings of IEEE ISBI, pp. 240–244 (2017)
3. Çiçek, Ö., Abdulkadir, A., Lienkamp, S.S., Brox, T., Ronneberger, O.: 3D U-Net: learning dense volumetric segmentation from sparse annotation. In: Ourselin, S., Joskowicz, L., Sabuncu, M.R., Unal, G., Wells, W. (eds.) MICCAI 2016. LNCS, vol. 9901, pp. 424–432. Springer, Cham (2016). https://doi.org/10.1007/978-3-319-46723-8_49

4. Goodfellow, I., Pouget-Abadie, J., Mirza, M., et al.: Generative adversarial nets. In: Advances in Neural Information Processing Systems, pp. 2672–2680 (2014)
5. Harrison, A.P., Xu, Z., George, K., Lu, L., Summers, R.M., Mollura, D.J.: Progressive and multi-path holistically nested neural networks for pathological lung segmentation from CT images. In: Descoteaux, M., Maier-Hein, L., Franz, A., Jannin, P., Collins, D.L., Duchesne, S. (eds.) MICCAI 2017. LNCS, vol. 10435, pp. 621–629. Springer, Cham (2017). https://doi.org/10.1007/978-3-319-66179-7_71
6. Isola, P., Zhu, J.Y., Zhou, T., Efros, A.A.: Image-to-image translation with conditional adversarial networks. In: Proceedings of IEEE CVPR, pp. 1125–1134 (2017)
7. Jin, D., Xu, Z., Harrison, A.P., George, K., Mollura, D.J.: 3D convolutional neural networks with graph refinement for airway segmentation using incomplete data labels. In: Wang, Q., Shi, Y., Suk, H.-I., Suzuki, K. (eds.) MLMI 2017. LNCS, vol. 10541, pp. 141–149. Springer, Cham (2017). https://doi.org/10.1007/978-3-319-67389-9_17
8. Karwoski, R.A., Bartholmai, B., Zavaletta, V.A., et al.: Processing of ct images for analysis of diffuse lung disease in the lung tissue research consortium. In: Proceedings of SPIE, vol. 6916 (2008)
9. Kingma, D.P., Ba, J.: Adam: a method for stochastic optimization. arXiv preprint arXiv:1412.6980 (2014)
10. Mirza, M., Osindero, S.: Conditional generative adversarial nets. arXiv preprint arXiv:1411.1784 (2014)
11. Nie, D., et al.: Medical image synthesis with context-aware generative adversarial networks. In: Descoteaux, M., Maier-Hein, L., Franz, A., Jannin, P., Collins, D.L., Duchesne, S. (eds.) MICCAI 2017. LNCS, vol. 10435, pp. 417–425. Springer, Cham (2017). https://doi.org/10.1007/978-3-319-66179-7_48
12. Pathak, D., Krahenbuhl, P., Donahue, J., et al.: Context encoders: Feature learning by inpainting. In: Proceedings of IEEE CVPR, pp. 2536–2544 (2016)
13. Radford, A., Metz, L., Chintala, S.: Unsupervised representation learning with deep convolutional generative adversarial networks. arXiv preprint arXiv:1511.06434 (2015)
14. Wang, X., Peng, Y., Lu, L., et al.: Chestx-ray8: Hospital-scale chest x-ray database and benchmarks on weakly-supervised classification and localization of common thorax diseases. In: Proceedings of IEEE CVPR, pp. 3462–3471 (2017)
15. Wolterink, J.M., Dinkla, A.M., Savenije, M.H.F., Seevinck, P.R., van den Berg, C.A.T., Išgum, I.: Deep MR to CT synthesis using unpaired data. In: Tsaftaris, S.A., Gooya, A., Frangi, A.F., Prince, J.L. (eds.) SASHIMI 2017. LNCS, vol. 10557, pp. 14–23. Springer, Cham (2017). https://doi.org/10.1007/978-3-319-68127-6_2

Fast CapsNet for Lung Cancer Screening

Aryan Mobiny and Hien Van Nguyen[✉]

Department of Electrical and Computer Engineering, University of Houston,
Houston, USA
hvnguy35@central.uh.edu

Abstract. Lung cancer is the leading cause of cancer-related deaths in
the past several years. A major challenge in lung cancer screening is
the detection of lung nodules from computed tomography (CT) scans.
State-of-the-art approaches in automated lung nodule classification use
deep convolutional neural networks (CNNs). However, these networks
require a large number of training samples to generalize well. This paper
investigates the use of capsule networks (CapsNets) as an alternative to
CNNs. We show that CapsNets significantly outperforms CNNs when
the number of training samples is small. To increase the computational
efficiency, our paper proposes a consistent dynamic routing mechanism
that results in 3× speedup of CapsNet. Finally, we show that the original
image reconstruction method of CapNets performs poorly on lung nodule
data. We propose an efficient alternative, called convolutional decoder,
that yields lower reconstruction error and higher classification accuracy.

1 Introduction

Lung cancer is consistently ranked as the leading cause of the cancer-related
deaths all around the world in the past several years, accounting for more than
one-quarter (26%) of all cancer-related deaths [1]. The stage at which diagnosis
is made largely determines the overall prognosis of the patient. The five-year
relative survival rate is over 50% in early-stage disease, while survival rates
drop to less than 5% for late-stage disease [1]. A major challenge in lung cancer
screening is the detection of lung nodules [2].

Convolutional neural networks (CNNs) [3,4] are the state-of-the-art methods
in lung nodule classification. However, CNNs have a number of important drawbacks mostly due to their procedure of routing data. Routing is the process of
relaying the information from one layer to another layer. CNNs perform routing
via pooling operations such as max-pooling and average-pooling. These pooling
operations discard information such as location and pose of the objects which
can be valuable for classification purposes.

Recently, Sabour et al. [5] introduced a new architecture, called Capsule
Network, to address CNNs' shortcomings. The idea is to encode the relative
relationships (e.g., locations, scales, orientations) between local parts and the
whole object. Encoding these relationships equips the model with a built-in

© Springer Nature Switzerland AG 2018
A. F. Frangi et al. (Eds.): MICCAI 2018, LNCS 11071, pp. 741–749, 2018.
https://doi.org/10.1007/978-3-030-00934-2_82

understanding of the 3D space. This enables CapsNet to recognize objects from different 3D views that were not seen in the training data.

CapsNets employ a dynamic routing mechanism to determine where to send the information. Sabour et al. [5] successfully used this algorithm for training the network on hand-written images of digits (MNIST) and achieved state-of-the-art performance. However, it remains unclear how CapsNets perform on medical image analysis tasks. In addition, the dynamic routing operations are computationally expensive making them significantly slower than other modern deep networks. This prevents the use of CapsNet for higher dimensional data such as 3D computed tomography (CT) scans. It is also unclear how CapsNet will compare to state-of-the-art methods on medical imaging tasks.

Motivated by these observations, this paper makes the following contributions: (i) We investigate the performance of CapsNet on 3D lung nodule classification task. We show that CapsNets compare favorably to CNNs when the training size is large, but significantly outperform CNNs for small size datasets. (ii) We propose a consistent dynamic routing mechanism to speed up CapsNets. The proposed network runs 3× faster than the original CapsNets on 3D lung data. (iii) We develop an efficient method, called convolutional decoder, that is more powerful in reconstructing the input from the final capsules. The proposed decoder serves as a regularizer to prevent over-fitting issue, and yields higher classification accuracy than the original CapsNets.

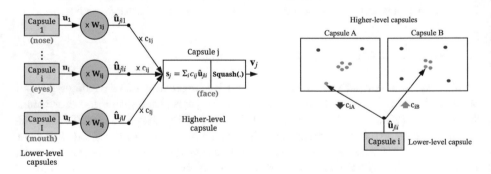

Fig. 1. Left: connections between the lower and higher-level capsules, **Right:** dynamic routing for sending information from a lower-level capsule to higher-level ones.

2   Capsule Network

Capsule Computation: In this architecture, a capsule is defined as a group of neurons (whose outputs form an *activation vector*). They predict the presence and the pose parameters of a particular object at a given pixel location. The direction of an activation vector captures the object's pose information, such as location and orientation, while the length (a.k.a norm or magnitude) of the activation vector represents the estimated probability that an object of interest exists. For instance, if we rotate an image, the activation vectors also change accordingly, but their lengths stay the same. Figure 1 illustrates the way CapsNets route the information from one layer to another layer, using face detection as an example. Lengths of the outputs of the lower-level capsules $(\mathbf{u}_1, \mathbf{u}_2, \ldots, \mathbf{u}_I)$ encode the existence probability of their corresponding entity (e.g. eyes, nose, and mouth). Directions of the vectors also encodes various properties of a particular entity, such as its size, orientation, position, etc.

The relationship between i-th capsule in a lower layer and j-th capsule in the next higher layer is encoded using a linear transformation matrix $\mathbf{W}_{ij}$. The information is propagated as: $\hat{\mathbf{u}}_{j|i} = \mathbf{W}_{ij}\mathbf{u}_i$. The vector $\hat{\mathbf{u}}_{ij}$ represents the belief of i-th capsule in a lower layer about j-th capsule in the higher layer. In our example, $\hat{\mathbf{u}}_{j|1}$ represents the predicted pose of the face according to the detected pose of the nose. During the training, the network will gradually learn a transformation matrix for each capsule pair to encode the corresponding part-whole relationship.

Dynamic Routing: Having computed the prediction vectors, the lower-level capsules then route their information to parent capsules that agree the most with their predictions. The mechanism that ensures that the outputs of the child capsules get sent to the proper parent capsules is named *Dynamic Routing*. Let c_{ij} denotes the routing coefficient from i-th capsule in the lower layer to j-th capsule in the higher layer, where $\sum_j c_{ij} = 1$ and $c_{ij} > 0$, $\forall j$. When $c_{ij} = 1$, all information from i-capsule will be sent to j-capsule, whereas when $c_{ij} = 0$, there is no information flowing between the two capsules. Dynamic routing method iteratively tunes the c_{ij} coefficients and routes the child capsules' outputs to the appropriate capsule in the next layer so that they get a cleaner input, thus determining the pose of the objects more accurately.

The right panel of Fig. 1 shows a lower-level capsule (e.g. nose capsule) making decision to send its output to the parent capsules. This decision is made by adjusting the routing coefficients, c_{ij}, that will be multiplied by the prediction vectors before sending it to high level capsules. CapsNets compute the parent capsules and routing coefficients as follows:

$$\mathbf{v}_j = \frac{||\mathbf{s}_j||^2}{1 + ||\mathbf{s}_j||^2} \frac{\mathbf{s}_j}{||\mathbf{s}_j||}, \quad \mathbf{s}_j = \sum_i c_{ij}\hat{\mathbf{u}}_{j|i}, \tag{1}$$

$$c_{ij} = \frac{\exp(b_{ij})}{\sum_k \exp(b_{ik})}, \quad b_{ij} \leftarrow b_{ij} + \hat{\mathbf{u}}_{j|i}.\mathbf{v}_j. \tag{2}$$

The output of each parent capsule $\mathbf{v}_j$ is computed as the weighted sum of all predictions from child capsules, then passed through a *squash* non-linearity. Squashing makes sure that the output vector has length no more than 1 (so that its length can be interpreted as the probability that a given feature being detected by the capsule) without changing its direction. Parent capsules receive predictions from all children. These vectors are represented by points in Fig. 1. The dynamic routing mechanism will increase the routing coefficient to j-parent capsule by a factor of $\hat{\mathbf{u}}_{j|i}.\mathbf{v}_j$. Thus a child capsule will send more information to the parent capsule whose output $\mathbf{v}_j$ is more similar to its prediction $\hat{\mathbf{u}}_{j|i}$.

Network Architecture: The network contains two main parts: *encoder* and *decoder*, depicted in the first two figures of [5]. The encoder contains three layers: two convolution and one fully-connected. The first layer is a standard convolution layer with 256 filters of size 9×9 and stride 1, followed by ReLU activation. The next layer is a convolutional capsule layer called the *PrimaryCaps* layer. Capsules are arranged in 32 channels where each primary capsule applies 8 convolutional filters of size 9×9 and stride 2 to the whole input volume. In this setting, all PrimaryCaps in each 32 channels share their weights with each other and each capsule outputs an 8-dimensional vector of activations. The last layer is called *DigitCaps* layer which has one 16D capsule per class. Routing takes place in between these capsules and all PrimaryCaps, encoding the input into 16-dimensional activation vector of instantiation parameters. The lengths of these prediction vectors are used to determine the predicted class.

The decoder tries to reconstruct the input from the final capsules, which will force the network to preserve as much information from the input as possible across the whole network. This effectively works as a regularizer that reduces the risk of over-fitting and helps generalize to new samples. In decoder, the 16D outputs of the final capsules are all masked out (set to zero) except for the ones corresponding to the target (while training) or predicted (while testing) class. They proposed using a three layer feed forward neural network with 512, 1024, and 784 units to reconstruct the input image.

3   Fast Capsule Network

Consistent Dynamic Routing: Dynamic routing has been showed to improve the classification accuracy of CapsNet [5]. However this operation is computationally expensive and does not scale well to high dimensional data, such as 3D CT scans with a large number of pixels. We propose a consistent dynamic routing mechanism to address this problem. Specifically, we enforce all capsules in the PrimaryCaps layer corresponding to the same pixels to have the same routing coefficients:

$$c_{ij} = c_{kj}, \quad \forall i, k \in \mathcal{S} = \{i, k \mid loc(i) = loc(k)\} \tag{3}$$

where $loc()$ is the function converting a capsule index to its pixel location. This strategy will dramatically reduce the number of routing coefficients. For example, the original CapsNet has 32 capsules for each pixel location in PrimaryCaps layer. The proposed method will therefore reduce the number of routing coefficients by a factor of 32. The iterative routing procedure is a bottleneck of CapsNets. Through reducing the number of routing operations, we expect to dramatically increase the network's efficiency. There are many possible ways to enforce the constraint in Eq. (3). In this paper, we use a simple strategy that allows only one capsule at each pixel location. To compensate for the reduction of number of capsules, we increase the dimension of each capsule to 256D instead of 8D as in the original CapsNet. Our results show that the proposed architecture achieves the similar classification accuracy, and is 3× faster than CapsNet.

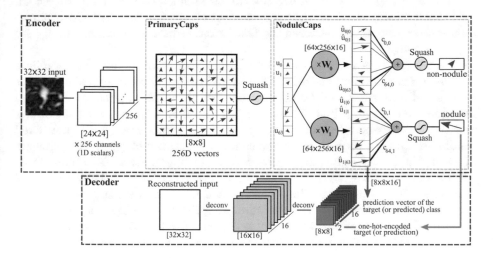

Fig. 2. Visual representation of Fast Capsule Network

Convolutional Decoder: CapsNet uses an additional reconstruction loss as a regularization to prevent over-fitting during learning the network's parameters [5]. This encourages the digit capsules to encode as much information from the input as possible. The reconstruction is done by feeding 16D output of the final capsules to a three-layer feed-forward neural network. Unfortunately, our experiments show that lung nodule data cannot be reconstructed well from the final capsules. This could be due to the high visual variability within the data. To this end, we propose a different reconstruction mechanism to serve as the training regularization. Instead of using the masked outputs of the NoduleCaps, we used the PrimaryCaps prediction vectors ($\hat{\mathbf{u}}_{j|i}$) only for the target (or predicted) class. For the example in Fig. 2, it is $8 \times 8 \times 16$ tensor. We also concatenated the one-hot-encoded target (predicted) vector replicated over the space to form a final tensor of $8 \times 8 \times 18$ as the decoder's input. This tensor is then fed to two consecutive fractionally-strided convolution layers (also known as deconvolution [6] or transposed convolution layers) with 16 and 1 filters of size 4×4 and stride 2. This structure have much fewer parameters (about 5K) and significantly outperforms the feed-forward network in the reconstruction task. Figure 3 shows examples of reconstructed images using CapsNet and the proposed method. Similar to [5], we used margin loss for classification and L2 for reconstruction.

4 Experiments

Dataset: The study included 226 unique Computed Tomography (CT) Chest scans (with or without contrast) captured by General Electric and Siemens scanners. The data was preprocessed by an automated segmentation software in order to identify structures to the organ level. From within the segmented lung tissue, a set of potential nodule point is generated based on the size and shape of regions within the lung which exceeds the air Hounsfield Unit (HU) threshold. Additional filters, based on symmetry and other common morphological characteristics, are applied to decrease the false positive rate while maintaining very high sensitivity.

Bounding boxes with at least 8 voxels padding surrounding the candidate nodules are cropped and resized to $32 \times 32 \times 32$ pixels. Each generated candidate is reviewed and annotated by at least one *board certified radiologist*. From all the generated images (about 7400 images), around 56% were labeled as nodules and the rest non-nodules. The first row of Fig. 3 shows examples of extracted candidates and the corresponding labels provided by radiologists. These images illustrate the highly challenging task of distinguishing nodules from non-nodule lesions. One reason is that the pulmonary nodules come with large variations in shapes, sizes, types, etc. The second reason which hinders the identification process is the non-nodule candidates mimicking the morphological appearance of the real pulmonary nodules. For all these reasons, the detection and classification of lung nodules is a challenging task, even for experienced radiologists.

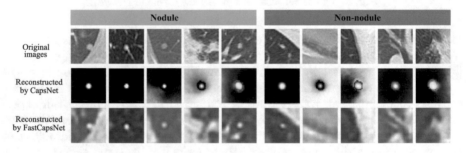

Fig. 3. Sample images of nodules (left) and non-nodules (right) and their reconstructions using the original CapsNet (middle row) and the FastCapsNet (last row)

2D CapsNet: Figure 2 provides an illustration of the proposed architecture, which consists of 3 different layers. To prepare the required 2D images, we used the middle slices of the 3D volumes along the x-axis (as x-axis contains more information according to radiologist's feedback). The first layer is a 3D convolution layer with 256 filters of size 9 and stride 1. Given our 32×32 pixel inputs, this layer outputs $24 \times 24 \times 256$ tensor which are the basic features extracted from input image. The next layer is the *PrimaryCaps* layer which applies 256 convolutional filters on the input to obtain $8 \times 8 \times 256$ tensor. We consider this tensor to be $8 \times 8 = 64$ capsules, each with 256D. This results in only one capsule at each pixel, therefore effectively enforces consistent dynamic routing. These vectors will then be passed through a squashing non-linearity to get the final output of the lower-level capsules (*i.e.* $\mathbf{u}_i$). The proposed architecture is a departure from from the original CapsNet, which divides the tensor into $8 \times 8 \times 32 = 2048$ capsules, each of 8D, resulting in 32 capsules for each pixel locations. While the total number of parameters of the two networks are the same, our network drastically reduces the number of PrimaryCaps from 2048 to 64, thereby decreases the number of voting coefficients by 32 times.

In the final layer, called *NoduleCaps*, 256D output from PrimaryCaps layer are multiplied with its own 256×16 transformation matrix which maps the output to the 16D space (results in $\hat{\mathbf{u}}_{j|i}$). Finally, the routing parameter tunes the coupling coefficients and decides about the amount of contribution they make to the NoduleCaps. During training, the coefficients are initialized uniformly, meaning that the output from the PrimaryCaps layer is sent equally to all the capsules in the NoduleCaps layer. Then the routing between the two layers is learned iteratively.

Table 1. Comparison of the performance, number of trainable parameters (M is for millions), and required training time per epoch of the Deep Networks

	precision	recall	error rate	#params	sec/epoch
Automated software	73.65	82.13	25.34	-	-
2D AlexNet	88.09	85.52	13.09	7.6M	6.9
2D ResNet-50	89.14	85.52	12.51	23.5M	16.3
2D CapsNet	89.44	85.98	12.16	7.4M	18.8
2D FastCapsNet	**89.71**	**87.41**	**11.45**	5.8M	6.2
3D AlexNet	91.05	87.92	10.42	7.8M	175.1
3D ResNet-50	90.51	**90.42**	9.58	48.2M	341.5
3D FastCapsNet	**91.84**	89.11	**9.52**	52.2M	320.0

3D Capsule Network: The 3D version of the proposed architecture is structurally similar to the explained 2D version. In the first two layers, 2D convolutions are replaced by 3D convolution operators capturing the cross-correlation of the voxels. The number and size of the filters and the strides are the same as before. This results in an $8 \times 8 \times 8$ volume of primary capsules, each sees the output of all $256 \times 9 \times 9 \times 9$ units of the previous convolution layer. Therefore, our proposed faster architecture gives 512 PrimaryCaps, compared with 23328 of the original network. This will limit the number of required routing coefficients, help the dynamic routing perform faster and perform significantly better. NodulesCaps are the same as in the 2D network, fully-connected to PrimaryCaps with the dynamic routing happening in the middle. Similar to the proposed 2D FastCapsNet, the decoder takes the prediction vectors of all *PrimaryCaps* (only the ones routed to the correct class), concatenates it with the one-hot-encoded label of the target to form a tensor of shape $8 \times 8 \times 8 \times 18$. It then reconstruct the input from this tensor by applying two consecutive 3D fractionally-strided convolution layers with 16 and 1 filters, respectively. Obviously, a feed-forward architecture wouldn't scale well for reconstructing the 3D images (it requires 32 × 32 × 32 output units which drastically increases the number of parameters).

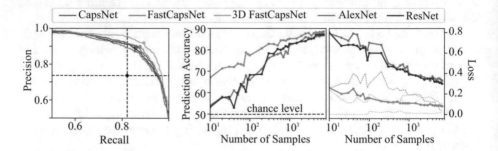

Fig. 4. Left: test precision-recall curves, **Center:** test prediction accuracy of models trained on different number of training samples, **Right:** train (dashed) and test (solid) loss of models trained on different number of training samples.

Results: 2D version of the proposed faster CapsNet was trained and compared with two well-known deep network architectures, AlexNet [3] and ResNet-50 [4], as well as the original Capsule network. Trying both 2D and 3D architectures helps testing the network's performance in both settings, as well as enabling us to quantify the contribution of the third dimension. All analyses are done using a desktop machine equipped with 128 GB of memory, 4 NVidia GTX 1080 with 8 GB of video memory each, and Intel Xeon CPU 2.40 GHz with 16 cores.

The test prediction results are presented in Table 1. Capsule networks achieve relatively lower error rates compared to AlexNet and ResNet. FastCapsNet has fewer parameters than other models, thus is more than 3 times faster than the regular CaspNet in both training and test runs. For 3D images, the 3D implementation of the original CapsNet failed to converge. The prediction accuracy remains close at the chance level with the validation loss increasing gradually. However, our proposed 3D FastCapsNet converges relatively fast (reaching less than 20% test loss after only 3 training epochs).

The precision-recall curve of the models are presented in the left panel of Fig. 4 confirming the superior performance of the proposed FastCapsNets compared to the other models. The 3D FastCapsNet performs significantly better than the rest, beating the 2D version by almost 2% accuracy indicating the contribution of the third dimension. We also trained the 2D models using different number of training samples. The prediction accuracy and loss values of different models are presented in the middle and right panel of Fig. 4, respectively. Capsule network performs comparatively more robust. For very few number of samples, AlexNet and ResNet-50 go almost to chance level while capsule network stays about 70%.

5   Conclusions

Our work shows that CapsNet is a promising alternative to CNN. Experimental results demonstrate that CapsNets compare favorably to CNNs when the training size is large, but significantly outperform CNNs on small size datasets. We showed that, by modifying the routing mechanism, we can speed up CapsNets 3 times while maintaining the same accuracy. In the future, we will explore unsupervised learning with CapsNets.

References

1. Siegel, R.L., Miller, K.D., Jemal, A.: Cancer statistics. CA Cancer J. Clin. **67**(1), 7–30 (2017)
2. Team, N.L.S.T.R.: Reduced lung-cancer mortality with low-dose computed tomographic screening. N Engl. J. Med. **365**, 395–409 (2011)
3. Krizhevsky, A., Sutskever, I., Hinton, G.E.: Imagenet classification with deep convolutional neural networks. In: Advances in Neural Information Processing Systems, pp. 1097–1105 (2012)
4. He, K., Zhang, X., Ren, S., Sun, J.: Deep residual learning for image recognition. In: Proceedings of the IEEE Conference on Computer Vision and Pattern Recognition, pp. 770–778 (2016)
5. Sabour, S., Frosst, N., Hinton, G.E.: Dynamic routing between capsules. In: Advances in Neural Information Processing Systems (2017)
6. Zeiler, M.D., Krishnan, D., Taylor, G.W., Fergus, R.: Deconvolutional networks. In: 2010 IEEE Conference on Computer Vision and Pattern Recognition (CVPR), pp. 2528–2535. IEEE (2010)

Mean Field Network Based Graph Refinement with Application to Airway Tree Extraction

Raghavendra Selvan[1]([✉]), Max Welling[2,3], Jesper H. Pedersen[4], Jens Petersen[1], and Marleen de Bruijne[1,5]

[1] Department of Computer Science, University of Copenhagen,
Copenhagen, Denmark
`raghav@di.ku.dk`
[2] Informatics Institute, University of Amsterdam, Amsterdam, Netherlands
[3] Canadian Institute for Advanced Research, Toronto, Canada
[4] Department of Cardio-Thoracic Surgery RT, University Hospital of Copenhagen,
Copenhagen, Denmark
[5] Departments of Medical Informatics and Radiology, Erasmus Medical Center,
Rotterdam, Netherlands

Abstract. We present tree extraction in 3D images as a graph refinement task, of obtaining a subgraph from an over-complete input graph. To this end, we formulate an approximate Bayesian inference framework on undirected graphs using mean field approximation (MFA). Mean field networks are used for inference based on the interpretation that iterations of MFA can be seen as feed-forward operations in a neural network. This allows us to learn the model parameters from training data using back-propagation algorithm. We demonstrate usefulness of the model to extract airway trees from 3D chest CT data. We first obtain probability images using a voxel classifier that distinguishes airways from background and use Bayesian smoothing to model individual airway branches. This yields us joint Gaussian density estimates of position, orientation and scale as node features of the input graph. Performance of the method is compared with two methods: the first uses probability images from a trained voxel classifier with region growing, which is similar to one of the best performing methods at EXACT'09 airway challenge, and the second method is based on Bayesian smoothing on these probability images. Using centerline distance as error measure the presented method shows significant improvement compared to these two methods.

Keywords: Mean field network · Tree extraction · Airways · CT

1 Introduction

Markov random field (MRF) based image segmentation methods have been successfully used in several medical image applications [2,10]. Pixel-level MRF's

© Springer Nature Switzerland AG 2018
A. F. Frangi et al. (Eds.): MICCAI 2018, LNCS 11071, pp. 750–758, 2018.
https://doi.org/10.1007/978-3-030-00934-2_83

are commonly used for segmentation purposes to exploit the regular grid nature of images. These models become prohibitively expensive when dealing with 3D images, which are commonly encountered in medical image analysis. However, there are classes of methods that work with supervoxel representations to reduce the density of voxels by abstracting local information as node features [3,11]. Image segmentation, in such models, can be interpreted as connecting voxels/supervoxels to extract the desired structures of interest.

In this work, we present a novel approach to tree extraction by formulating it as a graph refinement procedure on MRF using mean field networks (MFN). We recover a subgraph corresponding to the desired tree structure from an over-complete input graph either by retaining or removing edges between pairs of nodes. We use supervoxel-like representation to associate nodes in the graph with features that make the input graph sparser. We formulate a probabilistic model based on unary and pairwise potential functions that capture nodes and their interactions. The inference is performed using mean field networks which implement the mean field approximation (MFA) [1] iteration as a feed-forward operation in a neural network [9]. The MFN interpretation enables us to learn the model parameters from training data using back-propagation algorithm; this allows our model to be seen as an intermediate between entirely model-based and end-to-end learning based approaches. The proposed model is exploratory in nature and, hence, not sensitive to local anomalies in data. We evaluate the method to extract airway trees in comparison with two methods: the first uses probability images from a trained voxel classifier with region growing [6], which is similar to one of the best performing methods in EXACT airway challenge [7], and the second method is based on Bayesian smoothing on probability images obtained from the voxel classifier [11].

2   Method

2.1   The Graph Refinement Model

Given a fully connected, or over-complete, input graph, $\mathcal{G} : \{\mathcal{N}, \mathcal{E}\}$ with nodes $i \in \mathcal{N}$ and edges in $(i, j) \in \mathcal{E}$, we are interested in obtaining a subgraph, $\mathcal{G}' : \{\mathcal{N}', \mathcal{E}'\}$, that in turn corresponds to a structure of interest like vessels or airways in an image. We assume each node $i \in \mathcal{N}$ to be associated with a set of d-dimensional features, $\mathbf{x}_i \in \mathbb{R}^d$, and collected into a random vector, $\mathbf{X} = [\mathbf{x}_1, \ldots, \mathbf{x}_N]$. We introduce a random variable, $\mathbf{S} = [\mathbf{s}_1 \ldots \mathbf{s}_N]$, to capture edge connections between nodes. Each node connectivity variable, $\mathbf{s}_i = \{s_{ij}\} : j = 1 \ldots N$, is a collection of binary random variables, $s_{ij} \in \{0, 1\}$, indicating absence or presence of an edge between nodes i and j. Each instance of $\mathbf{S}$ can be seen as an $N \times N$ adjacency matrix. We are interested in recovering $\mathbf{S}'$ corresponding to $\mathcal{G}'$.

The model described by the conditional distribution, $p(\mathbf{S}|\mathbf{X})$, bears similarities with hidden MRF models that have been used for image segmentation [2,10]. Based on this connection, we use the notion of node, $\phi_i(\mathbf{s}_i)$, and pairwise,

$\phi_{ij}(\mathbf{s}_i, \mathbf{s}_j)$, potentials to write the logarithm of joint distribution and relate it to the conditional distribution as,

$$\ln p(\mathbf{S}|\mathbf{X}) \propto \ln p(\mathbf{S}, \mathbf{X}) = -\ln Z + \sum_{i \in \mathcal{N}} \phi_i(\mathbf{s}_i) + \sum_{(i,j) \in \mathcal{E}} \phi_{ij}(\mathbf{s}_i, \mathbf{s}_j), \qquad (1)$$

where $\ln Z$ is the normalisation constant. For ease of notation, explicit dependence on observed data in these potentials is not shown.

Next we focus on formulating node and pairwise potentials introduced in (1) to reflect the behaviour of nodes and their interactions in the subgraph $\mathcal{G}'$, which can consequently yield good estimates of $p(\mathbf{S}|\mathbf{X})$. First, we propose a node potential that imposes a prior degree on each node and learns a per-node feature representation that can be relevant to nodes in the underlying subgraph, $\mathcal{G}'$. For each node $i \in \mathcal{N}$, it is given as,

$$\phi_i(\mathbf{s}_i) = \sum_{v=0}^{D} \beta_v \mathbb{I}\Big[\sum_j s_{ij} = v\Big] + \mathbf{a}^T \mathbf{x}_i \sum_j s_{ij}, \qquad (2)$$

where $\sum_j s_{ij}$ is the degree of node i and $\mathbb{I}[\cdot]$ is the indicator function. The parameters $\beta_v \in \mathbb{R}, \forall v = [0, \dots, D]$, can be seen as a prior on the degree per node. We explicitly model and learn this term for upto 2 edges per node and assume uniform prior for $D > 2$. Further, individual node features, $\mathbf{x}_i$, are combined with $\mathbf{a} \in \mathbb{R}^{d \times 1}$ and captures a combined node feature representation that is characteristic to the desired subgraph $\mathcal{G}'$. The degree of each node, $\sum_j s_{ij}$, controls the extent of each node's contribution to the node potential.

Secondly, we model the pairwise potential such that it captures interactions between pairs of nodes and is crucial in deciding the existence of edges between nodes. We propose a potential that enforces symmetry in connections, and also has terms that derive joint features for each pair of nodes that are relevant in prediction of edges, and is given as,

$$\phi_{ij}(\mathbf{s}_i, \mathbf{s}_j) = \lambda\big(1 - 2|s_{ij} - s_{ji}|\big) + (2s_{ij}s_{ji} - 1)\Big[\boldsymbol{\eta}^T |\mathbf{x}_i - \mathbf{x}_j| + \boldsymbol{\nu}^T (\mathbf{x}_i \mathbf{x}_j)\Big]. \quad (3)$$

The function parameterised by $\lambda \in \mathbb{R}$ in (3) ensures symmetry in connections between nodes, i.e., for nodes i, j it encourages $s_{ij} = s_{ji}$. The parameter $\boldsymbol{\eta} \in \mathbb{R}^{d \times 1}$ combines the absolute difference between each feature dimension. The element-wise feature product term $(\mathbf{x}_i \mathbf{x}_j)$ with $\boldsymbol{\nu} \in \mathbb{R}^{d \times 1}$ is a weighted, non-stationary polynomial kernel of degree 1 that computes the dot product of node features in a weighted feature space. Under these assumptions, the posterior distribution, $p(\mathbf{S}|\mathbf{X})$, can be used to extract $\mathcal{G}'$ from $\mathcal{G}$. However, except for in trivial cases, it is intractable to estimate $p(\mathbf{S}|\mathbf{X})$ and we must resort to making some approximations. We take up the variational mean field approximation (MFA) [1], which is a structured approach to approximating $p(\mathbf{S}|\mathbf{X})$ with candidates from a class of simpler distributions: $q(\mathbf{S}) \in \mathcal{Q}$. This approximation is performed by minimizing the exclusive Kullback-Leibler divergence [1], or equivalently maximising the evidence lower bound (ELBO) or the variational free energy, given as

$$\mathcal{F}(q_{\mathbf{S}}) = \ln Z + \mathbb{E}_{q_{\mathbf{S}}}\Big[\ln p(\mathbf{S}|\mathbf{X}) - \ln q(\mathbf{S})\Big], \tag{4}$$

where $\mathbb{E}_{q_{\mathbf{S}}}$ is the expectation with respect to the distribution $q_{\mathbf{S}}$. In MFA, the class of distributions, $\mathcal{Q}$, are constrained such that $q(\mathbf{S})$ can be factored further. In our model, we assume the existence of each edge is independent of the others, which is enforced as the following factorisation:

$$q(\mathbf{S}) = \prod_{i=1}^{N}\prod_{j=1}^{N} q_{ij}(s_{ij}), \text{ where } q_{ij}(s_{ij}) = \begin{cases} \alpha_{ij} & \text{if } s_{ij} = 1 \\ (1-\alpha_{ij}) & \text{if } s_{ij} = 0 \end{cases}, \tag{5}$$

where $\alpha_{ij} \in [0,1]$ is the probability of an edge existing between nodes i and j.

Using the potentials from (2) and (3) in (4) and taking expectation with respect to $q_{\mathbf{S}}$, we obtain the ELBO in terms of $\alpha_{ij} \; \forall \; i,j = [1,\ldots,N]$. By differentiating this ELBO with respect to any individual α_{kl}, we obtain the following update equation for performing MFA iterations. At iteration $t+1$:

$$\alpha_{kl}^{(t+1)} = \sigma(\gamma_{kl}) = \frac{1}{1 + \exp^{-\gamma_{kl}}} \; \forall \; k = \{1\ldots N\}, \; l \in \mathcal{N}_k \; : \; |\mathcal{N}_k| = L, \tag{6}$$

where $\sigma(\;)$ is the sigmoid activation function, $\mathcal{N}_k$ are the L nearest neighbours of node k based on positional Euclidean distance, and

$$\gamma_{kl} = \prod_{j \in \mathcal{N}_k \backslash l} \left(1 - \alpha_{kj}^{(t)}\right)\Bigg\{ \sum_{m \in \mathcal{N}_k \backslash l} \frac{\alpha_{km}^{(t)}}{(1 - \alpha_{km}^{(t)})}\Big[(\beta_2 - \beta_1) - \beta_2 \sum_{n \in \mathcal{N}_k \backslash l,m} \frac{\alpha_{kn}^{(t)}}{(1 - \alpha_{kn}^{(t)})}\Big]$$
$$+ (\beta_1 - \beta_0)\Bigg\} + \mathbf{a}^T\mathbf{x}_i + (4\alpha_{lk}^{(t)} - 2)\lambda + 2\alpha_{lk}^{(t)}\big(\boldsymbol{\eta}^T|\mathbf{x}_i - \mathbf{x}_j| + \boldsymbol{\nu}^T(\mathbf{x}_i\mathbf{x}_j)\big). \tag{7}$$

After each iteration t, MFA outputs $N \times N$ edge predictions, denoted by $\boldsymbol{\alpha}^{(t)}$, with entries $\alpha_{kl}^{(t)}$. MFA iterations are performed until convergence, and a reasonable stopping criteria is when the increase in ELBO is below a small threshold between successive iterations. Note that an estimate of the connectivity variable $\mathbf{S}$ at iteration t can be recovered as $\mathbf{S}^{(t)} = \mathbb{I}[\boldsymbol{\alpha}^{(t)} > 0.5]$.

2.2   Mean Field Network

The MFA update equations in (6) and (7) resemble the computations in a feed-forward neural network. The predictions from iteration t, $\boldsymbol{\alpha}^{(t)}$, are combined and passed through a non-linear activation function, a sigmoid in our case, to obtain predictions at iteration $t+1$, $\boldsymbol{\alpha}^{(t+1)}$. This interpretation can be used to map T iterations of MFA to a T-layered neural network, based on the underlying graphical model, and is seen as the mean field network (MFN) [9]. The parameters of our model form weights of such a network and are shared across all layers. Given this setting, parameters for the MFN model can be learned using back-propagation on the binary cross entropy (BCE) loss:

$$\mathcal{L}(\mathbf{S}', \boldsymbol{\alpha}^{(T)}) = \frac{1}{N^2} \sum_{i=1}^{N} \sum_{j=1}^{N} \Big(s_{ij} \log(\alpha_{ij}) + (1 - s_{ij}) \log(1 - \alpha_{ij}) \Big), \quad (8)$$

where $\boldsymbol{\alpha}^{(T)}$ is the predicted probability of edge connections at the last iteration (T) of MFA and $\mathbf{S}'$ is the ground truth adjacency of the desired subgraph $\mathcal{G}'$.

2.3   Airway Tree Extraction as Graph Refinement

Depending on the input features of observed data, $\mathbf{X}$, the MFN presented above can be applied to different applications. Here we present extraction of airway tree centerlines from CT images as a graph refinement task and show related experiments in Sect. 3. To this end, the image data is processed to extract useful node features to input to the MFN. We assume that each node is associated with a 7-dimensional Gaussian density comprising of location (x, y, z), local radius (r), and orientation (v_x, v_y, v_z), such that $\mathbf{x}_i = [\mathbf{x}_\mu^i, \mathbf{x}_{\sigma^2}^i]$, comprising of mean, $\mathbf{x}_\mu^i \in \mathbb{R}^{7 \times 1}$, and variance for each feature, $\mathbf{x}_{\sigma^2}^i \in \mathbb{R}^{7 \times 1}$. We obtain these features by performing Bayesian smoothing on probability images obtained from the voxel classifier [6], with process and measurement models that model individual branches in an airway tree using the method of [11].

The node and pairwise potentials in Eqs. (2) and (3) are general and applicable to commonly encountered trees. The one modification we make due to our feature-based representation is to one of the terms in (3), where we normalise the absolute difference in node positions, $\mathbf{x}_p = [x, y, z]$, with the average radius of the two nodes, i.e., $|\mathbf{x}_p^i - \mathbf{x}_p^j|/(r^i + r^j)$, as the relative positions of nodes are proportional to their scales in the image.

For evaluation purposes, we convert the refined graphs into binary segmentations by drawing spheres in 3D volume along the predicted edges using location and scale information from the corresponding node features.

3   Experiments and Results

Data. The experiments were performed on 32 low-dose CT chest scans from a lung cancer screening trial [5]. All scans have voxel-resolution of approximately $0.78 \times 0.78 \times 1\,\text{mm}^3$. The reference segmentations consist of expert-user verified union of results from two previous methods: first method uses a voxel classifier to distinguish airway voxels from background to obtain probability images and extracts airways using region growing and vessel similarity [6], and the second method continually extends locally optimal paths using costs computed using the voxel classification approach [4]. We extract ground truth adjacency matrices for training the MFN using Bayesian smoothing to extract individual branches from the probability images obtained using the voxel classifier, then connect only the branches within the reference segmentation to obtain a single, connected tree structure using a spanning-tree algorithm.

Error Measure. To evaluate the proposed method along with the comparison methods in a consistent manner, we extract centerlines using a 3D-thinning algorithm from the generated binary segmentations. The error measure used is based on centerline distance, defined as $d_{\mathrm{err}} = (d_{\mathrm{FP}} + d_{\mathrm{FN}})/2$, where d_{FP} is average minimum Euclidean distance from segmented centerline points to reference centerline points and captures false positive error, and d_{FN} is average minimum Euclidean distance from reference centerline points to segmentation centerline points and captures false negative error.

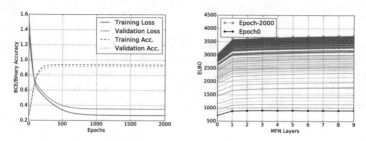

Fig. 1. Training and validation losses for MFN along with binary accuracy averaged over the four-folds of cross-validation procedure are shown in the figure to left. Binary accuracy is obtained by thresholding predicted probability, i.e., $\mathbf{S}^{(t)} = \mathbb{I}[\boldsymbol{\alpha}^{(t)} > 0.5]$. Figure to the right shows the ELBO computed at each layer within an epoch and across epochs averaged over four folds.

Learning of Parameters. We create batches of sub-images comprising of 500 nodes from each image and derive the corresponding adjacency matrices to reduce memory footprint during the training procedure. Parameters of the MFN are learned by minimising the BCE loss in (8) computed on all the training data using back-propagation with Adam optimiser with recommended settings [8]. To further reduce computational overhead we restrict the neighbourhood of each node to be $L = 10$ nearest neighbours based on Euclidean distance of their locations in the image data. Based on initial investigations of ELBO we set the number of layers in MFN, $T = 10$. The learning curves for loss and binary accuracy are shown in Fig. 1, along with the ELBO plot showing the successive increase in ELBO with each iteration within an epoch (as guaranteed by MFA) and with increasing epochs (due to gradient descent).

Table 1. Performance comparison based on 4-fold cross validation.

Method	d_{FP}(mm)	d_{FN}(mm)	d_{err}(mm)
Voxel Classifier	0.792	4.807	2.799 ± 0.701
Bayesian Smoothing	0.839	2.812	1.825 ± 0.232
MFN	0.835	2.571	1.703 ± 0.186

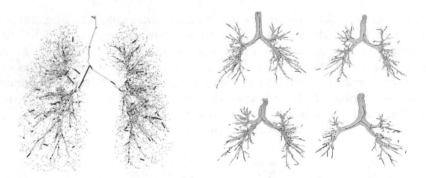

Fig. 2. Figure on left: Predicted connections by MFN for one case: Yellow edges are true positives, red edges are false positives and blue are false negatives. Figure on right: Airway tree centerlines for four cases obtained from MFN predictions (blue) overlaid with the reference segmentations (pink surface) and the centerlines from the voxel-classifier based region growing method (yellow).

Results. We compare performance of the proposed MFN method with a method close to the voxel classifier approach that uses region growing on probability images [6] which was one of the best performing methods in the EXACT'09 challenge [7], and Bayesian smoothing method used in tandem with the voxel classifier approach [11]. We perform 4-fold cross validation using the 32 images on all three methods and report centerline distance based performance measure, d_{err}, in Table 1 based on the cross validation predictions. Our method shows an improvement in d_{err} with significant gains ($p < 0.05$) by reducing the false negative error d_{FN}, implying extraction of more complete trees, when compared to both methods. The results were compared based on paired-sample t-test.

In Fig. 2, we first present the predicted subgraph for one of the images. The gray dots are nodes of the over-complete graph with features, $\mathbf{x}_i$, extracted using Bayesian smoothing; the edges are colour-coded providing an insight into the performance of the method: yellow edges are true positives, red edges are false positives and blue edges are false negatives compared to the ground truth connectivity derived from the reference segmentations. Several of the false negatives are spaced closely, and in fact, do not contribute to the false negative error, d_{FN}, after generating the binary segmentations. The figure to the right in Fig. 2 shows four predicted centerlines overlaid with the reference segmentation and centerlines from the voxel-classifier approach. Clearly, the MFN method is able to detect more branches as seen in most of the branch ends, which is also captured as the reduction in d_{FN} in Table 1. Some of the false positive predictions from MFN method appear to be missing branches in the reference, as seen in first of the four scans. However, there are few other false positive predictions that could be due to the model using only pairwise potentials; this can be alleviated either by using higher order neighbourhood information or with basic post-processing. The centerlines extracted from MFN are slightly offset from the center of airways at larger scales; this could be due to the sparsity of the nodes at those scales and can be overcome by increasing resolution of the input graph.

4   Discussion and Conclusion

We presented a novel method to perform tree extraction by posing it as a graph refinement task in a probabilistic graphical model setting. We performed approximate probabilistic inference on this model, to obtain a subgraph representing airway-like structures from an over-complete graph, using mean field approximation. Further, using mean field networks we showed the possibility of learning parameters of the underlying graphical model from training data using back-propagation algorithm. The main contribution within the presented MFN framework is our formulation of unary and pairwise potentials in (2) and (3). By designing these potentials to reflect the nature of tasks we are interested in, the model can be applied to a diverse set of applications. We have shown its application to extract airway trees with significant improvement in the error measure, when compared to the two comparison methods. However, tasks like tree extraction can benefit from using higher order potentials that take more than two nodes jointly into account. This limitation is revealed in Fig. 2, where the resulting subgraph from MFN is not a single, connected tree. While we used a linear data term in the node potential, $\mathbf{a}^T \mathbf{x}_i$ in (2), and a polynomial kernel of degree 1 in the pairwise potential to learn features from data, $\nu^T(\mathbf{x}_i \mathbf{x}_j)$ in (3), there are possibilities of using more complex data terms to learn more expressive features, like using a Gaussian kernel as in [10]. Another interesting direction could be to use a smaller neural network to learn pairwise or higher-order features from the node features. On a GNU/Linux based standard computer with 32 GB of memory running one full cross validation procedure on 32 images takes upto 6 h. Predictions using a trained MFN takes less than a minute per image.

Our model can be seen as an intermediate between an entirely model-based solution and an end-to-end learning approach. It can be interpreted as a structured neural network where the interactions between layers are based on the underlying graphical model, while the parameters of the model are learned from data. This, we believe, presents an interesting link between probabilistic graphical models and neural network-based learning.

Acknowledgements. This work was funded by the Independent Research Fund Denmark (DFF) and Netherlands Organisation for Scientific Research (NWO).

References

1. Jaakkola, T.S., Jordan, M.I.: Improving the mean field approximation via the use of mixture distributions. In: Jordan, M.I. (ed.) Learning in Graphical Models. NATO ASI Series (Series D: Behavioural and Social Sciences), vol.D 89. Springer, Dordrecht (1998). https://doi.org/10.1007/978-94-011-5014-9_6
2. Zhang, Y., et al.: Segmentation of brain MR images through a hidden Markov random field model and the expectation-maximization algorithm. IEEE Trans. Med. Imaging **20**(1), 45–57 (2001)
3. Wang, X.F., Zhang, X.-P.: A new localized superpixel Markov random field for image segmentation. In: IEEE International Conference on Multimedia and Expo. IEEE (2009)
4. Lo, P., Sporring, J., Pedersen, J.J.H., de Bruijne, M.: Airway tree extraction with locally optimal paths. In: Yang, G.-Z., Hawkes, D., Rueckert, D., Noble, A., Taylor, C. (eds.) MICCAI 2009. LNCS, vol. 5762, pp. 51–58. Springer, Heidelberg (2009). https://doi.org/10.1007/978-3-642-04271-3_7
5. Pedersen, J.H., et al.: The Danish randomized lung cancer CT screening trial - overall design and results of the prevalence round. J. Thoracic Oncol. **4**(5), 608–614 (2009)
6. Lo, P., et al.: Vessel-guided airway tree segmentation: a voxel classification approach. Med. Image Anal. **14**(4), 527–538 (2010)
7. Lo, P., et al.: Extraction of airways from CT (EXACT'09). IEEE Trans. Med. Imaging **31**(11), 2093–2107 (2012)
8. Kingma, D.P., Ba, J.: Adam: a method for stochastic optimization. arXiv preprint arXiv:1412.6980 (2014)
9. Li, Y., Zemel, R.: Mean-field networks. arXiv preprint arXiv:1410.5884 (2014)
10. Orlando, J.I., Blaschko, M.: Learning fully-connected CRFs for blood vessel segmentation in retinal images. In: Golland, P., Hata, N., Barillot, C., Hornegger, J., Howe, R. (eds.) MICCAI 2014. LNCS, vol. 8673, pp. 634–641. Springer, Cham (2014). https://doi.org/10.1007/978-3-319-10404-1_79
11. Selvan, R., Petersen, J., Pedersen, J.H., de Bruijne, M.: Extraction of airways with probabilistic state-space models and bayesian smoothing. In: Cardoso, M.J. (ed.) GRAIL/MFCA/MICGen -2017. LNCS, vol. 10551, pp. 53–63. Springer, Cham (2017). https://doi.org/10.1007/978-3-319-67675-3_6

Automated Pulmonary Nodule Detection: High Sensitivity with Few Candidates

Bin Wang[1,3], Guojun Qi[2], Sheng Tang[1(✉)], Liheng Zhang[2], Lixi Deng[1,3], and Yongdong Zhang[1]

[1] Key Lab of Intelligent Information Processing, Institute of Computing Technology, Chinese Academy of Sciences, Beijing, China
ts@ict.ac.cn
[2] University of Central Florida, Orlando, FL, USA
[3] University of the Chinese Academy of Sciences, Beijing, China

Abstract. Automated pulmonary nodule detection plays an important role in lung cancer diagnosis. In this paper, we propose a pulmonary detection framework that can achieve high sensitivity with few candidates. First, the Feature Pyramid Network (FPN), which leverages multi-level features, is applied to detect nodule candidates that cover almost all true positives. Then redundant candidates are removed by a simple but effective Conditional 3-Dimensional Non-Maximum Suppression (Conditional 3D-NMS). Moreover, a novel Attention 3D CNN (Attention 3D-CNN) which efficiently utilizes contextual information is proposed to further remove the overwhelming majority of false positives. The proposed method yields a sensitivity of 95.8% at 2 false positives per scan on the LUng Nodule Analysis 2016 (LUNA16) dataset, which is competitive compared to the current published state-of-the-art methods.

1 Introduction

Lung cancer is one of the most lethal diseases worldwide [1]. It can be early diagnosed among high-risk individuals through screening with low-dose computed tomography (LDCT). Compared with traditional chest radiography screening, LDCT has reduced the mortality of lung cancer by 20% in seven years with early diagnosis [3]. The prevalence of CT technology has generated enormous CT data. However, it is challenging for radiologists to accurately localize every pulmonary nodule appearing on all CT slices.

Over the past two decades, researchers have developed many Computer-Aided Diagnosis (CAD) systems for automatical detection of lung nodules [2,3]. The performances of these CAD systems have been improved significantly over previous systems. However, these techniques still have a long way to enable practical applications. These CAD systems are often designed by using hand-craft features that

This work was supported by the National Natural Science Foundation of China under Grant (61525206, 61572472, U1703261, 61571424).

© Springer Nature Switzerland AG 2018
A. F. Frangi et al. (Eds.): MICCAI 2018, LNCS 11071, pp. 759–767, 2018.
https://doi.org/10.1007/978-3-030-00934-2_84

are based on some low-level features such as size, shape, texture and intensity. They cannot deal with the large variations of nodules, thus may fail to distinguish nodules from those ambiguous regions. Fortunately, the development of deep learning enables us to engineer representative features to recognize various appearances of pulmonary nodules, which shows promising detection accuracy with significantly improved performances. Over the past two years, many deep learning based systems have been proposed and delivered exciting results [3–6]. However, it is still a challenging task to detect small pulmonary nodules from CT slices. Detecting small or even tiny nodules plays an important role in early diagnosis and treatment, which can effectively lower the risk of lung cancers before they develop into worse stages. This inspires us to develop a high sensitive CAD system.

Conventional pulmonary nodule detection systems usually consist of two stages: proposing nodule candidates and removing false positives. In this paper, we carefully design Convolutional Neural Network (CNN) structures to address the challenge of detecting small pulmonary nodules at each stage: First of all, in order to ensure detecting all the nodules without missing those small nodules, we design the *candidate detection network* (see Fig. 1-Stage 1) by exploring the property of Feature Pyramid Networks (FPN) [7]. This detection network could cover almost all nodules with only very few nodules missed ($16/1186 \approx 1.3\%$). Then, we propose an effective Conditional 3D-NMS to remove the redundant candidates. Moreover, we propose a novel Attention 3D-CNN model (see Fig. 1-Stage 2) allowing the model to focus on the most relevant regions for reducing false positives. We will demonstrate that the proposed pulmonary nodule detection architecture achieves as high as 95.8% sensitivities with only two false positives per scan on LUNA16 dataset, which is very competitive compared to the current state-of-the-art methods.

2   Methods

As shown in Fig. 1, the proposed framework consists of two main parts: (1) the detection of nodule candidates by using FPN and (2) false positive reduction with the Attention 3D-CNN.

2.1   High Sensitivity Candidate Detection with FPN

Candidate detection is a crucial stage for pulmonary nodule detection. The purpose of this step is to recall all possible nodules subject to a reasonable number of candidates. In principle, sliding windows of various scales can cover all possible nodules. However, it is practically impossible because of a too large number of candidates which bring great challenges for subsequent operations. On the contrary, Region Proposal Network (RPN) [8] makes a better balance between the computational cost and the amount of recalled candidates. By using the RPN, Ding *et al.* [5] showed a higher sensitivity with even fewer candidates compared with traditional CAD systems. However, small nodules are still hard to detect

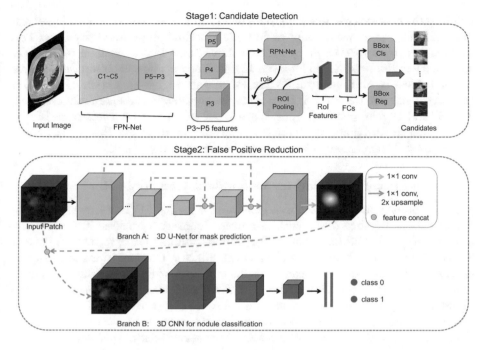

Fig. 1. The framework of proposed pulmonary nodule detection system.

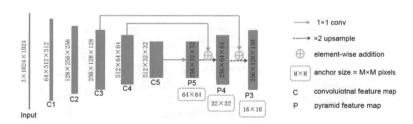

Fig. 2. Feature pyramid networks in our candidate detection architecture.

with the original RPN. To this end, we propose the FPN-based detection architecture in detail below.

Like [5], we take three consecutive layers of CT slices as input and resize them to $3 \times 1024 \times 1024$ before feeding into the network. To detect candidates, we design the FPN-based architecture as illustrated in Fig. 2. The C1~C5 layers in the proposed network correspond to the VGG16 network [9], just adding a new 2×2 pooling layer with stride 2 after Conv5_3 of the original VGG16 network. In most cases, the C5 feature map is already effective for object detection in general natural image. However, since nodules in CT are usually very small (3~30 mm in LUNA 2016 [3]), after passing through several pooling layers, the features of small nodules would become too weak or even disappear. We then take P3~P5 as the final features instead of C5. A 1×1 convolutional layer is attached on C5 to produce the coarsest resolution map P5 of 256 channels. Since P5 has a lower resolution feature map, we attempt to find larger nodule proposals of size 64×64 on it. Then, we upsample the P5 by a factor of two and add it to channel-reduced C4 to obtain a middle-resolution P4 layer. In a similar way, we can obtain the P3 layer at the highest resolution. Both P3 and P4 contain higher-resolution information (which comes from C3 and C4) than P5 layer for detecting smaller nodules. Thus, 32×32 and 16×16 nodule proposals are found at P4 and P3 layers respectively. With these feature maps at different resolutions, we use RPN-Net to get nodule proposals and then classify them into nodule candidates or not.

2.2   Conditional 3D-NMS for Redundant Candidate Removal

Most pulmonary nodule candidates generated from the FPN may be repetitively detected because they often exist in multiple consecutive slices. To reduce the unnecessary computational burden, we propose a simple yet effective Conditional 3D-NMS method to remove redundant candidates. The basic idea is to divide candidates of the same CT scan into different sets of highly overlapped candidates based on their positions and radius. Then we choose the candidate with the highest mean pixel value as the final candidate of the current set. The reason we use pixel mean value as the condition is that the mean value corresponds to the Hounsfield unit (HU) value which reflects the characteristics (pulmonary nodule or lung parenchyma) of the current region. The overview of the algorithm is summarized in Algorithm 1.

Algorithm 1. Conditional 3D Non-Maximum Suppression.

Input:
- The set of candidates which belong to the same CT scan: C
  $C = \{C_1, ..., C_N\}; C_i = (C_i^w, C_i^v, r_i^w, r_i^v, s_i)$, in which
  $C^w = (x^w, y^w, z^w)$ represents world coordinates,
  $C^v = (x^v, y^v, z^v)$ represents voxel coordinates,
  r and s represent the radius and the confidence of the candidate respectively.
- The image array of the CT scan: I

Output:
- The set of remaining candidates after Conditional 3D-NMS: L;

1: Initialize L = {}
   Note $V(z, y, x, r) = I[z, y - \frac{r}{2} : y + \frac{r}{2}, x - \frac{r}{2} : x + \frac{r}{2}]$; which means the mean pixel value of the square area with (y, x) as center and $r/2$ as length in the z-th slice.
2: **repeat**
3:    Initialize temporary set T = {};
4:    Sort all the candidates in C by confidence s in descending order, mark the first candidate as C_h;
5:    For any $C_i \in C$:if $\|C_i^w - C_h^w\|_2 \leq r_h^w$, Do $T = T \cup \{C_i^v\}, C = C - \{C_i\}$;
6:    Conditional Selection: Find the minimum z_{min} and the maximum z_{max} of coordinate z in T,
      $z_{choose} = \arg\max_{z_i} V(z_i^v, y_h^v, x_h^v, r_h^v), i \in [z_{min}, z_{min+1}, ..., z_{max}]$,
7:    $L = L \cup \{(x_h^v, y_h^v, z_{choose})\}$
8: **until** C={}

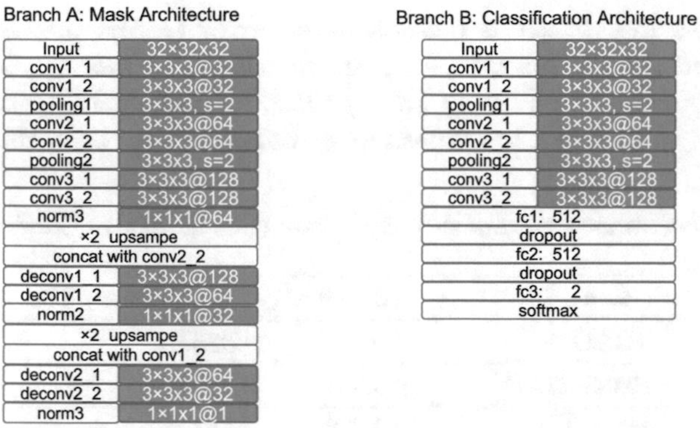

Branch A: Mask Architecture

Input	32×32x32
conv1_1	3×3x3@32
conv1_2	3×3x3@32
pooling1	3×3x3, s=2
conv2_1	3×3x3@64
conv2_2	3×3x3@64
pooling2	3×3x3, s=2
conv3_1	3×3x3@128
conv3_2	3×3x3@128
norm3	1×1x1@64
×2 upsampe	
concat with conv2_2	
deconv1_1	3×3x3@128
deconv1_2	3×3x3@64
norm2	1×1x1@32
×2 upsampe	
concat with conv1_2	
deconv2_1	3×3x3@64
deconv2_2	3×3x3@32
norm3	1×1x1@1

Branch B: Classification Architecture

Input	32×32x32
conv1_1	3×3x3@32
conv1_2	3×3x3@32
pooling1	3×3x3, s=2
conv2_1	3×3x3@64
conv2_2	3×3x3@64
pooling2	3×3x3, s=2
conv3_1	3×3x3@128
conv3_2	3×3x3@128
fc1: 512	
dropout	
fc2: 512	
dropout	
fc3: 2	
softmax	

Fig. 3. The network structure of attention 3D-CNN.

2.3 Attention 3D-CNN for False Positive Reduction

The proposed candidate detection method can recall almost all of the nodules. Nevertheless, a large number of false positives exist among those candidates since it is difficult to distinguish true nodules from highly similar false positives without using three-dimensional spatial contextual information. Some researchers take advantage of 3D CNN for false positive reduction [5,6,10]. By contrast, to use spatial information more effectively, we propose a novel Attention 3D-CNN architecture for false positive reduction.

As shown in Fig. 1 (Stage2), the Attention 3D-CNN has two components: Branch A is the attention subnet (U-net structure [11]), which produces a 3D mask that is supposed to have a high response near the nodule. We apply the resultant 3D mask to the source patch before it is fed into the 3D CNN classification network. This allows the network to focus on the lesion area while ignoring the noisy irrelevant background. The detailed architecture of this Attention 3D-CNN network is presented in Fig. 3, where the convolutional layers are followed by batch normalization and ReLU activation.

While Branch A produces a mask of the nodule's Gaussian distribution, its ground truth used to train the network is calculated below:

$$V = \frac{K}{\sqrt[3]{2\pi\sigma^3}} \cdot exp(-\frac{(x-\overline{x})^2 + (y-\overline{y})^2 + (z-\overline{z})^2}{2\sigma^2}) \qquad (3\sigma = 1.5r) \qquad (1)$$

where $(\overline{x}, \overline{y}, \overline{z})$ represents the nodule centroid, (x, y, z) represents the voxel point of the mask in the CT scan, V is the mask value, and K is a constant term. We adopt $3\sigma = 1.5r$ instead of r, because we aim to consider context information in the model to better recognize nodules. Finally, Branch B outputs a classification probability to decide whether the current voxel is a nodule or not. We use a multi-task loss L to jointly train the network:

$$L = \lambda L_{mask} + L_{cls} \qquad (2)$$

where the mask loss L_{mask} is mean squared error (MSE) between the ground truth mask and the prediction mask, the classification loss L_{cls} is focal loss [7] that is more effective than cross entropy loss to classify hard examples on an imbalanced set, and λ is a hyperparameter balancing between the two losses.

Table 1. Detection performance comparison (Sensitivity vs Candidates/scan)

System	Sensitivity	Candidates/scan
ISICAD	0.856	335.9
SubsolidCAD	0.361	290.6
LargeCAD	0.318	47.6
M5L	0.768	22.2
ETROCAD	0.929	333.0
FUSION	0.983	850.2
FRCNN	0.817	22.7
FRCNN+3DCNN [5]	0.946	15.0
FCN+OSF [6]	0.971	219.1
Cand-Det	**0.987**	179.6
3D-NMS	0.967	103.3
Conditional 3D-NMS	0.981	91.5
3D-CNN	0.946	8.5
Attention 3D-CNN	0.958	**6.6**

3   Experiments

We evaluate the proposed framework on the LUNA16 [3] dataset. It contains 888 CT scans whose pulmonary nodules have been well annotated by four experienced radiologists. The LUNA16 dataset is divided into ten subsets for ten-fold cross validation. The performances of detection algorithms are evaluated by sensitivity and average number of false positives per scan (FPs/scan). The overall score (CPM score) is defined as the average of sensitivity at seven predefined false positive rates – 1/8, 1/4, 1/2, 1, 2, 4 and 8 FPs per scan.

3.1   Implementation Details

On the candidate detection stage, we normalize the values of CT scans (Houndsfield Unit between −1000 and 400) to the range (0, 1). In the stage of false positive reduction, we crop $36 \times 36 \times 36$ voxels from the detected candidates that are preprocessed by Conditional 3D-NMS. Then, data augmentation is used for training the Attention 3D-CNN network: we flip the voxels from coronal, sagittal and axial dimensions and crop $32 \times 32 \times 32$ patches as the input into the network. The constant term K in generating Gaussian masks is set to 1000 and the hyper-parameter λ is set based on the cross-validation result.

3.2 Ablation Study and Results

To check the contribution of each step in the proposed framework, we perform an ablation study. As shown in Table 1, our candidate detection network (Cand-Det) can achieve a sensitivity of 98.7% with an average of 179.6 detected candidate nodules per scan. Compared with the 'FUSION' result that combines five traditional CAD systems (ISICAD∼ETROCAD), the proposed candidate detection method can achieve higher sensitivity with fewer candidates.

After candidate detection, the Conditional 3D-NMS (Cand-Det-CNMS) method is adopted to remove redundant candidates. From the table, we can see that, compared with the normal 3D-NMS, the Conditional 3D-NMS is more effective for removing redundancy. Finally, we use the Attention 3D-CNN to remove massive false positives and reach a sensitivity of 95.8% with only 6.6 detected nodules per scan. By comparison, if we remove the branch A from the Attention 3D-CNN network, it becomes a typical 3D CNN, and the result would reduce to 94.6% sensitivity with 8.5 detections per scan. This shows that adding attention branch can help improve the sensitivity as well as reduce false detections. The FROC curve for each step is plotted in Fig. 4. We can see that the performance of the proposed framework is improved by combining these steps.

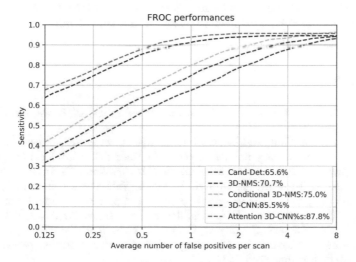

Fig. 4. FROC performances in each stage of the proposed method

To further analyze the performance of the proposed framework, we compared with state-of-the-art methods [5, 6, 10] by using CPM score. In Table 2, we can see that the CPM score of the proposed system is 87.8%, which is better than the methods proposed in [6, 10], and only a little lower than the FRCN+3DCNN. However, in clinical practice, radiologists are more concerned with the sensitivities when the FPs per scan rates vary from 1 to 4 [5, 6], where the proposed architecture achieves the best performance.

Table 2. Comparison with state-of-art methods on LUNA16 dataset [3] (CPM score). We achieve best results when FPs per scan vary from 1 to 4 which is more worth noting in clinical practice.

Sensitivity FPs/scan Teams	0.125	0.25	0.5	1	2	4	8	CPM score
MultiLevel[10]	0.677	0.737	0.815	0.848	0.879	0.907	0.922	0.827
FCN+OSF [6]	0.659	0.745	0.819	0.865	0.906	0.933	0.946	0.839
FRCN+3DCNN[5]	**0.748**	**0.853**	**0.887**	0.922	0.938	0.944	0.946	**0.891**
Ours	0.676	0.776	0.879	**0.949**	**0.958**	**0.958**	**0.958**	0.878

4   Conclusion

In this work, we propose an architecture for the detection of pulmonary nodules. The architecture can first produce nodule candidates with high sensitivity using a FPN-based detection network. Then, a simple and effective Conditional 3D-NMS method removes the redundant candidates. Finally, a novel Attention 3D-CNN network is proposed to reduce the abundance of false positives. Experiments show that our architecture can achieve a high sensitive result with few candidates. The architecture can also be extended to other similar object detection tasks in CT scans.

References

1. Siegel, R.L., Miller, K.D., Jemal, A.: Cancer statistics, 2018. CA Cancer J. Clin. **68**(1), 7–30 (2018)
2. Murphy, K., van Ginneken, B., Schilham, A.M.R., et al.: A large-scale evaluation of automatic pulmonary nodule detection in chest CT using local image features and k-nearest-neighbour classification. Med. Image Anal. **13**(5), 757–770 (2009)
3. Setio, A.A.A., Traverso, A., De Bel, T., et al.: Validation, comparison, and combination of algorithms for automatic detection of pulmonary nodules in computed tomography images: the LUNA16 challenge. Med. Image Anal. **42**, 1–13 (2017)
4. Setio, A.A.A., Ciompi, F., Litjens, G., et al.: Pulmonary nodule detection in CT images: false positive reduction using multi-view convolutional networks. IEEE Trans. Med. Imaging **35**(5), 1160–1169 (2016)
5. Ding, J., Li, A., Hu, Z., Wang, L.: Accurate pulmonary nodule detection in computed tomography images using deep convolutional neural networks. In: Descoteaux, M., Maier-Hein, L., Franz, A., Jannin, P., Collins, D.L., Duchesne, S. (eds.) MICCAI 2017. LNCS, vol. 10435, pp. 559–567. Springer, Cham (2017). https://doi.org/10.1007/978-3-319-66179-7_64
6. Dou, Q., Chen, H., Jin, Y., Lin, H., Qin, J., Heng, P.-A.: Automated pulmonary nodule detection via 3d convnets with online sample filtering and hybrid-loss residual learning. In: Descoteaux, M., Maier-Hein, L., Franz, A., Jannin, P., Collins, D.L., Duchesne, S. (eds.) MICCAI 2017. LNCS, vol. 10435, pp. 630–638. Springer, Cham (2017). https://doi.org/10.1007/978-3-319-66179-7_72

7. Lin, T.Y., Dollár, P., Girshick, R., et al.: Feature pyramid networks for object detection. In: CVPR, vol. 1, no. 2, p. 4 (2017)
8. Ren, S., He, K., Girshick, R., et al.: Faster R-CNN: towards real-time object detection with region proposal networks. In: Advances in Neural Information Processing Systems, pp. 91–99 (2015)
9. Simonyan, K., Zisserman, A.: Very deep convolutional networks for large-scale image recognition. arXiv preprint arXiv:1409.1556 (2014)
10. Dou, Q., Chen, H., Yu, L., et al.: Multilevel contextual 3-D CNNs for false positive reduction in pulmonary nodule detection. IEEE Trans. Biomed. Eng. **64**(7), 1558–1567 (2017)
11. Ronneberger, O., Fischer, P., Brox, T.: U-Net: convolutional networks for biomedical image segmentation. In: Navab, N., Hornegger, J., Wells, W.M., Frangi, A.F. (eds.) MICCAI 2015. LNCS, vol. 9351, pp. 234–241. Springer, Cham (2015). https://doi.org/10.1007/978-3-319-24574-4_28

Deep Learning from Label Proportions for Emphysema Quantification

Gerda Bortsova[1(✉)], Florian Dubost[1], Silas Ørting[2], Ioannis Katramados[3],
Laurens Hogeweg[3], Laura Thomsen[4], Mathilde Wille[5],
and Marleen de Bruijne[1,2]

[1] Biomedical Imaging Group Rotterdam, Erasmus MC, Rotterdam, The Netherlands
gerdabortsova@gmail.com
[2] Department of Computer Science, University of Copenhagen,
Copenhagen, Denmark
[3] COSMONiO, Groningen, The Netherlands
[4] Department of Respiratory Medicine, Hvidovre Hospital, Hvidovre, Denmark
[5] Department of Diagnostic Imaging, Bispebjerg Hospital, Copenhagen, Denmark

Abstract. We propose an end-to-end deep learning method that learns
to estimate emphysema extent from proportions of the diseased tissue.
These proportions were visually estimated by experts using a standard
grading system, in which grades correspond to intervals (label example:
1–5% of diseased tissue). The proposed architecture encodes the knowledge that the labels represent a volumetric proportion. A custom loss
is designed to learn with intervals. Thus, during training, our network
learns to segment the diseased tissue such that its proportions fit the
ground truth intervals. Our architecture and loss combined improve the
performance substantially (8% ICC) compared to a more conventional
regression network. We outperform traditional lung densitometry and
two recently published methods for emphysema quantification by a large
margin (at least 7% AUC and 15% ICC), and achieve near-human-level
performance. Moreover, our method generates emphysema segmentations
that predict the spatial distribution of emphysema at human level.

Keywords: Emphysema quantification · Weak labels
Multiple instance learning · Learning from label proportions

1 Introduction

Estimating the volume of abnormalities is useful for evaluating disease progression and identifying patients at risk [1,2,11,12]. For example, emphysema extent
is useful for monitoring COPD [12] and predicting lung cancer [11].

One common approach to automating the volume estimation is to segment
the target abnormalities and subsequently measure their volume. This requires
expensive manual annotations, often making it infeasible to train and validate
on large datasets. Another approach is to directly regress the volume estimate

© Springer Nature Switzerland AG 2018
A. F. Frangi et al. (Eds.): MICCAI 2018, LNCS 11071, pp. 768–776, 2018.
https://doi.org/10.1007/978-3-030-00934-2_85

(or, equivalently, a proportion of the abnormal voxels in an image). This only needs relatively cheap weak labels (e.g. image-level visual scoring).

In this paper, we explore the weakly-labeled approach and consider it a learning from label proportions (LLP) problem [9]. LLP is similar to multiple instance learning (MIL) in that training samples are labeled group-wise. However, in MIL the label only signifies the presence of positive samples, whereas in LLP it is a proportion of positive samples in a group (i.e. a "bag").

We propose a deep LLP approach for emphysema quantification that leverages proportion labels by incorporating prior knowledge on the nature of these labels. We consider a case where emphysema is graded region-wise using a common visual scoring system [12], in which grades correspond to intervals of the proportion of region tissue affected by emphysema. Our method consists of a custom loss for learning from intervals and an architecture specialized for LLP. This architecture has a hidden layer that segments emphysema, followed by a layer that computes its proportion in the input region.

Our architecture is similar to architectures proposed for MIL [10]. These methods, however, use different pooling methods and loss functions. Very few neural-network based methods specialized for LLP were proposed [3,6]. [3] learns to classify particles in high-energy physics from label proportions using a fully-connected network with one hidden layer. [6] applies LLP to ice-water classification in natural images. This method, however, is not end-to-end: it optimizes pixel labels and network parameters in an alternating fashion. In the case of image labeling, LLP can also be addressed more simply by using a CNN (e.g., [4,5]) together with a regression loss (e.g., root mean square or RMS).

Our **methodological contribution** is that we propose the first (to our knowledge) end-to-end deep learning based LLP method for image labeling. We compare the proposed interval loss to RMS and our architecture to a conventional CNN (similar to [4,5]). We perform the latter comparison in the MIL setting (when only emphysema presence labels are used for training) and in the LLP setting. Our **application-wise contributions** are three-fold. Firstly, we substantially outperform previous works [7,8] in emphysema presence and extent prediction. Secondly, we achieve near-human performance level in these tasks. Thirdly, despite being trained only using emphysema proportions, our method generates emphysema segmentations that can be used to classify the spatial distribution of emphysema (paraseptal or centrilobular) at human level.

2   Methods

In both MIL and LLP scenarios, a dataset consists of bags of instances $\mathcal{X} = \{x_i \mid i = 1...m\}$ (m is a number of instances). In MIL, each bag $\mathcal{X}$ has a binary label signifying a presence of at least one positive instance. In LLP, this label is a proportion of positive instances in a bag. In our case, the bag label is an ordinal variable $y \in [0, \text{ncat} - 1]$ (with an interpretation of emphysema grade; grade 0 corresponds to the absence of emphysema). Values of y correspond to intervals of proportion $[\text{thresh}_{y+1}, \text{thresh}_{y+2})$, where thresh is a vector of thresholds with the first element $\text{thresh}_1 = 0$ and the last element $\text{thresh}_{\text{ncat}+1} = 1$.

2.1   Architectures

We call our proposed and baseline architectures "ProportionNet" and "GAP-Net", respectively (see Fig. 1). The first layers of these architectures are the same: they both take a 3D image X of a lung region as input and convert it to a set of 3D feature maps $\{F_1..F_k\}$. The only difference between them is in how these feature maps are converted into the final output – a proportion $\hat{y}$.

ProportionNet first maps the features $\{F_1..F_k\}$ to a single 3D emphysema probability map $p(X)$ and then averages the probabilities within a given region mask R using "ProportionLayer" to obtain the emphysema proportion. When supervised with region label proportions, ProportionNet learns to classify every instance (an image patch, in our case) in such a way that the average label in the bag (i.e. the region) is close to the ground truth proportion.

GAPNet first pools the feature maps $\{F_1..F_k\}$ using a global average pooling (GAP) layer (it thus aggregates instance features into bag features) and then combines these averages into the proportion prediction using a fully-connected layer. We also consider a variation of GAPNet where GAP is replaced by masked GAP (MGAP), which averages every feature individually using R as a mask.

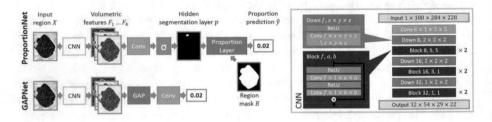

Fig. 1. (a) "Conv": $1 \times 1 \times 1$ convolution with one output feature; "GAP": global average pooling; σ: sigmoid. (b) "Conv": valid convolutions with parameters "{# of output features}, {kernel size} / {stride}"; "Block": residual blocks [5].

2.2   A Loss for Learning from Proportion Intervals (LPI)

A good LPI loss would be near-constant when the predicted proportion $\hat{y}$ is inside the ground truth interval $[\text{thresh}_{y+1}, \text{thresh}_{y+2})$ and would increase as $\hat{y}$ goes outside the interval's boundaries. We propose a loss that approximates those properties: $\text{LPI}_{\text{ncat}}(\hat{y}, y) = \sum_{c=1}^{\text{ncat}-1} w_c \text{CrossEntropy}(\sigma_\alpha(\hat{y} - \text{thresh}_{c+1}), \mathbb{I}(y \geq c))$, where $\sigma_\alpha(x) = (1 + e^{-\alpha x})^{-1}$ is a sharper version of the sigmoid function, w are tunable weights and ncat is a number of categories (see Fig. 2, left). A cth term enforces that for images of grade $y \geq c$ the network predicts $\hat{y} > \text{thresh}_{c+1}$ and images of grade $y < c$ get $\hat{y} < \text{thresh}_{c+1}$. Loss function LPI_2 that contains only the first term can be used as a MIL loss needing only binary labels (thresh_2 will be used to classify a bag into positive or negative).

In the case of ProportionNet, to the above loss we add a term enforcing the MIL assumption that in a negative bag ($y = 0$ means no emphysema) there are no positive instances: $\mathsf{MILA}(\hat{y}, y) = \mathbb{I}(y = 0) w_{\mathsf{MILA}} \left(\frac{1}{m} \sum_i \mathsf{CrossEntropy}(p(X)_i, 0) \right)$.

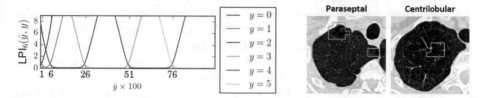

Fig. 2. *Left*: $\mathsf{LPl_6}$ loss with all $w_c = 1$, $\alpha = 120$ and **thresh** $= (0, 0.005, 0.055, 0.255, 0.505, 0.755, 1)$. *Right*: images with different predominant emphysema patterns. Green: ProportionNet segmentations; red: region mask; blue: the 10px margin for separating near-boundary detections from the rest.

3 Experimental Setting

Dataset and Preprocessing. Two low-dose CT scans (the baseline and follow up) were acquired from 1990 participants of the Danish Lung Cancer Screening Trial [12]. Lungs were automatically segmented and divided into 6 regions (roughly corresponding to lobes). The image resolution was 0.78mm × 0.78mm and slice thickness was 1 mm. In every region, emphysema extent and the predominant pattern (paraseptal, centrilobular, panlobular) were independently identified by two observers. The extent was assessed as a categorical grade ranging from 0 to 5 and corresponding to 0%, 1–5%, 6–25%, 26–50%, 51–75% and 76–100% of emphysematous tissue, respectively (as in [12]). We only used images of the right upper region and scores of one observer to train our networks (the interobserver agreement was highest in this region). For our experiments, we randomly sampled 7 training sets of 50, 75, 100, 150, 200, 300 and 700 subjects with validation sets of the same size, except that for the largest training set the validation set contained 300 subjects. The remaining images were assigned to the test sets. The sampling was stratified to ensure similar inter-rater agreement in the training, validation and testing sets.

Using the region masks, we cropped images to select the target region and set all voxels outside of this region to a constant of −800 HU. We used shifting and flipping in the axial plane to augment our training and validation sets.

Network Training and Application. All networks were trained using the Adadelta algorithm for a maximum of 150 epochs, with every epoch consisting of 600 batch iterations. The batch size was 3. The images were sampled in a such way that in every batch there was one healthy image (grade 0), one grade 1 image and one image of grade 2 to 5 sampled uniformly at random (meaning that e.g. grade 5 images appeared with the same frequency as grade 2). This sampling strategy ensures that higher grade images, which are much rarer, are sufficiently represented. For our LPI loss we used thresholds thresh $= (0, 0.005, 0.055, 0.165, 0.385, 0.605, 1)$, which are slightly different from the ones defined by the scoring system (given in the "Dataset" subsection and illustrated in Fig. 2, left). This was because with the standard thresholds our method systematically underestimated the extent of emphysema in grade 3–5 regions, implying that these thresholds might be biased (they were not validated to correspond to real proportions). The weights of the loss $w = (0.5, 0.1, 0.005, 0.005, 0.005)$ were chosen to prioritize accurate emphysema presence classification and account for the poorer inter-rater agreement for higher grade classification. w_{MILA} was set to 0.5 and $\alpha = 120$.

4   Results

Performance Metrics. We evaluated our networks using these two metrics, averaged among the two annotators: (1) area under the receiver operating characteristic curve (AUC) measuring discrimination between grade 0 (no emphysema) and grades 1–5, and (2) average of the AUCs measuring discrimination of grades 1 vs. 2, 2 vs. 3, 3 vs. 4 and 4 vs. 5. These metrics represent emphysema presence and extent prediction performances, respectively. In Table 1 we report means and standard deviations of these metrics computed over multiple test sets.

In Table 2, we use different metrics to be able to compare with other methods. Intraclass correlation (ICC) was computed between predictions of a method converted to interval midpoints and average interval midpoints of the two raters (same as in [8]). Spearman's r was computed between raw predictions and the averaged midpoints of the raters. AUC was computed with respect to the maximum of the presence labels of the raters (as in [7]).

Learning from Emphysema Presence Labels (MIL). First, we trained GAPNet and ProportionNet for 75 epochs using LPI_2 and $LPI_2 + MILA$ losses, respectively. These losses only need binary presence labels, which makes it a MIL problem. ProportionNet outperformed GAPNet in both presence and extent prediction by a large margin when trained on the small sets (see Table 1). When trained on the medium and large sets, ProportionNet was similar to GAPNet in presence detection and better in extent estimation by 2–3% of mean AUC.

To understand the contribution of region masking to the performance of ProportionNet, we also trained MGAPNet, in which GAP was replaced by region-masked GAP, using LPI_2 (on our small sets only due to limited computational resources). MGAPNet performed better than GAPNet in both presence (AUC 0.90 ± 0.06) and extent (AUC 0.71 ± 0.03) prediction. ProportionNet still substantially outperformed MGAPNet.

Table 1. Performance of emphysema presence detection and extent estimation (measured in average AUC over multiple test sets) of networks trained on sets of different size (in patients) and using different labels.

	Architecture	GAPNet		ProportionNet	
	Training set size\Task	Presence	Extent	Presence	Extent
MIL	Small sets (50, 75, 100)	0.87 ± 0.05	0.68 ± 0.06	$\mathbf{0.95 \pm 0.01}$	$\mathbf{0.74 \pm 0.02}$
	Medium sets (150, 200, 300)	$\mathbf{0.96 \pm 0.01}$	0.72 ± 0.02	$\mathbf{0.96 \pm 0.01}$	$\mathbf{0.74 \pm 0.02}$
	Large set (700)	**0.96**	0.76	**0.96**	**0.79**
LLP	Small sets (50, 75, 100)	0.90 ± 0.04	0.74 ± 0.06	$\mathbf{0.94 \pm 0.01}$	$\mathbf{0.79 \pm 0.02}$
	Medium sets (150, 200, 300)	$\mathbf{0.96 \pm 0.01}$	0.80 ± 0.02	$\mathbf{0.96 \pm 0.01}$	$\mathbf{0.84 \pm 0.01}$
	Large set (700)	0.96	0.79	**0.97**	**0.86**

Learning from Emphysema Proportion Labels (LLP). We fine-tuned the GAPNet and ProportionNet previously trained in the MIL setting (see previous subsection) for another 75 epochs using LPI_6 and LPI_6+MILA losses, respectively. ProportionNet outperformed GAPNet in both presence and extent prediction tasks in all cases, except for the medium sets, on which the presence detection performance of both networks was the same.

We also compared LPI_6 with a more conventional RMS loss. We trained GAPNet from scratch for 150 epochs with RMS loss to regress emphysema scores (not proportions, as in this case there would be a relatively very little cost for confusing 0% and 1–5% grades) using the largest training set. RMS did substantially worse than LPI_6 and worse than ProportionNet in both presence (AUC 0.94) and extent (AUC 0.72) prediction (see also Table 2).

Comparison to Other Methods and Human Experts. We compare our methods to two published methods, which are the most recent works that use the same dataset. [8] is an LLP method based on cluster model selection. [7] is a MIL method (trained using only presence labels) based on logistic regression. To compare with each one of these methods, we chose a split having the same number of images or fewer for training and validation (100 and 700 subjects to compare with [8] and [7], respectively). We also evaluated several traditional densitometric methods [11] and report the best result (LAA%-950). As can be seen from Table 2, ProportionNet and GAPNet substantially outperformed densitometry and the methods of [7,8].

When compared with the expert raters, ProportionNet trained using the largest training set achieves ICCs of 0.84 and 0.81 between its predictions and raters' annotations, whereas the inter-rater ICC is 0.83. It is slightly worse than the second rater in predicting the first rater's emphysema presence labels (sensitivity 0.92 vs. 0.93 when specificity is 0.9) and is as good as the first rater in predicting the second rater's labels (sensitivity 0.73, specificity 0.98).

Table 2. Comparison of our networks with densitometry and machine learning approaches [8] and [7] (they use the same dataset). "LLP" stands for training using extent labels and "MIL" – using presence labels. "RU" and "LU" stand for right and left upper regions. Metrics used are ICC, Spearman's r and AUC.

Labels	LLP								MIL	
Training set size	100 subjects				700 subjects				700 subjects	
Region	RU		LU		RU		LU		RU	LU
Metric:	ICC	r_s	ICC	r_s	ICC	AUC	ICC	AUC	AUC	AUC
Densitometry [11]	–	0.23	–	0.14	–	0.59	–	0.54	0.59	0.54
[8] and [7]	0.72	–	0.63	–	–	–	–	–	0.89	0.87
GAPNet+RMS	–	–	–	–	0.79	0.93	0.76	0.90	–	–
GAPNet+LPI$_6$	0.77	0.62	0.74	0.52	0.82	0.96	0.76	0.94	**0.96**	**0.94**
ProportionNet	**0.87**	**0.73**	**0.81**	**0.66**	**0.87**	**0.97**	**0.85**	**0.95**	**0.96**	**0.94**

Emphysema Pattern Prediction. The most common emphysema patterns are centrilobular and paraseptal (around 90% cases in upper regions). Paraseptal emphysema is located adjacent to lung pleura, whereas centrilobular can be anywhere in the lungs. We designed a simple feature to discriminate between the two, given an emphysema segmentation: a ratio between the foreground volume near the boundary and inside the region (see Fig. 2). We computed this feature using segmentations of ProportionNet trained on the largest training set. On the test set, we obtained AUC 0.89 using the first rater (sensitivity 0.65 and specificity 0.95, same as the inter-rater ones) and AUC 0.92 using the second rater as the ground truth (sensitivity 0.61 and specificity 0.96 vs. inter-rater 0.61 and 0.91). This performance is thus on a par with both raters.

5   Discussion and Conclusion

We compared two architectures for MIL and LLP (ProportionNet and GAPNet) under fair conditions: the only differences were in the few final layers that aggregated instance features into bag label predictions. ProportionNet outperformed GAPNet in both MIL and LLP settings. We can attribute this to two factors. Firstly, from our comparison between GAPNet and MGAPNet we learned that region masking is beneficial, probably because it acts as a location prior and makes compensating for variable region sizes unnecessary. However, it was not the main contributor to the performance boost. The second factor is that ProportionNet in a combination with LPI loss reflects the prior assumptions of our problem better. When ProportionNet is trained using our MIL loss (LPI$_2$+MILA with $\mathsf{thresh}_2 = 0.005$), the assumption is that even a very small (>0.5% volume) pathological area makes the image positive. When trained using our LLP loss (LPI$_6$ + MILA) and proportion labels, the network is guided on approximately how much of the abnormality is in the images. This loss also captures the interval nature of our labels better, as it allows for different predictions for same grade images. RMS loss, for example, tries to map all examples of one grade into one value, whereas in reality same grade images often have different proportions of emphysema. This is a probable reason for LPI outperforming RMS.

We are aware of only one work [10] that performed a fair comparison of different network architectures for MIL. In their case, a GAPNet-like network performed better than a ProportionNet-like network. We think that to achieve a regularization effect using ProportionNet, it is crucial to select a pooling strategy and a loss that match the prior assumptions of the target problem well.

Another important advantage of ProportionNet compared to GAPNet is that it localizes the target abnormality. In our case, the localization was good enough to classify spatial distribution of emphysema with human-level accuracy.

While in this work we focused on emphysema quantification, we expect using the proposed architecture and loss to be beneficial in other problems as well. ProportionNet can be a good regularizer for learning from visual scores related to the volume of abnormalities. It might be a good fit for estimating the volume of intracranial calcification [1] and lung abnormalities [2]. Our LPI loss can be useful when labels have interval nature (e.g., [2]).

Acknowledgment. This research is financed by the Netherlands Organization for Scientific Research (NWO) and COSMONiO.

References

1. Bos, D., et al.: Intracranial carotid artery atherosclerosis and the risk of stroke in whites: the Rotterdam study. JAMA Neurol. **71**(4), 405–411 (2014)
2. De Jong, P.A., Tiddens, H.A.: Cystic fibrosis-specific computed tomography scoring. Proc. Am. Thorac. Soc. **4**(4), 338–342 (2007)
3. Dery, L.M., Nachman, B., Rubbo, F., Schwartzman, A.: Weakly supervised classification in high energy physics. JHEP **2017**(5), 145 (2017)
4. Dubost, F., et al.: GP-Unet: lesion detection from weak labels with a 3D regression network. In: Descoteaux, M., Maier-Hein, L., Franz, A., Jannin, P., Collins, D.L., Duchesne, S. (eds.) MICCAI 2017. LNCS, vol. 10435, pp. 214–221. Springer, Cham (2017). https://doi.org/10.1007/978-3-319-66179-7_25
5. He, K., Zhang, X., Ren, S., Sun, J.: Deep residual learning for image recognition. In: CVPR 2016, pp. 770–778. IEEE (2016)
6. Li, F., Taylor, G.: Alter-CNN: an approach to learning from label proportions with application to ice-water classification. In: NIPSW (2015)
7. Ørting, S.N., Petersen, J., Thomsen, L.H., Wille, M.M.W., De Bruijne, M.: Detecting emphysema with multiple instance learning. In: ISBI (2018)
8. Ørting, S.N., Petersen, J., Wille, M.M.W., Thomsen, L.H., De Bruijne, M.: Quantifying emphysema extent from weakly labeled CT scans of the lungs using label proportions learning. In: Proceedings of Sixth International Workshop on Pulmonary Image Analysis (2016)
9. Patrini, G., Nock, R., Rivera, P., Caetano, T.: (Almost) No Label No Cry. NIPS 2014 (c), 1–9 (2014)

10. Wang, X., Yan, Y., Tang, P., Bai, X., Liu, W.: Revisiting multiple instance neural networks. Pattern Recognit. **74**, 15–24 (2018)
11. Wille, M.M.W., et al.: Visual assessment of early emphysema and interstitial abnormalities on CT is useful in lung cancer risk analysis. Eur. Radiol. **26**(2), 487–494 (2016)
12. Wille, M.M.W., Thomsen, L.H., Dirksen, A., Petersen, J., Pedersen, J.H., Shaker, S.B.: Emphysema progression is visually detectable in low-dose CT in continuous but not in former smokers. Eur. Radiol. **24**(11), 2692–2699 (2014)

Tumor-Aware, Adversarial Domain Adaptation from CT to MRI for Lung Cancer Segmentation

Jue Jiang[1], Yu-Chi Hu[1], Neelam Tyagi[1], Pengpeng Zhang[1], Andreas Rimner[2], Gig S. Mageras[1], Joseph O. Deasy[1], and Harini Veeraraghavan[1(✉)]

[1] Medical Physics, Memorial Sloan Kettering Cancer Center, New York, USA
veerarah@mskcc.org
[2] Radiation Oncology, Memorial Sloan Kettering Cancer Center, New York, USA

Abstract. We present an adversarial domain adaptation based deep learning approach for automatic tumor segmentation from T2-weighted MRI. Our approach is composed of two steps: (i) a tumor-aware unsupervised cross-domain adaptation (CT to MRI), followed by (ii) semi-supervised tumor segmentation using Unet trained with synthesized and limited number of original MRIs. We introduced a novel target specific loss, called tumor-aware loss, for unsupervised cross-domain adaptation that helps to preserve tumors on synthesized MRIs produced from CT images. In comparison, state-of-the art adversarial networks trained without our tumor-aware loss produced MRIs with ill-preserved or missing tumors. All networks were trained using labeled CT images from 377 patients with non-small cell lung cancer obtained from the Cancer Imaging Archive and unlabeled T2w MRIs from a completely unrelated cohort of 6 patients with pre-treatment and 36 on-treatment scans. Next, we combined 6 labeled pre-treatment MRI scans with the synthesized MRIs to boost tumor segmentation accuracy through semi-supervised learning. Semi-supervised training of cycle-GAN produced a segmentation accuracy of 0.66 computed using Dice Score Coefficient (DSC). Our method trained with only synthesized MRIs produced an accuracy of 0.74 while the same method trained in semi-supervised setting produced the best accuracy of 0.80 on test. Our results show that tumor-aware adversarial domain adaptation helps to achieve reasonably accurate cancer segmentation from limited MRI data by leveraging large CT datasets.

1 Introduction

MRI-guided radiotherapy is an emerging technology for improving treatment accuracy over conventional CT-based radiotherapy due to better soft-tissue con-

---

H. Veeraraghavan—Equal contributing.

Electronic supplementary material The online version of this chapter (https:// doi.org/10.1007/978-3-030-00934-2_86) contains supplementary material, which is available to authorized users.

© Springer Nature Switzerland AG 2018
A. F. Frangi et al. (Eds.): MICCAI 2018, LNCS 11071, pp. 777–785, 2018.
https://doi.org/10.1007/978-3-030-00934-2_86

trast in MR compared to CT images. Real-time and accurate tumor segmentation on MRI can help to deliver high dose to tumors while reducing normal tissue dose. However, as MRI-guided radiotherapy is not used in standard-of-care, only very few MRIs are available for training. Therefore, we developed an adversarial domain adaptation from large CT datasets for tumor segmentation on MRI.

Although deep neural networks excel in learning from large amounts of (labeled) data, their accuracy is reduced when applied to novel datasets or domains [1]. Differences between source and target domain distribution is called *domain shift*. Typically used fine-tuning methods require prohibitively large labeled data in the target domain. As an alternative, domain adaptation methods attempt to minimize domain shift either by feature sharing [2] or by learning to reconstruct the target from source domain [3,4]. In essence, domain adaptation methods learn the marginal distributions [5] to transform source to target domain.

The problems of domain shift are exacerbated in medical images, where imaging modalities capture physical properties of the underlying anatomy differently (eg. CT vs. MRI). For example, whereas bones appear hyper-dense on CT and dark on MRI, tumors appear with similar contrast as normal soft-tissue on CT but have a distinct appearance on MRI (Fig. 1(a) and (b)). Consequently, learning the marginal distributions of the domains alone may not be sufficient.

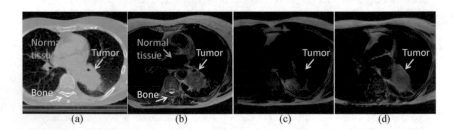

Fig. 1. MRI synthesized from a representative (a) CT image using (c) cycle-GAN [5] and (d) proposed method. The corresponding MRI scan for (a) is shown in (b). As shown, the proposed method (d) using tumor-aware loss helps to fully preserve tumor in the synthesized MRI compared with (c).

Cross-domain adaptation of highly different modalities, has been applied in medical image analysis for image synthesis using paired images [6] and unpaired images [7], as well as for segmentation [8,9]. However, all aforementioned approaches aim to only synthesize images that match the marginal but not the structure-specific conditional distribution such as tumors. Therefore, segmentation/classification using such synthetic images will lead to lower accuracy.

Therefore, we introduced a novel target specific loss, called tumor-aware loss, for unsupervised cross-domain adaptation that helps to preserve tumors on synthesized MRIs produced from CT images (Fig. 1(d)), which cannot be captured with just the cycle loss (Fig. 1(c)).

2   Method

Our objective is to solve the problem of learning to segment tumors from MR images through domain adaptation from CT to MRI, where we have access to a reasonably sized labeled data in the source domain (X_{CT}, y_{CT}) but are provided with very limited number of target samples $X_{MRI} \ll X_{CT}$ and fewer labels y_{MR}. Our solution first employs tumor-aware unsupervised cross-domain adaptation to synthesize a reasonably large number of MRI from CT through adversarial training. Second, we combine the synthesized MRI with a fraction of real MRI with corresponding labels and train a Unet [10] for generating tumor segmentation as outlined in Fig. 2.

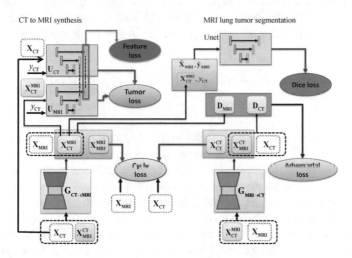

Fig. 2. Approach overview. X_{CT} and X_{MRI} are the real CT and MRI; X_{CT}^{MRI} and X_{MRI}^{CT} are the synthesized MR and CT images; y_{CT} is the CT image label; $G_{CT \rightarrow MRI}$ and $G_{MRI \rightarrow CT}$ are the CT and MRI transfer networks; $\tilde{X}_{MRI}$ and $\tilde{y}_{MRI}$ are a small sample set from the real MRI, used to train semi-supervised segmentation.

2.1   Step 1: MRI Synthesis Using Tumor-Aware Unsupervised Cross Domain Adaptation

The first step is to learn a mapping $G_{CT \rightarrow MRI}$ that synthesizes MRI from the CT images to fool a discriminator D_{MRI} using adversarial training [11]. Additionally, we compute an adversarial loss L_{adv}^{CT} for synthesizing CT from MRI by simultaneously training a network that learns a mapping $G_{MRI \rightarrow CT}$. The adversarial loss,

L_{adv}^{MRI}, for synthesizing MRI from CT, and L_{adv}^{CT}, for synthesizing CT from MRI, are computed as:

$$L_{adv}^{MRI}(G_{CT \to MRI}, D_{MRI}, X_{MRI}, X_{CT}) = \mathbb{E}_{x_m \sim X_{MRI}}[log(D_{MRI}(x_m))]$$
$$+\mathbb{E}_{x_c \sim X_{CT}}[log(1 - (D_{MRI}(G_{CT \to MRI}(x_c))]$$
$$L_{adv}^{CT}(G_{MRI \to CT}, D_{CT}, X_{CT}, X_{MRI}) = \mathbb{E}_{x_c \sim X_{CT}}[log(D_{CT}(x_c))]$$
$$+\mathbb{E}_{x_m \sim X_{MRI}}[log(1 - (D_{CT}(G_{MRI \to CT}(x_m))]$$

(1)

where x_c and x_m are real images sampled from the CT (X_{CT}) and MRI (X_{MRI}) domains, respectively. The total adversarial loss (Fig. 2 (purple ellipse)) is then computed as the summation of the two losses as $L_{adv} = L_{adv}^{MRI} + L_{adv}^{CT}$. We also compute a cycle consistency loss [5] to regularize the images synthesized through independent training of the two networks. By letting the synthesized images be $x_m' = G_{CT \to MRI}(x_c)$ and $x_c' = G_{MRI \to CT}(x_m)$, the cycle consistency loss L_{cyc} is calculated as:

$$L_{cyc}(G_{CT \to MRI}, G_{MRI \to CT}, X_{CT}, X_{MRI}) = \mathbb{E}_{x_c \sim X_{CT}} \left[\left\| G_{MRI \to CT}(x_m') - x_c \right\|_1 \right]$$
$$+ \mathbb{E}_{x_m \sim X_{MRI}} \left[\left\| G_{CT \to MRI}(x_c') - x_m \right\|_1 \right].$$

(2)

The cycle consistency and adversarial loss only constrain the model to learn a global mapping that matches the marginal distribution but not the conditional distribution pertaining to individual structures such as the tumors. Therefore, a model trained using these losses does not need to preserve tumors, which can lead to either deterioration or total loss of tumors in the synthesized MRIs (Fig. 1(c)). Therefore, we introduced a tumor-aware loss that forces the network to preserve the tumors. To be specific, the tumor-aware loss is composed of a tumor loss (Fig. 2 (red ellipse)) and a feature loss (Fig. 2 (orange ellipse)). We compute the tumor loss by training two parallel tumor detection networks using simplified models of the Unet [10] for CT (U_{CT}) and the synthesized MRI (U_{MRI}). The tumor loss constrains the CT and synthetic MRI-based Unets to produce similar tumor segmentations, thereby, preserving the tumors and is computed as:

$$L_{tumor} = \mathbb{E}_{x_c \sim X_{CT}, y_c \sim y_{CT}}[log P(y_c | G_{CT \to MRI}(x_c))]$$
$$+ \mathbb{E}_{x_c \sim X_{CT}, y_c \sim y_{CT}}[log P(y_c | X_{CT})].$$

(3)

On the other hand, the tumor feature loss L_{feat} forces the high-level features of X_{CT} and X_{CT}^{MRI} to be shared by using a constraint inspired by [12] as:

$$L_{feat}(x_c \sim X_{CT}) = \frac{1}{C \times H \times W} \left\| \phi_{CT}(x_c) - \phi_{MRI}(G_{CT \to MRI}(x_c)) \right\|^2.$$ (4)

where ϕ_{CT} and ϕ_{MRI} are the high-level features extracted from the U_{CT} and U_{MRI}, respectively; C, H and W indicate the size of the feature. The total loss is then expressed as:

$$L_{total} = L_{adv} + \lambda_{cyc}L_{cyc} + \lambda_{tumor}L_{tumor} + \lambda_{feat}L_{feat},$$ (5)

where λ_{cyc}, λ_{tumor} and λ_{feat} are the weighting coefficients for each loss. During training, we alternatively update the domain transfer or generator network G, the discriminator D, and the tumor constraint network U with the following gradients, $-\Delta_{\theta_G}(L_{adv} + \lambda_{cyc}L_{cyc} + \lambda_{tumor}L_{tumor} + \lambda_{feat}L_{feat})$, $-\Delta_{\theta_D}(L_{adv})$ and $-\Delta_{\theta_U}(L_{tumor} + \lambda_{feat}L_{feat})$.

2.2   Step 2: Semi-supervised Tumor Segmentation from MRI

The synthesized MRI from the first step were combined with a small set of real MRI with labels ($\tilde{X}_{MRI}$ and $\tilde{y}_{MRI}$ in Fig. 2) to train a U-net [10] using Dice loss [13] (Fig. 2 (blue ellipse)) to generate tumor segmentation. Adversarial network optimization for MRI synthesis was frozen prior to semi-supervised tumor segmentation training to prevent leakage of MRI label information.

2.3   Network Structure and Implementation

The generators G and discriminators D for CT and MRI synthesis networks were implemented similar to that in [5]. We tied the penultimate layer in U_{MRI} and U_{CT}. The details of all networks are shown in the supplementary documents. Pytorch library [14] was used for implementing the proposed networks, which were trained on Nvidia GTX 1080Ti of 12 GB memory with a batch size of 1 during image transfer and batch size of 10 during semi-supervised segmentation. The ADAM algorithm [15] with an initial learning rate of 1e-4 was used during training. We set $\lambda_{cyc} = 10$, $\lambda_{tumor} = 5$ and $\lambda_{feat} = 1$.

3   Experiments and Results

3.1   Ablation Tests

We tested the impact of adding tumor-aware loss to the cycle loss (proposed vs. cycle-GAN [5] vs. masked-cycle-GAN [8]). Images synthesized using aforementioned networks were trained to segment using semi-supervised learning by combining with a limited number of real MRI. We call adversarial synthesis [8] that combined tumor labels as an additional channel with the original images as masked-cycle-GAN. We also evaluated the effect of adding a limited number of original MRI to the synthesized MRI on segmentation accuracy (tumor-aware with semi-supervised vs. tumor-aware with unsupervised training). We benchmarked the lowest achievable segmentation accuracy by training a network with only the pre-treatment (or week one) MRI.

3.2   Datasets

The image synthesis networks were trained using contrast-enhanced CT images with expert delineated tumors from 377 patients with non-small cell lung cancer (NSCLC) [16] available from The Cancer Imaging Archive (TCIA) [17], and

782   J. Jiang et al.

an unrelated cohort of 6 patients scanned with T2w MRI at our clinic before and during treatment every week (n = 7) with radiation therapy. Masked cycle-GANs used both tumor labels and the images as additional channels even for image synthesis training. Image regions enclosing the tumors were extracted and rescaled to 256 × 256 to produce 32000 CT image slices and 9696 T2w MR image slices. Only 1536 MR images from pre-treatment MRI were used for semi-supervised segmentation training of all networks. Segmentation validation was performed on the subsequent on-treatment MRIs (n = 36) from the same 6 patients. Test was performed using 28 MRIs consisting of longitudinal scans (7, 7, 6) from 3 patients and pre-treatment scans from 8 patients not used in training. Tumor segmentation accuracy was evaluated by comparing to expert delineations using the Dice Score Coefficient (DSC), and the Hausdorff Distance 95% (HD95).

3.3   MR Image Synthesis Results

Figure 3 shows the representative qualitative results of synthesized MRI produced using only the cycle-GAN (Fig. 3(b)), masked cycle-GAN (Fig. 3(c)) and using our method (Fig. 3(d)). As seen, our method best preserves the anatomical details between CT and MRI. Quantitative evaluation using the Kullback - Leibler (KL) divergence computed from tumor regions between synthesized and original MRI, used for training, confirmed that our method resulted in the best match of tumor distribution with the lowest KL divergence of 0.069 compared with those obtained using the cycle-GAN (1.69) and masked cycle-GAN (0.32).

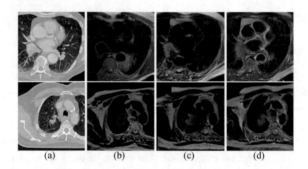

Fig. 3. MRI synthesized from CT using different deep learning methods. The red contour indicates the manually delineated tumor region in the NSCLC datasets [16]. (a) CT image; (b) Cycle-GAN [5]; (c) Masked cycle-GAN [8]; (d) Proposed.

3.4   Segmentation Results

Figure 4 shows the segmentations generated using the various methods (yellow contours) for three representative cases from the test and validation sets, together with the expert delineations (red contours). As shown in Table 1, our approach outperformed cycle GAN irrespective of training without (unsupervised) or with (semi-supervised) labeled target data. Semi-supervised segmentation outperformed all methods in both test and validation datasets.

Table 1. Segmentation accuracy

Method	Validation		Test	
	DSC	HD95 mm	DSC	HD95 mm
Week one only	0.63 ± 0.27	7.22 ± 7.19	0.55 ± 0.25	13.23 ± 0.75
Cycle-GAN [5]	0.57 ± 0.24	11.41 ± 5.57	0.66 ± 0.16	11.91 ± 4.44
Masked cycle-GAN [8]	0.67 ± 0.21	7.78 ± 4.40	0.63 ± 0.24	11.65 ± 6.53
Tumor aware unsupervised	0.62 ± 0.26	7.47 ± 4.66	0.74 ± 0.15	8.88 ± 4.83
Tumor aware semi-supervised	$\mathbf{0.70 \pm 0.19}$	$\mathbf{5.88 \pm 2.88}$	$\mathbf{0.80 \pm 0.08}$	$\mathbf{7.16 \pm 4.52}$

4   Discussion

In this work, we introduced a novel target-specific, tumor-aware loss for synthesizing MR images from unpaired CT datasets using unsupervised cross-domain adaptation. The tumor-aware loss forces the network to retain tumors that are typically lost when using only the cycle-loss and leads to accurate tumor segmentation. Although applied to lung tumors, our method is applicable to other

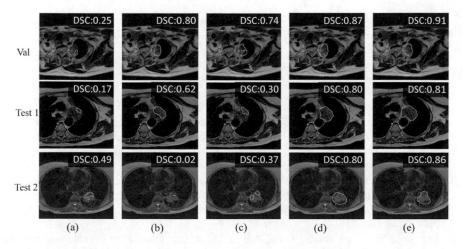

Fig. 4. Segmentation results on the representative examples from the validation and test set of different methods. The red contour stands for the expert delineations and the yellow contour stands for the segmentation results. (a) segmentation with only week 1 MRI; (b) segmentation using MRI synthesized by cycle-GAN [5]; (c) segmentation using MRI synthesized by masked cycle-GAN [8]; (d) tumor-aware unsupervised learning; (e) tumor-aware semi-supervised learning

structures and organs. Segmentation accuracy of our approach trained with only synthesized MRIs exceeded other methods trained in a semi-supervised manner. Adding small set of labeled target domain data further boosts accuracy. The validation set produced lower but not significantly different ($p = 0.1$) DSC accuracy than the test set due to significantly smaller ($p = 0.0004$) tumor volumes in validation (mean 37.66cc) when compared with the test set (mean 68.2cc). Our results showed that masked-cycle-GAN produced lower test performance compared to basic cycle-GAN, possibly due to poor modeling from highly unbalanced CT and MR datasets. As a limitation, our approach only forces the synthesized MRIs to preserve tumors but not the MR intensity distribution within tumors. Such modeling would require learning the mapping for individual scan manufacturers, magnet strengths and coil placements which was outside the scope of this work. Additionally, synthesized images irrespective of the chosen method do not produce a one-to-one pixel mapping from CT to MRI similar to [8]. There is also room for improving the segmentation accuracy by exploring more advanced segmentation models, e.g. boundary-aware fully convolutional networks (FCN) [18].

5   Conclusions

In this work, we proposed a tumor-aware, adversarial domain adaptation method using unpaired CT and MR images for generating segmentations from MRI. Our approach preserved tumors on synthesized MRI and generated the best segmentation performance compared with state-of-the-art adversarial cross-domain adaptation. Our results suggest feasibility for lung tumor segmentation from MRI trained using MRI synthesized from CT.

Acknowledgement. This work was funded in part through the NIH/NCI Cancer Center Support Grant P30 CA008748.

References

1. Tzeng, E., Hoffman, J., Saenko, K., Darrell, T.: Adversarial discriminative domain adaptation. In: 2017 IEEE Conference on Computer Vision and Pattern Recognition, CVPR 2017, Honolulu, HI, USA, 21–26 July 2017, pp. 2962–2971 (2017)
2. Ganin, Y., Lempitsky, V.: Unsupervised domain adaptation by backpropagation. In: International Conference on Machine Learning (ICML), pp. 1180–1189 (2015)
3. Shrivastava, A., Pfister, T., Tuzel, O., Susskind, J., Wang, W., Webb, R.: Learning from simulated and unsupervised images through adversarial training. In: IEEE Conference on Computer Vision and Pattern Recognition (CVPR), vol. 3, pp. 2107–2116 (2017)
4. Yoo, D., Kim, N., Park, S., Paek, A.S., Kweon, I.S.: Pixel-level domain transfer. In: Leibe, B., Matas, J., Sebe, N., Welling, M. (eds.) ECCV 2016. LNCS, vol. 9912, pp. 517–532. Springer, Cham (2016). https://doi.org/10.1007/978-3-319-46484-8_31
5. Zhu, J.Y., Park, T., Isola, P., Efros, A.: Unpaired image-to-image translation using cycle-consistent adversarial networks. In: International Conference on Computer Vision (ICCV), pp. 2223–2232 (2017)

6. Nie, D., et al.: Medical image synthesis with context-aware generative adversarial networks. In: Descoteaux, M., Maier-Hein, L., Franz, A., Jannin, P., Collins, D.L., Duchesne, S. (eds.) MICCAI 2017. LNCS, vol. 10435, pp. 417–425. Springer, Cham (2017). https://doi.org/10.1007/978-3-319-66179-7_48
7. Wolterink, J.M., Dinkla, A.M., Savenije, M.H.F., Seevinck, P.R., van den Berg, C.A.T., Išgum, I.: Deep MR to CT synthesis using unpaired data. In: Tsaftaris, S.A., Gooya, A., Frangi, A.F., Prince, J.L. (eds.) SASHIMI 2017. LNCS, vol. 10557, pp. 14–23. Springer, Cham (2017). https://doi.org/10.1007/978-3-319-68127-6_2
8. Chartsias, A., Joyce, T., Dharmakumar, R., Tsaftaris, S.A.: Adversarial image synthesis for unpaired multi-modal cardiac data. In: Tsaftaris, S.A., Gooya, A., Frangi, A.F., Prince, J.L. (eds.) SASHIMI 2017. LNCS, vol. 10557, pp. 3–13. Springer, Cham (2017). https://doi.org/10.1007/978-3-319-68127-6_1
9. Huo, Y., Xu, Z., Bao, S., Assad, A., Abramson, R.G., Landman, B.-A.: Adversarial synthesis learning enables segmentation without target modality ground truth. In: IEEE International Symposium on Biomedical Imaging (2018)
10. Ronneberger, O., Fischer, P., Brox, T.: U-Net: convolutional networks for biomedical image segmentation. In: Navab, N., Hornegger, J., Wells, W.M., Frangi, A.F. (eds.) MICCAI 2015. LNCS, vol. 9351, pp. 234–241. Springer, Cham (2015). https://doi.org/10.1007/978-3-319-24574-4_28
11. Goodfellow, I., et al.: Generative adversarial nets. In: Advances in Neural Information Processing Systems (NIPS), pp. 2672–2680 (2014)
12. Johnson, J., Alahi, A., Fei-Fei, L.: Perceptual losses for real-time style transfer and super-resolution. In: Leibe, B., Matas, J., Sebe, N., Welling, M. (eds.) ECCV 2016. LNCS, vol. 9906, pp. 694–711. Springer, Cham (2016). https://doi.org/10.1007/978-3-319-46475-6_43
13. Milletari, F., Navab, N., Ahmadi, S.A.: V-net: fully convolutional neural networks for volumetric medical image segmentation. In: 2016 Fourth International Conference on 3D Vision (3DV), pp. 565–571. IEEE (2016)
14. Paszke, A., et al.: Automatic differentiation in Py Torch (2017)
15. Kingma, D.P., Ba, J.: Adam: a method for stochastic optimization. In: Proceedings of the 3rd International Conference on Learning Representations (ICLR) (2014)
16. Aerts, H., et al.: Data from NSCLC-radiomics. The Cancer Imaging Archive (2015)
17. Clark, K., et al.: The cancer imaging archive (TCIA): maintaining and operating a public information repository. J. Digital Imaging 26(6), 1045–1057 (2013)
18. Shen, H., Wang, R., Zhang, J., McKenna, S.J.: Boundary-aware fully convolutional network for brain tumor segmentation. In: Descoteaux, M., Maier-Hein, L., Franz, A., Jannin, P., Collins, D.L., Duchesne, S. (eds.) MICCAI 2017. LNCS, vol. 10434, pp. 433–441. Springer, Cham (2017). https://doi.org/10.1007/978-3-319-66185-8_49

From Local to Global: A Holistic Lung Graph Model

Yashin Dicente Cid[1,2](✉), Oscar Jiménez-del-Toro[1,2,3], Alexandra Platon[3],
Henning Müller[1,2], and Pierre-Alexandre Poletti[3]

[1] University of Applied Sciences Western Switzerland (HES-SO), Sierre, Switzerland
`yashin.dicente@hevs.ch`
[2] University of Geneva, Geneva, Switzerland
[3] University Hospitals of Geneva (HUG), Geneva, Switzerland

Abstract. Lung image analysis is an essential part in the assessment
of pulmonary diseases. Through visual inspection of CT scans, radiologists detect abnormal patterns in the lung parenchyma, aiming to establish a timely diagnosis and thus improving patient outcome. However,
in a generalized disorder of the lungs, such as pulmonary hypertension,
the changes in organ tissue can be elusive, requiring additional invasive studies to confirm the diagnosis. We present a graph model that
quantifies lung texture in a holistic approach enhancing the analysis
between pathologies with similar local changes. The approach extracts
local state-of-the-art 3D texture descriptors from an automatically generated geometric parcellation of the lungs. The global texture distribution is encoded in a weighted graph that characterizes the correlations
among neighboring organ regions. A data set of 125 patients with suspicion of having a pulmonary vascular pathology was used to evaluate
our method. Three classes containing 47 pulmonary hypertension, 31
pulmonary embolism and 47 control cases were classified in a one vs.
one setup. An area under the curve of up to 0.85 was obtained adding
directionality to the edges of the graph architecture. The approach was
able to identify diseased patients, and to distinguish pathologies with
abnormal local and global blood perfusion defects.

Keywords: Lung graph model · Texture analysis
Pulmonary perfusion

1 Introduction

An important task in the radiology workflow is detecting subtle alterations in
patient scans that could help to correctly identify and diagnose diseases. However, when there is a widespread distribution of the disease in an organ, i.e.
the lungs, the pathological changes can be so elusive that require more (invasive) studies to establish a diagnosis [16]. Particularly in the case of pulmonary
hypertension (PH), an invasive catheterization procedure is the gold standard

© Springer Nature Switzerland AG 2018
A. F. Frangi et al. (Eds.): MICCAI 2018, LNCS 11071, pp. 786–793, 2018.
https://doi.org/10.1007/978-3-030-00934-2_87

for diagnosis and allows the differentiation of PH from pulmonary embolism (PE) [12]. A correct interpretation of the cases in their early stages is relevant since both pathologies have similar local manifestations, despite requiring different treatments [10]. Moreover, the pulmonary perfusion changes in PH and PE might not only be present in small regions, but also have a profound impact on the entire pulmonary circulatory network [11]. A holistic lung blood perfusion analysis, instead of local independent assessments of haemodynamic alterations, could improve the clinical evaluation of a patient by providing a global pathological status of the lungs.

Graph modeling is a complete framework that has been previously proposed for brain connectivity analysis, but has rarely been applied to other organs [14]. In short, graph methods divide the brain into fixed anatomical regions, and compare neural activations between different regions [15]. Based on these approaches, we propose a graph model of the lungs built from 3D local texture descriptors extracted on an atlas-based parcellation, with the purpose of encoding pulmonary blood perfusion relations between neighboring regions. An early version of this method was proposed in [8], combining simple intensity features in a 30 patients dataset of dual energy CT scans, combining 11 energy levels. The approach was also compared against 8 other methods, including deep learning approaches in the ImageCLEF tuberculosis challenge 2017 [4], obtaining the 3 top scores for the lung image analysis task in drug resistance detection [7].

In this paper we exploit the graph architecture for the analysis of the whole pulmonary circulatory network in a relatively large and heterogeneous dataset of patients with pulmonary vascular pathologies. The global analysis of the lungs was refined to detect and differentiate between PH and PE, relying only on the CT scans taken in an emergency radiology service. A novel visual interpretation of the biomedical tissue texture is presented as well, which can help radiologists to promptly interpret and localize 3D textural changes in anatomical structures.

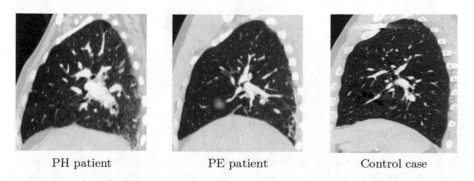

PH patient   PE patient   Control case

Fig. 1. Examples of the three classes in the dataset. Iodine maps showed that both PH and PE cases presented hypo- and hyper-perfused regions, not apparent in the CT scans.

2   Methods

2.1   Dataset

Experiments were carried out on contrast-enhanced chest CT images at 70 KeV of 125 patients: 31 with diagnosed PE, 47 with diagnosed PH and 47 control cases (CC) (see Fig. 1). The resolution of the CT slices in x- and y-directions varied from 0.5742 to 0.9766 mm, while the inter-slice distance was 1.00 mm. Since 3D rotation-invariant texture features were used in our approach, all CT images were converted into isometric volumes, with a voxel size of $1 \times 1 \times 1$ mm^3.

2.2   Holistic Graph Model of the Lungs

A pipeline composed of four steps was developed for building a distinctive graph per patient (see Fig. 2). Initially, the lung fields were automatically extracted using the method explained in [6]. Then, the lung masks were geometrically divided into a 36-region atlas [3,5] derived from the 3D model of the human lung presented by Zrimec et al. [17]. For each region r of this atlas two texture-based feature descriptors were extracted: the Fourier histograms of oriented gradients (FHOG) [13] and the locally-oriented 3D Riesz-wavelet transform (3DRiesz) [9]. These descriptors have been successful for multiple biomedical texture analysis applications [1,2]. FHOG was computed using 28 3D directions for the histogram, obtaining a 28-dimensional feature vector per image voxel v ($\mathbf{f}_H(v) \in \mathbb{R}^{28}$). For 3DRiesz we used the 3rd-order Riesz-wavelet transform, with 4 scales and 1st-order alignment (see [9]). The feature vector for a single voxel was defined as the weighted sum of the absolute Riesz response along the 4 scales, obtaining a 10-dimensional feature vector ($\mathbf{f}_\mathcal{R}(v) \in \mathbb{R}^{10}$). Finally, the average and standard deviation of these descriptors were obtained for each region r: $\boldsymbol{\mu}_H(r)$, $\boldsymbol{\sigma}_H(r)$, $\boldsymbol{\mu}_\mathcal{R}(r)$, and $\boldsymbol{\sigma}_\mathcal{R}(r)$.

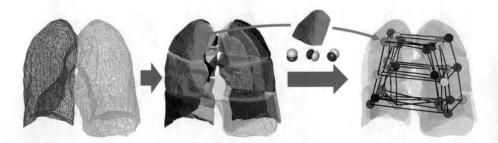

Fig. 2. Construction of the graph model: First the lungs were automatically segmented. Then they were divided using the geometric atlas with 36 regions. Finally, the graph was built based on the 3D adjacency of the regions (including left-right lung connections). The edges contained the similarities between 3D texture descriptors computed in the regions.

2.3   Undirected Weighted Graph Model of the Lung

In [4] Dicente et al. tested several graph configurations for lung modeling of tuberculosis cases using the 36-regions atlas. The graph architecture obtaining the best scores contained 84 edges, based on a region adjacency defined on the atlas. Formally, there exists an undirected edge $E_{i,j}$ between nodes N_i and N_j if regions r_i and r_j are 3D adjacent in the atlas or symmetric with respect the left-right division of the lungs (see Fig. 2). Considering $\mathbf{f}_i$ and $\mathbf{f}_j$ the feature vectors of regions r_i and r_j respectively, the weight $w_{i,j}$ of an edge $E_{i,j}$ was defined as: $w_{i,j} = 1 - corr(\mathbf{f}_i, \mathbf{f}_j) \in [0, 2]$. The use of rotation-invariant texture descriptors where each component corresponds to a texture-direction implies that regions with similar texture will be highly correlated, and thus, with $w_{i,j} \approx 0$. Since the edges used for this graph were undirected, then $w_{i,j} = w_{j,i}$ and this graph has 84 weights. For a patient p this graph will be referred as G_p^U.

2.4   Directed Weighted Graph-Model of the Lungs

Using the same graph architecture (36 nodes and 84 edges), we introduce the notion of directionality. let $\mathbf{f}_i$ and $\mathbf{f}_j$ be the feature vectors of regions r_i and r_j, respectively. The weight of an edge $E_{i,j}$ between nodes N_i and N_j is then defined as $w_{i,j} = 1 - corr(\mathbf{f}_i, \mathbf{f}_j)$ if $||\mathbf{f}_i|| \leq ||\mathbf{f}_j||$, and 0 otherwise. Since $w_{i,j} \neq w_{j,i}$ (except when $||\mathbf{f}_i|| = ||\mathbf{f}_j||$), this graph contains 168 weights, of which 84 are equal to 0. However, for each patient these 84 weights equal to 0 may be at different positions since the condition for being 0 relies on the properties of each patient lung tissue. The idea of this approach is to better exploit the same graph architecture adding more information about the texture in the regions (nodes), i.e. which node contained more/less texture than its neighbors For a patient p this graph is referred as G_p^D.

2.5   Graph-Based Patient Descriptor

As mention before, the undirected graph G_p^U of a patient p only contained 84 weights. Then, we defined the graph-based patient descriptor $\boldsymbol{w}_p^U$ as the vector containing the 84 weights ordered by their location in the graph. For the directed graph, $\boldsymbol{w}_p^D$ contained the 168 weights ordered by their graph location.

Patient Descriptor Normalization. The descriptor vectors $\boldsymbol{w}_p$ were normalized based on the training set, obtaining $\hat{\boldsymbol{w}}_p$. However, since each component of $\boldsymbol{w}_p$ corresponded to a weight in the graph, these can not be seen independently and the normalization was done for all components simultaneously.

Concatenation of Patient Descriptors. As mentioned before, four different feature vectors were computed in each atlas region $r(\boldsymbol{\mu}_H(r), \boldsymbol{\sigma}_H(r), \boldsymbol{\mu}_R(r),$ and $\boldsymbol{\sigma}_R(r))$ providing complementary information about the texture and its variability. Given a patient p, a different graph was obtained from each of these feature vectors. The final patient descriptor vector $\boldsymbol{W}_p$ used in our experiments was defined as the concatenation of the four normalized graph-based descriptors: $\boldsymbol{W}_p = (\hat{\boldsymbol{w}}_{\mu_H,p} \| \hat{\boldsymbol{w}}_{\sigma_H,p} \| \hat{\boldsymbol{w}}_{\mu_R,p} \| \hat{\boldsymbol{w}}_{\sigma_R,p})$. After this concatenation, $\boldsymbol{W}_p^U \in \mathbb{R}^{336}$ when using the undirected graph and $\boldsymbol{W}_p^D \in \mathbb{R}^{672}$ for the directed approach.

3   Experimental Setup

Four binary classification experiments were performed: (a) PH vs. PE, (b) PH vs. CC, (c) PE vs. CC, and (d) (PH+PE) vs. CC. In experiment (d) PH and PE patients were considered to belong to same class. The dataset was divided in each experiment in ~70% for training and ~30% for testing. This results in 34 PH, 22 PE and 34 CC for training and 13 PH, 9 PE and 13 CC for testing. As the classes were not balanced in the test sets, the random accuracy (when assigning the most frequent label to all the patients) was 59.09% for experiments (a) and (c), 50.00% for experiment (b) and 62.86% for experiment (d). 2-class SVM classifier with Gaussian kernel was used in each experiment. The parameter optimization was performed using 10-fold cross-validation on the training set. All experiments were performed using both the undirected and the directed graph models.

The descriptor vectors for a given patient $\boldsymbol{W}_p^U$ and $\boldsymbol{W}_p^D$ had a dimension significantly higher than the size of our dataset (336 and 672 vs. 125). To avoid the known overfitting problems when using large feature spaces, feature dimensionality reduction was performed in the training phase. This consisted on selecting those dimensions that correlate above the average with the training labels. This method reduced the feature space dimension approximately by two, both when using the undirected and directed graph models. Moreover, since the random split of the dataset in training and test sets may have a strong effect in the classification performance, we ran each experiment using five different random splits to ensure the robustness of our models.

4   Results

Figure 3 shows the average and standard deviation of the accuracy and the AUC over the five random splits for each of the four experiments. The accuracy and the confusion matrices in Fig. 4 are reported using the standard classification decision threshold of 0.5, and not in the optimal threshold provided by the ROC curves. The results of each experiment were above the random performance in all cases (see red line in Fig. 3). When analyzing all the performance measures, the directed graph model performed better than the undirected in the experiments (b) and (c). However, both models performed almost equivalent in experiments (a) and (b). The highest benefit of the directed graph among the undirected is shown in experiment (b), where the true positive rate increases from 69.23% and 75.38% to 76.92% and 81.54% in the PH and CC classes respectively. In experiment (d) the increment is similar, however, the directed graph is still not able to identify the CC class above random. These results suggest that PH and PE do not form a clear cluster in the feature space.

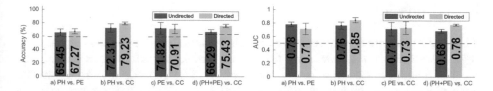

Fig. 3. Average accuracy and AUC over the five random splits of the dataset (both training and test set). The error bars show the standard deviation. The red line indicates the random performance in each measure and experiment.

a) PH vs. PE

Und.	PH	PE
PH	70.77	29.23
PE	42.22	57.78

Dir.	PH	PE
PH	73.85	26.15
PE	42.22	57.78

b) PH vs. CC

Und.	PH	CC
PH	69.23	30.77
CC	24.62	75.38

Dir.	PH	CC
PH	76.92	23.08
CC	18.46	81.54

c) PE vs. CC

Und.	PE	CC
PE	64.44	35.56
CC	23.08	76.92

Dir.	PE	CC
PE	64.44	35.56
CC	24.62	75.38

d) (PH+PE) vs. CC

Und.	PH+PE	CC
PH+PE	80.91	19.09
CC	58.46	41.54

Dir.	PH+PE	CC
PH+PE	89.09	10.91
CC	47.69	52.31

Fig. 4. Confusion matrices with the % of TP, FP, TN and FN for the four experiments over the 5 random dataset splits.

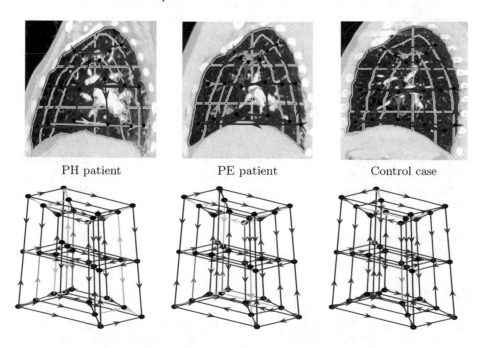

Fig. 5. 3D visualization of the graphs obtained for the three patients shown in Fig. 1. The first row contains the subgraph corresponding to the regions in the 2D slice. All six graphs are depicted using the same color code. This example has been generated using the $\mu_{\mathcal{R}}$ feature. In this case, heterogenous edge connections can be seen in PH and PE patients.

5   Discussion

This work presents a comprehensive graph model of the lungs that connects 3D regional texture nodes enclosing the whole circulatory network of lungs. The method was evaluated in a large dataset of 125 CT thorax scans from patients with clinical symptoms commonly associated to vascular pathologies, such as pulmonary hypertension and pulmonary embolism. Even for experienced radiologists detecting and differentiating pulmonary hypertension is a challenging task diagnosed only by using a catheterization procedure. The proposed approach was able to correctly identify most of the patients with these pulmonary perfusion defects in a standard CT scan, even without any prior clinical information.

The proposed composite interpretation of the lung circulatory network was able to distinguish between local defects (PE) and elusive global pathological patterns (PH). By analyzing the confusion matrices in Fig. 4, it can be seen that the method had the worse classification scores with the control class. Nonetheless, it is important to highlight that all the patients in the dataset were obtained from an emergency department and may well have other lung malfunctions. A straightforward 3D visualization of the textural changes in the lungs was additionally generated from the obtained graph architectures. The graph depicting both lungs could be useful for radiologists to understand intrinsic parenchymal texture distributions that might not be apparent in 2D renderings of the organ.

6   Conclusions and Future Work

A precise assessment of pulmonary perfusion can lead to a fast diagnosis and optimal treatment in the presence of haemodynamic changes. A directed weighted graph model of the lungs encoding blood perfusion relations from an automatically generated geometric atlas of the lungs was evaluated. The approach was able to not only recognize diseased patients, but also to classify correctly similar abnormal local and global patterns in the pulmonary parenchymal texture. This holistic graph descriptor can be expanded to include more lung pathologies and potentially be applied to other anatomical structures as well.

Acknowledgments. This work was partly supported by the Swiss National Science Foundation in the PH4D project (grant agreement 320030-146804).

References

1. Chalkidou, A., O'Doherty, M.J., Marsden, P.K.: False discovery rates in PET and CT Studies with texture features: a systematic review. PLOS ONE **10**(5), 1–18 (2015)
2. Depeursinge, A., Al-Kadi, O.S., Mitchell, J.R.: Biomedical Texture Analysis: Fundamentals, Applications and Tools. Elsevier-MICCAI Society Book series. Elsevier, October 2017. https://www.elsevier.com/books/title/author/9780128121337

3. Depeursinge, A., Zrimec, T., Busayarat, S., Müller, H.: 3D lung image retrieval using localized features. In: Medical Imaging 2011: Computer-Aided Diagnosis, vol. 7963, p. 79632E. SPIE, February 2011
4. Dicente Cid, Y., Batmanghelich, K., Müller, H.: Textured graph-model of the lungs for tuberculosis type classification and drug resistance prediction: participation in ImageCLEF 2017. In: CLEF2017 Working Notes. CEUR Workshop Proceedings, CEUR-WS.org, Dublin, Ireland, 11–14 September 2017 (2017). http://ceur-ws.org
5. Dicente Cid, Y., Depeursinge, A., Foncubierta-Rodríguez, Platon, A., Poletti, P.A., Müller, H.: Pulmonary embolism detection using localized vessel-based features in dual energy CT. In: SPIE Medical Imaging. International Society for Optics and Photonics (2015)
6. Dicente Cid, Y., Jimenez-del-Toro, O., Depeursinge, A., Müller, H.: Efficient and fully automatic segmentation of the lungs in CT volumes. In: Goksel, O., Jimenez-del-Toro, O., Foncubierta-Rodriguez, A., Müller, H. (eds.) Proceedings of the VIS-CERAL Challenge at ISBI, pp. 31–35. No. 1390 in CEUR Workshop Proceedings, April 2015
7. Dicente Cid, Y., Kalinovsky, A., Liauchuk, V., Kovalev, V., Müller, H.: Overview of ImageCLEFtuberculosis 2017 - predicting tuberculosis type and drug resistances. In: CLEF 2017 Labs Working Notes. CEUR Workshop Proceedings, CEUR-WS.org, Dublin, Ireland, 11–14 September 2017 (2017). http://ceur-ws.org
8. Dicente Cid, Y., et al.: A lung graph–model for pulmonary hypertension and pulmonary embolism detection on DECT images. In: Müller, H. (ed.) MCV/BAMBI -2016. LNCS, vol. 10081, pp. 58–68. Springer, Cham (2017). https://doi.org/10.1007/978-3-319-61188-4_6
9. Dicente Cid, Y., Müller, H., Platon, A., Poletti, P.A., Depeursinge, A.: 3-D solid texture classification using locally-oriented wavelet transforms. IEEE Trans. Image Process. **26**(4), 1899–1910 (2017)
10. Farber, H.: Pulmonary circulation: diseases and their treatment. Eur. Respir. Rev. **21**(123), 78 (2012). 3rd edition
11. Galiè, N., et al.: Treatment of patients with mildly symptomatic pulmonary arterial hypertension with bosentan (early study): a double-blind, randomised controlled trial. Lancet **371**(9630), 2093–2100 (2008)
12. Lador, F., Herve, P.: A practical approach of pulmonary hypertension in the elderly. Semin. Respir. Crit. Care Med. **34**(5), 654–664 (2013)
13. Liu, K., et al.: Rotation-invariant hog descriptors using fourier analysis in polar and spherical coordinates. Int. J. Comput. Vis. **106**(3), 342–364 (2014)
14. Richiardi, J., Bunke, H., Van De Ville, D., Achard, S.: Machine learning with brain graphs. IEEE Signal Process. Mag. **30**, 58 (2013)
15. Richiardi, J., Eryilmaz, H., Schwartz, S., Vuilleumier, P., Van De Ville, D.: Decoding brain states from fMRI connectivity graphs. NeuroImage **56**(2), 616–626 (2011)
16. Tuder, R.M.: Relevant issues in the pathology and pathobiology of pulmonary hypertension. J. Am. Coll. Cardiol. **62**(25 SUPPL.), D4–D12 (2013)
17. Zrimec, T., Busayarat, S., Wilson, P.: A 3D model of the human lung with lung regions characterization. In: ICIP 2004 Proceedings of the IEEE International Conference on Image Processing, vol. 2, pp. 1149–1152 (2004)

S4ND: Single-Shot Single-Scale Lung Nodule Detection

Naji Khosravan[(⊠)] and Ulas Bagci

Center for Research in Computer Vision (CRCV), School of Computer Science,
University of Central Florida, Orlando, FL, USA
naji.khosravan@gmail.com

Abstract. The most recent lung nodule detection studies rely on computationally expensive multi-stage frameworks to detect nodules from CT scans. To address this computational challenge and provide better performance, in this paper we propose S4ND, a new deep learning based method for lung nodule detection. Our approach uses a single feed forward pass of a single network for detection. The whole detection pipeline is designed as a single $3D$ Convolutional Neural Network (CNN) with dense connections, trained in an end-to-end manner. S4ND does not require any further post-processing or user guidance to refine detection results. Experimentally, we compared our network with the current state-of-the-art object detection network (SSD) in computer vision as well as the state-of-the-art published method for lung nodule detection (3D DCNN). We used publicly available 888 CT scans from LUNA challenge dataset and showed that the proposed method outperforms the current literature both in terms of efficiency and accuracy by achieving an average FROC-score of 0.897. We also provide an in-depth analysis of our proposed network to shed light on the unclear paradigms of tiny object detection.

Keywords: Object detection · Deep learning
Lung nodule detection · Dense CNN · Tiny object detection

1   Introduction

Successful diagnosis and treatment of lung cancer is highly dependent on early detection of lung nodules. Radiologists are analyzing an ever increasing amount of imaging data (CT scans) every day. Computer Aided Detection (CAD) systems are designed to help radiologists in the screening process. However, automatic detection of lung nodules with CADs remains a challenging task. One reason is the high variation in texture, shape, and position of nodules in CT scans, and their similarity with other nearby structures. Another reason is the discrepancy between the large search space (i.e., entire lung fields) and respectively tiny nature of the nodules. Detection of tiny/small objects has remained a very challenging task in computer vision, which so far has only been solved using

© Springer Nature Switzerland AG 2018
A. F. Frangi et al. (Eds.): MICCAI 2018, LNCS 11071, pp. 794–802, 2018.
https://doi.org/10.1007/978-3-030-00934-2_88

computationally expensive multi-stage frameworks. Current sate of art methods for lung nodule detection follow the same multi-stage detection frameworks as in other computer vision areas.

The literature for lung nodule detection and diagnosis is vast. To date, the common strategy for all available CAD systems for lung nodule detection is to use a candidate identification step (also known as region proposal). While some of these studies apply low-level appearance based features as a prior to drive this identification task [8], others use shape and size information [5]. Related to deep learning based methods, Ypsilantis et al. proposed to use recurrent neural networks in a patch based strategy to improve nodule detection [11]. Krishnamurthy et al. proposed to detect candidates using a $2D$ multi-step segmentation process. Then a group of hand-crafted features were extracted, followed by a two-stage classification of candidates [5]. In a similar fashion, Huang et al. proposed a geometric model based candidate detection method which followed by a $3D$ CNN to reduce number of FPs [4]. Golan et al. used a deep $3D$ CNN with a small input patch of $5 \times 20 \times 20$ for lung nodule detection. The network was applied to the lung CT volume multiple times using a sliding window and exhaustive search strategy to output a probability map over the volume [3].

There has, also, been detailed investigations of high-level discriminatory information extraction using deep networks to perform a better FP reduction [10]. Setio et al. used 9 separate $2D$ convolutional neural networks trained on 9 different views of candidates, followed by a fusion strategy to perform FP reduction [10]. Another study used a modified version of Faster R-CNN, state of the art object detector at the time, for candidate detection and a patch based $3D$ CNN for FP reduction step [1]. However, all these methods are computationally inefficient (e.g., exhaustive use of sliding windows over feature maps), and often computed in 2D manner, not appreciating the 3D nature of the nodule space. It is worth mentioning that patch based methods are 3D but they suffer from the same computational burdens, as well as missing the entire notion of 3D nodule space due to limited information available in the patches.

Our Contributions: We resolve the aforementioned issues by proposing a completely $3D$ deep network architecture designed to detect lung nodules in a single shot using a single-scale network. To the best of our knowledge, this is the first study to perform lung nodule detection in one step. Specific to the architecture design of the deep network, we make use of convolution blocks with dense connections for this problem, making one step nodule detection computationally feasible. We also investigate and justify the effect of different down-sampling methods in our network due to its important role for tiny object detection. Lastly, we argue that lung nodule detection, as opposed to object detection in natural images, can be done with high accuracy using only a single scale network when network is carefully designed with its hyper-parameters.

2 Method

Figure 1 shows the overview of the proposed method for lung nodule detection in a single shot. The input to our network is a $3D$ volume of a lung CT scan. The proposed $3D$ densely connected Convolutional Neural Network (CNN) divides the input volume into a grid of size $S \times S \times T$ cells. We model lung nodule detection as a cell-wise classification problem, done simultaneously for all the cells. Unlike commonly used region proposal networks, our proposed network is able to reason the presence of nodule in a cell using global contextual information, based on the whole 3D input volume.

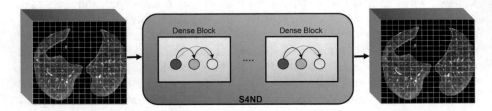

Fig. 1. Our framework, named S4ND, models nodule detection as a cell-wise classification of the input volume. The input volume is divided by a $16 \times 16 \times 8$ grid and is passed through a newly designed $3D$ dense CNN. The output is a probability map indicating the presence of a nodule in each cell.

2.1 Single-Scale Detection

As opposed to object detection in natural scenes, we show that lung nodule detection can be performed efficiently and with high accuracy in a single scale. Current literature reports the most frequently observed nodule sizes fall within 32 mm by 32 mm [9], most of which are less than 9 mm and are considered as small (def. American Thoracic Society). Nodules less than 3 mm in size are the most difficult to detect due to their tiny nature and high similarities to vessels. Based on the statistics of nodule size and the evidence in literature, we hypothesize that a single scale framework with the grid size that we defined ($16 \times 16 \times 8$ leading to the cell sized of $32 \times 32 \times 8$ on a volume of size $512 \times 512 \times 8$) is sufficient to fit all the expected nodule sizes and provide good detection results without the need to increase the algorithmic complexity to multi-scale. This has been partially proven in other multi-scale studies [2].

2.2 Dense and Deeper Convolution Blocks Improve Detection

The loss of low-level information throughout a network causes either a high number of false positives or low sensitivity. One efficient way that helps the flow of information in a network and keeps this low level information, combining it with the high level information, is the use of dense connections inside the convolution blocks. We empirically show that deeper densely-connected blocks provide better detection results. This, however, comes with the cost of more computation. In our experiments we found that dense blocks with 6 convolution layers provide a good balance of detection accuracy and computational efficiency.

2.3 Max-Pooling Improves Detection

As we go deeper in a CNN, it is desired to pick the most descriptive features and pass only those to the next layers. Recently, architectures for object detection in natural images preferred the use of convolutions with stride 2 instead of pooling [7]. In the context of tiny object detection, this feature reduction plays an important role. Since our objects of interest are small, if we carelessly pick the features to propagate we can easily lose the objects of interest through the network and end up with a sub-optimal model. In theory, the goal is to have as less pooling as possible. Also, it is desired to have this feature sampling step in a way that information loss is minimized. There are multiple approaches for sampling information through the network. Average pooling, max pooling and convolutions with stride 2 are some of the options. In our experiments, we showed that max pooling is the best choice of feature sampling for our task as it selects the most discriminative feature in the network. Also, we showed that convolution layers with stride of 2 are performing better compared to average pooling. The reason is that convolution with stride 2 is very similar in its nature to weighted averaging with the weights being learned in a data driven manner.

2.4 Proposed 3D Deep Network Architecture

Our network architecture consists of 36, $3D$ convolution layers, 4 max-pooling layers and a sigmoid activation function at the end. 30 of convolution layers form 5 blocks with dense connections and without pooling, which enhance low-level information along with high-level information, and the remainder form the transition layers. The details of our architecture can be seen in Fig. 2. The input to our network is $512 \times 512 \times 8$ and the output is a $16 \times 16 \times 8$ probability map. Each cell in the output corresponds to a cell of the original image divided by a $16 \times 16 \times 8$ grid and decides whether there is a nodule in that cell or not.

Densely Connected Convolution Blocks: As stated, our network consists of 5 densely connected blocks, each block containing 6 convolution layers with an output channel of g, which is the growth rate of that block. Inside the blocks, each layer receives all the preceding layers' feature maps as inputs. Figure 2 (top right) illustrates the layout of a typical dense block. Dense connections help the flow of information inside the network. Assume x_0 is the input volume to the block and x_i is the output feature map of layer i inside the block. Each layer is a non-linear function F_i, which in our case is a composition of convolution, batch normalization (BN) and rectifier linear unit (ReLU). With dense connections, each layer receives a concatenation of all previous layers' feature maps as

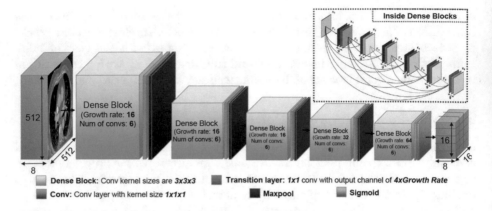

Fig. 2. Input to the network is a $512 \times 512 \times 8$ volume and output is a $16 \times 16 \times 8$ probability map representing likelihood of nodule presence. Our network has 5 dense blocks each having 6 conv. layers. The growth rates of blocks 1 to 5 is $16, 16, 16, 32, 64$ respectively. The network has 4 transition layers and 4 max-pooling layers. The last block is followed by a convolution layer with kernel size $1 \times 1 \times 1$ and output channel of 1 and a sigmoid activation function.

input $x_i = F_i([x_0, x_1, ..., x_{i-1}])$, where x_i is the output feature map from layer i and $[x_0, x_1, ..., x_{i-1}]$ is the channel-wise concatenation of previous layers' feature maps.

Growth Rate (GR): is the number of feature maps that each layer F_i produces in the block. This number is fixed for each block but it can change from one block to the other. Assume the number of channels in the input layer of a block is c_0 and the block has i convolution layers with a growth rate of g. Then the output of the block will have $c_0 + (i - 1)g$ channels.

Transition Layers: as can be seen in the above formulations, the number of feature maps inside each dense block increases dramatically. Transition layers are $1 \times 1 \times 1$ convolution layers with $4 \times g$ output channels, where g is the growth rate of previous block. Using a convolution with kernel size of $1 \times 1 \times 1$ compresses the information channel-wise and reduces the total number of channels throughout the network.

Training the Network: The created ground truths for training our network are $3D$ volumes with size $16 \times 16 \times 8$. Each element in this volume corresponds to a cell in the input image and has label 1 if a nodule exists in that cell and 0 otherwise. The design of our network allows for an end-to-end training. We model detection as a cell wise classification of input which is done in one feed forward path of the network in one shot. This formulation detects all the nodules in the given volume simultaneously. The loss function for training our network is weighted cross-entropy defined as:

$$L(Y^{(n)}, f(X^{(n)})) = \sum_{i=1}^{k_n} -y_i \log(f(x_i)), \tag{1}$$

where Ys are the labels and Xs are the inputs.

3   Experiments and Results

Data and Evaluation: To evaluate detection performance of S4ND, we used Lung Nodule Analysis (LUNA16) Challenge dataset (consisting of a total of 888 chest CT scans, slice thickness <2.5 mm, with ground truth nodule locations). For the training, we performed a simple data augmentation by shifting the images in 4 directions by 32 pixels. We sampled the 3D volumes for training so that nodules appear in random locations to avoid bias toward location of nodules. We performed 10-fold cross validation to evaluate our method by following the LUNA challenge guidelines. Free-Response Receiver Operating Characteristic (FROC) analysis has been conducted to calculate sensitivity and specificity [6]. Suggested by the challenge organizers, sensitivity at 7 FP/scan rates (i.e. $0.125, 0.25, 0.5, 1, 2, 4, 8$) was computed. The overall *score* of system (Competition Performance Metric-CPM) was defined as the average sensitivity for these 7 FP/scan rates.

Building Blocks of S4ND and Comparisons: This subsection explains how we build the proposed S4ND network and provides a detailed comparison with several baseline approaches. We compared performance of S4ND with state-of-the-art algorithms, including SSD (single-shot multi-box object detection) [7], known to be very effective for object detection in natural scenes. We show that SSD suffers from low performance in lung nodule detection, even though trained from scratch on LUNA dataset. A high degree of scale bias and known difficulties of the lung nodules detection (texture, shape, etc.) in CT data can be considered as potential reasons. To address this poor performance, we propose to replace the convolution layers with *dense* blocks to improve the information flow in the network. Further, we experimentally tested the effects of various down sampling techniques. Table 1 shows the results of different network architectures along with the number of parameters based on these combinations. We implemented the SSD based architecture with 3 different pooling strategies: (1) average pooling (2D Dense Avepool), (2) replacing pooling layers with convolution layers with kernel size 3×3 and stride 2 (2D Dense Nopool) and (3) max pooling (2D Dense Maxpool). Our experiments show that max pooling is the best choice of feature sampling for tiny object detection as it selects the most discriminating feature in each step. *2D Dense Nopool* outperforms the normal average pooling (*2D Dense Avepool*) as it is in concept a learnable averaging over 3×3 regions of our network, based on the way we defined kernel size and stride.

3D Networks, Growth Rate (GR), and Comparisons: We implemented S4ND in a completely 3D manner. Growth rate for all the blocks inside the network was initially fixed to 16 (3D Dense). However, we observed that increasing the growth rate in the last 2 blocks of our network, where the computational expense is lowest, (from 16 to 32 and 64, respectively) improved the performance of detection (3D Increasing GR in Table 1). Also, having deeper blocks, even with a fixed growth rate of 16 for all the blocks, help the information flow in the network and improved the results further (3D Deeper Blocks in Table 1). The final proposed method benefits from both deeper blocks and increasing growth rate in its last two blocks. Figure 3 (left) shows the FROC comparison of proposed method with the baselines. The 10-fold cross validation results were compared with the current state of the art lung nodule detection method (3D DCNN which is the best published results on LUNA dataset) [1]. Our proposed method outperformed the best available results both in sensitivity and FROC score, while only using as less as a third of its parameters, and without the need for multi-stage refinements.

Table 1. Comparison of different models with varying conditions.

	Model	Sensitivity%	Num of parameters	CPM
Randomly selected 1-fold	2D SSD	77.8%	59,790,787	0.649
	2D Dense Avepool	84.8%	67,525,635	0.653
	2D Dense Nopool	86.4%	70,661,955	0.658
	2D Dense Maxpool	87.5%	67,525,635	0.672
	3D Dense	93.7%	694,467	0.882
	3D Increasing GR	95.1%	2,429,827	0.890
	3D Deeper Blocks	94.2%	1,234,179	0.913
	Proposed (S4ND)	**97.2%**	4,572,995	**0.931**
10-fold	3D DCNN [1]	94.6%	11,720,032	0.891
	Proposed (S4ND)	**95.2%**	4,572,995	**0.897**

Major Findings: (1) We obtained 0.897 FROC rate in 10-fold cross validation, and consistently outperformed the state of the art methods as well as other alternatives. (2) SSD (the state of the art for object detection in natural images) resulted in the lowest accuracy in all experiments. Proposed S4ND, on the other hand, showed that single scale single shot algorithm performs better and more suited to tiny object detection problem. (3) The proposed method achieved better sensitivity, specificity, and CPM in single fold and 10-fold throughout experiments where S4ND used less than the half parameters of 3D DCNN (current state of the art in lung nodule detection). (4) A careful organization of the architecture helps avoiding computationally heavy processing. We have shown that maxpooling is the best choice of feature selection throughout the network amongst current available methods. (5) Similarly, dense and deeper connections improve the detection rates through better information flow through layers. It should be noted that the runtime of our algorithm for the whole scan, on the test phase, varies from 11 *secs* to 27 *secs* based on the number of slices in the scan on a single NVIDIA TITAN Xp GPU workstation with RAM of 64 GBs.

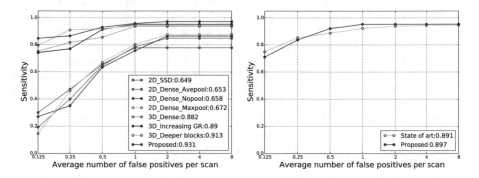

Fig. 3. Comparison of base line as well as comparison with the state of the art. Numbers in front of each method in the legend show Competition Performance Metric (CPM).

4   Conclusion

This paper introduces a single-shot single-scale fast lung nodule detection algorithm without the need for additional FP removal and user guidance for refinement of detection process. Our proposed deep network structure is fully 3D and densely connected. We also critically analyzed the role of densely connected layers as well as maxpooling, average pooling and fully convolutional down sampling in detection process. We present a fundamental solution to address the major challenges of current region proposal based lung nodule detection methods: candidate detection and feature resampling stages. We experimentally validate the proposed network's performance both in terms of accuracy (high sensitivity/specificity) and efficiency (less number of parameters and speed) on publicly available LUNA data set, with extensive comparison with the natural object detector networks as well as the state of the art lung nodule detection methods. A promising future direction will be to combine diagnosis stage with the detection.

References

1. Ding, J., Li, A., Hu, Z., Wang, L.: Accurate pulmonary nodule detection in computed tomography images using deep convolutional neural networks. In: Descoteaux, M., Maier-Hein, L., Franz, A., Jannin, P., Collins, D.L., Duchesne, S. (eds.) MICCAI 2017. LNCS, vol. 10435, pp. 559–567. Springer, Cham (2017). https://doi.org/10.1007/978-3-319-66179-7_64
2. Dou, Q., Chen, H., Yu, L., Qin, J., Heng, P.A.: Multilevel contextual 3-D CNNs for false positive reduction in pulmonary nodule detection. IEEE Trans. Biomed. Eng. **64**(7), 1558–1567 (2017)

3. Golan, R., Jacob, C., Denzinger, J.: Lung nodule detection in ct images using deep convolutional neural networks. In: 2016 International Joint Conference on Neural Networks (IJCNN), pp. 243–250. IEEE (2016)
4. Huang, X., Shan, J., Vaidya, V.: Lung nodule detection in ct using 3d convolutional neural networks. In: 2017 IEEE 14th International Symposium on Biomedical Imaging (ISBI 2017), pp. 379–383. IEEE (2017)
5. Krishnamurthy, S., Narasimhan, G., Rengasamy, U.: An automatic computerized model for cancerous lung nodule detection from computed tomography images with reduced false positives. In: Santosh, K.C., Hangarge, M., Bevilacqua, V., Negi, A. (eds.) RTIP2R 2016. CCIS, vol. 709, pp. 343–355. Springer, Singapore (2017). https://doi.org/10.1007/978-981-10-4859-3_31
6. Kundel, H., Berbaum, K., Dorfman, D., Gur, D., Metz, C., Swensson, R.: Receiver operating characteristic analysis in medical imaging. ICRU Report **79**(8), 1 (2008)
7. Liu, W., et al.: SSD: single shot multibox detector. In: Leibe, B., Matas, J., Sebe, N., Welling, M. (eds.) ECCV 2016. LNCS, vol. 9905, pp. 21–37. Springer, Cham (2016). https://doi.org/10.1007/978-3-319-46448-0_2
8. Lopez Torres, E., et al.: Large scale validation of the M5L lung cad on heterogeneous CT datasets. Med. Phys. **42**(4), 1477–1489 (2015)
9. Setio, A.A.A., et al.: Validation, comparison, and combination of algorithms for automatic detection of pulmonary nodules in computed tomography images: The LUNA16 challenge. Med. Image Analy. **42**(Supplement C), 1–13 (2017). http://www.sciencedirect.com/science/article/pii/S1361841517301020
10. Setio, A.A.A., et al.: Pulmonary nodule detection in ct images: false positive reduction using multi-view convolutional networks. IEEE Trans. Med. Imaging **35**(5), 1160–1169 (2016)
11. Ypsilantis, P.P., Montana, G.: Recurrent convolutional networks for pulmonary nodule detection in CT imaging. arXiv preprint arXiv:1609.09143 (2016)

Vascular Network Organization via Hough Transform (VaNgOGH): A Novel Radiomic Biomarker for Diagnosis and Treatment Response

Nathaniel Braman$^{(\boxtimes)}$, Prateek Prasanna, Mehdi Alilou, Niha Beig, and Anant Madabhushi

Department of Biomedical Engineering, Case Western Reserve University, Cleveland, OH 44106, USA
nmb60@case.edu

Abstract. As a "hallmark of cancer", tumor-induced angiogenesis is one of the most important mechanisms of a tumor's adaptation to changes in nutrient requirement. The angiogenic activity of certain tumors has been found to be predictive of a patient's ultimate response to therapeutic intervention. This then begs the question if there are differences in vessel arrangement and corresponding convolutedness, between tumors that appear phenotypically similar, but respond differently to treatment. Even though textural radiomics and deep learning-based approaches have been shown to distinguish disease aggressiveness and assess therapeutic response, these descriptors do not specifically interpret differences in vessel characteristics. Moreover, most existing approaches have attempted to model disease characteristics just within tumor confines, or right outside, but do not consider explicit parenchymal vessel morphology. In this work, we introduce VaNgOGH (Vascular Network Organization via Hough transform), a new descriptor of architectural disorder of the tumor's vascular network. We demonstrate the efficacy of VaNgOGH in two clinically challenging problems: (a) Predicting pathologically complete response (pCR) in breast cancer prior to treatment (BCa, $N = 76$) and (b) distinguishing benign nodules from malignant non-small cell lung cancer (LCa, $N = 81$). For both tasks, VaNgOGH had test area under the receiver operating characteristic curve ($AUC_{BCa} = 0.75$, $AUC_{LCa} = 0.68$) higher than, or comparable to, state of the art radiomic approaches ($AUC_{BCa} = 0.75$, $AUC_{LCa} = 0.62$) and convolutional neural networks ($AUC_{BCa} = 0.67$, $AUC_{LCa} = 0.66$). Interestingly, when a

N. Braman and P. Prasanna—Equal contribution. Research was supported by 1U24CA199374-01, R01CA202752-01A1, R01CA208236-01A1, R21CA179327-01, R21CA195152-01, R01DK098503-02, 1C06-RR12463-01, PC120857, LC130463, T32EB007509, the DOD Prostate Cancer Idea Development Award, W81XWH-16-1-0329, the CCCC Pilot Grant, CCF VelaSano Grant, I-Corps program, OTF Program, and the Wallace H. Coulter Foundation Program in BME, CWRU. The content is solely the responsibility of the authors and does not necessarily represent the official views of the National Institutes of Health.

© Springer Nature Switzerland AG 2018
A. F. Frangi et al. (Eds.): MICCAI 2018, LNCS 11071, pp. 803–811, 2018.
https://doi.org/10.1007/978-3-030-00934-2_89

known radiomic signature was used in conjunction with VaNgOGH, AUC_{BCa} increased to 0.79.

1 Introduction

Angiogenesis, the process by which a tumor hijacks the body's machinery for creating new vasculature in order to redirect blood flow to itself [1], plays an important role in determining tumor response to chemo- and radiotherapy. Stimulatory signals, such as vascular endothelial growth factor (VEGF) expression, result in neovascularization [2], ultimately leading to sprouting and irregular branching of blood vessels, or erratic angiogenesis. The associated tortuosity and leakiness directly affects the course of disease progression, and possibly its response to therapeutic interventions. For example, it has been qualitatively shown that temporal changes in vessel tortuosity on brain magnetic resonance imaging (MRI) are indicative of a favorable response to therapy [3]. A more convoluted tumor vasculature might constrict the delivery of therapeutic drugs to the lesion, thereby resulting in potentially worse prognosis and treatment response.

These qualitative observations therefore beg the question as to whether computerized analysis of tumor vasculature could (a) reveal differences in malignant and benign tumors as well as patients who undergo differential treatment response (see Fig. 1) and (b) whether these measurements could be translated into new imaging biomarkers of tumor diagnosis and treatment response.

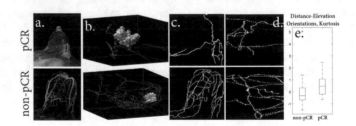

Fig. 1. Differences in tumor vascular network from baseline DCE-MRI scans for two different breast cancer patients (upper row: pCR and bottom row: non-pCR) who received neoadjuvant chemotherapy.

In this work, we present a new image-based descriptor, Vascular Network Organization via Hough transform (VaNgOGH), which attempts to model the architectural disorder of a tumor's vascular network by computing local measures of vessel-curvature in the Hough parameter space. VaNgOGH first looks at projections of vascular segmentations along different planes, in cartesian, as well as spherical coordinates. This is followed by localized Hough transforms to identify dominant peaks in the accumulator space. The applicability is demonstrated in two clinically challenging tasks: (a) predicting pathologic complete response (pCR) from non-response (non-pCR) to chemotherapy in breast cancer from pre-treatment dynamic contrast-enhance (DCE) MRI and (b) distinguishing benign granulomas from malignant adenocarcinomas from non-contrast computed tomography (CT) scans.

2 Previous Work and Novel Contributions

While there has been substantial interest in both radiomics and deep learning approaches for disease diagnosis as well as treatment response of tumors, most of these feature analysis approaches have been limited either to the tumor [4,5] or the associated parenchyma [6,7]. Recent work such as [6], which leveraged textural features of the tumor and the surrounding peri-tumoral tissue to predict therapeutic response from breast MRI, suggests the discriminating nature of the tumor microenvironment on imaging and the potential of extra-tumoral quantitative analysis. However, there is a lack of radiomic features capable of directly targeting biological aspects of the microenvironment, such as vascularity. VaNgOGH represents a novel approach for the characterization of chaotic vasculature associated with tumor-induced angiogenesis. In capturing morphology of the tumor-associated vascular network, VaNgOGH implicitly captures functional attributes of the tumor.

A unique advantage of VaNgOGH over other state-of-the-art quantitative metrics of vessel architecture is its capability to define abnormal vessel arrangement across multiple planes and projections, and relative to the tumor core and boundary itself. Specifically, VaNgOGH invokes Hough transformation to characterize the vessel network across multiple spatial representations, operating both in the cartesian domain, to capture disorder in the plane of image acquisition, and in the spherical domain, to capture deflections of neighboring vasculature towards the tumor centroid due to angiogenesis. In the latter operation, we further leverage the spherical coordinate space by computing VaNgOGH beyond the tumor within annular bands of increasing radius and summarize across regions in order to capture the magnitude of the tumor's angiogenic influence. VaNgOGH features consist of the first order statistics of maximum Hough peak orientations computed in a sliding fashion across vessel projections summarizing vasculature orientation in the following domains: the XY-plane, distance from the tumor vs. azimuthal rotation, distance from the tumor vs. elevation angle, and azimuthal rotation vs. elevation angle.

In this work, we evaluated the approach on $N = 157$ breast and lung cancer patients in predicting treatment response and cancer presence, also comparing the approach against a convolutional neural network (CNN) and state-of-the-art textural radiomic measures of tumoral and peri-tumoral regions.

3 Methodology

3.1 Notation

We define an image scene $\mathcal{I}$ as $\mathcal{I} = (C, f)$, where $\mathcal{I}$ is a spatial grid C of voxels $c \in C$, in a 3-dimensional space, $\mathbb{R}^3$. Each voxel, $c \in C$ is associated

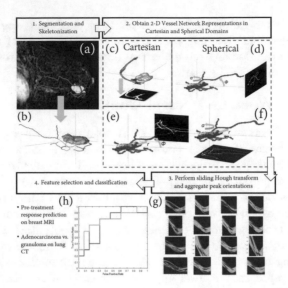

Fig. 2. Overview of VaNgOGH computational workflow.

with an intensity value $f(c)$. $\mathcal{I}_T$, and $\mathcal{I}_P$ correspond to the intra-tumoral and surrounding peritumoral parenchyma sub-volumes within every $\mathcal{I}$ respectively, such that $[\mathcal{I}_T, \mathcal{I}_P] \subset \mathcal{I}$. We further divide the sub-volume $\mathcal{I}_P$ into uniformly sized annular sub-volumes $\mathcal{I}_N^j$, where j is the number of uniformly-sized annular bands, such that $j \in \{1, \ldots, k\}$, and k is an user-defined proximity parameter dependent on the distance g from the tumor margin. For each $\mathcal{I}$, there exists a corresponding tumor segmentation $\mathcal{T}$ and vessel segmentation $\mathcal{V}$.

3.2   VaNgOGH Descriptor

1. **Segmentation and skeletonization of tumor and vasculature**
   A segmentation algorithm is applied to $\mathcal{I}$, yielding a volume $\mathcal{T}$ containing the tumor, and a volume $\mathcal{V}$ containing the surrounding tumor-associated vasculature (Fig. 2(a)). $\mathcal{T}$ is subtracted from $\mathcal{V}$ to ensure that there are no residual tumor voxels within the segmented vasculature. A fast marching approach is employed to compute the centerlines of vessels within $\mathcal{V}$, forming $\mathcal{S}$: a series of points in 3-dimensional cartesian space comprising the medial axis skeleton of $\mathcal{V}$ (Fig. 2(b)). Segmentation algorithms utilized for each dataset are described in greater detail in Sects. 4.3 and 4.4.
2. **Obtain 2-Dimensional vessel network representations in cartesian and spherical domains.**
   (a) *Cartesian domain:* $\mathcal{S}$ is projected along the plane of image acquisition, z, in order to obtain a 2-dimensional representation of the vasculature, $\mathcal{V}_{xy}$, which depicts the vascular network in the XY plane (Fig. 2(c)).
   (b) *Spherical domain:* The vascular network is converted to spherical coordinates and projected along each spherical axis to yield three 2-D

representations of 3-D vessel orientation with respect to the tumor centroid. Each point within S is converted to its spherical coordinates relative to the tumor centroid, D. Let x_D, y_D, and z_D represent distance from D of a point S_i within S along the corresponding cartesian axes. Each S_i then corresponds to an azimuth α and an elevation ϕ, indicating rotation around the z-axis and angle from the XY-plane, respectively, such that $\alpha = \arctan(\frac{y_D}{x_D})$ and $\phi = \arctan(\frac{z_D}{\sqrt{x_D^2 + y_D^2}})$. A third spherical coordinate, r, given by $argmin(\sqrt{(x_D - T_x^j)^2 + (y_D - T_y^j)^2 + (z_D - T_z^j)^2})$ defines the Euclidean distance between S_i and the nearest voxel within $\mathcal{T}$. This conversion is repeated for each S_i in S, yielding a 3-D skeleton within the spherical coordinate space, $\mathcal{S}_{r\alpha\phi}$. $\mathcal{S}_{r\alpha\phi}$ is projected along each spherical dimension to yield the following 2-dimensional representations of 3-D vessel orientation relative to the tumor centroid in spherical space: $V_{r\alpha}^j$, azimuth angle with respect to Euclidean distance from the tumor (Fig. 2(f)); $V_{r\phi}^j$, elevation angle with respect to Euclidean distance from the tumor (Fig. 2(e)); and $V_{\alpha\phi}^j$, elevation angle with respect to azimuth angle (Fig. 2(d)).

3 **Sliding Hough transforms and aggregate peak orientations.**

(a) *Computation and aggregation of localized Hough transforms in the cartesian space:* Using a $\mathcal{N} \times \mathcal{N}$ sliding window $\mathcal{W}$ with an offset of k pixels, each pixel in $\mathcal{V}_{xy}$ is mapped to an accumulator space using the Hough Transform, where the equation of a line is represented by $y = (-\frac{\cos\theta}{\sin\theta})x + (\frac{\rho}{\sin\theta})$. This transforms the spatial coordinate system (x, y) to the polar coordinate system (ρ, θ), such that for every point on the medial axis representation $\mathcal{V}_{xy}$, there exists a unique sinusoid in the Hough accumulator space (Fig. 2(g)). The five grid locations accumulating the most sinusoid crossings are identified for each $\mathcal{W}$. Feature set $\mathcal{F}_{xy}$ then comprises the θ values associated with the five most prominent peak orientations such that $\mathcal{F}_{xy} = [\theta_1, \theta_2, ...\theta_5]$.

(b) *Computation of localized Hough transforms on spherical projections within annular sub-volumes*: For a given annular sub-volume outside the tumor $\mathcal{I}_N^j$, 2-D spherical representations are obtained from vessels only within the sub-volume, denoted as $V_{r\alpha}^j$, $V_{r\phi}^j$, and $V_{\alpha\phi}^j$. Peaks are computed from 2-D spherical representations using the above approach. This is repeated for all annular bands $j \in \{1, ..., k\}$. Peak orientations are concatenated for all annular bands, yielding a single feature vector, i.e. $\mathcal{F}_{r\alpha} = [\mathcal{F}_{r\alpha}^1, \mathcal{F}_{r\alpha}^2, ... \mathcal{F}_{r\alpha}^k]$, $\mathcal{F}_{r\phi} = [\mathcal{F}_{r\phi}^1, \mathcal{F}_{r\phi}^2, ... \mathcal{F}_{r\phi}^k]$, and $\mathcal{F}_{\alpha\phi} = [\mathcal{F}_{\alpha\phi}^1, \mathcal{F}_{\alpha\phi}^2, ... \mathcal{F}_{\alpha\phi}^k]$.

4. **Computation of VaNgOGH descriptor**
The final VaNgOGH feature set, $\mathcal{F}_V$, is a concatenation of the first order statistics, mean, median, standard deviation, skewness, and kurtosis, of $\mathcal{F}_{xy}$, $\mathcal{F}_{r\alpha}^k$, $\mathcal{F}_{r\phi}^k$, and $\mathcal{F}_{\alpha\phi}^k$

4   Experimental Results and Discussion

4.1   Data Description

Dataset 1 included axial breast DCE-MRIs, collected prior to administration of neoadjuvant chemotherapy with a 1.5/3T magnet. Dataset 2 included non-contrast lung CT scans, collected from two sites. Patients were divided at random into training and testing cohorts as shown in Table 1. All studies were acquired as part of an Institutional Review Board-approved, HIPAA-compliant protocol.

4.2   Comparative Strategies and Classifier Construction

Intra- and Peri-tumoral Radiomics: For Experiment 1, VaNgOGH was compared against four radiomic features capable of predicting response on pre-treatment DCE-MRI, previously published in [6]. The feature comprised 2 intra-tumoral features (CoLlAGe Info1 [8], Laws S5R5) and 2 peri-tumoral features (Laws L5S5, CoLlAGe Entropy). In Experiment 2, we used the same list of features described in [6], with the most important features being three intranodular low frequency Gabor and a perinodular Laws W5E5 feature.

Convolutional Neural Network: We used a multi-layer 2D LeNet-like architecture [9], comprising three sets of convolutional, activation (ReLU), and pooling layers, followed by a fully-connected layer, activation, another fully-connected, and finally a softmax classifier. In this patch-based classification approach, the softmax classifier returns the probability of each patch belonging to the two classes of interest. The model was trained over 100 epochs.

Feature Selection and Classifier Construction: Once the VaNgOGH and other radiomic features were extracted, a set of 4 top features were selected by Wilcoxon rank-sum test and training of a linear discriminant analysis classifier was performed in a 3-fold cross-validation setting across 100 iterations. The locked-down model was then applied to the independent validation cohorts. Performance of individual classifiers was assessed by the area under the receiver operating characteristic curve (AUC) (Fig. 2(h)).

4.3   Experiment 1: Pre-treatment Response Prediction in Breast Cancer DCE-MRI

Implementation Details. Subtraction images were derived from MRI scans prior to, and immediately following contrast agent injection. Multi-scale vessel enhancement [10] was performed to emphasize the vasculature, which was then isolated by thresholding. A series of morphological operations were performed to remove noise and join adjacent vascular regions. Tumor boundaries were delineated by an expert radiologist. Hough transforms were applied to image projections using a sliding window size of $\mathcal{N} = 30$ pixels with a step size $k = 5$ pixels. Spherical projections were performed within annular sub-volumes with a radial width of 25 pixels out to a maximum radial distance of 100 pixels, with a step size $= 12.5$ pixels.

Table 1. Dataset for the two experiments

	Experiment 1 (N = 76)	Experiment 2 (N = 81)
Training	14 pCR, 39 non-pCR	20 Adenocarcinoma, 21 Granuloma
Testing	10 pCR, 13 non-pCR	20 Adenocarcinoma, 20 Granuloma

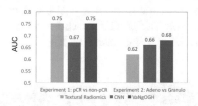

Fig. 3. Performance AUC on independent validation sets using VaNgOGH, textural radiomics and CNN.

Results: pCR demonstrates a less chaotic vascular network, potentially evidenced by projection images in Fig. 1(c) on the cartesian plane and a distance-elevation image in Fig. 1(d) on the spherical plane. Hough transformation on (c) and (d) further accentuates the differences in vessel arrangement by detecting the orientation of straight line segments in the accumulator grid. The best discriminating VaNgOGH features comprised the standard deviation and kurtosis of $\mathcal{F}^1_{\alpha\phi}$ and skewness and kurtosis of $\mathcal{F}^1_{r\phi}$. Kurtosis of $\mathcal{F}^1_{r\phi}$ was elevated in pCR (Fig. 1(e)), indicating a reduced disorder of vessel orientation in the $\mathcal{V}_{r\phi}$ space. The training AUCs were .63 ± .06 and .64 ± .07 using VaNgOGH and texture features, respectively. Combining VaNgOGH and texture resulted in an improved testing AUC of .79. Testing AUCs have are shown in Fig. 3.

4.4 Experiment 2: Malignancy Diagnosis for Lung Nodules

Implementation Details. Distinguishing granulomas from adenocarcinomas is amongst the most challenging clinical problems for lung radiologists. Nodules were manually segmented by a cardiothoracic radiologist. To obtain the vasculature, lung regions were first isolated from the surrounding anatomy using a multi-threshold based algorithm [11]. This was followed by region growing [12]. The center of gravity of the segmented nodules was used as the initial seed point for the region growing algorithm [13]. Within the nodule volume, seed points were initialized at random locations. Based off the intensity similarity of the seed points and surrounding pixels, an initial region was iteratively grown to encompass the nodule and associated vasculature. VaNgOGH features were extracted using the approach described in Sect. 4.3.

Results: As may be observed from Fig. 4, although both nodules are highly vascularized, spherical projections (below) accentuate the elevated disorder of the vascular network in adenocarcinoma, whereas granuloma vessel orientations are predominantly linear in the $V_{\alpha\phi}^j$ (d) and $V_{r\alpha}^j$ (e) spaces. VaNgOGH successfully separated adenocarcinomas and granulomas with an AUC of .65 ± .06 in the training set. The top feature set included one statistic for each view (standard deviation of $\mathcal{F}_{r\phi}^1$, median of $\mathcal{F}_{\alpha\phi}^1$, kurtosis of $\mathcal{F}_{xy}^1$, and skewness of $\mathcal{F}_{r\alpha}^1$). Figure 4 shows elevated vascular disorder in adeno, e.g. increased standard deviation of $\mathcal{F}_{r\phi}^1$ in (d). Performance of VaNgOGH in the independent validation set was comparable to that of the CNN, as shown in Fig. 3.

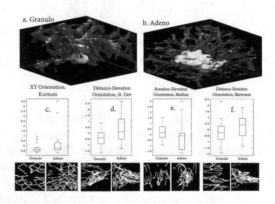

Fig. 4. VaNgOGH distinguishes similarly appearing granulolomas and adenocarcinoma on CT. (a) Vessel segmentations and centerlines for a representative adenocarcinoma and granuloma with high vascularity. (b–e) Box plots corresponding to top VaNgOGH features.

5   Concluding Remarks

In this work, we presented a new radiomic descriptor, VaNgOGH, that quantifies disorder of the tumor-associated vascular network by assessing the morphology of vessel orientation across multiple spatial domains. To the best of our knowledge, VaNgOGH is the first radiomic descriptor of tumor-associated vascular morphology. We demonstrated the ability of VaNgOGH to (a) predict benefit of neoadjuvant chemotherapy in breast cancer patients on DCE-MRI (N = 76), and (b) distinguish malignant adenocarcinoma from visually confounding granuloma on lung CT (N = 81). VaNgOGH performed comparably to deep learning and state of the art radiomic approaches, and provides greater biological interpretability. When considered in conjunction with an established radiomic response signature in breast MRI, VaNgOGH further improved pCR identification. Future work will entail larger validation studies and also evaluation on other use cases.

References

1. Yamazaki, K., et al.: Tumor angiogenesis in human lung adenocarcinoma. Cancer **74**, 2245–2250 (1994)
2. Grunewald, M., et al.: VEGF-induced adult neovascularization: recruitment, retention, and role of accessory cells. Cell **124**, 175–189 (2006)
3. Bullitt, E., et al.: Tumor therapeutic response and vessel tortuosity: preliminary report in metastatic breast cancer. In: Larsen, R., Nielsen, M., Sporring, J. (eds.) MICCAI 2006. LNCS, vol. 4191, pp. 561–568. Springer, Heidelberg (2006). https://doi.org/10.1007/11866763_69
4. Aerts, H.J.W.L., et al.: Decoding tumour phenotype by noninvasive imaging using a quantitative radiomics approach. Nat. Commun. **5**, 4006 (2014)
5. Li, H., et al.: Quantitative MRI radiomics in the prediction of molecular classifications of BCA subtypes in the TCGA/TCIA data set. NPJ Breast Cancer **2**, 16012 (2016)
6. Braman, N.M., et al.: Intratumoral and peritumoral radiomics for the pretreatment prediction of pathological complete response to neoadjuvant chemotherapy based on breast DCE-MRI. Breast Cancer Res. **19**, 57 (2017)
7. Zheng, Y., et al.: Parenchymal texture analysis in digital mammography: A fully automated pipeline for breast cancer risk assessment. Med Phys. **42**, 4149–4160 (2015)
8. Prasanna, P., Tiwari, P., Madabhushi, A.: Co-occurrence of local anisotropic gradient orientations (CoLlAGe): distinguishing tumor confounders and molecular subtypes on MRI. In: Golland, P., Hata, N., Barillot, C., Hornegger, J., Howe, R. (eds.) MICCAI 2014. LNCS, vol. 8675, pp. 73–80. Springer, Cham (2014). https://doi.org/10.1007/978-3-319-10443-0_10
9. LeCun, Y., et al.: Gradient-based learning applied to document recognition. IEEE **86**, 2278–2324 (1998)
10. Frangi, A.F., Niessen, W.J., Vincken, K.L., Viergever, M.A.: Multiscale vessel enhancement filtering. In: Wells, W.M., Colchester, A., Delp, S. (eds.) MICCAI 1998. LNCS, vol. 1496, pp. 130–137. Springer, Heidelberg (1998). https://doi.org/10.1007/BFb0056195
11. Hu, S., et al.: Automatic lung segmentation for accurate quantitation of volumetric x-ray CT. IEEE TMI **20**, 490–498 (2001)
12. Adams, R., et al.: Seeded region growing. IEEE PAMI **16**, 641–647 (1994)
13. Sethian, J.A.: Fast marching methods. SIAM Rev. **41**, 199–235 (1999)

DeepEM: Deep 3D ConvNets with EM for Weakly Supervised Pulmonary Nodule Detection

Wentao Zhu[1]([✉]), Yeeleng S. Vang[1], Yufang Huang[2], and Xiaohui Xie[1]

[1] University of California, Irvine, USA
{wentaoz1,ysvang,xhx}@uci.edu
[2] Lenovo Research, Beijing, China
huangyf8@lenovo.com

Abstract. Recently deep learning has been witnessing widespread adoption in various medical image applications. However, training complex deep neural nets requires large-scale datasets labeled with ground truth, which are often unavailable in many medical image domains. For instance, to train a deep neural net to detect pulmonary nodules in lung computed tomography (CT) images, current practice is to manually label nodule locations and sizes in many CT images to construct a sufficiently large training dataset, which is costly and difficult to scale. On the other hand, electronic medical records (EMR) contain plenty of partial information on the content of each medical image. In this work, we explore how to tap this vast, but currently unexplored data source to improve pulmonary nodule detection. We propose DeepEM, a novel deep 3D ConvNet framework augmented with expectation-maximization (EM), to mine weakly supervised labels in EMRs for pulmonary nodule detection. Experimental results show that DeepEM can lead to 1.5% and 3.9% average improvement in free-response receiver operating characteristic (FROC) scores on LUNA16 and Tianchi datasets, respectively, demonstrating the utility of incomplete information in EMRs for improving deep learning algorithms (https://github.com/uci-cbcl/DeepEM-for-Weakly-Supervised-Detection.git).

Keywords: Deep 3D convolutional nets
Weakly supervised detection · DeepEM (deep 3D ConvNets with EM)
Pulmonary nodule detection

1 Introduction

Lung cancer is the most common cause of cancer-related death in men. Low-dose lung computed tomography (CT) screening provides an effective way for early diagnosis and can sharply reduce the lung cancer mortality rate. Advanced computer-aided diagnosis (CAD) systems are expected to have high sensitivities while maintaining low false positive rates to be truly useful. Recent advance in

© Springer Nature Switzerland AG 2018
A. F. Frangi et al. (Eds.): MICCAI 2018, LNCS 11071, pp. 812–820, 2018.
https://doi.org/10.1007/978-3-030-00934-2_90

deep learning provides new opportunities to design more effective CAD systems to help facilitate doctors in their effort to catch lung cancer in their early stages.

The emergence of large-scale datasets such as the LUNA16 [12] has helped to accelerate research in nodule detection. Typically, nodule detection consists of two stages: nodule proposal generation and false positive reduction. Traditional approaches generally require hand-designed features such as morphological features, voxel clustering and pixel thresholding [6,9]. More recently, deep convolutional architectures were employed to generate the candidate bounding boxes. Setio et al. proposed multi-view convolutional network for false positive nodule reduction [11]. Several work employed 3D convolutional networks to handle the challenge due to the 3D nature of CT scans. The 3D fully convolutional network (FCN) was proposed to generate region candidates and deep convolutional network with weighted sampling was used in the false positive reduction stage [3,8,13,14]. CASED proposed curriculum adaptive sampling for 3D U-net training in nodule detection [7,10]. Ding et al. used Faster R-CNN to generate candidate nodules, followed by 3D convolutional networks to remove false positive nodules [2]. Due to the effective performance of Faster R-CNN [14], Faster R-CNN with a U-net-like encoder-decoder scheme was proposed for nodule detection [14].

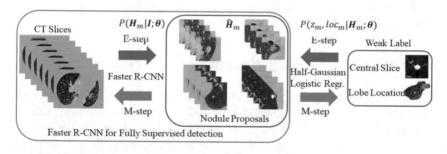

Fig. 1. Illustration of DeepEM framework. Faster R-CNN is employed for nodule proposal generation. Half-Gaussian model and logistic regression are employed for central slice and lobe location respectively. In the E-step, we utilize all the observations, CT slices, and weak label to infer the latent variable, nodule proposals, by maximum a posteriori (MAP) or sampling. In the M-step, we employ the estimated proposals to update parameters in the Faster R-CNN and logistic regression.

A prerequisite to utilization of deep learning models is the existence of an abundance of labeled data. However, labels are especially difficult to obtain in the medical image analysis domain. There are multiple contributing factors: (a) labeling medical data typically requires specially trained doctors; (b) marking lesion boundaries can be hard even for experts because of low signal-to-noise ratio in many medical images; and (c) for CT and magnetic resonance imaging (MRI) images, the annotators need to label the entire 3D volumetric data, which can be costly and time-consuming. Due to these limitations, CT medical image datasets are usually small, which can lead to over-fitting on the training set and, by extension, poor generalization performance on test sets [16].

By contrast, medical institutions have large amount of weakly labeled medical images. In these databases, each medical image is typically associated with an electronic medical report (EMR). Although these reports may not contain explicit information on detection bounding box or segmentation ground truth, it often includes the results of diagnosis, rough locations and summary descriptions of lesions if they exist. We hypothesize that these extra sources of weakly labeled data may be used to enhance the performance of existing detector and improve its generalization capability.

There are previous attempts to utilize weakly supervised labels to help train machine learning models. Deep multi-instance learning was proposed for lesion localization and whole mammogram classification [15]. Different pooling strategies were proposed for weakly supervised localization and segmentation respectively [1,4]. Self-transfer learning co-optimized both classification and localization networks for weakly supervised lesion localization [5]. Different from these works, we consider nodule proposal as latent variable and propose DeepEM, a new deep 3D convolutional nets with Expectation-Maximization optimization, to mine the big data source of weakly supervised label in EMR as illustrated in Fig. 1. Specifically, we infer the posterior probabilities of the proposed nodules being true nodules, and utilize the posterior probabilities to train nodule detection models.

2   DeepEM for Weakly Supervised Detection

Notation. We denote by $I \in \mathbb{R}^{h \times w \times s}$ the CT image, where h, w, and s are image height, width, and number of slices respectively. The nodule bounding boxes for I are denoted as $H = \{H_1, H_2, \ldots, H_M\}$, where $H_m = \{x_m, y_m, z_m, d_m\}$, the (x_m, y_m, z_m) represents the center of nodule proposal, d_m is the diameter of the nodule proposal, and M is the number of nodules in the image I. In the weakly supervised scenario, the nodule proposal H is a latent variable, and each image I is associated with weak label $X = \{X_1, X_2, \ldots, X_M\}$, where $X_m = \{loc_m, z_m\}$, $loc_m \in \{1, 2, 3, 4, 5, 6\}$ is the location (right upper lobe, right middle lobe, right lower lobe, left upper lobe, lingula, left lower lobe) of nodule H_m in the lung, and z_m is the central slice of the nodule.

For fully supervised detection, the objective function is to maximize the loglikelihood function for observed nodule ground truth H given image I as

$$\mathcal{L}(\theta) = \log P(H \cup \bar{H} | I; \theta) = \frac{1}{M} \sum_{m=1}^{M} \log P(H_m | I; \theta) + \frac{1}{N} \sum_{n=1}^{N} \log P(\bar{H}_n | I; \theta),$$

(1)

where $\bar{H} = \{\bar{H}_1, \bar{H}_2, \ldots, \bar{H}_N\}$ are hard negative nodule proposals [14], θ is the weights of deep 3D ConvNet. We employ Faster R-CNN with 3D Res18 for the fully supervised detection because of its superior performance.

For weakly supervised detection, nodule proposal $\boldsymbol{H}$ can be considered as a latent variable. Using this framework, image $\boldsymbol{I}$ and weak label $\boldsymbol{X} = \{(loc_1, z_1), (loc_2, z_2), \ldots, (loc_M, z_M)\}$ can be considered as observations. The joint distribution is

$$
\begin{aligned}
P(\boldsymbol{I}, \boldsymbol{H}, \boldsymbol{X}; \boldsymbol{\theta}) &= P(\boldsymbol{I}) \prod_{m=1}^{M} \big(P(\boldsymbol{H}_m | \boldsymbol{I}; \boldsymbol{\theta}) P(\boldsymbol{X}_m | \boldsymbol{H}_m; \boldsymbol{\theta}) \big) \\
&= P(\boldsymbol{I}) \prod_{m=1}^{M} \big(P(\boldsymbol{H}_m | \boldsymbol{I}; \boldsymbol{\theta}) P(loc_m | \boldsymbol{H}_m; \boldsymbol{\theta}) P(z_m | \boldsymbol{H}_m; \boldsymbol{\theta}) \big).
\end{aligned}
\tag{2}
$$

To model $P(z_m | \boldsymbol{H}_m; \boldsymbol{\theta})$, we propose using a half-Gaussian distribution based on nodule size distribution because z_m is correct if it is within the nodule area (center slice of $\boldsymbol{H}_m$ as $z_{\boldsymbol{H}_m}$, and nodule size σ can be empirically estimated based on existing data) for nodule detection in Fig. 2(a). For lung lobe prediction $P(loc_m | \boldsymbol{H}_m; \boldsymbol{\theta})$, a logistic regression model is used based on relative value of nodule center $(x_{\boldsymbol{H}_m}, y_{\boldsymbol{H}_m}, z_{\boldsymbol{H}_m})$ after lung segmentation. That is

$$
P(z_m, loc_m | \boldsymbol{H}_m; \boldsymbol{\theta}) = \frac{2}{\sqrt{2\pi\sigma^2}} \exp\left(-\frac{|z_m - z_{\boldsymbol{H}_m}|^2}{2\sigma^2}\right) \frac{\exp(\boldsymbol{f}(\boldsymbol{H}_m)\boldsymbol{\theta}_{loc_m})}{\sum_{loc_m=1}^{6} \exp(\boldsymbol{f}(\boldsymbol{H}_m)\boldsymbol{\theta}_{loc_m})},
\tag{3}
$$

where $\boldsymbol{\theta}_{loc_m}$ is the associated weights with lobe location loc_m for logistic regression, feature $\boldsymbol{f}(\boldsymbol{H}_m) = (\frac{x_{\boldsymbol{H}_m}}{r_I}, \frac{y_{\boldsymbol{H}_m}}{y_I}, \frac{z_{\boldsymbol{H}_m}}{z_I})$, and (x_I, y_I, z_I) is the total size of image $\boldsymbol{I}$ after lung segmentation. In the experiments, we found logistic regression converges quickly and is stable.

The expectation-maximization (EM) is a commonly used approach to optimize the maximum log-likelihood function when there are latent variables in the model. We employ the EM algorithm to optimize deep weakly supervised detection model in Eq. 2. The expected complete-data log-likelihood function given previous estimated parameter $\boldsymbol{\theta}'$ in deep 3D Faster R-CNN is

$$
\begin{aligned}
Q(\boldsymbol{\theta}; \boldsymbol{\theta}') = \frac{1}{M} \sum_{m=1}^{M} &\mathbb{E}_{P(\boldsymbol{H}_m | \boldsymbol{I}, z_m, loc_m; \boldsymbol{\theta}')} \big[\log P(\boldsymbol{H}_m | \boldsymbol{I}; \boldsymbol{\theta}) \\
&+ \log P(z_m, loc_m | \boldsymbol{H}_m; \boldsymbol{\theta}) \big] + \mathbb{E}_{Q(\bar{\boldsymbol{H}}_n | z)} \big[\log P(\bar{\boldsymbol{H}}_n | \boldsymbol{I}; \boldsymbol{\theta}) \big],
\end{aligned}
\tag{4}
$$

where $z = \{z_1, z_2, \ldots, z_m\}$. In the implementation, we only keep hard negative proposals far away from weak annotation z to simplify $Q(\bar{\boldsymbol{H}}_n | z)$. The posterior distribution of latent variable $\boldsymbol{H}_m$ can be calculated by

$$
P(\boldsymbol{H}_m | \boldsymbol{I}, z_m, loc_m; \boldsymbol{\theta}') \propto P(\boldsymbol{H}_m | \boldsymbol{I}; \boldsymbol{\theta}') P(z_m, loc_m | \boldsymbol{H}_m; \boldsymbol{\theta}').
\tag{5}
$$

Because Faster R-CNN yields a large number of proposals, we first use hard threshold (-3 before sigmoid function) to remove proposals of small confident probability, then employ non-maximum suppression (NMS) with intersection over union (IoU) as 0.1. We then employ two schemes to approximately infer the latent variable $\boldsymbol{H}_m$: maximum a posteriori (MAP) or sampling.

Algorithm 1. DeepEM for Weakly Supervised Detection

Input: Fully supervised dataset $D_F = \{(\boldsymbol{I}, \boldsymbol{H})_i\}_{i=1}^{N_F}$, weakly supervised dataset $D_W = \{(\boldsymbol{I}, \boldsymbol{X})_i\}_{i=1}^{N_W}$, 3D Faster R-CNN and logistic regression parameters $\boldsymbol{\theta}$.

1: *Initialization*: Update weights $\boldsymbol{\theta}$ by maximizing Eq. 1 using data from D_F.
2: *for epoch = 1 to #TotalEpochs*:
      ▷▷▷ **Weakly supervised training**
3:     Use Faster R-CNN model $\boldsymbol{\theta}'$ to obtain proposal probability $P(\boldsymbol{H}_m|\boldsymbol{I};\boldsymbol{\theta}')$ for weakly supervised data sampled from D_W.
4:     Remove proposals with small probabilities and NMS.
5:     *for m = 1 to M*:   ▷▷▷ Each weak label
6:          Calculate $P(z_m, loc_m|\boldsymbol{H}_m;\boldsymbol{\theta})$ for each proposal by Eq. 3.
7:          Estimate posterior distribution $P(\boldsymbol{H}_m|\boldsymbol{I}, z_m, loc_m;\boldsymbol{\theta}')$ by Eq. 5 with normalization.
8:          Employ MAP by Eq. 6 or Sampling to obtain the inference of $\boldsymbol{H}_m$.
9:     Obtain the expect log-likelihood function by Eq. 4 using the estimated proposal (MAP) or by Eq. 7 (Sampling).
10:    Update parameter by equation 8.
      ▷▷▷ **Fully supervised training**
11:    Update weights $\boldsymbol{\theta}$ by maximizing Eq. 1 using fully supervised data D_F.

DeepEM with MAP. We only use the proposal of maximal posterior probability to calculate the expectation.

$$\hat{\boldsymbol{H}}_m = \arg\max_{\boldsymbol{H}_m} P(\boldsymbol{H}_m|\boldsymbol{I};\boldsymbol{\theta}')P(z_m, loc_m|\boldsymbol{H}_m;\boldsymbol{\theta}') \tag{6}$$

DeepEM with Sampling. We approximate the distribution by sampling $\hat{M}$ proposals $\hat{\boldsymbol{H}}_m$ according to normalized Eq. 5. The expected log-likelihood function in Eq. 4 becomes

$$Q(\boldsymbol{\theta};\boldsymbol{\theta}') = \frac{1}{M\hat{M}} \sum_{m=1}^{M} \sum_{\hat{\boldsymbol{H}}_m}^{\hat{M}} \left(\log P(\hat{\boldsymbol{H}}_m|\boldsymbol{I};\boldsymbol{\theta}) + \log P(z_m, loc_m|\hat{\boldsymbol{H}}_m;\boldsymbol{\theta}) \right)$$
$$+ \mathbb{E}_{Q(\bar{\boldsymbol{H}}_n|z)}\left[\log P(\bar{\boldsymbol{H}}_n|\boldsymbol{I};\boldsymbol{\theta}) \right]. \tag{7}$$

After obtaining the expectation of complete-data log-likelihood function in Eq. 4, we can update the parameters $\boldsymbol{\theta}$ by

$$\hat{\boldsymbol{\theta}} = \arg\max Q(\boldsymbol{\theta};\boldsymbol{\theta}'). \tag{8}$$

The M-step in Eq. 8 can be conducted by stochastic gradient descent commonly used in deep network optimization for Eq. 1. Our entire algorithm is outlined in Algorithm 1.

3   Experiments

We used 3 datasets, LUNA16 dataset [12] as fully supervised nodule detection, NCI NLST[1] dataset as weakly supervised detection, Tianchi Lung Nodule Detection[2] dataset as holdout dataset for test only. LUNA16 dataset is the largest publicly available dataset for pulmonary nodules detection [12]. LUNA16 dataset removes CTs with slice thickness greater than 3 mm, slice spacing inconsistent or missing slices, and consist of 888 low-dose lung CTs which have explicit patient-level 10-fold cross validation split. NLST dataset consists of hundreds of thousands of lung CT images associated with electronic medical records (EMR). In this work, we focus on nodule detection based on image modality and only use the central slice and nodule location as weak supervision from the EMR. As part of data cleansing, we remove negative CTs, CTs with slice thickness greater than 3 mm and nodule diameter less than 3 mm. After data cleaning, we have 17,602 CTs left with 30,951 weak annotations. In each epoch, we randomly sample $\frac{1}{16}$ CT images for weakly supervised training because of the large numbers of weakly supervised CTs. Tianchi dataset contains 600 training low-dose lung CTs and 200 validation low-dose lung CTs for nodule detection. The annotations are location centroids and diameters of the pulmonary nodules, and do not have less than 3 mm diameter nodule, which are the same with those on LUNA16 dataset.

Parameter Estimation in $P(z_m|\boldsymbol{H}_m;\boldsymbol{\theta})$. If the current z_m is within the nodule, it is a true positive proposal. We can model $|z_m - z_{\boldsymbol{H}_m}|$ using a half-Gaussian distribution shown as the red dash line in Fig. 2(a). The parameters of the half-Gaussian is estimated from the LUNA16 data empirically. Because LUNA16 removes nodules of diameter less than 3 mm, we use the truncated half-Gaussian to model the central slice z_m as $\max(|z_m - z_{\boldsymbol{H}_m}| - \mu, 0)$, where μ is the mean of related Gaussian as the minimal nodule radius with 1.63.

Performance Comparisons on LUNA16. We conduct 10-fold cross validation on LUNA16 to validate the effectiveness of DeepEM. The baseline method is Faster R-CNN with 3D Res18 network denoted as **Faster R-CNN** [14]. Then we employ it to model $P(\boldsymbol{H}_m|\boldsymbol{I};\boldsymbol{\theta}')$ for weakly supervised detection scenario. Two inference scheme for $\boldsymbol{H}_m$ are used in DeepEM denoted as **DeepEM (MAP)** and **DeepEM (Sampling)**. In the proposal inference of DeepEM with Sampling, we sample two proposals for each weak label because the average number of nodules each CT is 1.78 on LUNA16. The evaluation metric, Free receiver operating characteristic (FROC), is the average recall rate at the average number of false positives at 0.125, 0.25, 0.5, 1, 2, 4, 8 per scan, which is the official evaluation metric for LUNA16 and Tianchi [12].

From Fig. 2(b), DeepEM with MAP improves about 1.3% FROC over Faster R-CNN and DeepEM with Sampling improves about 1.5% FROC over Faster R-CNN on average on LUNA16 when incorporating weakly labeled data from NLST. We hypothesize the greater improvement of DeepEM with Sampling over

---

[1] https://biometry.nci.nih.gov/cdas/datasets/nlst/.
[2] https://tianchi.aliyun.com/.

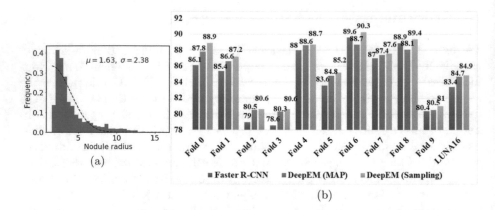

Fig. 2. (a)Empirical estimation of half-Gaussian model for $P(z_m | \boldsymbol{H}_m; \boldsymbol{\theta})$ on LUNA16. (b) FROC (%) comparison among Faster R-CNN [14], DeepEM with MAP, DeepEM with Sampling on LUNA16.

DeepEM with MAP is that MAP inference is greedy and can get stuck at a local minimum while the nature of sampling may allow DeepEM with Sampling to escape these local minimums during optimization.

Performance Comparisons on Holdout Test Set from Tianchi. We employed a holdout test set from Tianchi to validate each model from 10-fold cross validation on LUNA16. The results are summarized in Table 1. We can see DeepEM utilizing weakly supervised data improves 3.9% FROC on average over Faster R-CNN. The improvement on holdout test data validates DeepEM as an effective model to exploit potentially large amount of weak data from electronic medical records (EMR) which would not require further costly annotation by expert doctors and can be easily obtained from hospital associations (Fig. 3).

Table 1. FROC (%) comparisons among Faster R-CNN with 3D ResNet18 [14], DeepEM with MAP, DeepEM with Sampling on Tianchi.

Fold	0	1	2	3	4	5	6	7	8	9	Average
Faster R-CNN	72.8	70.8	69.8	71.9	76.4	73.0	71.3	74.7	72.9	71.3	72.5
DeepEM (MAP)	77.2	75.8	75.8	74.9	77.0	75.5	77.2	75.8	76.0	74.7	76.0
DeepEM (Sampling)	77.4	75.8	75.9	75.0	77.3	75.0	77.3	76.8	77.7	75.8	76.4

Visualizations. We compare Faster R-CNN with the proposed DeepEM visually in Fig. 3. We randomly choose nodules from Tianchi. From Fig. 3, DeepEM yields better detection for nodule center and tighter nodule diameter which demonstrates DeepEM improves the existing detector by exploiting weakly supervised data.

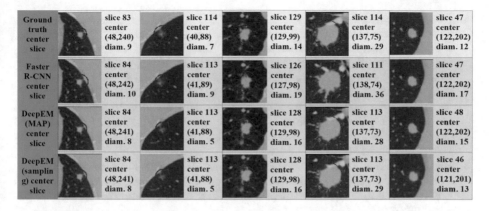

Fig. 3. Detection visual comparison among Faster R-CNN [14], DeepEM with MAP and DeepEM with Sampling on nodules randomly sampled from Tianchi. DeepEM provides more accurate detection (central slice, center and diameter) than Faster R-CNN.

4   Conclusion

In this paper, we have focused on the problem of detecting pulmonary nodules from lung CT images, which previously has been formulated as a supervised learning problem and requires a large amount of training data with the locations and sizes of nodules precisely labeled. Here we propose a new framework, called DeepEM, for pulmonary nodule detection by taking advantage of abundantly available weakly labeled data extracted from EMRs. We treat each nodule proposal as a latent variable, and infer the posterior probabilities of proposal nodules being true ones conditioned on images and weak labels. The posterior probabilities are further fed to the nodule detection module for training. We use an EM algorithm to train the entire model end-to-end. Two schemes, maximum a posteriori (MAP) and sampling, are used for the inference of proposals. Extensive experimental results demonstrate the effectiveness of DeepEM for improving current state of the art nodule detection systems by utilizing readily available weakly supervised detection data. Although our method is built upon the specific application of pulmonary nodule detection, the framework itself is fairly general and can be readily applied to other medical image deep learning applications to take advantage of weakly labeled data.

References

1. Bilen, H., et al.: Weakly supervised deep detection networks. In: CVPR (2016)
2. Ding, J., Li, A., Hu, Z., Wang, L.: Accurate pulmonary nodule detection in computed tomography images using deep convolutional neural networks. In: Descoteaux, M., Maier-Hein, L., Franz, A., Jannin, P., Collins, D.L., Duchesne, S. (eds.) MICCAI 2017. LNCS, vol. 10435, pp. 559–567. Springer, Cham (2017). https://doi.org/10.1007/978-3-319-66179-7_64

3. Dou, Q., Chen, H., Jin, Y., Lin, H., Qin, J., Heng, P.-A.: Automated pulmonary nodule detection via 3D ConvNets with online sample filtering and hybrid-loss residual learning. In: Descoteaux, M., Maier-Hein, L., Franz, A., Jannin, P., Collins, D.L., Duchesne, S. (eds.) MICCAI 2017. LNCS, vol. 10435, pp. 630–638. Springer, Cham (2017). https://doi.org/10.1007/978-3-319-66179-7_72

4. Feng, X., Yang, J., Laine, A.F., Angelini, E.D.: Discriminative localization in CNNs for weakly-supervised segmentation of pulmonary nodules. In: Descoteaux, M., Maier-Hein, L., Franz, A., Jannin, P., Collins, D.L., Duchesne, S. (eds.) MICCAI 2017. LNCS, vol. 10435, pp. 568–576. Springer, Cham (2017). https://doi.org/10.1007/978-3-319-66179-7_65

5. Hwang, S., Kim, H.-E.: Self-transfer learning for weakly supervised lesion localization. In: Ourselin, S., Joskowicz, L., Sabuncu, M.R., Unal, G., Wells, W. (eds.) MICCAI 2016. LNCS, vol. 9901, pp. 239–246. Springer, Cham (2016). https://doi.org/10.1007/978-3-319-46723-8_28

6. Jacob, C., et al.: Automatic detection of subsolid pulmonary nodules in thoracic computed tomography images. Med. Image Anal. **18**, 374–384 (2014)

7. Jesson, A., Guizard, N., Ghalehjegh, S.H., Goblot, D., Soudan, F., Chapados, N.: CASED: curriculum adaptive sampling for extreme data imbalance. In: Descoteaux, M., Maier-Hein, L., Franz, A., Jannin, P., Collins, D.L., Duchesne, S. (eds.) MICCAI 2017. LNCS, vol. 10435, pp. 639–646. Springer, Cham (2017). https://doi.org/10.1007/978-3-319-66179-7_73

8. Liao, F., et al.: Evaluate the malignancy of pulmonary nodules using the 3d deep leaky noisy-or network. arXiv preprint (2017)

9. Lopez Torres, E., et al.: Large scale validation of the M5L lung cad on heterogeneous ct datasets. Med. Phys. **42**, 1477–1489 (2015)

10. Ronneberger, O., Fischer, P., Brox, T.: U-Net: convolutional networks for biomedical image segmentation. In: Navab, N., Hornegger, J., Wells, W.M., Frangi, A.F. (eds.) MICCAI 2015. LNCS, vol. 9351, pp. 234–241. Springer, Cham (2015). https://doi.org/10.1007/978-3-319-24574-4_28

11. Setio, A.A.A., et al.: Pulmonary nodule detection in CT images: false positive reduction using multi-view convolutional networks. IEEE TMI **35**, 1160–1169 (2016)

12. Setio, A.A.A., et al.: Validation, comparison, and combination of algorithms for automatic detection of pulmonary nodules in computed tomography images: the luna16 challenge. Med. Image Anal. **42**, 1–13 (2017)

13. Tang, H., Kim, D., Xie, X.: Automated pulmonary nodule detection using 3D deep convolutional neural networks. In: ISBI (2018)

14. Zhu, W., Liu, C., Fan, W., Xie, X.: Deeplung: deep 3d dual path nets for automated pulmonary nodule detection and classification. In: IEEE WACV (2018)

15. Zhu, W., Lou, Q., Vang, Y.S., Xie, X.: Deep multi-instance networks with sparse label assignment for whole mammogram classification. In: Descoteaux, M., Maier-Hein, L., Franz, A., Jannin, P., Collins, D.L., Duchesne, S. (eds.) MICCAI 2017. LNCS, vol. 10435, pp. 603–611. Springer, Cham (2017). https://doi.org/10.1007/978-3-319-66179-7_69

16. Zhu, W., et al.: Adversarial deep structured nets for mass segmentation from mammograms. In: IEEE ISBI (2018)

Statistical Framework for the Definition of Emphysema in CT Scans: Beyond Density Mask

Gonzalo Vegas-Sánchez-Ferrero[✉] and Raúl San José Estépar

Applied Chest Imaging Laboratory (ACIL), Brigham and Women's Hospital, Harvard Medical School, Boston, MA, USA
{gvegas,rsanjose}@bwh.harvard.edu

Abstract. Lung parenchyma destruction (emphysema) is a major factor in the description of Chronic Obstructive Pulmonary Disease (COPD) and its prognosis. It is defined as an abnormal enlargement of air spaces distal to the terminal bronchioles and the destruction of alveolar walls. In CT imaging, the presence of emphysema is observed by a local decrease of the lung density and the diagnose is usually set as more than 5% of the lung below −950 HU, the so-called emphysema density mask. There is still debate, however, about the definition of this percentage and many researchers set it depending on the population under study. Additionally, the −950 HU threshold may vary depending on factors as the slice thickness or the respiratory phase of the acquisition. In this paper we propose (1) a statistical framework that provides an automatic definition of the density threshold based on the statistical characterization of air and lung parenchyma; (2) the definition of a statistical test for emphysema detection that accounts for the CT noise characteristics. Results show that this novel statistical framework improves the quantification of emphysema against a visual reference and improves the association of emphysema with the pulmonary function tests.

Keywords: CT scans · Emphysema · Lung disease
Statistical characterization

1 Introduction

Emphysema is one of the most common disease manifestations that causes airflow limitation due to the destruction of alveolar walls and loss of elastic recoil. It is a common component of Chronic Obstructive Pulmonary Disease (COPD), a lung condition defined by expiratory airflow limitation associated with an inflammatory response to noxious particles such as cigarette smoke. COPD is currently the 3rd leading cause of death in the U.S. and represents an enormous

This study was supported by the National Institutes of Health NHLBI awards R01HL116931, R01HL116473 and R21HL140422.

© Springer Nature Switzerland AG 2018
A. F. Frangi et al. (Eds.): MICCAI 2018, LNCS 11071, pp. 821–829, 2018.
https://doi.org/10.1007/978-3-030-00934-2_91

societal burden. Recent evidences suggest a rapid decline in lung function occurs and may be prevented if acted upon [1]. Early diagnosis is, therefore, essential.

Although pulmonary function tests remain the standard diagnostic tool for COPD, image-based diagnosis of CT scans are increasingly used in diagnosing and categorizing COPD. The detection of emphysema is generally performed by visual inspection of CT images for Low-Attenuation Areas (LAA) [2]. Quantitatively, CT is a well-validated technique to assess the in vivo presence and extent of emphysema [3]. The identification of emphysema areas is usually prescribed to areas under a density level set to −950 Hounsfield Units (HU), the so-called *density mask*. This threshold has been selected by the community as the one with the highest correlation with microscopic emphysema analyzed though biopsies [4]. This threshold, however, may vary with the slice thickness (the original study was confined to scans with 1 cm), exposure dose and respiratory phase during the acquisition.

This work proposes to reduce the confounding factors that affect the emphysema detection by defining a statistical framework that provides a characterization of both lung parenchyma and air. The characterization will lead to the definition of an adaptive threshold that fits the particular conditions of the scan. The adaptive threshold will be defined as the one that reduces both type I and type II errors in a statistical hypothesis testing problem where the air probability distribution is acquired in the trachea, and the parenchyma distribution is inferred from the lung. This way, we palliate effect of the noise caused by lower effective radiation due to body mass, reconstruction deviations or respiratory phase. The statistical framework will also lead to define a statistical test for emphysema detection. Results show a significant improvement in the correlation with functional respiratory parameters used for the diagnosis of COPD.

2   Characterization of Emphysema in CT Scans

The definition of a statistical framework for the characterization of emphysema will require the determination of the probability distribution of air and lung parenchyma. In the case of air, the estimation of the probability distribution becomes easy since apparent anatomical structures like the trachea provide a suitable set of samples for the estimation. On the other hand, the parenchyma characterization is far more intricate because the lung tissue is a heterogeneous composition of tissues (connective tissue, capillaries, blood, and air). The intrinsic relationship between air and lung parenchyma is a critical factor that takes place in the variation of lung densities throughout the respiratory cycle due to the volume change.

We will disentangle the parenchyma composition of air by adopting a mixture model in the statistical description of emphysema proposed in [5]. This model is defined as a finite non-central Gamma Mixture Model (nc-ΓMM) whose probability density function (PDF) is:

$$p(x) = \sum_{j=1}^{J} \pi_j f_X(x|\alpha_j, \beta_j, \delta) \tag{1}$$

for J components, where π_j are the weights of the mixture and α_j, β_j and δ are the shape, scale and location parameters of a non-central Gamma distribution with probability density function defined as:

$$f_X(x|\alpha,\beta,\delta) = \frac{(x-\delta)^{\alpha-1}}{\beta^\alpha \Gamma(\alpha)} e^{-\frac{x-\delta}{\beta}}, \qquad x \geq \delta \text{ and } \alpha,\beta > 0 \tag{2}$$

The characterization of the air component of the mixture can be accurately calculated considering anatomical structures such as the trachea. The δ parameter estimated for air can be extended for the rest of components since the CT numbers are all relative to the lowest density level (air). Once the parameters of the air component are estimated, one can calculate the rest of components for the lung constraining the air to the parameters already derived. This will lead to a more accurate estimate of the air component that is not affected by the number of tissues of different densities.

Many methodologies can be applied for the estimation of the mixture model. Among them, probably the simplest is achieved with the Expectation Maximization method, which reduces the problem to solve a non-linear equation in each iteration, as proposed in [5]. In our work, we propose a modification of this Expectation Maximization methodology which comprises the following steps:

Estimation of the Air Component. Let $x = \{x_i\}_{i=1}^N$ be the set of samples acquired in the trachea (following a nc-Γ distribution). The parameters of the air component (α_{air}, β_{air}, δ) are calculated as the maximum log-likelihood estimates:

$$\{\alpha_{\text{air}}, \delta\} = \underset{\alpha,\delta \leq \min x}{\operatorname{argmax}} \, \mathcal{L}(\alpha,\delta|x) \tag{3}$$

where

$$\mathcal{L}(\alpha,\delta|x) = (\alpha-1)\sum_{i=1}^N \log(x_i-\delta) - N\alpha - N\alpha \log\left(\frac{1}{\alpha N}\sum_i^N (x_i - \delta)\right) - N\log(\Gamma(\alpha)) \tag{4}$$

and

$$\beta_{\text{air}} = \frac{1}{\alpha_{\text{air}} N} \sum_{i=1}^N (x_i - \delta) \tag{5}$$

Characterization of Lung Parenchyma. Once the parameters of the air component are known, the mixture model can be estimated constrained to the air parameters. To ensure that the heterogeneous composition of the lung is properly described in the mixture model, we set components from -950 to -750 HU in steps of 50 HU, and from -700 to -400 HU in steps of 100 HU. This is more than a reasonable range of attenuations considering that the normal lung attenuation is between -600 and -700 HU. So, the mixture model will be constrained to the mean values $\mu_j \in \{\mu_{\text{air}}, -950, \ldots, -400\}$.

The estimation of the shape parameters for each component, α_j (except the air component), are obtained by solving the following non-linear equation [5]:

$$\log(\alpha_j) - \psi(\alpha_j) = \frac{\sum_{i=1}^N \gamma_{i,j}(x_i - \delta)/\mu_j}{\sum_{i=1}^N \gamma_{i,j}} - \frac{\sum_{i=1}^N \gamma_{i,j}\log((x_i-\delta)/\mu_j)}{\sum_{i=1}^N \gamma_{i,j}} - 1 \tag{6}$$

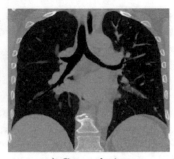
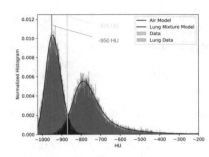

a) Coronal view   b) Histogram of trachea and lung parenchyma

Fig. 1. Coronal view of a chest CT scan and histogram. Trachea and lung segmentations are shown in red and lung blue, respectively. Note that the density mask (-950 HU) underestimates the emphysema (more than 50% of trachea is classified as parenchyma).

where $\psi(\cdot)$ is the digamma function, $\psi(\cdot) = \Gamma'(x)/\Gamma(x)$, and $\gamma_{i,j} = P(j|x_i)$ are the posterior probabilities for the j-th tissue class:

$$\gamma_{i,j} = \frac{\pi_j f_X(x_i|\alpha_j,\beta_j,\delta)}{\sum_{j=1}^{J} \pi_j f_X(x_i|\alpha_j,\beta_j,\delta)} \tag{7}$$

Finally, the scale factor is trivially calculated as $\beta_j = \mu_j/\alpha_j$ and the priors π_j are updated as $\pi_j = \frac{1}{N}\sum_{i=1}^{N}\gamma_{i,j}$.

The fitting is performed iteratively until convergence in the parameters is reached. This is usually achieved in very few iterations since the shape parameter α_j is already constrained to the mean μ_j, which ensures the robustness of the convergence. A suitable initialization of parameters for the iterative optimization is $\pi_j = 1/J$, $\alpha_j = 2$ and $\beta_j = \mu_j/\alpha_j$ for each component, $J = 2, \ldots, J$ with the exception of the air component, $j = 1$, which is set to $\alpha_1 = \alpha_{\text{air}}$ and $\beta_1 = \beta_{\text{air}}$.

Figure 1a shows a real CT scan where the lung and trachea masks are superimposed in blue and red respectively. In Fig. 1b, the histograms obtained from the trachea and lung parenchyma are depicted along with the nc-Γ distribution fitted with Eqs. (3–5) plotted in solid red line, and the ΓMM fitted to the parenchyma data in solid blue line.

Air Component Removal. We can now disentangle the air component from the parenchyma description by imposing $\pi_{\text{air}} = \pi_1 = 0$ and updating the priors as $\pi_j^* = \pi_j/\sum_{k=2}^{J}\pi_k$ for $j = 2, \ldots, J$. The resulting mixture model now describes the composition of tissue without air:

$$p_{\text{tissue}}(x) = \sum_{j=2}^{J} \pi_j^* f_X(x|\alpha_j\beta_j,\delta) \tag{8}$$

3 Adaptive Threshold for Emphysema Detection

To improve the performance of the density mask threshold recommendation $(-950\ \mathrm{HU})$, we will consider the minimization of type I and type II errors of the statistical hypothesis testing for air and normal tissue for each subject. With the statistical framework established in the previous section, we can effectively characterize the air and parenchyma in each patient and a more accurate threshold can be established for emphysema detection. Formally speaking, let us consider the PDFs of air and tissue:

$$p_{\mathrm{air}}(x) = f_X(x|\alpha_{\mathrm{air}}, \beta_{\mathrm{air}}, \delta); \qquad p_{\mathrm{tissue}}(x) = \sum_{j=2}^{J} \pi_j^* f_X(x|\alpha_j, \beta_j, \delta), \qquad (9)$$

where $f_X(\cdot|\alpha, \beta, \delta)$ is the nc-Γ PDF of Eq. (1). The optimal threshold is derived as:

$$t = \operatorname*{argmin}_{x} \left| 1 - F_X(x, |\alpha_{\mathrm{air}}, \beta_{\mathrm{air}}, \delta) - \sum_{j=2}^{J} \pi_j^* F_X(x|\alpha_j, \beta_j, \delta) \right|, \qquad (10)$$

where $F_X(x, |\alpha, \beta, \delta)$ is the cumulative distribution function (CDF) of a nc-Γ distribution:

$$F_X(x|\alpha_j, \beta_j, \delta) = \int_{\delta}^{x} \frac{(y-\delta)^{\alpha-1}}{\beta^\alpha \Gamma(\alpha)} e^{-\frac{y-\delta}{\beta}} dy = \frac{1}{\Gamma(\alpha)} \gamma\left(\alpha, \frac{x-\delta}{\beta}\right), \ x \geq \delta \text{ and } \alpha, \beta > 0$$
$$(11)$$

The monotonic behavior of Eq. (11) ensures the existence of t in Eq. (10).

The statistical framework introduced in the previous section in combination to the definition of the optimal threshold in Eq. (10) allows us to define a statistical test for the detection of emphysema on a certain region of interest. The statistic will be defined as the *degree of implication of emphysema*, $\hat{p}$, i.e. the percentage of emphysema within the region under study. According to the statistical model here derived, samples will have a probability of being emphysema $p_{\mathrm{emph}} = F_X(t, |\alpha_{\mathrm{air}}, \beta_{\mathrm{air}}, \delta)$. Then, $\hat{p}$ is distributed as a Binomial, $\mathcal{B}(p_{\mathrm{emph}}, n)$, of parameters p_{emph} and the number of samples, n. Note that, as $n \to \infty$, $\hat{p} \xrightarrow{\mathcal{L}} \mathcal{N}\left(p_{\mathrm{emph}}, \sqrt{\frac{p_{\mathrm{emph}}(1-p_{\mathrm{emph}})}{n}}\right)$. Therefore, we can set a statistical test with null hypothesis $\mathrm{H_0}$: *"The region under study is normal parenchyma"* whose critical point from which the null hypothesis is rejected if $\hat{p} > p_0 + z_\alpha \sqrt{\frac{p_{\mathrm{emph}}(1-p_{\mathrm{emph}})}{n}}$, with $P(Z \leq z_\alpha) = \alpha$ and $Z \sim \mathcal{N}(0,1)$.

4 Results

The air and lung parenchyma were statistically characterized in 48 inspiratory scans acquired from subjects with diagnosed COPD with all the different severity levels according to the GOLD guidelines classification of patients[1]. 5 Different

---

[1] The data was acquired at three centers as part of a COPD study and with the approval of their ethics committee and the informed consent of each subject.

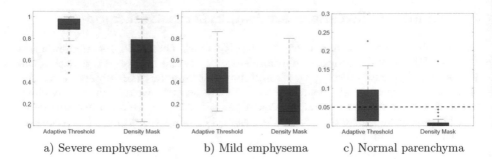

a) Severe emphysema   b) Mild emphysema   c) Normal parenchyma

Fig. 2. Boxplots for the implication of emphysema detected in segmentations. The adaptive threshold detects more implication in severe and mild emphysema, while maintaining the normal parenchyma significantly below 5%.

devices from 2 different manufacturers were used: GE VCT-64, Siemens Definition Flash, Siemens Definition, Siemens Sensation-64, and Siemens Definition AS+. The dose was set to 200 mAs in all the acquisitions.

Lung segmentations and trachea segmentations were automatically obtained with an automatic method as implemented in the Chest Imaging Platform (www.chestimagingplatform.org). The distribution of air was defined by adjusting nc-Γ statistical model as exposed in Eqs. (3–5) for the trachea samples, while the distribution of lung parenchyma was obtained by fitting the ΓMM to the lung parenchyma samples, Eqs. (6 and 7), and the tissue PDF is calculated by removing the air component, Eq. (8). The optimal threshold was computed as the optimal CT number that minimizes both type I and type II errors, Eq. (10).

We performed two different validations of the proposed methodology. First, we compareed the proposed method and the density mask within regions already labeled by an expert as *severe emphysema*, meaning most of the region affected; *mild emphysema*, where the tissue shows a mild low attenuation density; and *normal parenchyma*, where no parenchymal damage was perceived. The expert was free to select as many regions as necessary for each group on each subject. We used the *degree of implication of emphysema* as the validation metric defined as the percentage of voxels within the region that were considered emphysema according to each method. Finally, we provided an indirect validation of our method with a correlation analysis with respiratory function. We correlated the emphysema score obtained in each subject with FEV1%, a standard functional respiratory measure used for COPD diagnose. This measure is defined as the ratio between the volume of air that can forcibly be blown out in one second after full inspiration (the so-called Forced Expiratory Volume in 1 second, FEV1) and the volume of air that can forcibly be blown out after full inspiration (the so-called Forced Vital Capacity, FVC). Emphysema affects pulmonary function by compromising the lung elastic recoil and restricting flow by small airway collapse during expiration. Therefore, improved correlation with FEV1% can be seen as a functional validation of any approach that aims at quantifying emphysema.

Quantitative Validation in Classified Regions. The implication of emphysema was studied in the segmentations provided by the expert for all the 48 subjects. In Fig. 2 we show the boxplots for the three classes. Note that the implication of emphysema in regions labeled as severe and mild emphysema remarkably increases. We test the differences with a paired Wilcoxon signed-rank test at a significance level $\alpha = 0.05$ resulting in statistically significant differences for both severe and mild emphysema (p-values $< 10^{-7}$ for both cases) between the proposed adaptive threshold and density masking. Additionally, Fig. 2c evidences that the increase in the sensitivity to emphysema detection still maintains a low type I error below 5% involvement (p-values > 0.3), meaning that the null hypothesis H_0: *"normal parenchyma"* cannot be rejected.[2]

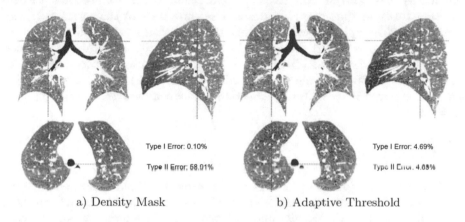

a) Density Mask   b) Adaptive Threshold

Fig. 3. Emphysema classification for the density mask (-950 HU) and for the Adaptive Threshold of subject shown in Fig. 1. Density Mask underestimates the emphysema composition (a): Most of the samples in the trachea are labeled as tissue. (b) The Adaptive Threshold successfully labels the trachea samples. Besides, a prominent region of low attenuation density is now detected as emphysema.

Table 1. Linear-log regression analysis for the FEV1% with respect the emphysema for the density mask (-950 HU) and the adaptive threshold.

	Density Mask ($R^2 = 0.25$)		Adaptive Threshold ($R^2 = 0.44$)	
	Beta [95% CI]	p-value	Beta [95% CI]	p-value
Log-Emph.	-23.80 [-35.98, -11.62]	$p < 0.001$	-17.03 [-22.78, -11.286]	$p < 0.001$

As an example of the performance of the proposed threshold, we show in Fig. 3 the density mask threshold at -950 HU and the optimal adaptive threshold

---

[2] 5% involvement is the level of implication that the clinical community uses as consensus to define presence of disease on CT scans.

$t = -870$ HU calculated with Eq. (10) for the same subject shown in Fig. 1. The density mask obtains a Type I error of 0.10% and a Type II error 58.91%. Note that the -950 HU threshold is far below the extreme of the air and implies an unnecessary increase of type II error. This threshold is clearly underestimating the emphysema in this subject and, paradoxically, classifying more than 50% of the trachea samples as tissue. On the other hand, the proposed threshold provides an optimal balance between both types of error, achieving a type I and type II errors equal to 4.69%. Note that the increase of type I error is still below the 5% while the type II error is dramatically reduced to more reasonable values.

Physiological Validation. We performed a linear-log regression analysis of the FEV1% with respect to the emphysema detected in inspiratory scans for both the density mask and the adaptive threshold. Results are shown in Table 1 where the superiority of the adaptive threshold explains 44% of the variance in contrast to the 25% explained with the -950 HU one. We used the William's test for dependent samples to test differences in correlations [6]. The statistic obtained for our dataset was $T = 2.024$, for $N = 48$ and correlation between dependent variables $\rho = 0.756$, implying that the adaptive threshold significantly improves the correlation with respiratory function when compare to density masking ($p = 0.024$).

5   Conclusion

In this work, we show the problems derived from the definition of emphysema in CT scans by the density mask approach. As shown in Fig. 1, the threshold set by the density mask usually underestimates the distribution of air as a consequence of confounding factors such as slice thickness, device calibration, and noise due to body mass. The underestimation originates an important bias in the detection of emphysema that hinders the association with functional respiratory measures and early disease detection. Our work defines a statistical framework to circumvent this problem. We characterize both trachea and lung parenchyma, and derive a statistical test based on the optimal threshold that adapts to each acquisition and reduces type I and type II errors. Results show a consistent reduction of type II error in severe and mild emphysema regions while confines type I error to rates below 5% in normal parenchyma. Our adaptive threshold also shows a statistically significant improvement in association with pulmonary function. This result evidences the suitability of our methodology for clinical applications.

References

1. Csikesz, N.G., Gartman, E.J.: New developments in the assessment of COPD: early diagnosis is key. Int. J. COPD **9**, 277–286 (2014)
2. Lynch, D.A., et al.: CT-definable subtypes of chronic obstructive pulmonary disease: a statement of the Fleischner Society. Radiology **277**(1), 141579 (2015)

3. Müller, N.L., Staples, C.A., Miller, R.R., Abboud, R.T.: Density mask. an objective method to quantitate emphysema using computed tomography. Chest **94**(4), 782–787 (1988)
4. Gevenois, P.A., et al.: Comparison of computed density and microscopic morphometry in pulmonary emphysema. Am. J. Respir. Crit. Care Med. **154**(1), 187–192 (1996)
5. Vegas-Sánchez-Ferrero, G., Ledesma-Carbayo, M.J., Washko, G.R., San José Estépar, R.: Statistical characterization of noise for spatial standardization of CT scans: enabling comparison with multiple kernels and doses. Med. Image Anal. **40**, 44–59 (2017)
6. Steiger, J.H.: Tests for comparing elements of a correlation matrix. Psychol. Bull. **87**(2), 245–251 (1980)

Cardiac, Chest and Abdominal Applications: Breast Imaging Applications

Conditional Generative Adversarial and Convolutional Networks for X-ray Breast Mass Segmentation and Shape Classification

Vivek Kumar Singh[1]([✉]), Santiago Romani[1], Hatem A. Rashwan[1], Farhan Akram[2], Nidhi Pandey[3,4], Md. Mostafa Kamal Sarker[1], Saddam Abdulwahab[1], Jordina Torrents-Barrena[1], Adel Saleh[1], Miguel Arquez[4], Meritxell Arenas[4], and Domenec Puig[1]

[1] DEIM, Universitat Rovira i Virgili, Tarragona, Spain
vivekkumar.singh@urv.cat
[2] Imaging Informatics Division, Bioinformatics Institute, Singapore, Singapore
[3] Kayakalp Hospital, New Delhi 110084, India
[4] Hospital Universitari Sant Joan de Reus, Tarragona, Spain

Abstract. This paper proposes a novel approach based on conditional Generative Adversarial Networks (cGAN) for breast mass segmentation in mammography. We hypothesized that the cGAN structure is well-suited to accurately outline the mass area, especially when the training data is limited. The generative network learns intrinsic features of tumors while the adversarial network enforces segmentations to be similar to the ground truth. Experiments performed on dozens of malignant tumors extracted from the public DDSM dataset and from our in-house private dataset confirm our hypothesis with very high Dice coefficient and Jaccard index (>94% and >89%, respectively) outperforming the scores obtained by other state-of-the-art approaches. Furthermore, in order to detect portray significant morphological features of the segmented tumor, a specific Convolutional Neural Network (CNN) have also been designed for classifying the segmented tumor areas into four types (irregular, lobular, oval and round), which provides an overall accuracy about 72% with the DDSM dataset.

Keywords: cGAN · CNN · Mammography · Mass segmentation
Mass shape classification

1 Introduction

Mammography screening is the most reliable method for early detection of breast carcinomas [1]. Among diverse types of breast abnormalities, such as micro-calcifications or architectural distortion, breast masses are the most important findings since they may be pointing out the presence of malignant tumors [2].

© Springer Nature Switzerland AG 2018
A. F. Frangi et al. (Eds.): MICCAI 2018, LNCS 11071, pp. 833–840, 2018.
https://doi.org/10.1007/978-3-030-00934-2_92

However, to locate masses and discern mass borders are difficult tasks because of their high variability, low contrast and high similarity with the surrounding healthy tissue, as well as their low signal-to-noise ratio [3].

Therefore, Computer-Aided Diagnosis (CAD) systems are highly recommended for helping radiologists in detecting masses, outlining their borders (mass segmentation) and suggesting their morphological features, such as shape type (irregular, lobular, oval and round) and margin type (circumscribed, obscured, ill-defined, spiculated). Recent studies point out some loose correlations between mass features and molecular subtypes, i.e., Luminal-A, Luminal-B, HER-2 (Human Epidermal growth factor receptor 2) and Basal-like (triple negative), which are key for prescribing the best oncological treatment [4–6].

Although it is impossible for an expert radiologist to discern the molecular subtypes from the mammography. Recently, a Convolutional Neural Network (CNN) was used to classify molecular subtypes using texture based descriptors of image crops of mass area [7], which yielded an overall accuracy of 67%.

In this paper, we present a novel approach for (1) breast mass segmentation based on conditional Generative Adversarial Networks (cGAN) [8], (2) to predict the mass shape type (irregular, lobular, oval and round) from the binary mask of the mass area. Beside these two contributions, this paper provides a study of the correlation between the mass shape and molecular subtypes.

2   Related Work

Numerous methods have been proposed to solve the problem of breast mass segmentation from a classical point of view, including techniques based on thresholding, iterative pixel classification, region growing, region clustering, edge detection, template matching and stochastic relaxation [1,9].

For the segmentation problem, some proposals rely on classic statistical models, such as structured Support Vector Machines, using Deep Belief Network or CNN features as their potential functions [10]. On the other hand, it is also possible to perform image segmentation based on the Fully Convolutional Network (FCN) approach [11]. However, the classical FCN pipeline does not accurately preserve the objects boundaries. To overcome this drawback, an FCN network has been concatenated with a CRF layer taking into account the pixel position to enforce the compactness of the output segmentation [12].

In [13], a conditional Generative Adversarial Network (cGAN) has been used to segment the human liver in 3D CT images. However, this architecture is based on 3D filters, thus it is not suitable for mammography segmentation.

3   Proposed Model

3.1   System Overview

Figure 1 represents the training phase of the proposed cGAN network for mass segmentation (left) as well as the full predicting workflow (right), defined by two stages. The first stage uses the generator part of the trained cGAN to automatically obtain a binary mask that selects the pixels (in white) that are supposed to correspond to the area of the breast mass, while ignores the pixels (in black) corresponding to healthy tissue. The input image is a squared crop of the mammogram containing the mass ROI. The input is reshaped to 256×256 pixels size and the value of each pixel is scaled into a $[0,1]$ range. For noise removal, we have regularized the image with Gaussian filter of 0.5 standard deviation. The second stage of the workflow uses a regular CNN trained to classify the obtained binary mask into one out of four classes of mass shape, which are irregular, lobular, oval and round.

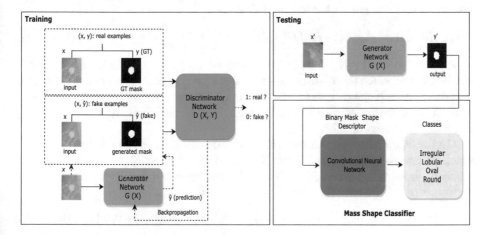

Fig. 1. Proposed framework for breast mass segmentation and shape classification

3.2 Mass Segmentation Model (with cGAN)

We hypothesized that the cGAN structure proposed in [8] would be perfect for segmentation, mainly for two reasons:

1. The Generator network of the cGAN is an FCN network composed of two networks: encoders and decoders. Encoders can learn the intrinsic features of the masses and normal breast parenchyma (gray-level, texture, gradients, edges, shape, etc.), in turn decoders can learn how to mark up the binary mask according to the input features of the two output classes (mass/normal).
2. The Discriminative network of the cGAN compares the generated binary mask with the corresponding ground truth to make them as similar as possible. Therefore, including the adversarial score in the loss computation of the generator strengthens its capabilities to provide a valid segmentation.

This combination of generator/discriminator networks allows robust learning with very few training samples. Since both generative and discriminative networks are conditioned by observing the input image, thus the resulting segmentation is a "function" over the input pixels. Otherwise, regular GAN (unconditional) will infer the segmentation just from random noise, which obviously will not bind the mass appearance gathered by the x-ray with the output binary mask.

Let x represents a mass ROI image, y the corresponding ground truth segmentation, z a random variable, $G(x, z)$ is the predicted mask, $\|y - G(x, z)\|_1$ is the L1 normalized distance between ground truth and predicted masks, λ is an empirical weighting factor and $D(x, G(x, z))$ is the output score of the discriminator, the generator loss is defined as:

$$\ell_{Gen}(G, D) = E_{x,y,z}\big(-log(D(x, G(x, z)))\big) + \lambda E_{x,y,z}\big(\|y - G(x, z)\|_1 \big), \quad (1)$$

As pointed out in [8], if we only use the L1 term, the obtained binary masks will be blurred since the distance metric averages all pixel differences. Therefore, including the adversarial term allows the generator to learn how to transform input images at fine-grained details (high frequencies), which results in sharp and realistic binary masks.

On the other hand, the L1 term is also necessary to boost the learning process, which otherwise may be too slow because the adversarial loss term may not properly formulate the gradient towards the expected mask shape. The loss computation of the discriminator network is defined as:

$$\ell_{Dis}(G, D) = E_{x,y}\big(-log(D(x, y))\big) + E_{x,y,z}\big(-log(1 - D(x, G(x, z)))\big), \quad (2)$$

Hence, the optimizer will fit the discriminator network in order to maximize the real mask predication (by minimizing $-log(D(x, y))$) and to minimize the generated masks predication (by minimizing $-log(1 - D(x, G(x, z)))$).

3.3   Shape classification model (with CNN)

For this stage, we have chosen a CNN approach instead of other classical approaches of extracting shape features (e.g. HOG, shape context) mainly because of the recent success of Deep Neural Networks in object recognition and segmentation tasks [14]. Nevertheless, the input images for this stage (binary masks) do not render complex distribution of pixel values, just morphological structure, hence we hypothesized that a rather simple CNN (i.e., two convolutional layers plus two fully connected layers) will be sufficient to learn a generalization of the four mass shapes.

4   Experiments

To evaluate the performance of the proposed models, two datasets have been used: Digital Database for Screening Mammography (DDSM) [15] and our private in-house dataset of mammograms obtained from Hospital Universitari Sant

Joan de Reus-Spain. For numerical assessment of the performance of the proposed mass segmentation, we have computed Accuracy, Dice Coefficient, Jaccard index (i.e., Intersection over Union (IoU)), Sensitivity and Specificity [16].

4.1 Datasets

DDSM Dataset: It is a publicly available database including about 2500 benign and malignant breast tumor masses, with ground truths of different shape classes. From malignant cases, we have selected 567 mammography images (330, 108, 90 and 39 images of irregular, lobular, oval and round shapes, respectively). We have used this dataset for training both segmentation and shape classification models.

Reus Hospital Dataset: It contains 194 malignant masses distributed into four molecular subtypes of breast cancer: 64 Luminal-A, 59 Luminal-B, 34 Her-2 and 37 Basal-like. This dataset is used to test the segmentation model and to make an analysis between shape mass and molecular subtype distributions.

4.2 Experimental Results

For the first stage, we have trained two versions of the proposed cGAN architecture, Auto-Encoder (i.e., without skip connections) and U-Net (i.e., with skip connections), and compared them with three models: FCN [11], U-Net [17] and CRFCNN [10] retrained for our data. For all experiments, the DDSM dataset is divided into training, validation and testing by 70%, 15% and 15%, respectively. In turn, whole in-house private dataset samples are used for testing (see Table 1). After segmentation, we have applied a post-processing morphological filtering (i.e., erosion and dilation) to remove the artifacts and small white regions from the binary masks generated by all compared methods.

Table 1. Accuracy, Dice coefficient, Jaccard index, Sensitivity and Specificity from the two architectures of cGAN (Auto-Encoder and Unet), FCN, U-Net and CRFCNN evaluated on DDSM and our private dataset. Best results are marked in bold.

Dataset	Methods	Accuracy	Dice	Jaccard	Senstivity	Specificity
DDSM	FCN	0.9114	0.8480	0.7361	0.8193	0.9511
	U-Net	0.9308	0.8635	0.7896	0.8365	0.9552
	CRFCNN	0.8245	0.8457	0.7925	0.8421	0.8975
	cGAN-AutoEnc	0.9469	0.9061	0.8283	0.8975	0.9666
	cGAN-Unet	**0.9716**	**0.9443**	**0.8944**	**0.9274**	**0.9871**
Private	FCN	0.9484	0.8698	0.7799	0.8002	**0.9905**
	U-Net	0.8647	0.7442	0.6622	0.6921	0.8641
	CRFCNN	0.7542	0.6135	0.5247	0.7126	0.7458
	cGAN-AutoEnc	0.9481	**0.8894**	**0.8008**	**0.9726**	0.9414
	cGAN-Unet	**0.9555**	0.8648	0.7618	0.8576	0.9750

The cGAN-Unet provides the best results of all computed metrics on the DDSM test samples, with very remarkable Accuracy, Dice and Jaccard scores (around 97%, 94% and 89%, respectively). On the in-house private dataset, however, the cGAN-AutoEnc yields better results than the cGAN-Unet in terms of Dice, Jaccard and Sensitivity (+2%, +4% and +12%, respectively), which indicates that the cGAN-AutoEnc has learned a more generalized representation of tumor features since it performs better on the dataset not used for training. Although the accuracy of cGAN-AutoEnc (94.81%) is not higher than FCN (94.84%) and cGAN-Unet (95.55%), the former has obtained an impressive rate of true positives (97.26%), which leads to the highest values of Dice and Jaccard (88.94% and 80.08%, respectively). The FCN model obtains the highest rate of true negatives (99.05%) but its Sensitivity is poorer (80.02%) than both cGAN versions, which indicates that it misses more real tumor area than the cGAN proposals. On the other hand, U-Net and CRFCNN provided even poorer results in both Sensitivity and Specificity for the private dataset, although the U-Net and FCN methods performed relatively well on the DDSM dataset. Some qualitative examples using our in-house private dataset are shown in Fig. 2.

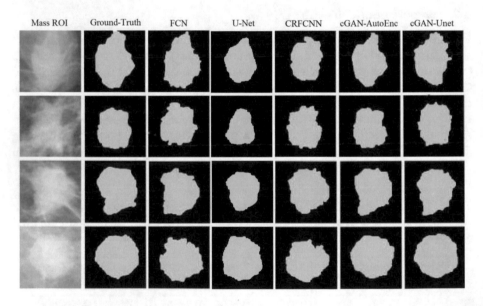

Fig. 2. Examples of hospital dataset mammographic mass ROI images (col 1), ground truth masks (col 2), and generated masks with FCN (col 3), CRFCNN (col 4), cGAN-AutoEnc (col 5), cGAN-Unet (col 6) and U-Net (col 7).

For training the second stage of shape classification, 80% of the selected images from the DDSM dataset are used in training our classifier with their corresponding ground truth of mass shape labels, using a stratified 10 fold cross validation with 50 epochs per fold. The remaining 20% of images are used for testing, obtaining an overall accuracy around 72%.

Tumor shape could play an important role to predict the breast cancer molecular subtypes [18]. Thus, we have computed the correlation between breast cancer molecular subtypes classes of our in-house private dataset with the four shape classes. As shown in Table 2, Luminal-A and -B groups are mostly assigned to irregular and lobular shape classes. In addition, some images related to Luminal-A are assigned to oval shape. In turn, oval and round masses give indications to the Her-2 and Basal-like groups, as well as some images related to Basal-like are moderately assigned to the lobular class.

Table 2. Distribution of breast cancer molecular subtypes samples from the hospital dataset with respect to its predicted mask shape.

Shape classes/molecular subtypes	Irregular	Lobular	Oval	Round	Total
Luminal A	24	19	19	2	64
Luminal B	23	27	8	1	59
Her-2	7	3	10	14	34
Basal-like	2	13	4	18	37

5   Conclusions

In this paper, we propose two versions of cGAN networks for breast mass segmentation: cGAN-AutoEnc and cGAN-Unet. The generative network of both versions follows similar structures compared to FCN and U-Net networks, respectively. However, experimental results confirm that the inclusion of an adversarial network significantly improves the performance of the segmentation, about +6% and +9% in terms of Dice coefficient and Jaccard index, respectively on the public DDSM dataset. In turn, on our in-house private dataset, it yields an improvement of +2% and +2% with the two metrics. The CRFCNN provided worse test results in general. In addition, we have also proved that a rather simple CNN architecture is enough for distinguishing shape-related classes of the mass shapes from their binary masks. Future work aims to improve the overall accuracy (72%) by using a large dataset and using a robust loss function, such as negative log likelihood and dice loss function for improving the convergence and accuracy of the proposed system.

Acknowledgement. This research has been partly supported by the Spanish Government through project DPI2016-77415-R.

References

1. Cheng, H., Shi, X., Min, R., Hu, L., Cai, X., Du, H.N.: Approaches for automated detection and classification of masses in mammograms. Pattern Recognit. **39**(4), 646–668 (2006)
2. Kopans, D.: Breast Imaging. Lippincott, New York (1998)

3. Elmore, J.G., et al.: Variability in interpretive performance at screening mammography and radiologists' characteristics associated with accuracy. Radiology **253**(3), 641–651 (2009)
4. Cho, N.: Molecular subtypes and imaging phenotypes of breast cancer. Ultrasonography **35**(4), 281 (2016)
5. Liu, S., Wu, X.D., Xu, W.J., Lin, Q., Liu, X.J., Li, Y.: Is there a correlation between the presence of a spiculated mass on mammogram and luminal a subtype breast cancer? Korean J. Radiol. **17**(6), 846–852 (2016)
6. Tamaki, K., et al.: Correlation between mammographic findings and corresponding histopathology: potential predictors for biological characteristics of breast diseases. Cancer Sci. **102**(12), 2179–2185 (2011)
7. Singh, V.K., et al.: Classification of breast cancer molecular subtypes from their micro-texture in mammograms using a VGGNet-based convolutional neural network. In: Recent Advances in Artificial Intelligence Research and Development - Proceedings of the 20th International Conference of the Catalan Association for Artificial Intelligence, pp. 76–85 (2017)
8. Isola, P., Zhu, J.Y., Zhou, T., Efros, A.A.: Image-to-image translation with conditional adversarial networks. arXiv preprint (2017)
9. Oliver, A., et al.: A review of automatic mass detection and segmentation in mammographic images. Med. Image Anal. **14**(2), 87–110 (2010)
10. Dhungel, N., Carneiro, G., Bradley, A.P.: Deep learning and structured prediction for the segmentation of mass in mammograms. In: Navab, N., Hornegger, J., Wells, W.M., Frangi, A.F. (eds.) MICCAI 2015. LNCS, vol. 9349, pp. 605–612. Springer, Cham (2015). https://doi.org/10.1007/978-3-319-24553-9_74
11. Long, J., Shelhamer, E., Darrell, T.: Fully convolutional networks for semantic segmentation. In: Proceedings of the IEEE Conference on Computer Vision and Pattern Recognition, pp. 3431–3440 (2015)
12. Zhu, W., Xie, X.: Adversarial deep structural networks for mammographic mass segmentation. arXiv preprint arXiv:1612.05970 (2016)
13. Yang, D., et al.: Automatic liver segmentation using an adversarial image-to-image network. In: Descoteaux, M., Maier-Hein, L., Franz, A., Jannin, P., Collins, D.L., Duchesne, S. (eds.) MICCAI 2017. LNCS, vol. 10435, pp. 507–515. Springer, Cham (2017). https://doi.org/10.1007/978-3-319-66179-7_58
14. Litjens, G., et al.: A survey on deep learning in medical image analysis. Med. Image Anal. **42**, 60–88 (2017)
15. Heath, M., Bowyer, K., Kopans, D., Moore, R., Kegelmeyer, P.: The digital database for screening mammography. In: Digital Mammography, pp. 431–434 (2000)
16. Vacavant, A., Chateau, T., Wilhelm, A., Lequièvre, L.: A benchmark dataset for outdoor foreground/background extraction. In: Park, J.-I., Kim, J. (eds.) ACCV 2012. LNCS, vol. 7728, pp. 291–300. Springer, Heidelberg (2013). https://doi.org/10.1007/978-3-642-37410-4_25
17. Ronneberger, O., Fischer, P., Brox, T.: U-Net: convolutional networks for biomedical image segmentation. In: Navab, N., Hornegger, J., Wells, W.M., Frangi, A.F. (eds.) MICCAI 2015. LNCS, vol. 9351, pp. 234–241. Springer, Cham (2015). https://doi.org/10.1007/978-3-319-24574-4_28
18. Zhang, L., et al.: Identifying ultrasound and clinical features of breast cancer molecular subtypes by ensemble decision. Sci. Rep. **5**, 11085 (2015)

A Robust and Effective Approach Towards Accurate Metastasis Detection and pN-stage Classification in Breast Cancer

Byungjae Lee[✉] and Kyunghyun Paeng

Lunit Inc., Seoul, South Korea
{jaylee,khpaeng}@lunit.io

Abstract. Predicting TNM stage is the major determinant of breast cancer prognosis and treatment. The essential part of TNM stage classification is whether the cancer has metastasized to the regional lymph nodes (N-stage). Pathologic N-stage (pN-stage) is commonly performed by pathologists detecting metastasis in histological slides. However, this diagnostic procedure is prone to misinterpretation and would normally require extensive time by pathologists because of the sheer volume of data that needs a thorough review. Automated detection of lymph node metastasis and pN-stage prediction has a great potential to reduce their workload and help the pathologist. Recent advances in convolutional neural networks (CNN) have shown significant improvements in histological slide analysis, but accuracy is not optimized because of the difficulty in the handling of gigapixel images. In this paper, we propose a robust method for metastasis detection and pN-stage classification in breast cancer from multiple gigapixel pathology images in an effective way. pN-stage is predicted by combining patch-level CNN based metastasis detector and slide-level lymph node classifier. The proposed framework achieves a state-of-the-art quadratic weighted kappa score of 0.9203 on the Camelyon17 dataset, outperforming the previous winning method of the Camelyon17 challenge.

Keywords: Camelyon17 · Convolutional neural networks
Deep learning · Metastasis detection · pN-stage classification
Breast cancer

1 Introduction

When cancer is first diagnosed, the first and most important step is staging of the cancer by using the TNM staging system [1], the most commonly used system. Invasion to lymph nodes, highly predictive of recurrence [2], is evaluated by pathologists (pN-stage) via detection of tumor lesions in lymph node histology slides from a surgically resected tissue. This diagnostic procedure is prone to misinterpretation and would normally require extensive time by pathologists

© Springer Nature Switzerland AG 2018
A. F. Frangi et al. (Eds.): MICCAI 2018, LNCS 11071, pp. 841–850, 2018.
https://doi.org/10.1007/978-3-030-00934-2_93

because of the sheer volume of data that needs a thorough review. Automated detection of lymph node metastasis and pN-stage prediction has the potential to significantly elevate the efficiency and diagnostic accuracy of pathologists for one of the most critical diagnostic process of breast cancer.

In the last few years, considerable improvements have been emerged in the computer vision task using CNN [3]. Followed by this paradigm, CNN based computer assisted metastasis detection has been proposed in recent years [4–6]. However, recent approaches metastasis detection in whole slide images have shown the difficulty in handling gigapixel images [4–6]. Furthermore, pN-stage classification requires handling multiple gigapixel images.

In this paper, we introduce a robust method to predict pathologic N-stage (pN-stage) from whole slide pathology images. For the robust performance, we effectively handle multiple gigapixel images in order to integrate CNN into pN-stage prediction framework such as balanced patch sampling, patch augmentation, stain color augmentation, 2-stage fine-tuning and overlap tiling strategy. We achieved patient-level quadratic weighted kappa score 0.9203 on the Camelyon17 test set which it yields the new state-of-the-art record on Camelyon17 leaderboard [7].

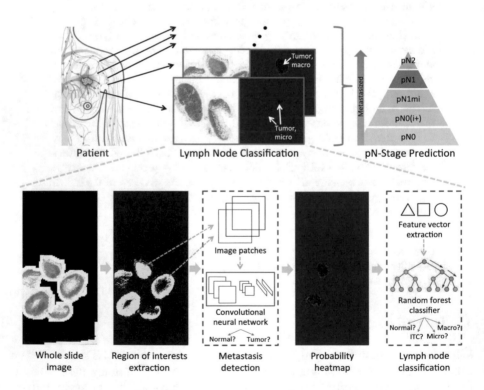

Fig. 1. Overall architecture of our pN-stage prediction framework.

2   Methodology

Figure 1 shows the overall scheme of our proposed framework. First, ROI extraction module proposes candidate tissue regions from whole slide images. Second, CNN-based metastasis detection module predicts cancer metastasis within extracted ROIs. Third, the predicted scores extracted from ROI are converted to a feature vector based on the morphological and geometrical information which is used to build a slide-level lymph node classifier. Patient-level pN-stage is determined by aggregating slide-level predictions with given rules [7].

2.1   Regions of Interests Extraction

A whole slide image (WSI) is approximately 200000×100000 pixels on the highest resolution level. Accurate tissue region extraction algorithms can save computation time and reduce false positives from noisy background area. In order to extract tissue regions from the WSIs, Otsu threshold [8] or gray value threshold is commonly used in recent studies [4–6]. We decide to use gray value threshold method which shows superior performance in our experiments.

2.2   Metastasis Detection

Some annotated metastasis regions include non-metastasis area since accurate pixel-level annotation is difficult in gigapixel WSIs [5]. We build a large scale dataset by extracting small patches from WSIs to deal with those noisy labels. After the ROIs are found from WSIs as described in Sect. 2.1, we extract 256×256 patches within ROIs with stride 128 pixels. We label a patch as tumor if over 75% pixels in the patch are annotated as a tumor. Our metastasis detection module is based on the well-known CNN architecture ResNet101 [3] for patch classification to discriminate between tumor and non-tumor patches.

Although the proposed method seems straightforward, we need to effectively handle gigapixel WSIs to integrate CNN into pN-stage prediction framework for the robust performance, as described below.

Balanced Patch Sampling. The areas corresponding to tumor regions often covered only a minor proportion of the total slide area, contributing to a large patch-level imbalance. To deal with this imbalance, we followed similar patch sampling approach used in [5]. In detail, we sample the same number of tumor/normal patches where patches are sampled from each slide with uniform distribution.

Patch Augmentation. There are only 400 WSIs in Camelyon16 dataset and 500 WSIs in Camelyon17 train set. Patches sampled from same WSI exhibit similar data property, which is prone to overfitting. We perform extensive data augmentation at the training step to overcome small number of WSIs. Since the classes of histopathology image exhibit rotational symmetry, we include patch augmentation by randomly rotating over angles between 0 and 360, and random left-right flipping. Details are shown in Table 1.

Table 1. Patch augmentation details.

Methods	Details
Translation	random x, y offset in $[-8, 8]$
Left/right flip	with 0.5 probability
Rotation	random angle in $[0, 360)$

Stain Color Augmentation. To combat the variety of hematoxylin and eosin (H&E) stained color because of chemical preparation difference per slide, extensive color augmentation is performed by applying random hue, saturation, brightness, and contrast as described in Table 2. CNN model becomes robust against stain color variety by applying stain color augmentation at the training step.

Table 2. Stain color augmentation details.

Methods	Details
Hue	Random delta in $[-0.04, 0.04]$
Saturation	Random saturation factor in $[0.75, 1.25]$
Brightness	Random delta in $[-0.25, 0.25]$
Contrast	Random contrast factor in $[0.25, 1.75]$

2-Stage Fine-Tuning. Camelyon16 and Camelyon17 dataset are collected from different medical centers. Each center may use different slide scanners, different scanning settings, difference tissue staining conditions. We handle this multi-center variation by applying the 2-stage fine-tuning strategy. First, we fine-tune CNN with the union set of Camelyon16 and Camelyon17 and then fine-tune CNN again with only Camelyon17 set. The fine-tuned model becomes robust against multi-center variation between Camelyon16 and Camelyon17 set.

Overlap Tiling Strategy. In the prediction stage, probability heatmap is generated by the trained CNN based metastasis detector. A straightforward way to generate a heatmap from WSI is separating WSI into patch size tiles and merging patch level predictions from each tile. However, this simple strategy provides insufficient performance. Instead, we

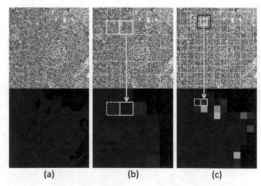

(a)   (b)   (c)

Fig. 2. Tiling strategy for dense heatmap. (a) A ground truth; (b) Straightforward tiling strategy; (c) Overlap-tile strategy.

use similar overlap-tile strategy [9] for dense heatmap from tiled WSI. As shown in Fig. 2, the probability heatmap generated by overlap-tile strategy provides denser heatmap than straightforward tiling strategy even though the same classifier is used. By default, we used 50% overlapped tiles shown in Fig. 2(c).

2.3 Lymph Node Classification

To determine each patient's pN-stage, multiple lymph node slides should be classified into four classes (Normal, Isolated tumor cells (ITC), Micro, Macro). For each lymph node WSI, we obtain the $128\times$ down-sampled tumor probability heatmap through the CNN based metastasis detector (Sect. 2.2). Each heatmap is converted into a feature vector which is used to build a slide level lymph node classifier. We define 11 types of features based on the morphological and geometrical information. By using converted features, random forest classifier [10] is trained to automatically classify the lymph node into four classes. Finally, each patient's pN-stage is determined by aggregating all lymph node predictions with the given rule [7]. We followed the Camelyon17's simplified version of the pN-staging system (pN0, pN0(i+), pN1mi, pN1, pN2) [7].

3   Experiments

3.1   Dataset

We evaluate our framework on Camelyon16 [6] and Camelyon17 [7] dataset. The Camelyon16 dataset contains 400 WSIs with region annotations for all its metastasis slides. The Camelyon17 dataset contains 1000 WSIs with 5 slides per patient: 500 slides for the **train** set, 500 slides for the **test** set. The **train** set consists of the slide level metastasis annotation. There are 3 categories of lymph node metastasis: Macro (Metastases greater than 2.0 mm), Micro (metastasis greater than 0.2 mm or more than 200 cells, but smaller than 2.0 mm), and ITC (single tumor cells or a cluster of tumor cells smaller than 0.2 mm or less than 200 cells).

Since the Camelyon17 set provides only 50 slides with lesion-level annotations in **train** set, we split 100 patients (total 500 WSIs since each patient provides 5 WSIs) into 43 patients for the Camelyon17 **train-M** set to train metastasis detection mod-

Table 3. Details of our Camelyon17 dataset split.

Dataset	# of patients per each pN-stage					
	pN0	pN0(i+)	pN1mi	pN1	pN2	Total
Camelyon17 train-M	0	9	11	14	9	43
Camelyon17 train-L	24	3	9	11	10	57
Dataset	# of patients per each medical center					
	Center1	Center2	Center3	Center4	Center5	Total
Camelyon17 train-M	7	8	9	10	9	43
Camelyon17 train-L	13	12	11	10	11	57
Dataset	# of WSIs per each metastasis type				
	Negative	ITC	Micro	Macro	Total
Camelyon17 train-M	110	26	35	44	215
Camelyon17 train-L	203	9	29	44	285

ule, 57 patients for the Camelyon17 **train-L** set to train lymph node classification module. In detail, if patient's any slide include lesion-level annotation, we allocate that patient as a Camelyon17 train-M set. Other patients are allocated as a Camelyon17 train-L set. As shown in Table 3, our split strategy separates similar data distribution between them in terms of the medical centers and metastasis types.

3.2   Evaluation Metrics

Metastasis Detection Evaluation. We used the Camelyon16 evaluation metric [6] on the Camelyon16 dataset to validate metastasis detection module performance. Camelyon16 evaluation metric consists of two metrics, the area under receiver operating characteristic (AUC) to evaluate the slide-level classification and the FROC to evaluate the lesion-level detection and localization.

pN-stage Classification Evaluation. To evaluate pN-stage classification, we used the Camelyon17 evaluation metric [7], patient-level five-class quadratic weighted kappa where the classes are the pN-stages. Slide-level lymph node classification accuracy is also measured to validate lymph node classification module performance.

3.3   Experimental Details

ROI Extraction Module. For the type of ROI extraction between Otsu threshold and gray value threshold, we determined to use gray value threshold method which is obtained a better performance on Camelyon16 train set. In detail, we convert RGB to gray from 32× down-sampled WSI and then extract tissue regions by thresholding gray value >0.8.

Metastasis Detection Module. During training and inference, we extracted 256 × 256 patches from WSIs at the highest magnification level of 0.243 µm/pixel resolution. For training of the patch-level CNN based

Table 4. Number of training WSIs for metastasis detection module.

Training data	# of tumor slides	# of normal slides
Camelyon16 train	110	160
Camelyon16 test	50	80
Camelyon17 train-M	50*	110

* only 50 slides include region annotations from total 105 tumor slides in Camelyon17 train-M set

classifier, 400 WSIs from Camelyon16 dataset and 160 WSIs from Camelyon17 train set are used as shown in Table 4. Total 1,430K tumor patches and 43,700K normal patches are extracted.

We trained ResNet101 [3] with initial parameters from ImageNet pretrained model to speed up convergence. We updated batch normalization parameters during fine-tuning because of the data distribution difference between the ImageNet dataset and the Camelyon dataset. We used the Adam optimization method with a learning rate 1e-4. The network was trained for approximately 2 epoch (500K iteration) with a batch size 32 per GPU.

To find hyperparameters and validate performance, we split Camelyon16 `train` set into our train/val set, 80% for train and 20% for validation. For AUC evaluation, we used maximum confidence probability in WSI. For FROC evaluation, we followed connected component approach [11] which find connected components and then report maximum confidence probability's location within the component. After hyperparameter tuning, we finally train CNN with all given training dataset in Table 4.

Table 5. Feature components for predicting lymph node metastasis type.

No.	Feature description	No.	Feature description
1	Largest region's major axis length	7	Maximum confidence probability in WSI
2	Largest region's maximum confidence probability	8	Average of all confidence probability in WSI
3	Largest region's average confidence probability	9	Number of regions in WSI
4	Largest region's area	10	Sum of all foreground area in WSI
5	Average of all region's averaged confidence probability	11	Foreground and background area ratio in WSI
6	Sum of all region's area		

Lymph Node Classification Module. We generated the tumor probability heatmap from WSI using the metastasis detection module. For the post-processing, we thresholded the heatmap with a threshold of $t = 0.9$. We found hyperparameters and feature designs for random forest classifier in Camelyon17 `train-L` set with 5-fold cross-validation setting. Finally, we extracted 11 features described in Table 5. We built a random forest classifier to discriminate lymph node classes using extracted features. Each patient's pN-stage was determined by the given rule [7] with the 5 lymph node slide prediction results.

3.4 Results

Metastasis Detection on Camelyon16. We validated our metastasis detection module on the Camelyon16 dataset. For the fair comparison with the state-of-the-art methods,

Table 6. Metastasis detection results on Camelyon16 **test set**

Method	Ensemble	AUC	FROC
Lunit Inc.		0.985	0.855
Liu et al. ensemble-of-3 [5]	✓	0.977	0.885
Liu et al. 40X [5]		0.967	0.873
Harvard & MIT [11]	✓	0.994	0.807
Pathologist* [6]	–	0.966	0.724

*expert pathologist who assessed without a time constraint

Table 7. Top-10 pN-stage classification result on the Camelyon17 leaderboard [7]. The kappa score is evaluated by the Camelyon17 organizers. Accessed: 2018-03-02.

Team	Affiliation	Kappa score
Lunit Inc.*	**Lunit Inc.**	**0.9203**
HMS-MGH-CCDS	Harvard Medical School, Mass. General Hospital, Center for Clinical Data Science	0.8958
DeepBio*	Deep Bio Inc.	0.8794
VCA-TUe	Electrical Engineering Department, Eindhoven University of Technology	0.8786
JD*	JD.com Inc. - PCL Laboratory	0.8722
MIL-GPAT	The Univercity of Tokyo, Tokyo Medical and Dental University	0.8705
Indica Labs	Indica Labs	0.8666
chengshenghua*	Huazhong University of Science and Technology, Britton Chance Center for Biomedical Photonics	0.8638
Mechanomind*	Mechanomind	0.8597
DTU	Technical University of Denmark	0.8244

*Submitted result after reopening the challenge

our model is trained on the 270 WSIs from Camelyon16 `train` set and evaluated on the 130 WSIs from Camelyon16 `test` set using the same evaluation metrics provided by the Camelyon16 challenge. Table 6 summarizes slide-level AUC and lesion-level FROC comparisons with the best previous methods. Our metastasis detection module achieved highly competitive AUC (0.9853) and FROC (0.8552) without bells and whistles.

pN-stage Classification on Camelyon17. For validation, we first evaluated our framework on Camelyon17 `train-L` set with 5-fold cross-validation setting. Our framework achieved 0.9351 slide-level lymph node classification accuracy and 0.9017 patient-level kappa score using single CNN model in metastasis detection module. We trained additional CNN models with different model hyperparameters and fine-tuning setting. Finally, three model was ensembled by averaging probability heatmap and reached 0.9390 slide-level accuracy and 0.9455 patient-level kappa score with the 5-fold cross-validation.

Next, we evaluated our framework on the Camelyon17 `test` set and the kappa score has reached 0.9203. As shown in Table 7, our proposed framework significantly outperformed the state-of-the-art approaches by large-margins where it achieves better performance than the previous winning method (HMS-MGH-CCDS) of the Camelyon17 challenge.

Table 8. Slide-level lymph node classification confusion matrix comparison on the Camelyon17 **test** set. The confusion matrix is generated by the Camelyon17 organizers.

		Predicted							Predicted			
		Negative	ITC	Micro	Macro				Negative	ITC	Micro	Macro
Reference	Negative	**96.15%**	3.08%	0.77%	0.00%		Reference	Negative	**95.38%**	0.38%	4.23%	0.00%
	ITC	55.88%	**11.76%**	32.35%	0.00%			ITC	76.47%	**14.71%**	8.82%	0.00%
	Micro	9.64%	2.41%	**85.54%**	2.41%			Micro	13.25%	1.20%	**78.31%**	7.23%
	Macro	3.25%	0.00%	5.69%	**91.06%**			Macro	1.63%	0.00%	12.20%	**86.18%**
(a) **Lunit Inc.**							(b) HMS-MGH-CCDS					

Furthermore, the accuracy of our algorithm not only exceeded that of current leading approaches (bold black color in Table 8) but also significantly reduced false-negative results (red color in Table 8). This is remarkable from a clinical perspective, as false-negative results are most critical, likely to affect patient survival due to consequent delay in diagnosis and appropriate timely treatment.

4   Conclusion

We have introduced a robust and effective method to predict pN-stage from lymph node histological slides, using CNN based metastasis detection and random forest based lymph node classification. Our proposed method achieved the state-of-the-art result on the Camelyon17 dataset. In future work, we would like to build an end-to-end learning framework for pN-stage prediction from WSIs.

References

1. Sobin, L.H., Gospodarowicz, M.K., Wittekind, C.: TNM Classification of Malignant Tumours. Wiley, Hoboken (2011)
2. Saadatmand, S., et al.: Influence of tumour stage at breast cancer detection on survival in modern times: population based study in 173 797 patients. Bmj **351**, h4901 (2015)
3. He, K., Zhang, X., Ren, S., Sun, J.: Deep residual learning for image recognition. In: Proceedings of the IEEE Conference on Computer Vision and Pattern Recognition, pp. 770–778 (2016)
4. Paeng, K., Hwang, S., Park, S., Kim, M.: A unified framework for tumor proliferation score prediction in breast histopathology. In: Cardoso, M.J., et al. (eds.) DLMIA/ML-CDS -2017. LNCS, vol. 10553, pp. 231–239. Springer, Cham (2017). https://doi.org/10.1007/978-3-319-67558-9_27
5. Liu, Y., et al.: Detecting cancer metastases on gigapixel pathology images. arXiv preprint arXiv:1703.02442 (2017)
6. Bejnordi, B.E., et al.: Diagnostic assessment of deep learning algorithms for detection of lymph node metastases in women with breast cancer. Jama **318**(22), 2199–2210 (2017)
7. Camelyon 2017. https://camelyon17.grand-challenge.org/. Accessed 02 Feb 2018
8. Otsu, N.: A threshold selection method from gray-level histograms. IEEE Trans. Syst. Man Cybern. **9**(1), 62–66 (1979)

9. Ronneberger, O., Fischer, P., Brox, T.: U-Net: convolutional networks for biomedical image segmentation. In: Navab, N., Hornegger, J., Wells, W.M., Frangi, A.F. (eds.) MICCAI 2015. LNCS, vol. 9351, pp. 234–241. Springer, Cham (2015). https://doi.org/10.1007/978-3-319-24574-4_28

10. Breiman, L.: Random forests. Mach. Learn. **45**(1), 5–32 (2001)

11. Wang, D., Khosla, A., Gargeya, R., Irshad, H., Beck, A.H.: Deep learning for identifying metastatic breast cancer. arXiv preprint arXiv:1606.05718 (2016)

3D Anisotropic Hybrid Network: Transferring Convolutional Features from 2D Images to 3D Anisotropic Volumes

Siqi Liu[1(✉)], Daguang Xu[1], S. Kevin Zhou[1], Olivier Pauly[2], Sasa Grbic[1],
Thomas Mertelmeier[2], Julia Wicklein[2], Anna Jerebko[2], Weidong Cai[3],
and Dorin Comaniciu[1]

[1] Medical Imaging Technologies, Siemens Healthineers, Princeton, NJ, USA
`siqi.liu@siemens-healthineers.com`
[2] X-Ray Products, Siemens Healthineers, Erlangen, Germany
[3] School of Information Technologies, University of Sydney, Sydney, Australia

Abstract. While deep convolutional neural networks (CNN) have been successfully applied to 2D image analysis, it is still challenging to apply them to 3D medical images, especially when the within-slice resolution is much higher than the between-slice resolution. We propose a 3D Anisotropic Hybrid Network (AH-Net) that transfers convolutional features learned from 2D images to 3D anisotropic volumes. Such a transfer inherits the desired strong generalization capability for within-slice information while naturally exploiting between-slice information for more effective modelling. We experiment with the proposed 3D AH-Net on two different medical image analysis tasks, namely lesion detection from a Digital Breast Tomosynthesis volume, and liver and liver tumor segmentation from a Computed Tomography volume and obtain state-of-the-art results.

1 Introduction

3D volumetric images (or volumes) are widely used for clinical diagnosis, intervention planning, and biomedical research. However, given the additional dimension, it is more time consuming and sometimes harder to interpret 3D volumes than 2D images by machines. Many imaging modalities come with anisotropic voxels, meaning not all of the three dimensions have equal resolutions, for example the Digital Breast Tomosynthesis (DBT) and sometimes Computed Tomography (CT). Directly applying 3D CNN to such images remains challenging due to the following reasons: (1) It may be hard for a small $3 \times 3 \times 3$ kernel to learn useful features from anisotropic voxels. (2) The capability of 3D networks is bounded by the GPU memory, constraining both the width and depth of the networks. (3) 3D tasks mostly have to train from scratch, and hence suffer from the lack of large 3D datasets. In addition, the high data biases make the 3D

D. Xu—Equal contribution.

© Springer Nature Switzerland AG 2018
A. F. Frangi et al. (Eds.): MICCAI 2018, LNCS 11071, pp. 851–858, 2018.
https://doi.org/10.1007/978-3-030-00934-2_94

networks harder to generalize. Besides the traditional 3D networks built with $1 \times 1 \times 1$ and $3 \times 3 \times 3$ kernels, there are other methods for learning representations from anisotropic voxels. Some studies process 2D slices separately with 2D networks [9]. To make a better use of the 3D context, more than one image slice is used as the input for 2D networks [8]. The 2D slices can also be viewed sequentially by combining a fully convolutional network (FCN) architecture with Convolutional LSTM [1]. Anisotropic convolutional kernels were used to distribute more learning capability on the xy plane [7].

In this paper, we propose the 3D Anisotropic Hybrid Network (AH-Net) to learn informative features for object detection and segmentation tasks in 3D medical images. To obtain the 3D AH-Net, we firstly train a 2D fully convolutional ResNet [10] which is initialized with pre-trained weights and uses multiple 2D image slices as inputs. The feature encoder of such a 2D network is then transformed into a 3D network by extending the 2D kernel with one added dimension. Then we add a feature decoder sub-network to extract the 3D context. The feature decoder consists of anisotropic convolutional blocks with $3 \times 3 \times 1$ and $1 \times 1 \times 3$ convolutions. Different anisotropic convolutional blocks are combined with dense connections [5]. Similar to the U-Net [11], we use skip connections between the feature encoder and the decoder. A pyramid volumetric pooling module [13] is stacked at the end of the network before the final output layer for extracting multiscale features. Since the AH-Net can make use of 2D networks pre-trained with large 2D general image datasets such as ImageNet [12], it is easier to train as well as to generalize. The anisotropic convolutional blocks enable the exploiting of 3D context. With end-to-end inference as a 3D network, the AH-Net runs much faster than the conventional multi-channel 2D networks regarding the GPU time required for processing each 3D volume.

2   Anisotropic Hybrid Network

The AH-Net is designed for the object detection and the segmentation tasks in 3D medical images. It is able to transfer learnt 2D networks to 3D learning problems and further exploit 3D context information. As an image-to-image network, the AH-Net consists of a feature encoder and a feature decoder as shown in Fig. 1. The encoder, transformed from a fine-tuned 2D network, is designed for extracting the deep representations from 2D slices with high resolution. The decoder built with densely connected blocks of anisotropic convolutions is responsible for exploiting the 3D context and maintaining the between-slice consistency. The network training is performed in two stages: the 2D encoder is firstly trained and transformed into a 3D encoder; then the 3D decoder is added and fine-tuned with the encoder parameters locked.

2.1   Pre-training a Multi-Channel 2D Feature Encoder

To obtain a pre-trained 2D image-to-image network, we train a 2D multi-channel global convolutional network (MC-GCN) similar to the architecture in [10] to

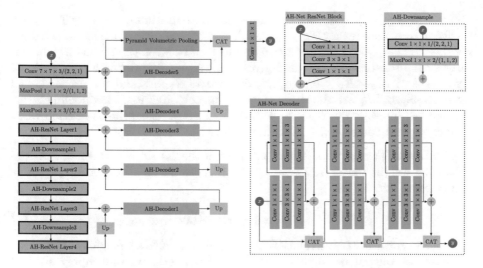

Fig. 1. The architecture of 3D AH-Net. We hide the batch normalization and ReLu layers for brevity. The parameters of the blocks with bold boundaries are transformed from the pre-trained 2D ResNet50 encoder.

extract the 2D within-slice features at different resolutions. We choose the 2D ResNet50 model [4] as the backbone network, which is initialized by pre-training with the ImageNet images [12]. The network is then fine-tuned with 2D image slices extracted from the 3D volumes. The inputs to this network are three neighbouring slices (as RGB channels). Thus, the entire architecture of the ResNet50 remains unchanged. With a 2D decoder upscaling the responses to the original resolution as described in [10], the MC-GCN outputs response maps with the same dimensions as the input slices. To fine tune this network, the scaled L2 loss is used for object detection and weighted cross entropy is used for segmentation.

2.2 Transferring the Learned 2D Features into 3D AH-Net

We extract the parameters of the trained ResNet50 encoder from the 2D MC-GCN and transfer them to the corresponding encoder layers of the AH-Net. The decoder of the MC-GCN is thus discarded. The input and output of AH-Net are now 3D volumes. The transformation of the convolution tensors from 2D to 3D aims to perform 2D convolutions on 3D volumes slice by slice in the encoder of the AH-Net. Overall, we permute the weight tensors of the first convolution layer so the channel dimension becomes the z-dimension. For the rest of the encoder, we treat 2D filters as 3D filters by setting the extra dimension as 1.

Notations. A 2D convolutional tensor is denoted by $T^i_{n \times m \times h \times w}$, where n, m, h, and w respectively represent the number of output channels, the number of input channels, the height and width of the ith convolution layer. Similarly, a 3D weight tensor is denoted by $T^i_{n \times m \times h \times w \times d}$ where d is the filter depth. We use

$P^{(b,a,c,d)}(T_{a\times b\times c\times d})$ to denote the dimension permutation of a tensor $T_{a\times b\times c\times d}$, resulting in a new tensor $T_{b\times a\times c\times d}$ with the 1st and 2nd dimensions switched. $P^{(a,*,b,c,d)}(T_{a\times b\times c\times d})$ adds an identity dimension between the 1st and 2nd dimensions of the tensor $T_{a\times b\times c\times d}$ and gives $T_{a\times 1\times b\times c\times d}$. We define a convolutional layer as Conv $K_x \times K_y \times K_z/(S_x, S_y, S_z)$, where K_x, K_y and K_z are the kernel sizes; S_x, S_y and S_z are the stride step size in each direction. Max pooling layers are denoted by MaxPool $K_x \times K_y \times K_z/(S_x, S_y, S_z)$. The stride is omitted when a layer has a stride size of 1 in all dimensions.

Input Layer Transform. The input layer of the 2D ResNet50 contains a convolutional weight tensor $T^1_{64\times 3\times 7\times 7}$. The 2D convolutional tensor $T^1_{64\times 3\times 7\times 7}$ is transformed into 3D as

$$P^{(1,*,3,4,2)}(T^1_{64\times 3\times 7\times 7}) = T^1_{64\times 1\times 7\times 7\times 3} \tag{1}$$

in order to form a 3D convolution kernel that convolves 3 neighbouring slices. To keep the output consistent with the 2D network, we only apply stride-2 convolutions on the xy plane and stride 1 on the third dimension. This results in the input layer Conv $7 \times 7 \times 3/(2,2,1)$. To downsample the z dimension, we use a MaxPool $1 \times 1 \times 2/(1,1,2)$ to fuse every pair of the neighbouring slices. An additional MaxPool $2 \times 2 \times 2/(2,2,2)$ is used to keep the feature resolution consistent with the 2D network.

ResNet Block Transform. All the 2D convolutional tensors $T^i_{n\times m\times 1\times 1}$ and $T^i_{n\times m\times 3\times 3}$ in the ResNet50 are transformed as

$$P^{(1,2,3,4,*)}(T^i_{n\times m\times 1\times 1}) = T^i_{n\times m\times 1\times 1\times 1} \tag{2}$$

and

$$P^{(1,2,3,4,*)}(T^i_{n\times m\times 3\times 3}) = T^i_{n\times m\times 3\times 3\times 1}. \tag{3}$$

In this way, all the ResNet Conv $3 \times 3 \times 1$ blocks only perform 2D slice-wise convolutions on the 3D volume within the xy plane. The original downsampling between ResNet blocks is performed with Conv $1 \times 1/(2,2)$. However, in a 3D volume, a Conv $1 \times 1 \times 1/(2,2,2)$ skips a slice for every step on the z dimension. This would miss important information when the image only has a small z-dimension. We therefore use a Conv $1 \times 1 \times 1/(2,2,1)$ following by a MaxPool $1\times 1\times 2/(1,1,2)$ to downsample the 3D feature maps between the ResNet blocks.

2.3   Anisotropic Hybrid Decoder

Accompanying the transformed encoder, an anisotropic 3D decoder sub-network is added to exploit the 3D anisotropic image context with chained separable convolutions as shown in Fig. 1. In the decoder, anisotropic convolutional blocks with Conv $1 \times 1 \times 1$, Conv $3 \times 3 \times 1$ and Conv $1 \times 1 \times 3$ are used. The features are passed into an xy bottleneck block at first with a Conv $3 \times 3 \times 1$ surrounded by two layers of Conv $1 \times 1 \times 1$. The output is then forwarded to another bottleneck block with a Conv $1 \times 1 \times 3$ in the middle and summed with itself before being forwarded to the next block. This anisotropic convolution block decomposes a 3D convolution into 2D and 1D convolutions. It receives the inputs from the previous layers using a 2D convolution at first, preserving the detailed 2D features. Conv $1 \times 1 \times 3$ mainly fuses the within-slice features to keep the z dimension output consistent.

Three anisotropic convolutional blocks are connected as the densely connected neural network [5] using feature concatenation for each resolution of encoded features. The features received from each resolution of the encoder are firstly projected to match the number of features of the higher encoder feature resolution using a Conv $1 \times 1 \times 1$. They are then upsampled using the 3D tri-linear interpolation and summed with the encoder features from a higher resolution. The summed features are forwarded to the decoder blocks in the next resolution.

At the end of the decoder network, we add a pyramid volumetric pooling module [13] to obtain multi-scaled features. The output features of the last decoder block are firstly down-sampled using 4 different Maxpooling layers, namely Max-Pool $64 \times 64 \times 1$, MaxPool $32 \times 32 \times 1$, MaxPool $16 \times 16 \times 1$ and MaxPool $8 \times 8 \times 1$ to obtain a feature map pyramid. Conv $1 \times 1 \times 1$ layers are used to project each resolution in the feature pyramid to a single response channel. The response channels are then interpolated to the original size and concatenated with the features before downsampling. The final outputs are obtained by applying a Conv $1 \times 1 \times 1$ projection layer on the concatenated features.

2.1 Training the AH-Net

Training the AH-Net using the same learning rate on both the pre-trained encoder and the randomly initialized decoder would make the network difficult to optimize. To train the 3D AH-Net, all the transferred parameters are locked at first. Only the decoder parameters are fine-tuned in the optimization. All the parameters can be then fine-tuned altogether afterwards to the entire AH-Net jointly. Though it is optional to unlock all the parameters for fine-tuning afterwards, we did not observe better performance. We use the scaled L2 loss for training the network for object detection tasks and the weighted cross entropy for segmentation tasks. We use ADAM [6] to optimise all the compared networks with $\beta_1 = 0.9$, $\beta_2 = 0.999$ and $\epsilon = 10^{-8}$. We use the initial learning-rate 0.0005 to fine-tune the 2D MC-GCN. Then, the learning rate is increased to 0.001 to fine-tune the AH-Net after the 2D network is transferred.

3 Experimental Results

To demonstrate the efficacy and efficiency of the proposed 3D AH-net, we conduct two experiments, namely lesion detection from a DBT volume and liver tumor segmentation from a CT volume. All the evaluated networks are implemented in Pytorch (https://github.com/pytorch).

3.1 Breast Lesion Detection from DBT

We use an in-house database containing 2809 3D DBT volumes acquired from 12 sites globally. The DBT volume has an anisotropic resolution of 0.085 mm × 0.085 × 1 mm. We have experienced radiologists annotate and validate the lesions in DBT volumes as 3D bounding boxes. To train the proposed networks for lesion detection, we generate 3D multi-variant Gaussian heatmaps based on the annotated 3D boxes that have the same sizes as the original images. We randomly split the database into the training set with 2678 volumes (1111 positives) and the testing sets with 131 volumes (58 positives). We ensure the images from the same patient could only be found either in the training or the testing set. For training, we extract 256×256×32 3D patches. 70% of the training patches are sampled as positives with at least one lesion included, considering the balance between the voxels within and without a breast lesion. The patches are sampled online asynchronously to form the mini-batches.

Along with the proposed networks, we also train 2D and 3D U-Nets with the identical architecture and parameters [2,11] as the two baselines. The 2D U-Net is also trained with input having three input channels. The 3D U-Net is trained with the same patch sampling strategies as the AH-Net. We measure the GPU inference time of networks by forwarding a 3D DBT volume of size 384 × 256 × 64 1000 times on an NVIDIA GTX 1080Ti GPU respectively. The GPU inference of the AH-Net (17.7 ms) is 43 times faster than that of the 2D MC-GCN (775.2 ms) though the AH-Net has more parameters. The speed gain could be achieved mostly by avoiding repetitive convolutions on the same slices required by multi-channel 2D networks.

By altering a threshold to filter the response values, we can control the balance between the False Positive Rate (FPR) and True Positive Rate (TPR). TPR represents the percentage of lesions that have been successfully detected by the network. FPR represents the percentage of lesions that the network predicted that are false positives. The lesion detected by the network is considered a true

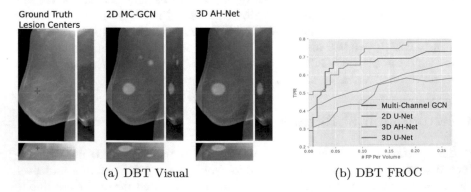

(a) DBT Visual   (b) DBT FROC

Fig. 2. Left: The visual comparisons of the network responses on a DBT volume from 2D MC-GCN and the 3D AH-Net with the encoder weights transferred from it. Right: FROC curves of the compared networks on the DBT dataset.

positive finding if the maximal point resides in a 3D bounding box annotated by the radiologist. Similarly, if a bounding box contains a maximal point, we consider it is detected by the network. They are otherwise considered as false positives. We evaluate the lesion detection performance by plotting the Free Response Operating Characteristic (FROC) curves as shown in Fig. 2(b). The proposed AH-Net outperforms both the 2D and 3D U-Net with large margins. Compared to the performance of the 2D MC-GCN, the 3D AH-Net generates higher TPR for a majority of thresholds, except the region around 0.05 per volume false positives. It is noticeable that AH-Net also obtains nearly 50% TPR even when only 0.01 false positive findings are allowed per volume.

3.2   Liver and Liver Tumor Segmentation from CT

The second evaluation dataset was obtained from the liver lesion segmentation challenge in MICCAI 2017 (lits-challenge.com), which contains 131 training and 70 testing 3D contrast-enhanced abdominal CT scans. The ground truth masks contain both liver and lesion labels. Most CT scans consist of anisotropic resolution: the between-slice resolution ranges from 0.45 mm to 6.0 mm while the within-slice resolution varies from 0.55 mm to 1.0 mm. In preprocessing, the abdominal regions are truncated from the CT scans using the liver center landmark detected by a reinforcement learning based algorithm [3]. Due to the limited number of training data, we applied random rotation (within $\pm 20°$ in the xy plane), random scaling (within $+0.2$ in all directions), and random mirror (within xy plane) to reduce overfitting.

The performance of the AH-Net is listed in Table 1, together with other top-ranked submissions retrieved from the LITS challenge leaderboard. These submissions employ various types of neural network architectures: 2D, 3D, 2D-3D hybrid, and model fusion. Two evaluation metrics are adapted: (1) Dice Global (DG) which is the dice score combining all the volumes into one; (2) Dice per Case (DPC) which averages the dice scores of every single case. The Dice score between two masks is defined as $DICE(A, B) = 2|A \cap B|/(|A| + |B|)$. Our results achieve state-of-the-art performance in three of the four metrics.

Table 1. The liver lesion segmentation (LITS) challenge results with the dice global (Dice-G) and dice per case (Dice-PC). The compared results were obtained from the LITS challenge leaderboard (lits-challenge.com/#results) before the paper submission.

Method	Lesion		Liver	
	Dice-G	Dice-PC	Dice-G	Dice-PC
leHealth	0.794	**0.702**	0.964	0.961
H-DenseNet [8]	0.829	0.686	0.965	0.961
deepX	0.820	0.657	0.967	**0.963**
MC-GCN	0.788	0.593	0.963	0.951
3D AH-Net	**0.834**	0.634	**0.970**	**0.963**

4   Conclusion

In this paper, we propose the 3D Anisotropic Hybrid Network (3D AH-Net) which is capable of transferring the convolutional features of 2D images to 3D volumes with anisotropic resolution. By evaluating the proposed methods on both a large-scale in-house DBT dataset and a highly competitive open challenge dataset of CT liver and lesion segmentation, we show our network obtains state-of-the-art results. The GPU inference of the AH-Net is also much faster than piling the results from a 2D network.

Disclaimer: This feature is based on research, and is not commercially available. Due to regulatory reasons, its future availability cannot be guaranteed.

References

1. Chen, J., Yang, L., Zhang, Y., Alber, M.S., Chen, D.Z.: Combining fully convolutional and recurrent neural networks for 3D biomedical image segmentation. In: NIPS (2016)
2. Çiçek, Ö., Abdulkadir, A., Lienkamp, S.S., Brox, T., Ronneberger, O.: 3D U-Net: Learning Dense Volumetric Segmentation from Sparse Annotation. ArXiv eprints arXiv:1606.06650 (2016)
3. Ghesu, F.C., Georgescu, B., Grbic, S., Maier, A.K., Hornegger, J., Comaniciu, D.: Robust multi-scale anatomical landmark detection in incomplete 3D-CT data. In: Descoteaux, M., Maier-Hein, L., Franz, A., Jannin, P., Collins, D.L., Duchesne, S. (eds.) MICCAI 2017. LNCS, vol. 10433, pp. 194–202. Springer, Cham (2017). https://doi.org/10.1007/978-3-319-66182-7_23
4. He, K., Zhang, X., Ren, S., Sun, J.: Deep residual learning for image recognition. In: Proceedings of CVPR, pp. 770–778 (2016)
5. Huang, G., Liu, Z., Weinberger, K.Q., van der Maaten, L.: Densely Connected Convolutional Networks. ArXiv eprints arXiv:1608.06993 (2016)
6. Kingma, D.P., Ba, J.: Adam: A Method for Stochastic Optimization. ArXiv eprints arXiv:1412.6980 (2014)
7. Lee, K., Zung, J., Li, P., Jain, V., Seung, H.S.: Superhuman Accuracy on the SNEMI3D Connectomics Challenge. ArXiv e-prints arXiv:1706.00120 (2017)
8. Li, X., Chen, H., Qi, X., Dou, Q., Fu, C.W., Heng, P.A.: H-DenseUNet: Hybrid Densely Connected UNet for Liver and Liver Tumor Segmentation from CT Volumes. ArXiv e-prints arXiv:1709.07330 (2017)
9. Liu, F., Zhou, Z., Jang, H., Samsonov, A., Zhao, G., Kijowski, R.: Deep convolutional neural network and 3D deformable approach for tissue segmentation in musculoskeletal MR imaging. Magn. Reson. Med. (2017)
10. Peng, C., Zhang, X., Yu, G., Luo, G., Sun, J.: Large Kernel Matters - Improve Semantic Segmentation by Global Convolutional Network. ArXiv eprints arXiv:1703.02719 (2017)
11. Ronneberger, O., Fischer, P., Brox, T.: U-Net: Convolutional Networks for Biomedical Image Segmentation. ArXiv eprints arXiv:1505.04597 (2015)
12. Russakovsky, O., et al.: ImageNet large scale visual recognition challenge. IJCV **115**(3), 211–252 (2015)
13. Zhao, H., Shi, J., Qi, X., Wang, X., Jia, J.: Pyramid Scene Parsing Network. ArXiv eprints arXiv:1612.01105 (2016)

Deep Generative Breast Cancer Screening and Diagnosis

Shayan Shams, Richard Platania, Jian Zhang, Joohyun Kim,
and Seung-Jong Park[✉]

Louisiana State University, Baton Rouge, USA
sjpark@cct.lsu.edu

Abstract. Mammography is the primary modality for breast cancer screening, attempting to reduce breast cancer mortality risk with early detection. However, robust screening less hampered by misdiagnoses remains a challenge. Deep Learning methods have shown strong applicability to various medical image datasets, primarily thanks to their powerful feature learning capability. Such successful applications are, however, often overshadowed with limitations in real medical settings, dependency of lesion annotations, and discrepancy of data types between training and other datasets. To address such critical challenges, we developed DiaGRAM (Deep GeneRAtive Multi-task), which is built upon the combination of Convolutional Neural Networks (CNN) and Generative Adversarial Networks (GAN). The enhanced feature learning with GAN, and its incorporation with the hybrid training with the region of interest (ROI) and the whole images results in higher classification performance and an effective end-to-end scheme. DiaGRAM is capable of robust prediction, even for a small dataset, without lesion annotation, via transfer learning capacity. DiaGRAM achieves an AUC of 88.4% for DDSM and even 92.5% for the challenging INbreast with its small data size.

1 Introduction

Breast cancer is the most common and fatal cancer among adult women [12]. According to the National Cancer Institute, approximately one in eight women will develop an invasive form of this cancer at some point in their lives [11]. Frequent screenings through mammograms can help detect early signs of breast cancer. However, certain challenges, such as false negatives, unnecessary biopsies, and low screening rate in some rural areas, overshadow the effectiveness of mammogram screening [8,9]. We believe deep learning aided software is a promising direction to achieve highly accurate screening, reducing the number of false negatives and unnecessary biopsies, while at the same time expanding screening capacity and coverage. Deep learning makes this possible by learning hidden features and correlations that might not be visible to humans [5]. Towards this goal, our work aims to provide an end-to-end deep learning system. There are several challenges that we need to overcome.

© Springer Nature Switzerland AG 2018
A. F. Frangi et al. (Eds.): MICCAI 2018, LNCS 11071, pp. 859–867, 2018.
https://doi.org/10.1007/978-3-030-00934-2_95

Firstly, limited training data makes it difficult to achieve highly accurate diagnosis. Secondly, not all data have lesion annotations because making the annotations is a very expensive and time consuming task. Therefore, developing an accurate model that can conduct inference on whole images without annotation is very important. Lastly, it is desirable that models should be robust and adaptable to heterogeneous datasets.

To address these challenges, we propose DiaGRAM (Deep GeneRAtive Multi-task), an end-to-end system that combines a Generative Adversarial Networks (GANs) [4] with discriminative learning using a multi-task learning strategy, to enhance classification performance when training data is limited. We also employ transfer learning to adapt a model trained with one type of data to another.

Generative Adversarial Networks (GANs) are often used to produce data when the analytic form of the data distribution is hard to obtain. Instead of using GAN as a data augmenting device, we use GAN to enhance feature learning. Insights from deep learning show us that features that capture the characteristics of the data, that are learned without label information by unsupervised methods, can still be helpful for discriminative tasks such as classification. For example, stacked autoencoders or deep belief network (DBN) can be used to pre-train the weights of a discriminative model in an unsupervised fashion, then fine-tune the model using the label information. DiaGRAM's design follows this insight with some modification. Rather than taking a two-stage process, DiaGRAM is end-to-end. It extracts features that are good both for the discriminative tasks (i.e., patch and image classification) and for the GAN's generative task (i.e., differentiate the real patches from the generated ones). The latter task ensures that the learned features capture the data characteristics, and thus can help classification, in a way similar to pre-training by autoencoders or DBNs.

Previously, there have been several works related to applying deep learning towards mammogram classification [1–3, 10, 13, 14]. Most of these works focus on either mass segmentation, detection, or classification. A recent survey regarding deep learning in medical imaging analysis mentioned the lack of GAN-based approaches, pointing out the absence of any peer-reviewed papers regarding this subject [7]. Our proposed framework, DiaGRAM, is capable of both mass and whole image classification and inherently agonistic for the mentioned above challenges and thus allows an end-to-end solution for breast cancer screening and diagnosis purposes.

2   Methods

2.1   Model Overview

Figure 1(a) shows our model architecture which consists of four components: generator network, feature extraction network, discriminator network, and extended classification network. The feature extraction network and the extended classification network form a path for mammogram classification. The generator network, the feature extraction network, and the discriminator network form a GAN. (Note that the "discriminator" of the original GAN paper [4] corresponds to the combination of both our feature extraction network and our discriminator). The main novel feature of our model is that it fuses, using a multi-task learning strategy, part of the image classification path with part of the GAN path to extract features that can help both tasks.

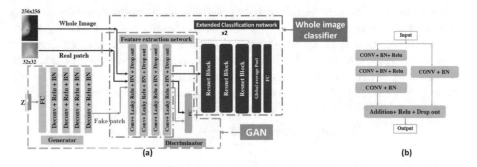

Fig. 1. (a) DiaGRAM architecture (b) Residual block in DiaGRAM

2.2   GAN-Enhanced Deep Classification

Two types of images are considered in our model. One is the whole mammogram images and the other is patches from mammograms. Let $\{(\mathbf{I}_i, \mathbf{t}_i)\}_{i=1}^{N}$ be a collection of N mammogram images ($\mathbf{I}_i$) and their labels ($\mathbf{t}_i$). Some mammogram datasets (such as DDSM) include regions of interest (ROI) on the image. These regions of interest serve as image patches in our learning. Since ROIs may differ in size, we resize them to the same size, $s \times s$. We denote by $\{(\mathbf{C}_j, \mathbf{t}_j)\}_{j=1}^{M}$ a set of M patch images and their labels. In both cases, the label $\mathbf{t}_i$ is an indicator vector (i.e., if the i-th image belongs to class k, the k-th entry of the corresponding label vector has value 1 ($\mathbf{t}_i^{(k)} = 1$) and all other entries have value 0). We describe the components of our model in the following:

Generator: The generator is a deep neural network that takes as input a random vector and produces an image patch. It comprises of one fully connected and four deconvolution layers. We denote by $\mathcal{G}$ the generator network and $\boldsymbol{\theta}_g$ its parameters. Let $\mathbf{z} \in \mathbb{R}^n$ be a random vector whose entries are drawn uniformly in the range $[-1, 1]$. Also, let $\mathcal{G}(\mathbf{z}; \boldsymbol{\theta}_g) \in \mathbb{R}^{s \times s}$ be the size ($s \times s$) image patch generated. For a set of random vectors $\{\mathbf{z}_1, \mathbf{z}_2, \ldots, \mathbf{z}_M\}$, the generator can produce a set of patches $\{\mathcal{G}(\mathbf{z}_1; \boldsymbol{\theta}_g), \mathcal{G}(\mathbf{z}_2; \boldsymbol{\theta}_g), \ldots, \mathcal{G}(\mathbf{z}_M; \boldsymbol{\theta}_g)\}$.

Feature Extraction Network: The purpose of the feature extraction network is to discover features that may be present in both a patch and a whole mammogram image and that can be useful in the classification of both. This is the common component between the GAN and the image classifiers. We employ a four-layered CNN as the feature extraction network. We denote by $\mathcal{F}$ the feature extraction network and $\boldsymbol{\theta}_f$ its parameters. Given an input x, we denote by $\mathcal{F}(x; \boldsymbol{\theta}_f)$ the output (features maps) from the network. The feature extraction network may take an image $\mathbf{I}$ as input and give output $\mathcal{F}(\mathbf{I}; \boldsymbol{\theta}_f)$, or it may take a patch $\mathbf{C}$ (or generated patch $\mathcal{G}(\mathbf{z})$) as input and give output $\mathcal{F}(\mathbf{C}; \boldsymbol{\theta}_f)$ (or $\mathcal{F}(\mathcal{G}(\mathbf{z}); \boldsymbol{\theta}_f)$). Note that since $\mathbf{C}$ and $\mathcal{G}(\mathbf{z})$ are of the same size, the feature maps of $\mathcal{F}(\mathbf{C}; \boldsymbol{\theta}_f)$ and $\mathcal{F}(\mathcal{G}(\mathbf{z}); \boldsymbol{\theta}_f)$ have the same size, whereas the feature maps of $\mathcal{F}(\mathbf{I}; \boldsymbol{\theta}_f)$ have a size different from them.

Discriminator: The discriminator network takes features produced by the feature extraction network and performs patch classification. It consists of a single fully connected layer that has $m+1$ neurons, where m is the number of classes in the patch images. We denote by $\mathcal{D}$ the network and $\boldsymbol{\theta}_d$ its parameters. The first m neurons of $\mathcal{D}$ are softmax units. Given a patch $\mathbf{C}$, the output from the i-th neuron $(\mathcal{D}^{(i)}(\mathcal{F}(\mathbf{C}; \boldsymbol{\theta}_f); \boldsymbol{\theta}_d))$ computes the probability that the patch belongs to class i. Let y be the variable for the patch's label. We have:

$$P(y = i|\mathbf{C}) = \mathcal{D}^{(i)}(\mathcal{F}(\mathbf{C}; \boldsymbol{\theta}_f); \boldsymbol{\theta}_d). \tag{1}$$

The $(m+1)$-th neuron is a sigmoid neuron and computes the probability that a patch is from a real image (not generated). We denote its output by $\mathcal{D}^{(m+1)}(\mathcal{F}(x; \boldsymbol{\theta}_f); \boldsymbol{\theta}_d)$ and have:

$$P(r = 1|x) = \mathcal{D}^{(m+1)}(\mathcal{F}(x; \boldsymbol{\theta}_f); \boldsymbol{\theta}_d) \tag{2}$$

where x is a patch (real or generated) and r is the variable that takes value 1 if the patch is from a real image and 0 otherwise.

Extended Classification Network: Features produced by the feature extraction network are local features from a small region. Deep CNNs often contain many layers and neurons in higher layers that respond to larger-size features that are constructed from small-size features reacted to by lower layer neurons. We follow the same idea, taking the feature maps produced by the feature extraction network and passing them through more layers of the CNN before the final classification. We call the additional layers the extended classification network. It consists of six Residual network blocks [6] and an output layer that gives the class probability. We denote by $\mathcal{E}$ the extended classification network and by $\boldsymbol{\theta}_e$ its parameters. For a whole image $\mathbf{I}$, the i-th output of $\mathcal{E}$ is the probability that the image belongs to the i-th class:

$$P(y = i|\mathbf{I}) = \mathcal{E}^{(i)}(\mathcal{F}(\mathbf{I}; \boldsymbol{\theta}_f); \boldsymbol{\theta}_e) \tag{3}$$

2.3   Training

Our model combines multiple network components together for better feature extraction and classification. To train the model, we employ multiple loss functions. Given a random vector $\mathbf{z}$, the generator loss is:

$$\mathcal{L}_g(\mathbf{z}) = -log P(r = 1|\mathcal{G}(\mathbf{z}; \boldsymbol{\theta}_g)) \tag{4}$$

Our discriminator performs two tasks and thus involves two losses: the loss for distinguishing the real patches from the generated ones and the loss for patch classification. Given a patch $\mathbf{C}$ and a random vector $\mathbf{z}$, the loss for distinguishing the real from the generated is:

$$\mathcal{L}_d(\mathbf{C}, \mathbf{z}) = -\big[\log P(r = 1|\mathbf{C}) + \log P(r = 0|\mathcal{G}(\mathbf{z}; \boldsymbol{\theta}_g))\big]. \tag{5}$$

For patch classification, we use the cross-entropy loss. Given a patch $\mathbf{C}$ and its label indicator vector $\mathbf{t}$, the loss is as follows:

$$\mathcal{L}_c(\mathbf{C}, \mathbf{t}) = -\sum_k \mathbf{t}^{(k)} \log P(y = k|\mathbf{C}) \tag{6}$$

Finally the cross-entropy loss for whole image classification, given an image $\mathbf{I}$ and its label indicator vector $\mathbf{t}$, is:

$$\mathcal{L}_i(\mathbf{I}, \mathbf{t}) = -\sum_k \mathbf{t}^{(k)} \log P(y = k|\mathbf{I}) \tag{7}$$

The overall training process is presented in Algorithm 1. During a training iteration, we update the parameters of the model components using stochastic gradient descending on the related losses.

Algorithm 1. Training algorithm

---

for number of training iterations **do**
    for k *steps* **do**
        $S_C \leftarrow$ *Sample a minibatch of m patches*
        $S_I \leftarrow$ *Sample a minibatch of n images*
        $S_z \leftarrow$ *Sample a minibatch of m random vectors*
        Update the feature extract network and the discriminator by descending on their parameter gradients:

$$\nabla_{(\boldsymbol{\theta}_f, \boldsymbol{\theta}_d)} \frac{1}{m} \bigg(\sum_{\mathbf{C} \in S_C, \mathbf{z} \in S_z} \mathcal{L}_d(\mathbf{C}, \mathbf{z}) + \sum_{(\mathbf{C},\mathbf{t}) \in S_C} \mathcal{L}_c(\mathbf{C}, \mathbf{t}) \bigg)$$

        Update the feature extract network and the extended classifier by descending on their parameter gradients:

$$\nabla_{(\boldsymbol{\theta}_f, \boldsymbol{\theta}_e)} \frac{1}{n} \sum_{(\mathbf{I},\mathbf{t}) \in S_I} \mathcal{L}_i(\mathbf{I}, \mathbf{t})$$

    end for
    $S_z \leftarrow$ *Sample a minibatch of m random vectors*
    Update the generator by descending on its parameter gradient:

$$\nabla_{\boldsymbol{\theta}_g} \frac{1}{m} \sum_{\mathbf{z} \in S_z} \mathcal{L}_g(\mathbf{z})$$

end for

2.4   Transfer Learning

Digital mammography has been widely adopted in modern hospitals, providing a clearer image in comparison with the film mammography of the past. For example, INbreast is a digital mammography dataset. To build an accurate model for small-size datasets such as INbreast, we utilize transfer learning. We train a DiaGRAM model using a larger dataset with region annotations (DDSM). Then, we take out the classification path (the feature extraction and the extended classification networks) from the model, fine-tune it in a supervised mode with INbreast training data, and use it as a classifier for INBreast data.

3   Experiments and Results

In this section, we present the experimental results of DiaGRAM for the DDSM and INbreast datasets and discuss the benefit of combining the GAN with discriminative learning using a multi-task learning strategy. For fair comparisons, we use 5-fold cross validation to evaluate DiaGRAM. The reported AUC is the result from 5-fold cross validation.

Since the DDSM dataset is used for multi-task learning, we use annotated lesion and whole mammogram images, which are 3,500 images in total, divided into cancer and benign. We utilize several common data augmentation methods to reduce over-fitting and improve overall accuracy. For instance, we rotate and mirror images across the y-axis randomly. We use the overlay files to extract the region of interests, which have various shapes. We crop the smallest possible square that can fully contain a ROI and resize it to 32×32. Thus, we generate 25,000 cropped images of ROIs. For the INbreast dataset, we convert BI-RADS 4, 5, and 6 to cancerous samples and 1 and 2 to negative samples. Since it is not clear that BI-RADS 3 samples are benign or cancerous, we exclude 23 mammograms, which were labeled as BI-RADS 3.

Since the INbreast dataset is not large enough to train a model from scratch, we use transfer learning, which is explained in Sect. 2.4, and fine-tune DiaGRAM

Table 1. Comparison with other works for whole image classification.

Paper	End-to-end	Dataset	Accuracy	AUC
Ball and Bruce [1]	✗	DDSM	87%	N/A
Varela et al. [13]	✗	DDSM	81%	N/A
Domingues et al. [3]	✗	INbreast	89%	N/A
Dhungel et al. [2]	✗	INbreast	$(95 \pm 5)\%$	(91 ± 12)
Dhungel et al. [2]	✓	INbreast	$(91 \pm 2)\%$	(76 ± 23)
Zhu et al. [14]	✓	INbreast	$(90 \pm 2)\%$	$(89 \pm 4)\%$
DiaGRAM	✓	DDSM	$89 \pm 3.4\%$	$88.4 \pm 2.9\%$
	✓	INbreast	$93.5 \pm 2.9\%$	$92.5 \pm 2.4\%$

for 20 epochs using the dataset. In Table 1, the best results of previous works using DDSM or INbreast are reported. DiaGRAM achieves a mean AUC of 92.5% and 88.4% for INbreast and DDSM datasets, respectively, and provides superior AUC and accuracy over other previous works for both datasets. ROC curves for both datasets are plotted in Fig. 2.

3.1   Performance Enhanced by GAN

To investigate whether the GAN is effective in enhancing classification performance, we created a model variant that does not include GAN and compare the performance of DiaGRAM to that of the variant. The variant without GAN contains the feature extraction network, the discriminator (without the neuron that outputs the probability whether a patch is real or generated), and the extended classification network. It performs two tasks: patch classification (combining the feature extraction network and the discriminator) and whole image classification (combining the feature extraction network and the extended classification network). The variant was trained in a multi-task learning fashion using the losses in Eqs. 6 and 7.

As shown in Fig. 3, the model variant without GAN suffered a drop of 2.9% on AUC (85.5% compared to DiaGRAM's 88.4%) for the DDSM dataset. This indicates that having the GAN in the model indeed contributes to the model's high performance. It demonstrates that the task of discriminating fake data from real data can be leveraged to learn latent and hidden features that will improve classification performance.

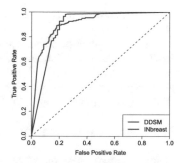

Fig. 2. ROC curves for DDSM and INbreast.

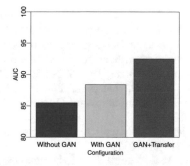

Fig. 3. AUC for different configurations.

4   Conclusion

In this work, we introduced DiaGRAM (Deep GeneRAtive Multi-task), an end-to-end deep learning solution for breast cancer screening and diagnosis purposes. DiaGRAM employs two main approaches to achieve highly accurate mammogram diagnosis: (1) it combines a GAN with a deep classifier to learn features that benefit both, (2) and transfer learning is used to adapt the model trained with one type of data to another. We conducted a set of experiments using the DDSM and the INbreast datasets. The results showed better performance of DiaGRAM on both the accuracy and the AUC measures when compared to prior works. DiaGRAM also demonstrated transfer learning capacity as the model trained on DDSM dataset and adapted to the INbreast dataset showed good performance. In future works, we plan to extend the techniques used in this paper for real medical settings, focusing on usabilities for screening and diagnosis procedure.

Acknowledgments. This work was partially funded by NIH grants (P20GM103458-10, P30GM110760-03, P20GM103424), NSF grants (MRI-1338051, IBSS-L-1620451, SCC-1737557, RAPID-1762600), LA Board of Regents grants (LEQSF(2016-19)-RD-A-08 and ITRS), and IBM faculty awards.

References

1. Ball, J.E., Bruce, L.M.: Digital mammographic computer aided diagnosis (CAD) using adaptive level set segmentation. In: 2007 29th Annual International Conference of the IEEE Engineering in Medicine and Biology Society, EMBS 2007, pp. 4973–4978. IEEE (2007)
2. Dhungel, N., Carneiro, G., Bradley, A.P.: The automated learning of deep features for breast mass classification from mammograms. In: Ourselin, S., Joskowicz, L., Sabuncu, M.R., Unal, G., Wells, W. (eds.) MICCAI 2016. LNCS, vol. 9901, pp. 106–114. Springer, Cham (2016). https://doi.org/10.1007/978-3-319-46723-8_13
3. Domingues, I., et al.: Inbreast-database masses characterization. XXIII CBEB (2012)
4. Goodfellow, I., et al.: Generative adversarial nets. In: Advances in Neural Information Processing Systems, pp. 2672–2680 (2014)
5. He, K., et al.: Delving deep into rectifiers: surpassing human-level performance on imagenet classification. In: Proceedings of the IEEE International Conference on Computer Vision, pp. 1026–1034 (2015)
6. He, K., et al.: Deep residual learning for image recognition. In: Proceedings of the IEEE Conference on Computer Vision and Pattern Recognition, pp. 770–778 (2016)
7. Litjens, G.: A survey on deep learning in medical image analysis. Med. Image Anal. **42**, 60–88 (2017)
8. Ong, M.S., Mandl, K.D.: National expenditure for false-positive mammograms and breast cancer overdiagnoses estimated at $4 billion a year. Health Aff. **34**(4), 576–583 (2015)
9. Orwat, J.: Comparing rural and urban cervical and breast cancer screening rates in a privately insured population. Soc. Work Publ. Health **32**(5), 311–323 (2017)
10. Platania, R., et al.: Automated breast cancer diagnosis using deep learning and region of interest detection (BC-DROID). In: Proceedings of the 8th ACM International Conference on Bioinformatics, Computational Biology, and Health Informatics, pp. 536–543. ACM (2017)
11. Siegel, R.: Cancer statistics, 2014. CA Cancer J. Clin. **64**(1), 9–29 (2014)
12. Teh, Y.C.: Opportunistic mammography screening provides effective detection rates in a limited resource healthcare system. BMC Cancer **15**(1), 405 (2015)

13. Varela, C.: Use of border information in the classification of mammographic masses. Physics Med. Biol. **51**(2), 425 (2006)

14. Zhu, W., Lou, Q., Vang, Y.S., Xie, X.: Deep multi-instance networks with sparse label assignment for whole mammogram classification. In: Descoteaux, M., Maier-Hein, L., Franz, A., Jannin, P., Collins, D.L., Duchesne, S. (eds.) MICCAI 2017. LNCS, vol. 10435, pp. 603–611. Springer, Cham (2017). https://doi.org/10.1007/978-3-319-66179-7_69

Integrate Domain Knowledge in Training CNN for Ultrasonography Breast Cancer Diagnosis

Jiali Liu[1,2], Wanyu Li[3], Ningbo Zhao[4], Kunlin Cao[3(✉)],
Youbing Yin[3(✉)], Qi Song[3], Hanbo Chen[3], and Xuehao Gong[1,2(✉)]

[1] Shenzhen Second People's Hospital, Shenzhen, Guangdong, China
fox_gxh@sina.com
[2] Anhui Medical University, Heifei, Anhui, China
[3] Shenzhen Keya Medical Technology Corporation,
Shenzhen, Guangdong, China
{cao,yin}@keyayun.com
[4] The Third People's Hospital of Shenzhen, Shenzhen, Guangdong, China

Abstract. Breast cancer is the most common cancer in women, and ultrasound imaging is one of the most widely used approach for diagnosis. In this paper, we proposed to adopt Convolutional Neural Network (CNN) to classify ultrasound images and predict tumor malignancy. CNN is a successful algorithm for image recognition tasks and has achieved human-level performance in real applications. To improve the performance of CNN in breast cancer diagnosis, we integrated domain knowledge and conducted multi-task learning in the training process. After training, a radiologist visually inspected the class activation map of the last convolutional layer of trained network to evaluate the result. Our result showed that CNN classifier can not only give reasonable performance in predicting breast cancer, but also propose potential lesion regions which can be integrated into the breast ultrasound system in the future.

Keywords: Breast cancer · Ultrasound · BI-RADS assessments
Convolutional neural network · Multi-task learning

1 Introduction

Breast cancer is the most common cancer in women. According to statistics in 2013, breast cancer caused approximately 8.2–14.94 million death worldwide [2]. The corresponding morbidity rate is 15.1%, while the death rate is about 6.9%. Detection and diagnosis in the early stage are essential for its treatment, which could improve survival rate. One of the most efficient diagnostic methods is mammographic screening. However, mammographic sensitivity can be relatively low in dense breasts (less than 50%) [2], which may lead to unnecessary breast biopsies (65–85%) [3]. Whereas, with the interpretation of skilled radiologists, ultrasonography presents a higher accuracy in distinguishing benign breast lumps from malignant tumors. A US population study has

---

J. Liu and W. Li — Have equal contribution.

© Springer Nature Switzerland AG 2018
A. F. Frangi et al. (Eds.): MICCAI 2018, LNCS 11071, pp. 868–875, 2018.
https://doi.org/10.1007/978-3-030-00934-2_96

demonstrated that by using brightness mode ultrasound, the overall sensitivity could reach 97.2% (281 of 289). The specificity can achieve 61.1% (397 of 650) and the accuracy could be 72.2% (678 of 939) [4]. In addition, ultrasound is radiation free, easily accessible, economical and convenient in practice. Therefore, ultrasonography has gradually become an alternative to mammography in clinical diagnosis of breast cancer.

The Breast Imaging Reporting and Data System (BI-RADS) [5] offered standardized terminology to depict features, and to provide assessments as well as recommendations. Features including shape, orientation, margin, echo pattern, and posterior features of masses are compiled in the BI-RADS lexicon for ultrasound. Based on the particular features of the lesion, radiologists would recommend one BI-RADS category (Table 1). Radiologists would finally issue a clinical recommendation according to these categories, which suggested an annual examination for categories 1 and 2, an extra test six months later for category 3, and a biopsy for categories 4, 5 and 6 [6]. But the image-based diagnosis was dependent on practitioners' experience and thus relatively subjective. A computer aided diagnosis system is of great demands to resolve this issue.

Table 1. Table of BI-RADS categories and the number of images acquired for each category

BI-RADS	Description	# of images	# of patients
1	Negative finding	1016	243
2	Benign	54	47
3	Probably benign	55	27
4a	Low suspicion	352	139
4c	Moderate suspicion	61	31
5	Highly suggestive of malignancy	205	99
6	Known Biopsy-Proven malignancy	190	35

Thanks to the emerging deep learning technique such as convolutional neural network (CNN) [7], computer aided automatic detection system can now achieve comparable or even better performance than radiologists in detecting lesion or diagnosing medical conditions from image data. For instance, with CNN, computers achieved 90% sensitivity and 85% specificity in predicting brain hemorrhage, mass effect, or hydrocephalus from CT images [8], successfully predicted diabetic retinopathy patients among 11711 retinal fundus photographs with 96% sensitivity and 93% specificity [9], or even can diagnose skin cancer with only photos taken by smartphone [10]. In previous works, based on CNN, breast cancer diagnosis systems have also been proposed to classify breast cancer in mammogram images [11] or segment breast tumor regions in histopathological images [12]. Thus, this paper seeks feasibility of utilizing CNN to predict breast cancer in ultrasound images into one of the three malignancy categories: malignant tumor, benign lump, or normal tissue. We adopted BIRADS categories as a "domain knowledge" to improve the classification of ultrasound images. Specifically, two different classifiers have been proposed. One directly classifies the malignancy and the other one simultaneously predicts BI-RADS category. By this means, BIRADS categories, which can be interpreted as doctors' visual interpretation of image features, can guide the training of image features obtained by CNN to improve the performance of malignancy claasification. The performance of each classifier and the cause of failures were then examined in details. We will show that CNN classifier can not only give reasonable performance in predicting breast cancer but also propose potential lesion regions.

2 Method

2.1 Data Acquisition

We retrospectively collected 1933 breast ultrasound images from 608 patients. Eligibility criteria excluded patients who received breast implants or surgeries on the ipsilateral breast, and those who were pregnant or breastfeeding. All images were reviewed by experienced radiologists and BI-RADS assessments [5] were recorded (Table 1). Based on BI-RADS categories, images were then classified as malignant tumor (BI-RADS categories 5, 6, and part of 4), benign lump (BI-RADS categories 2, 3 and part of 4), and normal tissue (BI-RADS category 1). Since radiologists cannot directly verify the malignancy of lumps classified as BI-RADS category 4 with ultrasound images, a pathological test was conducted by ultrasound-guided core needle biopsy (CNB) or a surgery following the clinical procedures to confirm the malignancy. In total, 96 BI-RADS category 4 images were classified as malignant. To summary, among the images acquired, 491 show malignant tumor, 426 show benign lump, and 1016 are normal tissues.

2.2 Image Preprocessing

After collecting data, we pre-processed the data following the steps below:

Cropping Images. The ultrasound images collected had uninformative parts, such as screen background, acquisition parameters and hospital name. Since these are not helpful and may even introduce bias, we manually cropped all the images to remove them. In addition, since the shape of ultrasound images may vary across devices and imaging settings – some are in horizontal rectangle while others are in vertical rectangle shape, we cropped the images into square shape for the training convenience. This may remove useful information in the image. To avoid that, we ensured to keep the complete lump which is critical for the prediction, and the skin tissues whose contrast is more accurate than deep tissues and more uniform across devices.

Removing Makers: In some ultrasound images radiologists left markers to indicate or quantify tumor position (e.g. cross symbol, rectangle box, dash line). These markers, colorized or black-and-white, may introduce bias to the training of classifier. For instance, classifier may likely take cross symbols as a tumor indicator since no such symbols appear on normal tissues. Hence, we adopted a semi-automatic approach to clean those symbols. Considering that the ultrasound images we collected are in gray color, we first detected all the colored or pure black-or-white pixels in the image as a mask of potential markers. The mask was reviewed and cleaned manually with in-house image annotation tools. Then, the masked pixels were restored by linear inter-polation with the surrounding pixels. All images were reviewed after processing to ensure that no obvious artifacts were left and the failed ones were excluded.

2.3   Training Multi-task CNN

We adopted the convolutional layers in VGG16 [7] to extract image features for the classifier. VGG16 contains 13 convolutional layers and 5 max pooling layers. It is a well-established CNN classifier for image recognition tasks and has been utilized in many applications. Though there are other deeper and more advanced CNN classifiers, we decided to choose VGG16 to avoid potential overfitting issues considering the limited training data in our experiments. Following this philosophy, a dense layer that is small than the original VGG16 network was cascaded after flattened convolutional layers (Fig. 1).

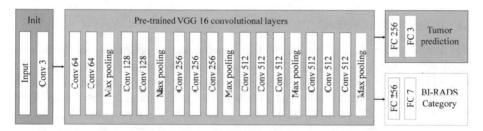

Fig. 1. Illustration of the multi-task CNN applied. The numbers of hidden units/convolutional kernels applied in each layer were shown in the figure.

When training the classifier, we applied the weights pre-trained based on ImageNet database as the initial weights. Notably, since our ultrasound images are monochrome but pre-trained VGG16 network takes colorful images with 3 channels as input, we need to first convert the monochrome image to colorful images. One typical approach that is widely used by others is to use the same image in all 3 channels. However, in our view, the redundant information introduced in those approaches does not fully embrace the power of CNN. Instead, we inserted a convolutional layer with three 3×3 kernels between the input layer and VGG16 convolution layers. This layer will be trained to convert input monochrome images into the three channel images that best fits the pre-trained VGG16 network.

In our baseline method, the network proposed above only classified the image into 3 classes: malignant tumor, benign lump, and normal tissue. We wondered if the per-formance of this task can be further improved by introducing clinical domain knowledge into the training process. Thus, when training the network, another logistic regression classifier was appended after the convolution layers to classify the image into the BI-RADS categories (Fig. 1). Though this might add an extra burden to the network and BI-RADS categories are highly coupled with tumor prediction, our rationale of this design is as follows: (1) BI-RADS assessment is based on professionals' visual inspection of the image features. It might help guide the training of the tumor related features. (2) BI-RADS categories are finer than the 3 maliginacy classes we want to predict and thus may offer better guidance. (3) Additional burden in the training process may help to reduce the chance of overfitting.

3   Results

In our experiments, data was evenly split into five folds. Since multiple ultrasound images may be acquired for each patient, we ensured that the images from the same patient will be assigned to the same fold. Also, we tried to keep the distribution of each class as the same as possible in each fold. To fully utilized the data to examine our proposed method, the training process follows cross-validation training scheme – each time take four folds as training set and test on the rest fold. Five independent trainings and testings were conducted on both the baseline network and the multi-task network.

3.1   Classification Result

We combined the testing results of five independent experiments and conducted quantitative analyses accordingly. Table 2 shows the number of images in each category. Though the result is not perfect, both classifiers worked reasonably well in classifying images. With the baseline method, the prediction accuracy is 82.9%. By using the multi-task network, the prediction accuracy slightly increased to 83.3%. Notably, both methods have high sensitivity in differentiating abnormal cases from normal ones (baseline: 95%, multi-task: 96.7%). The major error comes from separating malignant tumors and benign lumps. For the proposed multi-task approach, only 74.3% malignant (baseline: 71.9%) tumors were correctly classified. This is reasonable since the malignancy level of BI-RADS category 4 tumor is also difficult for experts to tell based on an ultrasound image only. About half of the errors between malignant tumor and benign lump prediction happened in BI-RADS category 4 images (baseline: 57.5%, multi-task: 54.9%). Overall, despite the reduced sensitivity in predicting normal tissues (baseline: 93.7%, multi-task: 91.2%), better performance has been achieved by the proposed multi-task approach.

Table 2. Number of images in each category. Table on the top shows the result from the baseline method. Table on the bottom shows the result of the multi-task network.

Baseline	Predict malignant	Predict benign	Predict normal
Truth malignant	353	101	37
Truth benign	120	298	8
Truth normal	20	44	952
Multi-task	Predict malignant	Predict benign	Predict normal
Truth malignant	365	101	25
Truth benign	103	318	5
Truth normal	30	59	927

3.2 Examples of Correct and Wrong Predictions

To further examine the performance of each classifier and understand why this classification task is challenging, we selected some example images. In order to understand what happened inside the CNN classifier, class activation map (CAM) of the last convolutional layer was visualized [13]. CAM is a heat map highlights the attention of a classifier when making the decision and thus can reveal the regions associated with the prediction. Specifically, two groups of examples were selected and shown. (1) The tumors/lumps correctly predicted by the multi-task method only and the normal tissues correctly predicted by the baseline method only were shown (Fig. 2). (2) A considerable number of images were wrongly classified by both methods, examples of those images were shown (Fig. 3). The images and the corresponding CAM were examined by experienced radiologists.

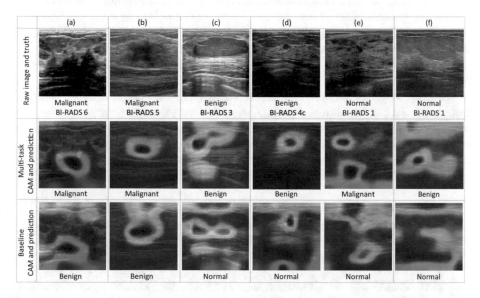

Fig. 2. Examples of images that were correctly predicted by one method only. Red color highlights the activation region associated with the class predicted by the classifier.

As shown in Fig. 2a–d, when the classification is correct, CAM accurately highlighted the malignant masses (Fig. 2a–b) and benign lumps (Fig. 2c–d). When the baseline method wrongly classified malignant tumors as benign, the network pays attention to both CAM area as well as the adjacent normal tissues. As for the normal cases which were correctly predicted by the baseline only, the attention is on the normal shallow skin tissues while the multi-task method wrongly regarded the decay resulted from deep location or dense superficial tissues and some cellulite that extended into the glandular layer as masses (Fig. 2e–f).

As for the cases failed by both methods, some of them belongs to BI-RADS category 4, which is also difficult for radiologists to decide and requires pathological verifications (Fig. 3b–c). Nevertheless, for these cases, CAM still accurately highlighted lumps in the image. Figure 3d was predicted as normal tissues due to the tiny volume of the mass. Some radiologists may consider it as normal ducts while others may think of cysts. The interpretation on this kind of images is relatively subjective, and the lesion has little impact on patients. In Fig. 3e, a malignant label was given to normal tissues, as the area was a centralized point of mammary ducts and thus was difficult to be distinguished from lesions even by senior doctors, if the location is unclear. Another misdiagnosis example was Fig. 3f, in which normal tissues were deemed as benign lumps. The interpretation identified the cellulite as a hypoechoic mass. It was difficult to tell the exact nature of this mass, since ultrasound radiologists also depended on whether the mass continued with normal tissues to determine its character. Due to the complex structures of breasts, such as the cellulite penetrating into the glands, the collection of vasa efferentia under the nipples, the common features of benign and malignant lumps, together with the different features of each section, it is difficult to determine the relationship between lumps and its surrounding tissues, as well as its overall situation. More complete patient-based videos might be required to obtain better results.

Notably, in our preliminary results, we found some intriguing malignant cases that were classified as normal (e.g. Fig. 3a). After reviewing the cases, we found that some of them came from the patients which were diagnosed as cancer. But the tumor was not captured in the image and the tissues shown in the image are normal findings. Those cases were eliminated with a second review. This also suggests that CNN is a powerful tool to learn the generalized pattern even when there are noises in the training data.

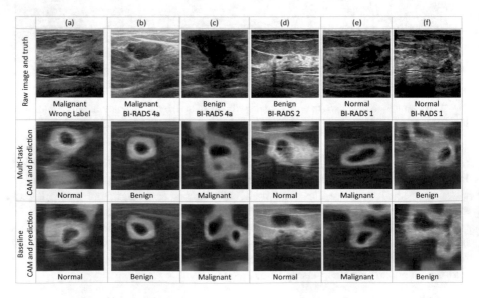

Fig. 3. Examples of images that were wrongly predicted by both methods. Red color highlights the activation region associated with the class predicted by the classifier.

4   Conclusion

In this paper, we adopted CNN to predict breast tumors in ultrasound images. Domain knowledge was integrated into the training process. Promising results were obtained in separating images with lump and normal findings. Moreover, though this is not a segmentation task, the activation map of the trained classifier can still correctly highlight the mass regions in images. In addition, reasonable results were also obtained in differentiating malignant tumors and benign lumps. In the future, more data will be collected to fine-tune the network. And the system will be extended to process video data for better classification and prediction of the tumor malignancy. The correlation between BI-RADS categories and the classification results will be then investigated such that the whole system can be integrated into current breast cancer diagnosis procedure.

Acknowledgement. The work received supports from Shenzhen Municipal Government under the grants JCYJ20170413161913429 and KQTD2016112809330877.

References

1. Fitzmaurice, C., et al.: The global burden of cancer 2013. JAMA Oncol. **1**(4), 505 (2015)
2. Kolb, T.M., Lichy, J., Newhouse, J.H.: Comparison of the performance of screening mammography, physical examination, and breast US and evaluation of factors that influence them: an analysis of 27,825 patient evaluations. Radiology **225**(1), 165 (2002)
3. Jesneck, J.L., Lo, J.Y., Baker, J.A.: Breast mass lesions: computer-aided diagnosis models with mammographic and sonographic descriptors. Radiology **244**(2), 390 (2007)
4. Berg, W.A., et al.: Shear-wave elastography improves the specificity of breast US: the BE1 multinational study of 939 masses. Int. J. Med. Radiol. **262**(2), 435 (2012)
5. Mendelson, E., et al.: Breast imaging reporting and data system, BI-RADS: ultrasound (2003)
6. D'Orsi, C., et al.: ACR BI-RADS® Atlas, Breast Imaging Reporting and Data System (2013)
7. Simonyan, K., Zisserman, A.: Very Deep Convolutional Networks for Large-Scale Image Recognition. arXiv:1409.1556 (2014)
8. Prevedello, L.M., et al.: Automated critical test findings identification and online notification system using artificial intelligence in imaging. Radiology **285**(3), 162664 (2017)
9. Gulshan, V., et al.: Development and validation of a deep learning algorithm for detection of diabetic retinopathy in retinal fundus photographs. JAMA **316**(22), 2402 (2016)
10. Esteva, A., et al.: Corrigendum: dermatologist-level classification of skin cancer with deep neural networks. Nature **542**(7639), 115 (2017)
11. Sun, W., et al.: Enhancing deep convolutional neural network scheme for breast cancer diagnosis with unlabeled data. Comput. Med. Imaging Graph. **57**, 4–9 (2017)
12. Su, H., et al.: Region segmentation in histopathological breast cancer images using deep convolutional neural network. In: IEEE 12th International Symposium on Biomedical Imaging (ISBI), pp. 55–58 (2015)
13. Kotikalapudi, Raghavendra and contributors: https://github.com/raghakot/keras-vis (2017)

Small Lesion Classification in Dynamic Contrast Enhancement MRI for Breast Cancer Early Detection

Hao Zheng[1,2], Yun Gu[1,2,3], Yulei Qin[1,2], Xiaolin Huang[1,2], Jie Yang[1,2(✉)], and Guang-Zhong Yang[3]

[1] Institute of Image Processing and Pattern Recognition,
Shanghai Jiao Tong University, Shanghai, China
jieyang@sjtu.edu.cn
[2] Medical Robotics Institute, Shanghai Jiao Tong University, Shanghai, China
[3] Hamlyn Centre for Robotic Surgery, Imperial College London, London, UK

Abstract. Classification of small lesions is of great importance for early detection of breast cancer. The small size of lesion makes handcrafted features ineffective for practical applications. Furthermore, the relatively small data sets also impose challenges on deep learning based classification methods. Dynamic Contrast Enhancement MRI (DCE-MRI) is widely-used for women at high risk of breast cancer, and the dynamic features become more important in the case of small lesion. To extract more dynamic information, we propose a method for processing sequence data to encode the DCE-MRI, and design a new structure, dense convolutional LSTM, by adding a dense block in convolutional LSTM unit. Faced with the huge number of parameters in deep neural network, we add some semantic priors as constrains to improve generalization performance. Four latent attributes are extracted from diagnostic reports and pathological results, and are predicted together with the classification of benign or malignant. Predicting the latent attributes as auxiliary tasks can help the training of deep neural network, which makes it possible to train complex network with small size dataset and achieve a satisfactory result. Our methods improve the accuracy from 0.625, acquired by ResNet, to 0.847.

1 Introduction

Breast cancer is the most common cancer among women cancer worldwide. The high risk for breast cancer has attracted extensive efforts to early examination and diagnosis with medical imaging systems. Among them, the dynamic contract enhancement MRI (DCE-MRI) is a popular screening methodology, which presents higher sensitivity [9] compared to mammography. The small size of lesions which are normally less than 15 mm in diameter, requires well-trained

This research is partly supported by Committee of Science and Technology, Shanghai, China (No. 17JC1403000) and 973 Plan, China (No. 2015CB856004).

© Springer Nature Switzerland AG 2018
A. F. Frangi et al. (Eds.): MICCAI 2018, LNCS 11071, pp. 876–884, 2018.
https://doi.org/10.1007/978-3-030-00934-2_97

clinicians to manually exam the imaging data which is very expensive and time-cosuming. In order to reduce the manual efforts, the Computer-aided Diagnosis systems have been developed to automatically detect and classify the potential regions of breast cancers that provides references for diagnosis. The main challenges in small lesion breast cancer classification are three-folded: (1) the small size of lesion leads to some diagnostic basis difficult to describe by handcraft features; (2) Different protocols create difficulties in data preprocessing and normalization; (3) The small size of dataset leads to poor generalization capability when trained end to end using deep learning methods.

(a)   (b)

Fig. 1. Examples of two small breast cancer lesions. (a) a benign lesion with irregular shape; (b) a malignant lesion with clear edge and homogeneous enhancement.

Traditional machine learning methods which use manually designed features for breast cancer DCE-MRI classification are reviewed as [5]. The problem is that some handcraft features become obscure especially the morphological features in the case of small lesions. This can be improved by deep learning methods which are popular in recent years and can learn features from low level to high level by computers. [2] compares the performance of deep learning and segmentation based radiomic methods for breast cancer DCE-MRI classification, and gets a better result using segmentation based methods. The bad performance of deep learning is because the input to their CNN model is only a 2D-slice at the first post-contrast time point. Using only morphological features is not sufficient to complete the classification of benign and malignant lesions. Figure 1 shows two examples whose morphological features may lead to misclassification. In this case, the dynamic contrast enhanced features should be carefully considered. DCE-MRI is a series of three-dimensional images acquired along time axis for recording the change of intensity after the injection of contrast agent, and the time-intensity curve is a key diagnostic feature [11]. In previous works, the dynamic contrast enhanced property is used to highlight the lesion part. [8] uses the first DCE-MRI subtraction volume and [1] selects three sequences to represent the whole DCE-MRI. The number of time sequences they used is no more than three, which may be enough for detection but not sufficient for classification. To achieve a high classification accuracy, it is necessary to consider the intensity changes in all time sequences.

Taking into account that the number of time sequences varies with the protocol, we propose to process the DCE-MRI as sequential data. Convolutional LSTM (ConvLSTM) [10] is a nature choice for encoding sequential image data.

However, the ability of a few layers of ConvLSTM is not capable of extracting enough information, while stacking more layers makes the training significantly slower, harder, and brings redundant gate operations. To improve the network's ability for extracting more information from DCE-MRI, inspired by DenseNet [7] which achieves a good feature reuse, we propose a new structure, dense convolutional LSTM (DC-LSTM) by adding a dense block in ConvLSTM unit. But even with the simplest structure, the number of parameters of deep neural network is so huge in the case of our medical image dataset. This makes the training of network unstable, and the final results unsatisfactory. Thus, more constrains should be added to improve the network's generalization performance. It is observed that semantic priors are critical in breast cancer classification, for example, diagnostic reports and pathological results, which can be easily taken with the progress of hospital database management. In previous studies, [12] uses attention mechanism to combine the text information of diagnostic reports and image, while [4] learns a text-image mapping model. Considering that the size of medical dataset is not enough for a natural language processing model, we extract labels from the text rather than using the textual information directly. We leverage the latent attributes learning methods to predict these labels as auxiliary tasks, in which the textual information is only needed during training. With these auxiliary tasks, the neural networks converge faster, which is of great importance to train our complex network with small sample, and achieve better generalization performance.

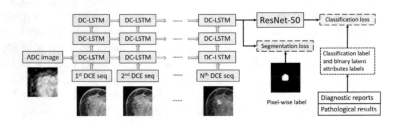

Fig. 2. Architectural details of our framework.

Generally, as shown in Fig. 2, we propose a new method for classification of small lesions in breast cancer. Our work comprises four major contributions: (1) a new approach to encode DCE-MRI, processing DCE-MRI as sequence data; (2) a new structure, DC-LSTM, which is more effective to encode the sequential image data, in this paper, extracting more time-intensity information from DCE-MRI, with matching training method to solve the hard-training problem; (3) a new way to use diagnostic reports and pathological results, extracting labels directly from the text, and feeding the labels into a latent attributes learning framework which can help the training of network and achieve high generalization performance; (4) examed in our dataset, the method achieved an accuracy of 0.847, a precision of 0.782 and a recall of 0.815, which is much higher than the baselines.

2   Methods

2.1   Datasets

Our data sets are obtained through a project with Renji Hospital Affiliated to Shanghai Jiao Tong University School of Medicine, Shanghai, China. MRI units by 2 vendors are comprised: GE (18 examples) and Philips (54 examples). We use two types of MRI in this study: Dynamic contrast enhanced (DCE) MRI and Diffusion Weighted Imaging (DWI) MRI. Two experienced breast radiologists make pixel-wise labels on 72 lesions (benign = 45 and malignant = 27) in DCE-MRI from 72 female patients. Based on the edge of breast, we make a rough registration of DWI-MRI and DCE-MRI. Then the DCE-MRI is cropped into $40 \times 40 \times 40 \times t$ where t is the number of time sequences, according to the labels, and the DWI-MRI is cropped into $40 \times 40 \times 40$ at the same location. Diagnostic reports and pathological results are collected together with the image, while the labels of benign or malignant is extracted from the pathological results.

2.2   DC-LSTM

DCE-MRI is sequence of 3D images along the time axis. In order to extract more time-intensity information, we propose to process DCE-MRI as sequence data, for which convolutional LSTM is a nature choice. But in the experiment, we find that the proposed network is hard to train only using the category label. The accuracy is low while the variance is high. So we add a segmentation loss on the output of ConvLSTM to help training and restrict the network's attention on lesion part. But as seen in Fig. 3, the segmentation result of ConvLSTM is not satisfactory. This is because the lack of capacity of a three-layer ConvLSTM to pick up so much information. However, stacking more layers leads the training more difficult and brings a lot redundant gate operations, which is not a wise choice. DenseNet achieves the same capability as ResNet [6] with better feature reuse. Inspired by the dense block in DenseNet, we add a simplified dense block in ConvLSTM unit. As shown in Fig. 4, our dense block is composed of four convolutional layers and works in the cell state of ConvLSTM. The first three

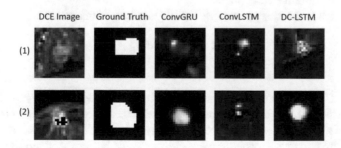

Fig. 3. The DCE image at the second post-contrast time point, the ground truth and the segmentation results of ConvGRU, ConvLSTM and DC-LSTM in test set.

layers use kernels sized of $3 \times 3 \times 3$ while the final layer is $1 \times 1 \times 1$ convolution. The input of each layer is concatenated by the original input and the outputs of previous layers. In our experiments, the number of output channels of each convolution operator is set to 16.

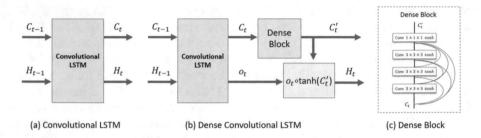

(a) Convolutional LSTM   (b) Dense Convolutional LSTM   (c) Dense Block

Fig. 4. Comparison between ConvLSTM and DC-LSTM. C is the cell state. H is the hidden state and o is the output gate.

2.3 Latent Attributes Learning

After encoding the DCE-MRI by DC-LSTM, we use ResNet50 as the classification network. But faced with the huge number of parameters, our dataset is not big enough to achieve a satisfactory generalization performance. Thus, more constrains should be added. A good choice is the diagnostic features summarized in medical research. These features are latent attributes of the lesions, containing dynamic features, morphological features and so on [11]. In this paper, we select four diagnostic basis as latent attributes from the diagnostic reports and pathological results. They are: (1) Interference Diseases; (2) Nodule Mass; (3) Boundary Smoothness; (4) Homogeneous Enhancement. Interference diseases are marked as breast disease in the patholofical results in our dataset when doctor found no evidence of cancer in the tissue sent to biopsy, although this part is likely to be a cancer lesion when examined from the image. The latter three attributes are all important morphological features reported in [11] and are marked in diagnostic reports.

Summarizing the discussion, we define the loss function as

$$\ell = \ell_{\text{cla}} + \lambda \ell_{\text{seg}} \tag{1}$$

$$\ell_{\text{cla}} = \ell_{\text{cancer}} + \mu \left(\ell_{\text{disease}} + \ell_{\text{mass}} + \ell_{\text{edge}} + \ell_{\text{enhance}} \right), \tag{2}$$

where μ and λ are the parameters controlling the weights between the classification for lesion and the predictions of latent attributes. ℓ_{cla} is the classification loss. ℓ_{cancer} is weighted sigmoid cross-entropy loss for classification of benign and malignant, in which the weight we used between benign and malignant is 1:2.

ℓ_{disease}, ℓ_{mass}, ℓ_{edge} and ℓ_{enhance} are softmax cross-entropy losses for the prediction of interference diseases, nodule mass, boundary smoothness and homogeneous enhancement. ℓ_{seg} is the dice loss for segmentation defined as

$$\ell_{\text{seg}} = 1 - \sum_{i=1}^{N} p_i g_i / \left(\sum_{i=1}^{N} p_i^2 + \sum_{i=1}^{N} g_i^2 \right), \tag{3}$$

where p_i is the volume of the average of DC-LSTM's output channels and g_i is the volume of ground truth.

3   Experiments

In this section, we describe the details of our experiments and analyze the results. The Apparent Diffusion Coefficient (ADC) map is calculated same as [3] by DWI-MRI to initialise the DC-LSTM states. The parameters are optimized by stochastic gradient descent with a learning rate of 0.001, a decay of 0.0005 with a decay steps of 50, a momentum of 0.9 and a batch size of 8. We use $\lambda = 0.7$ and $\mu = 1.0$ in all experiments. Data augmentation is applied during the training, which contains random flip and random crop ($24 \times 24 \times 24$). When testing, data are cropped in the middle $24 \times 24 \times 24$ part. We use cross-validation ($k = 3$) to test the performance of the network, training sets and test sets are extracted from benign and malignant samples respectively. The framework is implemented in TensorFlow and running on 4 Titan Xp GPUs.

3.1   DC-LSTM

When training the proposed network, we first use the ADC image as the initial state of the DC-LSTM cell. Then train the DC-LSTM only with the segmentation loss to initialize the parameters. Finally, train the network with all losses.

The classification results are shown in Table 1. ResNet is treated as the baseline. Using the ConvLSTM or ConvGRU to encode the DCE-MRI, the accuracy, precision, and recall are all improved, which shows that processing DCE-MRI as sequential data really makes sense. The best result is achieved by our DC-LSTM, and the increases are obvious.

Table 1. The classification results of benign or malignant. ResNet(single) is ResNet-50 trained only for the main task while ResNet(multi) is for all tasks. The filters' number of the 3-layer ConvGRU and ConvLSTM is 24 and 32.

Network	Accuracy	Precision	Recall
ResNet(single)	0.625	0.500	0.556
ResNet(multi)	0.667	0.566	0.556
ConvGRU+ResNet	0.736	0.617	0.778
ConvLSTM+ResNet	0.750	0.650	0.778
DC-LSTM+ResNet	**0.847**	**0.782**	**0.815**

3.2   Latent Attributes Learning

In order to test the ability of the latent attributes, we train ResNet with different combinations of attributes. The input DCE-MRI to ResNet is pre-processed same as [1]. The main classification task and the prediction of latent attributes share parameters except the final layer. During training, we check the results on training set (middle cropped) and test set every 100 steps, and record the number of steps by which the result on training set exceeds a threshold (accuracy >0.9, precision >0.8 and recall >0.8). We run each combinations five times then take the average.

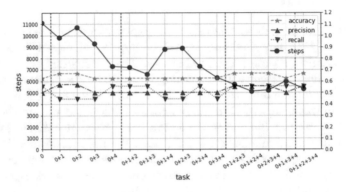

Fig. 5. The results of training ResNet-50 with category label and different combination of latent attribute labels. '0' denotes the classification of benign or malignant and '1', '2', '3', '4' denote the prediction of the four latent attributes.

As shown in Fig. 5, as the number of latent attributes increase, the number of steps required to reach the threshold drops significantly, while the classification results also have minor increases. Thus, the most significant effect of the latent attributes is that they can accelerate convergence. We summarize two main reasons why the latent attributes can help converge. (1) When trained by a small dataset, ResNet may make the prediction based on some background information. All the latent attributes are related to the lesion, so that they can help to concentrate the network's attention on the lesion part. As a result, they speed up the training of network. (2) Some useful features are difficult to learn from the main task while they are easy to learn from the auxiliary tasks, which is called 'eavesdropping'. Each task owns a fc-layer which is a 2048 × 2 matrix in ResNet-50. We substract the second column from the first column and take the absolute value to denote the weights of each feature for each task. Then select the largest 10 weights for the main task and the related weights for the other tasks. As shown in the left chart in Table 2, the important weights for the main task are also important for some auxiliary tasks. We also check the largest 10 weights of the auxiliary tasks. Almost all the weights are large for the main task as well. That shows a high relatedness between the main task and the auxiliary tasks. We also analyze the weights of DC-LSTM+ResNet, as seen in the

Table 2. The largest 10 weights for the main task and the related weights for the other tasks, the left chart is from ResNet-50 and the right chart is from DC-LSTM+ResNet.

Weights of ResNet-50

task \ feature	0	1	2	3	4
1	4.310	3.144	0.664	0.105	1.119
2	3.305	0.596	0.943	0.044	0.614
3	3.514	2.352	0.168	1.433	1.042
4	3.672	0.451	2.694	0.227	1.222
5	5.067	0.284	2.184	0.035	0.152
6	6.097	0.480	3.549	0.357	0.247
7	3.416	2.147	2.207	0.129	0.728
8	2.911	0.525	3.175	0.075	1.085
9	2.863	2.680	0.135	0.923	0.052
10	2.743	0.675	1.060	0.436	0.985

Weights of DC-LSTM+ResNet

task \ feature	0	1	2	3	4
1	1.361	0.111	0.073	0.045	0.005
2	1.398	0.044	0.041	0.114	0.101
3	1.373	0.013	0.035	0.094	0.076
4	1.286	0.105	0.096	0.143	0.108
5	1.310	0.065	0.058	0.052	0.031
6	1.202	0.143	0.178	0.128	0.074
7	1.347	0.017	0.115	0.120	0.028
8	1.366	0.027	0.000	0.076	0.063
9	1.239	0.126	0.122	0.009	0.036
10	1.173	0.002	0.039	0.016	0.163

right chart. The weights of DC-LSTM+ResNet are obviously smaller than these of ResNet, which implies an improvement on generaliztion ability. The biggest difference is that the largest 10 weights in the main task are not large in the auxiliary tasks. This is a reasonable results because some features such as the time-intensity curve and the ADC value are critical diagnostic features in the main task but are not valuable in the auxiliary tasks.

4   Conclusion

In this work we propose a method to classify the benign and malignant of small lesions in breast cancer DCE MRI. The method consists of two parts. To extract more time-intensity information, we propose to encode DCE-MRI as sequential data and design a new structure DC-LSTM. Examed in our dataset, our DC-LSTM improves the accuracy from 0.625 to 0.847. Faced with the hard-training problem, we propose a latent attributes learning method. Our latent attributes learning method efficiently uses the information in diagnostic reports and pathological results, and accelerates the convergence of our network.

References

1. Amit, G., et al.: Hybrid mass detection in breast MRI combining unsupervised saliency analysis and deep learning. In: Descoteaux, M., Maier-Hein, L., Franz, A., Jannin, P., Collins, D.L., Duchesne, S. (eds.) MICCAI 2017. LNCS, vol. 10435, pp. 594–602. Springer, Cham (2017). https://doi.org/10.1007/978-3-319-66179-7_68
2. Antropova, N., et al.: Performance comparison of deep learning and segmentation-based radiomic methods in the task of distinguishing benign and malignant breast lesions on DCE-MRI. In: Medical Imaging 2017: Computer-Aided Diagnosis, 101341G (2017)
3. Bickel, H., et al.: Diffusion-weighted imaging of breast lesions: region-of-interest placement and different ADC parameters influence apparent diffusion coefficient values. Eur Radiol. **27**(5), 1883–1892 (2017)
4. Dai, L., et al.: Retinal microaneurysm detection using clinical report guided multi-sieving CNN. In: Descoteaux, M., Maier-Hein, L., Franz, A., Jannin, P., Collins, D.L., Duchesne, S. (eds.) MICCAI 2017. LNCS, vol. 10435, pp. 525–532. Springer, Cham (2017). https://doi.org/10.1007/978-3-319-66179-7_60

5. Fusco, R., et al.: Pattern recognition approaches for breast cancer DCE-MRI classification: a systematic review. JMBE **36**, 449–459 (2016)
6. He, K., et al.: Deep residual learning for image recognition. In: CVPR (2016)
7. Huang, G., et al.: Densely connected convolutional networks. In: CVPR (2017)
8. Maicas, G., Carneiro, G., Bradley, A.P., Nascimento, J.C., Reid, I.: Deep reinforcement learning for active breast lesion detection from DCE-MRI. In: Descoteaux, M., Maier-Hein, L., Franz, A., Jannin, P., Collins, D.L., Duchesne, S. (eds.) MICCAI 2017. LNCS, vol. 10435, pp. 665–673. Springer, Cham (2017). https://doi.org/10.1007/978-3-319-66179-7_76
9. Peters, N.: Meta-analysis of MR imaging in the diagnosis of breast lesions. Radiology **246**(1), 116–124 (2008)
10. Shi, X., et al.: Convolutional LSTM network: a machine learning approach for precipitation nowcasting. In: NIPS (2015)
11. Woitek, R.: A simple classification system (the Tree flowchart) for breast MRI can reduce the number of unnecessary biopsies in MRI-only lesions. Eur Radiol. **27**(9), 3799–3809 (2017)
12. Zhang, Z., Chen, P., Sapkota, M., Yang, L.: TandemNet: distilling knowledge from medical images using diagnostic reports as optional semantic references. In: Descoteaux, M., Maier-Hein, L., Franz, A., Jannin, P., Collins, D.L., Duchesne, S. (eds.) MICCAI 2017. LNCS, vol. 10435, pp. 320–328. Springer, Cham (2017). https://doi.org/10.1007/978-3-319-66179-7_37

Thermographic Computational Analyses of a 3D Model of a Scanned Breast

Alisson Augusto Azevedo Figueiredo[1], Gabriela Lima Menegaz[1],
Henrique Coelho Fernandes[2](✉) ⓘ, and Gilmar Guimaraes[1]

[1] School of Mechanical Engineering, Federal University of Uberlandia,
Uberlandia 38408-100, Brazil
[2] School of Computer Science, Federal University of Uberlandia,
Uberlandia 38408-100, Brazil
henrique.fernandes@ufu.br

Abstract. Breast cancer is the most common type of cancer among women. Cancer cells are characterized by having a higher metabolic activity and superior vascularization when compared to healthy cells. The internal heat generated by tumors travels to the skin surface where an infrared camera is capable of detecting small temperatures variations on the dermal surface. Breast cancer diagnosis using only thermal images is still not accepted by the medical community which makes necessary another exam to confirm the disease. This work presents a methodology which allows identification of breast cancer using only simulated thermal images. Experiments are performed in a three-dimensional breast geometry obtained with a 3D digital scanning. The procedure starts with the 3D scanning of a model of a real female breast using a "Picza LPX-600RE 3D Laser Scanner" to generate the breast virtual geometry. This virtual 3D model is then used to simulate the heat transfer phenomena using Finite Element Model (FEM). The simulated thermal images of the breast surface are obtained via the FEM model. Based on the temperature difference of a healthy breast and a breast with cancer it is possible to identify the presence of a tumor by analyzing the biggest thermal amplitudes. Results obtained with the FEM model indicate that it is possible to identify breast cancer using only infrared images.

Keywords: Breast cancer · 3D scanning · Thermal images
Numerical simulation · Inverse problem

1 Introduction

Breast cancer and the most common type of cancer among women in the United States and around the world [14]. This disease is characterized by the disordered growth of cells from different parts of the breast, which may invade other tissues, until the appearance of a malignant tumor [15]. Early detection of breast cancer can significantly reduce the mortality rates caused by the disease [16].

© Springer Nature Switzerland AG 2018
A. F. Frangi et al. (Eds.): MICCAI 2018, LNCS 11071, pp. 885–892, 2018.
https://doi.org/10.1007/978-3-030-00934-2_98

There are several medical imaging techniques that are used for the detection of breast cancer. Mammography still is the main exam. However, magnetic resonance imaging and ultrasound are also useful for the evaluation of the disease [13]. Infrared thermography, capable of capture temperature changes in skin surface, has also been explored as a possible screening tool for detection of mammary tumors [11]. Although, the medical authorities in the subject do not yet allow the use of only thermal imaging as a substitute for mammography [7].

As it is generally assumed that tumor tissue has a higher vascularity and metabolism than healthy tissue, the heat produced by the tumor can propagate through the tissues to the surface of the body where it can produce a temperature pattern variation in the skin [8]. Thus, an infrared thermal camera can detect these changes in the surface of the body.

The strategy of using an optimization algorithm together with an infrared camera can be a useful diagnostic tool for characterizing cancer and reducing unnecessary biopsy testing [3]. Computational simulations allow the increase of data processing capacity, it can assist in the numerical modeling of complex geometries, it can facilitate the automatic search by abnormal thermal patterns in thermographic images [10].

Many papers in the literature present several methodologies to aid in the identification of tumors using only surface temperatures of human skin. Most of them deal with heat transfer simulations in simplified breast geometries, and, the calculated temperatures on the surface are used to detect the presence of tumors [1,2].

The main objective of this work is to detect the presence of breast cancer through the simulation of thermographic images of a three-dimensional model of a breast obtained by digital scanning. Previous works available in the literature simulate temperatures in simplified models of the breast while in this work a real 3D model is used. Temperatures are calculated using the numerical solution of the Pennes equation using the finite element method through commercial software COMSOL. Then, the thermal superficial images of the breast are analyzed using the MATLAB commercial software for the exact identification of the point of greatest temperature increase caused by the presence of the tumor which can be used for the identification of the position of the tumor.

2   Materials and Methods

2.1   Heat Biotransference Equation

The thermal images obtained in the simulations depend on the solution of the Pennes equation by the finite element method using commercial software COMSOL. The pioneering work of Pennes has proposed a quantitative relationship that describes the heat transfer in human tissues and organs, performing the energy balance within the biological tissues through the interaction of blood perfusion and metabolism. Equation 1 represents Pennes' heat biotransference equation [12].

$$\rho c \frac{\partial T}{\partial t} = k\nabla^2 T + w\rho_s c_s (T_a - T) + Q_m \tag{1}$$

where ρ, c, w and k are the specific mass, the specific heat, the blood perfusion rate and the thermal conductivity of the tissue, respectively. ρ_s, c_s and T_a are the specific mass, the specific heat and the temperature of the arterial blood, respectively. Q_m represents the volumetric metabolic heat generation rate of the tissue.

The blood perfusion effect was considered homogeneous and isotropic. It was also considered that thermal equilibrium occurs in the capillaries microcirculatory networks. In these circumstances, the blood enter the capillaries and the difference of temperature due to the arterial blood temperature causes an exchange of temperature with the surrounding tissue until it reaches thermal equilibrium. At this point, there is not heat transfer, either before or after the passage of the blood thorough the capillaries, so that the temperature at which the blood enters the venous circulation is that of the local tissue [5].

2.2 3D Scanned Computational Model and Numerical Solution

Figure 1 shows in schematic form the procedure to obtain the numerical model of the breast used in the simulated thermal analyzes. A real breast model was purchased from the company 3B Scientific and the Picza LPX-600RE 3D Laser Scanner was used to scan the sample, thus obtaining a representative 3D model of the breast. This procedure may be analogous to a possible future capture of the breast geometry of a patient who wishes to be diagnosed.

The numerical solution of the Pennes equation was obtained with the objective of analyzing the thermal behavior of energy transport in the breast. The mesh used in the COMSOL simulations is composed of 66220 tetrahedral elements and 5742 triangular elements.

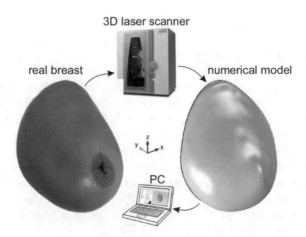

Fig. 1. Procedure for obtaining the 3D geometry of the breast.

2.3   Case of Simulated Breast Cancer

To obtain the simulated thermographic images, only one case of breast cancer was analyzed. This choice was made based on the statics of breast cancer occurrence found in the literature. Figure 2 shows that most breast cancers are found in the upper right quadrant. Therefore, two simulations were performed. In the first, no tumor was inserted in to the breast. In the second, a tumor was inserted in the upper right quadrant. Later the permanent thermal problem will be solved for both cases.

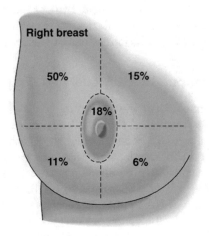

Fig. 2. Breast quadrants and breast cancer occurrence [4].

3   Results and Discussions

At this stage, temperatures on the skin surface of the breast are obtained by solving the Pennes equation in a steady state regime using COMSOL. The tumor inserted has a diameter equal to 1 cm and it was located 10 mm from the skin surface. To solve the equation, in addition to the inclusion of a tumor in the upper right quadrant of the breast, it is necessary to know the bio-thermal properties of the phenomenon. These properties are presented in the Table 1. The boundary conditions considered in the problem are prescribe temperature of $T_a = 37$ °C in the internal surface of the breast, thermal convection in the skin surface with temperature ambient of 25 °C and convective coefficient of 5 W/m^{2}K. These conditions were considered to solve the equation.

Figure 3 shows a thermal image of the simulated surface for a healthy breast, i.e., without tumor. The superficial temperatures in the skin of the breast have a normal thermal behavior, where the maximum temperature of 37 °C observed is still related to the internal surface of the breast that is influenced by the

Table 1. Tissues thermal and biological properties [6,9].

Properties	Value	Layer
Thermal conductivity, k	0.21 W/mK	Healthy tissue
	0.62 W/mK	Tumor
Blood perfusion, w	0.00022 1/s	Healthy tissue
	0.016 1/s	Tumor
Specific mass, ρ	920 kg/m^3	Everywhere
Specific heat, c	3000 J/kgK	Everywhere
Volumetric metabolic heat generation, Q_m	420 W/m^3	Healthy tissue
	300000 W/m^3	Tumor

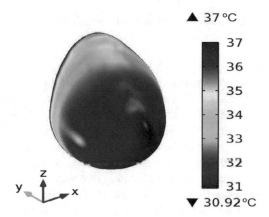

Fig. 3. Thermal image of the surface of a healthy breast.

arterial temperature of the body. The minimum temperature found is in the region of the areola of the breast, because this is the region farthest from the inner part of the body, therefore, being less influenced by the heat transferred from inside the breast, and, more influenced by the thermal convection of the external environment.

The other simulation performed involves a scanned breast with a tumor in the upper right quadrant. The thermal behavior at the skin surface for this particular case of breast cancer is presented in Fig. 4. It can be observed in the Figure that there was temperature changes in almost the entire surface of the breast, however, a greater thermal disturbance is found in the upper right quadrant where a tumor was internally inserted.

The values of temperature variations observed only through the thermal images are not accurate, but it can be seen that in the region of the areola there has been a temperature increase of around 2 °C.

After simulating two distinct conditions in the breast, it was possible to observe an alteration in the skin temperature profile. However, for a better con-

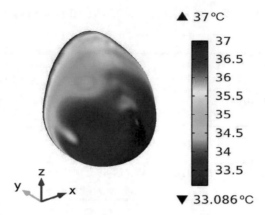

Fig. 4. Surface thermal image of a breast with tumor in the upper right quadrant.

clusion about what occurred in the breast after the appearance of the tumor, the subtraction of the skin surface temperatures between the breast with the tumor and the breast without the tumor is performed. Figure 5a shows only the temperature difference of the skin surface of the breast. Now, one can observe only the temperature variation caused by breast cancer. Thus, it is possible to observe that the maximum temperature variation occurred in the right upper quadrant. The peripheral regions also had a change in their temperature values.

Finally, a temperature curve is obtained by creating a 'cut line' that intercepts the point of greatest thermal variation in the skin caused by the tumor as shown in Fig. 5a. This curve is showed in Fig. 5b which characterizes the ther-

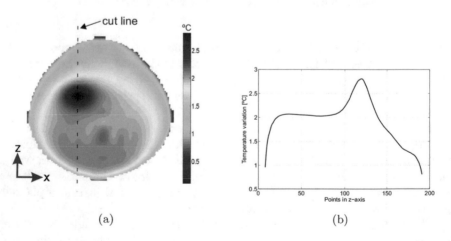

Fig. 5. (a) Skin surface temperature variation caused by the presence of a tumor in the breast right upper quadrant and (b) Temperature profile variation in the breast skin surface caused by the tumor.

mal pattern caused by breast cancer. The idea of this work is that other profiles could be obtained for several other cases of the disease, creating a database that in the future could allow doctors to evaluate patients with and without breast cancer.

4   Conclusions

In this work, the detection of temperature increase caused by the presence of breast cancer was performed using simulated thermographic images.

Unlike other works available in the literature where simplify geometries are considered, in this work, a real breast sample was acquired and a three-dimensional digital scan of the geometry was performed to obtain the 3D computational model. A numerical model of the breast was simulated using COMSOL, and temperatures were calculated for a case without and with tumor using the Pennes equation.

The superficial temperatures in the skin of the breast were obtained for the two studied cases. After, only the difference between the thermal profiles was analyzed. From the obtained temperature changes, it was possible to find the point on the surface where the greatest thermal change occurred and to determined a characteristic thermal profile for the evaluated breast cancer case. In this sense, it is possible to acquire characteristic profiles for several cases making it possible to make a correlation between breast cancers and observed thermal profiles.

Therefore, this work indicates that it is possible to acquire thermal images to identify mammary tumors through the identification of thermal patterns. Experiments are currently being performed to experimentally validate the proposed approach involving thermal images of real breast models acquired by an infrared camera.

Acknowledgments. The authors would like to gratefully acknowledge the support of the following Brazilian agencies: FAPEMIG, Minas Gerais Research Funding Foundation; CNPq, National Council for Scientific and Technological Development; and CAPES, Coordination for the Improvement of Higher Education Personnel.

References

1. Agnelli, J.P., Barrea, A., Turner, C.V.: Tumor location and parameter estimation by thermography. Math. Comput. Model. **53**(7–8), 1527–1534 (2011)
2. Amri, A., Pulko, S.H., Wilkinson, A.J.: Potentialities of steady-state and transient thermography in breast tumour depth detection: a numerical study. Comput. Methods Programs Biomed. **123**, 68–80 (2016)
3. Bhowmik, A., Repaka, R.: Estimation of growth features and thermophysical properties of melanoma within 3-D human skin using genetic algorithm and simulated annealing. Int. J. Heat Mass Transf. **98**, 81–95 (2016)
4. Byer, C.O., Galliano, G., Shriver, S.P.: Dimensions of Human Sexuality. McGraw-Hill Humanities Social, New York (2002)

5. Chato, J.: Heat transfer to blood vessels. J. Biomech. Eng. **102**(2), 110–118 (1980)
6. Gautherie, M.: Thermopathology of breast cancer: measurement and analysis of in vivo temperature and blood flow. Ann. New York Acad. Sci. **335**(1), 383–415 (1980)
7. Gourd, E.: Breast thermography alone no substitute for mammography. Lancet Oncol. **19**(2), E78–E78 (2018)
8. Han, F., Liang, C., Shi, G., Wang, L., Li, K.: Clinical applications of internal heat source analysis for breast cancer identification. Gent. Mol. Res. **14**(1), 1450–60 (2015)
9. Hossain, S., Mohammadi, F.A.: Tumor parameter estimation considering the body geometry by thermography. Comput. Biol. Med. **76**, 80–93 (2016)
10. Ng, E.Y., Sudharsan, N.: Computer simulation in conjunction with medical thermography as an adjunct tool for early detection of breast cancer. BMC Cancer **4**(1), 17 (2004)
11. Pavithra, P., Ravichandran, K., Sekar, K., Manikandan, R.: The effect of thermography on breast cancer detection. Syst. Rev. Pharm. **9**, 10–16 (2018)
12. Pennes, H.H.: Analysis on tissue arterial blood temperature in the resting human forearm. Appl. Physiol. **1**(2), 93–122 (1948)
13. Shah, R., Rosso, K., Nathanson, S.D.: Pathogenesis, prevention, diagnosis and treatment of breast cancer. World J. Clin. Oncol. **5**(3), 283 (2014)
14. Siegel, R.L., et al.: Colorectal cancer statistics, 2017. CA Cancer J. Clin. **67**(3), 177–193 (2017)
15. Society, A.C.: What is breast cancer? (2017). https://www.cancer.org/cancer/breast-cancer/about/what-is-breast-cancer.html
16. Wang, L.: Early diagnosis of breast cancer. Sensors **17**(7), 1–20 (2017). https://doi.org/10.3390/s17071572. Article number 1572

Y-Net: Joint Segmentation and Classification for Diagnosis of Breast Biopsy Images

Sachin Mehta[1]($\boxtimes$), Ezgi Mercan[1], Jamen Bartlett[2], Donald Weaver[2], Joann G. Elmore[3], and Linda Shapiro[1]

[1] University of Washington, Seattle, WA 98195, USA
{sacmehta,ezgi,shapiro}@cs.washington.edu
[2] University of Vermont, Burlington 05405, USA
{jamen.bartlett,donald.weaver}@uvmhealth.org
[3] University of California, Los Angeles, CA 90095, USA
jelmore@mednet.ucla.edu

Abstract. In this paper, we introduce a conceptually simple network for generating discriminative tissue-level segmentation masks for the purpose of breast cancer diagnosis. Our method efficiently segments different types of tissues in breast biopsy images while simultaneously predicting a discriminative map for identifying important areas in an image. Our network, Y-Net, extends and generalizes U-Net by adding a parallel branch for discriminative map generation and by supporting convolutional block modularity, which allows the user to adjust network efficiency without altering the network topology. Y-Net delivers state-of-the-art segmentation accuracy while learning 6.6× fewer parameters than its closest competitors. The addition of descriptive power from Y-Net's discriminative segmentation masks improve diagnostic classification accuracy by 7% over state-of-the-art methods for diagnostic classification. Source code is available at: https://sacmehta.github.io/YNet.

1 Introduction

Annually, millions of women depend on pathologists' interpretive accuracy to determine whether their breast biopsies are benign or malignant [4]. Diagnostic errors are alarmingly frequent, lead to incorrect treatment recommendations, and can cause significant patient harm [2]. Pathology as a field has been slow to move into the digital age, but in April 2017, the FDA authorized the marketing of the Philips IntelliSite Pathology Solution (PIPS), the first whole slide imaging system for interpreting digital surgical pathology slides on the basis of biopsy tissue samples, thus changing the landscape[1].

---

[1] https://www.fda.gov/NewsEvents/Newsroom/PressAnnouncements/ucm552742.htm.

© Springer Nature Switzerland AG 2018
A. F. Frangi et al. (Eds.): MICCAI 2018, LNCS 11071, pp. 893–901, 2018.
https://doi.org/10.1007/978-3-030-00934-2_99

Convolutional neural networks (CNNs) produce state-of-the-art results in natural [6,12] and biomedical classification and segmentation [8,11] tasks. Training CNNs directly on whole slide images (WSIs) is difficult due to their massive size. Sliding-window-based approaches for classifying [5,8] and segmenting [10,11] medical images have shown promising results. Segmentation and classification are usually separate steps in automated diagnosis systems.

Segmentation-based methods consider tissue structure, such as size and distribution, to help inform class boundary decisions. However, these segmentation methods suffer from two major drawbacks. First, labeled data is scarce because the labeling of biopsy images is time-consuming and must be done by domain experts. Second, segmentation-based approaches are not able to weigh the importance of different tissue types. The latter limitation is particularly concerning in biopsy images, because not every tissue type in biopsy images is relevant for cancer detection. On the other hand, though classification-based methods fail to provide structure- and tissue-level information, they can identify regions of interest inside the images that should be used for further analysis.

In this paper, we combine the two different methods, segmentation and classification, and introduce a new network called Y-Net that simultaneously generates a tissue-level segmentation mask and a discriminative (or saliency) map. Y-Net generalizes the U-Net network [11], a well-known segmentation network for biomedical images. Y-net includes a *plug-and-play* functionality that enables the use of different types of convolutional blocks without changing the network topology, allowing users to more easily explore the space of networks and choose more efficient networks. For example, Y-Net delivers the same segmentation performance as that of [10] while learning 6.6× fewer parameters. Furthermore, the discriminative tissue-level segmentation masks produced using Y-Net provide powerful features for diagnosis. Our results suggest that Y-Net is 7% more accurate than state-of-the-art segmentation and saliency-based methods [5,10].

Statement of Problem: The problem we wish to solve is the simultaneous segmentation and diagnosis of whole slide breast cancer biopsy images. For this task, we used the breast biopsy dataset in [2,10] that consists of 240 whole slide breast biopsy images with heamatoxylin and eosin (H&E) staining. A total of 87 pathologists diagnosed a randomly assigned subset of 60 slides into four diagnostic categories (benign, atypia, ductal carcinoma *in situ*, and invasive cancer), producing an

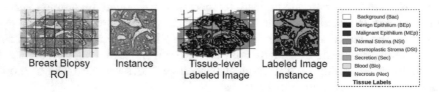

Fig. 1. This figure shows (at left) the breast biopsy ROI with H&E staining broken into multiple instances with one instance enlarged to show more detail. On the right are the pixel-wise tissue-level labelings of the ROI and the instance.

average of 22 diagnostic labels per case. Then, each slide was carefully interpreted by a panel of three expert pathologists to assign a consensus diagnosis for each slide that we take to be the gold standard ground truth. Furthermore, the pathologists have marked 428 regions of interest (ROIs) on these slides that helped with diagnosis and a subset of 58 of these ROIs have been hand segmented by a pathology fellow into eight different tissue classifications: *background, benign epithelium, malignant epithelium, normal stroma, desmoplastic stroma, secretion, blood,* and *necrosis.* The average size of these ROIs is $10,000 \times 12,000$. We use these 428 ROIs for our data set.

In this work, we break each ROI into a set (or bag) of equal size patches that we will call *instances*, as shown in Fig. 1. Each ROI X has a known groundtruth diagnostic label Z. There are no separate diagnostic labels for the instances; they all have the same groundtruth label Z, but some of them contribute to the diagnosis of Z and others do not. Our system, therefore, will learn the *discriminativeness* of each instance during its analysis. Furthermore, each pixel of each of these instances has a known tissue classification into one of the eight categories; tissue classification must be learned from the groundtruth ROIs. Using the groundtruth diagnostic labels Z of the ROIs and the groundtruth tissue labels Y from the 58 labeled ROIs, our goal is to build a classification system that can input a ROI, perform simultaneous segmentation and classification, and output a diagnosis. Our system, once trained, can be easily applied to WSIs.

Related Work: Biomedical images are difficult to classify and segment, because their anatomical structures vary in shape and size. CNNs, by virtue of their representational power and capacity for capturing structural information, have made such classification and segmentation tasks possible [8,11]. The segmentation-based method in [10] and saliency map-based method in [5] are most similar to our work. Mehta *et al.* [10] developed a CNN-based method for segmenting breast biopsy images that produces a tissue-level segmentation mask for each WSI. The histogram features they extracted from the segmentation masks were used for diagnostic classification. Geçer [5] proposed a saliency-based method for diagnosing cancer in breast biopsy images that identified relevant regions in breast biopsy WSIs to be used for diagnostic classification. Our main contribution in this paper is a method for *joint learning* of both segmentation and classification. Our experiments show that joint learning improves diagnostic accuracy.

2   A System for Joint Segmentation and Classification

Our system (Fig. 2) is given an ROI from a breast biopsy WSI and breaks it into instances that are fed into Y-Net. Y-Net produces two different outputs: an instance-level segmentation mask and an instance-level probability map. The instance-level segmentation masks have, for each instance, the predicted labels of the eight different tissue types. These are combined to produce a segmentation mask for the whole ROI. The instance-level probability map contains (for every pixel) the maximum value of the probability of that instance being in one of the four diagnostic categories. This map is thresholded to binary and combined

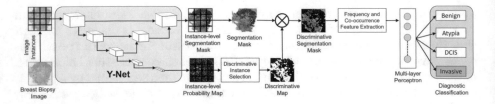

Fig. 2. Overview of our method for detecting breast cancer.

with the segmentation mask to produce the discriminative segmentation mask. A multi-layer perceptron then uses the frequency and co-occurrence features extracted from the final mask to predict the cancer diagnosis.

2.1 Y-Net Architecture

Y-Net is conceptually simple and generalizes U-Net [11] to joint segmentation and classification tasks. U-Net outputs a single segmentation mask. Y-Net adds a second branch that outputs the classification label. The classification output is distinct from the segmentation output and requires feature extraction at low spatial resolutions. We first briefly review the U-Net architecture and then introduce the key elements in the Y-Net architecture.

U-Net: U-Net is composed of two networks: (1) encoding network and (2) decoding network. The encoding network can be viewed as a stack of encoding and down-sampling blocks. The encoding blocks learn input representations; down-sampling helps the network learn scale invariance. Spatial information is lost in both convolutional and down-sampling operations. The decoder can be viewed as a stack of up-sampling and decoding blocks. The up-sampling blocks help in inverting the loss of spatial resolution, while the decoding blocks help the network to compensate for the loss of spatial information in the encoder. U-Net introduces skip-connections between the encoder and the decoder, which enables the encoder and the decoder to share information.

Y-Net: Y-Net (Fig. 3a) adopts a two-stage procedure. The first stage outputs the instance-level segmentation mask, as U-Net does, while the second stage adds a parallel branch that outputs the instance-level classification label. In spirit, our approach follows Mask-RCNN [7] which jointly learns the segmentation and classification of natural images. Unlike Mask-RCNN, Y-Net is fully convolutional; that is, Y-Net does not have any region proposal network. Furthermore, training Y-Net is different from training Mask-RCNN, because Mask-RCNN is trained with object-level segmentations and classification labels. Our system has diagnostic labels for entire ROIs, but not for the instance-level.

   Y-Net differs from the U-Net in the following aspects:

Abstract Representation of Encoding and Decoding Blocks: At each spatial level, U-Net uses the same convolutional block (a stack of convolutional

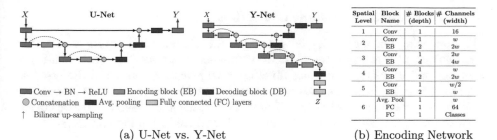

(a) U-Net vs. Y-Net   (b) Encoding Network

Fig. 3. (a) Comparison between U-Net and Y-Net architectures. (b) The encoding network architecture used in (a). U-Net in (a) is a generalized version of U-Net [11].

layers) in both the encoder and the decoder. Instead, Y-Net abstracts this representation and represents convolutional blocks as general encoding and decoding blocks that can be used anywhere, and are thus not forced to be the same at each spatial level. Representing Y-Net in such a modular form provides it a *plug-and-play* functionality and therefore enables the user to try different convolutional block designs without changing the network topology.

Width and Depth Multipliers: Larger CNN architectures tend to perform better than smaller architectures. We introduce two hyper-parameters, a width multiplier w and a depth-multiplier d, that allow us to vary the size of the network. These parameters allow Y-Net to span the network space from smaller to larger networks, allowing identification of better network structures.

Sharing Features: While U-Net has skip-connections between the encoding and decoding stages, Y-net adds a skip-connection between the first and last encoding block at the same spatial resolution in the encoder, as shown in Fig. 3 with a dashed arrow, to help improve segmentation.

Implementation Details: The encoding network in Y-Net (Fig. 3a) consists of the repeated application of the encoding blocks and 3×3 convolutional layers with a stride of 2 for down-sampling operations, except for the first layer which is a 7×7 standard convolution layer with a stride of 2. Similarly, the decoding network in Y-Net consists of the repeated application of the decoding blocks and bilinear up-sampling for up-sampling operations. We first train Y-Net for segmentation and then attach the remaining encoding network (spatial levels 4, 5 and 6 in Fig. 3b) to jointly train for segmentation and classification. We define a multi-task loss on each instance as $\mathcal{L} = \mathcal{L}_{seg} + \mathcal{L}_{cls}$, where $\mathcal{L}_{seg}$ and $\mathcal{L}_{cls}$ are the multi-nominal cross-entropy loss functions for the segmentation and classification tasks, respectively. All layers and blocks, except the classification and fully connected (FC) layers, are followed by a batch normalization and ReLU non-linearity. An average pooling layer with adaptive kernel size enables Y-Net to deal with arbitrary image sizes.

2.2   Discriminative Instance Selection

The encoding network in Y-Net generates a C-dimensional output vector $\mathbf{z}$ of real values; C represents the number of diagnostic classes. The real-values in $\mathbf{z}$ are normalized using a softmax function σ to generate another C-dimensional vector $\bar{\mathbf{z}} = \sigma(\mathbf{z})$. It is reasonable to assume that instances with low probability will have low discriminativeness. If $\max(\bar{\mathbf{z}}) > \tau$, then the instance is considered *discriminative*, where τ is the threshold selected using the method in [8].

2.3   Diagnostic Classification

Segmentation masks provide tissue-level information. Since training data with tissue-level information is limited and not all tissue types contribute equally to diagnostic decisions, our system combines the segmentation mask with the discriminative map to obtain a *tissue-level discriminative segmentation mask*. Frequency and co-occurrence histograms are extracted from the discriminative segmentation mask and used to train a multi-layer perceptron (MLP) with 256, 128, 64, and 32 hidden nodes to predict the diagnostic class.

3   Experiments

In this section, we first study the effect of the modular design in Y-Net. We then compare the performance of Y-Net with state-of-the-art methods on tissue-level segmentation as well as on diagnostic classification tasks. For evaluation, we used the breast biopsy dataset [2, 10] that consists of 428 ROIs with classification labels and 58 ROIs with tissue-level labels.

3.1   Segmentation Results

We used residual convolutional blocks (RCB) [6] and efficient spatial pyramid blocks (ESP) [9] for encoding and decoding. Based on the success of PSPNet for segmentation [12], we added pyramid spatial pooling (PSP) blocks for decoding.

Training Details: We split the 58 ROIs into nearly equal training (# 30) and test (# 28) sets. For training, we extracted 384×384 instances with an over-lap of 56 pixels at different image resolutions. We used standard augmentation strategies, such as random flipping, cropping, and resizing, during training. We used a 90:10 ratio for splitting training data into training and validation sets. We trained the network for 100 epochs using SGD with an initial learning rate of 0.0001, decaying the rate by a factor of 2 after 30 epochs. We measured the accuracy of each model using mean Region Intersection over Union (mIOU).

Segmentation Studies: Segmentation results are given in Tables 1 and 2a. We make the following observations:

Feature Sharing: (Table 1a) When features were shared between the encoding blocks at the same spatial level, the accuracy of the network improved by about

Table 1. Ablation studies on Y-Net. In (a), we used $d = 5$. In (b), we used $w = 64$. The experimental settings in (b) were the same as for R3 and R6 in (a).

Row #	Encoding Block ESP	RCB	Decoding Block ESP	RCB	PSP	Feature Sharing Add	Concat	# Params (in million) $w = 64$	mIOU	# Params (in million) $w = 128$	mIOU
R1	✓		✓					0.49	30.39	1.95	35.23
R2	✓		✓			✓		0.49	32.12	1.95	36.19
R3	✓		✓				✓	0.57	34.58	2.25	38.03
R4		✓		✓				1.72	33.05	6.84	37.93
R5		✓		✓		✓		1.72	36.34	6.84	39.21
R6		✓		✓			✓	1.81	38.75	7.16	40.23
R7	✓				✓		✓	0.69	37.12	2.75	44.03
R8		✓			✓		✓	1.91	**41.96**	7.62	**44.19**

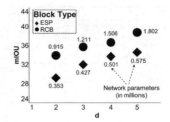

(a) Network width vs. accuracy   (b) Network depth vs. accuracy

2% (R2 and R5) with element-wise addition operations and about 4% (R3 and R6) with concatenation operations for both ESP and RCB blocks. The increase in number of parameters due to concatenation operations was not significant.

Network Depth: (Table 1b) The value of d was varied from 2 to 5 in Y-Net for both ESP and RCB types of convolutional blocks. The accuracy of the network increased with the depth of the network. When we increased d from 2 to 5, the accuracy improved by about 4% while the network parameters were increased by about $1.6\times$ and $1.9\times$ for Y-Net with ESP and RCB respectively. In the following experiments, we used $d = 5$.

Network Width: (Table 1a) When the value of w changed from 64 to 128, the accuracy of Y-Net with ESP (R1–R3) and RCB (R4–R6) increased by about 4%. However, the number of network parameters increased drastically.

PSP as Decoding Block: (Table 1a) Changing the decoding block from ESP and RCB to PSP helped improve the accuracy by about 3%. This is because the pooling operations in PSP modules helped the network learn better global contextual information. Surprisingly, when the value of w increased from 64 to 128, Y-Net with ESP and PSP delivered accuracies similar to PCB and PSP. This is likely due to the increased number of kernels per branch in the ESP blocks, which helps to learn better representations. Y-Net with ESP blocks learns about $3\times$ fewer parameters and is therefore more efficient.

Joint Training: (Table 2a) Training Y-Net jointly for both classification and segmentation tasks dropped the segmentation accuracy by about 1%. This is likely because we trained the network using an instance-based approach and we did not have classification labels at instance-level.

Comparison with State-of-the-Art: (Table 2a) Y-Net outperformed the plain [1] and residual [3] encoder-decoder networks by 7% and 6% respectively. With the same encoding block (RCB) as in [10], Y-Net delivered a similar accuracy while learning $2.85\times$ fewer parameters. We note that Y-Net with ESP and PSP blocks also delivered a similar performance while learning $6.6\times$ fewer parameters than [10] and $2.77\times$ fewer parameters than Y-Net with RCB and

Table 2. Comparison with state-of-the-art methods. seg: training Y-Net only for the segmentation task; joint: joint learning for segmentation and classification tasks.

Network	mIOU	# Params (in million)
Superpixel + SVM [10]	25.8	NA
Badrinarayanan *et al.* [1]	37.6	12.8
Fakhry *et al.* [3]	38.1	12.8
Mehta *et al.* [10]	**44.20**	26.03
YNet (ESP-PSP) - seg	44.03	**2.75**
YNet (RCB-PSP) - seg	44.19	7.62
YNet (ESP-PSP) - joint	43.24	3.91
YNet (RCB-PSP) - joint	43.11	9.11

(a) Segmentation results

Feature Type	Accuracy (in %)
Pathologists (# 44)	70.0
LAB + LBP features [5]	45.0
Segmentation mask [10]	54.5
Saliency map [5]	55.0
Y-Net with different choices	
Segmentation mask	53.25
-background	52.22
-stroma	48.06
Discriminative mask	**62.50**

(b) Diagnostic classification results

PSP blocks. Therefore, the modular architecture of Y-Net allowed us to explore different convolutional blocks with a minimal change in the network topology to find a preferred network design.

3.2   Diagnostic Classification Results

For classification experiments, we split the 428 ROIs in the dataset into almost equal training (# 209) and test (# 219) sets while maintaining the same class distribution across both the sets. We note that the 30 ROIs used for training the segmentation part were part of the training subset during the classification task. The tissue-level segmentation mask and discriminative map were first generated using Y-Net with ESP as encoding blocks and PSP as decoding blocks, which were then used to generate the discriminative segmentation mask. A 44-dimensional feature vector (frequency and co-occurrence histogram) was then extracted from the discriminative mask. These features were used to train a MLP that classifies the ROI into four diagnoses (benign, atypia, DCIS, and invasive cancer).

A summary of results is given in Table 2b. The classification accuracy improved by about 9% when we used discriminative masks instead of segmentation masks. Our method outperformed state-of-the-art methods that use either the segmentation features [10] or the saliency map [5] by a large margin. Our method's 62.5% accuracy is getting closer to the 70% accuracy of trained pathologists in a study [2]. This suggests that the discriminative segmentation masks generated using Y-Net are powerful.

4   Conclusion

The Y-Net architecture achieved good segmentation and diagnostic classification accuracy on a breast biopsy dataset. Y-Net was able to achieve the same segmentation accuracy as state-of-the-art methods while learning fewer parameters. The features generated using discriminative segmentation masks were shown to be powerful and our method was able to attain higher accuracy than state-of-the-art methods. Though we studied breast biopsy images in this paper, we believe that Y-Net can be extended to other medical imaging tasks.

Acknowledgements. Research reported in this publication was supported by the National Cancer Institute awards R01 CA172343, R01 CA140560, and RO1 CA200690. We would also like to thank NVIDIA Corporation for donating the Titan X Pascal GPU used for this research.

References

1. Badrinarayanan, V., Kendall, A., Cipolla, R.: SegNet: a deep convolutional encoder-decoder architecture for image segmentation. TPAMI **39**(12), 2481–2495 (2017)
2. Elmore, J.G., et al.: Diagnostic concordance among pathologists interpreting breast biopsy specimens. JAMA **313**(11), 1122–1132 (2015)
3. Fakhry, A., Zeng, T., Ji, S.: Residual deconvolutional networks for brain electron microscopy image segmentation. IEEE Trans. Med. Imaging **36**(2), 447–456 (2017)
4. Fine, R.E.: Diagnostic Techniques, 2nd edn. B. C. Decker Inc, Ontario (2006)
5. Geçer, B.: Detection and classification of breast cancer in whole slide histopathology images using deep convolutional networks. Ph.D. thesis, Bilkent University (2016)
6. He, K., et al.: Deep residual learning for image recognition. In: CVPR (2016)
7. He, K., et al.: Mask R CNN. In: ICCV (2017)
8. Hou, L., et al.: Patch-based convolutional neural network for whole slide tissue image classification. In: CVPR (2016)
9. Mehta, S., et al.: ESPNet: Efficient Spatial Pyramid of Dilated Convolutions for Semantic Segmentation. arXiv preprint arXiv:1803.06815 (2018)
10. Mehta, S., et al.: Learning to segment breast biopsy whole slide images. In: WACV (2018)
11. Ronneberger, O., Fischer, P., Brox, T.: U-net: Convolutional networks for biomedical image segmentation. In: MICCAI (2015)
12. Zhao, H., et al.: Pyramid scene parsing network. In: CVPR (2017)

Cardiac, Chest and Abdominal Applications: Other Abdominal Applications

AutoDVT: Joint Real-Time Classification for Vein Compressibility Analysis in Deep Vein Thrombosis Ultrasound Diagnostics

Ryutaro Tanno[1,2], Antonios Makropoulos[1], Salim Arslan[1,3], Ozan Oktay[1,3],
Sven Mischkewitz[1], Fouad Al-Noor[1], Jonas Oppenheimer[1],
Ramin Mandegaran[1,4], Bernhard Kainz[1,3(✉)], and Mattias P. Heinrich[1,5]

[1] ThinkSono Ltd., London, UK
{ryutaro,antonios,salim,ozan,sven,fouad,jonas,
ramin,bernhard,mattias}@thinksono.com
[2] Department of Computer Science, University College London, London, UK
[3] Department of Computing, Imperial College London, London, UK
[4] Department of Radiology, Guy's and St Thomas' NHS Foundation Trust,
London, UK
[5] Institute of Medical Informatics, University of Lübeck, Lübeck, Germany

Abstract. We propose a dual-task convolutional neural network (CNN) to fully automate the real-time diagnosis of deep vein thrombosis (DVT). DVT can be reliably diagnosed through evaluation of vascular compressibility at anatomically defined landmarks in streams of ultrasound (US) images. The combined real-time evaluation of these tasks has never been achieved before. As proof-of-concept, we evaluate our approach on two selected landmarks of the femoral vein, which can be identified with high accuracy by our approach. Our CNN is able to identify if a vein fully compresses with a F1 score of more than 90% while applying manual pressure with the ultrasound probe. Fully compressible veins robustly rule out DVT and such patients do not need to be referred to further specialist examination. We have evaluated our method on 1150 5–10 s compression image sequences from 115 healthy volunteers, which results in a data set size of approximately 200k labelled images. Our method yields a theoretical inference frame rate of more than 500 fps and we thoroughly evaluate the performance of 15 possible configurations.

1 Introduction

Deep vein thrombosis (DVT) is caused by the formation of a blood clot within a deep vein, that most commonly takes place in the leg. If left untreated, DVT may lead to serious complications, including pulmonary embolism, which develops when pieces of blood clot break loose into the bloodstream and block vessels in the lungs. Typically, an average of one in a thousand people will be affected by DVT and related conditions during their lifetime. 20% of patients die because of DVT-related complications. Worldwide, approximately 10 million people suffer from DVT or related conditions, estimates suggest that 100,000 Americans alone

© Springer Nature Switzerland AG 2018
A. F. Frangi et al. (Eds.): MICCAI 2018, LNCS 11071, pp. 905–912, 2018.
https://doi.org/10.1007/978-3-030-00934-2_100

die of DVT each year [1]. Patients are referred for DVT-specific tests by front line medical professionals, or following surgery. As the risk of DVT leading to serious complications, including death, is high, development of DVT-focused point-of-care diagnostics is of great importance.

There are two major challenges in diagnosing DVT. First, DVT does not necessarily show evident symptoms and the symptoms may overlap with other less serious conditions, making it impossible to discover DVT without clinical tests. Second, the clinical routine method used to diagnose DVT is a D-dimer blood test [2], which determines the concentration of a small protein fragment in the blood that occurs when a blood clot is degraded by fibrinolysis. The D-dimer blood test can with high certainty rule out a pulmonary embolism (PE), the main DVT-related complication leading to death. However, while this test shows a high sensitivity to PE it has a low specificity to early DVT and returns a high number of false positives. Patients with false-positive D-dimer results are referred to unnecessary further expert examinations, which is costly and time consuming. Furthermore, the consequently introduced workload is very large relative to the number of specialist DVT radiologists.

A more accurate screening method is the manual evaluation of vein compressibility during ultrasound (US) examination of standardised anatomical locations (usually at three specified landmarks on the femoral and popliteal veins [3], C-US method). However, for front line medical professionals, it is currently difficult to assess DVT using US since training is required to navigate to anatomically defined landmarks on the veins where compressibility has to be evaluated.

Contribution: To solve this problem we propose an automatic, point-of-care ultrasound (POCUS) image-based method to make DVT diagnostics accessible for front-line non-specialists. We propose a dual-task convolutional neural network (CNN) that jointly classifies the anatomical landmark plane in the current field-of-view and scores vein compressibility. Thus, the proposed AutoDVT network can intrinsically learn to interpret video data to perform localisation, segmentation, local deformation estimation and classification from weak global labels. Furthermore, it is designed to require few floating point operations to enable real-time performance and its accuracy is thoroughly evaluated on over 100 real, manually annotated ultrasound sequences from DVT examinations.

Related Work: Automated methods for DVT screening using ultrasound have been subject to some research. They can be roughly categorised in image segmentation and tracking approaches. Early approaches used specialised ultrasound probe extensions to provide external tracking and pressure measurements [4]. Vessel segmentation has been achieved using semi-automatic initialisation (seed-points) and heuristic intensity-based algorithms [5]. These approaches need manual intervention, suffer from lack of robustness and real-time capabilities. More recently Doppler flow measurements have been added to heuristically define compressibility parameters derived from vessel segmentation masks [6]. While providing a high sensitivity of over 90% they generally suffer from low specificity around 50% and are not fully automatic.

Machine learning, especially deep learning, has recently shown to be highly useful for ultrasound image analysis [7,8]. End-to-end training from clinical data, high accuracy and real-time performance during model evaluation are essential for tasks like POCUS DVT diagnostics. While vessel localisation has been shown to be achievable through deep learning [9] we propose the first, fully automatic deep learning vessel compressibility evaluation that enables a semantic under-standing of anatomy based on only weakly-labelled ultrasound images.

2   Method

AutoDVT aims to automate the compression-based examination of DVT [10], in which predefined landmarks on the femoral and popliteal veins are examined with regards to their compressibility by manually applying pressure with the US probe. DVT is suspected if any of the landmark veins is not fully compressible, indicating the potential presence of a clot in the vein. We propose AutoDVT, an end-to-end multi-task deep learning approach, which processes a stream of freehand US images in real-time, and simultaneously determines the type of relevant vessel landmark in the current frame and inspects its compressibility during the exam. The synopsis of the proposed method is shown in Fig. 1.

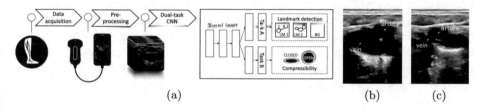

(a)   (b)   (c)

Fig. 1. Overview of the proposed approach (a): A dual-task CNN evaluates a stream of free-hand US frames in real-time and determines landmark type and compressibility. Example for an uncompressed (b) and compressed (c) vein as seen at a landmark position during diagnosis. Note that arteries do not compress during examination as seen in (c).

Preprocessing: Our network is trained on ultrasound sequences acquired with probes from different vendors. This makes inference more robust and more widely applicable, but requires preprocessing. We automatically remove text informa-tion from the frames, pad or crop to a common size of 600×600 pixels, and downsample by a factor of 4 in each dimension to the size of 150×150 pixels.

The **AutoDVT model** is a deep CNN that jointly solves two classification problems: (1) *landmark (LM) detection i.e.* a 3-way classification that discrim-inates, whether a given frame shows either one of the two major landmarks located on the femoral veins (FOVs), called LM1 and LM2 or any other anatomy, which we refer to as BG (background); (2) *open or closed (O/C) classification* *i.e.* a binary classification if the present vein is open or closed. Based on the predictions of the two classification tasks from an ultrasound video, AutoDVT evaluates the vein compressibility of the two key landmarks in FOVs.

There are two important architectural choices that enable AutoDVT to accurately perform these tasks. Firstly, the network operates on a stack of consecutive frames and takes temporal information in a sequence into account through 3D convolutions. The network is thereby able to learn motion and deformation features, which enhances the temporal consistency of the predicted landmarks and open/closed state labels, particularly in the presence of noise and artifacts, ubiquitous issues with handheld US probes. Secondly, we employ a multi-task learning approach that shares the majority of convolutional layers across landmark localisation and vein compressibility. It branches out into task specific layers only for the last layers (see Fig. 1). This enables us to leverage sequences with partially missing labels (i.e. only for one task) and increases the amount of overall training data. Our joint training therefore improves generalisation via inductive transfer, where cues from one task regularise and improve the representation for another related task [11].

The details of the shared layers and task-specific layers are given in Table 1. All convolution layers (both 3D and 2D) are followed by rectified linear (ReLU) non-linearity. We apply batch-normalisation after each convolution for improved convergence and accuracy. In the task specific branches, dropout is used for every convolution layer with a rate of 0.5 for regularisation. For each task, the feature maps of the last convolution layers are spatially averaged, and fed into a linear classifier with softmax output. We use relatively few feature map channels and an aggressive progression of strided convolutions to limit both network capacity and floating point operations. This enables us to avoid overfitting and realise realtime performance for inference.

Table 1. Million floating point operations per second (MFlops, fused multiply-adds) performance for each layer in our network model and Global average pooling (GAP).

Layer	Shared layers					Task-specific layers			
	Conv3d	Conv3d	Conv3d	Conv3d	Conv2d	Conv2d	Conv2d	GAP	Linear
Channels	32	32	64	64	128	128	128	128	#classes
Kernel	$3 \times 3 \times 3$	$3 \times 3 \times 3$	$3 \times 3 \times 3$	$3 \times 3 \times 3$	3×3	3×3	3×3	2×2	1×1
Stride	(2,2,1)	(2,2,1)	(2,2,1)	(2,2,1)	(1,1)	(1,1)	(1,1)	N/A	N/A
Size	$150 \times 150 \times 9$	$74 \times 74 \times 7$	$36 \times 36 \times 5$	$17 \times 17 \times 3$	8×8	6×6	4×4	2×2	1
MFlops	23.7	107.5	5.3	2.4	2.7	2.4	0.6	0.1	0.0

Model Training. Unless otherwise stated, we employ a common protocol for the training of networks and determine best performing parameters experimentally. The loss is defined as the sum of the cross-entropy from O/C and LM classification, plus the L2 weight norm (weight decay) with a factor of 10^{-5}. We optimise the parameters by minimising the loss using ADAM for 50 epochs with an initial learning rate of 10^{-3}, exponential decay every epoch, and a momentum parameter $\beta = [0.9, 0.999]$. ADAM was chosen because it is known for its stable and efficient optimisation performance. Values of β are chosen close to 1 to provide robustness to sparse gradients. The model from the last epoch is used for evaluation. We adopt a data-augmentation scheme where training images are randomly scaled, rotated, horizontally flipped and intensity-augmented.

3 Data and Experiments

Data Collection and Annotation: We have trained our model on manually labelled data from 115 healthy volunteers. Images have been acquired using a Clarius L7 Handheld Wireless Ultrasound Scanner, a Phillips iU22, a GE Logiq E9, and a Toshiba Aplio 500. The dataset is comprised of 1150 videos of length 5–10 s. Each sequence contains between 100 to 200 frames. In this paper we focus on landmark labels from a subset of 240 annotated sequences from the groin area. In each sequence, images have been labelled by 25 skilled annotators (medical students) and one radiologist as one of four landmark labels. We sample background from random frames without labels in these 240 videos and from additional 340 sequences that have been acquired from areas surrounding the femoral vein. We use two of the four available locations, thus, landmarks are located at the saphenofemoral junction (LM1) and great saphenous vein (LM2). Open/close binary labels are manually obtained for every frame by labelling and counting the number of vein pixels, i.e. measuring the area and a defined threshold. The O/C labels have been reviewed by an experienced radiologist. 60% of the volunteer examinations have been used for training, 20% for validation and 20% for testing. We split the data on subject level and not per sequence to avoid unfair testing.

Classification Performance Experiments: We evaluate the predictive performance of AutoDVT in O/C and LM image classification (O/C, LM1, LM2 vs. background BG). We measure the performance on standard metrics used for classification tasks: precision, recall and F1 score, and perform an ablation study to quantify the effects of the main three proposed features of our approach: data-augmentation, modelling temporal information with 3D convolutions and dual-task formulation. Table 2 summarises the results of this analysis.

To demonstrate the benefits of the dual-task architecture of AutoDVT, we constructed two task-specific baseline networks for O/C classification and LM classification by only retaining the shared layers and the individual branch for the chosen task. The two baseline networks have the same target classes for respective tasks as the AutoDVT model, enabling a direct evaluation of the regularisation effect gained from shared representation.

We also assessed the effect of modelling temporal information on classification performance. We implemented variants of the dual-task AutoDVT architecture and the task-specific networks in which every 3D convolution layer is replaced by a 2D convolution with appropriately increased number of kernels (keeping overall numbers of parameters the same).

4 Results and Discussion

Table 2 shows that the best average F1 scores (the harmonic mean of precision and recall) of 91% and 78% are achieved by the dual-task model with +Aug. +Temp. on O/C and LM classification, respectively. It is evident that our dual-task approach outperforms the single-task baselines (+Aug. +Temp.), in particular for the clinically most relevant compressibility analysis (O/C).

It is also clear that analysing a stack of nine consecutive frames with 3D convolutions (denoted by +Temp.) improves the F1 score compared to a static 2D image analysis, which also results in temporally more consistent classification in the presence of artefacts and noise. This indicates that the temporal network alleviates these challenges by augmenting the missing information using temporal context from the previous frames and estimates useful deformation features.

Table 2. Average performance of different models with best results in bold. +Temp. denotes the integration of spatial-temporal convolutions on nine frames (*i.e.* 3D convolutions) and +Aug. denotes the use of data augmentation during training. For single-task baselines, the results for two task-specific networks (one for O/C classification and the other for LM classification) are shown in each row of the table. AutoDVT corresponds to the dual-task model +Aug.+Temp.

	Precision				Recall				F1 score			
	O/C	LM1	LM2	BG	O/C	LM1	LM2	BG	O/C	LM1	LM2	BG
Separate models	0.78	**0.70**	0.54	0.94	0.92	0.60	0.35	**0.97**	0.84	0.64	0.43	0.95
+Aug.	0.85	0.63	0.53	0.93	0.88	0.86	**0.67**	0.94	0.88	0.73	0.59	0.96
+Aug.+Temp.	0.85	0.69	**0.63**	0.96	0.92	0.82	0.61	0.96	0.88	0.75	**0.62**	0.96
Dual-task models	0.77	0.41	0.41	0.97	**0.97**	**0.91**	0.34	0.90	0.86	0.57	0.37	0.93
+Aug.	0.83	0.66	0.53	0.95	0.92	0.68	0.41	0.96	0.88	0.67	0.46	0.96
+Aug.+Temp.	**0.89**	0.67	0.56	**0.97**	0.92	0.87	0.64	0.96	**0.91**	**0.76**	0.60	**0.97**

Runtime Performance: Table 1 shows the number of million floating point operations (MFlops) for AutoDVT for each layer. Current mobile GPUs can provide up to 384 GFlops (e.g. PowerVR GT7600 Plus), while AutoDVT only requires 148 MFlops, which would result in a theoretical computational overhead of 0.002 s when accounting for approximately 60% overhead for memory transfers and caching. Practically the frame-rate is limited by the image acquisition rate of the ultrasound probe, which is ~20 fps. Thus, using our K80 GPU yields an application performance of ~20 fps and ~14 fps when using a Xeon E5-2686v4 CPU without GPU. We observed real-time frame rates for the implementations of AutoDVT model in two deep-learning frameworks, Theano and PyTorch. The dual-task architecture requires 50% fewer computations than running two separate task-specific networks (which amounts to 290 MFlops vs. 148 MFlops of AutoDVT).

Visual Exploration of Results: We used Gradient-weighted Class Activation Mapping (Grad-CAM) [12] to gain insight into which areas are considered by AutoDVT to make predictions. Figure 2 shows the obtained saliency maps, which qualitatively confirms that the model focuses on the relevant anatomy and makes the correct O/C and LM classifications in the example frames.

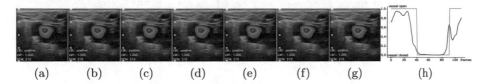

(a)   (b)   (c)   (d)   (e)   (f)   (g)   (h)

Fig. 2. Visualisation of saliency maps of AutoDVT (MT+A.+T.) for O/C classification, obtained by applying Grad-CAM [12] to sample frames in a compression sequence at LM1. The super-imposed heatmaps (red is high, blue is low) indicate that AutoDVT prediction is most excited by the anatomically relevant areas around the femoral vein. (a–c) shows uncompressed state, (d, e) show compressed state, (f, g) show release of manual pressure. (h) shows a summary for a random example compression sequence with the predicted vessel compression state in red and the ground truth label in green. Note that, when the vessel is entirely closed, i.e. invisible, our method predicts the 'closed' state from spatio-temporal information and other structures in the image.

Limitations: This work focuses on DVT diagnosis in the groin area. Further evaluation will be required to confirm similar performance for all possible landmarks used during DVT examination especially in the area of the popliteal veins. Like most deep learning methods, domain shift is still a challenge despite having trained on data from four different devices. We are aware of the option to use Doppler ultrasound as additional source of information. However, the aim of this work is to make DVT diagnostics available for point-of-care applications. Doppler reduces the image acquisition frame rate significantly, needs to be adjusted by an experienced operator and does not necessarily increase detection rate of asymptomatic DVT [10]. Furthermore, not all POCUS transducers support Doppler imaging. A pure image-based approach is therefore desirable for POCUS DVT diagnostics and potential applications in ODE countries.

Conclusion: We have proposed a novel dual-task CNN to assist the real-time diagnosis of DVT. Our approach enables non-expert health practitioners to reliably support DVT diagnosis using machine learning guidance. Previous work [6] shows that 100% sensitivity and specificity can be reached for semi-automatic DVT classification and that also venous pressure can be determined [13]. Our approach can automate several of the currently required manual steps to achieve this level of diagnostic accuracy on a range of different devices. AutoDVT evaluates vascular compressibility at two anatomically classified landmark positions on the femoral vein. Landmark detection and compression state inference can be combined in a joint dual-path network and the tasks can be trained end-to-end. Our approach shows promising performance at accuracies greater than 90%, which is well within the expected performance of expert examinations [3]. Three architectural choices: joint learning of open/close discrimination and landmark detection; data augmentation and careful restriction of model capacity as well as spatio-temporal convolutions, enabled substantial improvements in accuracy compared to baseline models. Our approach provides real-time performance and the potential to be used directly on mobile devices for POCUS diagnostics with significant impact on patient care and health care costs. In future work, we will evaluate our method on a more comprehensible dataset including patients with pathologies and generalise landmark classification to all relevant areas along the femoral vein.

References

1. Beckman, M.G., et al.: Venous thromboembolism: a public health concern. Am. J. Prev. Med. **38**(4, Supplement), S495–S501 (2010)
2. Stein, P.D., et al.: D-dimer for the exclusion of acute venous thrombosis and pulmonary embolism: a systematic review. Ann. Intern. Med. **140**(8), 589–602 (2004)
3. Schellong, S.M., et al.: Complete compression ultrasonography of the leg veins as a single test for the diagnosis of deep vein thrombosis. Thromb. Haemost. **89**(2), 228–234 (2003)
4. Guerrero, J., et al.: System for deep venous thrombosis detection using objective compression measures. IEEE Trans. Biomed. Eng. **53**(5), 845–854 (2006)
5. Friedland, N., Adam, D.: Automatic ventricular cavity boundary detection from sequential ultrasound images using simulated annealing. IEEE Trans. Med. Imaging **8**(4), 344–353 (1989)
6. Guerrero, J., et al.: Deep venous thrombosis identification from analysis of ultrasound data. Int. J. Comput. Assist. Radiol. Surg. **10**(12), 1963–1971 (2015)
7. Baumgartner, C.F., et al.: SonoNet: real-time detection and localisation of fetal standard scan planes in freehand ultrasound. IEEE Trans. Med. Imaging **36**(11), 2204–2215 (2017)
8. Prevost, R., Salehi, M., Sprung, J., Bauer, R., Wein, W.: Deep learning for sensorless 3D freehand ultrasound imaging. In: Descoteaux, M., Maier-Hein, L., Franz, A., Jannin, P., Collins, D.L., Duchesne, S. (eds.) MICCAI 2017. LNCS, vol. 10434, pp. 628–636. Springer, Cham (2017). https://doi.org/10.1007/978-3-319-66185-8_71
9. Smistad, E., Løvstakken, L.: Vessel detection in ultrasound images using deep convolutional neural networks. In: Carneiro, G. (ed.) LABELS/DLMIA-2016. LNCS, vol. 10008, pp. 30–38. Springer, Cham (2016). https://doi.org/10.1007/978-3-319-46976-8_4
10. Lensing, A., et al.: A comparison of compression ultrasound with color doppler ultrasound for the diagnosis of symptomless postoperative deep vein thrombosis. Arch. Intern. Med. **157**(7), 765–768 (1997)
11. Caruana, R.: Multitask learning: a knowledge-based source of inductive bias. In: International Conference on Machine Learning (ICML) (1993)
12. Selvaraju, R.R., et al.: Grad-Cam: visual explanations from deep networks via gradient-based localization. CoRR abs/1610.02391 v3 **7**(8) (2016)
13. Crimi, A., et al.: Automatic measurement of venous pressure using B-mode ultrasound. IEEE Trans. Biomed. Eng. **63**(2), 288–299 (2016)

MRI Measurement of Placental Perfusion and Fetal Blood Oxygen Saturation in Normal Pregnancy and Placental Insufficiency

Rosalind Aughwane[1,2], Magdalena Sokolska[3], Alan Bainbridge[3],
David Atkinson[4], Giles Kendall[2], Jan Deprest[2,5], Tom Vercauteren[1,6],
Anna L. David[2,5,7], Sébastien Ourselin[1,6], and Andrew Melbourne[1,6(✉)]

[1] Department of Medical Physics and Biomedical Engineering,
University College London, London, UK
a.melbourne@ucl.ac.uk
[2] Institute for Women's Health, University College London, London, UK
[3] Medical Physics, UCH, London, UK
[4] Centre for Medical Imaging, UCL, London, UK
[5] University Hospital KU Leuven, Leuven, Belgium
[6] BMEIS, Kings College London, London, UK
[7] NIHR University College London Hospitals Biomedical Research Centre,
London, UK

Abstract. The placenta is essential for successful pregnancy outcome. Inadequate placenta development leads to poor placental perfusion and placental insufficiency, responsible for one third of antenatal stillbirths. Current imaging modalities provide poor clinical assessment of placental perfusion and pregnancy outcome. In this work we propose a technique to estimate the vascular properties of retro-placenta myometrial and placental perfusion. The fetal blood saturation is a relative unknown, thus we describe a method to simultaneously estimate the fetal blood volume in addition to the fetal blood T2 relaxation time from which we can estimate this parameter. This information may prove useful for predicting if and when a placenta will fail, and thus when a small baby must be delivered to have the best neurological outcome. We report differences in vascular compartments and saturation values observed between 5 normal pregnancies, and two complicated by placental insufficiency.

1 Introduction

The placenta is a unique organ, being perfused simultaneously by two or more individuals. Assessing placental perfusion is key to understanding and diagnosing placental insufficiency (PI), which is a significant cause of morbidity and mortality, accounting for one third of antenatal, and one quarter of intrapartum stillbirths in high income countries [1]. PI occurs when the maternal spiral arteries fail to remodel normally in early pregnancy. This leads to inadequate maternal

© Springer Nature Switzerland AG 2018
A. F. Frangi et al. (Eds.): MICCAI 2018, LNCS 11071, pp. 913–920, 2018.
https://doi.org/10.1007/978-3-030-00934-2_101

perfusion of the placenta, the fetus becomes hypoxic affecting cognitive development and if not delivered prematurely may ultimately die.

Evaluating placental function using magnetic resonance imaging (MRI) is a growing research area [2–4]. Several MRI modalities have been investigated to monitor placental blood flow and function, each with their own advantages and disadvantages [4]. Diffusion weighted imaging (DWI) is becoming increasingly widespread in abdominal and placental imaging. When combined with the intra-voxel incoherent motion model (IVIM [5]) of blood flow in capillaries, it provides a non-invasive method of measuring tissue properties relating to flow and perfusion. T2 relaxometry, made possible by the acquisition of images with variable echo-time, provides additional information on the static tissue composition, and T2 relaxation times have been shown to be significantly shorter in placenta insufficiency [3]. Both techniques have been proposed for placental imaging [2,3] but how best to measure the microstructural and microvascular properties of placental tissue remains an open question. The retro-placental myometrium is the closest tissue to the placenta from which to estimate maternal perfusion and blood relaxation time without the influence of signal from fetal perfusion, which may also give interesting information on the pathophysiology of PI. We also explore the theory that fitting fetal blood T2 will allow us to estimate fetal blood saturation, and that this may be a valuable measurement of placental function.

2   Methods

Data. The study was approved by the local research ethics committee and all participants gave written informed consent. Five women in mid-pregnancy (between $28 + 4$ to $34 + 0$ gestational weeks) with normal pregnancies, and two complicated by placental insufficiency ($25 + 0$ and $27 + 2$ gestational weeks) were included. Obstetric ultrasound confirmed normal fetal growth ($>$10th centile) and Dopplers in the control group. Ultrasound in the PI group showed estimated fetal weight $<$1st centile, and abnormal fetal umbilical artery Doppler.

Imaging was performed on 1.5T Siemens Avanto, at 7 b-values (**b**) (0, 50, 100, 150, 200, 400, 600 s.mm^{-2}) and ten echo times (**t**) (81, 90, 96, 120, 150, 180, 210, 240, 270, 300 ms). All echo times were acquired at b-value 0, to allow T2 fitting, and all b-values at **t** = 96 ms. In addition, data was acquired at b-value 50, 200 for **t** = (81, 90, 120, 150, 180, 210, 240) ms. Voxel resolution was $1.9 \times 1.9 \times 6$ mm. To minimise the effect of motion we first used an open-source non-rigid registration routine to align all images. Masks were then drawn manually within the tissue bounadry for the placenta and retro-placental myometrium in multiple slices.

DECIDE - Multi-compartment Placenta Modelling. The Diffusion-rElaxation Combined Imaging for Detailed Placental Evaluation (DECIDE) model is a multi-compartment model of placental perfusion that combines T2 relaxometry and diffusion weighted imaging [6]. Intercapillary fetal blood has high pseudo-diffusivity, d^*, and long T2 relaxation time, $T_2^{fb} = 1/r_2^{fb}$ and volume fraction f. Maternal blood with volume fraction ν, is in the intervillous space, as opposed to intravascular, and therefore has lower diffusivity d, and slow relaxation r_2^{mb}. Finally, the remaining signal from the tissue has low diffusivity d, and rapid relaxation, r_2^t, associated with dense tissue.

Extending the DECIDE Model to Fit T2 Relaxation Times. Estimating T2 relaxation values from the literature as in [6] may add bias to the model, as both maternal and fetal blood characteristics are different from the normal, healthy adult. It is normal for pregnant women to have a physiological anaemia, and therefore reduced haematocrit. This may affect the T2 relaxation time of blood, which is known to be sensitive to haematocrit and oxygen saturation [7]. We adapt the DECIDE model [6] to compare typical T2 values of the maternal and fetal blood [7]. Fetal blood has higher hematocrit and lower oxygen saturation than adult blood. Deoxygenated fetal blood in the umbilical artery (supplying the placenta) at 30 weeks gestational age is estimated to be 65% saturated, and oxygenated blood returning to the fetus in the umbilical vein is estimated to be 85% saturated [8]. This is much lower than adult saturations of 97–100%.

Model-Fitting Routine. We develop a bespoke fitting routine for this data to improve model-fitting performance with two key features:
ROI Parameter Initialisation. In the presense of noisy data, non-linear models with several free parameters can be prone to fitting to local minima. We avoid this situation by making use of model-fitting results obtained from average ROI signal curves. This has the effect of boosting the signal-to-noise ratio, yielding robust ROI parameter estimates from the average signal curve which make reasonable starting estimates for fitting at the voxel-level within the ROI. We thus initialise our non-linear fitting routines with parameter estimates from larger placental and myometrial regions of interest.

Fitting of Independent Parameters. Models often contain parameters which are dependent only weakly on some parts of the underlying data. A good example of this is in diffusion MRI where ADC measurements can be robustly obtained from high b-value mono-exponential data entirely separate from low b-value perfusion effects. This technique is a common approach for IVIM model-fitting and we make use of this constraint when fitting our data. We also make use of this technique when applying the standard IVIM model to both the myometrial and placenta data sets.

Myometrium Model-Fitting. The myometrium is maternal-perfused, highly-vascular, muscular tissue and is not expected to have a significant pooled-fluid compartment. Thus it is reasonable to assume that there are two-compartments representing an IVIM-like blood pool at high oxygen saturation and a dense tissue space of much lower T2 (Eq. 1).

$$S(b,t) = S_0 \left[f e^{-\mathbf{b}d^* - \mathbf{t}r_2^{mb}} + (1-f)e^{-\mathbf{b}d - \mathbf{t}r_2^t} \right] \tag{1}$$

1. *ADC d fitting.* We apply log-linear fitting of both whole-ROI and voxel-wise d values to the data with b-value $b > 100$ for fixed echo-time.

2. *Estimation of myometrial maternal blood T2.* Equation 1 is fitted to the high
   SNR average signal curve from the whole myometrial ROI. Average whole-
   placenta estimates of f, d^*, r_2^{mb} and r_2^t are obtained. ADC, d is constrained as
   in step 1.
3. *Estimation of myometrial volume fractions.* For each voxel we fix the local value
   of the ADC (step 1) and obtain non-linear fits of f, d^*, r_2^{mb} and r_2^t, initialised
   with the global tissue estimates from step 2.

Placenta Model-Fitting. We apply the DECIDE model to fit placental tissue
(Eq. 2) with variables as defined above.

$$S(b,t) = S_0\left[fe^{-\mathbf{b}d^*-\mathbf{t}r_2^{fb}} + (1-f)e^{-\mathbf{b}d}\left(\nu e^{-\mathbf{t}r_2^{mb}} + (1-\nu)e^{-\mathbf{t}r_2^t}\right)\right] \qquad (2)$$

We apply the same fitting approach described as for the myometrium, modiying
step 2 accordingly so that we may fit fetal blood relaxation r_2^{fb}. r_2^{mb} and r_2^t are held
fixed at literature values of $(240\,\mathrm{ms})^{-1}$ and $(46\,\mathrm{ms})^{-1}$ respectively, whilst all other
parameters are fitted.

Estimation of *in Utero* Fetal Blood Oxygen Saturation. Fitting an emperi-
cal curve to the data in [7] of the form $a/(1+e^{-b(s-c)})$ enables us to estimate oxygen
saturation values for known T2. Fitted parameters for this curve, given fractional
saturation s, are a $= 386\,\mathrm{ms}$, b $= 0.36$, c $= 0.88$. Thus we are able to find approximate saturation values for each known T2 blood pool (Fig. 4).

3   Results

DECIDE Fitting of Retro-placental Myometrium and Placenta.   One
case was excluded from the control dataset due to motion artefact as the
myometrium is very thin and therefore sensitive to motion. Figure 1 shows histograms of the voxel-by-voxel fit for the IVIM and DECIDE models of the
myometrium in the four included control cases. Table 1 shows the mean and standard deviation for f, d^*, d, T2 maternal blood and T2 myometrium using the IVIM
and DECIDE fit. These values are plausible given that myometrium is very vascular in normal pregnancy [9]. Mean T2 of maternal blood was $202.17 \pm 92.98\,\mathrm{ms}$,
and mean T2 of myometrium $123.63 \pm 6.71\,\mathrm{ms}$. Given that T2 blood was in keeping with the literature value of $240\,\mathrm{ms}$, the maternal blood T2 was fixed at $240\,\mathrm{ms}$
for all subsequent placental DECIDE fits.

Figure 2 shows histograms of the voxel-by-voxel fit for the placenta for the five
control cases. Table 1 shows the mean ($\pm$ standard deviation) for f, d^*, d, and T2
fetal blood using the IVIM and DECIDE model fit. Mean T2 of fetal blood was
$164.86 \pm 26.66\,\mathrm{ms}$.

**Comparing Control and Placental Insufficiency Myometrium and Pla-
centa.** Figure 3 shows histograms for the voxel-wise fit of all control and PI data
for the myometrium and the placenta. Table 1 presents control and PI mean parameter estimates of f, d^*, d, ν, and T2 relaxation times. Both the IVIM and DECIDE

Table 1. Mean ($\pm$ standard deviation) values for the voxel wise fit of all included datasets (n = 4 control, n = 2 PI) for myometrial and placental IVIM and DECIDE.

	Myometrium					Placenta			
	IVIM Fit (mean ($\pm$ SD))		T2 IVIM Fit (mean ($\pm$ SD))			IVIM Fit (mean ($\pm$ SD))		DECIDE Fit (mean ($\pm$ SD))	
Parameter	Control	PI	Control	PI	Parameter	Control	PI	Control	PI
f	0.480 (0.087)	0.285 (0.176)	0.443 (0.008)	0.149 (0.031)	f	0.260 (0.019)	0.240 (0.024)	0.218 (0.028)	0.293 (0.083)
d* (mm^2s^{-1})	0.051 (0.013)	0.048 (0.018)	0.044 (0.008)	0.037 (0.008)	d* (mm^2s^{-1})	0.034 (0.003)	0.044 (0.008)	0.073 (0.097)	0.060 (0.022)
d (mm^2s^{-1})	0.0016 (0.0003)	0.0017 (0.0001)	0.0016 (0.0003)	0.0017 (0.0001)	d (mm^2s^{-1})	0.0017 (0.0001)	0.0014 (0.0001)	0.0017 (0.0001)	0.0014 (0.0001)
T2 Blood (ms)			202.17 (92.98)	243.78 (74.32)	v			0.314 (0.068)	0.288 (0.028)
T2 Myometrium (ms)			123.63 (6.71)	87.93 (24.24)	T2 Fetal Blood (ms)			164.86 (26.66)	136.90 (42.05)

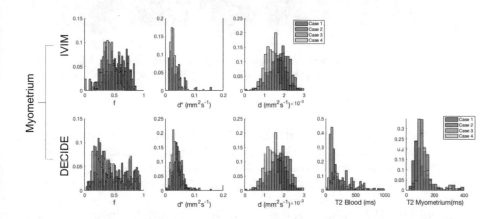

Fig. 1. Voxel-wise parameter histograms of maternal blood and myometrium.

mean f for myometrium, representing maternal perfusion, is lower in PI compared to control cases. Placental d was lower in the PI compared to control placenta with both models. Placental IVIM f was lower in PI compared to control, whereas the DECIDE f was higher in PI compared to control. However, in the DECIDE fit ν was lower in PI compared to control, and the T2 of fetal blood was also lower in PI.

Estimating Fetal Blood Saturation. Figure 4 shows the combined control and PI histograms for estimated fetal blood saturation, based on voxel-wise fetal blood T2 fit. Mean control fetal blood saturation was $69.14 \pm 20.12\%$, whereas mean PI fetal blood saturation was $46.36 \pm 31.71\%$.

4 Discussion

This work investigates MR imaging of placental perfusion, and the potential to estimate fetal blood saturation non-invasively for the first time. The model divides the

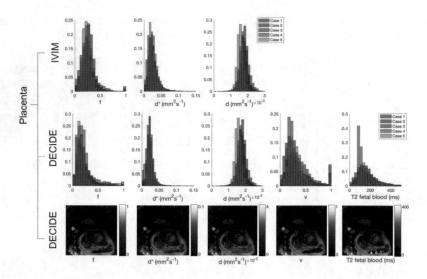

Fig. 2. Voxel-wise placenta parameter histograms for the five control dataset, showing f, d^*, d, ν and T2 of fetal blood. Row one; IVIM model, Row two; DECIDE model, with free fitting for fetal blood T2.

placental signal into three compartments, relating to maternal and fetal perfusion of the placenta and the placental tissue. This work extends this model by fitting T2 relaxation values for fetal and maternal blood alongside data from [7] to estimate blood saturation showing differences between pregnancies complicated by PI and controls.

Maternal blood T2 relaxation time was investigated within the retro-placental myometrium. This was chosen as it is a simplified model, only needing to fit two compartments. In addition, this is likely to be a relevant tissue in investigating placental function, as differences in spiral artery perfusion are known to be an important factor in developing PI. Both the IVIM and DECIDE model gave high value for f and d^*, which is feasible given that the myometrium is highly vascular in normal pregnancy, providing low resistant, high volume perfusion to the placenta. The DECIDE model found a mean maternal blood T2 relaxation time of $(202.17 \pm 92.98\,\text{ms})$, and a mean tissue T2 relaxation time of $123.63 \pm 6.71\,\text{ms}$. These relaxation times are consistent with those in the literature [9].

In the placenta, the DECIDE model gave a lower f value than the IVIM model (0.218 DECIDE vs 0.260 IVIM). This was expected given that previous work in liver has shown addition of T2 to the IVIM model reduces the value of f [5]. There was a significant ν fraction in placenta, which is expected, given that it is thought to represent maternal placental perfusion. Fetal blood T2 was lower than the value attributed to adult blood in the literature (240 ms), however given the dependence of T2 relaxation time on haematrocrit and saturation, which are known to be different in the fetus, it is a feasible value.

When comparing control and PI myometrial parameters, f was lower in PI compared to control cases. This is expected given the pathophysiology of PI, with minimal spiral artery remodelling, and therefore reduced placental perfusion.

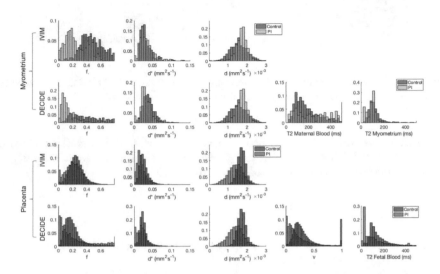

Fig. 3. Combined voxel-wise parameter histograms for the control and PI data. The first two rows show the myometrial data for maternal blood and myometrium, using the IVIM model (row 1) and DECIDE model (row 2). The last two rows show the placenta data using the IVIM model (row 1) and DECIDE model (row 2).

When comparing control and PI placental parameters, f was reduced in PI compared to control placenta with the IVIM model, but not the DECIDE model. This is unexpected, given that histology has shown reduced feto-placental vascular density in PI. We hypothesise this may be due to f measuring flow, rather than volume, which may be increased within the vasoconstricted fetal vasculature. ν was reduced in PI compared to control cases, in keeping with the myometrial results. The T2 of fetal blood within the placenta is also reduced in PI compared to control cases, which related to a reduced fetal blood saturation in PI compared to control cases. The reduction in fetal blood saturation in PI is reasonable, given the poor placental function. What is particularly interesting is the histogram, showing a peak in PI at 10–20% saturation. The control data histogram shows little data with a saturation less than 50%. This suggests a greater degree of heterogeneity within the PI placenta, with areas of poorly oxygenated tissue, which may relate to areas of poor maternal perfusion.

In conclusion, we present an extension of the three compartment DECIDE model, with T2 blood and tissue fitting. We applied this to a cohort of control and PI myometrial and placental image data, and showed differences in parameters that may have potential to measure placental pathology. We then presented the use of fetal blood T2 relaxation values for estimating fetal blood saturation non-invasively for the first time *in utero*.

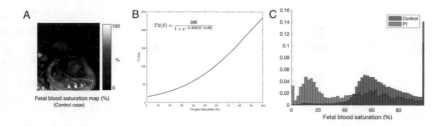

Fig. 4. (A) Parametric map of estimated oxygen saturation [7]. (B) T2/Sat curve (C) Histogram of fetal blood saturation distribution in the placenta.

Acknowledgements. We would like to acknowledge the Wellcome Trust (210182/ Z/18/Z, 101957/Z/13/Z), the National Institute for Health Research (NIHR), the EPSRC (NS/A000027/1) and the Radiological Research Trust.

References

1. Lawn, J.E., et al.: Stillbirths: where? when? why? how to make the data count? Lancet **377**(9775), 1448–1463 (2011)
2. Derwig, I., et al.: Association of placental perfusion, as assessed by magnetic resonance imaging and uterine artery doppler ultrasound, and its relationship to pregnancy outcome. Placenta **34**(10), 885–891 (2013)
3. Derwig, I., et al.: Association of placental t2 relaxation times and uterine artery doppler ultrasound measures of placental blood flow. Placenta **34**(6), 474–479 (2013)
4. Siauve, N., et al.: Functional imaging of the human placenta with magnetic resonance. Am. J. Obstet. Gynecol. **213**(4 Suppl), S103–S114 (2015)
5. Jerome, N., et al.: Extended T2-IVIM model for correction of te dependence of pseudo-diffusion volume fraction in clinical diffusion-weighted magnetic resonance imaging. Phys. Med. Biol. **61**(24), N667 (2016)
6. Melbourne, A., et al.: Decide: diffusion-relaxation combined imaging for detailed placental evaluation. In: ISMRM (2017)
7. Portnoy, S., Osmond, M., Zhu, M.Y., Seed, M., Sled, J.G., Macgowan, C.K.: Relaxation properties of human umbilical cord blood at 1.5 Tesla. Magn. Reson. Med. **77**(4), 1678–1690 (2017)
8. Siggaard-Andersen, O., Huch, R.: The oxygen status of fetal blood. Acta Anaesthesiol. Scand. **39**(s107), 129–135 (1995)
9. De Bazelaire, C.M., Duhamel, G.D., Rofsky, N.M., Alsop, D.C.: MR imaging relaxation times of abdominal and pelvic tissues measured in vivo at 3.0 T: preliminary results. Radiology **230**(3), 652–659 (2004)

Automatic Lacunae Localization in Placental Ultrasound Images via Layer Aggregation

Huan Qi[1](✉), Sally Collins[2], and J. Alison Noble[1]

[1] Institute of Biomedical Engineering (IBME), University of Oxford, Oxford, UK
huan.qi@eng.ox.ac.uk

[2] Nuffield Department of Women's and Reproductive Health, University of Oxford, Oxford, UK

Abstract. Accurate localization of structural abnormalities is a precursor for image-based prenatal assessment of adverse conditions. For clinical screening and diagnosis of abnormally invasive placenta (AIP), a life-threatening obstetric condition, qualitative and quantitative analysis of ultrasonic patterns correlated to placental lesions such as placental lacunae (PL) is challenging and time-consuming to perform even for experienced sonographers. There is a need for automated placental lesion localization that does not rely on expensive human annotations such as detailed manual segmentation of anatomical structures. In this paper, we investigate PL localization in 2D placental ultrasound images. First, we demonstrate the effectiveness of generating confidence maps from weak dot annotations in localizing PL as an alternative to expensive manual segmentation. Then we propose a layer aggregation structure based on iterative deep aggregation (IDA) for PL localization. Models with this structure were evaluated with 10-fold cross-validations on an AIP database (containing 3,440 images with 9,618 labelled PL from 23 AIP and 11 non-AIP participants). Experimental results demonstrate that the model with the proposed structure yielded the highest mean average precision (mAP $= 35.7\%$), surpassing all other baseline models (32.6%, 32.2%, 29.7%). We argue that features from shallower stages can contribute to PL localization more effectively using the proposed structure. To our knowledge, this is the first successful application of machine learning to placental lesion analysis and has the potential to be adapted for other clinical scenarios in breast, liver, and prostate cancer imaging.

1 Introduction

Abnormally invasive placenta (AIP) refers to a life-threatening obstetric condition in which the placenta adheres to or invades into the uterine wall. Depending on the degree of adherence or invasion, any attempt to forcibly remove the

Electronic supplementary material The online version of this chapter (https://doi.org/10.1007/978-3-030-00934-2_102) contains supplementary material, which is available to authorized users.

© Springer Nature Switzerland AG 2018
A. F. Frangi et al. (Eds.): MICCAI 2018, LNCS 11071, pp. 921–929, 2018.
https://doi.org/10.1007/978-3-030-00934-2_102

embedded tissue may lead to catastrophic maternal hemorrhage during child-birth [1]. Ultrasonography is widely used to identify women at high risk of AIP. However, recent population studies have shown that the rate of successful prenatal diagnosis of AIP remains unsatisfactory: merely between half and two-thirds [2,3]. In a recent review [1], Jauniaux *et al.* evaluated the pathophysiology of different ultrasound signs associated with AIP to better understand their relevance to prenatal screening and diagnosis, among which placental lacunae are of particular interest. Placental lacunae (PL) are sonolucent spaces within the placenta that appear to be randomly distributed with irregular shapes and have unpredictable size and number in a placental ultrasound image (Fig. 1(a)). PL occur in almost all pregnancy. However, as shown in Fig. 1, numerous, large, and irregular PL are more likely to occur in AIP cases than in non-AIP cases [4].

The contributions of this paper are twofold. First, we introduce an automatic method that generates confidence maps from expert dot annotations for subsequent training, as an alternative to detailed yet expensive manual segmentation of PL. This method harnesses over-segmentation techniques to generate Gaussian-like confidence maps centered at PL by taking into account local information, such as size, shape, and texture of PL. Second, we compare three layer aggregation structures: deep supervision (DS), feature pyramid network (FPN) and iterative deep aggregation (IDA) and then propose an IDA-based fully convolutional network (FCN) for PL localization in 2D grayscale placental ultrasound images. We demonstrate its effectiveness in localizing PL by running experiments on an AIP database.

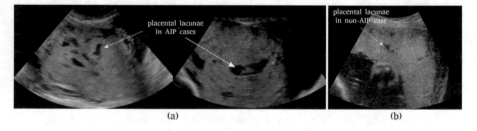

(a)   (b)

Fig. 1. Placental lacunae (PL) in placental ultrasound images. Red dots refer to expert dot annotations. (a) two AIP cases containing numerous PL of irregular shapes and sizes, (b) a placenta (with normal pregnancy outcome) containing only a few PL.

2   Methods

2.1   From Dot Annotation to Confidence Map

Detailed human labelling, such as manual segmentation of anatomical structures, is sometimes too expensive to carry out in large-scale medical image analysis studies. In this work, we investigate a *weak* way of annotating images, which is referred to as *dot annotation* [5]. The annotation protocol requires that the centroid of the observed PL is pinpointed by the annotator and the spatial coordinates stored. As shown in Fig. 1, dot annotations pinpoint the most reasonable locations of PL in expert opinion. Learning these coordinates directly would generally require computational complexity proportional to the number of PL in the image. Instead, we present a bottom-up approach that dissociates runtime complexity from the number of PL by generating a confidence map for each image, encoding the belief that PL would occur at each pixel location. Intuitively, dot annotations correspond to peaks in confidence maps.

Previous map generation approaches tend to fit a standard, isotropic Gaussian function at each annotated dot [5,6]. Here we propose an alternative by considering the size, shape, and texture of PL in order to improve localization performance. For each labelled PL, a local patch is first cropped, centering at the dot annotation location P, as shown in Fig. 2(a). Then the simple linear iterative clustering (SLIC) algorithm is applied on the patch to cluster pixels that are close to each other in a 3-D space spanned by pixel intensity and spatial coordinates [7], as shown in Fig. 2(b). A simple cluster expansion is then performed by recursively grouping adjacent clusters of similar average pixel intensity. The resulting grouped clusters form a binary mask, as shown in Fig. 2(c). In the final step (Fig. 2(d)), a 2D Gaussian function is fit that centered at P, whose covariance matrix Σ is determined by the ellipse that has the same variance as the binary mask, such that the eigenvalues of Σ are the lengths of the major and minor axes of the ellipse, scaled by a factor $l - \frac{1}{3}$ in order to control its spread. We rescale the Gaussian function by a factor of 50 as suggested in [5], yielding the peak to be larger than 45 for most PL. By repeating this process for all PL within an ultrasound image, we generate a smoothed confidence map. Where two or more Gaussian functions spatially overlap with each other, we take the pixel-wise *maximum* of the overlapping regions.

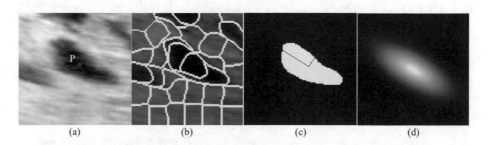

(a)   (b)   (c)   (d)

Fig. 2. The analysis pipeline that generates a local confidence map around PL given only a dot annotation. (a) a cropped PL image with the dot annotation in the center, (b) the SLIC over-segmentation of the region, (c) a cluster expansion algorithm yielding a binary mask around the dot annotation, (d) a local confidence map is generated by fitting a Gaussian function at the labelled PL.

2.2   Lacunae Localization: Layer Aggregation Approaches

Layer Aggregation: For convenience, we put layers that yield the same feature resolution into the same *stage*. FCN's natural pyramidal feature hierarchy enables aggregations of both spatial (i.e. where) and semantic (i.e. what) information from shallower stages to deeper ones. To achieve more accurate spatial inference of PL, whose size is essentially much smaller than the placenta itself, we propose to build up *non-linear* pathways that explicitly aggregate multi-scale semantics and resolutions. Specifically, we investigate two generic FCN architectures that have been widely used in medical image analysis: (1) a downsampling network (DN) and (2) a U-shape network (UN). As shown in Fig. 3, DN sequentially down-samples stages, leading to semantically richer but spatially coarser features [8]. UN follows an encoder-decoder architecture, with the encoder part being a DN and the decoder part an up-sampling network that gradually restores resolution via 2×2 transposed convolution [9]. We consider three layer aggregation approaches: deep supervision (DS) [10], feature pyramid network (FPN) [11], and iterative deep aggregation (IDA) [12]. As shown in Fig. 3(a), DS concatenates intermediate side-outputs and makes the final prediction. Here a side-output is a prediction made by the output of a stage. FPN intends to enhance semantically stronger features (from deeper stages) with weaker ones (from shallower stages) via skip connection and *linear* pixel-wise addition. In FPN, the shallowest stage will be aggregated last. IDA, on the other hand, starts from the shallowest stage and iteratively merges deeper ones. All feature channel mismatches in Fig. 3 are resolved by 1×1 convolution and resolution mismatches by bilinear upsampling.

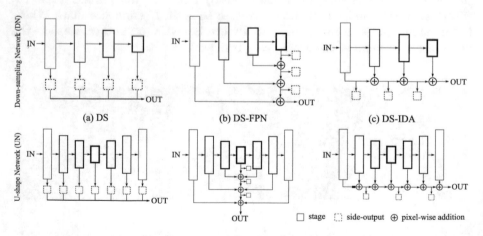

Fig. 3. Two generic FCN architectures: DN and UN with three layer aggregation structures: (a) deep supervision (DS), (b) deeply supervised feature pyramid network (DS-FPN), and (c) deeply supervised iterative deep aggregation (DS-IDA). Intuitively, the box size is proportional to the spatial resolution and the box linewidth to the feature channel number.

To achieve accurate PL localization, we propose two layer aggregation structures, namely deeply supervised feature pyramid network (DS-FPN, Fig. 3(b)) and deeply supervised iterative deep aggregation (DS-IDA, Fig. 3(c)). We introduce a non-linear pixel-wise addition in both structures for input feature maps $\{\mathbf{x_i}\}$. The output is $\sigma(\text{BN}(\sum_i \mathbf{w_i}\mathbf{x_i}))$, where σ is a non-linearity (e.g. ReLU), BN is a batch normalization layer, and $\mathbf{w_i}$ are convolutional weights to be learnt. Side-outputs are produced in both structures to cast additional supervision alongside the aggregation pathways. Intuitively, DS-FPN focuses more on semantically stronger features from deeper stages while DS-IDA progressively enhances spatially finer features from shallower stages. This comparison allows us to investigate the importance of features from shallower versus deeper stages in PL localization. The model output looks like a 'heatmap' that encodes PL localization confidence. PL centroid predictions are obtained by performing non-maximum suppression at a certain confidence level.

Loss Function: The objective function of DS-FPN and DS-IDA are the same, which is given by $\mathcal{L}(\mathbf{W}) = \ell(S_{OUT}, \hat{S}) + \frac{1}{N}\sum_{i=1}^{N} \ell(S_i, \hat{S})$. Here $\hat{S}$ is the reference confidence map, S_{OUT} is the final output of the model, and $\{S_i\}_{i=1}^{N}$ are N side-outputs. We cast supervision not only on the final output, but also on all the side-outputs to improve localization performance. $\mathbf{W}$ represents all the learnable parameters. $\ell(\cdot, \cdot)$ denotes the L-2 loss between the inputs.

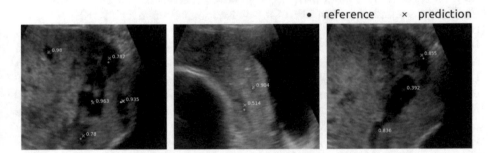

Fig. 4. Example images illustrating the use of SOKS to score PL localization. In each image, a dot denotes the dot annotation (reference) and a cross denotes the prediction. The value next to a pair of dot and cross is the SOKS score between them.

3   Experiments

Dataset: 34 placental ultrasound scans from 34 participants (23 AIP and 11 non-AIP) were collected as part of a large obstetrics research project [13]. Written consent was obtained with local research ethics approval. Static transabdominal 3D ultrasound volumes of the placental bed were obtained according to the predefined protocol with participants in semi-recumbent position and a full bladder using a 3D curved array abdominal transducer. Each 3D volume was sliced along the sagittal plane into 2D images and annotated by Huan Qi under the guidance of Dr. Sally Collins. The database contains 3,440 2D images with 9,618 labelled PL in total, from 60 to 140 slices per volume. A subject-level 10-fold cross-validation was performed for each model. In each fold, test data consisting of 2D image slices from 3–4 volumes were held out while images from the remaining volumes were used for training and validation.

Implementation Details: All models were trained end-to-end using the Adam optimizer. Pre-trained models were loaded for DN as well as the encoder part of UN. The decoder part of UN was initialized by sampling from a Gaussian distribution $\mathcal{N}(0, \sqrt{2/n})$, where n is the number of trainable parameters for each layer. The inputs were normalized to have zero mean and unit variance and resized to have the dimension of $384 \times 384 \times 3$. Horizontal flip was used for data augmentation. The hyper-parameters were: mini-batch size 8; weight decay 0.0005; initial learning rate 0.0001. All models reached convergence after 20 epochs. All experiments were implemented in PyTorch. A 10-fold training took around 30 h on a 12 GB NVIDIA graphic card.

Evaluation Metrics: Our task requires simultaneous detection and localization. For each PL, we already have its dot annotation (x_i, y_i), i.e. coordinates of its centroid. Each PL also has a scale s_i which we define as the square root of its SLIC cluster area. Following the evaluation metrics of the COCO Keypoint Challenge, we define a Simplified Object Keypoint Similarity (SOKS) score for each prediction-reference pair indexed by j: $\text{SOKS}(j) = \exp(-d_j^2/2s_j^2k^2)$. d_j is the Euclidean distance between reference and prediction and k is a constant that controls the overall falloff, which is empirically set to 0.424[1]. The intuition behind SOKS is that larger tolerance is given to PL of larger sizes. In practice, we found SOKS ≥ 0.3 generally yields a perceptually acceptable localization, as shown in Fig. 4. For evaluation, we compare AP_x, which denotes the average precision by thresholding SOKS at x. Specifically, any prediction with SOKS $\geq x$ would be marked as true positive (TP) and otherwise false positive (FP). Any undetected PL would be marked as false negative (FN). AP_x is the mean of precision over the recall interval at $[0, 1]$. To achieve a high score of AP_x, a model needs to have high precision at *all* levels of recall (or sensitivity), which is practically difficult in PL localization. We report four metrics: $\text{AP}_{0.3}$, $\text{AP}_{0.5}$, $\text{AP}_{0.75}$, and mAP. mAP is the mean of $\{\text{AP}_x\}$ for $x \in [0.3 : 0.05 : 0.95]$, measuring the overall localization performance at different SOKS levels. We use mAP as the primary metrics. Please refer to [6] for more details.

Performance Evaluation: As shown in Table 1, we chose ResNet18 and VGG16 as model backbones and ran tests for three layer aggregation structures: DS, DS-FCN, DS-IDA. We removed the first 7×7 convolutional layer and

---

[1] Please refer to cocodataset.org for details.

Table 1. The performance of different PL localizers on the test set via 10-fold cross validation. All results (%) are in the format of *median [first, third quartile]*. AP_x at three SOKS thresholds ($x \in \{0.3, 0.5, 0.75\}$) are reported. mAP is the primary metrics. Models are named in the format of *A-B*, where *A* is its generic architecture (DN or UN) and *B* its layer aggregation structure (DS or DS-FCN or DS-IDA)

Model	Backbone	mAP	$AP_{0.3}$	$AP_{0.5}$	$AP_{0.75}$
DN-DS	ResNet18	22.8 [20.2, 26.5]	33.0 [30.3, 36.3]	29.6 [27.1, 33.8]	19.7 [16.9, 23.9]
DN-DS-FCN		28.7 [22.0, 30.0]	42.7 [34.5, 43.6]	37.5 [30.6, 39.3]	24.0 [16.9, 25.7]
DN-DS-IDA		29.7 [25.3, 34.8]	38.6 [33.8, 46.0]	36.3 [31.0, 43.9]	28.5 [24.1, 32.5]
UN-DS	VGG16	32.6 [24.1, 37.5]	41.4 [35.2, 47.2]	39.6 [31.4, 44.1]	31.3 [22.0, 36.5]
UN-DS-FCN		32.2 [28.4, 37.4]	42.3 [39.7, 46.0]	40.2 [35.7, 44.1]	31.0 [24.8, 36.8]
UN-DS-IDA		**35.7** [28.4, 40.7]	**44.7** [40.9, 50.1]	**42.3** [36.5, 48.5]	**35.3** [26.4, 37.8]

the max-pooling layer from ResNet18 such that all models contain three down-sampling operations. We also introduced skip connections in all UN models in the same way as U-Net [9]. Performances of different PL localizers are given in Table 1. The median, first, and third quartile of 10-fold results are presented. The proposed UN-DS-IDA surpasses all other PL localizers in all AP metrics. Two-tailed paired t-tests showed that mAP from UN-DS-IDA is significantly higher than those from the rest PL localizers (with p-value < 0.001).

Generating Confidence Maps. In this paper, we proposed to use a SLIC-based approach to generate confidence maps that take into account the size, shape, and texture of PL, instead of fitting an isotropic Gaussian at each dot annotation with a fixed falloff σ. We compared these two approaches in experiments. For the latter, an isotropic Gaussian function was fit at each PL to generate confidence maps. Let $\mathbf{p_i}$ be the position of a dot annotation. The value at location $\mathbf{x}$ in the map was defined as: $C(\mathbf{x}) = A \exp(-\|\mathbf{x} - \mathbf{p_i}\|_2^2 / \sigma^2)$, where A was set to 50 as before. With this method, the best localization was achieved by a UN-DS-IDA model at $\sigma = 5$ with mAP $= 29.9\%$, being outperformed by the proposed SLIC-based approach. This is because the size and shape of PL are variable. There is no σ that would achieve good localization for all PL. Our proposed approach uses local information, which makes it well-suited to PL localization. Moreover, our approach leads to better visualization that learns the size and shape automatically, as shown in Fig. 5, which can be beneficial for clinical use.

4 Discussion

We further investigated the effectiveness of DS-IDA by probing the localization performance of side-outputs $\{S_i\}_{i=1}^{N}$. Let the side-outputs (from left to right) in DN-DS and UN-DS be $\{S_i\}_{i=1}^{4}$ and $\{\tilde{S}_i\}_{i=1}^{7}$ respectively. In the 10-fold cross validation experiment, the mAP score (median) of S_1, S_2, $\tilde{S}_1$, and $\tilde{S}_2$ are 0. Starting from S_3 and $\tilde{S}_3$, mAP scores start to increase as expected. From this, we argue that features from shallower stages are not effectively aggregated via either concatenation (DS) or skip connection (FPN). For instance, features from the shallowest stage in DS-FPN are aggregated last, with little room for adaption and improvement. On the contrary, DS-IDA structure progressively aggregates features from shallower stages. Our experimental results indicate that features from shallower stages can indeed contribute to PL localization effectively with the proposed DS-IDA structure. One reasonable explanation is that down-sampling operation would lose certain PL-related spatial information. Aggregating shallower features compensate such loss to some extent. In addition to use in placenta assessment such as lesion detection, we believe the analysis approach could be adapted for other clinical scenarios in breast, liver, and prostate cancer imaging.

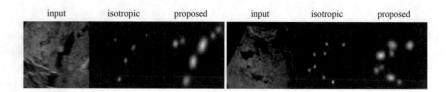

Fig. 5. Example results showing two model outputs, trained using isotropic Gaussian confidence map and the proposed SLIC-based confidence map respectively.

Acknowledgements. Huan Qi is supported by a China Scholarship Council doctoral research fund (grant No. 201608060317). The NIH Eunice Kennedy Shriver National Institute of Child Health and Human Development Human Placenta Project UO1 HD 087209, EPSRC grant EP/M013774/1, and ERC-ADG-2015 694581 are also acknowledged.

References

1. Jauniaux, E., et al.: The placenta accreta spectrum: pathophysiology and evidence-based anatomy for prenatal ultrasound imaging. AJOG **218**(1), 75–87 (2018)
2. Fitzpatrick, K., et al.: The management and outcomes of placenta accreta, increta, and percreta in the UK: a population-based descriptive study. BJOG **121**(1), 62–71 (2014)
3. Thurn, L., et al.: Abnormally invasive placenta - prevalence, risk factors and antenatal suspicion: results from a large population-based pregnancy cohort study in the Nordic countries. BJOG **123**(8), 1348–1355 (2016)
4. Collins, S., et al.: Proposal for standardized ultrasound descriptors of abnormally invasive placenta (AIP). Ultrasound Obstet. Gynecol. **47**(3), 271–275 (2016)
5. Xie, W., et al.: Microscopy cell counting with fully convolutional regression networks. In: MICCAI Deep Learning Workshop (2015)
6. Cao, Z., et al.: Realtime multi-person 2d pose estimation using part affinity fields. In: IEEE CVPR (2017)
7. Achanta, R., et al.: Slic superpixels compared to state-of-the-art superpixel methods. IEEE T-PAMI **34**(11), 2274–2282 (2012)

8. Zhou, Y., Xie, L., Fishman, E.K., Yuille, A.L.: Deep supervision for pancreatic cyst segmentation in abdominal CT scans. In: Descoteaux, M., Maier-Hein, L., Franz, A., Jannin, P., Collins, D.L., Duchesne, S. (eds.) MICCAI 2017. LNCS, vol. 10435, pp. 222–230. Springer, Cham (2017). https://doi.org/10.1007/978-3-319-66179-7_26

9. Ronneberger, O., Fischer, P., Brox, T.: U-Net: convolutional networks for biomedical image segmentation. In: Navab, N., Hornegger, J., Wells, W.M., Frangi, A.F. (eds.) MICCAI 2015. LNCS, vol. 9351, pp. 234–241. Springer, Cham (2015). https://doi.org/10.1007/978-3-319-24574-4_28

10. Xie, S., et al.: Holistically-nested edge detection. In: IEEE ICCV (2015)

11. Lin, T.Y., et al.: Feature pyramid networks for object detection. In: IEEE CVPR (2017)

12. Yu, F., et al.: Deep layer aggregation. In: IEEE CVPR (2018)

13. Collins, S., et al.: Influence of power doppler gain setting on virtual organ computer-aided analysis indices in vivo: can use of the individual sub-noise gain level optimize information? Ultrasound Obstet. Gynecol. **40**(1), 75–80 (2012)

A Decomposable Model for the Detection of Prostate Cancer in Multi-parametric MRI

Nathan Lay[1(✉)], Yohannes Tsehay[1], Yohan Sumathipala[1], Ruida Cheng[2], Sonia Gaur[3], Clayton Smith[3], Adrian Barbu[4], Le Lu[1], Baris Turkbey[3], Peter L. Choyke[3], Peter Pinto[3], and Ronald M. Summers[1]

[1] Imaging Biomarkers and Computer-Aided Diagnosis Laboratory, Clinical Center, National Institutes of Health, Bethesda, MD 20892, USA
nathan.lay@nih.gov
[2] Image Science Laboratory, Center of Information Technology, National Institutes of Health, Bethesda, MD 20892, USA
[3] Urologic Oncology Branch and Molecular Imaging Program, National Cancer Institute, National Institutes of Health, Bethesda, MD 20892, USA
[4] Department of Statistics, Florida State University, Tallahassee, FL 32306, USA

Abstract. Institutions that specialize in prostate MRI acquire different MR sequences owing to variability in scanning procedure and scanner hardware. We propose a novel prostate cancer detector that can operate in the absence of MR imaging sequences. Our novel prostate cancer detector first trains a forest of random ferns on all MR sequences and then decomposes these random ferns into a sum of MR sequence-specific random ferns enabling predictions to be made in the absence of one or more of these MR sequences. To accomplish this, we first show that a sum of random ferns can be exactly represented by another random fern and then we propose a method to approximately decompose an arbitrary random fern into a sum of random ferns. We show that our decomposed detector can maintain good performance when some MR sequences are omitted.

1 Introduction

The use of multi-parametric MRI (mpMRI) is the most effective way to detect and biopsy prostate cancer [4]. However, institutions specializing in prostate MRI have different scanning procedures and hardware resulting in different MR images. This particularly poses a challenge for computer-aided detection (CAD) of prostate cancer as many existing CAD methods (e.g. [7,9,12]) were developed for specific MR sequences coming from a single institution and will not function in the absence of expected MR images. To address this problem, we propose a novel prostate CAD that is capable of making predictions in the absence of one or more MR sequences it was trained on. This might include sequences like Dynamic

© Springer Nature Switzerland AG 2018
A. F. Frangi et al. (Eds.): MICCAI 2018, LNCS 11071, pp. 930–939, 2018.
https://doi.org/10.1007/978-3-030-00934-2_103

Contrast Enhancement (DCE) or high b-value (e.g. B1500) diffusion images that may not be acquired owing to patient comfort or limitations of scanner hardware respectively. Our CAD uses T2 weighted (T2W), apparent diffusion coefficient (ADC) and B1500 MR sequences and first builds several random ferns that use features computed on T2W, ADC and B1500 images combined. Then we present a method to decompose the trained random ferns into a sum of random ferns that each individually operate on one of T2W, ADC and B1500 images. The result is a prostate CAD that can simply exclude MR sequence-specific models from the sum during prediction. We show that the decomposed model exhibits similar performance to the original model. We also explore the performance consequences of missing information. Furthermore, we show that our prostate CAD can maintain good performance when omitting several combinations of MR sequences.

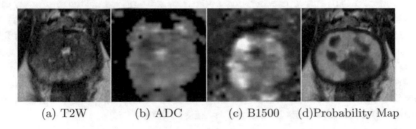

(a) T2W   (b) ADC   (c) B1500   (d)Probability Map

Fig. 1. Examples of T2W, ADC and calculated B1500 images with corresponding CAD probability map. Hypointense regions in T2W and ADC can indicate the presence of prostate cancer, while hyperintense regions in B1500 indicate the presence of prostate cancer. Probability map colors range from blue (low score) to red (high score). There is a clinically significant (Gleason $3 + 4$ or higher) transition zone lesion in this example that is correctly predicted by the CAD.

2   Related Works

There are several examples of prostate CAD systems in the literature. The general workflow for these systems is to read in several images from mpMRI and then produce a colorized confidence or probability map indicating voxel-by-voxel suspicious regions. Some systems [9] further process these probability maps to extract lesion segmentations. The probability maps can then be interpreted by radiologists or used in guided biopsy procedures. Figure 1 shows a few examples of mpMRI images and probability maps. A few recent examples of CAD include the works of [7,9,12]. The system in [7] uses Support Vector Machine (SVM) with local binary pattern features computed on T2W and B2000 images. The work of [9] uses random forest, Gentle Boost, and LDA each using a combination of T2W, ADC, B800 and DCE images with features based on pixel intensity, relative location in the prostate, texture, blobness and pharmacokinetic heuristics. This work further segments and classifies lesions based on the output from the voxel classifier. The system proposed in [12] picks candidate locations based on a multi-scale Hessian-based blobness filter which are then each classified with an LDA classifier. The LDA classifier uses statistics-based features computed on T1W, T2W, ADC, DCE and Ktrans images. Although not applied to mpMRI or prostate cancer detection, the work of [6] develops a deep learning system that can train and test in the absence of images. Their system uses a set of disjoint neural network (NN) pipelines that individually process different kinds of images. The output of these pipelines are then averaged to produce the prediction. When an image is missing, the average omits the output from the corresponding pipeline.

Our system is fundamentally different to existing prostate CAD systems in that it does not require the availability of all MR sequences used to train the model and can still make predictions even if operating on a single image. Other differences to existing prostate CAD systems include the use of a different classifier, the use of a transition zone segmentation, as well as the use of different features. We additionally introduce a new way to train random ferns and a way to decompose them into a sum of random ferns. While the work of [6] can also operate in the absence of images, our method infers sequence-specific classifiers through an explicit model decomposition while [6] jointly optimizes the modality-specific pipelines in an end-to-end fashion.

3   Methods

The proposed prostate CAD operates on 2D image slices and is comprised of pixel-wise random fern classifiers [11] employing intensity statistics and Haralick texture features [5]. The random ferns are first trained on features calculated on all T2W, ADC and B1500 MR images and then the resulting model is decomposed into a sum of random ferns that each operate individually on features calculated on T2W, ADC and B1500. Figure 1 shows an example of these MR sequences and corresponding CAD prediction. When one or more of these MR sequences are missing, the CAD excludes the corresponding random ferns from the evaluation and can still produce a probability map. We chose random ferns since they are similar to and *simpler than* decision trees and are thus robust and powerful learners while being intuitive to understand and manipulate.

3.1   Random Ferns

Random ferns [11] are constrained decision trees that behave like *checklists* of yes/no questions based on the input feature vector. The combination of yes/no answers are then used to lookup a prediction. As observed in [11], this checklist behavior is synonymous to a decision tree using the same decision criteria at each level of the tree.

Our method modifies random ferns in a number of ways. First, the binary decisions for each fern are selected by employing Feature Selection and Annealing (FSA) [2]. Second, we use mean aggregation instead of semi-naïve Bayes aggregation. Several independent random ferns are trained on randomly sampled data to produce a forest of random ferns.

Where decision tree training employs a simple recursive optimization strategy to select binary decisions, the constrained decision structure of random ferns make such recursive optimization strategies prohibitively expensive. We avoid this issue entirely by instead noting that a sum of decision stumps can be exactly represented as a random fern as illustrated in Fig. 2. We instead optimize a sum of decision stumps and assume the resulting model is approximately the unknown optimal random fern.

To select optimal binary decisions for the random fern, decision stumps are first exhaustively generated for each feature. This is done by discretizing the range of observed feature responses and using these as decision thresholds for each decision stump. Then a coefficient is associated with each leaf of every stump. The sum of these stumps forms a linear model for FSA to optimize. FSA simultaneously minimizes a loss function while selecting the most informative decision stumps. As in [2], we use the Lorenz loss function for FSA in this work. Lastly, the FSA-selected decisions are used to train the fern by passing examples down the fern and computing the label distribution $p(y|\mathbf{x})$ in each leaf where $y \in \{0,1\}$ is the class label and $\mathbf{x} \in \mathbf{R}^F$ is the feature vector. This process is repeated on several randomly sampled training sets to form a forest of jointly trained random ferns.

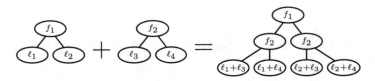

Fig. 2. Example of a sum of two decision stumps resulting in a random fern. This generalizes when summing more than two stumps. Note that an arbitrary random fern cannot be exactly represented by a sum of stumps in general.

3.2   Random Fern Decomposition

Each jointly trained random fern T is then decomposed into three MR sequence-specific random ferns by first forming empty random ferns each using only T2W, ADC and B1500 binary decisions from the original random fern. More specifically, if L represents a leaf of the original depth D random fern T with $L \in T$, then L represents a unique combination of yes/no answers that identify that specific leaf. We then augment $L = \{\ell_1 \mid \ell_2 \mid \ell_3\}$ where ℓ_m represents both a leaf of a random fern T_m specific to MR sequence m (T2W: $m = 1$, ADC: $m = 2$,

B1500: $m = 3$) as well as the outcome of decision criteria specific to that MR sequence. We additionally use the notation $I(\ell \subseteq L) \in \{0,1\}$ to indicate that a subset of the decision criteria outcomes ℓ match in L. We also further abuse notation by treating leaves $L \in T$, $\ell \in T_m$ as integers. Then we use specialized Artificial Prediction Market (APM) [1] to fit the sum of three MR sequence-specific random ferns to the jointly trained random fern. We chose specialized APM since it supports models that can abstain from participation (e.g. due to missing information). We treat random fern T as the ground truth and can thus exactly calculate the mass $p(L)$ of examples occurring in leaf L as well as the label distribution $p(y|L)$ in leaf L. We can then indirectly infer a linear aggregation $c(y|L)$ of the sequence specific random ferns T_1, T_2, T_3 by iterating the update rule (2) over each populated leaf $L \in T$.

$$c(y|L) = \frac{1}{Z} \sum_{m=1}^{3} \sum_{\ell \in T_m} I(\ell \subseteq L)\beta_{m,\ell,y} \quad \text{for } y = 0,1,\ L \in T \tag{1}$$

$$\beta_{m,\ell,y} \leftarrow \beta_{m,\ell,y} + \eta \left(-\beta_{m,\ell,y}I(\ell \subseteq L) + p(L)p(y|L)\frac{\beta_{m,\ell,y}I(\ell \subseteq L)}{c(y|L)} \right) \tag{2}$$

Here Z is a normalizer, η is the learning rate, $\beta_{m,\ell,y}$ the learned prediction of leaf ℓ. The update rule is repeatedly used for each leaf L from the jointly trained random fern until convergence. The result is 3 constituent random ferns with leaves ℓ predicting $\beta_{m,\ell,y}$. The resulting ferns can then be aggregated using a form similar to $c(y|L)$ as the predicted probability and this is given as

$$c(y|\mathbf{x}) = \frac{1}{Z} \sum_{I_m \text{ available}} \beta_{m,\ell_m,y} \tag{3}$$

where Z is a normalizer, $\ell_m = T_m(\mathbf{x})$ is the predicted leaf for feature vector $\mathbf{x}$ on MR image I_m.

3.3   Data

We train and evaluate the proposed method on a combination of cases from NIH and data made available through the recent ProstateX Challenge [9]. All MR sequences (T2W, ADC, B1500) were aligned, resampled to $0.35\,\text{mm} \times 0.35\,\text{mm} \times 3\,\text{mm}$, and normalized using a Rician-based normalization [8]. Cases from NIH feature 19 healthy patients and 49 pathology-corroborated hand-drawn lesions prepared by a radiologist. The ProstateX data featured a database of points with corresponding clinical significance binary label for 204 training cases.

3.4   Prostate Segmentation

This CAD relies on the presence of a prostate and transition zone segmentation as it trains separate transition zone and peripheral zone classifiers. Segmentations for the NIH cases were prepared manually by a radiologist while the 204

ProstateX cases were automatically segmented by an algorithm based on [3,10] with the possibility of manual correction. The method does depend on a *well bounded* prostate segmentation since it is liable to misclassify the background in T2W or ADC.

3.5 Training

Each fern was trained on an independent random subset of training cases without regard to annotation type. Positive and negative points were densely sampled inside the prostate for healthy cases and cases with hand-drawn lesion contours. Positives were densely sampled within 5 mm of clinically significant points in ProstateX cases. No negatives were sampled from ProstateX cases since lesion extent is not known and the reason for the points in the database are not known.

3.6 Statistical Analysis

The proposed CAD was analyzed on five sets of two fold cross validation experiments with each cross validation experiment generated on randomly shuffled data and thus resulting in 10 total distinct experiments. Our 10 experiments always train and test on $\approx 1/2$ and $\approx 1/2$ of data set and we believe this better characterizes the generalizability of the method than either 2 fold or 10 fold cross validation. Cross validation was used purely for assessing performance and no hyperparameters were picked using the test folds. The data were split so that approximately the same number of healthy, contour and ProstateX cases were used in each fold. We compared the original random fern model to the decomposed random fern model. We also considered the performance of the proposed CAD on a variety of combinations of T2W, ADC, and B1500 images. Performance was measured in terms of ROC curves for detection and clinical significance classification.

To demonstrate the difference between decomposing MR sequence-specific models and training directly on MR sequences we retrained the decomposed T2W, ADC and B1500 models on examples coming from each MR sequence. For the purpose of comparing the models, the decision criteria were kept constant and the fern predictions were directly recalculated on its training set. The resulting AUCs and margins were calculated for the two models over the five permutations of two fold cross validation. The margin was calculated in a weighted sense and is given by

$$\text{margin} = \frac{1}{2|N^+|} \sum_{x \in X^+} p(y=1|x) - \frac{1}{2|N^-|} \sum_{x \in X^-} p(y=1|x) \tag{4}$$

where X^+ and X^- are the positive and negative examples and $|\cdot|$ denotes cardinality.

Detection ROC. Detections and false positives were determined on the cases with lesion contour annotations. Probability maps and contour annotations were first stacked to define 3D probability maps and lesion masks. For each lesion, the 90th percentile of the probability scores occurring inside the lesion was taken to be the lesion's score. If the lesion score exceeded a threshold, then the lesion was said to be *detected*. False positives were determined by cutting the prostate into $3\,mm \times 3\,mm \times 3\,mm$ cubes. The 90th percentile of probabilities occurring inside each cube were determined and used as the cube's score. If a cube did not coincide with a lesion and its score exceeded a threshold, then cube was said to be a *false positive*.

ProstateX ROC. The ProstateX Challenge data includes an annotated database of image points and whether they correspond to clinically significant cancer or not. Each point was scored by the CAD by first stacking the probability maps into a 3D probability map. Then the 90th percentile of probability scores occurring inside a $5\,mm$ ball was taken to be the point's score. A classification ROC curve was then calculated against these scores and their ground truth.

4   Results

The ROC curves were calculated on each of the test sets from each of the cross validation experiments and were averaged with respect to false positive rate. These averaged ROC curves are displayed in Fig. 3. The curves compare the performance of the CAD using the random ferns trained on all MR sequences (Jointly Trained) to the CAD using decomposed random ferns evaluated on a combination of MR sequences.

Table 1 features AUCs and margins of the T2W, ADC and B1500 decomposed models and their retrained counterparts while Fig. 4 illustrates the margin's effects on the decomposed T2W model and retrained T2W model.

Table 1. Comparison of MR sequence-specific classifiers produced from decomposition (Ours) and the same classifier retrained on the corresponding MR sequence (Tuned). The columns are the average margin and AUC from the averaged ROC curves over the five permutations of two fold cross validation. Bold numbers indicate maximum value for the corresponding task.

MR Seq.	Detection ours		Detection tuned		ProstateX ours		ProstateX tuned	
	Margin	AUC	Margin	AUC	Margin	AUC	Margin	AUC
T2W	**0.17** (0.02)	0.84	0.09 (0.01)	**0.85**	**0.08** (0.02)	**0.72**	0.04 (0.02)	0.71
ADC	**0.24** (0.03)	0.91	0.09 (0.01)	0.91	**0.10** (0.03)	0.72	0.04 (0.01)	**0.74**
B1500	**0.21** (0.02)	0.90	0.13 (0.01)	0.90	**0.13** (0.03)	**0.84**	0.08 (0.01)	0.83

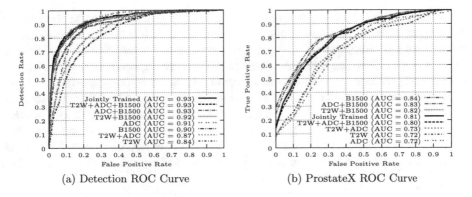

(a) Detection ROC Curve   (b) ProstateX ROC Curve

Fig. 3. ROC curves of the CAD system evaluated as a detector and a clinical significance classifier.

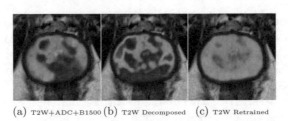

(a) T2W+ADC+B1500 (b) T2W Decomposed   (c) T2W Retrained

Fig. 4. An example of probability maps produced by the decomposed model using T2W+ADC+B1500 (a), the T2W model (b) and the retrained T2W model (c). The latter illustrates the reported low margin of the retrained model.

5 Discussion

The detection ROC in Fig. 3 reveals similar performance between the jointly trained model and the decomposed model using all sequences (T2W+ADC+B1500) demonstrating no loss in detection performance even after decomposing the jointly trained model. When some sequences are missing, the CAD is able to maintain similar or good detection performance with decomposed models ADC+B1500, T2W+B1500, ADC and B1500 achieving not less than 0.9 AUC in performance. When diffusion is completely excluded, we see that the decomposed CAD can still achieve a *good* AUC of 0.84, the lowest of all reported detection AUCs.

Similar ProstateX performance is also seen in Fig. 3 between the jointly trained model and decomposed model again showing little to no loss in performance. The ProstateX data set is comprised of outcomes of targeted biopsies which implies that the data set may be biased toward only suspicious prostate regions and many false positives such as artifacts or benign structures are likely to be already ruled out. For this reason and based on findings in the work of [7], it is not beyond expectation to find that B1500 achieved the highest ProstateX AUC of 0.84.

Table 1 shows the value of decomposition over training single sequence models. Importantly, both single-sequence models use identical features and decision criteria for fair comparison. While the detection and ProstateX AUCs of the two models are similar, the prediction margin of the decomposed models are higher and would produce more contrasting probability maps as seen in Fig. 4.

Lastly, owing to differing evaluation methodology, private data sets, and the lack of prostate CAD systems that can operate in the absence of MR sequences, it is difficult, perhaps even meaningless, to objectively compare our performance with other methods in the literature. However, this method did place third in the ProstateX competition with a test AUC of 0.83 tailing methods that achieved test AUCs of 0.84 and 0.87.

6   Conclusion

Decomposing random ferns to operate on individual MR sequences provides increased flexibility with little to no performance loss when working with data that may or may not include some MR sequences. Many combinations of MR sequences were also shown to provide similar performance to the CAD using all available MR sequences. The decomposed models also generally provide more contrasting positive and negative predictions while matching the performance of same models explicitly retrained on individual sequences.

Acknowledgements. This research was funded by the Intramural Research Program of the National Institutes of Health, Clinical Center. Data used in this research were obtained from The Cancer Imaging Archive (TCIA) sponsored by the SPIE, NCI/NIH, AAPM, and Radboud University.

References

1. Barbu, A., Lay, N.: An introduction to artificial prediction markets for classification. JMLR **13**(Jul), 2177–2204 (2012)
2. Barbu, A., She, Y., Ding, L., et al.: Feature selection with annealing for computer vision and big data learning. IEEE TPAMI **39**(2), 272–286 (2017)
3. Cheng, R., Roth, H.R., Lay, N.S., et al.: Automatic magnetic resonance prostate segmentation by deep learning with holistically nested networks. JMI **4**(4), 041302 (2017)
4. Costa, D.N., Pedrosa, I., Donato Jr., F., et al.: MR imaging-transrectal us fusion for targeted prostate biopsies: implications for diagnosis and clinical management. Radiographics **35**(3), 696–708 (2015)
5. Haralick, R.M., Shanmugam, K., et al.: Textural features for image classification. IEEE T-SMCA **3**(6), 610–621 (1973)
6. Havaei, M., Guizard, N., Chapados, N., Bengio, Y.: HeMIS: Hetero-Modal Image Segmentation. In: Ourselin, S., Joskowicz, L., Sabuncu, M.R., Unal, G., Wells, W. (eds.) MICCAI 2016. LNCS, vol. 9901, pp. 469–477. Springer, Cham (2016). https://doi.org/10.1007/978-3-319-46723-8_54

7. Kwak, J.T., Xu, S., Wood, B.J., et al.: Automated prostate cancer detection using T2-weighted and high-b-value diffusion-weighted magnetic resonance imaging. Med. Phys. **42**(5), 2368–2378 (2015)
8. Lemaître, G., Rastgoo, M., Massich, J., et al.: Normalization of T2W-MRI prostate images using Rician a priori. In: Medical Imaging 2016: Computer-Aided Diagnosis, vol. 9785, p. 978529. SPIE (2016)
9. Litjens, G., Debats, O., Barentsz, J., et al.: Computer-aided detection of prostate cancer in MRI. IEEE TMI **33**(5), 1083–1092 (2014)
10. Nogues, I., et al.: Automatic Lymph Node Cluster Segmentation Using Holistically-Nested Neural Networks and Structured Optimization in CT Images. In: Ourselin, S., Joskowicz, L., Sabuncu, M.R., Unal, G., Wells, W. (eds.) MICCAI 2016. LNCS, vol. 9901, pp. 388–397. Springer, Cham (2016). https://doi.org/10.1007/978-3-319-46723-8_45
11. Ozuysal, M., Calonder, M., Lepetit, V., et al.: Fast keypoint recognition using random ferns. IEEE TPAMI **32**(3), 448–461 (2010)
12. Vos, P., Barentsz, J., Karssemeijer, N., et al.: Automatic computer-aided detection of prostate cancer based on multiparametric magnetic resonance image analysis. PMB **57**(6), 1527 (2012)

Direct Automated Quantitative Measurement of Spine via Cascade Amplifier Regression Network

Shumao Pang[1], Stephanie Leung[2,3], Ilanit Ben Nachum[2,3], Qianjin Feng[1(✉)], and Shuo Li[2,3(✉)]

[1] Guangdong Provincial Key Laboratory of Medical Image Processing, School of Biomedical Engineering, Southern Medical University, Guangzhou 510515, China
qianjinfeng08@gmail.com
[2] Department of Medical Imaging, Western University, London, ON, Canada
slishuo@gmail.com
[3] Digital Imaging Group of London, London, ON, Canada

Abstract. Automated quantitative measurement of the spine (i.e., multiple indices estimation of heights, widths, areas, and so on for the vertebral body and disc) is of the utmost importance in clinical spinal disease diagnoses, such as osteoporosis, intervertebral disc degeneration, and lumbar disc herniation, yet still an unprecedented challenge due to the variety of spine structure and the high dimensionality of indices to be estimated. In this paper, we propose a novel cascade amplifier regression network (CARN), which includes the CARN architecture and local shape-constrained manifold regularization (LSCMR) loss function, to achieve accurate direct automated multiple indices estimation. The CARN architecture is composed of a cascade amplifier network (CAN) for expressive feature embedding and a linear regression model for multiple indices estimation. The CAN consists of cascade amplifier units (AUs), which are used for selective feature reuse by stimulating effective feature and suppressing redundant feature during propagating feature map between adjacent layers, thus an expressive feature embedding is obtained. During training, the LSCMR is utilized to alleviate overfitting and generate realistic estimation by learning the multiple indices distribution. Experiments on MR images of 195 subjects show that the proposed CARN achieves impressive performance with mean absolute errors of 1.2496 ± 1.0624 mm, 1.2887 ± 1.0992 mm, and 1.2692 ± 1.0811 mm for estimation of 15 heights of discs, 15 heights of vertebral bodies, and total indices respectively. The proposed method has great potential in clinical spinal disease diagnoses.

Keywords: Spine · Deep learning · Manifold regularization
Disc height measurement · Vertebral body height measurement

© Springer Nature Switzerland AG 2018
A. F. Frangi et al. (Eds.): MICCAI 2018, LNCS 11071, pp. 940–948, 2018.
https://doi.org/10.1007/978-3-030-00934-2_104

1   Introduction

The quantitative measurement of the spine (i.e., multiple indices estimation of heights, widths, areas, and so on for the vertebral body and disc) plays a significant role in clinical spinal disease diagnoses, such as osteoporosis, intervertebral disc degeneration, and lumbar disc herniation. Specifically, the vertebral body height (VBH) and intervertebral disc height (IDH) (as shown in Fig. 1) are the most valuable indices for the quantitative measurement of the spine. The VBHs are correlated with the bone strength, which is of great significance to the vertebral fracture risk assessment for the osteoporotic patients [1, 2]. Furthermore, the IDH reduction is associated with the intervertebral disc degeneration [3, 4] and lumbar disc herniation [5].

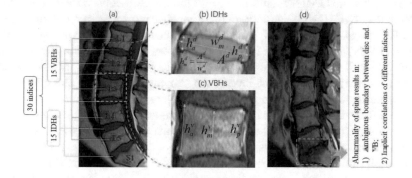

Fig. 1. (a) Illustration of 30 indices to be estimated; (b) Three heights for each disc (i.e., anterior IDH h_a^d, middle IDH h_m^d, and posterior IDH h_p^d); (c) Three heights for each vertebral body (i.e., anterior VBH h_a^v, middle VBH h_m^v, and posterior VBH h_p^v), where A^d denotes the disc area; (d) Ambiguous boundary between disc and VB and implicit correlations of different indices due to spinal abnormality.

Automated quantitative measurement of the spine is of significant clinical importance because it is reliable, time-saving, reproducible, and has higher consistency compared with manual quantitative measurement, which is usually obtained by manually detecting landmarks of the intervertebral disc (ID) and vertebral body (VB) from MR image [5, 6].

Direct automated quantitative measurement of the spine is an exceedingly intractable task due to the following challenges: (1) The high dimensionality of estimated indices (as shown in Fig. 1(a)), which leads to difficulty in expressive feature embedding for such complex regression problem. (2) The excessive ambiguity of the boundary between VB and ID for abnormal spine (as shown in Fig. 1(d)), which increases intractability of expressive feature embedding. (3) Implicit correlations between different estimated indices (as shown in Fig. 1(d), the heights of the abnormal disc and the heights of adjacent VB are correlated because disc abnormality leads to simultaneous changes of IDH and the adjacent

VBH), which is difficult to be captured. (4) Insufficient labelled data (as shown in Fig. 1(d)), which possibly results in overfitting.

In recent years, an increasing number of approaches emerged in the direct quantitative measurement of other organs (e.g., heart) [7,8]. Although these methods achieved promising performance in the quantification of the cardiac image, they are incapable of achieving quantitative measurement of the spine because they suffer from the following limitations. (1) Lack of expressive feature representation. Traditional convolutional neural network (CNN) [9] is incapable of generating an expressive feature for multiple indices estimation because CNN possibly loses effective feature due to the lack of an explicit structure for feature reuse. (2) Incapability of learning the estimated indices distribution, which will lead to unreasonable estimation and overfitting.

In this study, we propose a cascade amplifier regression network (CARN), which includes the CARN architecture and local shape-constrained manifold regularization (LSCMR) loss function, for quantitative measurement of the spine from MR images. The CARN architecture is comprised of a cascade amplifier network (CAN) for expressive feature embedding and a linear regression model for multiple indices estimation. In CAN, amplifier unit (AU) is used for selective feature reuse between adjacent layers. As shown in Fig. 2(b), the effective feature of the anterior layer is stimulated while the redundant feature is suppressed, thus generating the selected feature, which is reused in posterior layer by a concatenation operator. CAN reuses multi-level features selectively for representing complex spine, thus an expressive feature embedding is obtained. During training, the high dimensional indices can be embedded in a low dimensional manifold due to the correlations between these indices. LSCMR is employed to restrict the output of the CARN to the target output manifold. As a result, the distribution of the estimated indices is close to the real distribution, which reduces the impact of outliers and alleviates overfitting. Combining the expressive feature embedding produced by CAN with LSCMR, a simple linear regression model, i.e., fully connected network, is sufficient to produce accurate estimation results.

The main contributions of the study are three-fold. (1) To the best of our knowledge, it is the first time to achieve automated quantitative measurement of the spine, which will provide a more reliable metric for the clinical diagnosis of spinal diseases. (2) The proposed CAN provides an expressive feature map for automated quantitative measurement of the spine. (3) Overfitting is alleviated by LSCMR, which utilizes the local shape of the target output manifold to restrict the estimated indices to being close to the manifold, thus a realistic estimation of indices is obtained.

2   Cascade Amplifier Regression Network

The CARN employs the CARN architecture and LSCMR loss function to achieve accurate quantitative measurement of the spine. The CARN architecture is composed of the CAN for expressive feature embedding and the linear regression model for multiple indices estimation. As shown in Fig. 2, in CAN, AU is used for selective feature reuse between the adjacent layers by a gate, multiplier, adder and concatenate operator. In AU, the effective feature map is stimulated while the redundant feature map is suppressed. CAN provides expressive feature embedding via reusing multi-level features selectively. The linear regression model in CARN is a fully connected network without non-linear activation. During training, overfitting is alleviated by LSCMR, which is employed to oblige the output of CARN to lie on the target output manifold expressed by local linear representation [10], i.e., a sample on the manifold can be approximately represented as a linear combination of several nearest neighbors from the manifold. Local linear representation captures the local shape of the manifold, therefore, the distribution of estimated indices is close to the real distribution and the indices estimated by CARN are realistic.

2.1   Mathematical Formulation

Automated quantitative measurement of the spine is described as a multi-output regression problem. Given a training dataset $T = \{x_i, y_i\}_{i=1}^{N}$, we aim to train a multi-output regression model (i.e., the CARN) to learn the mapping $f : x \in R^{h \times w} \to y \in R^d$, where x_i and y_i denote the MR image and the corresponding multiple indices respectively, and N is the number of training samples. CARN should learn an effective feature and a reliable regressor simultaneously.

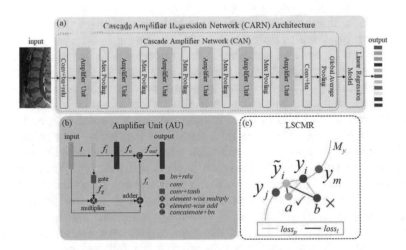

Fig. 2. (a) Overview of CARN architecture, including CAN for expressive feature embedding and a linear regression model for multiple indices estimation. (b) AU for selective feature reuse between adjacent layers. (c) LSCMR for obtaining realistic estimation and alleviating overfitting.

2.2 CARN Architecture

The CARN architecture is comprised of the CAN for expressive feature embedding and the linear regression model for multiple indices estimation.

CAN for Expressive Feature Embedding. The CAN consists of six AUs, two convolutional layers, five max pooling layers, and a global average pooling layer as shown in Fig. 2(a). AU is designed for selective feature reuse between adjacent layers. During feature selection, the selected feature is obtained by amplifying the input feature of AU using an amplifier, whose amplification factor is learned automatically (details in Section Feature Selection Mechanism). The effective low-level feature is stimulated and concatenated by the high-level feature while the redundant low-level feature is suppressed. The selective feature reuse is achieved by CAN level by level; then the multi-level selective reused feature generates an expressive feature embedding. The first convolutional layer with a 7×7 kernel size and stride of 2 reduces the resolution of feature maps from 512×256 to 256×128, while the last convolutional layer with a 1×1 kernel size and stride of 1 linearly combines the feature maps for information integration. The max pooling with a 2×2 kernel size and a stride of 2 is used to provide translation invariance to the internal representation. The global average pooling layer is utilized to reduce the dimensionality of feature maps.

The most crucial component of CAN is AU (as demonstrated in Fig. 2(b)), which is composed of a gate for controlling information propagation between adjacent layers, a convolutional layer with a 3×3 kernel size and stride of 1 for extracting a linear feature map, which is used to control the gate, a batch normalization layer with relu activation for producing non-linear feature map, a multiplier, an adder, and a concatenation operator with batch normalization for combining the selected feature map and non-linear feature map. The input t of AU goes through a convolutional layer and produces the linear feature map $f_l(t) = w_l * t + b_l$ for guiding feature selection, where w_l and b_l are the convolution kernel weight and bias of the convolutional layer respectively, and $*$ is the convolutional operator. Then the $f_l(t)$ flows into two paths. One path consists of batch normalization and relu activation, which is analogous to the traditional CNN to generate non-linear feature map $f_n(t) = relu(bn(f_l(t)))$, where bn and $relu$ denote the batch normalization and relu activation respectively. The other path is a gate composed of a convolutional layer and tanh activation, which generates output $f_g(t) = tanh(w_g * f_l(t) + b_g)$, where w_g and b_g are the convolution kernel weight and bias in the gate respectively, for selecting feature map. The output of the gate flows into a multiplier followed by an adder, and generates the selected feature:

$$f_s(t) = t \odot f_g(t) + t = t \odot (f_g(t) + 1) \tag{1}$$

where $\odot$ denotes the element-wise multiplication. Finally, the f_n and f_s are concatenated along the channel axis and normalized by the batch normalization layer to generate a output feature map $f_{out}(t) = bn(f_n(t) \oplus f_s(t))$, where $\oplus$ denotes the concatenation operator.

Feature Selection Mechanism. In Eq. 1, the value of each pixel in the selected feature map f_s is obtained by multiplying an amplification factor with the corresponding value in the input feature map t. The amplification factor $[f_g(t) + 1]$ ranges from 0 to 2; substantially, the selected feature map f_s is equivalent to stimulating or suppressing the input feature map via an amplifier. When the amplification factor is less than 1, the input feature map is suppressed, vice versa. If the amplification factor is 1, the input feature map is directly propagated to the output, which is analogous to the denseNet [11].

Linear Regression Model for Multiple Indices Estimation. The linear regression model is a fully connected layer. The output of the linear regression model is: $f(x_i) = w_o h(x_i) + b_o$, where $h(x_i)$ is the output of the global average pooling (i.e., the feature embedding) as shown in Fig. 2(a), and w_o and b_o are the weights matrix and bias of the linear regression respectively.

2.3   Local Shape-Constrained Manifold Regularization Loss Function

The loss function is divided into two parts, including preliminary loss $loss_p$ and LSCMR loss $loss_m$. The preliminary loss is designed to minimize the distance between the estimation of indices and the ground truth, while the LSCMR loss is aimed at alleviating overfitting and generating realistic results by obliging the output of CARN to lie on the target output manifold using local linear representation. The total loss function is defined as follows;

$$loss_t(w) = loss_p(w) + \lambda_l loss_l(w) \qquad (2)$$

where the λ_l is a scaling factor controlling the relative importance of the LSCMR loss. The preliminary loss function is defined as follows:

$$loss_p(w) = \frac{1}{N \times d} \sum_{i=1}^{N} \|y_i - f(x_i)\|_1 + \lambda_p \sum_i \|w_i\|_2 \qquad (3)$$

where the first term is the mean absolute error (MAE) of the regression model; the second term is the l_2 norm regularization for the trainable weight w_i in CARN; λ_p is a hyper-parameter.

By using only the preliminary loss function, unreasonable multiple indices estimation may be obtained because the estimated result is possible to be out of their real distribution. For instance, as shown in Fig. 2(c), y_i, y_j, and y_m are the target outputs of samples. The points a and b are two possible estimations of y_i. The distances between the two estimations (the points a and b) and the target output y_i are the same, i.e., they have an identical preliminary loss. However, the loss of point a should be smaller than the point b as a is much closer to the local shape of the output space than b. Hence, a is a better estimation of y_i than b.

LSCMR is proposed to achieve a realistic and accurate estimation of multiple indices. Inspired by [12], y_i lies on a manifold M_y with an inherent dimension smaller than d as the elements of y_i are correlated. The manifold M_y is spanned by $\{y_i\}_{i=1}^N$. We introduce the local linear representation, i.e., a sample on manifold M_y can be approximately represented as a linear combination of several nearest neighbors from M_y [10]. A sample y_i on M_y is locally linearly represented as:

$$y_i = \sum_{j=1}^k y_j \alpha_j + \varepsilon \approx \sum_{j=1}^k y_j \alpha_j = \tilde{y}_i$$
$$s.t. \|\varepsilon\| < \tau, \sum_{j=1}^k \alpha_j = 1, \alpha_j \geq 0, y_j \in N(y_i) \tag{4}$$

where ε is the reconstruction error and τ is a small non-negative constant. $N(y_i)$ denotes the k-nearest neighbors of y_i on M_y and α_j is the reconstruction coefficient, which is calculated by LAE [13]. As shown in Fig. 2(c), $\tilde{y}_i$ is the local linear representation of y_i using its k-nearest neighbors (here k is equal to 2) y_j and y_m. The local linear representation of y_i reflects the local manifold shape. If the predicted indices is close to $\tilde{y}_i$, it will be near the manifold M_y. Therefore, the LSCMR loss is defined as:

$$loss_l(w) = \frac{1}{N \times d} \sum_{i=1}^N \|f(x_i) - \tilde{y}_i\|_1 \tag{5}$$

Using the $loss_l$, the prediction of y_i is restricted to being close to the manifold M_y, thus a more realistic result is obtained (e.g., the model generate the point a as the estimation of y_i instead of point b in Fig. 2(c)).

3 Experimental Results

Dataset. The dataset consists of 195 midsagittal spine MR images from 195 patients. The pixel spacings range from 0.4688 mm/pixel to 0.7813 mm/pixel. Images are resampled to 0.4688 mm/pixel and the ground truth values are obtained manually in this space. In our experiments, two landmarks, i.e., the left-top corner of the L1 VB and the left-bottom corner of the L5 VB, are manually marked for each image to provide reference for ROI cropping, in which five VBs, including L1, L2, L3, L4 and L5, and five IDs under them are enclosed. The cropped images are resized to 512×256.

Experimental Configurations. The network is implemented by Tensorflow. Four group experiments under different configurations, including CARN-$loss_p$, CNN-$loss_p$, CNN-$loss_t$, and CARN-$loss_t$, are used to validate the effectiveness of our proposed method. In CNN-$loss_p$ and CNN-$loss_t$, AU is replaced with a traditional convolutional layer, in which the output feature channels are the same as AU; the -$loss_p$ and -$loss_t$ denote the loss function defined in Eqs. 3 and 2 respectively used in the model.

Overall Performance. As shown in the last column of Table 1, the proposed CARN achieves low error for automated quantitative measurement of the spine, with MAE of 1.2496 ± 1.0624 mm, 1.2887 ± 1.0992 mm, and 1.2692 ± 1.0811 mm for IDHs, VBHs, and total indices respectively. These errors are small referring to the maximums of IDHs (20.9203 mm) and VBHs (36.7140 mm) in our dataset.

CAN and LSCMR Effectiveness. Combining CAN and LSCMR, the performance improved by 2.44%, 1.16%, and 1.80% for IDHs, VBHs, and total indices estimation respectively, which is clearly demonstrated by comparing the third and last columns of Table 1. Using CAN without LSCMR, the MAE decreased by 0.21%, 0.49%, and 0.36% for IDHs, VBHs, and total indices estimation respectively, as shown in the second and third columns of Table 1. These results indicate that the CAN improves the performance for total indices estimation, especially for VBHs. This results from the fact that CAN generates expressive feature embedding although pathological changes in the disc can reduce the intensity of the adjacent VB and lead to ambiguity in the boundary. Using LSCMR without CAN, the performance improved by 2.14%, 1.03% for IDHs, and total indices estimation respectively, as shown in the third and fourth columns of Table 1.

LSCMR alleviates overfitting as shown in Table 1, in which CARN-$loss_t$ and CNN-$loss_t$ have high training errors (0.8591 mm vs 0.5024 mm, 0.9059 mm vs 0.5224 mm) but low test errors (1.2692 mm vs 1.2878 mm, 1.2791 mm vs 1.2924 mm) for total indices estimation compared with CARN-$loss_p$ and CNN-$loss_p$.

Table 1. Performance of CARN in terms of MAE under different configurations for IDH (mm), VBH (mm), and total indices (mm) estimation. MAE is illustrated in each cell. Best results are bolded for each row.

Method		CARN-$loss_p$	CNN-$loss_p$	CNN-$loss_t$	CARN-$loss_t$
IDH	Train	0.4633 ± 0.4706	0.4920 ± 0.4574	0.8689 ± 0.7417	0.8265 ± 0.7012
	Test	1.2782 ± 1.1173	1.2809 ± 1.1172	1.2535 ± 1.0754	$\mathbf{1.2496 \pm 1.0624}$
VBH	Train	0.5414 ± 0.5846	0.5528 ± 0.5615	0.9429 ± 0.8383	0.8916 ± 0.8004
	Test	1.2974 ± 1.0922	1.3038 ± 1.1154	1.3047 ± 1.1215	$\mathbf{1.2887 \pm 1.0992}$
Total	Train	0.5024 ± 0.5321	0.5224 ± 0.5130	0.9059 ± 0.7923	0.8591 ± 0.7531
	Test	1.2878 ± 1.1049	1.2924 ± 1.1163	1.2791 ± 1.0990	$\mathbf{1.2692 \pm 1.0811}$

4   Conclusions

We have proposed a multi-output regression network CARN for automated quantitative measurement of spine. By taking advantage of expressive feature extracted from CAN, and employing LSCMR for alleviating overfitting, CARN is capable of achieving promising accuracy for all indices estimation.

Acknowledgements. This work was supported by China Scholarship Council (No. 201708440350), National Natural Science Foundation of China (No. U1501256), and Science and Technology Project of Guangdong Province (No. 2015B010131011).

References

1. McCloskey, E., Johansson, H., Oden, A., Kanis, J.A.: Fracture risk assessment. Clin. Biochem. **45**(12), 887–893 (2012)
2. Tatoń, G., Rokita, E., Korkosz, M., Wróbel, A.: The ratio of anterior and posterior vertebral heights reinforces the utility of DXA in assessment of vertebrae strength. Calcif. Tissue Int. **95**(2), 112–121 (2014)
3. Jarman, J.P., Arpinar, V.E., Baruah, D., Klein, A.P., Maiman, D.J., Muftuler, L.T.: Intervertebral disc height loss demonstrates the threshold of major pathological changes during degeneration. Eur. Spine J. **24**(9), 1944–1950 (2014)
4. Salamat, S., Hutchings, J., Kwong, C., Magnussen, J., Hancock, M.J.: The relationship between quantitative measures of disc height and disc signal intensity with Pfirrmann score of disc degeneration. SpringerPlus **5**(1), 829 (2016)
5. Tunset, A., Kjaer, P., Chreiteh, S.S., Jensen, T.S.: A method for quantitative measurement of lumbar intervertebral disc structures: an intra- and inter-rater agreement and reliability study. Chiropr. Man. Ther. **21**(1), 26 (2013)
6. Videman, T., Battié, M.C., Gibbons, L.E., Gill, K.: Aging changes in lumbar discs and vertebrae and their interaction: a 15-year follow-up study. Spine J. **14**(3), 469–478 (2014)
7. Zhen, X., Zhang, H., Islam, A., Bhaduri, M., Chan, I., Li, S.: Direct and simultaneous estimation of cardiac four chamber volumes by multioutput sparse regression. Med. Image Anal. **36**, 184–196 (2017)
8. Xue, W., Lum, A., Mercado, A., Landis, M., Warrington, J., Li, S.: Full quantification of left ventricle via deep multitask learning network respecting intra- and inter-task relatedness. In: Descoteaux, M., Maier-Hein, L., Franz, A., Jannin, P., Collins, D.L., Duchesne, S. (eds.) MICCAI 2017. LNCS, vol. 10435, pp. 276–284. Springer, Cham (2017). https://doi.org/10.1007/978-3-319-66179-7_32
9. Simonyan, K., Zisserman, A.: Very deep convolutional networks for large-scale image recognition. CoRR abs/1409.1556 (2014)
10. Pang, S., et al.: Hippocampus segmentation based on local linear mapping. Sci. Rep. **7**, 45501 (2017)
11. Huang, G., Liu, Z., van der Maaten, L., Weinberger, K.Q.: Densely connected convolutional networks. In: 2017 IEEE Conference on Computer Vision and Pattern Recognition (CVPR). IEEE, July 2017
12. Liu, G., Lin, Z., Yu, Y.: Multi-output regression on the output manifold. Pattern Recognit. **42**(11), 2737–2743 (2009)
13. Liu, W., He, J., Chang, S.F.: Large graph construction for scalable semi-supervised learning. In: Proceedings of the 27th International Conference on Machine Learning (ICML-2010), pp. 679–686 (2010)

Estimating Achilles Tendon Healing Progress with Convolutional Neural Networks

Norbert Kapinski[1]([✉]), Jakub Zielinski[1,3], Bartosz A. Borucki[1],
Tomasz Trzcinski[2,5], Beata Ciszkowska-Lyson[4], and Krzysztof S. Nowinski[1]

[1] University of Warsaw, Warsaw, Poland
n.kapinski@icm.edu.pl
[2] Warsaw University of Technology, Warsaw, Poland
[3] Medical University of Warsaw, Warsaw, Poland
[4] Carolina Medical Center, Warsaw, Poland
[5] Tooploox, Wrocław, Poland

Abstract. Quantitative assessment of a treatment progress in the Achilles tendon healing process - one of the most common musculoskeletal disorders in modern medical practice - is typically a long and complex process: multiple MRI protocols need to be acquired and analysed by radiology experts for proper assessment. In this paper, we propose to significantly reduce the complexity of this process by using a novel method based on a pre-trained convolutional neural network. We first train our neural network on over 500 000 2D axial cross-sections from over 3 000 3D MRI studies to classify MRI images as belonging to a healthy or injured class, depending on the patient's condition. We then take the outputs of a modified pre-trained network and apply linear regression on the PCA-reduced space of the features to assess treatment progress. Our method allows to reduce up to 5-fold the amount of data needed to be registered during the MRI scan without any information loss. Furthermore, we are able to predict the healing process phase with equal accuracy to human experts in 3 out of 6 main criteria. Finally, contrary to the current approaches to healing assessment that rely on radiologist subjective opinion, our method allows to objectively compare different treatments methods which can lead to faster patient's recovery.

Keywords: Achilles tendon trauma · Deep learning · MRI

1 Introduction

Injuries of the Achilles tendons are one of the most common musculoskeletal disorders in modern medical practice, with more than 18 case per 100,000 people per year [1]. A ruptured tendon undergoes a surgical reconstruction followed by a rehabilitation process. A risk of the tendon re-rupture is between 20–40% and proper oversight of the healing process is needed to increase the chances that

© Springer Nature Switzerland AG 2018
A. F. Frangi et al. (Eds.): MICCAI 2018, LNCS 11071, pp. 949–957, 2018.
https://doi.org/10.1007/978-3-030-00934-2_105

the tendon is not ruptured again. Furthermore, continuous monitoring of the healing process can be useful for perfecting treatment techniques and adjusting them to patient's personal conditions.

Recently, several works showed how quantitative methods based on deep neural networks can successfully be used to monitor the healing of the Achilles tendon [2,3]. However, those methods are dedicated to simple classification tasks and do not fully take advantage of the mid-level neural network representation. As suggested by [4], those representations can be useful, especially for medical image processing tasks [5,6].

In this paper, we introduce a novel method for continuous evaluation of reconstructed Achilles tendon healing based on the responses of intermediate convolutional neural network layers. First, we train a neural network to classify MRI data as 'healthy' or 'injured'. We then use the pre-trained network as a feature extractor and build the representation of the image data from the outputs of the first fully connected layer. After reducing the dimensionality of this representation with Principal Component Analysis (PCA), we use linear regression to fit the resulting representation to the scores assigned by human annotators that describe a healing phase. The obtained results indicate that the proposed approach allows to reduce the number of MRI protocols used for healing assessment from 10 to 2, without losing accuracy of the healing phase classification. Furthermore, using the responses of the proposed neural network, we are able to estimate the healing phase measured on a five-point scale with a mean square error of less then a half point, when compared with human experts.

2   Method

In this section, we present our method that relies on the outputs of the intermediate neural network layers to predict the healing process phase. We start by training the AlexNet architecture [7] for the binary classification task of assigning 'healthy' vs 'injured' label to the input MRI images. Once trained, we use the truncated version of this architecture as a feature extractor. More precisely, we use the outputs of the first fully connected layer (fc6) and apply a Principal Component Analysis to reduce the dimensionality of the resulting representation. Finally, we introduce a metric H which is a novel contribution of the paper, representing a score of the Achilles tendon condition, visible in a single 3D MRI study image of a given protocol:

$$H = TM(PC1(x_1), PC1(x_2), ..., PC1(x_n))$$ (1)

where TM is a truncated mean with 2.5 upper and lower hinges (a value we obtained in our initial set of experiments), $PC1(x_i)$ is the first principal component value for the network inference performed on the slice x_i where i is the index of the slice in the 3D MRI study.

Figure 1 shows the overview of our framework based on a neural network. We take the feature extractor (FE) and fully connected layer (FC) from the pre-trained AlexNet model. The network uses features extracted for healthy tendons

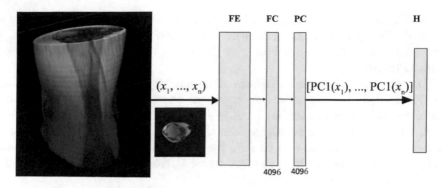

Fig. 1. The neural network topology used to generate tendon healing assessment.

and those after rupture in different time of the healing. The FC layer performs initial weighting of the features, yet avoiding strong discretization that increases with the subsequent fully connected layers of the binary trained AlexNet model. The PC layer, comprising of Principal Components, reduces the number of output parameters while preserving the differentiation of the tendons in different healing state. Finally, H reduces the number of outliers, as presented in details in Sect. 3.2, with the use of truncation and produces a single value output for the whole 3D MRI study of a given protocol.

3 Experiments

In this section, we present experimental results obtained with the proposed method. First, we describe the dataset used in our experiments and show the results obtained using classification algorithms based on several neural network architectures. We then verify if the H metric proposed in this work corresponds to the progress of the healing process. Finally, we evaluate our approach and present studies on minimal number of MRI protocols required for the healing process assessment.

3.1 Dataset

We acquired MRI data of a lower limb of healthy volunteers and patients after the Achilles tendon rupture with the use of a GE Signa HDxt 1.5T scanner with Foot & Ankle array coil.

To monitor the progress of the healing, each of the individuals was scanned with 10 MRI protocols, typically used in orthopaedics (and containing the most significant visual information) i.e. four 3D FSPGR Ideal [Fast Spoiled Gradient Echo] (In Phase, Out Phase, Fat, Water), PD [Proton Density], T1, T2, T2 mapping, T2* GRE [Gradient Echo] and T2* GRE TE_MIN [Minimal Time Echo]. The group of healthy patients was scanned only once, while the injured patients were scanned once before the tendon reconstruction surgery and 9 times afterwards (after 1, 3, 6, 9, 12, 20, 26, 40 and 52 weeks). As of March 2018, we collected 270 3D MRI scans of healthy individuals (including 27 volunteers, 10 protocols) and 2 772 of injured patients (including 60 patients, 10 protocols and up to 10 timesteps).

To overcome the possible artifacts of volumetric interpolation with spatially anisotropic data resolution and to represent the internal structure of tendon tissue, we performed an additional analysis only within axial slices of the 3D MRI scans. We augmented the healthy tendon slices number by mirroring and random rotations in the range of −10 to 10°. We also mirrored the slices representing injured tendons. The resulting dataset contains 234,502 slices labeled as healthy and 277,208 slices labeled as injured.

Table 1. 5-fold cross-validation accuracy results for the tendon binary classification.

	Average	Min	Max	SD
AlexNet	99.19	99.15	99.24	0.04
ResNet-18	95.98	92.78	99.04	2.5
GoogleNet	99.83	99.68	99.91	0.1

To determine the ground truth for our dataset we worked with a group of expert radiologists. More precisely, we prepared a survey that includes 6 parameters describing the tendon healing process, visible in the MRI scans:

1. Structural changes within the tendon (SCT) - informs about the loss of cohesion within the tendon area.
2. Tendon thickening (TT) - informs about the maximum dimension in the sagittal direction.
3. Sharpness of the tendon edges (STE) - informs about the edge fractality.
4. Tendon edema (TE) - informs about an abnormal accumulation of fluid in the interstitium of the tendon.
5. Tendon uniformity (TU) - informs about the level of similarity of subsequent cross-sections of the tendon.
6. Tissue edema (TisE) - informs about an abnormal accumulation of fluid and enlarged size of the fascial compartment.

We asked experts to assess the healing condition of Achilles tendons based on the MRI images from our dataset. For each of the parameters, the experts could select a single score in a 5 point scale, where 1 describes a healthy tendon and 5 describes severely injured one.

3.2   Tendon Healing Process Assessment

Binary Classification Task: We first evaluate neural networks on the task of binary classification of the dataset. Table 1 presents the comparison of 5-fold cross-validation accuracy results of AlexNet, ResNet-18 [8] and GoogleNet [9] models used to classify the tendon condition (healthy vs. injured). 3 folds were used for training, one for validation and one for testing.

The performance of all of the tested models on the classification task is satisfactory. Nevertheless, the average, minimum and maximum accuracy for both AlexNet and GoogleNet reaches over 99% and in case of ResNet-18 the results are scattered between 93 and 99%, giving an average accuracy of 96%.

The AlexNet is the least complex of the tested models and its training takes less than two hours, while in the case of ResNet-18 it takes over 20 h to train the network, for GoogleNet this time increases to around 48 h. All times were measured on a server station with NVIDIA V100 GPU. Taking into account the accuracy and the model complexity, we choose the AlexNet architecture for all the experiments in the remainder of this paper.

Most of the samples labeled as injured and misclassified by our network as healthy come from 3D MRI scans that focus on the area far away from the rupture. In this work, we eliminate those outliers by using a truncated mean of our H metric, but in future work we plan to address this problem by incorporating fuzzy logic or soft classification methods.

Principal Components Analysis: For this task, we use the feature extractor part of the binary trained AlexNet model and its first fully connected layer (see Fig. 1). We evaluate whether the number of outputs can be decreased while preserving the differentiation of the stages of the healing process. For this purpose we use 48,225 slices derived from 10 patients that concluded a full year of the rehabilitation and were monitored in 10 timesteps. We perform PCA and compare the amount of variance preserved by 1, 10 and 200 most significant principal components. First 1, 10 and 200 principal components preserve 50.2, 90.8 and 98.8% amount of variance respectively. This means that 4096 outputs of our modified AlexNet topology can be reduced to a single output while preserving over 50% of variance. We therefore decide to test our approach using only the most significant principal component PC1 and this approach is used in the remaining experiments. Further study of consecutive components is a part of our future work.

Healing Monitoring: In this task, we evaluate changes of the metric H in different stages of the tendon healing. Figure 2 presents the time curves of the average H metric for 9 patients, monitored in 10 timesteps distributed over the year of the tendon recovery, for all of the 10 MRI protocols.

Except for the T2 mapping (T2MAP) with slices acquired from the raw signal data, all other protocols show a decreasing trend that can be interpreted as a negative difference between H value before the reconstruction and at the end of the recovery period. According to the feedback provided by radiologists and medical professionals, all 9 curves correspond well with the real-life healing process assessment. In most cases the progress of healing is more pronounced at the beginning than in the following stages. However, one can also observe the fluctuations related to patient activity, diet and their obedience to the treatment prescription. Taking into account the above results, we select all 9 protocols in the following experiments.

Correlation of H with the Ground Truth: Table 2 presents the values of Pearson correlation of the assessment done by the expert radiologist with our results obtained for 9 MRI protocols (excluding T2 mapping). The coefficients marked in bold are statistically significant with $p < 0.01, N = 10$. For 4 protocols (i.e. PD, T1, T2, T2*GRE) we can observe relatively high correlation with the ground truth in terms of the tendon and tissue edema size (TE and TisE), as well as the sharpness of the tendon edges (STE). Those parameters reach their maximum before the reconstruction and decrease with time. When they stabilize, the patients reach the end of the healing process. We also see that the parameter saturation coincides with plateauing of H values for all 4 protocols.

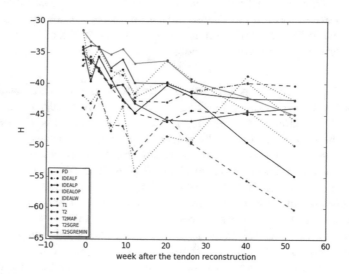

Fig. 2. Comparison of the curves of an average H value over 9 patients monitored over the year of the tendon recovery for all of the 10 MRI protocols.

Table 2. Pearson correlation between the ground truth parameters and the H measure. Coefficients with significance p < 0.01 are shown in bold.

	PD	IDELF	IDELP	IDELOP	IDELW	T1	T2	T2*GRE	T2*GREMIN
SCT	0.69	0.42	0.53	0.59	0.55	0.66	0.60	0.74	0.4
TT	0.52	0.71	0.46	0.30	0.37	0.55	0.40	0.38	0.45
STE	**0.87**	0.74	0.60	0.50	0.54	**0.84**	**0.81**	0.72	0.64
TE	**0.89**	0.53	0.63	0.62	0.58	**0.81**	**0.82**	**0.82**	0.60
TU	0.45	0.19	0.48	0.59	0.50	0.44	0.26	0.64	0.56
TisE	**0.82**	0.51	0.61	0.65	0.58	**0.84**	0.67	**0.90**	0.73

The TU parameter is assessed with the use of the sagittal slices. Thus, our neural network model is not able to successfully assess the healing phase using this parameter, as it is trained on axial cross-sections, not sagittal ones. We plan to further investigate the results of SCT and TT correlations and extend their analysis using more principal components.

Inter-protocol Correlation: In this section, we analyse the correlation between results obtained with different MRI protocols to find a minimal subset of protocols that is needed by our method to provide satisfactory performance. We investigate 4 protocols that perform best in the previous task and present the inter-protocol correlations results in Table 3.

Table 3. Inter-protocol correlation of PD, T1, T2 and T2* GRE MRI protocols. The results marked in bold have a significance level p < 0.01.

	PD	T1	T2	T2*GRE
PD	1.00	**0.96**	**0.90**	**0.89**
T1	**0.96**	1.00	**0.85**	**0.92**
T2	**0.90**	**0.85**	1.00	0.71
T2*GRE	**0.89**	**0.92**	0.71	1.00

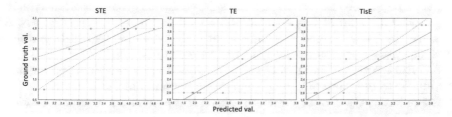

Fig. 3. Comparison of our model predictions with the ground truth. Our method predicts the correct outputs with error of less than a half of the score point.

The coefficients marked in bold are statistically significant with $p < 0.01, N = 10$. Due to the fact that the PD and T1 protocols correlate strongly with each other, it is sufficient to select only one of them for our experiments. We identify two least correlated protocols, namely PD and T2*GRE, and choose this pair. Although alternative methods for protocol selection exist, *e.g.* one can use backward feature elimination strategy, however, our initial experiments indicate that the performance of the proposed approach is sufficient.

Prediction of the Healing Parameters: Here, we test how accurate predictions of the ground truth we can obtain using a combination of the results for PD and T2*GRE-based inference. We use a linear regression of the results from both protocols and analyze the predictions of STE, TE and TisE parameters. Figure 3 presents the results of our study.

The prediction error is below 1 score point in a 5-point scale for every case. This result confirms the validity of our method and can justify using our method in the context of automatic assessment of the Achilles tendon healing.

4 Conclusions

In this paper, we proposed to use convolutional neural networks to automatically assess the Achilles tendon healing phase. Currently, radiologists spend significant amount of time on analysing MRI images to manually evaluate tendond's condition. The results presented in this paper prove that methods based on deep neural networks can provide automatic, quantitative analysis of the 3D MRI scans. This, in turn, can lead to significant time savings and increase the efficiency of healing assessment without losing its precision.

More precisely, we proposed a novel method for the tendon healing process assessment based on the pre-trained convolutional neural network. Our method allows to significantly improve the clinical workflow by minimizing the number of MRI protocols used to assess the healing and by providing objective, single value assessment for the current condition of the tendon.

In this paper, we also presented the results confirming that our method allows to approximate 3 out of 6 assessment criteria with a human expert accuracy. At the same time, our method uses only 2 out of 10 typically used MRI protocols which can also prove the efficiency of the proposed method.

As future work, we plan to focus on approximating the remaining parameters. Our idea is to use more principal components to compute the H metric, as well as test different types of regression methods and extend our neural network to process also the data from sagittal cross-sections.

Acknowledgments. The following work was part of *Novel Scaffold-based Tissue Engineering Approaches to Healing and Regeneration of Tendons and Ligaments (START)* project, co-funded by The National Centre for Research and Development (Poland) within STRATEGMED programme (STRATEGMED1/233224/10/NCBR/2014).

References

1. Raikin, S.M.: Epidemiology of Achilles tendon rupture in the US. Lower Extremity Review (2014)
2. Kapinski, N., Zielinski, J., Borucki, B., Nowinski, K.: MRI-based deep learning for in-situ monitoring of achilles tendon regeneration process. Int. J. Comput. Assist. Radiol. Surg. **12**(Supplement 1), 57–58 (2017)

3. Nowosielski, J., Zielinski, J., Borucki, B., Nowinski, K.: Multidimensional haralick feature space analysis for assessment of the achilles tendon in mr imaging. Int. J. Comput. Assist. Radiol. Surg. **12**(Supplement 1), 218–220 (2017)
4. Oquab, M., Bottou, L., Laptev, I., Sivic, J.: Learning and transferring mid-level image representations using convolutional neural networks. In: CVPR (2014)
5. Dou, Q., Chen, H., Jin, Y., Yu, L., Qin, J., Heng, P.: 3d deeply supervised network for automatic liver segmentation from CT volumes, CoRR, vol. abs/1607.00582 (2016)
6. Bar, Y., Diamant, I., Wolf, L., Greenspan, H.: Deep learning with non-medical training used for chest pathology identification. In: SPIE Medical Imaging (2015)
7. Krizhevsky, A., Sutskever, I., Hinton, G.E.: Imagenet classification with deep convolutional neural networks. In: NIPS (2012)
8. He, K., Zhang, X., Ren, S., Sun, J.: Deep residual learning for image recognition. CoRR, vol. abs/1512.03385 (2015)
9. Szegedy, C., et al.: Going deeper with convolutions. In: CVPR (2015)

Author Index

Printed in the United States
By Bookmasters